CHEST MEDICINE

ESSENTIALS OF PULMONARY AND CRITICAL CARE MEDICINE

CHEST MEDICINE

ESSENTIALS OF PULMONARY AND CRITICAL CARE MEDICINE

FOURTH EDITION

Editors

RONALD B. GEORGE, M.D.

Professor and Chairman
Department of Medicine
Louisiana State University School of Medicine
Shreveport, Louisiana

RICHARD W. LIGHT, M.D.

Professor of Medicine
Department of Medicine
Vanderbilt University
Director of Pulmonary Disease Program
Department of Medicine
St. Thomas Hospital
Nashville, Tennessee

MICHAEL A. MATTHAY, M.D.

Professor of Medicine and Anesthesia
Department of Medicine and Anesthesia
Senior Associate, Cardiovascular Research Institute
University of California, San Francisco
Associate Director, Intensive Care Unit
Cardiovascular Research Institute
University of California Medical Center
San Francisco, California

RICHARD A. MATTHAY, M.D.

Boehringer Ingelheim Professor of Medicine
Associate Director
Pulmonary and Critical Care Section
Department of Medicine
Yale University School of Medicine
Attending Physician
Internal Medicine, Section of Pulmonary Medicine
Yale-New Haven Hospital
New Haven, Connecticut

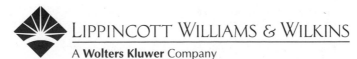

LIPPINCOTT WILLIAMS & WILKINS
A **Wolters Kluwer** Company
Philadelphia • Baltimore • New York • London
Buenos Aires • Hong Kong • Sydney • Tokyo

Acquisitions Editor: Joyce-Rachel John
Developmental Editor: Tanya Lazar
Production Editor: W. Christopher Granville
Manufacturing Manager: Colin Warnock
Cover Designer: Mark Lerner
Compositor: Maryland Composition
Printer: Maple Press

© 2000 by LIPPINCOTT WILLIAMS & WILKINS
530 Walnut Street
Philadelphia, PA 19106 USA
LWW.com

Printed in the USA

Library of Congress Cataloging-in-Publication Data

Chest medicine : essentials of pulmonary and critical care medicine / edited by Ronald B. George . . . [et al.].—4th ed.
    p. ; cm.
  Includes bibliographical references and index.
  ISBN 0-683-30667-7
    1. Chest—Diseases. 2. Respiratory intensive care. I. George, Ronald B.
  [DNLM: 1. Lung Diseases. 2. Critical Care. WF 600 C525 2000]
RC941.C5675 2000
616.2′4—dc 21

                                                    00-020038

10 9 8 7 6 5 4 3 2 1

CONTENTS

Contributing Authors vii
Preface xi

SECTION I: ANATOMY AND PHYSIOLOGY OF THE RESPIRATORY SYSTEM 1

1   Functional Anatomy of the Respiratory System 3
Donna L. Carden, Michael A. Matthay, and Ronald B. George

2   Mechanics of Respiration 26
Richard W. Light

3   Alveolar Ventilation, Gas Exchange, and Oxygen Delivery 44
Ronald B. George

SECTION II: GATHERING THE DATA BASE 57

4   The Respiratory History and Physical Examination 59
Ronald B. George and D. Keith Payne

5   Chest Imaging 68
H. Dirk Sostman, Frank M. Mele, and Richard A. Matthay

6   Clinical Pulmonary Function Testing, Exercise Testing, and Disability Evaluation 91
Richard W. Light

7   Invasive Diagnostic Procedures 117
Richard W. Light and R. Michael Rodriguez

SECTION III: MANAGEMENT OF RESPIRATORY DISEASES 131

8   Asthma 133
Mani S. Kavuru and Herbert P. Wiedemann

9   Chronic Obstructive Pulmonary Disease, Bronchiectasis, and Cystic Fibrosis 174
Ronald B. George, Gerardo S. San Pedro, and James K. Stoller

10   Lung Transplantation and Lung Volume Reduction Surgery 208
Stephanie M. Levine, Jay I. Peters, and Stephen G. Jenkinson

11   Pulmonary Thromboembolism and Other Pulmonary Vascular Diseases 233
Alejandro C. Arroliga, Michael A. Matthay, and Richard A. Matthay

12   Diffuse Interstitial and Alveolar Inflammatory Diseases 262
Herbert Y. Reynolds, Paul W. Noble, and Richard A. Matthay

13   Occupational and Environmental Lung Disease 314
Carrie A. Redlich and John R. Balmes

14   Lung Neoplasms 346
Richard A. Matthay, Lynn T. Tanoue, and Darryl C. Carter

15   Respiratory Tract Infections 377
Michael S. Niederman and George A. Sarosi

16   Pulmonary Complications in the Immunosuppressed Patient 430
Wendy J. Mangialardi and Robert J. Mangialardi

17   Diseases of the Pleura, Mediastinum, Chest Wall, and Diaphragm 441
Richard W. Light

18   Sleep-Related Breathing Disorders 478
Richard B. Berry

19   Pulmonary and Critical Care Problems in the Elderly 503
E. Wesley Ely

SECTION IV: THE CRITICALLY ILL PATIENT 515

20   Administrative, Nutritional, and Ethical Principles for the Management of Critically Ill Patients 517
Annette Stralovich-Romani, C. Kees Mahutte, Michael A. Matthay, and John M. Luce

21   General Principles of Managing the Patient with Respiratory Failure 539
James A. Frank, David Schwartz, Brian M. Daniel, Robert M. Jasmer, and Michael A. Matthay

22   Acute Hypercapnic Respiratory Failure: Neuromuscular and Obstructive Diseases 561
Michael A. Matthay and Kamran Atabai

23   Acute Hypoxemic Respiratory Failure: Pulmonary Edema and Acute Lung Injury 576
Lorraine B. Ware and Michael A. Matthay

24   Thoracic Trauma, Surgery, and Perioperative Management 592
Michael W. Owens, Muhammad S. Chaudry, Jane M. Eggerstedt, and Lou M. Smith

25   Managing the Patient with Hemodynamic Insufficiency, Shock, and Multiple Organ Failure 620
Michael A. Matthay and Paul M. Dorinsky

26   Prevention of Nonpulmonary Complications of Intensive Care 639
Mark D. Eisner, Michael A. Matthay, and Sanjay Saint

Subject Index 655

CONTRIBUTING AUTHORS

Alejandro C. Arroliga, M.D.   Head, Medical Intensive Care Unit, Pulmonary and Critical Care Department, The Cleveland Clinic, 9500 Euclid Avenue, Cleveland, Ohio 44106

Kamran Atabai, M.D.   Research Fellow, Cardiovascular Research Institute, Resident, Department of Medicine, University of California, 505 Parnassus Avenue, San Francisco, California 94143-0132

John R. Balmes, M.D.   Professor, Department of Medicine, University of California, San Francisco; Chief, Division of Occupational and Environmental Medicine, San Francisco General Hospital, 1001 Potrero Avenue, San Francisco, California 94110

Richard B. Berry, M.D.   Professor of Medicine, Department of Medicine, Division of Pulmonary and Critical Care Medicine, University of Florida, Box 100225, Health Sciences Center; Medical Director, Sleep Disorders Center, Shands at the University of Florida, 1600 Southwest Archer Road, Gainesville, Florida 32610

Donna L. Carden, M.D.   Professor, Department of Medicine, Molecular and Cellular Physiology, Louisiana State University, School of Medicine, 1501 Kings Highway, Shreveport, Louisiana 71130-3932

Darryl C. Carter, M.D.   Professor, Department of Pathology, Yale University School of Medicine, New Haven, Connecticut 06320; Attending Physician, Department of Pathology, Yale University Hospital, 20 York Street, New Haven, Connecticut 06510

Muhammad S. Chaudry, M.D.   Fellow, Pulmonary and Critical Care Medicine, Louisiana State University Health Sciences Center, 1501 Kings Highway, Shreveport, Louisiana 71130

Brian M. Daniel, RTT   Assistant Clinical Professor, Department of Physiological Nursing, Clinical Coordinator, Department of Respiratory Care, University of California, San Francisco, 505 Parnassus Avenue, San Francisco, California 94143-0120

Paul M. Dorinsky, M.D.   Clinical Associate Professor of Medicine, Department of Medicine, University of North Carolina, 420 Burnett Womack Buildingm, Chapel Hill, North Carolina 27554-7020; Principal Clinical Research Office Physician, U.S. Medical Affairs-Respiratory, Glaxowellcome, 5 Moore Drive, Research Triangle Park, North Carolina 27704

Jane M. Eggerstedt, M.D.   Associate Professor and Attending Surgeon, Department of Surgery, Division of Cardiothoracic Surgery, Louisiana State University Health Sciences Center, 1501 Kings Highway, Shreveport, Louisiana 71130

Mark D. Eisner, M.D.   Assistant Professor, Department of Medicine, Divisions of Occupational and Environmental Medicine, Pulmonary and Critical Care Medicine, University of California, San Francisco, 350 Parnassus Avenue, Suite 609, San Francisco, California 94143

E. Wesley Ely, M.D., M.P.H.   Assistant Professor of Medicine, Medical Co-Director of Lung Transplantation, Allergy, Pulmonary and Critical Care Medicine, Vanderbilt Lung Transplantation Program, Vanderbilt University Medical Center, Room 913 Oxford House, Nashville, Tennessee 37232-4760

James A. Frank, M.D.   Senior Pulmonary/Critical Care Fellow, Cardiovascular Research Institute, University of California, San Francisco, 505 Parnassus Avenue, San Francisco, California 94143-0132

Ronald B. George, M.D.   Professor and Chairman, Department of Medicine, Louisiana State University School of Medicine, 1501 Kings Highway, PO Box 33932, Shreveport, Louisiana 71130-3932

Robert M. Jasmer, M.D.   Assistant Professor, Department of Medicine, University of California, San Francisco; Staff Physician, Department of Medicine, Pulmonary and Critical Care Division, San Francisco General Hospital and SFVAMC, 1001 Potrero Avenue, San Francisco, California 94110

Stephen G. Jenkinson, M.D.   Professor of Medicine and Director, Division of Pulmonary Diseases/Critical Care Medicine, Department of Medicine, The University of Texas Health Service Center of San Antonio, 7703 Floyd Curl Drive, San Antonio, Texas 78229

Mani S. Kavuru, M.D.   Director, Pulmonary Function Laboratory, Pulmonary and Critical Care Medicine, Cleveland Clinic Foundation, 9500 Euclid Avenue, Cleveland, Ohio 44195

Stephanie M. Levine, M.D.   Associate Professor of Medicine, Division of Pulmonary Diseases/Critical Care Medicine, The University of Texas Health Sciences Center, 7703 Floyd Curl Drive, San Antonio, Texas 78229; Staff Physician, Pulmonary Diseases Section (111E), South Texas Veterans Health Care System, Audie Murphy VA Medical Center, 7400 Merton Minter Boulevard, San Antonio, Texas 78284

Richard W. Light, M.D.   Professor of Medicine, Department of Medicine, Vanderbilt University; Director of Pulmonary Disease Program, Saint Thomas Hospital, 4220 Harding Road, Nashville, Tennessee 37202

John M. Luce, M.D.   Professor, Department of Medicine and Anesthesia, University of California, San Francisco; Professor, Department of Medicine, Division of Pulmonary and Critical Care Medicine, San Francisco General Hospital, 1001 Potrero Avenue, San Francisco, California 94110-3518

C. Kees Mahutte, M.D., Ph.D.   Professor of Medicine, University of California, Irvine, College of Medicine, Irvine, California 92717; Chief, Pulmonary/Critical Care Section, Veterans Administration Medical Center, Long Beach, California 90822

Robert J. Mangialardi, M.D.   Center for Lung Research, Vanderbilt University School of Medicine, B-1308 Medical Center North, Nashville, Tennessee 37232-2650

Wendy J. Mangialardi, M.D.   Center for Lung Research, Vanderbilt University School of Medicine, B-1308 Medical Center North, Nashville, Tennessee 37232-2650

Michael A. Matthay, M.D.   Professor of Medicine and Anesthesia, University of California, San Francisco; Senior Associate, Cardiovascular Research Institute, Associate Director, Intensive Care Unit, University of California Medical Center, 505 Parnassus Avenue, San Francisco, California 94143-0120

Richard A. Matthay, M.D.   Boehringer Ingelheim Professor of Medicine, Associate Director, Pulmonary and Critical Care Section, Department of Medicine, Yale University School of Medicine, PO Box 208057, New Haven, Connecticut 06520; Attending Physician, Internal Medicine, Section of Pulmonary Medicine, Yale-New Haven Hospital, 20 York Street, New Haven, Connecticut 06504

Frank M. Mele, M.D.   Attending Radiologist, Department of Diagnostic Radiology, Hopital of Saint Raphael, 1450 Chapel Street, New Haven, Connecticut 06311

Michael S. Niederman, M.D.   Professor of Medicine, Department of Medicine, State University of New York at Stony Brook, Stony Brook, New York, 11794; Chief, Pulmonary and Critical Care, Winthrop-University Hospital, 222 Station Plaza North, Mineola, New York 11501

Paul W. Noble, M.D.   Pulmonary and Critical Care Medicine, Yale University School of Medicine, PO Box 208057, New Haven, Connecticut 06520

Michael W. Owens, M.D.   Associate Professor of Medicine, Department of Medicine, Louisiana State University School of Medicine; Chief, Medical Service (111), Department of Medicine, Overton Brooks VA Medical Center, 510 East Stoner Avenue, Shreveport, Louisiana 71101

D. Keith Payne, M.D.   Professor of Medicine, Department of Medicine, Section of Pulmonary and Critical Care Medicine, Louisiana State University Medical Center, 1501 Kings Highway, Shreveport, Louisiana 71130-3932

Jay I. Peters, M.D.   Professor of Medicine, Division of Pulmonary Diseases/Critical Care Medicine, Department of Medicine, The University of Texas Health Science Center at San Antonio, 7703 Floyd Curl Drive, San Antonio, Texas 78229

Carrie A. Redlich, M.D., M.P.H.   Associate Professor of Medicine, Yale Occupational and Environmental Medicine Program and Section of Pulmonary and Critical Care Medicine, Department of Internal Medicine, Yale University School of Medicine; Staff Physician, Internal Medicine, Yale-New Haven Hospital, 135 College Street, New Haven, Connecticut 06510

Herbert Y. Reynolds, M.D.   Professor of Medicine, Department of Medicine, Pennsylvania State University; Staff Physician, Department of Medicine, Milton S. Hershey Medical Center, 500 University Drive, Hershey, Pennsylvania 17033

R. Michael Rodriguez, M.D.   Associate Professor of Medicine, Department of Medicine, Vanderbilt University, 203 Light Hall, Nashville, Tennessee 37232; Director of Medical Education, St. Thomas Intensive Care Unit, Saint Thomas Hospital, 4220 Harding Road, Nashville, Tennessee 37202

Sanjay Saint, M.D. Assistant Professor of Internal Medicine, Department of Internal Medicine, University of Michigan Medical School, 3116 Taubman Center, 1500 East Medical Center Drive, Ann Arbor, Michigan 48109-0376

Gerardo S. San Pedro, M.D. Associate Professor of Clinical Medicine, Department of Internal Medicine, Section of Pulmonary and Critical Care Medicine, Louisiana State University Health Sciences Center, 1501 Kings Highway, Shreveport, Louisiana 71130-3932

George A. Sarosi, M.D. Professor of Medicine, Department of Medicine, Indiana University School of Medicine; Chief, Medical Service, Department of Medicine, Richard L. Roudebush VAMC, 1481 West Tenth Street, Indianapolis, Indiana 46202

David Schwartz, M.D. Anesthesiology Department, University of Illinois at Chicago, 1740 West Taylor, Suite 3200W, Chicago, Illinois 60612

Lou M. Smith, M.D. Assistant Professor, Department of Surgery; Director, Trauma and Surgical Critical Care, Louisiana State University School of Medicine, 1501 Kings Highway, Shreveport, Louisiana 71130

H. Dirk Sostman, M.D. Professor and Chairman, Department of Radiology, Joan and Sanford I. Weill Medical College of Cornell University, New York, New York, 10021; Radiologist in Chief, Department of Radiology, New York Presbyterian Hospital, 525 East 68th Street, New York, New York 10021

James K. Stoller, M.D. Professor of Medicine, Department of Pulmonary/Critical Care Medicine, Vice Chairman, Division of Medicine, Section of Respiratory Therapy, Cleveland Clinic Foundation, 9500 Euclid Avenue, Cleveland, Ohio 44122

Annette Stralovich-Romani, RD, CNSD Adult Critical Care Nutritionist, Department of Nutrition and Dietetics, University of California, San Francisco Medical Center, 505 Parnassus Avenue, M-294, San Francisco, California 94143-0212

Lynn T. Tanoue, M.D. Associate Professor of Medicine, Department of Medicine, Yale University School of Medicine, PO Box 208057, New Haven, Connecticut 06520; Medical Director, Department of Respiratory Care, Yale-New Haven Hospital, 20 York Street, New Haven, Connecticut 06504

Lorraine B. Ware, M.D. Post Doctoral Fellow, Cardiovascular Research Institute, Pulmonary and Critical Care Medicine, 505 Parnassus Avenue, Box 0130, San Francisco, California 94143-0130

Herbert P. Wiedemann, M.D. Professor, Department of Internal Medicine, Cleveland Clinic Health Sciences Center of Ohio State University; Chairman, Department of Pulmonary and Critical Care Medicine, Cleveland Clinic Foundation, 9500 Euclid Avenue, Cleveland, Ohio 44106

PREFACE

It is hard to believe that we first began to develop the idea for *Chest Medicine* almost 20 years ago. After two years of planning and development, the First Edition was published in 1983. Our goal was to provide a concise, easy to read textbook which would allow the busy trainee and practitioner to obtain the essentials of the subject without having to resort to the large, multi-volume textbooks of the day. Since then, other concise texts have appeared in our field, but when we survey the field (and we often do) what we hear is, "this is the book I used to prepare for my board examination." In fact, we are told that this book is most often selected by fellows for review during the weeks prior to taking their board exams.

Through the years, we have striven to produce a distillate of the latest and most important knowledge in the field. This is a more difficult task than it may sound. We have agonized over removing and combining a number of sections in favor of adding more clinical information. Since most of our readers are in the pulmonary/critical care specialty, we have expanded the critical care section of the text with each new edition.

The Fourth Edition of *Chest Medicine* is a complete, chapter-by-chapter revision of the Third Edition. We have combined and eliminated chapters, added new chapters and authors, and updated all the material and references. We have preserved a number of figures from the last edition, but only if they were pertinent and useful. As always, we have concentrated on the important new advances in our field—in pathogenesis, diagnosis, and therapy. For the millenium edition of *Chest Medicine,* we have accomplished our goals by providing a compendium of the essentials of modern pulmonary/critical care medicine that will appeal to the busy trainee and practitioner.

We want to express our sincere thanks to our contributors for their hard work, and to apologize for the constant badgering they received during the preparation period. We also thank the many devoted editors at Lippincott Williams & Wilkins, especially Tanya Lazar, Joyce-Rachel John, and Sharon Zinner. They have kept our e-mail folders full with ideas and suggestions, as well as urgent reminders about impending deadlines. We are indebted to our secretaries and administrative staff, who have done much of the work in obtaining figures, finding material, and helping with manuscript preparation. We thank our fellow faculty members and clinicans, who have assisted us with advice and critiques. We also appreciate the support of our families, who have allowed us to work on weekends and holidays without interruption.

We wish to repeat the dedication from the previous editions: "Most of all we thank our students, housestaff physicians, and fellows, who force us to be current and who make our task a pleasant one." Many of those students and residents are now teachers and practitioners themselves, and we hope that this text continues to be useful to them.

Ronald B. George, M.D.
Richard W. Light, M.D.
Michael A. Matthay, M.D.
Richard A. Matthay, M.D.

CHEST MEDICINE

ESSENTIALS OF PULMONARY AND CRITICAL CARE MEDICINE

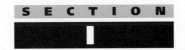

SECTION

I

ANATOMY AND PHYSIOLOGY OF THE RESPIRATORY SYSTEM

1

FUNCTIONAL ANATOMY OF THE RESPIRATORY SYSTEM

DONNA L. CARDEN
MICHAEL A. MATTHAY
RONALD B. GEORGE

VENTILATORY PUMP
Chest Wall
Respiratory Muscles
Pleura

DISTRIBUTION OF AIR
Nose
Paranasal Sinuses
Pharynx
Larynx
Trachea
Bronchi
Bronchioles

METABOLIC AND SECRETORY FUNCTIONS OF THE RESPIRATORY MUCOSA

DISTRIBUTION OF BLOOD
Right Ventricle
Pulmonary Arteries and Veins
Pulmonary Capillaries

ALVEOLAR–CAPILLARY BARRIER
Alveolar–Epithelial Barrier
Capillary–Endothelial Barrier

PHYSIOLOGY OF THE PULMONARY CIRCULATION
Pulmonary Vascular Pressures
Pulmonary Vascular Resistance
Distribution of Pulmonary Blood Flow
Regulation of the Pulmonary Circulation

METABOLIC, NONRESPIRATORY FUNCTIONS OF THE LUNG
Vasoactive Substances

GAS EXCHANGE AREA
Terminal Respiratory Unit

LUNG CLEARANCE AND DEFENSES
Particle Deposition in the Respiratory Tract
Transport Systems of the Lungs
Mucociliary Escalator
Alveolar Macrophage
Lymphohematogenous Drainage
Pulmonary Lymphatics

The lungs perform many important functions, including the filtering of systemic venous blood prior to its entry into the left ventricle and the production and metabolism of vasoactive substances. Their most important function, however, is the exchange of carbon dioxide—a byproduct of cellular metabolism—for oxygen, which is necessary for cellular activity. The respiratory system is ideally designed to perform this vital function 24 hours a day with a minimum amount of work (1).

During a lifetime of breathing the delicate tissues of the lung periphery are constantly exposed to environmental toxins and irritants of varying potency, including viruses, bacteria, and other living organisms as well as cigarette smoke, dust particles, and toxic chemicals. This constant exposure to a hostile environment has resulted in the development of an elaborate defense mechanism for the purpose of maintaining the integrity of the lung periphery.

Table 1.1 outlines the functional components of respiration and lung defenses and the structures involved. This chapter provides an overview of these structures as they relate to the functions for which they were designed.

VENTILATORY PUMP

The ventilatory pump consists of the chest wall, the respiratory muscles, and the pleural space, which connects the lungs to the chest wall. The chest wall acts as a rigid cylinder

TABLE 1.1 RESPIRATORY STRUCTURES AS RELATED TO THEIR FUNCTION

Function	Structures
Ventilatory pump	Chest wall and pleura
	Respiratory muscles
Distribution of ventilation	Upper respiratory tract
	Conducting airways
	Respiratory bronchioles
Distribution of blood	Pulmonary arteries and veins
	Pulmonary capillaries
Gas exchange	Terminal respiratory unit
Bronchial clearance	Mucociliary escalator
	Macrophages
Alveolar clearance and defense	Pulmonary lymphatics
	Alveolar macrophages
	Humoral mediators
	Inflammatory cells

within which the lungs are expanded and deflated by the action of the respiratory muscles. The diaphragm, the principal muscle of quiet breathing, moves like a piston within the cylinder, and the movement of this wide-bore piston over relatively short distances represents an efficient method of moving large volumes of air with minimum work. Air moves into and out of the lungs in a to-and-fro manner like the tides of the ocean; thus, it is called *tidal* flow.

Chest Wall

The bony thorax consists of the spine, ribs, and sternum. The basic shape of the thorax is that of a truncated cone (Fig. 1.1). Both the superior and inferior ends of the cone are inclined anteriorly so that the posterior portion of the cone, the spine, is longer than the anterior portion, the

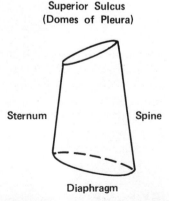

FIGURE 1.1. Simplified diagram of the cone-shaped thorax (lateral view). There is anterior-posterior compression, so the thorax is widened laterally; the anterior wall is shorter than the posterior wall, and the superior and inferior planes are inclined anteriorly.

sternum. These structures are innervated and may be a source of chest pain. The ribs are hinged on the spine by ligaments and cartilage in such a way that the ribs move upward and outward during inspiration and downward and inward during expiration. This hinging movement results in a change in thoracic volume. In addition, the connective tissue components of the chest wall function as a spring storing mechanical energy. This elastic property of the chest wall is a function both of the geometry of chest wall structures and of their composition. The extracellular matrix components that determine the mechanical properties of the chest include both the calcified bony ribs and the proteoglycans, elastin, and collagen of the cartilaginous ribs.

The expansion of the chest wall driven by respiratory muscles causes a fall in pressure of the air contained within the lungs, which in turn causes the flow of gas into the lungs. Air continues to flow into the lungs until the intrapulmonary gas pressure equals the atmospheric pressure. As the respiratory muscles relax, expiration begins and the elastic recoil of the chest wall and lungs compresses the air contained within the lungs, resulting in a pressure greater than atmospheric. This causes gas to flow out of the lungs. The movement of the chest wall and lungs during inspiration and expiration is shown in Figure 1.2.

Respiratory Muscles

The respiratory muscles are the only skeletal muscles that are essential to life; they have been called "the vital pump" by Macklem and associates (2). Clinical investigations have shown that weakness or fatigue of the respiratory muscles is a common cause of hypercapnic respiratory failure and difficulty of weaning from mechanical ventilation (3,4).

Inspiration requires active work, which is provided by the muscles of inspiration. These include the diaphragm, the inspiratory intercostal muscles, and the accessory muscles of inspiration (the scalenes and sternomastoids). Expiration under normal, quiet conditions is passive and requires no work; however, when ventilatory needs increase because of exertion or when the lungs are abnormal, as in asthma or chronic obstructive pulmonary disease (COPD), expiration often becomes an active process. The muscles of expiration include the internal intercostal muscles and the muscles of the abdominal wall (Fig. 1.3). In quadriplegic patients the pectoralis major and serratus anterior muscles may be used during expiration (5).

Like all skeletal muscle, and unlike the smooth muscle that lines airways, the muscles of respiration have no basal tone. Release of acetylcholine at the neuromuscular junction is required to initiate the contraction process. Binding of acetylcholine to the N_2 nicotinic cholinergic receptor on the target muscle cell initiates a depolarization that in turn releases calcium from the T-tubule system into the cytoplasm. This calcium then activates the adenosinetriphos-

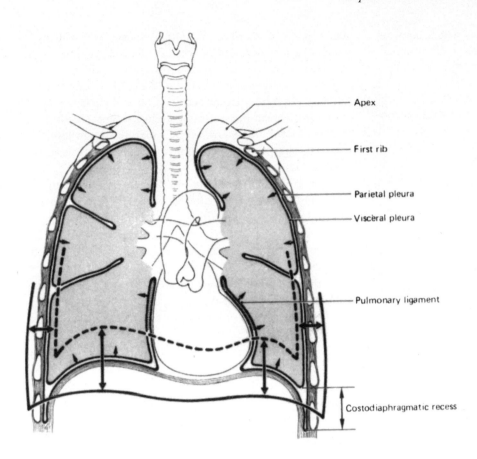

FIGURE 1.2. Frontal section of chest and lung showing pleural space. *Single arrows* indicate retractive force, and *double arrows* show the excursion of the lung bases and periphery between deep inspiration and expiration.

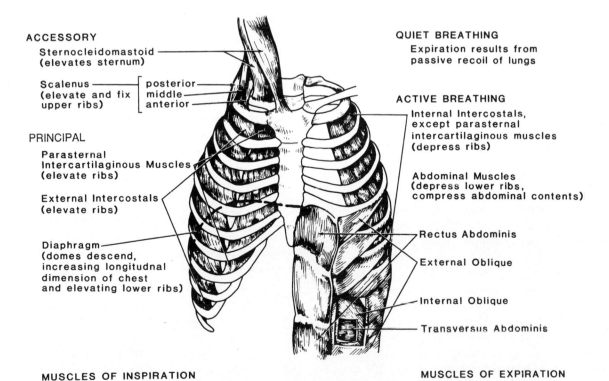

FIGURE 1.3. Diagram of the anatomy of the major respiratory muscles. Left side, inspiratory muscles; right side, expiratory muscles. (Reprinted with permission from Garrity ER, Sharp JT. Respiratory muscles: function and dysfunction. In: *Pulmonary and Critical Care Update*, vol. 2. Park Ridge, IL: American College of Chest Physicians, 1986.)

phatase (ATPase) of myosin heavy chain, which converts adenosine triphosphate (ATP) to adenosine diphosphate (ADP); causing the myosin to move along the actin fibers present within the cellular cytoplasm. This movement results in cellular shortening, and in this manner chemical energy is converted from ATP to the mechanical energy needed to drive ventilation. The ATP, in turn, is generated by the mitochondria of the muscle cell by oxidative metabolism or, for brief intervals, from glycolysis. Repolarization of the cell membrane, resequestration of calcium, and cleavage of acetylcholine by acetylcholinesterase results in relaxation of the muscle cell and readies it for another round of contraction.

Resting tidal breathing depends on the diaphragm, which is composed of two distinct portions. The costal and crural diaphragm have separate functions and innervations. The motor innervation to the diaphragm is via the phrenic nerve, which is derived from the third, fourth, and fifth cervical nerves. Sensory nerves to the crural portion of the diaphragm are also carried in the phrenic nerve; thus, irritation of the center of the diaphragm may cause pain that is referred to the ipsilateral neck or shoulder areas, which are also innervated by the third, fourth, and fifth cervical segments. Sensory innervation of the costal portion of the diaphragm is via the intercostal nerves from the adjacent chest wall, which they also innervate, and pain from the lateral portion of the diaphragm is referred to the chest wall.

The dome of the diaphragm moves downward with contraction, displacing abdominal contents; therefore, during inspiration the abdomen normally moves outward. Because of the fulcrum effect of the relatively fixed abdominal contents, diaphragm contraction also elevates and increases the diameter of the lower rib cage (Fig. 1.2). The accessory muscles of inspiration become important only during high levels of ventilation and with hyperinflation of the thorax associated with obstructive lung disease. The accessory muscles move the cage upward so that the ribs themselves lie in a more horizontal plane, thus increasing the diameter of the thoracic cage.

Fatigue of the inspiratory muscles occurs when the energy supply is exceeded as a result of increased ventilatory demands (vigorous exercise), increased work of breathing (asthma or COPD), or inadequate energy generation by the muscles (hypoxemia, congestive heart failure). Dyspnea is the major complaint when the respiratory muscles become fatigued. The sensation of dyspnea has not been completely explained, but it may be related to a disproportion between the amount of work required and the amount of work the respiratory muscles can perform. Healthy respiratory muscles can increase minute ventilation from a normal resting level of 6 to 7 L/min to a maximum of over 100 L/min with voluntary effort. However, this maximum level of ventilation cannot be sustained over long periods, and with vigorous exercise minute ventilation is more often maintained at five to six times the normal resting level. The body adapts to the increased ventilatory demand by increasing the circulation to the muscles of inspiration and by increasing the extraction of oxygen from the diaphragmatic capillaries. Lactate production occurs in normal persons only as a result of breathing against a high resistance, leading to fatigue, or breathing low-oxygen mixtures. High levels of blood lactate have been found in patients during severe asthma attacks (6).

Hyperinflation, which occurs in patients with emphysema and during asthma attacks, places the diaphragm at a distinct disadvantage. With hyperinflation the diaphragm is already low and flat; contraction neither moves the diaphragm downward nor moves the lower rib cage outward. In fact, with severe hyperinflation diaphragm contraction may pull the lower rib cage inward *(Hoover's sign),* causing an expiratory effect on the rib cage (7).

The clinical signs of inspiratory muscle fatigue have been summarized by Macklem's group (2,3,8). During early muscle fatigue the ratio of high-frequency to low-frequency electrical activity of the diaphragm as recorded on an electromyogram decreases. This is manifested by an increased respiratory rate; rapid, shallow breathing; and an early fall in the measured arterial P_{CO_2}. As muscle fatigue increases, the diaphragm movement diminishes and the accessory muscles assume a greater role. The contraction of accessory muscles produces a negative pressure in the thorax that may actually pull the flaccid diaphragm upward, causing the abdomen to move inward during inspiration; this is called *paradoxical respiration* and indicates significant diaphragm fatigue (3). Respiration may also shift back and forth from predominantly diaphragmatic breathing to predominantly accessory muscle breathing *(respiratory alternans).* In summary, the clinical signs of inspiratory muscle fatigue include rapid, shallow respiration with an initial increase in minute ventilation; an initial fall in Pa_{CO_2}; often paradoxical respiration and respiratory alternans; and finally, a decrease in respiratory rate and minute ventilation leading to hypoventilation and respiratory acidosis.

Tobin and associates have compared the clinical findings used to assess the state of the respiratory muscles prior to weaning from mechanical ventilation (9). The ratio of the respiratory rate to the tidal volume (f/VT) is the most useful of the bedside measurements of respiratory muscle function. They also found that although respiratory muscle dysfunction is a primary cause of ventilatory failure in patients with neuromuscular disorders, respiratory muscle fatigue per se is not a primary cause of ventilatory failure in patients with chronic obstructive pulmonary disease (COPD); rather, the increased demands on the respiratory muscles by airway obstruction and hyperinflation seem to be the primary factor in ventilatory failure (10).

The Pleura

As the lungs grow laterally from the mediastinum during fetal development, they grow into a part of the celomic cavity that is lined with undifferentiated mesenchyme. As the lungs extend into the cavity, they are covered by these mesenchymal cells, which become the parietal pleura. The mesenchymal cells that line the chest wall and mediastinum become the visceral pleura. The visceral and parietal pleura join one another at the lung hila. The parietal pleura contains abundant pain fibers derived from the intercostal nerves, and irritation of this membrane produces a characteristic, well-localized type of chest pain, which is exacerbated by chest wall movement *(pleuritic pain)*.

The pleural space is airtight; the two pleural surfaces, parietal and visceral, are separated only by a thin film that contains hyaluronic acid and provides lubrication during lung movement. In the intact system at rest the lung has a natural tendency to become smaller and the chest wall has a natural tendency to become larger. They are thus pulling against each other across the pleural space and, because it is airtight and no air can enter, a negative pressure is produced. It is this negative pleural pressure that links the lung to the chest wall and transmits movements of the chest wall to the lung. At rest the average negative intrapleural pressure is about 4 cm H_2O. In the upright position this negative pressure is greater at the top of the lungs than at the lung bases because of the effects of gravity on the lungs themselves.

Fluid flows constantly through the pleural space, forming a lubricating film over the surface of the lungs. Recent studies show that approximately 100 mL of pleural fluid is formed each hour; because this fluid is rapidly absorbed, the pleural space contains a minimal amount of fluid at any given time. Previous theories proposed that pleural fluid was formed from the systemic capillaries adjacent to the parietal pleura and absorbed into the plexus of capillaries under the visceral pleura. However, recent studies suggest that the absorption of pleural fluid is more complicated than this and that the parietal pleural lymphatics play a role in the removal of liquid, protein, and other large particles from the pleural cavity (11,12). The visceral pleural capillaries drain via the pulmonary veins into the left atrium.

DISTRIBUTION OF AIR

Before atmospheric air reaches the alveolar–capillary membrane, the air must be conditioned so that it does not injure this delicate surface area. The *upper respiratory tract* is primarily designed to purify, warm, and humidify the air; it consists of the nose, paranasal sinuses, pharynx, and larynx.

Nose

The nose contains a layer of epithelial cells overlying a rich capillary plexus, all resting on thin bony plates, the turbinates. The vascular and epithelial structures are responsive to neural and humoral mediators. Therefore, the nasal tissues can provide for rapid heat exchange, transudation of fluid, or recruitment of inflammatory cells to the nose. The nasal mucosa is normally bathed by thin, watery secretions designed to trap foreign particles and to add moisture to the inspired air. With normal, quiet breathing, inspired air is heated to body temperature and the relative humidity is increased to over 90% during passage through the nose. Resistance to air flow is higher in the nose than in the mouth because of the intricate system of baffles. This is the explanation for mouth breathing during vigorous exercise; in this case the air conditioning function of the nose is lost and dry, cold air may enter the lower airways. In patients with abnormal irritability of the bronchial tree, inspiration of cold air through the mouth during exercise may initiate bronchospasm. Patients with tracheostomy and those being ventilated via endotracheal tubes also lose the function of the nose, and inspired gas must be artificially humidified and warmed to prevent drying and irritation of the lower airways.

Paranasal Sinuses

The sinuses are lined by ciliated columnar epithelium and communicate with the nasal passages by narrow openings, which may become occluded when they are inflamed. Cilia within the sinus cavities beat in a pattern that tends to propel secretions toward the opening into the nasal cavity. The function of paranasal sinuses is not completely clear, but they add resonance to voice sounds and may insulate the cranial vault. They also provide lightness to the skull without unduly compromising its protective function. The sinuses may become inflamed and cause drainage of material into the pharynx (postnasal drip). This material may be aspirated into the lower respiratory tract, especially during sleep, and this may be a source of chronic bronchial irritation.

Pharynx

The pharynx is divided by the soft palate into the nasopharynx and the oropharynx. The adenoids, tonsils, and eustachian tubes are located in the nasopharynx. The epiglottis, which protects the laryngeal opening during swallowing, is at the base of the tongue. In unconscious patients the base of the tongue may fall posteriorly and obstruct the laryngeal opening. To avoid this the head should be hyperextended and the lower jaw pulled forward. Alternatively, the patient may be placed in a position in which gravity causes the tongue to fall forward. The oropharynx is easily seen through the open mouth; it serves as an entryway to both the larynx and the esophagus.

Larynx

The larynx has evolved from a simple valve, designed to prevent aspiration in to the trachea, into a complex structure containing the vocal cords, capable of phonation (13). The larynx is also vital to the defense of the respiratory system because the vocal cords participate in coughing. Coughing is a major clearance mechanism for material that collects in the larger airways; it is initiated by irritation of nerves in the walls of the trachea and large bronchi. Coughing is produced by closure of the vocal cords combined with contraction of the respiratory and abdominal muscles, so that high pressures are created in the lower airways. Sudden opening of the vocal cords then allows a rush of air, carrying larger particles of mucus with it. Normally the respiratory tract is free of bacteria below the level of the larynx.

One or both vocal cords may become paralyzed by surgery or injury to the nerves in the neck or thorax. The left recurrent laryngeal nerve descends into the mediastinum and around the arch of the aorta before returning to the larynx. This nerve may become disrupted by cancer involving lymph nodes adjacent to the left hilum, and hoarseness is an ominous sign in patients with carcinoma of the lung. Other diseases such as granulomas, lymphomas, and aortic aneurysms may also interrupt the left recurrent laryngeal nerve in the mediastinum. The right recurrent laryngeal nerve descends only to the level of the subclavian artery; therefore, it is less often affected.

If both vocal cords are paralyzed, they become flaccid near the midline and breathing may be hindered. Large airway obstruction produces a characteristic combination of symptoms, signs, and pulmonary function abnormalities (14). Bilateral vocal cord paralysis causes a variable extrathoracic airway obstruction, which produces inspiratory stridor associated with hoarseness, dyspnea, and anxiety. Tests of ventilatory function, such as a flow-volume loop or a spirogram, may show relatively normal forced expiration; however, there is a decrease in peak air flow during inspiration. Carcinoma of the larynx also produces the combination of hoarseness and stridor. However, since this is a fixed obstruction, stridor occurs usually during both inspiration

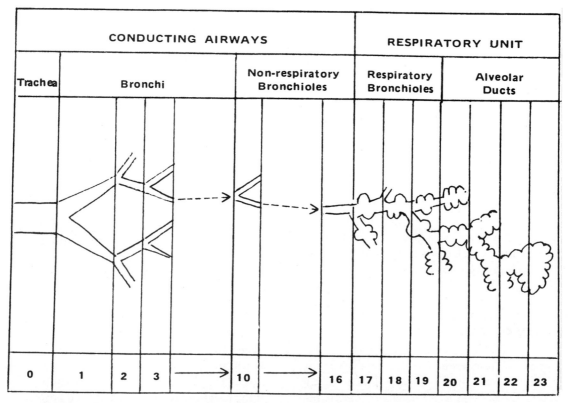

	CONDUCTING AIRWAYS			RESPIRATORY UNIT	
Trachea	Bronchi	Non-respiratory Bronchioles	Respiratory Bronchioles	Alveolar Ducts
0	1 2 3 → 10 →	16	17 18 19	20 21 22 23

FIGURE 1.4. Conducting airways and terminal respiratory unit of the lung. The relative size of the respiratory unit is greatly enlarged. Figures at the bottom indicate the approximate number of generations from trachea to alveoli. (Modified from Weibel ER. *Morphometry of the human lung.* Heidelberg: Springer-Verlag, 1963.)

and expiration, and pulmonary function tests show both inspiratory and expiratory flow limitation.

The *lower respiratory tract* begins at the junction of the larynx with the trachea and includes the trachea, bronchi, bronchioles, and alveoli. The air conduction system of the lungs is a series of dichotomously branching bronchi and bronchioles, ending blindly in some 300 million alveoli, which collectively form the gas exchange surface (Fig. 1.4). There are normally about 23 generations of airways, of which the first 16 or so are conducting airways, where no gas exchange occurs, and the last seven or so are respiratory airways, where alveoli appear in progressively larger numbers (15). The average diameter of a daughter branch is smaller than that of its parent branch, but the *total cross-sectional area* of each successive generation *increases* from trachea to alveoli; thus, the total area of the respiratory bronchioles is much greater than that of the trachea (Fig. 1.5).

Trachea

The trachea begins at the base of the neck and extends about 10 to 12 cm to its bifurcation into the right and left main bronchi. It lies immediately anterior to the esophagus and behind the aorta and often lies slightly to the right of the midline after entering the thorax. Its transverse diameter is greater than its anterior-posterior diameter, and it is held

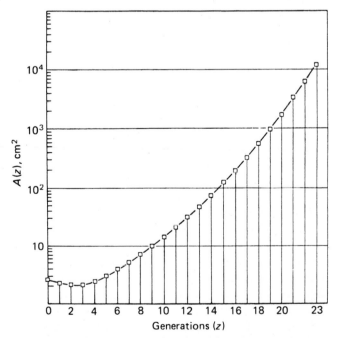

FIGURE 1.5. Total cross section of the airways in the human lung by generation. Although each generation of airways is smaller than its parent, the *total* cross-sectional area of each generation is greater than the *total* area of the previous generation. (From Weibel ER. *Morphometry of the human lung.* Heidelberg: Springer-Verlag, 1963.)

open by a series of anterior horseshoe-shaped cartilaginous rings bound posteriorly by fibrous bands. The position of the carina varies according to the position of the neck and the level of inspiration but is normally at about the level of the second anterior rib, just below the aortic arch. The angle between the right and left main bronchi is normally acute, varying from 50 to 100 degrees.

Bronchi

The right main bronchus divides almost immediately into the upper lobe bronchus and the intermediate bronchus. The left main bronchus is considerably longer, extending across the midline approximately 5 cm before it divides into the left upper-lobe and left lower-lobe bronchi. The major bronchi contain large numbers of mucous glands; their surface is innervated by branches of both the parasympathetic and the sympathetic nervous systems. These nerves are connected to the brain via the vagus nerves. Irritant receptors in large airways initiate the cough reflex, and resultant motor stimuli through the vagi cause bronchoconstriction and mucus secretion. Airway nerves also permit axon–axonal reflexes; therefore, irritation of one site in the airway can lead to bronchoconstriction or secretion diffusely. Neuropeptides, including substance P and the neurokinins, are thought to be important mediators released by these sensory nerves in the airways (16).

The right main bronchus is larger and less deviated from the axis of the trachea than the left; it thus may be considered an extension of the trachea itself. This is an explanation for the more frequent aspiration of foreign material into the right lung. The main bronchi divide into five lobar bronchi—the upper, middle, and lower on the right and the upper and lower on the left. The left upper lobe divides into the apical-posterior and anterior segments and the lingula, which developmentally corresponds to the right middle lobe. The lobes are separated from each other by fissures, which are lined by two layers of visceral pleura.

The lobar bronchi divide into segmental bronchi, 10 on the right and nine on the left (Fig. 1.6). Segments are usually separated by delicate connective tissue planes but not by fissures. There is some disagreement concerning the nomenclature of the bronchopulmonary segments; however, the classification of the Thoracic Society of Great Britain (shown in Fig. 1.10), is the one most commonly used. A thorough knowledge of the lung segments has become necessary in recent years because of the high incidence of bronchogenic carcinoma, one of the most common neoplasms. These neoplasms commonly occur in lobar and segmental bronchi and produce characteristic patterns, based on their anatomic location, on the chest x-ray film.

The epithelial cells that line the airways change in character from the proximal to the distal airways. In the trachea, the epithelium is pseudostratified with as many as four or five nuclei arranged above each other. Most of the surface

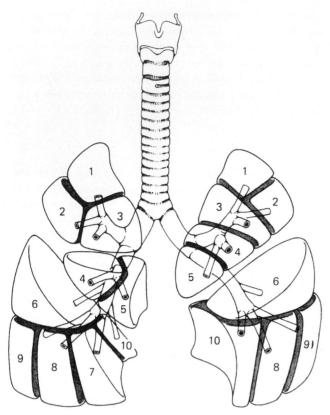

FIGURE 1.6. The bronchopulmonary segments. *Upper lobes:* (1) apical; (2) posterior; (3) anterior; (4) superior lingular; and (5) inferior lingular segments. *Middle lobe:* (4) lateral and (5) medial segments. *Lower lobes:* (6) apical (superior); (7) medial basal; (8) anterior basal; (9) lateral basal; and (10) posterior basal segments. The medial basal segment (7) is absent in the left lung. (From Weibel ER. Design and structure of the human lung. In: Fishman AP (ed). *Assessment of pulmonary function.* New York: McGraw-Hill, 1980.)

area of the basement membrane, however, is covered by basal cells. These small cells with scant cytoplasm have numerous hemidesmosomes, which anchor them to the basement membrane, as well as numerous desmosomes, which provide mechanical anchors for the columnar cells of the epithelium. It is currently thought that all columnar cells extend a slender process that contacts the basement membrane, hence the designation "pseudostratified." These processes may function to regulate the differentiated phenotype of the epithelial cells.

The columnar cells consist predominantly of ciliated cells, with smaller numbers of goblet cells and brush cells. *Ciliated cells* contain motile cilia, which beat in a coordinated manner to move the mucus layer toward the mouth. *Goblet cells,* interspersed among the ciliated epithelial cells, secrete mucus. *Brush cells* contain microvilli resembling those of basal cells in the gut and may function to control fluid balance in the airway lumen. These cells may also represent immature ciliated cells. Following injury, the epi-

thelial cellular components change, and goblet cells or squamous cells, which are usually nonkeratinizing and stratified, may replace the population of ciliated cells.

The columnar cells are connected by several types of junctions. Mechanical integrity is thought to depend on desmosomes formed with basal cells and with other columnar cells. Gap junctions between epithelial cells provide for exchange of nutrients and metabolites and may be important in permitting cell-to-cell exchange of mediators that coordinate epithelial functioning. Near the epithelial surface, the epithelial cells are linked by tight junctions. These junctions permit a fusion of the outer leaflet of the lipid bilayer cell membrane of adjacent cells. These junctions prevent exchange between the apical and basolateral membranes because they extend entirely around each cell. Tight junctions thus permit the airway epithelium to form a barrier segregating the airway lumen from the airway parenchyma. In addition, the apical cell surface is segregated from the basolateral cell surface. Many functions, particularly those involved in the regulation of secretion, depend on processes that are localized within the cell membranes.

The epithelium contains numerous glands with ducts that penetrate and empty into the airway lumen. In addition to the trachea, glands are particularly prevalent in the medium-sized bronchi but are sparse in the smaller bronchi. Glands contain two types of secretory cells: *serous cells,* which secrete a variety of peptides including lysozyme, lactoferrin, and the secretory leukoprotease inhibitor as well as ions and water, and *mucous cells,* which secrete mucins. Because the volume of glands is estimated to be 40-fold greater than that of the luminal goblet cells, they are thought to be the major sources of bronchial mucous secretions. Luminal secretory cells and glands, however, may be regulated differently and may make qualitatively different contributions to airway secretions. Hypertrophy of the mucous glands can occur in chronic bronchitis; the *Reid index* (a ratio of the depth of gland penetration to the thickness of the bronchial wall) is a measure of this hypertrophy.

The columnar cells are highly elongated in the proximal airways, and basal cells are common (Fig. 1.7). In more peripheral airways, the columnar cells gradually become shorter and basal cells become fewer, disappearing in the terminal airways. The total height of the epithelium diminishes as its character changes from pseudostratified to columnar. Ciliated cells become less numerous and glands gradually disappear in the smaller bronchi. *Clara cells* are often seen scattered between ciliated cells and may project into the airway lumen (17). These cells contribute, along with the type II alveolar cells, to the surface lining layer of the bronchioles and alveoli. Clara cells may also function as progenitors for ciliated cells, brush cells, and goblet cells. This may explain why there is a decrease in Clara cells with an increase in epithelial mucous cells in the bronchi of heavy smokers.

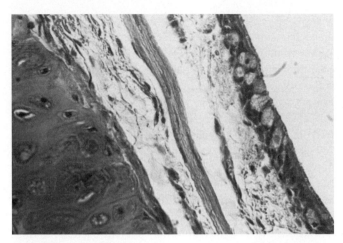

FIGURE 1.7. Section through the wall of a large bronchus (×400). The lumen (right) is lined with pseudostratified columnar epithelial cells containing tiny cilia, which propel mucus toward the trachea. The submucosa is surrounded by a thin layer of smooth muscle. To the left is a part of the cartilage that lends support to the bronchial wall. (Courtesy of Warren D. Grafton, MD.)

Bronchioles

The segmental bronchi continue to bifurcate for about 10 generations, until the nonrespiratory bronchiole is reached (Fig. 1.4). Bronchioles usually are 1 mm in diameter or smaller (18). Respiratory bronchioles, which are 0.5 mm or smaller in diameter, have alveoli in their walls and communicate directly with the alveolar ducts (Fig. 1.8). The bronchioles have a lining mucosa that contains Clara, ciliated, and basal cells. Clara cells are scattered between ciliated cells and may project into the airway lumen (17). Clara cells

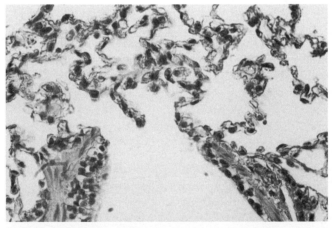

FIGURE 1.8. Section through a terminal bronchiole (×400). At the center of the picture the terminal bronchiole is dividing into two respiratory bronchioles whose walls contain alveoli. The respiratory bronchioles end in alveolar sacs. (Courtesy of Warren D. Grafton, MD.)

tend to disappear with an increase in epithelial mucous cells in the bronchi of heavy smokers. Surrounding the bronchiolar mucosal layer is a basement membrane, a lamina propria, an elastic tissue layer, a layer of smooth muscle, and an adventitial layer that is attached to the surrounding alveoli and perivascular interstitium. The total cross-sectional circumference of the terminal bronchioles in human lungs is nearly 2,000 times that of the trachea (Fig. 1.5) (15). Beyond the terminal bronchiole the airways contain progressively larger numbers of alveoli. As shown in Figure 1.4, *alveolar ducts* are found after approximately three generations of respiratory bronchioles. These are totally lined by alveolar type I cells.

Direct communications occur between bronchioles and surrounding alveoli *(canals of Lambert),* and it is through these canals that bronchiolar epithelium may grow into the alveoli in the healing phase of bronchiolitis (18). This has been called lambertosis or peribronchiolar metaplasia. Ventilation of the conducting airways ceases to be bulk flow at the level of the alveolar ducts. Farther distally, movement of gases is by gaseous diffusion. Ventilation of the gas-exchange surfaces, therefore, depends on how far the gases must travel from the alveolar duct to the alveolar wall. If small peripheral airways become partly or completely occluded, collateral ventilation of alveoli may occur via the *pores of Kohn,* holes in the alveolar walls that connect alveoli directly, or via the canals of Lambert. This collateral ventilation increases the physiologic dead space and adds to the ventilation-perfusion mismatching seen in diseases that affect the small airways (19). However, it prevents lung segments distal to obstructed airways from becoming atelectatic.

METABOLIC AND SECRETORY FUNCTIONS OF THE RESPIRATORY MUCOSA

In addition to their role as conducting airways, the respiratory bronchi and bronchioles have been shown to perform ever-expanding duties involving the production of secretory products and the transport of electrolytes and water. Surfactant is a highly heterogeneous mixture of phospholipid-protein aggregates. It is produced by the nonciliated cells of the bronchioles as well as the type II cells of the alveoli. In the adult lung, phosphatidylcholine and phosphatidylglycerol are the most abundant phospholipids; lesser amounts of sphingomyelin, neutral lipids, glycolipids, and other lipids are found in surfactant as well. Toward the end of fetal gestation, surfactant phospholipids increase markedly in the lungs, and are secreted into the amniotic fluid. The levels of phospholipids in amniotic fluid correlate with postnatal respiratory function. Four surfactant proteins, SP-A, SP-B, SP-C, and SP-D, are produced by respiratory epithelial cells (20). They play important roles in surfactant function and host defenses. Other proteins produced by the respiratory epithelieal cells include the Clara Cell Protein (CC16,

CC10) and mucin-associated antigens (KL-6, 17-Q2, 17-B1). These proteins are important for host defenses (20). Beyond this, the epithelial goblet cells and the mucous glands secrete the complex mucous blanket, which serves a vital role in the defense of the lungs and the removal of foreign particles.

The respiratory epithelium also serves an important role in the movement of solutes and water, contributing to the maintenance of lung fluid balance. The epithelial cells are joined at their apical surface by tight junctions, which have selective permeabilities to ions, other solutes, and water (21). Furthermore, the cells are polar, and the apical membrane, which faces the mucosal surface, is different from the basolateral membrane, which faces the submucosal space. This provides for selective celluar pathways for ion transport (Fig. 1.9). The apical membrane contains chloride channels, known as cystic fibrosis transmembrane conductance regulator (CFTR) chloride channels (22). Epithelial cells lack the CFTR chloride channels in patients with cystic

fibrosis. A variety of neurohumeral and pharmacologic agents regulate the transepithelial electrolyte transport; most of these tend to stimulate the chloride transepithelial channels. Less is known about the control of sodium transport in the airway epithelium; however, active sodium absorption appears to be responsible for fluid absorption, and when amiloride, which inhibits sodium absorption, is given, fluid secretion ensues. Normally, the fluid in the bronchi has a low salt concentration, with chloride levels of 80 to 90 mM. In patients with cystic fibrosis, surface fluid has higher chloride levels, in the range of 130 to 170 mM, suggesting that chloride absorption through CFTR channels tends to lower the salt concentration in the mucosal fluid. High salt concentrations in CF airway fluid may prevent bacterial killing by antibacterial factors from the epithelium, and may also affect the normal hydration of mucus (23).

DISTRIBUTION OF BLOOD

The lungs contain approximately 450 mL of blood, or 12% of the body's total blood volume. Seventy to one hundred milliliters of this blood are contained within the pulmonary capillaries, the rest is equally divided between the pulmonary arteries and veins (24).

The lungs are the only organ to receive essentially the entire cardiac output, a feature that facilitates their role in gas exchange and allows them to modify the blood before it is returned to the left ventricle. The lungs receive blood from two sources: the bronchial arteries, which contain oxygenated blood; and the pulmonary arteries, which contain systemic venous blood. The bronchial arteries are part of the systemic circulation and supply the supporting tissue of the lungs, including the walls of the bronchi and bronchioles to the level of the alveoli. In contrast, the pulmonary arteries are components of the low-pressure, highly compliant pulmonary circulation that originates from the right ventricle and supplies the dense capillary network surrounding the alveolar wall. The structure of this dense vascular meshwork facilitates the critical gas-exchange as well as metabolic functions of the lung.

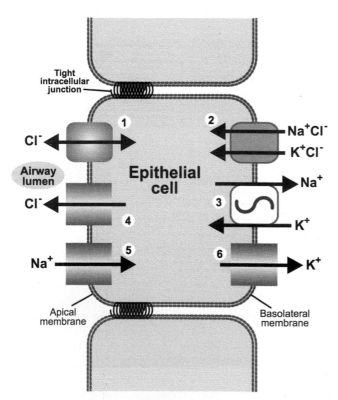

FIGURE 1.9. Mechanisms of electrolyte transport through the respiratory epithelium. Rounded boxes indicate passive pathways of ion exchange, whereas square boxes indicate active transport channels. (1) Cystic fibrosis transmembrane conductance regulatory (CFTR) chloride channel, which is powered by cAMP; patients with cystic fibrosis lack this pathway. (2) Electrically neutral co-transport channel moves Cl^- into the cell coupled with Na^+ and K^+. (3) The ATPase-powered sodium-potassium pump maintains high intracellular K^+ levels and low intracellular Na^+ levels. (4) Chloride exits passively into the mucosa via apical membrane channels. (5) Sodium enters the cell passively via epithelial Na^+ channels (ENaC). (6) Passive K^+ exit via basolateral K^+ channels.

Right Ventricle

The pulmonary circulation begins as the main pulmonary artery leaves the right ventricle. Because the left ventricle contracts with extreme force compared to the right ventricle, it assumes a globular shape and the septum protrudes into the right heart. Because both sides of the heart pump essentially the same quantity of blood, the external wall of the right ventricle bulges outward, surrounding a large portion of the left ventricle to accommodate the blood volume (Fig.

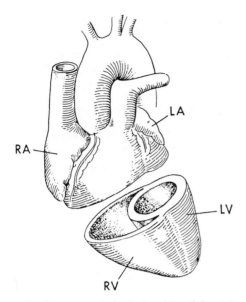

FIGURE 1.10. The anatomical relationship of the right ventricle to the left ventricle, demonstrating the globular-shaped left ventricle protruding into the right heart. LA, left atrium; LV, left ventricle; RA, right atrium; RV, right ventricle. (Adapted with permission from Guyton AC. The pulmonary circulation. In: *Textbook of medical physiology,* 9th ed. Philadelphia: Saunders, 1996.)

1.10) (24). As a result of the lower pressures generated by the right side of the heart, the right ventricular muscle is only one-third as thick as that of the left ventricle (24).

Pulmonary Arteries and Veins

The main pulmonary artery, carrying mixed venous blood from the right side of the heart, extends only 5 cm beyond the apex of the right ventricle before dividing into the right and left main branches, which supply the two respective lungs. The main pulmonary artery and its subdivisions are thin-walled, distensible vessels (24). Furthermore, the subdivisions of the pulmonary artery, including the small arteries and arterioles, have much larger diameters than the corresponding systemic arteries. This anatomic feature makes the pulmonary vascular tree extremely compliant, averaging 7 mL/mm Hg, which is almost equal to that of the entire systemic arterial tree. This large compliance allows the pulmonary arteries to accommodate the stroke volume output of the right heart (24).

Like the airways, the main pulmonary artery branches successively, the pulmonary arteries accompanying the bronchi through the centers of the primary lobules as far as the terminal bronchioles (25). Beyond that point, the pulmonary arterioles form a dense capillary network (Fig. 1.11) within the alveolar wall, an arrangement exceedingly efficient for gas exchange (25,26).

Oxygenated blood leaves the pulmonary capillaries in the short, distensible, pulmonary veins that form at the periph-

ery of the terminal respiratory unit and that later coalesce to form the four large pulmonary veins that empty into the left atrium. In addition to the alveolar capillaries, a portion of the bronchial system also empties into the pulmonary veins. The deoxygenated blood added to the pulmonary veins by the bronchial system accounts for a significant portion of the right-to-left anatomic shunt that normally occurs in the lungs.

Pulmonary Capillaries

The majority of lung vasculature consists of alveolar capillaries (27). The alveolar walls are occupied by a dense meshwork or sheet of capillaries and supporting tissue that together form a barrier to transvascular fluid exchange (Fig. 1.11). Arteriolar branches of the pulmonary artery feed at regular intervals into this dense capillary meshwork that then coalesce into venules (28). The pulmonary capillaries are surrounded by air rather than supported by tissue, as in the systemic circulation. Although this arrangement facilitates gas exchange, it exposes the pulmonary capillaries to stress failure or rupture if intravascular pressure becomes excessive (29).

The closely apposed epithelial and endothelial barriers of the alveolar-capillary membrane are both involved in the regulation of fluid and solute exchange in the lung (Fig. 1.12) (27). The alveolar capillary allows a net outward movement of fluid and small solutes from the vascular to the interstitial space. In contrast, the alveolar epithelium forms a highly restrictive barrier that limits the movement of water and ions into the alveolus. Although the vascular

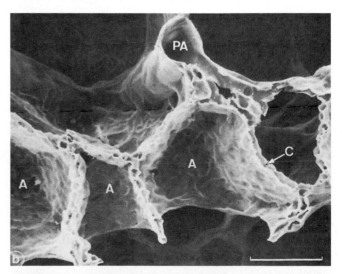

FIGURE 1.11. Blood flow in pulmonary capillaries (C) surrounds the alveoli (A) in a dense vascular network. PA, pulmonary arteriole; marker = 50 μm. (Reprinted with permission from Weibel ER. Design and morphometry of the pulmonary gas exchanger. In: Crystal RG, West JB, Weibel WR, et al, eds. *The lung: scientific foundations.* New York: Lippincott-Raven, 1997:1147–1159.)

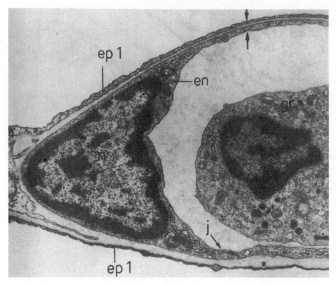

FIGURE 1.12. The alveolar–capillary membrane constitutes the primary barrier at the air–blood interface and consists of an endothelial cell (en) and the adjacent type I epithelial cell (ep1) with their fused basement membranes. (Reprinted with permission from Weibel ER. Lung cell biology. In: Fishman AP, ed. *Handbook of physiology, Vol 1, The respiratory system.* Baltimore: Williams & Wilkins; 1985:47–91.)

layer of the alveolus appears to be formed only by endothelial cells, the alveolar airspace is lined by at least two types of epithelial cells (Table 1.2) (30). Type I epithelial cells cover the majority of the alveolar lining, whereas type II cells cover a smaller percentage of the air space, but actively synthesize and secrete surfactant. The type II cells also appear to regenerate damaged type I cells. Interstitial cells provide support for the structures in the alveolar walls, whereas alveolar macrophages are an important component of the host defense and lung clearance mechanisms.

ALVEOLAR–CAPILLARY BARRIER

Although the major site of fluid exchange in the lung is in the alveolar capillaries, some fluid also leaks from the small

TABLE 1.2 CELLS OF THE ALVEOLAR REGION OF THE HUMAN LUNG

Cells	$n \times 10^9$	Total (%)
Alveolar epithelial cells		
Type I cells	19	8.3
Type II cells	37	15.9
Endothelial cells	68	30.2
Interstitial cells	84	36.1
Macrophages	23	9.4

Reprinted with permission from Crapo JD, Barry BE, Gehr P, et al. Cell number and cell characteristics of the normal human lung. *Am Rev Respir Dis* 1982;125:740–745.

arterioles and venules at the junctions of alveolar walls (31). The forces that govern microvascular fluid exchange are discussed in detail in Chapter 23, Acute Hypoxemic Respiratory Failure.

Alveolar–Epithelial Barrier

Once thought to be composed of passive, structural cells, the alveolar epithelium is now recognized as the primary barrier against fluid movement into the alveolus. In fact, current evidence suggests that the alveolar epithelium is at least an order of magnitude less permeable than the pulmonary endothelium; hence, it is the main regulator of fluid and solute exchange across the alveolar–capillary membrane (33,34). The restrictive properties of the epithelial barrier are thought to depend on the adhesion of several specialized proteins found in the tight and adherens junctions (35–37). Moreover, the alveolar epithelium plays an active role in the reabsorption of any fluid that leaks into the alveolus (38).

Capillary–Endothelial Barrier

The pulmonary vasculature is composed of continuous or nonfenestrated endothelium, characterized by organelle-free zones that provide an exceptionally thin barrier to gas exchange (39). Most of the exchange of fluid and solute across the vascular endothelium occurs at endothelial cell–cell junctions (Fig. 1.13) (40,41). The structural components of these junctions consist of *occludin,* a major component of tight junctions, and *cadherins,* which form the adherens junction (36,42).

Pulmonary endothelial cells express adhesion molecules that facilitate leukocyte–endothelial cell interaction and that contribute to enhanced transvascular fluid leak in response to a variety of lung insults (Fig. 1.13). The interaction of these endothelial cell adhesive proteins with specific white blood cell counter-receptors, mediates leukocyte slowing, arrest, and tissue migration in response to lung injury or inflammation (43,44).

PHYSIOLOGY OF THE PULMONARY CIRCULATION

Pulmonary Vascular Pressures

Because the pulmonary circulation supplies only one organ, the right ventricle is required to generate only enough pressure in the pulmonary artery to pump blood to the top of the lung. Consequently, pressures in the pulmonary circulation are approximately 10-fold less than pressures in the systemic circulation (Fig. 1.14) (25). As a result of the remarkably low pressures in the pulmonary vasculature, the walls of the pulmonary artery and its branches are extremely

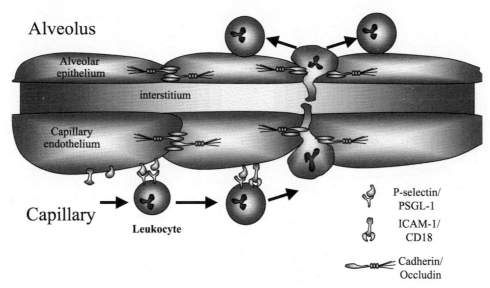

FIGURE 1.13. The interaction of the adhesion glycoprotein, P-selectin, on the alveolar endothelium with P-selectin glycoprotein ligand (PSGL-1) on white blood cells mediates leukocyte rolling along the vascular wall. The interaction of endothelial ICAM-1 with the leukocyte adhesive determinant, CD 18, contributes to firm leukocyte adhesion and extravascular migration. These events contribute to leukocyte trafficking in the lung and alter the barrier properties of the alveolar–capillary membrane.

thin, with little surrounding connective tissue and minimal smooth muscle.

Figure 1.14 illustrates that the pressure drop within the pulmonary vasculature is more uniform than in the systemic circulation. In addition, the capillaries are more important determinants of vascular resistance in the pulmonary circulation than in the systemic circulation, where the primary resistance vessels are the small, muscular arterioles (45).

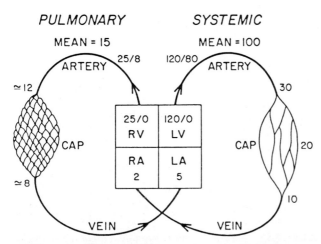

FIGURE 1.14. Comparison of pressure (in mm Hg) in the pulmonary and systemic circulations. LA, left atrium; LV, left ventricle; RA, right atrium; RV, right ventricle. (Reproduced with permission from West JB. *Respiratory physiology: the essentials,* 4th ed. Baltimore: Williams & Wilkins, 1989.)

Pulmonary Vascular Resistance

Pulmonary vascular resistance (PVR) can be described by the following relationship:

$$\text{PVR (mm Hg/L/min)} = \frac{\Delta P \text{ (mm Hg)}}{Q \text{ (L/min)}}$$

where ΔP is the pressure gradient between the pulmonary artery and the pulmonary veins or left ventricle and Q is pulmonary blood flow. The total pressure drop from the pulmonary artery to the left ventricle is about 10 mm Hg in contrast to a pressure gradient of about 100 mm Hg in the systemic circulation (Fig. 1.14). Since blood flow through the pulmonary and systemic circulations is essentially identical, PVR is only one-tenth systemic vascular resistance.

Resistance to blood flow through the vasculature is directly related to vessel length and inversely related to vessel diameter (24). Consequently, anything that increases pulmonary capillary diameter will decrease PVR. The unique arrangement of the pulmonary capillaries in dense sheets (Fig. 1.11) over the alveolar wall provides much less resistance than flow through systemic capillaries (46).

Although the PVR is normally low, it has an extraordinary capacity to become even lower as pressure within the pulmonary vasculature rises (25,47). Figure 1.15 demonstrates that an increase in either pulmonary arterial or venous pressure causes PVR to decrease. Two mechanisms contribute to this decrease. First, as pulmonary vascular pressure rises, previously collapsed vessels begin to conduct

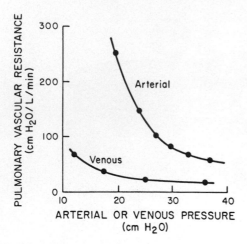

FIGURE 1.15. Fall in pulmonary vascular resistance as the pulmonary arterial or venous pressure is raised. Venous pressure was held constant at 12 cm H_2O when the arterial pressure was changed and arterial pressure was held at 37 cm H_2O when the venous pressure was changed. Data from an excised dog preparation. (Adapted with permission from West JB. *Respiratory physiology: the essentials,* 4th ed. Baltimore: Williams & Wilkins, 1989.)

blood, a process termed capillary *recruitment.* Recruitment is the primary mechanism responsible for the fall in PVR as pulmonary artery pressure rises. Second, as intravascular pressure rises, previously patent pulmonary capillaries become *distended,* thereby increasing their internal diameter and resulting in a decline in PVR.

Another important determinant of PVR is lung volume. As the lung expands, alveolar pressure rises and may exceed the intravascular pressure in *alveolar capillaries.* When alveolar pressure exceeds alveolar capillary intravascular pressure, these vessels collapse, resulting in an increase in their vascular resistance. In contrast, the connective tissue scaffolding surrounding *extra-alveolar capillaries* pulls them open as lung volume rises, causing vascular resistance in these vessels to fall (Fig. 1.16). Thus, changes in lung volume produce

opposing effects on vascular resistance in alveolar and extra-alveolar capillaries.

Distribution of Pulmonary Blood Flow

The distribution of blood flow throughout the pulmonary vasculature is not uniform (25). In the upright human lung, blood flow decreases from the bottom to the top of the lung, reaching the lowest levels at the lung apex (25). The effect of gravity on pulmonary vascular pressures is one of the major factors causing these regional inequalities in blood flow. The pulmonary arterial system behaves as a continuous column of blood with a hydrostatic pressure difference of about 30 cm H_2O (or 23 mm Hg) in the upright lung (25). This large pressure gradient has a significant impact on the low-pressure pulmonary circulation.

The effect of hydrostatic pressure gradients on regional lung blood flow is illustrated in Figure 1.17. In zone 1, at the top of the lung, pulmonary arterial pressure may fall below alveolar pressures, causing the capillaries to collapse and blood flow to cease. Under normal conditions, this does not occur because the pulmonary arterial pressure is sufficient to raise blood to the top of the lung. However, zone 1 conditions could occur if pulmonary arterial pressure falls (e.g., following severe hemorrhage) or if alveolar pressure is raised (e.g., during positive pressure ventilation).

Zone 2 occurs near the middle of the lung. Pulmonary arterial pressure rises in zone 2 because of the hydrostatic effect of gravity on the column of blood. In zone 2, pulmonary arterial pressure exceeds alveolar pressure. However, venous pressure remains lower than alveolar pressure because the veins in this zone may be below the level of the heart. In zone 2, the pressure gradient determining blood flow is the arterial–alveolar pressure difference, not the typi-

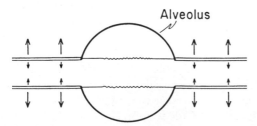

FIGURE 1.16. As lung volume and alveolar pressure rise, alveolar capillaries collapse causing vascular resistance in these vessels to increase. In contrast, extra-alveolar capillaries are pulled open by surrounding connective tissue as lung volume increases, resulting in a fall in vascular resistance. (Adapted with permission from Hughes JMB, Glazier JB, Maloney JE, et al. *Respir Physiol* 1968; 4:58.)

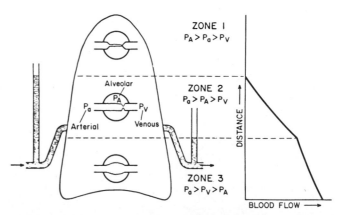

FIGURE 1.17. The zone model of regional inequalities in blood flow in the lung based on hydrostatic pressure differences affecting the capillaries. (Adapted with permission from West JB, Dollery CT, Naimark A. Distribution of blood flow in isolated lung: relation to vascular and alveolar pressure. *J Appl Physiol* 1964; 19:713.)

cal arterial–venous pressure gradient. Blood flow increases down zone 2 because the hydrostatic effect increases arterial pressure while alveolar pressure remains unchanged. Moreover, capillary *recruitment* occurs down zone 2 (25).

Zone 3 occurs near the bottom of the lung where the hydrostatic effect causes both arterial and venous pressure to exceed alveolar pressure. Blood flow in zone 3 is determined by the usual arterial–venous pressure gradient. Blood flow also increases down zone 3 because of *distention* of patent capillaries.

Some evidence suggests that blood flow decreases again in zone 4, at the very bottom of the lung. Excessive intravascular pressure resulting in interstitial edema and collapse of alveolar capillaries has been proposed as a possible mechanism for diminished blood flow in zone 4.

Regulation of the Pulmonary Circulation

The pulmonary circulation is regulated by *active* factors, such as the autonomic nervous system, circulating vasoactive substances, and alveolar oxygen content. However, it is also influenced by *passive* factors, such as changes in cardiac output and left atrial pressure as well as gravitational forces. It is likely that the normally low pulmonary vascular tone is maintained by a tightly regulated balance of locally and systemically produced vasoactive substances. The lung actively participates in the synthesis, storage, or degradation of these factors.

Resting Vascular Tone

Although the pulmonary circulation is a low-resistance system, some degree of resting vascular tone is maintained by the pulmonary vasculature, as evidenced by the fact that administration of vasodilators elicits a further decline in pulmonary artery pressure and resistance (48). It is likely that the sympathetic nervous system, as well as circulating catecholamines, prostaglandins, endothelins, and nitric oxide contribute to basal vascular tone in the pulmonary circulation.

Autonomic Nervous System

There are both α- and β-adrenergic receptors in the pulmonary vascular bed with a prevalence of α receptors (49,50). Evidence suggests that although there is some degree of basal sympathetic tone in the pulmonary circulation, it is less than in the systemic vascular bed (47).

Catecholamines and Other Vasoactive Substances

Release of substantial amounts of epinephrine or norepinephrine may elicit mild pulmonary vasoconstriction be-

cause of the prevalence of α receptors within the pulmonary vasculature (49). Other vasoactive substances also produce pulmonary vasoconstriction. For example, histamine—a mediator of type I (immediate) hypersensitivity reactions—is widely distributed throughout the lung parenchyma, pulmonary mast cells, and within the pulmonary circulation (52). In contrast to its vasodilating properties in the systemic circulation, histamine causes constriction of pulmonary vessels through interaction with H_1 receptors (53).

Other substances that are metabolically altered by the lung appear to contribute to basal or stimulated pulmonary vascular tone. For example, serotonin (5-hydroxytryptamine), released from argentaffin cells in the intestine or lung or from platelets, elicits a rise in pulmonary vascular resistance by increasing both pre- and postcapillary tone (47,54). Angiotensin II, prostaglandins of the F series, and the leukotrienes are also pulmonary vasoconstrictors. In contrast, bradykinin and prostaglandins of the E series elicit pulmonary vasodilation. PGI_2 (prostacyclin), one of the major eicosanoids produced by the lung, is also a vasodilator and platelet aggregation inhibitor that may contribute not only to low pulmonary vascular resistance, but also to the antithrombogenic properties of the pulmonary vasculature (55). The overall balance of vasodilating and vasoconstricting substances that are delivered to or metabolically altered by the lung, probably contributes to basal as well as stimulated pulmonary vascular tone.

Endothelial-Derived Vasoactive Factors

In addition to modifying vasoactive agents, the pulmonary vascular endothelium is capable of synthesizing substances that participate in the regulation of normal pulmonary vascular tone. These substances, such as endothelin-1 and nitric oxide, induce vasoconstriction or vasodilation, respectively (56,57).

Endothelins
Endothelin (ET)-1, ET-2, and ET-3 are members of a family of vasoconstrictor peptides that are synthesized as larger propeptides, termed big ETs. Pulmonary endothelial cells express an endothelin converting enzyme which converts big ET-1 to ET-1. Low concentrations of ET-1 elicit pulmonary vasodilation while larger concentrations produce significant and sustained vasoconstriction, mediated through ET_A receptors (58). A role for ET-1 in asthma and pulmonary hypertension has been suggested, because enhanced expression of this peptide has been identified in patients with these disorders (59,60).

Nitric Oxide
Nitric oxide (NO), previously known as endothelial-derived relaxing factor, is synthesized in pulmonary endothelial cells through the action of NO synthase on the amino acid pre-

cursor, L-arginine. NO diffuses to the underlying vascular smooth muscle cell where it activates the enzyme, guanylyl cyclase, thereby increasing intracellular concentrations of cGMP (cyclic guanosine monophosphate) and inducing smooth muscle relaxation (61). Not only does NO appear to contribute to basal pulmonary vascular tone, but also it may also contribute to pulmonary hypoxic vasoconstriction, because hypoxia has been shown to inhibit endothelial NO production (62,63).

Hypoxic Vasoconstriction

The most important mechanism that actively regulates blood flow in the lungs is hypoxic vasoconstriction. In contrast to the systemic circulation, where hypoxia induces vasodilation, hypoxia elicits vasoconstriction in the pulmonary circulation. The vasoconstriction occurs on the arterial side of the pulmonary circulation when *alveolar* oxygen tension approaches 60 mm Hg. Hypoxic pulmonary vasoconstriction is exaggerated in the presence of arterial acidosis (Fig. 1.18). In contrast to the effect of alveolar hypoxia, pulmonary arterial hypoxemia does not induce the vasoconstrictor response (49).

Pulmonary hypoxic vasoconstriction is beneficial in patients with pneumonia, pulmonary edema, or respiratory failure, in that blood flow is shunted away from poorly ventilated areas, thereby reducing the degree of venous admixture and hypoxemia. However, considerable attention has been given to the deleterious effects of hypoxic pulmonary vasoconstriction in chronic conditions such as severe COPD with hypoventilation. The marked increase in pulmonary vascular resistance resulting from the hypoxic vasoconstrictor response predisposes to cor pulmonale and right heart failure (64,65). Therapy with low-flow oxygen can relieve some of the pulmonary hypertension seen in hypoxic patients with COPD and prolong life (65).

Three mechanisms have been proposed to explain hypoxic vasoconstriction: (1) Hypoxia may stimulate the production of a vasoconstricting substance; (2) Hypoxia may inhibit the production of a vasodilating substance; and (3) Hypoxia may directly affect vascular smooth muscle (66). Although endothelin-1, histamine, angiotensin II, and prostaglandins of the F series have all been proposed as vasoconstrictors and NO as the vasodilator, the mechanism by which hypoxia elicits pulmonary vasoconstriction remains undefined (63).

Passive Forces

As described in the preceding, increased pulmonary arterial or venous pressure can elicit a decrease in PVR (Fig. 1.15) through capillary recruitment as well as capillary distention. In addition, the hydrostatic pressure effects on regional blood flow in the lung are significant (Fig. 1.17). Changes in cardiac output, left atrial pressure, and the effects of gravity all contribute to the regulation of the pulmonary circulation. In contrast to the effect of active factors such as vasoactive substances, passive factors change pulmonary vascular resistance or blood flow independent of changes in pulmonary vascular tone.

METABOLIC, NONRESPIRATORY FUNCTIONS OF THE LUNG

In addition to gas exchange, the lung performs a large number of metabolic functions in response to normal or inflammatory stimuli. The vast surface area of the pulmonary endothelium, strategically located to receive the entire output of the right ventricle, modifies the composition of the circulating blood before it returns to the left heart. The pulmonary microvascular endothelium has evolved elaborate systems for the synthesis, storage, degradation, or activation of inflammatory, chemical, and mechanical stimuli to accomplish these metabolic tasks.

The fate of several vasoactive substances during a single pass through the pulmonary circulation is indicated in Table 1.3. The extent of removal indicated applies only when the concentration of the substance in the pulmonary arteriolar blood is normal. In pathologic disturbances, when large amounts of compounds may be released or administered,

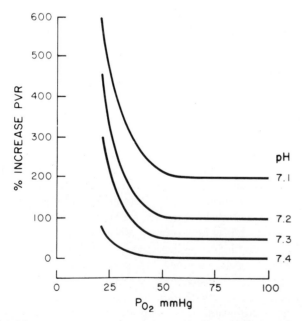

FIGURE 1.18. The effect of changes in inspired PO_2 on pulmonary vascular resistance (PVR) under conditions of different arterial blood pH in newborn calves. As inspired PO_2 is decreased, pulmonary vascular resistance increases; an effect exaggerated by acidosis. (Reproduced from Rudolph AM, Yuan S. Response of the pulmonary vasculature to hypoxia and H^+ ion concentration changes. *J Clin Invest* 1966;45:399–411, by copyright permission of the American Society for Clinical Investigation.)

TABLE 1.3 SUMMARY OF THE FATE OF CIRCULATING SUBSTANCES DURING A SINGLE PASS THROUGH THE INTACT PULMONARY CIRCULATION

Substance	Fate
Amines	
Acetylcholine	Uncertain
Serotonin	Almost completely removed
Norepinephrine	Up to 40% removed
Epinephrine	Unchanged
Dopamine	Unchanged
Histamine	Unchanged
Peptides	
Bradykinin	Up to 80% inactivated
Angiotensin I	Converted to angiotensin II
Angiotensin II	Unchanged
Vasopressin	Unchanged
Arachidonic acid metabolites	
Prostaglandin E_2	Almost completely removed
Prostaglandin F_2	Almost completely removed
Prostaglandin A_2	Unchanged
Prostaglandin I_2 (Prostacyclin)	Unchanged
Thromboxane	Unknown
Leukotrienes	Almost completely removed
Adenine Nucleotides	
Adenosine triphosphate	Almost completely removed
Adenosine monophosphate	Almost completely removed

Reproduced with permission from Murray JF. *The normal lung.* Philadelphia: Saunders, 1986.

the capacity of the lung to deal with them may be overwhelmed (47). Moreover, the efficacy of removal may be markedly altered in patients with lung disease (52,66).

Vasoactive Substances

Biogenic Amines

Pulmonary endothelial cells possess receptors for biogenic amines; however, the metabolism of these substances is not uniform. Some amines, such as serotonin, are rapidly internalized by endothelial cells and extensively degraded by monoamine oxidase (MAO) during a single pass through the lungs (70,71). Norepinephrine is also internalized and metabolized by the lungs, although less efficiently than serotonin. Biogenic amines such as propranolol are internalized and stored unchanged in lung endothelial cells, whereas others such as histamine, dopamine, and epinephrine pass through the pulmonary circulation without alteration (72). The fact that histamine is not removed from the pulmonary circulation is surprising given its widespread pulmonary distribution and the fact that most vascular beds metabolize histamine (72).

Proteins and Peptides

Many circulating peptides and proteins exhibit potent vasoactive properties that must be modified to function appro-

priately. The pulmonary endothelium contains enzymes that modulate circulating peptides, proteins, or amino acids as they traverse the pulmonary circulation under normal as well as pathologic conditions. For example, bradykinin, a potent endogenous vasodilator implicated in the pathogenesis of bronchial asthma and anaphylaxis, is almost completely removed during passage through the lungs by the action of enzymes and peptidases on the enodothelial cell surface (73,74). Furthermore, the pulmonary endothelial uptake of the NO precursor, L-arginine, as well as proteins required for antioxidant synthesis, are increased by inflammatory stimuli or oxidant injury (75–77).

One of the best characterized enzymes on the luminal surface of the pulmonary endothelium is angiotensin converting enzyme (ACE). ACE is uniformly distributed along the pulmonary endothelium and plays a critical role in the control of systemic vascular pressures and volume homeostasis by regulation of the renin–angiotensin system. Angiotensin I is formed in the circulation from an α-2 globulin precursor by the action of the enzyme renin. ACE converts the inactive decapeptide angiotensin I into the powerful vasoconstrictor, angiotensin II, in a single pass through the lung (78). No physiologically significant conversion of angiotensin I to angiotensin II has been demonstrated outside the lung (73).

Eicosanoids

Arachadonic acid (AA) is synthesized in the lung and other tissues from the cleavage of cellular membrane phospholipids (Fig. 1.19). The metabolites of AA, the *eicosanoids,* not only are synthesized by pulmonary endothelial cells, but also are inactivated to a large extent by the pulmonary vasculature. AA can be metabolized by either the cyclooxygenase

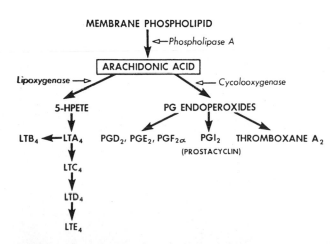

FIGURE 1.19. Pathways of arachidonic acid metabolism. Prostaglandins and thromboxane A_2 are generated by the cyclooxygenase pathway; the leukotrienes are generated by the lipoxygenase pathway. (Adapted with permission from Murray JF. *The normal lung.* Philadelphia: Saunders, 1986.)

pathway, resulting in the production of the *prostaglandins* and *thromboxanes,* or the lipoxygenase pathway, resulting in the production of the *leukotrienes* (Fig. 1.19).

Prostaglandins, specifically PGI_2 and PGE_2, are the major eicosanoids produced by the pulmonary endothelium (78). In general, prostaglandins of the F series constrict pulmonary and systemic blood vessels as well as bronchial smooth muscle, whereas prostaglandins of the E series elicit vasodilation and bronchodilation. The lungs inactivate AA and over 90% of prostanglandins of the E and F series but have little effect on prostaglandins of the A series and PGI_2 (80).

Leukotrienes induce enhanced microvascular permeability and marked bronchoconstriction, and contribute to the airway inflammatory response. The leukotrienes are almost entirely removed within a single pass by the pulmonary circulation.

Nucleotides

The pulmonary microvascular endothelium contributes significantly to the regulation of adenosine, a potent vasodilator, and its nucleotide derivatives by rapidly removing them from the circulation (81). In addition, pulmonary capillary endothelium has a high density of *caveolae intracellulare* that communicate with the vasculature and are the site of adenine nucleotide metabolism (Fig. 1.20) (82).

Endothelial-Derived Substances

Eighty percent of ET-1 and ET-3 are removed from the circulation by first-pass elimination by the lung (83). In contrast, there is basal production of NO that appears to contribute to normal pulmonary vascular tone. NO production in pulmonary endothelial cells is enhanced by changes in shear stress, blood flow, oxygen tension, and the binding of acetylcholine to specific endothelial receptors.

GAS EXCHANGE AREA

Terminal Respiratory Unit

In the past, different authors have used various names for the smaller divisions of the lung architecture. To prevent confusion, the *terminal respiratory unit* (TRU) is herein defined as the portion of lung distal to a terminal nonrespiratory bronchiole (84,85). The TRU has been called the acinus by Lauweryns and the primary lobule by Miller (86,87). Three to five TRUs together form a *pulmonary lobule,* which is separated from its neighboring lobules by an interlobular septum containing lymphatic channels; these interlobular septa may become visible as Kerley's "B" lines on the chest x-ray film when they are distended by fluid or fibrosis (88).

A stylized version of a TRU is illustrated in Figure 1.21. The unit is designed to perform its basic function of gas exchange efficiently. The terminal bronchiole enters the center of the TRU accompanied by a branch of the pulmonary artery carrying unoxygenated blood from the body tissues. The arteriole divides into a rich network of pulmonary capillaries that cover the alveolar walls and drain into pulmonary venules, which lie in the periphery of the TRU. These venules converge into larger branches situated in the interlobular septa. This arrangement results in the organized perfusion of a lobule from the center to the periphery.

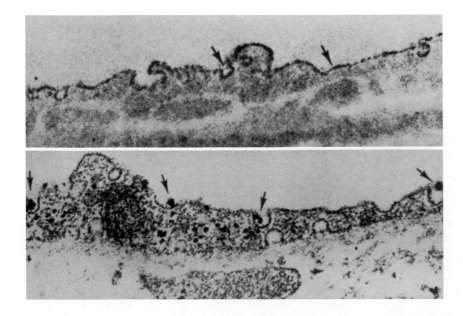

FIGURE 1.20. A: Section of rat pulmonary capillary endothelium demonstrating the location of angiotensin converting enzyme. The electron-dense reaction product (arrows) is located on the plasma membrane and caveolae intracellulare facing the vascular lumen (original magnification × 76,000). (Reprinted by permission from Ryan US, Ryan JW, Whitaker C, et al. Localization of angiotensin converting enzyme (Kinase II). II, Immunocytochemistry and immunoflurorescence. *Tissue cell* 1976;8:125–146.) **B:** Cytochemical localization of 5′ nucleotidase on rat pulmonary endothelial cell (arrows), (original magnification × 95,000). (Reprinted by permission from Smith U, Ryan JW. Pinocytotic vesicles of the pulmonary endothelial cell. *Chest* 1971;59:12S–15S.)

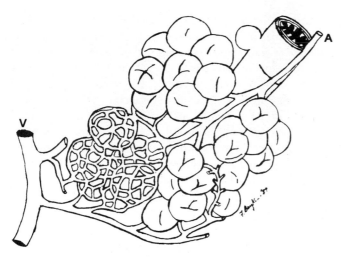

FIGURE 1.21. A terminal respiratory unit (TRU), the basic gas-exchanging unit of the lungs. The pulmonary arterial branch *(A)* enters the center of the TRU along with the terminal bronchiole. It anastomoses with the pulmonary venule in the alveolar walls, forming a dense capillary network for gas exchange. Venous drainage is to the periphery of the TRU, where the venous branches *(V)* lie. They coalesce to form the major pulmonary veins, which carry oxygenated blood.

LUNG CLEARANCE AND DEFENSES

The lung is at hazard for injury by virtue of its direct contact with the atmosphere, necessary for gas exchange. Major irritants that invade the respiratory tract include organic agents (e.g., bacteria, fungal spores, and viruses) and inorganic agents (e.g., industrial exhaust, dusts, and cigarette smoke). These infectious and noninfectious agents may act together to produce acute or chronic disease. Complicated and effective defense mechanisms have evolved to protect the respiratory tract from these inhaled substances (89).

Particle Deposition in the Respiratory Tract

The deposition of particles in the lungs depends on their size and density, the distance over which they must travel, and the relative humidity. The method of breathing (i.e., mouth breathing versus nose breathing), the rate of air flow, the minute ventilation, and the depth of breathing also influence the deposition of the aerosol. Defense mechanisms vary depending on where in the respiratory tract particles are deposited as well as on their size and composition. In general, particles larger than 10 μm in diameter are deposited by impaction in the upper respiratory passages. Particles between 2 and 10 μm are carried in the airstream into the lower respiratory tract, where they impact in the bronchial tree. Particles between 0.5 and 3 μm are too small to impact in the airways but are deposited in the gas exchange areas

of the lungs (the TRUs). Particles smaller than 0.2 μm are not efficiently deposited in the lung and may be exhaled. Modern nebulizers are capable of generating aerosols containing small particles of controlled size in high concentrations; thus, they are efficient means of depositing particles in the distal parts of the respiratory tract.

Transport Systems of the Lungs

Three transport systems are available for the removal of inhaled particles from the alveoli: the mucociliary escalator, the phagocytes, and the lymphohematogenous drainage system. These systems work together, although they operate through different pathways at different rates (89).

Mucociliary Escalator

The mucociliary escalator functions to transport deposited particles from the level of the terminal bronchioles to the major airways, where they are coughed up and either expectorated or swallowed. The transport rate of this system is about 3 mm/minute and becomes more rapid proximally, where the streams converge. Approximately 90% of the particles directly deposited on the mucus layer are cleared within 2 hours. In the main bronchi, the mucociliary apparatus is formed by the ciliated epithelial cells, the mucus-producing goblet cells, and the mucous glands, which open directly onto the mucosa. In the smaller bronchi and bronchioles mucus is formed from goblet cell secretions. In the smallest peripheral bronchioles, goblet cells are not normally seen, and the epithelium is lined by a thin layer of material containing surfactant that is derived from the Clara cells and the type II alveolar cells. This layer flows proximally and is continuous with the mucus layer of the mucociliary escalator.

The mucus, which is the transport medium, is a complex mucopolysaccharide arranged in a double layer on the surface of the epithelium (Fig. 1.22). The external layer is a

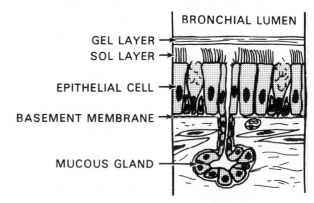

FIGURE 1.22. The mucociliary escalator. The gel layer of mucus is propelled toward the trachea by the movement of the cilia on the surface of the cells.

viscous gel, which acts as a trap to catch and transport deposited particles. The mucous gel is elastic, therefore, the mechanical beating of cilia is able to propel both mucus and any entrapped particulates proximally. Loss of mucus elasticity can impair clearance. The internal sol layer is a thin liquid in which the cilia are able to move easily. The cilia themselves move with a characteristic biphasic rhythm. Beating within the liquid layer and striking the gel layer with their tips, they exhibit a periodic movement, forming wave bands that move the mucus up the bronchial tree toward the larynx. Efficient beating of cilia requires that the sol layer have an appropriate viscosity. In addition, the sol layer must be of the proper thickness so that cilia tips contact the mucous gel on the forward beat, but release on the reverse beat. Effective clearance, therefore, requires a sol layer of appropriate composition and amount.

Many factors can alter clearance. Ciliary motion can be affected by exposure to a variety of substances. Toxic fumes and cigarette smoke, for example, may disrupt normal wave patterns or cause cilia to stop beating completely. Hereditary abnormalities of the cilia alter their movement and result in the "immotile cilia syndrome" (90). This syndrome can result from a variety of cilia defects, several of which can be recognized by electron microscopy of cilia. These hereditary diseases are associated with immotile cilia not only in the lung and upper respiratory tract, but also at other sites where cilia are present, such as sperm cells and cells lining the nasal sinuses. Immotile sperm and male infertility, therefore, may be associated with the immotile cilia syndromes. Cilia in the developing embryo are responsible for pushing the developing heart to the left. With immotile cilia, localization is nearly random, and approximately half of individuals have dextrocardia or situs inversus. The triad of situs inversus associated with bronchiectasis and sinusitis, associated with immotile cilia, is termed Kartagener's syndrome.

Chronic bronchitis, asthma, cystic fibrosis, and acute respiratory infections may cause loss of cilia or abnormal ciliary function. These conditions are also associated with altered mucus secretion. Deoxyribonucleic acid (DNA) derived from inflammatory cells can increase viscosity, and proteolytic enzymes can disrupt mucus elasticity; thus, these disorders are associated with impaired clearance for a number of reasons. It is likely that increased susceptibility to infection in these disorders results, at least in part, from these clearance defects.

The alveolar surface itself is protected to some extent by the normal movement of the surface lining layer into the peripheral bronchi. However, the alveolar phagocytes and the lymphohematogenous drainage system are more important to alveolar clearance.

Alveolar Macrophage

The principal resident phagocyte of the alveoli is the alveolar macrophage. Some replication of these cells may take place in the lung, but they are ultimately derived from precursors in bone marrow that migrate in the peripheral blood as monocytes. Compared to mononuclear phagocytes at other sites (e.g., peritoneal macrophages), alveolar macrophages possess adaptations for the aerobic environment of the lung. Macrophages can phagocytose surfactant and are probably involved in the metabolic turnover of many of the extracellular components of the alveoli. Macrophages also phagocytose both bacteria and nonliving particulates. This process can be augmented by both specific and nonspecific opsonins, which can bind to particulates and subsequently interact with specific macrophage receptors. Bacteria may be killed and particles digested by powerful enzymes in the cellular lysosomes following phagocytosis. Organic molecules may be further detoxified by oxidases and a variety of transferases.

Macrophages are also able to release a host of cytokines. Through the release of these mediators, macrophages are able to recruit and activate other inflammatory cells. Neutrophils, recruited in response to macrophage-derived chemotactic factors such as leukotriene B_4 or interleukin-8, can greatly augment the phagocytic defenses of the lung. Cytokines derived from macrophages can also recruit and activate lymphocytes and pulmonary parenchymal cells. Macrophages are likely, therefore, to play a central role in initiating and maintaining chronic inflammatory processes in the lungs. The ability of macrophages to regulate parenchymal cells, combined with their capability to release proteases capable of degrading all components of the extracellular matrix, suggests that they may also be crucial regulators of tissue repair and remodeling.

Lymphohematogenous Drainage

The third transport system of the lungs is the lymphohematogenous drainage system. The alveolar septum contains connective tissue and is a space that may potentially act as a vehicle for the exit of macrophages from the alveoli. From there macrophages may enter the pulmonary capillaries or the lymphatics of the lung periphery. Inhaled particles probably do not enter lymphatics directly unless inflammation is present, but are carried within phagocytic cells. The speed of transport via the lymphatic system is variable and may take months or years. Collections of macrophages containing large amounts of foreign particles are frequently seen in the lymph nodes of the lungs, where they may remain permanently.

Pulmonary Lymphatics

The lungs and pleura are richly supplied with lymphatics. The purpose of the large flow of lymph from the lungs is twofold. First, it forms a natural mechanism for the removal of excess fluid that moves into the interstitial spaces from the pulmonary capillaries, thus keeping the alveoli relatively free of fluid. Second, it forms an important part of the alveolar defense mechanism by transporting macrophages containing inhaled particles from distal areas of the lungs. It is largely because of this rich lymphatic system that bronchogenic carcinoma travels out of the lungs so readily. The lymphatics in the terminal respiratory units converge in the interlobular septa. Movement of lymph is increased by respiratory movements coupled with a series of valves in the lymphatic vessels, which ensures proximal flow. Chronic increased pulmonary capillary pressure, and presumably increased production of pulmonary lymph, can be associated with increased capacity for lymphatic clearance. The lymphatics line the pulmonary arteries and veins as well as the bronchi themselves and converge at the pulmonary hila, where the hilar lymph nodes are found. From here the thoracic duct drains the left lung, and the right lymphatic duct drains the right. These vessels enter the systemic venous circulation at the junctions of the subclavian and internal jugular veins.

The bronchopulmonary lymph nodes surround the divisions of the lobar bronchi, and hilar glands are clustered at the lung roots. The hilar lymph nodes occur around the upper and lower lobe bronchi and communicate richly via the subcarinal nodes with the opposite side. Paratracheal nodes are found on either side of the trachea and are most prominent on the right. The *azygos* node is found adjacent to the azygos vein at the junction of the right upper lobe bronchus and the right main bronchus. The pulmonary lymphatic system communicates with the lower deep cervical nodes above and with the abdominal lymphatics below. In addition to the hilar and mediastinal lymph nodes there are also lymphatics along the distribution of the internal mammary arteries, near the intercostal arteries adjacent to the posterior ribs, and in the anterior and posterior mediastinum, which receive drainage primarily from the chest wall.

There is some disagreement as to the drainage of the various lobes of the lung, and indeed drainage channels may vary among individuals. In general, the lower lobes drain into the hilar and subcarinal nodes, whereas the upper lobes more often drain directly to the paratracheal nodes. Thus, cancers arising in lower-lobe bronchi must traverse an extra set of lymph nodes, the hilar group, before reaching the paratracheal chain. The rich system of anastomoses among lymph node groups may account at least in part for the variation in lymphatic drainage of the lobes. Lymphocytes in intrapulmonary and regional nodes may become reactive, and the nodes may enlarge in a variety of inflammatory lung diseases, both infectious (e.g., granulomas) and noninfectious (e.g., silicosis).

Lymphocytes accumulate beneath the epithelium of airways, where they are termed bronchus-associated lymphoid tissue (BALT). These airway lymphocytes are thought to participate in the system of mucosal immunity and to be responsible for local responses to antigen with both local and generalized production of immunoglobulin, particularly IgA. Lymphocytes are also present in the pulmonary parenchyma, and their numbers may increase significantly in disease states. Although the mechanisms responsible are not fully elucidated, lymphocytes present in the lung are thought to be capable of migrating to regional nodes, circulating in the blood, and then relocalizing at specific tissue sites by virtue of the expression of specific "homing receptors."

ACKNOWLEDGMENT

This work was supported in part by a grant from the National Institutes of Health (NIDDK 2 PO1 DK 4378506).

REFERENCES

1. Staub NC, Albertine KH. The structure of the lungs relative to their principal function. In: Murray JF, Nadel JA, eds. *Textbook of respiratory medicine.* Philadelphia: Saunders, 1988:12–16.
2. Macklem PT. Respiratory muscles: the vital pump. *Chest* 1980; 78:753–758.
3. Cohen CA, Zagelbaum G, Gross D, et al. Clinical manifestations of inspiratory muscle fatigue. *Am J Med* 1982;73:308–316.
4. Garrity ER Jr, Shart JT. Respiratory muscles: function and dysfunction. *ACCP Pulm Crit Care Update* 1986;2:lesson 10.
5. De Troyer A, Estene M, Heilporn A. Mechanisms of active expiration in tetraplegic patients. *N Engl J Med* 1986;314:740–744.
6. Roncoroni AJ, Androgue HJA, DeObrutsky CW, et al. Metabolic acidosis in status asthmaticus. *Respiration* 1976;33:85–94.
7. Minh VD, Dolan GF, Konopka RF, et al. Effect of hyperinflation on inspiratory function of the diaphragm. *J Appl Physiol* 1976; 40:67–73.
8. Roussos C, Macklem PT. The respiratory muscles. *N Engl J Med* 1982;307:786–797.
9. Yang KL, Tobin MJ. A prospective study of indexes predicting the outcome of trials of weaning from mechanical ventilation. *N Engl J Med* 1991;325:1445–1450.
10. Tobin MJ. Respiratory muscles in disease. *Clin Chest Med* 1988; 9:263–286.
11. Weiner-Kronish JP, Albertine KH, Licko V, et al. Protein egress and entry rates in pleural fluid and plasma in sheep. *J Appl Physiol* 1984;56:459–463.
12. Broaddus VC, Wiener-Kronesh JP, Berthiaume Y, et al. Removal of pleural liquid and protein in lymphatics in awake sheep. *J Appl Physiol* 1988;64:384–390.
13. Armstrong WB, Netterville JL. Anatomy of the larynx, trachea, and bronchi. *Otolaryng Clin NA* 1995;28:685–699.
14. Light RW, George RB. Upper airway obstruction (editorial). *Arch Intern Med* 1977;137:281.
15. Weibel ER. *Morphometry of the lung.* New York: Academic Press, 1963:111.
16. Barnes PJ. Airway neuropeptides: roles in fine tuning and in disease? *News Physiol Sci* 1989;4:116–120.
17. Massaro G. Nonciliated bronchiolar epithelial (Clara) cells. In: Massaro D, ed. *Lung biology in health and disease, Vol 41, Lung cell biology.* New York: Marcel Dekker, 1989:81–114.
18. Colby TV. Bronchiolitis: pathological considerations. *Am J Clin Pathol* 1998;109:101–109.
19. Terry PB, Traystman RJ, Newball HH, et al. Collateral ventilation in man. *N Engl J Med* 1978;298:10.

20. Hermans C, Bernard A. Lung epithelium-specific proteins. *Am J Respir Crit Care Med* 1999;159:646–678.

21. Boucher RC. Human airway ion transport. *Am J Respir Crit Care Med* 1994;150:271–281.

22. Riordan JR. The cystic fibrosis transmembrane conductance regulator. *Ann Rev Physiol* 1993;55:609–630.

23. Smith JJ, Travis SM, Greenberg EP, et al. Cystic fibrosis airway epithelia fail to kill bacteria because of abnormal airway surface fluid. *Cell* 1996;85:229–236.

24. Guyton AC. The pulmonary circulation. In: *Textbook of medical physiology*, 9th ed. Philadelphia: Saunders, 1996:491–501.

25. West JB. *Respiratory physiology*, 4th ed. Baltimore: Williams & Wilkins, 1990:31–49.

26. Weibel ER. Design and morphometry of the pulmonary gas exchanger. In: Crystal RG, West JB, Weibel ER, et al, eds. *The lung: scientific foundations*. New York: Lippincott-Raven, 1997:1147–1159.

27. Weibel ER. Lung cell biology. In: Fishman AP, ed. *Handbook of physiology. Vol 1, The respiratory system*. Baltimore: Williams & Wilkins: 1985:47–91.

28. Weibel ER, Gil J. Structure-function relationships at the alveolar level. In: West JB, ed. *Bioengineering aspects of the lung. Vol 3, Lung biology health and disease series*. New York: Marcel Dekker, 1977:1–81.

29. West JB, Mathieu-Costell O. Structure, strength, failure and remodeling of the pulmonary blood-gas barrier. *Annu Rev Physiol* 1999;61:543–572.

30. Crapo JD, Barry BE, Gehr P, et al. Cell number and cell characteristics of the normal human lung. *Ann Rev Resp Dis* 1982;125:740–745.

31. Matthay MA, Matthay RA *Chest medicine: essentials of pulmonary and critical care medicine*. Baltimore: Williams & Wilkins, 1995:593–618.

32. Wood LD, Prewitt RM. Cardiovascular management in acute hypoxemic respiratory failure. *Am J Cardiol* 1981;47:963–972.

33. Taylor AE, Gaar KA. Estimation of equivalent pore radii of pulmonary capillary and alveolar membranes. *Am J Physiol* 1970;218:1133–1140.

34. Normand ICS, Olver RE, Reynolds EOR, et al. Permeability of lung capillaries and alveoli to non-electrolytes in the fetal lamb. *J Physiol* 1971;219:303–330.

35. Gumbiner B, Simons K. A functional assay for proteins involved in establishing an epithelial occluding barrier: identification of a uvomorulin-like polypeptide. *J Cell Biol* 1986;102:457–468.

36. Volk T, Geiger B. A-cam: A 135-kD receptor of intercellular adherens junctions. II. Antibody-mediated modulation of junction formation. *J Cell Biol* 1986;103:1451–1464.

37. Gumbiner B, Stevenson B, Grimaldi A. The role of the cell adhesion molecule uvomorulin in the formation and maintenance of the epithelial junctional complex. *J Cell Biol* 1988;107:1575–1587.

38. Matthay MA, Landolt CC, Staub NC. Differential liquid and protein clearance from the alveoli of anesthetized sheep. *J Appl Physiol* 1982;53:96–104.

39. Simionescu M. Lung endothelium: structure-function correlates. In: Crystal RG, West JB, Weibel ER, et al, eds. *The lung: scientific foundations*. New York: Lippincott-Raven, 1997;615–629.

40. Allport JR, Ding H, Collins T, et al. Endothelial dependent mechanisms regulate leukocyte transmigration: a process involving the proteasome and disruption of the vascular endothelial cadherin complex at endothelial cell to cell junctions. *J Exp Medicine* 1997;186:517–527.

41. Burns AR, Walker DC, Brown ES, et al. Neutrophil transendothelial migration is independent of tight junctions and occurs preferentially at tricellular corners. *J Immunol* 1997;159:2893–2903.

42. Lampugnani MF, Resnati M, Raiteri M, et al. A novel endothelial specific membrane protein is a marker of cell-cell contacts. *J Cell Biol* 1992;118:1511–1522.

43. Carden DL, Alexander JS, George RB. The pathophysiology of the acute respiratory distress syndrome. *Pathophysiology* 1998;5:1–13.

44. Diamond MS, Staunton DE, Marlin SD, et al. Binding of the integrin Mac-1 (CD11b/CD18) to the third Ig-like domain of ICAM-1 (CD54) and its regulation by glycosylation. *Cell* 1991;65:961–967.

45. Guyton AC. Overview of the circulation: medical physics of pressure, flow and resistance. In: *Textbook of medical physiology*, 9th ed. Philadelphia: Saunders, 1996:493.

46. Powell FL. Structure and function of the respiratory system. In: Johnson LR, ed. *Essential medical physiology*, 2nd ed. Philadelphia: Lippincott-Raven, 1998:248–249.

47. Murray JF. *The normal lung*. Philadelphia: Saunders, 1986:150.

48. Bergofsky EH, Bass BG, Ferretti R, et al. Pulmonary vasoconstriction in response to precapillary hypoxemia. *J Clin Invest* 1963;4:1201–1205.

49. Bergofsky EH. Active control of the normal pulmonary circulation. In: Moser KM, ed. *Pulmonary vascular disease*. New York: Marcel Dekker, 1979:1–18.

50. Widdicombe JG, Sterling G. The autonomic nervous system and breathing. *Ann Intern Med* 1970;126:311.

51. Murray PA, Lodato RF, Michael JR. Neural antagonists modulate pulmonary vascular pressure-flow plots in conscious dogs. *J Appl Physiol* 1986;60:1900–1907.

52. Gillis CN, Roth JA. Pulmonary disposition of circulation vasoactive hormones. *Biochem Pharmacol* 1976;25:2547–2553.

53. Tucker A, Weir EK, Reeves JT, et al. Histamine H_1 and H_2 receptors in the pulmonary and systemic vasculature of the dog. *Am J Physiol* 1975;229:1008–1013.

54. Bhattacharya JH, Nanjo S, Staub NC. Micropuncture measurement of lung microvascular pressure during 5-HT infusion. *J Appl Physiol* 1982;52:634–637.

55. Grygkewsju RJ, Korbut R, Ocetkiewicz A. Generation of prostacyclin by lungs in vivo and its release into the arterial circulation. *Nature* 1978;273:765–767.

56. Moncada S, Higgs A. The L-arginine-nitric oxide pathway. *N Engl J Med* 1993;329:2002–2012.

57. Dinh-Xuan AT. Endothelial modulation of pulmonary vascular tone. *Eur Respir J* 1992;5:757–762.

58. Bonvallet ST, Oka M, Yano M, et al. BQ123, an ET_A receptor antagonist, attenuates endothelin-1 induced vasoconstriction in rat pulmonary circulation. *J Cardiovas Pharmacol* 1993;22:39–43.

59. Mattoli S, Soloperto M, Marini M, et al. Levels of endothelin in the bronchalveolar lavage fluid of patients with symptomatic asthma and reversible airflow obstruction. *J Allergy Clin Immunol* 1991;88:376–384.

60. Stewart DJ, Levy RD, Cernacek P, et al. Increased plasma endothelin-1 in pulmonary hypertension: marker or mediator of disease? *Ann Intern Med* 1991;114:464–469.

61. Palmer RMJ, Ashton DS, Moncada S. Vascular endothelial cells synthesize nitric oxide from L-arginine. *Nature* 1988;333:664–666.

62. Stamler JS, Loh E, Roddy MA, et al. Nitric oxide regulates basal systemic and pulmonary vascular resistance in healthy humans. *Circulation* 1994;89:2035–2040.

63. Rodman DM, Yamaguchi T, Hasunuma K, et al. Effect of hypoxia on endothlium-dependent relaxation of rat pulmonary artery. *Am J Physiol* 1990;258:L207–L214.

64. Burrows B, Kettel LJ, Niden AH, et al. Patterns of cardiovascular dysfunction in chronic obstructive pulmonary disease. *N Engl J Med* 1972;286:912–918.

65. Nocturnal Oxygen Therapy Trial Group. Continuous or nocturnal oxygen therapy in hypoxemic chronic obstructive lung disease: a clinical trial. *Ann Intern Med* 1981;93:391–398.

66. Fishman AP. Hypoxia on the pulmonary circulation. *Circ Res* 1976;38:221–231.

67. Gillis CN, Catravas JD. Altered removal of vasoactive substances by the injured lung: detection by lung microvascular injury. *Ann NY Acad Sci* 1982;384:458–474.

68. Carlos WM, Bedrossian MD, Woo J, et al. Decreased ACE in adult respiratory distress syndrome. *Am J Clin Pathol* 1978;70: 244–247.

69. Oparis S, Low J, Koerner TJ. Altered angiotensin I conversion in pulmonary disease. *Clin Sci Mol Med* 1976;51:537–543.

70. Fisher A, Block ER, Pietra G. Environmental influences on uptake of serotonin and other amines. *Environ Health Perspect* 1980; 35:191–198.

71. Roth RA, Wallace KB, Alper RH, et al. Effect of paraquat treatment of rats on disposition of 5-hydroxytryptamine and angiotensin I by perfused lung. *Biochem Pharmacol* 1979;28: 2349–2355.

72. Youdim MBH, Bakhle YS, Ben-Harari RR. Inactivation of monoamines by the lung. *Ciba Found Symb* 1980;78:105–128.

73. Vane JR. The release and fate of vaso-active hormones in the circulation. *Br J Pharmacol* 1969;35:202–208.

74. Baker CRF Jr, Little AD, Little GH, et al. Kinin metabolism in the perfused ventilated rat lung. I: Bradykinin metabolism in a system modeling the normal, uninjured lung. *Circ Shock* 1991; 33:37–47.

75. Cendan JC, Moldawer LL, Souba WW, et al. Endotoxin-induced nitric oxide production in pulmonary artery endothelial cells is regulated by cytokines. *Arch Surg* 1994;129:1296–1300.

76. Souba WW, Salloum RM, Bode BP, et al. Cytokine modulation of glutamine transport by pulmonary artery endothelial cells. *Surgery* 1991;110:295–302.

77. Deneke SM, Baxter DF, Phelps DT, et al. Increase in endothelial cell glutathione and precursor amino acid uptake by diethyl maleate and hyperoxia. *Am J Physiol* 1989;257:L265–L271.

78. Bunning P, Budeck W, Escher R, et al. Characteristics of angiotensin converting enzyme and its role in the metabolism of angiotensis I by endothelium. *J Cardiovasc Pharmacol* 1986;8(suppl 10):S52–S57.

79. Hewitt PW, Murray JC. Human lung microvessel endothelial cells: isolation, culture, and characterization. *Microvasc Res* 1993; 46:89–102.

80. McGiff JC, Terragno NA, Strand JC, et al. Selective passage of prostaglandins across the lung. *Nature* 1969;216:762–766.

81. Pearson JD, Carleton JS, Hutchings A, et al. Uptake and metabolism of adenosine by pig aortic endothelial and smooth-muscle cells in culture. *Biochem J* 1978;170:265–271.

82. Smith U, Ryan JW. An electron microscopic study of the vascular endothelium as a site for bradykinin and adenosine-5′-triphosphate inactivation in rat lung. *Adv Exp Med Biol* 1979;8: 249–261.

83. De Nucci G, Thomas R, D'Orleans JP, et al. Presser effects of circulating endothelin are limited by its removal in the pulmonary circulation and by the release of protacyclin and endothelium derived relaxing factor. *Proc Natl Acad Sci USA* 1988;85: 9797–9800.

84. Von Hayek H. *The human lung* (trans. Krohl VE). New York: Hafner, 1960.

85. Staub NC. The interdependence of pulmonary structure and function. *Anesthesiology* 1963;24:831.

86. Lauweryns JM. The blood and lymphatic microcirculation of the lung. In Sommers SC, ed: *Pathology annual 1971*. New York: Appleton-Century-Crofts, 1971.

87. Miller WS. *The lung*. Baltimore: Charles C Thomas, 1937.

88. Reid L, Simon G. The peripheral pattern in the normal bronchogram and its relation to peripheral pulmonary anatomy. *Thorax* 1958;13:103.

89. Green GM. In defense of the lung. *Am Rev Respir Dis* 1970;102: 691.

90. Eliasson R, Mossberg B, Camner P, et al. The immotile cilia syndrome: a congenital ciliary abnormality as an etiologic function in chronic infection and male sterility. *N Engl J Med* 1977; 297:1–6.

2

MECHANICS OF RESPIRATION

RICHARD W. LIGHT

LUNG VOLUMES: THE DIMENSIONS OF THE RESPIRATORY SYSTEM

VOLUME-PRESSURE RELATIONS OF THE RESPIRATORY SYSTEM DURING RELAXATION
Pressure-Volume Curves for the Chest Wall, Lung, and Respiratory System

VOLUME-PRESSURE RELATIONS OF THE RESPIRATORY SYSTEM DURING MUSCULAR EFFORTS

Measurement of Pleural Pressure
Pleural Pressure Gradients
Factors Holding the Lung Against the Chest Wall
Factors Influencing the Pressure-Volume Curve of the Lung

DYNAMICS OF THE RESPIRATORY SYSTEM
Airway Resistances
Pressure–Flow Relationships
Density Dependence of Maximal Air Flow
Distribution of Ventilation
Work of Breathing

In this chapter, the factors that determine the volume of the lungs and hemithorax and the movement of air into and out of the lungs are described.

LUNG VOLUMES: THE DIMENSIONS OF THE RESPIRATORY SYSTEM

Figure 2.1 illustrates the subdivisions of the lungs during various respiratory maneuvers. The total lung capacity (TLC) is the total amount of air that is in the lungs after a maximal inspiration. The TLC is dependent on the height, age, and sex of the subject, being larger in taller, younger, and male individuals.

The vital capacity (VC) is the maximal amount of air that a subject is able to expire after a maximal inspiration. The residual volume (RV) of the lungs is the amount of air that is still in the lungs at the end of a maximal expiration. It is normally approximately 25% of the total lung capacity. The sum of the RV and the VC is equal to the TLC.

The functional residual capacity (FRC) is the quantity of air in the lungs and airways at the end of a spontaneous expiration. Therefore, it is the resting volume of the lungs. Normally, it is about 40% of the total lung capacity.

The tidal volume (V_T) is the volume of air that is breathed in during inspiration or out during expiration. It averages about 600 mL in normal subjects under resting conditions. The minute ventilation is the total amount of air moved into and out of the lungs during 1 minute. It is equal to the product of the V_T and the respiratory rate.

The inspiratory capacity (IC) is the maximal volume of air that can be inspired from the resting level (FRC). The IC is approximately 60% of the TLC. The inspiratory reserve volume (IRV) is the IC minus the V_T, or the maximal volume of air that can be inspired beyond the V_T. The expiratory reserve volume (ERV) is the maximal volume of air that can be expired beyond the FRC. The sum of the ERV and the IC is equal to the VC.

VOLUME-PRESSURE RELATIONS OF THE RESPIRATORY SYSTEM DURING RELAXATION

Everyone who has observed an autopsy realizes that when the chest is opened the lungs collapse and the thorax enlarges. This simple observation illustrates two fundamental static properties of the respiratory system: The lungs tend to recoil inward and the chest wall tends to recoil outward.

The lungs and the chest wall are distensible objects. As with any distensible object, their volume is dependent on their elastic properties and their distending pressure. The distending pressure is the pressure difference between the inner and outer surfaces. The distending pressures for the lungs and the chest are illustrated in Figure 2.2.

The distending pressure of the lung is termed the transpulmonary pressure (P_L) and is the alveolar pressure (P_A) minus the pleural pressure (Ppl).

$$P_L = P_A - Ppl \tag{2.1}$$

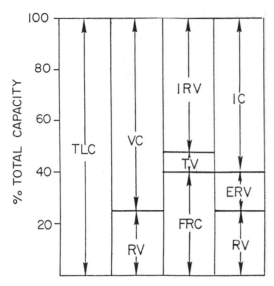

FIGURE 2.1. The subdivisions of the lung volume.

The distending pressure for the chest wall (Pw) is the pleural pressure minus the pressure at the body surface (Pbs).

$$Pw = Ppl - Pbs \qquad (2.2)$$

Note the importance of the pleural pressure in both of these expressions. The distending pressure for the entire respiratory system (Prs) is the sum of the distending pressures for the lung and the chest wall. Because the pleural pressures cancel out, it is the alveolar pressure minus the pressure at the body surface.

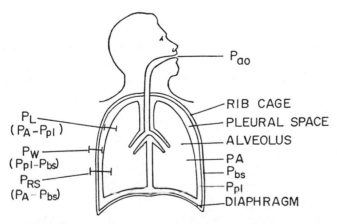

FIGURE 2.2. Respiratory pressures influencing ventilation. Pao, pressure at the airway opening; Ppl, pressure within the pleural space; PA, pressure within the alveoli; Pbs, pressure at the body surface; PL, pressure difference across the lung; Pw, pressure difference across the chest; Prs, pressure across the respiratory system.

$$Prs = PA - Pbs \qquad (2.3)$$

The elastic properties of a distensible object can be defined by means of a volume-pressure diagram for the object. To construct such a diagram, the volumes of the object at different distending pressures are determined. The relationship between changes in volume and changes in pressure define the *compliance* of the object, which is expressed as follows:

$$Compliance = change\ in\ volume/change\ in\ pressure \qquad (2.4)$$

Pressure-Volume Curves for the Chest Wall, Lung, and Respiratory System

If the respiratory muscles are completely relaxed and the heart and lungs removed from the thorax, the elastic properties of the thorax can be studied by adding or removing air from the thorax and observing the relationship between the distending pressure and the volume of the thorax. A pressure-volume curve obtained in this manner is depicted in Figure 2.3*A*. Note that the resting volume of the chest wall—that is, the volume at which the distending pressure is zero—is about 50% of the VC.

In a similar manner, if the lungs are removed from the thorax, a pressure-volume curve for them can be obtained. Such a curve is illustrated in Figure 2.3*B*. As the inflating pressure becomes higher, the volume increment with a given pressure increase becomes progressively smaller.

If the subject is relaxed, a pressure-volume curve for the respiratory system can be obtained by increasing or decreasing the alveolar pressures. The curve so obtained for a respiratory system is shown in Figure 2.3*C*. It is the sum of the curves for the chest wall and the lungs. The resting volume of the respiratory system is the volume at which PA is equal to Pbs and the distending pressure is zero. Note that it is the volume at which the distending pressures of the lungs and the chest wall are equal but opposite in sign. This resting volume is the FRC for the patient.

VOLUME-PRESSURE RELATIONS OF THE RESPIRATORY SYSTEM DURING MUSCULAR EFFORTS

For the volume of the respiratory system to be different than the FRC, muscular effort must be present if the glottis is open and if there is no air flow. In Figure 2.4 the alveolar pressures that can be generated at various lung volumes with maximal inspiratory (Pmax$_{insp}$) and expiratory (Pmax$_{exp}$) efforts are shown. Also shown are the alveolar pressures during relaxation at various lung volumes when there is no flow. The horizontal difference between Pmax$_{insp}$ or Pmax$_{exp}$ and

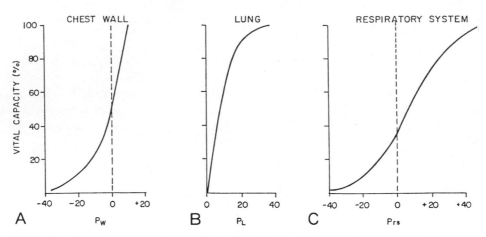

FIGURE 2.3. Static pressure-volume relationships for the chest wall **(A)**, the lungs **(B)**, and the respiratory system **(C)**.

the relaxation pressure gives the net maximal pressure generated by the inspiratory or expiratory muscles, respectively. Note that the higher the lung volumes, the lower the maximal inspiratory pressure and the higher the maximal expiratory pressure. At FRC, the maximal inspiratory pressure is about -100 cm H_2O, whereas the maximal expiratory pressure is about $+150$ cm H_2O.

From Figure 2.4 it is easy to see that the TLC is the volume at which the maximal negative pressure generated by the inspiratory muscles is equal to the relaxed positive pressure of the respiratory system. Accordingly, the total lung capacity is reduced if the lung or the chest wall becomes stiffer (less compliant) or if the inspiratory muscles become weaker. Conversely, the TLC is increased if the lungs or chest wall become more compliant or if the muscles become stronger.

In a similar fashion, the RV is the volume at which the maximal positive expiratory pressure is equal to the relaxed negative pressure of the respiratory system. The RV increases if there is expiratory muscle weakness or if the pressure-volume curve of the respiratory system is shifted to the left, which can occur with a noncompliant chest wall or a very compliant lung (Fig. 2.3). The RV decreases if the lower end of the pressure-volume curve for either the lung or the chest wall is shifted to the right.

Measurement of Pleural Pressure

Because the pleural pressure is the pressure at the inner surface of the chest wall and the outer surface of the lungs, it is an important pressure to measure when studying either normal subjects or patients with pulmonary disease. The

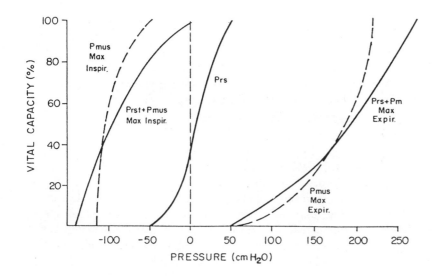

FIGURE 2.4. Schematic demonstrating the relationship between the alveolar pressures generated during maximal inspiratory and expiratory efforts. The dashed lines indicate the pressure contributed by the muscles.

pleural pressure can be measured directly by inserting needles, trocars, catheters, or balloons into the pleural space. However, direct measurement of the pleural pressure is not usually performed because of the danger of producing a pneumothorax or an infection of the pleural space. At the present time, pleural pressures are usually measured indirectly, using a fluid-filled catheter or a balloon positioned in the subject's esophagus. Because the esophagus is located between the two pleural spaces, esophageal pressure measurements provide a close approximation of the pleural pressure at the level of the device in the thorax (1). Estimation of pleural pressure by means of an esophageal balloon is not without its pitfalls (1). The volume of air within the balloon must be small so that the balloon is not stretched and the esophageal walls are not displaced; otherwise, falsely elevated pleural pressure measurements will be obtained. Moreover, the balloon must be short and must be placed in the lower part of the esophagus. If care is taken, reliable pressure-volume curves of the lung can be obtained by measuring esophageal pressure at different lung volumes while the subject holds his or her breath with the glottis open to eliminate the effect of changes in alveolar pressure. Reliable measurements of esophageal pressures can also be made with liquid-filled catheter manometer systems (2). Use of these devices circumvents some of the problems associated with esophageal balloons.

Pleural Pressure Gradients

Although estimation of the pleural pressure via an esophageal balloon gives a value for the pleural pressure, the pleural pressure is not uniform throughout the chest. There is a gradient in pleural pressure between the top and bottom of the lung, with the pleural pressure being lowest, or most negative, at the top and highest, or least negative, at the bottom. The main factors responsible for the pleural pressure gradient are probably gravity, mismatching of the shapes of the chest wall and lung, and the weight of the lungs and other intrathoracic structures (3).

The magnitude of the pleural pressure gradient is on the order of 0.50 cm H_2O per centimeter of vertical distance (3). Therefore, in the upright position the difference in the pleural pressure between the apex and the base of the lungs may be 12 cm H_2O or more. Because the alveolar pressure is constant throughout the lungs, the effect of the pleural pressure gradient is that different parts of the lungs have different distending pressures (PL). The transpulmonary pressure is approximately 12 cm H_2O higher in the uppermost than in the lowermost portion of the lungs.

It is thought that the pressure-volume curve is the same for different regions of the lung regardless of their location. Therefore, the variation in pleural pressure results in the alveoli in the superior parts of the lung being larger than those in the inferior parts. Moreover, since separate alveoli

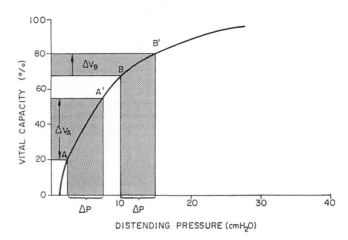

FIGURE 2.5. Pressure-volume curve of a normal lung. At functional residual capacity, the alveoli in the lower part of the lung *(A)* are at a smaller volume than those in the upper part of the lung *(B)* on account of the pleural pressure gradient. Then, when a given amount of distending pressure (ΔP) is applied to both sets of alveoli, the volume increase of those in the lower parts of the lung (ΔV_A) is much greater than that in the upper parts of the lung (ΔV_B) because of the shape of the pressure-volume curve.

are at different positions on their pressure-volume curves, a given change in distending pressure causes varying volume changes throughout the lung. For these reasons, at lung volumes above FRC, alveoli in the inferior parts expand considerably more than those at the top, as illustrated in Figure 2.5. At low lung volumes, the pleural pressure may become positive in the lower regions of the lung. This positive pressure can compress airways, resulting in alveoli that are not ventilated. This phenomenon is the basis for the closing volume test, which is described in Chapter 6, Clinical Pulmonary Function Testing, Exercise Testing, and Disability Evaluation.

Factors Holding the Lung Against the Chest Wall

The pleural pressure throughout most of the thorax is negative at FRC because the lungs and chest wall are, respectively, above and below their resting volumes. Why does the space between the lungs and chest wall (the pleural space) not become filled with either gas or liquid?

Gases move in and out of the pleural space from the capillaries in the visceral and parietal pleura. Because the sum of all the partial pressures in capillary blood (PH₂O = 47, PCO₂ = 46, PN₂ = 573, and PO₂ = 40 mm Hg) averages 706 mm Hg, there should be a net movement of gas into the pleural space only if the pleural pressure is below 706 mm Hg, or below −54 mm Hg relative to atmospheric pressure. Because mean pleural pressures this low virtually never occur, the pleural space does not fill up with gas unless there is a communication between the pleural space and either the lungs or the atmosphere, or unless there are gas-forming organisms in the pleural space. It is for the same reason that air from a pneumothorax is absorbed if the communication between the alveoli and the pleural space closes.

There is normally a small amount of liquid present in the pleural space. This liquid forms a very thin film of uniform thickness that couples the parietal and visceral pleural surfaces, enabling them to slide over each other with a minimum amount of friction. Normally, a small amount of fluid (~0.01 mL/kg/hr) continuously enters the pleural space from either the visceral or parietal pleura (4). Most liquid in the pleural space leaves via the lymphatics in the parietal pleura, which have a capacity of about 0.28 mL/kg/hr (5). The movement of fluid into and out of the pleural space is more fully discussed in Chapter 17, Diseases of the Pleura, Mediastinum, Chest Wall, and Diaphragm.

Factors Influencing the Pressure-Volume Curve of the Lung

Elastic Recoil of the Lungs

Pressure-volume curves for a lung of a normal individual, a lung from a patient with emphysema, and a lung from a patient with interstitial fibrosis are illustrated in Figure 2.6. As volume is added to the lung, pressure is generated within the system, owing to the tendency of the elastic component to recoil inward. As more volume is added, the pressure increase with each volume increment becomes larger. Eventually, the pressure-volume curve becomes almost flat as the elastic elements reach their limits of distensibility. If more

volume is then added, the lungs are liable to rupture because of the very high transpulmonary pressure.

Under static conditions, the pressure generated by the lung is determined solely by its elastic recoil pressure Pst(L). In other words, when the airways are open and there is no air flow, the Pst(L) is equal to PL. If the glottis is open so that the alveolar pressure is zero, the pleural pressure must be equal, but opposite in sign, to the recoil pressure:

$$Pst(L) = PL = PA - Ppl;$$
$$\text{but because } PA = 0, Pst(L) = -Ppl$$

The lungs of patients with emphysema are more distensible than normal lungs because many alveolar walls have been destroyed, resulting in a loss of elastic elements. As illustrated in Figure 2.6, the pressure-volume curve of the patient with emphysema is shifted to the left. The transpulmonary pressure at any given lung volume is less than it is for the normal lung. In contrast, the lungs of patients with interstitial fibrosis are less distensible than normal lungs because the tissue retractive forces are increased. Therefore, the pressure-volume curve of the patient with interstitial fibrosis is shifted to the right. The stiffness of the lung may also be increased when the pulmonary vessels are engorged with blood or when the interstitial spaces are filled with fluid.

Origin of Lung Elastic Recoil

The total force causing the inflated lung to recoil inward has two components: the first arises from the elastic properties of the lung tissue itself and the second arises from surface tension. In Figure 2.7, pressure-volume curves are shown for an excised lung when it is inflated with saline and then when it is inflated with air. When a normal excised lung is deflated and then inflated with air, the volume increases very little until a pressure of 8 cm H_2O is reached. At pressures above this, the volume increases rapidly until the TLC is approached at about 30 cm H_2O. The filling of the lung is uneven, as different areas of the lung are seen to inflate rapidly. Then if the pressure is decreased, the volume of air remaining in the lung remains much greater than at the same pressure during inflation, and the lung deflates evenly. Microscopic observations of subpleural air spaces show that these air spaces are recruited sequentially from largest to smallest during inflation from the gas-free state, but that they tend to deflate in parallel without extensive derecruitment (6). This difference between the inflation and deflation curves and the failure of the lung to return to its original state after deformation is called *hysteresis*.

When the lungs are filled with a liquid such as isotonic saline, they begin to expand at a lower pressure, fill uniformly, and require less pressure to fill completely. When the lung empties after being filled with liquid, very little hysteresis is noted. The differences in the pressure-volume

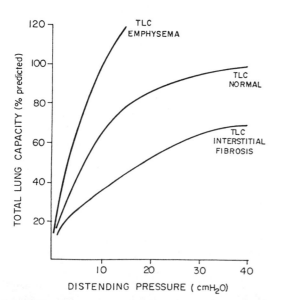

FIGURE 2.6. Representative pressure-volume curves from a normal subject, a patient with emphysema, and a patient with interstitial fibrosis.

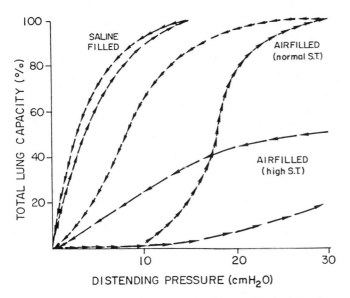

FIGURE 2.7. Pressure-volume curves of lungs filled with saline and with air with normal and high surface tension (ST). The arrows indicate whether the lung is being inflated or deflated. When the lung is filled with saline, the effects of surface forces at the air-liquid interfaces are eliminated. The differences between the curves of the saline-filled and air-filled lungs are owing to surface forces. The differences between the curve of the lung with normal surface tension and that of the lung with high surface tension are owing to the reduction of surface forces by surfactant.

curves with air and saline inflation are owing to differences in surface tension.

Surface tension does not represent a true force but arises because any surface has the tendency to decrease to a minimum. The molecules present at the surface of an air–liquid interface are pulled toward the liquid by molecules in the liquid, and this pull is not counterbalanced because the molecules lie on the surface. When one considers a spherical bubble, the surface tension (T) in the wall of the bubble tends to contract the bubble and the pressure (P) owing to the gas inside the bubble tends to expand it. At equilibrium:

$$P = 2T/r \qquad (2.5)$$

where r is the radius of the bubble.

From this equation (Laplace's equation) it can be seen that the larger the bubble, the smaller the pressure inside the bubble if T is constant. The lungs are actually two sets of millions of bubbles. Consider what would happen if T were the same throughout the lungs. At any given time, if all the alveoli were not exactly the same size, the pressure in the smaller alveoli would be greater than the pressure in the larger alveoli. Hence, air would flow from the smaller to the larger alveoli. This would exacerbate the pressure differences, and after a short period most alveoli would be collapsed or fully distended, obviously a less than ideal situation.

However, in the normal lung there is no such instability. The reason that the normal lung is stable is a substance called *surfactant* (7). Surfactant is a complex mixture composed of lipids, proteins, and carbohydrates, secreted by the type II pneumocytes that are present in all alveoli. The major surface-active component of pulmonary surfactant is the phospholipid dipalmitoyl phosphatidylcholine. Surfactant has two main functions. First, when it is present, the surface tension decreases dramatically as the surface area is decreased. The result of this is that the T in Laplace's equation becomes a variable depending on the radius of the alveoli, such that

$$P = 2T'/r = \text{constant} \qquad (2.6)$$

where T' is the varying surface tension in the presence of surfactant. In this manner, surfactant promotes alveolar stability. Its presence is partly responsible for the hysteresis observed with the inflating lung. It is difficult to open alveoli initially, but once they are inflated, the presence of surfactant allows them to empty evenly in parallel. The second characteristic of surfactant is that it markedly decreases surface tension. It has the lowest surface tension of any biologic substance ever measured and thereby reduces the transpulmonary pressure necessary to achieve a given lung volume. The presence of surfactant also increases the antibacterial capabilities of alveolar macrophages and modulates lymphocyte responsiveness (7).

The difference between the pressure-volume curves obtained with saline and with air indicate how much of the elastic recoil is owing to surface tension (Fig. 2.7). On the inflation part of the curve, much more elastic recoil is owing to surface tension than to the elastic properties of the lung. For example, to reach a volume of 50% TLC, a total pressure of 18 cm H_2O is necessary with air inflation, but only 3 cm H_2O with saline inflation, which indicates that 15 of the 18 cm H_2O of the elastic recoil is owing to surface tension. Alternatively, on the deflation limb of the curve with air inflation, a pressure of 8 cm H_2O is necessary for a volume of 50% TLC, and the elastic recoil owing to surface tension is only 5 cm H_2O.

The importance of surfactant in reducing the surface tension can be appreciated by comparing the pressure-volume curves of isolated lungs with and without surfactant (Fig. 2.7). In the lung with no surfactant and therefore high surface tension, the total lung capacity is not approached even with a distending pressure of 30 cm H_2O. Moreover, at 50% TLC, the distending pressure of the deflating lung devoid of surfactant is more than double that of the lung with normal surfactant.

Surfactant is important in several different clinical situations. The infant acute respiratory distress syndrome occurs in infants who are born prematurely, before they have developed sufficient ability to produce surfactant. As a result of the inadequate level of surfactant, their lungs are unstable and have very low compliance. The instability leads to complete atelectasis of many alveoli, which produces a right-to-left shunt and results in profound hypoxemia. The decreased compliance leads to alveolar hypoventilation. Surfactant production can be augmented by the administration of corticoids to the mother prenatally, which leads to a decreased incidence of the respiratory distress syndrome (8). Studies have consistently shown that the administration of exogenous surfactant therapy to premature babies with the infant respiratory distress syndrome results in improved gas exchange and lung mechanics as well as a reduced mortality rate. The administration of exogenous surfactant is now considered to be routine therapy for infants with the respiratory distress syndrome (9).

A lack of surfactant is also thought to play a role in producing the adult respiratory distress syndrome (ARDS) (Chapter 23, Acute Hypoxemic Respiratory Failure: Pulmonary Edema and Acute Lung Injury). This condition is characterized by diffuse pulmonary infiltrates and marked hypoxia refractory to high inspired concentrations of oxygen. The marked hypoxia is secondary to perfusion of atelectatic alveoli. On account of the atelectatic alveoli, the lungs are very noncompliant, as would be predicted from Figure 2.7. Therapy of the acute respiratory distress syndrome is directed in large part toward increasing lung volume to prevent alveoli from becoming atelectatic (Chapter 22, Acute Hypercapnic Respiratory Failure: Neuromuscular and Obstructive Disease). Despite several studies evaluating the therapeutic efficacy of exogenous surfactant, none has definitively shown that the surfactant therapy is efficacious. Further studies are necessary before exogenous surfactant can be recommended in the treatment of the adult respiratory distress syndrome (10).

DYNAMICS OF THE RESPIRATORY SYSTEM

The dynamics of breathing are discussed in this section. First, different types of air flow and resistances to air flow are described. Next, the relationship between alveolar pressures and air flow is reviewed, including the dynamic compression of the airways by positive pleural pressure on forced expiration. Finally, factors influencing the distribution of ventilation and the work of breathing are discussed.

Airway Resistances

Air moves into and out of the lungs whenever the alveolar pressure differs from the atmospheric pressure (assuming the airways are not obstructed). The airway resistance (Raw) is defined as the frictional resistance of the entire system of air passages to air flow from outside the body to within the alveoli. By definition:

$$Raw = (P_A - P_{ao})/\dot{V} \qquad (2.7)$$

where P_A is the alveolar pressure, P_{ao} is the pressure at the airway opening, and $\dot{V}$ is the flow rate. This system is analogous to an electrical circuit:

$$R = V/I \qquad (2.8)$$

where R is the electrical resistance, V is the voltage difference, and I is the current.

Patterns of Air Flow

The resistance to air flow in a tube depends on the type of flow, the dimensions of the tube, and the viscosity and density of the gas. Air flow through tubes can be either *laminar* or *turbulent*. Laminar flow is organized, and the streamlines are everywhere parallel to the sides of the tube and are capable of sliding over one another (Fig. 2.8). The streamlines at the center of the tube move faster than those closest to the walls, producing a flow profile that is parabolic. With laminar flow, the relation between pressure and flow is given by Poiseuille's equation:

$$P = 8\eta l\dot{V}/\pi r^4 = K_1\dot{V} \qquad (2.9)$$

or

$$\dot{V} = P\pi r^4/8\eta l \qquad (2.10)$$

where $\dot{V}$ is the flow rate, P is the driving pressure (pressure drop between the beginning and end of the tube), r and l are the radius and the length of the tube, respectively, and η is the viscosity of the gas. Because flow resistance (R) is the driving pressure divided by the flow [Eq. 2.7], the resistance with laminar flow is independent of the flow rate:

LAMINAR FLOW

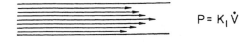

$$P = K_1\dot{V}$$

TURBULENT FLOW

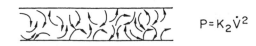

$$P = K_2\dot{V}^2$$

TRANSITIONAL FLOW

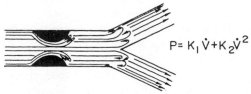

$$P = K_1\dot{V} + K_2\dot{V}^2$$

FIGURE 2.8. Patterns of air flow in tubes.

$$R = 8\eta l/\pi r^4 = K_1 \qquad (2.11)$$

Note the critical importance of the tube radius—if the radius of the tube is halved, the airway resistance increases 16-fold. Note also that laminar flow is dependent on the viscosity of a gas but is independent of its density.

Turbulent flow occurs at high flow rates and is characterized by a complete disorganization of the streamlines so that molecules of gas move laterally, collide with one another, and change their velocities (Fig. 2.8). Owing to this disorganization, the pressure drop across the tube is not proportionate to the flow rate as with laminar flow, but rather is proportional to the square of the flow rate:

$$P = K_2\dot{V}^2 \qquad (2.12)$$

It follows from Equation 2.7 that the resistance to air flow is proportional to the flow rate:

$$R = K\dot{V} \qquad (2.13)$$

in contrast with laminar flow. In addition, with turbulent flow an increase in gas density increases the pressure drop for a given flow, but the viscosity of the gas becomes unimportant.

Whether air flow is laminar or turbulent depends to a large extent on a dimensionless quantity called the Reynolds number, *Re*, which is given by:

$$Re = 2rvd/\eta \qquad (2.14)$$

where r is the radius of the tube, v is the average velocity, d is the density of the gas, and η is the viscosity of the gas. In straight, smooth, rigid tubes, turbulence occurs when *Re* exceeds 2,000.

In the lung, laminar flow occurs only in the small peripheral airways, where, owing to the large overall cross-sectional area, flow through any given airway is extremely slow. Turbulent flow occurs in the trachea. In the remainder of the lung, owing in large part to the multiple branchings of the tracheobronchial tree, flow is neither laminar nor turbulent, but rather mixed or transitional (Fig. 2.8). With a transitional flow pattern, flow is dependent on both the viscosity and the density of the gas.

Distribution of Airway Resistance

Toward the periphery in the tracheobronchial tree, the airways become successively narrower. Therefore, from Eq. 2.11 one would anticipate that the major part of the airway resistance would reside in the narrow peripheral airways. However, direct measurements of airway resistance have shown that less than 20% of the total airway resistance is confined to airways with diameters less than 2 mm. The explanation for this apparent paradox is that the progressive branching of the tracheobronchial tree results in an increased average cross-sectional diameter of the peripheral

airways; therefore, resistance does not increase disproportionately (11).

During nasal breathing, the resistance offered by the nose is the largest single component, constituting one-half to two-thirds of the total resistance at low flow rates. The nasal resistance increases disproportionately with increasing flow rates; therefore, during heavy exercise one switches from nasal breathing to mouth breathing. During quiet breathing the mouth, pharynx, larynx, and trachea provide 20% to 30% of the airway resistance. Most of the remainder of the airway resistance is in the bronchi with diameters greater than 2 mm. Less than 20% of the total airway resistance is in the bronchi with diameters less than 2 mm (12).

Factors Influencing Airway Resistance

Airway resistance depends on the number, length, and cross-sectional area of the conducting airways. Since resistance to air flow in a given airway changes according to the fourth power of its radius, the cross-sectional area within the tracheobronchial tree is by far the most important determinant of airway resistance. The airways, like the lung parenchyma, exhibit elasticity and are capable of being compressed or distended. Therefore, the diameter of an airway varies with the transmural pressure applied to that airway; that is, the difference between the pressure within the airway and the pressure surrounding the airway. The pressure surrounding the intrathoracic airways approximates pleural pressure.

As the lung volume increases, the traction applied to the walls of the intrathoracic airways also increases, widening the airways and decreasing their resistance to air flow. The relationship between the lung volume and airway resistance is not linear (Fig. 2.9*A*). However, the relationship between the reciprocal of the airway resistance, the *airway conductance* (*Gaw*), and lung volume is linear (Fig. 2.9*B*). The *specific airway conductance* (*SGaw*) is defined as:

$$SGaw = Gaw/V_L \qquad (2.15)$$

where V_L is the volume at which *Gaw* is measured. Since *SGaw* is nearly independent of the lung volume in a given patient, it is the index of airway resistance that should be used in the clinical situation. Furthermore, use of this index reduces the variations in resistance measurements from individual to individual owing to varying body size (13).

Contraction of the bronchial smooth muscles narrows the airways and increases airway resistance. Normally there is a small amount of resting smooth muscle tone in the bronchial smooth muscles. Administration of inhaled bronchodilator drugs to normal subjects leads to a significant decrease in the airway resistance (14). The tone of the bronchial smooth muscle is under the control of the autonomic nervous system. Sympathetic stimulation causes bronchodilation, whereas parasympathetic stimulation causes bronchoconstriction. Stimulation of the irritant receptors in the tracheobronchial tree induces bronchoconstriction reflexly

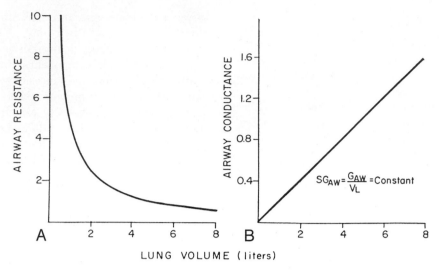

FIGURE 2.9. **A:** The relationship between airway resistance and lung volume. **B:** The relationship between airway conductance and lung volume. Note that the relationship between airway resistance and lung volume is not linear, whereas that between airway conductance and lung volume is linear.

via the parasympathetic nerve fibers contained in the vagus nerve (15). In patients with lung disease, mucosal edema, hypertrophy and hyperplasia of mucous glands, increased production of mucus, and hypertrophy of the bronchial smooth muscle all tend to decrease airway caliber and contribute to the increased airway resistance.

Pressure–Flow Relationships

It has been recognized for a long time that there is a limit to the flow rate that can be attained during expiration and that, once this limit is achieved, greater muscular effort does not augment flow. With both laminar flow (Eq. 2.10) and turbulent flow (Eq. 2.12), one would expect higher pressures to be associated with higher flows.

The limitation of flow at different lung volumes is best appreciated from the examination of isovolume pressure-flow curves at different lung volumes. Isovolume pressure-flow curves are constructed by simultaneously measuring the flow, volume, and pleural pressure as a subject inhales and exhales with varying amounts of effort that are reflected by changes in pleural pressure. Thus, for any given lung volume there is a set of pleural pressures and flow rates. Because at any given lung volume the elastic recoil pressure of the lung is constant, the pleural pressures can be converted to alveolar pressures by adding the elastic recoil pressure at the lung volume to the pleural pressure.

Figure 2.10 depicts a family of isovolume pressure-flow curves at different lung volumes. Two main characteristics of these curves should be noted. First, for a given alveolar pressure, the higher the lung volume, the greater the flow

rate during both inspiration (negative alveolar pressure) and expiration (positive alveolar pressure). The explanation for this on inspiration is that the higher the lung volume the lower the airway resistance. The explanation during expiration is not only the lower airway resistance but also the greater elastic recoil of the lung at higher lung volumes, since this latter pressure is important in determining expiratory flow rate (see discussion that follows).

Second, during expiration at all but the higher lung volumes, as alveolar pressure increases, flow rates increase until a certain alveolar pressure is reached. Then further increases in alveolar pressure do not result in increased flow. This flow limitation in view of increasing alveolar pressure is surprising, because with both laminar flow (Eq. 2.10) and turbulent flow (Eq. 2.12) one would expect higher pressures to be associated with higher flows. The explanation for this upper limit on expiratory flow is dynamic compression of the airways, which is discussed in the next section. Note that there is no similar limitation of flow on inspiration. Note also that the alveolar pressure necessary to generate the maximum flow is lower at lower lung volumes.

At volumes greater than 75% of the vital capacity, air flow increases progressively with increasing alveolar pressure and is considered *effort dependent*. In contrast, at lung volumes below 75% of the vital capacity, the flow rate reaches a maximum once a given alveolar pressure is reached. At these lung volumes, air flow is considered *effort independent*, but the critical alveolar pressure must be reached in order to have maximum flow.

The limitation of flow on expiration, demonstrated in Figure 2.10, is very important to the clinician. The majority

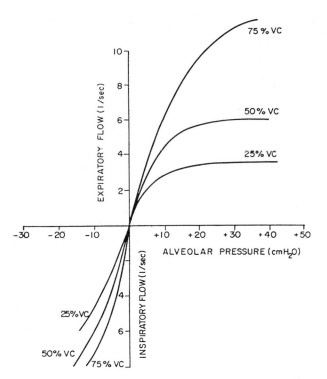

FIGURE 2.10. Isovolume pressure-flow curves at 25, 50, and 75% of the vital capacity. Note the limitation of air flow on expiration at alveolar pressures above 20 and 28 cm H₂O at 25 and 50% of the vital capacity, respectively.

of patients with lung disease have obstructive lung disease, which means that it takes them longer than normal to get the air out of their lungs. The two main tests used to diagnose and assess the response of these patients to therapy are the *forced expiratory spirogram* and the *flow-volume loop* (Chapter 6, Clinical Pulmonary Function Testing, Exercise Testing, and Disability Evaluation). With both of these tests, the patient takes a maximal inspiration and then exhales as hard and long as he or she can. From Figure 2.10 it can be seen that at lung volumes below about 75% of the vital capacity, these tests are independent of effort after the critical alveolar pressure is reached. Therefore, the tests are reproducible and are invaluable in the management of these patients. Because there is no flow limitation on inspiration, tests dependent on inspiratory flow rates are much less reproducible than are tests dependent on expiratory flow rates.

Dynamic Compression of the Airways

Limitation of flow on expiration results from dynamic compression of the airways. To illustrate the mechanisms involved in producing flow limitation during a maximal expiratory maneuver, it is useful to consider a model of the lung in which the alveoli are represented by an elastic sac

and the intrathoracic airways by a compressible tube, both of which are enclosed within a pleural space (Fig. 2.11).

At a given lung volume when there is no flow (Fig. 2.11*A*), the alveolar pressure is zero. The pleural pressure is subatmospheric and counterbalances the elastic recoil of the lung. To generate expiratory flow, the alveolar pressure must be increased above zero, which is accomplished by increasing the pleural pressure. Because the lung volume has not changed, the increase in the alveolar pressure is the same as the increase in the pleural pressure:

$$P_A = Ppl + Pst(L) \qquad (2.16)$$

The intrabronchial pressure decreases, moving downstream (toward the mouth) from the alveolus because of flow resistance. During quiet breathing, if the pleural pressure does not become positive, the intrabronchial pressure is always greater than the pleural pressure (Fig. 2.11*B*). When sufficient expiratory effort is generated, however, the pleural pressure becomes positive, and in this situation the intrabronchial pressure at some point along the airways is equal to the pleural pressure extrabronchial pressure (Fig. 2.11*C*). Mead and coworkers designated this point the *equal-pressure point* (EPP) (16). The EPP divides the airways into two components arranged in series: an *upstream segment* from the alveoli to the equal-pressure point, where the distending pressure of the bronchi is positive, and a *downstream segment* from the equal-pressure point to the airway opening, where the distending pressure of the bronchi is negative intratho-

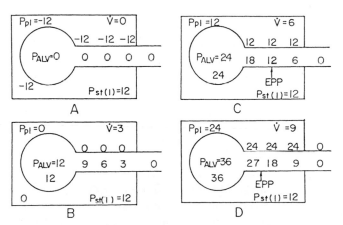

FIGURE 2.11. A schematic representation of the equal-pressure point (EPP) concept. **A:** the alveolar pressure is zero, so there is no flow. In **B:** the increase in the alveolar pressure is equal to the Pst(L), so the pleural pressure is zero. Here the equal-pressure point is at the airway opening. **C:** The alveolar pressure has increased more, so the pleural pressure must be positive. The pressure drops from the alveolus to different points along the airway are greater because V̇ is higher. Accordingly, the EPP moves closer to the alveolus. **D:** The Ppl has been increased even more and the EPP has moved farther upstream because flow has increased. When flow limitation occurs, the equal-pressure point becomes fixed, and Vmax is determined by Eq. 2.18.

racically. It is these downstream segments of the airways that are dynamically compressed during forced expiration.

Location of Equal-Pressure Point

When the pleural pressure is subatmospheric, there is no EPP (Fig. 2.11*A*). When the pleural pressure becomes atmospheric, the EPP is at the airway opening (Fig. 2.11*B*). As the pleural pressure becomes more positive, the EPP moves upstream (Fig. 2.11*C, D*)—but how far? When flow in the upstream segment is considered, the pressure drop from the alveolus to the EPP is the alveolar pressure minus the pleural pressure, which is the elastic recoil pressure of the lung. The resistance of the upstream segment is designated Rus. Therefore, it follows from Equation 2.7 that:

$$\dot{V} = Pst(L)/Rus \qquad (2.17)$$

At a constant lung volume $Pst(L)$ is constant. Therefore, the only way that $\dot{V}$ can be increased is for Rus to decrease, which can be accomplished only by having the EPP move upstream. With more and more effort, the EPP moves upstream (Fig. 2.11*B–D*) until the pleural pressure reaches a level at which further increases in it do not lead to further increases in $\dot{V}$. The $\dot{V}$ at this pleural pressure is called $\dot{V}$max and corresponds to the flat top at the isovolume pressure-flow curve.

Note by this analysis:

$$\dot{V}max = Pst(L)/Rus \qquad (2.18)$$

and therefore $\dot{V}$max is dependent on two factors: (a) the resistance of the upstream segment, and (b) the recoil pressure of the lung. In other words, a decreased elastic recoil of the lung is just as important in reducing $\dot{V}$max as is increased airway resistance.

Pride and coworkers (17) developed a different analysis of the mechanisms of forced expiration. Their analysis is similar to that of Mead but also takes into account the resistance to collapse of the intrathoracic airways. The analysis has not been publicized as much as the equal-pressure point analysis of Mead, but it better explains the mechanics of forced expiration.

In the model of Pride and coworkers (Fig. 2.12) the airways are divided into two rigid tubes connected in series by a short segment of a collapsible tube. They divided the airways into an upstream segment between the alveoli and the distal end of the collapsible segment, and a downstream segment from the end of the collapsible segment to the airway opening. Moreover, they defined the *critical closing pressure of the collapsible segment* (Ptm′) as the transmural pressure (Ptm), at which the segment collapsed. As with any distensible object, the transmural pressure is the pressure inside the wall minus the pressure outside the wall. Therefore, the value for Ptm′ indicates the distending pressure that must be maintained to keep the collapsible segment patent. They further assumed that the short, collapsi-

ble segment was fully open whenever its distending pressure exceeded Ptm′ and fully collapsed whenever Ptm fell below Ptm′.

The transmural pressure in the collapsible segment is given by the following:

$$Ptm = PA - (\dot{V} \times Rs) - Ppl \qquad (2.19)$$

where Rs is the resistance of the segment upstream from the collapsible segment. (Note the distinction from *Rus,* which is the resistance of the segment upstream from the EPP in the analysis of Mead et al.) Since:

$$PA = Pst(L) + Ppl \qquad (2.20)$$

then

$$Ptm = Pst(L) - (\dot{V} \times Rs) \qquad (2.21)$$

Therefore, as $\dot{V}$ increases, Ptm decreases. When $\dot{V}$ increases to a critical level (Vmax), Ptm drops to Ptm′. This is illustrated in Figure 2.12*B*, where $Ptm = 6 - 6 = 0$ and it is assumed that $Ptm′ = 0$. If flow rates increase more, as illustrated in Figure 2.12*C,* the Ptm would fall below Ptm′ (in the illustration Ptm = −4), but by our assumptions, the collapsible segment would be collapsed completely and there would be no flow (Fig. 2.12*D*). However, as soon as flow ceases, the intrabronchial pressure becomes the same as the alveolar pressure, and again Ptm exceeds Ptm′ and flow resumes. If the collapsible segment opens all the way, $\dot{V}$ again exceeds $\dot{V}$max, Ptm falls below Ptm′, and airflow ceases. Therefore, it is postulated that the collapsible segment acts as a variable resistor, as illustrated in Figure 2.12*E* and *F*. Once the pleural pressure is reached, at which dynamic compression of the airways occurs, the collapsible segment partially collapses; as a result, the pressure drop between the alveoli and the collapsible segment is such that the Ptm is equal to the Ptm′. As pleural pressures increase more and more (Fig. 2.12*F*), there is a larger and larger pressure drop across the collapsible segment. Note that by this analysis flow and intrabronchial pressures downstream from the collapsible segment do not change once flow limitation is achieved (Fig. 2.12*B,E,F*). From Equation 2.21, flow limitation occurs when Ptm = Ptm′. Therefore, when Ptm′ is substituted for Ptm in Equation 2.21,

$$Ptm′ = Pst(L) - \dot{V}max \times Rs \qquad (2.22)$$

which can be rewritten as follows:

$$\dot{V}max = (Pst(L) - Ptm′)/Rs \qquad (2.23)$$

Note that this analysis of respiratory mechanics is conceptually analogous to a waterfall. The height of the waterfall (i.e., the pressure drop across the collapsible segment) does not affect flow either above or below the waterfall. The flow above the waterfall is given by Equation 2.23 regardless of the height of the waterfall. The flow below the waterfall is determined by the flow above the waterfall. Since the resistance to flow below the waterfall is fixed, the pressure imme-

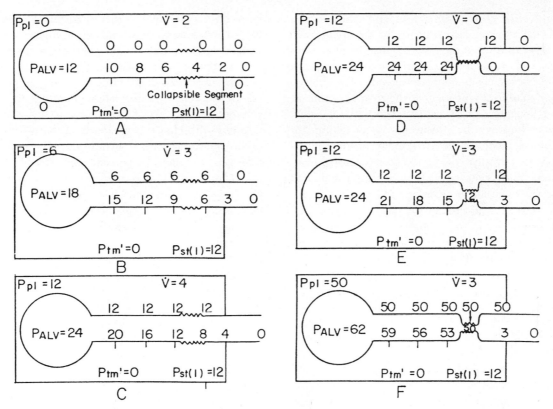

FIGURE 2.12. A schematic representation of the collapsible-segment concept. In these diagrams the lung volume is that giving a Pst(L) of 12 and it is assumed that Ptm′ is zero. **A:** Pressures along the airways when Ptm still exceeds Ptm′. There is no collapse. **B:** Pressures along the airways when Ptm approaches Ptm′. Note that the flow rate increases from **A**. **C:** Pressures along the airways when pleural pressures are increased more. Note that Ptm at the collapsible segment is now 8 − 12 = −4, which is below Ptm′ = 0, so this higher flow is impossible since the collapsible segment must collapse. **D:** Pressures along the airways when there is no flow. Now Ptm is 24 − 12 = 12, so the airways must open. **E:** Pressure along the airways when the collapsible segment is partially collapsed such that Ptm = Ptm′. **F.** Pressures along the airways when the alveolar pressure is raised much higher. Note that the collapsible segment is more collapsed than in **E** and that the flows in **B, E,** and **F** are also identical. The airway pressures downstream from the collapsible segment in **B, E,** and **F** are also identical.

diately downstream from the collapsible segment is equal to the product of V̇max and the resistance of the downstream segment.

When Equation 2.23 is analyzed, it is seen that V̇max depends on three different factors: (a) the elastic recoil of the lung (Pst(L)), (b) the tendency of the airways to collapse (Ptm′), and (c) the resistance of the upstream segment (Rs). Emphysema, chronic bronchitis, and asthma are the three main diseases that cause reduced flow rates on expiration. Analysis of Equation 2.23 reveals that the predominant mechanism causing reduced flow rates is different with each of these three diseases. With emphysema, the main abnormality is decreased elastic recoil of the lungs (Pst(L)); with chronic bronchitis, the predominant abnormality is increased resistance of the upstream segment (Rs), whereas with asthma the constriction of the bronchial smooth muscles greatly increases the tendency of the airways to collapse (Ptm′) and thereby reduces flow rates by this mechanism.

Of course with all three diseases, all the factors interact to some extent to produce reduced expiratory flow rates. An explanation for air trapping is also given by Equation 2.23. Air trapping occurs when the Pst(L) is less than Ptm′, for when this condition is met, V̇max is zero. Therefore, the lungs cannot empty at lung volumes below which Ptm′ exceeds Pst(L).

Experimental evidence supporting this analysis of flow limitation has been provided by Smaldone and Bergofsky [18]. They monitored intrabronchial pressures in excised lungs and demonstrated that the flow-limiting segment consisted of well-demarcated short lengths of the trachea at large lung volumes but of lobar or segmental bronchi at low lung volumes. There was a large pressure drop across the collapsible segment, which at any given lung volume was closely related to the driving pressure. Leaver and coworkers [19] investigated the contribution of the three factors in Equation 2.23 in producing decreased expiratory flow rates in 17 patients with chronic bronchitis and emphysema. They found that all three factors contributed to reduction in maximal flow. In three of their 17 patients, the reduction in expiratory flow rates could be entirely accounted for by loss of lung elastic recoil and enhanced airway collapsibility.

Although dynamic compression of the airways produces limitation of flow on expiration, it is not without value because it does improve the effectiveness of coughing. In the collapsible segment, the linear velocity of air flow is markedly increased owing to the smaller cross-sectional area. This increased linear velocity leads to a greater shearing force that serves to dislodge secretions and particles from the walls of airways. The shift of the collapsible segment from the trachea to the segmental bronchi as lung volumes get smaller increases the ease with which coughing can remove secretions from most of the larger airways.

Density Dependence of Maximal Air Flow

In the normal lung during forced expiration, flow in the peripheral airways is laminar, flow in the medium-sized airways is transitional, and flow in the large airways is turbulent. Only laminar flow is independent of gas *density*. Therefore, if maximal expiratory flow rates are measured with the patient breathing gases of varying densities, the flow rates should remain stable only if there is laminar flow in the flow-limiting segment. If there is either turbulent flow or transitional flow in this segment, breathing a gas with a lower density should result in increased flow rates at a given lung volume. In contrast, laminar flow is dependent on gas *viscosity*.

A mixture of 80% helium and 20% oxygen (He-O_2) has a viscosity very similar to that of air but a density that is approximately one-third that of air (20). Because the viscos-ity of He-O_2 is similar to that of air but the density of He-O_2 is much lower, one would expect higher maximal flows with the He-O_2 only if the flow in the flow-limiting segment were turbulent or transitional. Flow-volume loops from a normal subject obtained while breathing air and with He-O_2 are illustrated on the left in Figure 2.13. At all lung volumes above 15% of the vital capacity, the maximum flow rate with He-O_2 is greater than that with air. At 50% of the vital capacity the flow rate with He-O_2 is 50% higher than it is with air. The percent increase in flow rates with He-O_2 at 50% VC is termed the $\Delta\dot{V}max_{50}$. The point at which the flow rates with He-O_2 and with air become identical is termed the *isoflow volume* (Viso$\dot{v}$). The normal $\Delta\dot{V}max_{50}$ is 47.3 $\pm$ 27.4% (two standard deviations) and does not change with age. The normal Viso$\dot{v}$ at age 40 is 16.5 $\pm$ 13.8% and increases 0.3% for each additional year (21).

In normal subjects, flow at low lung volumes is density independent because the collapsible segment is more peripheral and flow rates are lower. Owing to the much smaller flow rates, the Reynolds number (Eq. 2.14) dictates that the flow will be laminar. Flow-volume loops for a smoker obtained with room air and with He-O_2 are illustrated on the right in Figure 2.13. Although the flow-volume loops with room air for the normal person and the smoker are virtually identical, the increases in the flow rates with He-O_2 are much less for the smoker. The $\Delta\dot{V}max_{50}$ for the smoker is only 15%, compared with 50% for the non-smoker, and the Viso$\dot{v}$ is 30% compared with 15% for the nonsmoker.

The use of He-O_2 flow-volume loops has its greatest utility in detecting disease of the small peripheral airways. Because the small airways usually contribute a minor portion to the total airway resistance, changes in these airways

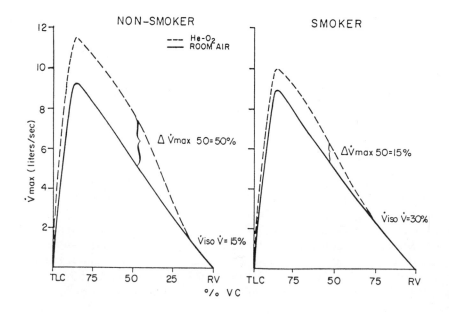

FIGURE 2.13. Flow-volume loops obtained with room air and He-O_2 on a normal nonsmoker and an asymptomatic smoker. Although the flow-volume loops on room air are identical, there is a substantially greater improvement in the flow rates with He-O_2 in the normal person than in the smoking individual.

may not be detectable by measurements of airway resistance. Increased resistance in the small airways should reduce maximal flow, but because of the great variability of flow-volume curves in normal individuals flows may not be reduced below the normal range. However, disease in the peripheral airways should decrease the relative contribution of density-dependent flow to the total pressure drop between the alveoli and the collapsible segment.

Dosman and coworkers obtained flow-volume loops with air and He-O_2 for 66 nonsmokers and 48 smokers whose forced expiratory volume in 1 second divided by the forced vital capacity (FEV$_1$/FVC%) ratios exceeded 70% (21). With air, only 12% of the smokers had a $\dot{V}max_{50}$ and only 2% had a $\dot{V}max_{25}$ that were more than two standard deviations below those of the nonsmokers. In contrast, with He-O_2 40% of the smokers had a $\Delta\dot{V}max_{50}$ that was more than two standard deviations below that of the nonsmokers and 52% had a Viso $\dot{v}$ that exceeded those of the nonsmokers by more than two standard deviations. These results show that use of He-O_2 during a forced expiratory maneuver allows the detection of functional abnormalities in smokers at a stage when their $\dot{V}max$ is still within the normal range while they are breathing room air. However, the significance of these functional abnormalities in terms of the patient eventually developing chronic obstructive pulmonary disease (COPD) remains to be proved.

Despite the theoretical considerations described in the preceding, there has not been widespread utilization of the He-O_2 flow-volume loops in clinical pulmonary disease. This is because they have proved difficult to use in healthy subjects and patients because of large intrasubject and intersubject variability and variability in interpretation of the same series of curves by different observers (22).

Distribution of Ventilation

The regional distribution of ventilation depends on the distensibility of the peripheral gas exchange units and the resistance of the airways leading to them. The emptying of an elastic reservoir such as the lung through a resistive conduit resembles the discharge of a capacitor through a resistor. If the volume V remaining in the reservoir as a fraction of the initial volume V_0 is plotted against time t, an exponential curve is obtained whose equation is:

$$V/V_0 = e^{-t/RC} \qquad (2.24)$$

where R is the resistance and C is the compliance of the system. When t is equal to RC, the exponent has a value of unity and $V/V_0 = e^{-1} = 0.37$. The product RC is the time that it takes the system to reach 37% of its original volume, and this product is termed the *time constant* of the respiratory unit.

When two or more parallel units are subjected to the same inflation or deflation pressure, they each fill or empty at a rate determined by their individual time constants. If their time constants are equal, the units fill and empty uniformly. If their time constants are unequal, the units fill or empty nonuniformly. From Equation 2.24 it can be seen that an increase in either the resistance or the compliance of a respiratory unit increases the time it takes the unit to empty or fill.

Frequency Dependence of Compliance

Since the time constants of the respiratory units are relatively small (0.01 sec), during quiet breathing equilibration between alveolar and mouth pressures occurs at both the end of expiration and the end of inspiration. Therefore, the dynamic compliance of the respiratory system (the change in volume divided by the change in pleural pressure) during quiet breathing is the same as the static compliance. In the normal lung, increases in the breathing frequency up to rates of 80/min do not affect the measured compliance, because the time constants are small and equilibration between alveolar and mouth pressure still occurs. However, in patients with peripheral airway disease, the time constants of at least some of the respiratory units are increased so that with more rapid breathing, equilibration between alveolar and mouth pressure does not occur at either end-inspiration or end-expiration. Accordingly, the volume change with a given pleural pressure change falls with increasing respiratory rate, and the compliance is said to be frequency dependent (23).

In patients with relatively normal expiratory flow rates, the decrease in dynamic compliance with increasing respiratory rates may be marked. Woolcock and coworkers found that the dynamic compliance of mild asthmatics breathing at a respiratory frequency of around 80/min was less than 50% of the static compliance (23). A large proportion of the decrease in dynamic compliance is owing to the fact that at times of zero flow at the mouth, air is flowing within the lung from one region to another *(pendelluft)*. The mechanism for this is illustrated in Figure 2.14. During inspiration, alveolus 1 fills more rapidly than alveolus 2 because of the increased airway resistance of the airways leading to alveolus 2 and hence its larger time constant. If the inspiratory time is short, alveolus 2 never becomes completely filled. Then on expiration, the pressure in alveolus 1 is higher than the pressure in alveolus 2 because of its larger volume; therefore flow goes not only from alveolus 1 to the mouth but also from alveolus 1 to alveolus 2. The higher the frequency, the lower the tidal volume to the abnormal region.

Tests of dynamic compliance are sensitive indicators of peripheral airway disease. The time constants of the lung units distal to airways 2 mm in diameter are on the order of 0.01 second. Fourfold increases in some time constants are necessary to cause dynamic compliance to become frequency dependent. However, measurements of frequency dependence of compliance are not performed in most pul-

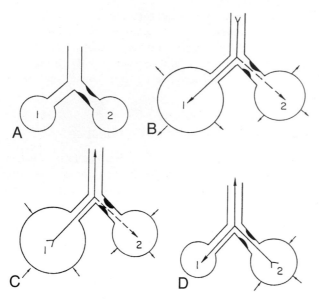

FIGURE 2.14. Effects of uneven time constants on ventilation. The airway leading to unit 2 is partially obstructed and therefore unit 2 has a longer time constant. After a slow expiration **(A)**, the units have the same size. With a rapid inspiration **(B)**, unit 1 fills more than unit 2 because it has a faster time constant. Shortly after the start of a rapid expiration **(C)**, air moves not only from unit 1 to the airway opening but also from unit 1 to unit 2 because the pressure in unit 2 is less than the pressure in unit 1. During the latter phases of expiration **(D)**, flow moves from unit 2 to unit 1. As the respiratory rate is progressively increased, the tidal volume of the abnormal region becomes smaller and smaller.

monary function laboratories because they are time consuming and technically difficult and require the patient to swallow an esophageal balloon.

From the preceding discussion it can be readily appreciated that the time constants of the respiratory units markedly influence the distribution of ventilation. A second factor that is influential is the regional differences in pleural pressures, as discussed earlier in this chapter. Owing to the regional difference in pleural pressure, dependent parts of the lung are ventilated better. Other factors that influence the distribution of ventilation are the *interdependence* that exists between adjacent lung units and the presence of collateral pathways for ventilation.

Interdependence

The lung has a connective tissue framework containing elastic elements. Because contiguous units are attached to each other, they are not free to move independently, but rather the behavior of one unit is influenced by the behavior of its neighbors. This dependence of one respiratory unit on the movements of its neighbors is termed *tissue interdependence.* Another factor that influences interdependence is the relationship between the lung and the adjacent chest wall. If on an inspiratory effort any part of the lung lags in its filling, the shape of the chest wall will be distorted. The

local distortion of the chest wall will produce a local decrease in pleural pressure over the slowly filling lung. This local decrease in pleural pressure will be transmitted to the alveoli, thereby producing a greater pressure differential between the mouth and the alveoli. This in turn augments the flow to the area that was lagging and promotes uniformity of ventilation. It has been shown that this interaction between the lung and the chest wall is more important for the preservation of homogeneous ventilation than is lung tissue interdependence (24).

Collateral Ventilation

Collateral ventilation is ventilation of the alveolar structures through passages that bypass the normal airways (25). Without collateral ventilation, alveoli distal to obstructed airways would become atelectatic. The possible pathways for collateral ventilation include interalveolar communications (pores of Kohn), bronchiole-alveolar communications (canals of Lambert), and the interbronchiolar communications of Martin. The relative contributions of these three different types of communications to collateral ventilation is unknown. In a normal human lung, the resistance to collateral ventilation is high and ventilation via collateral channels takes a long time in relation to the time taken for inspiration. However, in patients with emphysema the overall resistance to collateral ventilation is less than the airway resistance (25). Therefore, collateral ventilation may be very important in preserving the uniformity of ventilation in patients with emphysema and other lung diseases. In normal humans there is very little collateral ventilation between different lobes or different segments (26), but in patients with emphysema there is substantial collateral ventilation between adjacent segments via the interbronchiolar communications of Martin (25).

Work of Breathing

During breathing, the respiratory muscles must work to overcome the elastic, flow-resistive, and inertial forces of the lung and chest wall. In the respiratory system, work is expressed as the product of pressure and volume change according to the following equation:

$$\text{Work} = \int P \times \Delta V \qquad (25)$$

Therefore, to measure the mechanical work that is performed during breathing it is necessary to obtain simultaneous measurements of both the volume change and the pressure that is exerted across the respiratory system.

At the present there is no method available for measuring the total amount of work being done on the lung, the respired gases, the chest wall, the diaphragm, and the abdominal contents because no technique has been developed for determination of the nonelastic resistance of the chest wall. However, the mechanical work performed on the lungs during a breathing cycle can be estimated by simultaneously

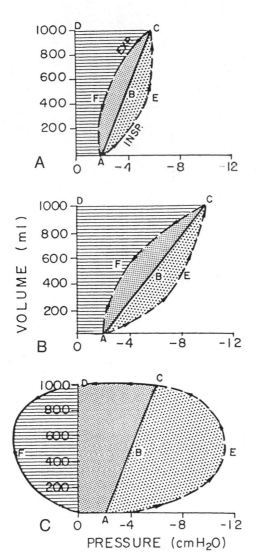

FIGURE 2.15. The mechanical work done during a respiratory cycle on a normal lung **(A)**, a lung with reduced compliance **(B)**, and a lung with increased airway resistance **(C)**. See text for explanation.

measuring the changes in the intrathoracic pressures and the volume of the lungs throughout a respiratory cycle (27).

Figure 2.15 illustrates the information concerning work on the lungs available from such measurements. In the figure the line *ABC* is the static inflation-deflation curve of the lung. The mechanical work necessary to overcome the elastic resistance of the lung is the trapezoidal area *OABCD*. The mechanical work required to overcome the nonelastic resistance is the area of the loop *AECF*. The portion of the loop that falls to the right of line *ABC (AECB)* represents the mechanical work necessary to overcome the nonelastic resistance during inspiration. The portion of the loop that falls to the left of line *ABC (ABCF)* represents the mechanical work required to overcome the nonelastic resistance during expiration. Note that in Fig. 2.15*A*, this area *(ABCF)*

lies entirely within area *OABCD*, which represents the elastic energy stored in the system during inspiration. The fact that the area *ABCF* lies within *OABCD* indicates that this stored energy is sufficient to overcome the flow-resistive forces of expiration and no work is required from the expiratory muscles.

When lung disease is present, the work of breathing can increase substantially. The mechanical work done on a lung in which the compliance is reduced by 50% is shown in Figure 2.15*B*. Note that the trapezoidal area *OABCD* is nearly doubled; hence, the work necessary to overcome the elastic resistance is nearly double that for the normal lung. The mechanical work necessary to overcome nonelastic resistance has not changed. In Figure 2.15*C* the mechanical work done on a lung in which the airway resistance is markedly increased is shown. Owing to the increased airway resistance, more negative pleural pressures must be generated to achieve the same inspiratory flow rates. Therefore, the distance between lines *ABC* and *AEC* is markedly increased and the inspiratory work *(OAECD)* is increased. Also on account of the increased airway resistance, positive pleural pressure occurs during expiration, indicating that muscular work is performed. No longer is the stored elastic energy sufficient. The net work during expiration is the area *DFO*. Therefore, the total work during the respiratory cycle is the inspiratory work *(OECD)* plus the expiratory work *(DFO)*, and this is increased substantially over the total work in Fig. 2.15*A*.

Relationship Between Mechanical Work and Alveolar Ventilation

The work of breathing at any given level of alveolar ventilation is dependent on the pattern of breathing. Large tidal volumes increase the elastic work of breathing, whereas rapid breathing frequencies increase the work against flow-resistive forces (Fig. 2.16). With small tidal volumes a higher total ventilation is required because more ventilation is wasted. Several studies have shown that both normal individuals and patients adopt the respiratory pattern at which work is minimal (Fig. 2.16). The respiratory rate at which the minimum work occurs increases progressively with increased alveolar ventilation. Individuals with pulmonary fibrosis, which is characterized by increased elastic work of breathing, tend to breathe rapidly and shallowly. Individuals with airway obstruction, which is characterized by increased nonelastic work of breathing, usually breathe more deeply and slowly.

Oxygen Cost of Breathing

To perform the mechanical work necessary for breathing, the respiratory muscles require oxygen. The oxygen cost of breathing provides an indirect measure of the work of breathing. The oxygen cost of breathing is measured by

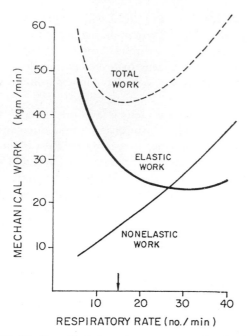

FIGURE 2.16. The effect of respiratory rate on the elastic, nonelastic, and total mechanical work of breathing at a given level of alveolar ventilation. Subjects tend to adopt the respiratory rate at which the total work of breathing is minimal (arrow).

determining the total oxygen consumption of the body at rest and at increased levels of ventilation produced by voluntary hyperventilation.

During quiet breathing, the total oxygen consumption of the body is between 200 and 300 mL/min. In normal subjects the oxygen cost of breathing is on the order of 1.0 mL/L of ventilation. If a minute ventilation of 10 L/min is assumed, the cost of breathing accounts for approximately 5% of the total oxygen consumption. When an individual exercises, the increase in the oxygen cost of breathing parallels the increase in the oxygen consumption and remains about 4% of the oxygen consumption (28). The oxygen cost of breathing is much greater in patients with lung disease. In one report the oxygen cost of breathing in patients with chronic obstructive pulmonary disease with a mean FEV_1 of 0.54 L was 16 mL/L of ventilation (29). In these patients the oxygen cost of breathing accounted for more that 50% of the total oxygen uptake; these patients had a markedly increased basal metabolic index (29).

REFERENCES

1. Milic-Emili J, Mead J, Turner JM, et al. Improved technique for estimating pleural pressure from esophageal balloons. *J Appl Physiol* 1964;19:207–211.
2. Hartford CG, Rogers GG, Turner MJ. Correctly selecting a liquid-filled nasogastric infant feeding catheter to measure intraesophageal pressure. *Pediatr Pulmonol* 1997;23:362–369.
3. Lai-Fook SJ, Rodarte JR. Pleural pressure distribution and its relationship to lung volume and interstitial pressure. *J Appl Physiol* 1991;70:967–978.
4. Wiener-Kronish JP, Albertine KH, Licko V, et al. Protein egress and entry rates in pleural fluid and plasma in sheep. *J Appl Physiol* 1984;56:459–463.
5. Broaddus VC, Wiener-Kronish JP, Berthiaume Y, et al. Removal of pleural liquid and protein by lymphatics in awake sheep. *J Appl Physiol* 1988;64:384–390.
6. Radford EP Jr. Mechanical factors determining alveolar configuration. *Am Rev Respir Dis* 1960;81:743–744.
7. Lewis JF, Jobe AH. Surfactant and the adult respiratory distress syndrome. *Am Rev Respir Dis* 1993;147:218–233.
8. Elimian A, Verma U, Canterino J, et al. Effectiveness of antenatal steroids in obstetric subgroups. *Obstet Gynecol* 1999;93:174–9.
9. Jobe AH. Pulmonary surfactant therapy. *N Engl J Med* 1993;328:861–868.
10. Warren WH. Is there a role for surfactant replacement therapy in adult pulmonary dysfunction? *Crit Care Med* 1998;26:1626–1627.
11. Hogg JC, Macklem PT, Thurlbeck WM. Site and nature of airway obstruction in chronic obstructive lung disease. *N Engl J Med* 1968;278:1355–1360.
12. Ferris BG Jr, Mead J, Opie LH. Partitioning of respiratory flow resistance in man. *J Appl Physiol* 1964;19:653–658.
13. Briscoe WA, Dubois AB. The relationship between airway resistance, airway conductance and lung volume in subjects of different age and body size. *J Clin Invest* 1958;37:1279–1285.
14. Skinner C, Palmer KNV. Changes in specific airways conductance and forced expiratory volume in one second after a bronchodilator in normal subjects and patients with airways obstruction. *Thorax* 1974;29:574–577.
15. Nadel JA. Autonomic control of airway smooth muscle and airway secretions. *Am Rev Respir Dis* 1977;115(Suppl):117–126.
16. Mead J, Turner JM, Macklem PT, et al. Significance of the relationship between lung recoil and maximum expiratory flow. *J Appl Physiol* 1967;22:95–105.
17. Pride NB, Permutt S, Riley RL, et al. Determinants of maximal expiratory flow from the lungs. *J Appl Physiol* 1967;23:646–662.
18. Smaldone GC, Bergofsky EH. Delineation of flow-limiting segment and predicted airway resistance by movable catheter. *J Appl Physiol* 1976;40:943–952.
19. Leaver DG, Tattersfield AE, Pride NB. Contributions of loss of lung recoil and of enhanced airways collapsibility to the airflow obstruction of chronic bronchitis and emphysema. *J Clin Invest* 1973;52:2117–2128.
20. Drazen JM, Loring SH, Ingram RH Jr. Distribution of pulmonary resistance: effects of gas density, viscosity, and flow rate. *J Appl Physiol* 1976;41:388–395.
21. Dosman J, Bode F, Urbanetti J, et al. The use of a helium-oxygen mixture during maximum expiratory flow to demonstrate obstruction in small airways in smokers. *J Clin Invest* 1975;55:1089–1090.
22. Lam S, Abboud RT, Chan-Yeung M, et al. Use of maximal expiratory flow-volume curves with air and helium-oxygen in the detection of ventilatory abnormalities in population survey. *Am Rev Respir Dis* 1981;123:234–237.
23. Woolcock AJ, Vincent NJ, Macklem PT. Frequency dependence of compliance as a test for obstruction in the small airways. *J Clin Invest* 1969;48:1097–1106.
24. Zidulka A, Sylvester JT, Nadler S, et al. Lung interdependence and lung-chest wall interaction of sublobar and lobar units in pigs. *J Appl Physiol* 1979;46:8–13.
25. Morrell NW, Wignall BK, Biggs T, et al. Collateral ventilation and gas exchange in emphysema. *Am J Respir Crit Care Med* 1994;150:635–641.

26. Morrell NW, Roberts CM, Biggs T, et al. Collateral ventilation and gas exchange during airway occlusion in the normal human lung. *Am Rev Respir Dis* 1993;147:535–539.

27. Milic-Emili J, Orzalesi MM. Mechanical work of breathing during maximal voluntary ventilation. *J Appl Physiol* 1998;85: 254–258.

28. Coast JR, Rasmussen SA, Krause KM, et al. Ventilatory work and oxygen consumption during exercise and hyperventilation. *J Appl Physiol* 1993;74:793–798.

29. Mannix ET, Manfredi F, Farber MO. Elevated O_2 cost of ventilation contributes to tissue wasting in COPD. *Chest* 1999;115: 708–713.

ALVEOLAR VENTILATION, GAS EXCHANGE, AND OXYGEN DELIVERY

RONALD B. GEORGE

NORMAL BLOOD GAS TENSIONS

ALVEOLAR-ARTERIAL OXYGEN GRADIENT

ALVEOLAR VENTILATION
Hypoventilation
The Bohr Equation
The Alveolar Air Equation

GAS TRANSFER (DIFFUSION)

VENTILATION-PERFUSION RELATIONSHIPS
Effects of Breathing 100% Oxygen

OXYGEN TRANSPORT
Cardiac Output

Oxygen Content and the Oxyhemoglobin Dissociation
　Curve
The Shunt Equation

ARTERIAL HYPOXEMIA
Low Inspired Oxygen Concentration
Hypoventilation
Diffusion Defect
Ventilation-Perfusion Mismatch
Right-to-Left Shunt
Low Mixed Venous Oxygen Tension

SYSTEMIC OXYGEN DELIVERY
The Circulatory System
The Erythropoietic System
The Respiratory System

The major function of the respiratory system is to provide gas exchange between the body and the environment. Oxygen is required for energy generation via oxidative phosphorylation, as well as for support of various metabolic processes. Carbon dioxide (CO_2) is produced as the endpoint of the metabolism of ingested food. The body is limited in its ability to store oxygen and CO_2; thus, there must be a continuous exchange of these gases with the environment to prevent hypoxemia and respiratory acidosis.

Gas exchange occurs by passive diffusion across a thin alveolar-capillary membrane, the functional unit of the lungs, which separates pulmonary capillaries from alveolar air spaces. The respiratory muscles bring in fresh air to the alveoli, creating an atmosphere of relatively high oxygen and low CO_2. The heart and pulmonary circulation deliver mixed venous blood from the tissues, which have low oxygen and relatively high CO_2 tensions. The gradients thus produced result in the passive transfer of CO_2 out of the blood and of oxygen into the blood.

One can determine if alveolar-capillary gas exchange is adequate by measuring arterial blood PO_2 and PCO_2; if these gas tensions are normal, the gas exchange apparatus is functioning adequately. However, much more can be learned about gas exchange by using a few simple formulas that allow an estimation of the efficiency of ventilation and perfusion. Information about the delivery of oxygen to the tissues where it is required can be gained by the careful use of additional tests, including the analysis of expired gas and mixed venous blood. This chapter demonstrates how this information can be used to assess the efficiency of gas exchange in the lungs and oxygen transport from the lungs to the tissues.

NORMAL BLOOD GAS TENSIONS

In normal subjects at sea level, the arterial PCO_2 is 35 to 45 mm Hg and the arterial PO_2 is 80 to 100 mm Hg. Normal arterial pH is 7.35 to 7.45. Average normal gas pressures at sea level for alveoli, arterial blood, and mixed venous blood are shown in Table 3.1. The development of reliable convenient pulse oximetry allows for the noninvasive monitoring of arterial hemoglobin saturation (SaO_2) levels. At a normal arterial PO_2 of 80 mm Hg or above, SaO_2 should be 95% or more. The effect of the oxyhemoglobin dissociation curve on the oxygen content of the blood is discussed in the section on oxygen transport.

TABLE 3.1 NORMAL GAS TENSIONS IN ALVEOLI AND ARTERIAL AND MIXED VENOUS BLOOD AT SEA LEVEL

	Alveoli	Arterial Blood	Mixed Venous Blood
P_{O_2}	100	95	40
P_{CO_2}	40	40	46
P_{H_2O}	47	47	47
P_{N_2}	573	573	573
P_{TOTAL}	760	755	706

In a resting adult, cardiac output, and thus pulmonary blood flow, is approximately 6 L/min. Alveolar ventilation is normally about 4.5 L/min, and the overall *ventilation-perfusion ratio* is approximately 0.8. Normal oxygen consumption ($\dot{V}_{O_2}$) is approximately 250 to 300 mL/min and normal CO_2 production ($\dot{V}_{CO_2}$) is approximately 200 to 250 mL/min; therefore, the average *respiratory exchange ratio* ($\dot{V}_{CO_2}/\dot{V}_{O_2}$) is also about 0.8. With a normal hemoglobin concentration of 15 g/dL, and a normal ratio of cardiac output to oxygen consumption, the mixed venous blood contains approximately 5 mL/dL less oxygen than the arterial blood under "steady-state" conditions.

ALVEOLAR-ARTERIAL OXYGEN GRADIENT

In Table 3.1, note that there is a small difference between alveolar and arterial P_{O_2} levels. This is the result of the normal anatomic shunts, through which 1% to 3% of mixed venous blood flows directly into the systemic circulation without perfusing the alveolar capillaries. This occurs mainly through the bronchial, mediastinal, and left thebesian veins. In normal young adults, the average alveolar-arterial gradient ($P_{A_{O_2}}$-$P_{a_{O_2}}$) is 5 to 10 mm Hg (1). With the normal aging process, there are gradually more and more lung units with uneven ventilation and perfusion. Thus, in a group of normal adults 61 to 75 years old, Mellemgaard found that the average $P_{A_{O_2}}$-$P_{a_{O_2}}$ was 16 mm Hg (1). The gradient may go up as high as 30 mm Hg in normal subjects over age 70.

ALVEOLAR VENTILATION

Of a resting tidal volume of 500 mL, approximately 150 mL (one-third) is required to fill the large airways in which no gas exchange occurs. Because this air is not involved in gas exchange, it is considered wasted and is a part of the *physiologic dead space*. This portion of the "wasted ventilation" is called the *anatomic dead space* and is present in all individuals. It is approximately equal to the body weight in pounds. Thus, at a resting minute ventilation of 7 L, if the tidal volume is 500 mL, the respiratory rate is 14/min,

and the physiologic dead space is composed of only the conducting airways (150 mL), the effective alveolar ventilation per minute will be 4.9 L. In normal young subjects the physiologic dead space is similar to the anatomic dead space; however, in the presence of aging or disease, the physiologic dead space is greatly increased by the presence of underperfused alveoli (*alveolar dead space*).

Hypoventilation

Overall hypoventilation of the lungs causes a decreased flow of inspired air relative to the venous blood perfusing the lungs. This results in a predictable fall in P_{O_2} and a rise in P_{CO_2} in alveolar gas and capillary blood. Although arterial P_{O_2} is dependent on several factors that affect gas exchange, arterial P_{CO_2} is dependent on the relationship of CO_2 production to alveolar ventilation. Thus, at a given level of CO_2 production ($\dot{V}_{CO_2}$), the volume of alveolar ventilation ($\dot{V}_A$) per minute may be calculated by using the *alveolar ventilation equation:*

$$\dot{V}_A = \dot{V}_{CO_2} \times 0.863/P_{A_{CO_2}} \qquad (3.1)$$

$\dot{V}_{CO_2}$ is the CO_2 production per minute and may be measured by collecting an expired gas sample. The factor 0.863 corrects for differences in measurement units and conversion from body temperature to standard temperature (BTPS to STPD). In practice, arterial pressure ($P_{a_{CO_2}}$) may be substituted for alveolar pressure ($P_{A_{CO_2}}$), because they are essentially equal.

The alveolar ventilation equation provides a means for relating inflow of fresh air ($\dot{V}_A$) to the rate of CO_2 production ($\dot{V}_{CO_2}$). In practice, it is seldom necessary to measure expired CO_2, and for practical purposes the equation may be simplified to express the inverse relationship between alveolar (and arterial) P_{CO_2} and alveolar ventilation:

$$P_{A_{CO_2}} \approx 1/\dot{V}_A \qquad (3.2)$$

The inverse relationship of alveolar and arterial P_{CO_2} to alveolar ventilation is shown in Figure 3.1. With a steady CO_2 output of 200 mL/min, halving the alveolar ventilation from 5 L/min to 2.5 L/min doubles the $P_{A_{CO_2}}$ to 80 mm Hg, and doubling alveolar ventilation to 10 L/min halves the $P_{A_{CO_2}}$ to 20 mm Hg. From the shape of this curve, it may be evident that relatively small increases in alveolar ventilation are associated with impressive reductions in $P_{a_{CO_2}}$ when the patient is hypercapnic. $P_{a_{CO_2}}$ can also rise quickly when alveolar ventilation changes by only a small amount in this setting. Conversely, in the setting of hypocapnia, relatively large changes are required to decrease $P_{a_{CO_2}}$ further. It is not uncommon to observe large fluctuations in $P_{a_{CO_2}}$ in hypercapnic patients responding to minor changes in ventilation. In response to metabolic acidosis, large increases in ventilation and work of breathing result in only modest changes in acid-base status. Obviously, if $\dot{V}_{CO_2}$ should change owing to increased metabolic activity,

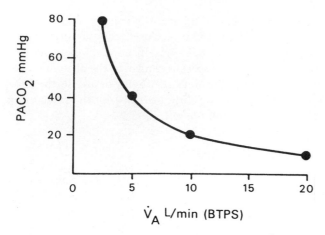

FIGURE 3.1. The relationship of alveolar ventilation ($\dot{V}A$) to alveolar CO_2 ($PACO_2$) at a given CO_2 production ($\dot{V}CO_2$) of 200 mL/min. Increased CO_2 production, as with exercise, shifts the curve to the right.

as with exercise, a new curve would be derived to the right of the one shown in Figure 3.1.

The Bohr Equation

Although the arterial PCO_2 provides a simple method of estimating effective alveolar ventilation, it is also useful in estimating the amount of dead space, or "wasted ventilation." This tells us how efficient a patient's breathing pattern is (i.e., how much of each breath is useful and how much is "wasted"). Figure 3.2 illustrates the variables used in calculating dead space ventilation. Note that *partial pressures* are used rather than *concentrations* of gases. The total minute ventilation ($\dot{V}E$) and expired carbon dioxide ($PECO_2$) are composed of the effective alveolar ventilation

($\dot{V}A$), which contains alveolar levels of CO_2 ($PACO_2$), and the dead space ventilation ($\dot{V}D$), which contains inspired levels of CO_2 ($PICO_2$). This sentence may be written in the form of an equation:

$$\dot{V}E \times PECO_2 = (\dot{V}A \times PACO_2) + (\dot{V}D \times PICO_2)$$
(3.3)

Rearranging and solving for $\dot{V}D/\dot{V}E$ (the portion of $\dot{V}E$ that is wasted), we have the *Bohr equation:*

$$\dot{V}D/\dot{V}E = PACO_2 - PECO_2/PACO_2 - PICO_2 \quad (3.4)$$

Furthermore, because $PICO_2$ breathing room air is zero, this factor can be eliminated and arterial CO_2 ($PaCO_2$) can be substituted for alveolar CO_2 as follows:

$$\dot{V}D/\dot{V}E = PaCO_2 - PECO_2/PaCO_2 \quad (3.5)$$

Arterial PCO_2 can be substituted for alveolar PCO_2 because they are assumed to be in complete equilibrium (and therefore identical). The CO_2 dissociation curve is relatively flat in the physiologic range (Fig. 3.3). Furthermore, the difference between the mixed venous and arterial PCO_2 is only about 6 mm Hg, and although venous admixture significantly affects PaO_2, it has relatively little effect on $PaCO_2$.

If you collect expired gas for a minute or two, mix it, and determine the partial pressure of CO_2, the normal value will be approximately 25 to 30 mm Hg. With a normal arterial PCO_2 of 40 and a $PECO_2$ of 25 mm Hg, the dead space is calculated as follows:

$$
\begin{aligned}
\dot{V}D/\dot{V}E &= 40 - 25/40 \\
&= 15/40 \\
&= 0.37 \text{ or } 37\%
\end{aligned}
$$

In patients with lung disease the difference between expired PCO_2 and arterial PCO_2 increases as the physiologic dead space increases. Comparison of expired PCO_2 with the

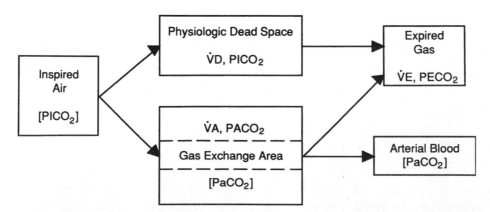

FIGURE 3.2. A gas exchange diagram, showing the variables that are measured for the Bohr equation. $PICO_2$, partial pressure of inspired CO_2 (normally zero); $PACO_2$, partial pressure of CO_2 in alveolar air (equal to arterial PCO_2); $PaCO_2$, partial pressure of CO_2 in arterial blood; $PECO_2$, partial pressure of CO_2 in expired gas; $\dot{V}D$, dead space ventilation; $\dot{V}E$, total minute ventilation; $\dot{V}A$, effective alveolar ventilation.

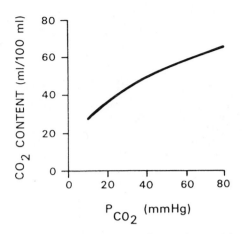

FIGURE 3.3. CO_2 dissociation curve for a subject with a normal level of saturated hemoglobin. The curve shifts to the right with polycythemia and to the left with anemia. Oxygenation shifts the curve to the right and hypoxemia shifts it to the left (Haldane effect).

arterial P_{CO_2} gives an estimate of the percentage of wasted ventilation (Eq. 3.5).

The Alveolar Air Equation

By comparing *arterial* blood gas values with *alveolar* gas values, one may estimate the impedance to gas transfer across the alveolar capillary membrane. End-expired alveolar gas may be sampled directly; however, the analysis of this expired gas sample includes both functional and nonfunctional alveoli (those that are and those that are not perfused). Although there is variation among alveoli depending on their relative ventilation and perfusion, the *average* alveolar P_{CO_2} so nearly equals arterial P_{CO_2} that Pa_{CO_2} may substitute for PA_{CO_2} in the alveolar ventilation equation (Eq. 3.1). Thus, $PA_{CO_2} - Pa_{CO_2}$ differences are not sensitive indicators of problems with gas exchange. On the other hand, large differences exist between mean alveolar *oxygen* tension and measured arterial oxygen tension, and the *alveolar-arterial oxygen difference* ($PA_{O_2} - Pa_{O_2}$) is a practical and relatively sensitive test for assessment of gas exchange. Fortunately, mean alveolar oxygen tension can be calculated with reasonable accuracy by using the *simplified alveolar air equation*:

$$PA_{O_2} = \frac{PI_{O_2} - Pa_{CO_2}}{R} \qquad (3.6)$$

where PA_{O_2} is the calculated alveolar PO_2, PI_{O_2} is the partial pressure of inspired oxygen, arterial P_{CO_2} is substituted for alveolar P_{CO_2}, and R is the respiratory exchange ratio.

This is a modification of the actual alveolar air equation. In practice, a respiratory exchange ratio of 0.8 is used in Equation 3.6. Begin and Renzetti have shown that these modifications using an R of 0.8 yield calculated values of PA_{O_2} that are accurate enough for clinical purposes (2). For example, a subject breathing room air at sea level has an arterial P_{CO_2} of 40 and an arterial PO_2 of 90. What are his calculated alveolar PO_2 and alveolar-arterial oxygen difference?

We must first calculate PA_{O_2}. With the patient breathing room air (21% O_2) at sea level (barometric pressure 760 mm Hg and body temperature 37°C), water vapor pressure is 47 mm Hg. Equation 3.6 becomes:

$$
\begin{aligned}
PA_{O_2} &= 0.21 \ (760 - 47) - 40/0.8 \\
&= 0.21 \ (713) - 50 \\
&= 150 - 50 \\
&= 100 \text{ mm Hg}
\end{aligned}
$$

This gives an estimate of the mean alveolar oxygen tension. The difference between alveolar and arterial oxygen tensions can then be calculated by subtracting the measured Pa_{O_2} (90 mm Hg) from the calculated PA_{O_2} (100 mm Hg) to give an alveolar-arterial oxygen difference of 10 mm Hg. The normal $PA_{O_2} - Pa_{O_2}$ in young adults averages about 8 mm Hg, and this increases gradually to a mean of 16 mm Hg in the 61 to 75 age group of healthy adults (1). Values significantly above this level indicate the presence of a lung abnormality causing a defect in gas transfer, and this may be assessed whether or not alveolar hypoventilation is present. The simplified alveolar air equation is extremely useful in clinical practice and should be committed to memory.

GAS TRANSFER (DIFFUSION)

Gas transfer across the alveolar-capillary membrane occurs by passive diffusion, which is related to the partial pressures of oxygen and carbon dioxide in the alveoli and in the pulmonary capillaries. The difference in oxygen and CO_2 tensions across the membrane represents the driving pressure for diffusion of each gas. It is impossible to measure diffusing capacity for oxygen because the capillary tension cannot be measured. In practice, carbon monoxide diffusion (D_{CO}) is measured, because the trace amounts of CO inhaled do not increase the P_{CO} in capillary blood. Diffusing capacity for oxygen (DO_2) is about 1.23 times the D_{CO}, or about 40 mL/min per mm Hg (3). During exercise, DO_2 may increase by more than three times through pulmonary capillary recruitment and an increase in capillary blood volume.

In the normal human capillary, equilibrium between alveolar and arterial PO_2 occurs in less than 0.25 second. Under normal resting conditions, blood spends about 0.75 second in the capillaries. Because it takes only one-third of this time for equilibration to occur, a wide safety margin exists, and even a large decrease in diffusion fails to affect gas exchange. The D_{CO} must fall to about 10% of the predicted value before any change in arterial oxygen at rest occurs because of an isolated diffusion defect.

The diffusion process may be affected by an abnormal resistance to diffusion, as in a thickened alveolar-capillary membrane; a decrease in the partial pressure gradient for oxygen across the membrane; or a shortened time for equilibration. At least two of these must coexist before arterial oxygen is affected. Thus, diffusion may become a factor in gas exchange during exercise (shortened equilibrium time) in a patient with interstitial fibrosis (thickened membrane) or at high altitude (decreased gradient).

For practical purposes, abnormal diffusion plays only a minor role in the hypoxemia seen in patients with lung diseases. This defect can easily be corrected by small increases in the inspired oxygen.

VENTILATION-PERFUSION RELATIONSHIPS

In the ideal gas exchange unit, ventilation and perfusion are equally matched and gas exchange is optimum. In real life, however, the situation is much more complex, and a *gradation* occurs from well-ventilated but underperfused areas, to equally ventilated and perfused areas, to areas that are well perfused but underventilated. In diseases that affect the lungs, the areas of equal matching are relatively small, and areas of mismatching of ventilation and perfusion are more important.

Using radioactive xenon scans, West and colleagues demonstrated that normally, in the upright position, blood flow increases progressively from the top to the bottom of the lungs, and blood flow per unit of lung area is increased approximately 10-fold from apex to base (4). Because of the movement of the diaphragm and larger pressure changes with inspiration around the lower lobe, *ventilation* also increases from top to bottom but not as much as perfusion. The bases are ventilated approximately three times as well as the apices. Thus, there is normally a gradient of both ventilation and perfusion from the top to the bottom of the lungs, in the upright position. When lying supine, these gradients occur from the anterior to the posterior portions of the lungs.

Because blood flow increases relatively more from apex to lung base than does ventilation, there is a decreasing *ratio* of ventilation to perfusion on descending from the apex to the base of the lungs. This is illustrated by the O_2-CO_2 diagram in Figure 3.4, which is taken from West's monograph. Using the figures from the O_2-CO_2 diagram, West has estimated that in normal resting humans in the upright position, the $\dot{V}/\dot{Q}$ ratio in the lung apices is about 3.3, whereas near the lung bases is only about 0.63. For this reason, oxygen tension in the alveoli at the apex is around 130 mm Hg, whereas in those at the lung base it is only about 90 mm Hg.

Note that according to the principles outlined in the preceding, the majority of the blood flows to the lung bases. Thus, areas at the apices, which are relatively well ventilated and have high $\dot{V}/\dot{Q}$ ratios, are poorly perfused, thus contributing relatively little to the measured PaO_2 in the systemic

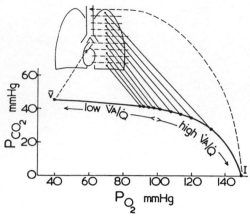

FIGURE 3.4. The O_2-CO_2 diagram showing normal ventilation-perfusion ratios in upright humans, from the top of the lungs to the bottom. The high $\dot{V}/\dot{Q}$ ratio at the apex results in a high PO_2 and low PCO_2 there. A low PO_2 and a high PCO_2 are found at the lung base. (Reprinted from West JB. *Ventilation/blood flow and gas exchange,* 4th ed. Oxford: Blackwell Scientific Publications, 1985. With permission of the author and publisher.)

arterial blood. The gas exchange units near the lung bases, where perfusion is relatively high and $\dot{V}/\dot{Q}$ ratios relatively low, contribute much more to the arterial blood, and because their effects predominate, arterial PO_2 primarily reflects areas with relatively low $\dot{V}/\dot{Q}$ relationships. This is a second reason why in normal humans arterial PO_2 is slightly less than alveolar PO_2. The remainder of the normal PAO_2 − PaO_2 gradient is explained by the normal anatomic shunts discussed in the preceding. Note in Figure 3.4 that the PCO_2 also varies normally from lung apices to lung bases. Because of relative hyperventilation, the PCO_2 at the top of the lungs is about 30 mm Hg, whereas that at the lung bases is around 40 mm Hg.

The $\dot{V}/\dot{Q}$ mismatching discussed in the preceding is that which occurs normally in the upright position. Patients with abnormal lungs have much more severe mismatching of ventilation to perfusion. Moreover, at the same horizontal level a lung lobule may contain terminal respiratory units that are adequately ventilated adjacent to underventilated terminal lung units whose bronchioles are completely occluded. Collateral ventilation may occur from a well-ventilated to a poorly ventilated pulmonary lobule, thus increasing the distance that the air must travel and increasing the dead space. The mismatching of ventilation to perfusion in disease occurs throughout the lungs and is difficult to measure with such gross tests of ventilation and perfusion as lung scans and arteriograms. In clinical practice, the amount of $\dot{V}/\dot{Q}$ mismatch is estimated from the amount of hypoxemia that remains after the effects of hypoventilation and true shunting are removed. The effects of hypoventilation are determined from the arterial PCO_2 (Eq. 3.1), and the effects of true shunts are estimated by measuring the PaO_2 while the patient breathes 100% oxygen.

Effects of Breathing 100% Oxygen

The portion of venous admixture caused by true right-to-left shunts can be separated from that caused by poorly ventilated lung units by having the subject breathe 100% oxygen for at least 15 minutes and then calculating the resultant change in shunt fraction (see Eq. 3.9). It is important that the patient take deep breaths during this procedure so that even poorly ventilated alveoli receive oxygen. The principle of this maneuver is that breathing 100% oxygen ultimately replaces the nitrogen in all functional lung units, even those that are poorly ventilated. Thus, the hemoglobin in the perfusing capillaries becomes completely saturated. These poorly ventilated alveoli then function as normal lung units as far as oxygen exchange is concerned. Alveolar oxygen tension is calculated from the alveolar air equation (using a respiratory exchange ratio of 1.0), and from that, capillary oxygen content is estimated. Arterial and mixed venous oxygen tensions are measured and oxygen contents are then calculated. Because defects in gas transfer owing to $\dot{V}/\dot{Q}$ inequality are eliminated by breathing 100% oxygen, the remaining $\dot{Q}s$ is owing solely to true right-to-left shunting. Subtracting the true shunt fraction from the total venous admixture (measured while breathing room air) yields an estimate of the contribution of $\dot{V}/\dot{Q}$ mismatching to arterial hypoxemia.

It should be noted that the alveolar-arterial oxygen tension difference normally increases as the F_{IO_2} is increased because the effects of poorly oxygenated blood from the normal right-to-left shunts on the PaO_2 become more pronounced. It is also common for the breathing of pure oxygen to cause absorption atelectasis. This phenomenon occurs when nitrogen from poorly ventilated alveoli is replaced by oxygen, which is subsequently absorbed into the pulmonary capillary blood.

OXYGEN TRANSPORT

The pulmonary venous blood leaves the pulmonary capillaries after equilibration with the alveolar gases, as arterial or oxygenated blood. It goes to the left atrium and ventricle, and from there to the systemic arteries. Arterial blood gas levels reflect the ability of the lungs to oxygenate the blood and remove excess CO_2. The oxygenated blood is distributed to the tissues via the systemic arteries and capillaries.

Cardiac Output

The cardiac output is the total amount of blood leaving the heart and going to the tissues. The normal resting cardiac output in an adult is about 6 L/min. The cardiac output may be measured by several techniques, including thermodilution using a pulmonary artery catheter; dye dilution using pulmonary and systemic arterial catheters; or Doppler

flow analysis. Cardiac output can be calculated using the Fick principle. The Fick principle states simply that the rate at which oxygen enters the blood during its passage through the lungs is a product of the blood flow and the difference between the oxygen content in the mixed venous blood and that of the arterial blood:

$$\dot{V}O_2 = \dot{Q}t \, (CaO_2 - C\bar{v}O_2) \qquad (3.7)$$

where $\dot{Q}t$ is the total blood flow from the right ventricle (i.e., the cardiac output). Solving for $\dot{Q}t$, we can rewrite this equation as follows:

$$\dot{Q}t = \dot{V}O_2/CaO_2 - C\bar{v}O_2 \qquad (3.8)$$

Oxygen Content and The Oxyhemoglobin Dissociation Curve

It should be emphasized that we are now dealing with oxygen *content* in arterial and mixed venous blood rather than with oxygen *tension,* and thus blood hemoglobin levels and the shape of the oxyhemoglobin dissociation curve must be considered. Because hemoglobin is the major oxygen carrier in the blood and because of the sigmoid shape of the oxyhemoglobin dissociation curve, we must calculate oxygen content from PaO_2 using the dissociation curve and measured levels of hemoglobin.

At this point it is reasonable to review the oxyhemoglobin dissociation curve. A few numbers are worth keeping in mind (Fig. 3.5). At a normal pH of 7.4 and a normal PaO_2 of 100 mm Hg, the hemoglobin is approximately 97% saturated. At the shoulder of the oxyhemoglobin dissociation

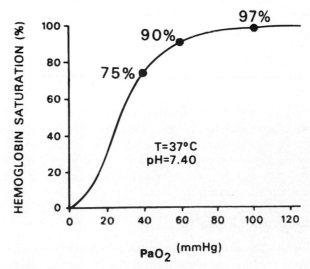

FIGURE 3.5. The normal oxyhemoglobin dissociation curve at pH 7.4 and temperature 37°C. Saturations at three key points are marked. Hyperthermia shifts the curve to the right and hypothermia shifts it to the left. Acidemia shifts it to the right and alkalemia to the left (Bohr effect).

curve, with a Pa_{O_2} of 60 and pH of 7.4, the hemoglobin is about 90% saturated. From here saturation drops quickly, and at a Pa_{O_2} of 40 (the normal mixed venous oxygen tension) the hemoglobin is only about 75% saturated.

The vast majority of the oxygen contained in blood is carried on the hemoglobin molecule. One gram of hemoglobin fully saturated carries 1.34 mL of oxygen (5). For example, with a hemoglobin content of 15 g/dL and a saturation of 97%, the oxygen content of arterial blood that is attached to hemoglobin is:

$$15 \text{ g/dL} \times 0.97 \times 1.34 \text{ mL/g} = 19.5 \text{ mL/dL}$$

In addition to the oxygen attached to hemoglobin, a small quantity is dissolved in arterial plasma, according to the solubility of oxygen in plasma (0.003 mL/dL per mm Hg P_{O_2}). At a normal Pa_{O_2} of 100 mm Hg, the dissolved content is:

$$100 \times 0.003 = 0.3 \text{ mL/dL}$$

The oxygen content of arterial blood for the normal patient in this example would be 19.8 (or about 20) mL/dL. In the normal range of Pa_{O_2}, the amount of dissolved oxygen is relatively minute and can be ignored; however, in situations where the F_{IO_2} is high, the amount of dissolved oxygen may become significant.

The blood normally loses about 25% of its oxygen content as it passes through the tissues. With a hemoglobin content of 15 g/dL the arterial blood carries about 20 mL of oxygen/dL. With a normal $P\bar{v}_{O_2}$ of 40 mm Hg and a mixed venous saturation of 75%, this same blood carries 15 mL of oxygen/dL. Thus, the normal *a-v̄ oxygen difference* is 5 mL/dL, and this difference may increase as tissue demands increase in relation to oxygen delivery. With an increase in metabolic demand, the a-v̄ oxygen difference increases at the same time the cardiac output increases, thus increasing oxygen delivery simultaneously by two mechanisms.

If cardiac output is insufficient to meet the body's needs, there is a drop in the $P\bar{v}_{O_2}$, because more oxygen must be extracted from the same amount of hemoglobin. In certain situations (e.g., sepsis syndrome), mixed venous oxygen content may increase in the face of low oxygen delivery, owing to inability of the tissues to utilize oxygen adequately. Thus, the measurement of mixed venous oxygen (saturation or tension) by indwelling catheters must be interpreted with caution in patients with gas exchange problems. In general, serial measurements are more useful for comparison than are single measurements.

The Shunt Equation

Although calculation of the alveolar-arterial oxygen gradient ($PA_{O_2} - Pa_{O_2}$) yields an assessment of gas transfer and therefore tells us whether there is wasted perfusion, the actual *percent* of the cardiac output that is shunted through the lungs and unavailable for gas transport may be estimated by using the *shunt equation:*

$$\frac{\dot{Q}s}{\dot{Q}t} = \frac{Cc'_{O_2} - Ca_{O_2}}{Cc'_{O_2} - C\bar{v}_{O_2}} \tag{3.9}$$

where $\dot{Q}s/\dot{Q}t$ is the shunt fraction or venous admixture and Cc'_{O_2}, Ca_{O_2}, and $C\bar{v}_{O_2}$ are the oxygen contents of end-capillary, arterial, and mixed venous blood, respectively. The Cc'_{O_2} is estimated by assuming that end-capillary P_{O_2} is the same as PA_{O_2} (calculated from the alveolar air equation). Ca_{O_2} is calculated from the measured arterial P_{O_2} and the oxyhemoglobin dissociation curve. The $C\bar{v}_{O_2}$ may be estimated by assuming a normal a-v̄ oxygen content difference of 5 mL/dL. This estimate of $C\bar{v}_{O_2}$ is not valid unless the cardiac output is adequate and stable, and tissue utilization is intact. If left ventricular function fails to meet the oxygen needs of the tissues, the a-v̄ difference is widened; conversely, if tissue utilization is impaired, the a-v̄ difference may be narrowed.

At a normal PA_{O_2} of 100 mm Hg and a hemoglobin of 15 g, the hemoglobin is 97% saturated and Cc'_{O_2} is 19.5 mL/dL. If the measured Pa_{O_2} is 80 mm Hg, the hemoglobin is 96% saturated and the Ca_{O_2} is 19.3 mL/dL. Assuming a normal cardiac output, and therefore an a-v̄ oxygen content difference of 5 mL/dL, we can calculate the shunt fraction as follows:

$$\begin{aligned} \frac{\dot{Q}s}{\dot{Q}t} &= \frac{Cc'_{O_2} - Ca_{O_2}}{Cc'_{O_2} - C\bar{v}_{O_2}} \\ &= \frac{19.5 - 19.3}{19.5 - 14.5} \\ &= \frac{0.2}{5.0} = 0.04 \text{ or } 4\% \end{aligned} \tag{3.10}$$

This relatively small percentage of the cardiac output that represents the normal shunting of blood in healthy people is made up of two components: blood that is perfusing relatively underventilated alveoli, and true shunts that perfuse areas that are not ventilated at all.

ARTERIAL HYPOXEMIA

The potential causes of arterial hypoxemia are listed in Table 3.2. In patients who are seen for evaluation of lung disease, arterial hypoxemia is usually the result of an increase in mismatching of ventilation to perfusion, and the causes of

TABLE 3.2 POTENTIAL CAUSES OF ARTERIAL HYPOXEMIA

Low F_{IO_2}
Hypoventilation
Diffusion defect
Ventilation-perfusion mismatch
Right-to-left shunt
Low mixed venous oxygen tension

hypoxemia not related to $\dot{V}/\dot{Q}$ mismatch (low inspired oxygen concentration, alveolar hypoventilation, diffusion defect, and low $P\bar{v}O_2$) are usually readily identifiable. This discussion addresses the differential diagnosis of arterial hypoxemia using a few simple observations and calculations to differentiate among the causes listed in Table 3.2. However, it should be noted that several causes often coexist in the same patient. For instance, the patient who is admitted with an acute exacerbation of COPD may have a combination of alveolar hypoventilation and a defect in gas transfer owing to mismatching of ventilation to perfusion. The relative contribution to the arterial hypoxemia should be determined for each of the factors when possible, as the various causes are treated differently and respond differently to an increase in inspired oxygen.

Low Inspired Oxygen Concentration

A review of the simplified alveolar air equation emphasizes the importance of FIO_2 and barometric pressure on the partial pressure of alveolar oxygen. In the example given in the preceding, the barometric pressure at sea level (760 mm Hg) was used; however, people frequently live at higher altitudes and are able to adapt quite well to living at altitudes as high as 2500 m (8,200 ft). Nearly 30 million people live at altitudes even higher, in the Rocky Mountains of North America, the Andes of South America, the Himalayas of Asia, and elsewhere (7). At 8,000 ft barometric pressure is approximately 565 mm Hg, the inspired PO_2 is about 120 mm Hg, and the alveolar oxygen is approximately 80 mm Hg. In subjects with normal lungs the PaO_2 remains high enough to achieve nearly complete hemoglobin saturation so that oxygen content is not severely affected.

In people living at altitudes above 8,000 ft, compensation occurs with increased hemoglobin levels and a shift in the oxygen-hemoglobin dissociation curve to the right so that oxygen is unloaded more efficiently to the tissues. Cardiac output increases in response to hypoxemia; however, this decrease in red cell transit time through the pulmonary capillaries in addition to a decrease in mixed venous PO_2 tends to emphasize existing $\dot{V}/\dot{Q}$ inequalities. Furthermore, pulmonary hypertension occurs at very high altitudes, and this is associated with an alteration in ventilation-perfusion relationships, which may result in further arterial hemoglobin desaturation. For a further discussion of altitude physiology and adaptation to high altitudes, the reader is referred to the work of West, Hackett, and associates (7).

Patients undergoing mechanical ventilation because of diffuse lung disease with severe defects in gas exchange (e.g., pneumonia, pulmonary edema, adult respiratory distress syndrome) may suffer rapid worsening of hypoxemia if the delivered FIO_2 falls because of ventilator malfunction or manipulation of the ventilator controls. Such patients are often maintained at the lowest FIO_2 that results in nearly complete saturation of the arterial hemoglobin. At levels of PaO_2 below 60 mm Hg a small decrease in FIO_2 results in a severe decline in SaO_2 and arterial oxygen content, owing to the steep slope of the oxyhemoglobin dissociation curve. Constant monitoring of SaO_2 with pulse oximetry alerts the clinician to such sudden and potentially dangerous decreases in oxygen content.

Hypoventilation

As noted in the preceding, alveolar PCO_2 is inversely related to alveolar ventilation; thus, if alveolar ventilation is halved, alveolar and arterial PCO_2 values double. The hallmark of alveolar hypoventilation is an increase in $PaCO_2$. Alveolar hypoventilation decreases alveolar PO_2 because as CO_2 accumulates in the alveoli it displaces oxygen; therefore, the displaced oxygen is not available for gas exchange. If the arterial PCO_2 is normal or low, hypoxemia cannot be explained by alveolar hypoventilation.

In normal patients, alveolar ventilation ($\dot{V}A$) is a fixed proportion of minute ventilation ($\dot{V}E$), because dead space ventilation is limited mainly to the anatomic dead space (conducting airways). Thus, we can consider the $\dot{V}E$ and $PaCO_2$ to be inversely proportional (Eq. 3.2). In patients with respiratory problems, the ventilatory pattern may change so that breathing becomes rapid and shallow; thus, a greater part of each breath is composed of dead space ventilation. In such patients, $\dot{V}A$ may decrease and $PaCO_2$ may rise without a change in measured minute ventilation ($\dot{V}E$). A change to slow, deep breaths results in a decrease of $PaCO_2$ without a change in $\dot{V}E$. In patients with chronic lung disease, minute ventilation may be increased, although $PaCO_2$ is elevated, because of an increase in the alveolar dead space and $\dot{V}/\dot{Q}$ mismatching.

Hypoventilation causes hypoxemia owing to its effects on the alveolar PO_2, a relationship described in the *alveolar air equation* (Eq. 3.6). Any rise in $PaCO_2$ causes a drop in the alveolar and thus the arterial PO_2. Thus, with moderate degrees of alveolar hypoventilation, the $PAO_2 - PaO_2$ remains normal. It has been shown that marked hypercapnia reduces the increased $PAO_2 - PaO_2$ that might otherwise exist because of abnormalities in gas exchange (8).

In patients who are hypoxemic and retaining CO_2, the relative contribution to the hypoxemia of alveolar hypoventilation can be determined by calculating $PAO_2 - PaO_2$. If this is normal, one can assume that the observed hypoxemia can be corrected by achieving adequate alveolar ventilation. If, however, the $PAO_2 - PaO_2$ is elevated, there is a defect in gas transfer (usually a $\dot{V}/\dot{Q}$ mismatch) in addition to the hypoventilation. In comatose patients who have no associated lung disease, the $PAO_2 - PaO_2$ is within normal limits and the hypoxemia can be corrected completely with adequate ventilation. If, however, the $PAO_2 - PaO_2$ is elevated in the presence of a high $PaCO_2$, there is an additional defect in gas transfer, and an increased FIO_2 or the addition of positive end-expiratory pressure (PEEP) may be necessary.

Diffusion Defect

A defect in gas transfer because of diffusion limitation does not occur in normal humans at sea level because even at high cardiac outputs the blood remains in the capillaries long enough for adequate equilibrium. However, during exercise at high altitudes the driving pressure (PA_{O_2}) of oxygen in the alveoli may be low enough and the transit time of blood in the capillaries so short that a limitation of diffusion of oxygen into the blood may become a factor in the development of hypoxemia (9). As noted, three factors may decrease oxygen diffusion and cause hypoxemia: (a) a defect in the lung diffusion capacity of oxygen; (b) a decrease in the oxygen gradient between alveoli and capillary blood; and (c) a decrease in equilibration time. Two or more of these abnormalities must occur for diffusion defects to become a factor in hypoxemia; however, defects in diffusion may play a minor role in patients with other problems. Diffusion defects are easily corrected by increasing the FI_{O_2}.

Ventilation-Perfusion Mismatch

Ventilation-perfusion mismatching is the most common cause of hypoxemia in patients with lung disease. Marked $\dot{V}/\dot{Q}$ mismatching is manifested by hypoxemia in the presence of a normal, low, or high Pa_{CO_2}. By definition, wasted ventilation ($\dot{V}D/\dot{V}T$) and wasted perfusion ($\dot{Q}s/\dot{Q}t$) are both increased. Measurement of $\dot{V}D/\dot{V}T$ yields an estimate of the amount of wasted ventilation, whereas calculating the shunt fraction indicates the amount of wasted perfusion.

The $PA_{O_2} - Pa_{O_2}$ is a useful index of the degree of $\dot{V}/\dot{Q}$ inequality in the lungs. Because the distribution of lung abnormalities is not uniform in the presence of disease, various units of the lungs are affected to different degrees. Thus, some areas have relatively high $\dot{V}/\dot{Q}$ ratios and others relatively low ratios. Arterial blood reflects areas with relatively high blood flow, and thus areas with relatively low $\dot{V}/\dot{Q}$ ratios. The majority of diffuse lung diseases, including those affecting the airways (e.g., chronic bronchitis and asthma) and those affecting the alveoli (e.g., emphysema and interstitial fibrosis), all result in increased $PA_{O_2} - Pa_{O_2}$ owing to $\dot{V}/\dot{Q}$ mismatching. Furthermore, therapeutic measures (e.g., administration of bronchodilators) may actually hinder the physiologic attenuation of perfusion to areas of localized hyperventilation, resulting in more severe shunting and a further drop in $PA_{O_2} - Pa_{O_2}$ (10).

The greater the degree of $\dot{V}/\dot{Q}$ inequality present, the higher the $\dot{V}E$ must be to maintain a normal or reduced Pa_{CO_2}. An elevated $\dot{V}E$ with a normal Pa_{CO_2} is evidence for the presence of a $\dot{V}/\dot{Q}$ abnormality. This is owing to an increase in the dead space ventilation. The overventilation of normal lung units required to compensate for low $\dot{V}/\dot{Q}$ units results in an increased gradient between the expired P_{CO_2} and the Pa_{CO_2}, and thus an increase in the $\dot{V}D/\dot{V}T$.

At some point, the work of increasing $\dot{V}E$ becomes too great to sustain, and any further increase in $\dot{V}/\dot{Q}$ mismatch results in a rise in Pa_{CO_2}. This may be slow (e.g., COPD), or rapid (e.g., acute asthma attacks). The respiratory center and the respiratory muscles determine the point at which Pa_{CO_2} begins to rise. The increased Pa_{CO_2} that occurs is a method of boosting the efficiency of a compromised ventilatory system. The higher the concentration of CO_2 in the alveolar gas, and thus in each expired breath, the lower the $\dot{V}E$ required to remove a specific amount of CO_2. The effect of the rise in Pa_{CO_2} on blood pH and central nervous system function limits the extent of this compensatory mechanism. However, with renal compensation, chronic elevations of Pa_{CO_2} are well tolerated.

During acute hypercapnic exacerbations of COPD, oxygen therapy almost always leads to a further rise in the Pa_{CO_2}. Although this has been thought to be caused by further depression of the respiratory drive, Aubier et al. showed that Pa_{CO_2} may rise without a significant reduction in $\dot{V}E$ (11). Other investigators have disputed their findings; at any rate, other factors seem to be active in causing the further rise in Pa_{CO_2} associated with oxygen administration. There is a further increase in $\dot{V}/\dot{Q}$ mismatching owing to vasodilation and increased perfusion of poorly ventilated lung units; and the hemoglobin affinity for CO_2 is reduced as oxygen saturation increases (Haldane effect). Because the increase in Pa_{CO_2} is not entirely due to respiratory center depression, progressively worsening hypercapnia is not inevitable.

A moderate increase in Pa_{CO_2} without mental changes requires no intervention. If hypercapnia progresses and CO_2 narcosis ensues, mechanical ventilation may be required. A common practice is to decrease the FI_{O_2} slightly, to "stimulate the respiratory center." This is a mistake because it may result in severe hypoxemia. Progressive hypercapnia rarely kills a patient; severe hypoxemia often does. A reasonable approach is to increase the FI_{O_2} in small increments while monitoring with a pulse oximeter, using only the FI_{O_2} necessary to achieve a hemoglobin saturation of about 90%.

Right-To-Left Shunt

The other potential cause of arterial hypoxemia is a true right-to-left shunt. Shunting may occur in conjunction with $\dot{V}/\dot{Q}$ mismatching or hypoventilation, in which case it adds to the severity of the hypoxemia. The contribution of shunting in patients with arterial hypoxemia may be assessed by calculating the shunt fraction with the patient breathing 100% oxygen, as outlined in the preceding. The $\dot{Q}s/\dot{Q}t$ that remains after breathing oxygen (correcting that portion caused by $\dot{V}/\dot{Q}$ mismatching) is the percentage of the cardiac output actually shunted through unventilated areas.

When breathing mixtures high in oxygen, the amount of oxygen dissolved in the plasma must be included in the estimation of Cc'_{O_2}, Ca_{O_2}, and $C\bar{v}_{O_2}$. This is calculated by multiplying the Pa_{O_2} by the solubility coefficient of oxygen in plasma at body temperature, which is 0.003 mL/dL/mm Hg. On breathing 100% oxygen at sea level, about 2 mL oxygen is dissolved in each 100 mL plasma. It should also be noted that the calculation of $PA_{O_2} - Pa_{O_2}$ whereas breathing 100% oxygen does not require the usual correction for R, since only oxygen and carbon dioxide are left in the alveoli, the nitrogen having been washed out.

Acute lung injuries, such as the adult respiratory distress syndrome (ARDS), cause severe hypoxemia mostly as a result of shunting. Serial changes in gas transfer cannot be determined using the $PA_{O_2} - Pa_{O_2}$ gradient, because the increased FI_{O_2} required to treat the hypoxemia is associated with a variable effect on the calculated gradient. An estimate of serial changes in gas transfer can be obtained by comparing the ratio of Pa_{O_2} to the FI_{O_2} (12). A Pa_{O_2}/FI_{O_2} of 250 or greater is indicative of a relatively mild defect in gas transfer in patients with ARDS; a ratio of 100 or less is a grave prognostic sign, indicating severe lung damage.

Low Mixed Venous Oxygen Tension

A reduction in $P\bar{v}_{O_2}$ may result in worsening arterial hypoxemia in patients with $\dot{V}/\dot{Q}$ mismatching, right-to-left shunts, or low hemoglobin levels (13). The drop in $P\bar{v}_{O_2}$ may result from a decrease in cardiac output or from an increase in oxygen uptake by the tissues. The lower $P\bar{v}_{O_2}$ increases the effects of right-to-left shunts on arterial PO_2 (depending on the intensity of hypoxemic vasoconstriction), further limiting oxygen delivery. In patients with limited cardiac output who require mechanical ventilation, factors such as fever, anxiety, and increased work of breathing may be corrected by such measures as lowering the temperature, administering sedation, or adjusting the ventilator. Decreasing oxygen uptake then results in an increased $P\bar{v}_{O_2}$ (assuming oxygen delivery is unchanged); this in turn increases arterial oxygen.

SYSTEMIC OXYGEN DELIVERY

In a normal adult approximately 300 mL of oxygen is used per minute at rest. During exercise, oxygen delivery is related linearly to oxygen uptake. The amount of oxygen delivered to the tissues per minute can be calculated by multiplying the arterial blood oxygen content (Ca_{O_2}) in mL/dL by the cardiac output ($\dot{Q}$) in L/min. The arterial oxygen content depends on the concentration of functional hemoglobin in arterial blood and the saturation of that hemoglobin with oxygen. The saturation of hemoglobin is dependent on the partial pressure of oxygen in the arterial blood. Thus, systemic oxygen delivery depends on the interaction of the *circulatory system* (delivery of arterial blood), *erythropoietic system* (hemoglobin in red blood cells), and *respiratory system* (gas exchange area) according to the following equation:

Systemic oxygen transport (mL/min)
$$= \dot{Q} \text{ (L/min)} \times Ca_{O_2} \text{ (mL/L)}$$
$$= \dot{Q} \times (\text{g hemoglobin} \times 1.34) \times Sa_{O_2} \quad (3.11)$$

| circulatory | erythropoietic | respiratory |
| system | system | system |

where $\dot{Q}$ is the cardiac output and Sa_{O_2} is the percent saturation of the hemoglobin. The respiratory system provides the oxygen tension in the pulmonary capillaries, which in turn determines hemoglobin saturation. The preceding equation does not include the (normally inconsequential) volume of oxygen that is dissolved in the blood.

The Circulatory System

With a normal resting cardiac output ($\dot{Q}$) of about 6 L/min, because each 100 mL of arterial blood contains about 20 mL oxygen, the total amount of oxygen delivered per minute to the tissues at rest is about 1200 mL. The cells use only about 300 mL of this oxygen, which means that about 900 mL remains in the mixed venous blood. The percent of oxygen remaining in the mixed venous blood represents the *average* extraction of oxygen from blood by all the tissues. It is important to understand that although the average oxygen extraction is about 25% of the oxygen present in the arterial blood, oxygen use differs markedly from one organ system to another. For instance, the heart uses essentially all the oxygen it receives, whereas the kidneys use only a small percentage. It is physiologically appropriate to have a surplus of oxygen available in case sudden changes in availability or use occur. Thus, the oxygen remaining in the mixed venous blood represents a reservoir for the tissues to call on should the normal adjustments to demand be temporarily inadequate.

The oxygen extracted from the blood during its passage through the tissues determines the *arterial-mixed venous difference* in oxygen tension ($Pa_{O_2} - P\bar{v}_{O_2}$). The $P\bar{v}_{O_2}$ is normally about 40 mm Hg, so that with a normal arterial PO_2 of 90 mm Hg and an adequate delivery of blood to the tissues, the a-v̄ oxygen difference is about 50 mm Hg. A fall in mixed venous PO_2 with an increase in the a-v̄ oxygen tension difference occurs during exercise, and whenever the oxygen delivery system is stressed. When an abnormal a-v̄ difference occurs in the absence of normal stress mechanisms, it is evidence for failure of the circulatory system (14–16).

The Erythropoietic System

Each 100 mL of blood normally contains about 15 g of hemoglobin. It is this hemoglobin content that allows for the remarkable oxygen-carrying ability of the blood, normally about 20 mL/dL. This is possible because 1 g of hemoglobin when fully saturated carries 1.34 mL of oxygen. At a normal PaO_2 of over 80 mm Hg, the hemoglobin molecule is almost completely saturated, whereas at a mixed venous PO_2 of 40 mm Hg, the hemoglobin is only about 75% saturated. The ability of hemoglobin to bind oxygen at normal values of arterial PO_2 and to give it up at lower values of PO_2 is described by the oxyhemoglobin dissociation curve (see Fig. 3.5).

To calculate arterial oxygen content, the percent saturation of the hemoglobin (SaO_2) must be determined. The SaO_2 may be estimated from the oxyhemoglobin dissociation curve, provided the PaO_2 and pH are known and the hemoglobin is normal. This is the procedure used in most blood gas laboratories, where SaO_2 is calculated rather than measured. Alternatively, SaO_2 may be measured by using a cooximeter for *in vitro* measurement or a pulse oximeter for *in vivo* measurement. Actual measurement is necessary if the shape or position of the oxyhemoglobin dissociation curve is abnormal because of changes in the hemoglobin molecule.

Normally, the relationship of SaO_2 to PO_2 is not static but changes with differing conditions, usually to the benefit of the individual. A decrease in blood pH is associated with a shift in the curve toward the right, as shown in Figure 3.6; thus, at the higher pH levels found in the lungs, oxygen is bound more easily, whereas at lower pH levels found in the tissues, oxygen is freed more easily (the Bohr effect). Lower temperatures shift the curve to the left, whereas higher temperatures shift the curve to the right.

The binding capacity for oxygen is also affected by an increase or decrease in the 2,3-diphosphoglycerate (2,3-DPG) content of the red cells. Because the 2,3-DPG competes with oxygen for sites on the hemoglobin molecule, increased levels of 2,3-DPG shift the curve to the right and allow for improved oxygen delivery. Carbon monoxide (CO) binds extremely readily with hemoglobin to form carboxyhemoglobin. This decreases the ability of the hemoglobin to carry oxygen. Some inherited abnormal types of hemoglobin are associated with marked changes in the oxyhemoglobin dissociation curve, with either an increased or decreased affinity of hemoglobin for oxygen.

Although almost all the oxygen in arterial blood is carried on the hemoglobin molecule, a small amount is also carried in the plasma as dissolved oxygen. Because the solubility of oxygen in plasma is very low, this portion of the oxygen content is insignificant except in unusual situations, such as in the breathing of high concentrations of oxygen. In patients with carbon monoxide poisoning, CO replaces oxygen on the hemoglobin molecule because its affinity for hemoglobin is greater, producing tissue hypoxia in the presence of a normal hemoglobin level and a normal PaO_2. In such cases, ventilation with high-oxygen mixtures may prevent hypoxic tissue damage and will augment the elimination of CO.

The affinity of hemoglobin for oxygen and its ability to give up oxygen at the tissue level are commonly assessed by calculating the P_{50}, the partial pressure of oxygen at which the hemoglobin is 50% saturated. The P_{50} can be calculated by equilibrating the patient's blood in a tonometer at various PO_2 levels and then measuring the saturation of the hemoglobin and plotting a dissociation curve. The normal P_{50} of human blood is about 26 mm Hg, with a fairly large variability around this level in the presence of disease. The P_{50} may be estimated from a random venous blood sample according to a formula proposed by Lichtman and coworkers (17). In a group of 38 healthy subjects, the mean P_{50} calculated by using their technique was 26 ± 1.3 mm Hg. It is important to note that most values of SaO_2 reported from the blood gas laboratory are calculated from a nomogram that assumes a normal hemoglobin dissociation curve. For estimation of P_{50}, saturation of the hemoglobin must be measured directly, for obvious reasons.

The Respiratory System

The respiratory system is assessed by measurement of PaO_2 while breathing room air. If the arterial blood is not adequately oxygenated, there is a defect in gas transfer at the pulmonary capillary level. This may be owing to precapillary shunting within the lungs, to mismatching of ventilation with perfusion in the gas transfer units of the lungs, or to hypoventilation. Frequently, several of these factors are abnormal in the same patient. Factors outside the lungs can also affect PaO_2. These include extrapulmonary right-to-left

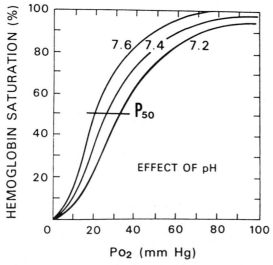

FIGURE 3.6. The oxyhemoglobin dissociation curve. The effects of shifts in pH on the affinity of hemoglobin for oxygen (the Bohr effect) are shown. Acidosis shifts the curve toward the right and thus increases oxygen delivery at the tissue level. The affinity of hemoglobin for oxygen is expressed as the P_{50} (the PaO_2 at which the hemoglobin is 50% saturated).

shunts, in which case blood never gets to the lungs to be oxygenated, and a decrease in mixed venous PO_2.

Inadequate oxygen delivery affects arterial oxygen content by decreasing the mixed venous PO_2. In patients with intrapulmonary shunts, because the mixed venous blood is added directly to the arterial blood, there is a dramatic fall in PaO_2 secondary to the decrease in $P\bar{v}O_2$ (13). Thus, when the PaO_2 deteriorates in a patient with multiple organ system failure, factors other than those directly related to abnormal gas exchange in the lungs must be considered.

REFERENCES

1. Mellemgaard K. The alveolar-arterial oxygen difference: its size and components in normal man. *Acta Physiol Scand* 1966;67: 10–20.
2. Begin R, Renzetti AD. Alveolar-arterial oxygen pressure gradient. Comparison between an assumed and actual respiratory quotient in stable chronic pulmonary disease. *Respir Care* 1977;22: 491–500.
3. Dantzker DR. Pulmonary gas exchange. In: Bone RE, Dantzker DR, George RB, et al (eds). *Pulmonary and critical care medicine.* St Louis: Mosby, 1993:B-1–13.
4. West JB. *Ventilation/blood flow and gas exchange,* 4th ed. Oxford, Blackwell Scientific Publications, 1985:17–29.
5. Murray JF. *The normal lung,* 2nd ed. Philadelphia: Saunders, 1986:201–209.
6. Baker PT. The adaptive fitness of high altitude populations. In: Baker PT (ed). *The biology of high altitude peoples.* Cambridge: Cambridge University Press, 1978:317–346.
7. West JB, Hackett PH, Maret KH, et al. Pulmonary gas exchange on the summit of Mount Everest. *J Appl Physiol* 1983;55: 678–687.
8. Gray BA, Blalock JM. Interpretation of the alveolar-arterial oxygen difference in patients with hypercapnia. *Am Rev Respir Dis* 1991;143:4–8.
9. West JB, Lahiri S, Gill MB, et al. Arterial oxygen saturation during exercise at high altitude. *J Appl Physiol* 1962;17:617–621.
10. Tai E, Reid J. Response of blood gas tensions to aminophylline and isoprenaline in patients with asthma. *Thorax* 1967;22: 543–549.
11. Aubier M, Marviano D, Millic-Emili J, et al. Effects of the administration of O_2 on ventilation and blood gases in patients with chronic obstructive pulmonary disease during acute respiratory failure. *Am Rev Respir Dis* 1980;122:747–754.
12. Murray JF, Matthay MA, Luce JM, et al. An expanded definition of the adult respiratory distress syndrome. *Am Rev Respir Dis* 1988;138:720–723.
13. Dantzker DR. The influence of cardiovascular function on gas exchange. *Clin Chest Med* 1983;4:149–159.
14. Kandel G, Aberman A. Mixed venous oxygen saturation. Its role in the assessment of the critically ill patient. *Arch Intern Med* 1983;143:1400–1402.
15. Kasnitz P, Druger GL, Yorra F, et al. Mixed venous oxygen tension and hyperlactatemia. *JAMA* 1976;236:570–574.
16. Bell RC, Coalson JJ, Smith JD, et al. Multiple organ system failure and infection in adult respiratory distress syndrome. *Ann Intern Med* 1983;99:293–298.
17. Lichtman MS, Murphy MS, Adamson JW. Detection of mutant hemoglobins with altered affinity for oxygen: a simplified technique. *Ann Intern Med* 1976;84:517–520.

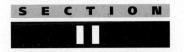

GATHERING THE DATA BASE

4

THE RESPIRATORY HISTORY AND PHYSICAL EXAMINATION

RONALD B. GEORGE AND D. KEITH PAYNE

OBTAINING A USEFUL HISTORY
Occupational and Exposure History

SYMPTOMS OF RESPIRATORY DISEASES
Upper Respiratory Tract Symptoms
Chest Pain
Breathlessness
Cough
Sputum Expectoration
Hemoptysis

PHYSICAL EXAMINATION

Inspection and Palpation
Percussion
Auscultation
Extrapulmonary Signs

OFFICE AND HOME TESTING OF PATIENTS WITH RESPIRATORY DISEASE

The process of obtaining a meaningful history, performing a good physical examination, and putting the information together to form an initial impression is an art that must be learned by experience. The history and physical examination should lead to a reasonable list of differential diagnoses. This list of impressions, in turn, forms the basis for a diagnostic plan, whereby the number of possible diagnoses is gradually decreased by the results of selected laboratory tests, radiographs, and specialized procedures. This chapter includes some guidelines for this important task.

OBTAINING A USEFUL HISTORY

The interview is designed to identify the important symptoms and determine their duration. To do this without being led into blind areas of discussion is an important step toward identifying the problem. The interviewer must lead the discussion, avoiding lengthy digressions; on the other hand, the patient must have the freedom to mention items that may prove important as the history unfolds. The patient should not be badgered, but should be made to feel that the interviewer is truly interested in his or her problems. The interviewer should not yawn or act bored, but should instead appear interested in the patient's story.

The chief complaint—the symptom that caused the patient to seek help—and its duration should be identified. Frequently the patient will say that he or she was referred because of an abnormal finding on a chest film or some other laboratory test. However, it is important to determine why that test was made and, if it was part of a routine examination, what changes from previous films resulted in referral.

Once the major complaint and its duration are identified, the development of the patient's symptoms should be investigated chronologically, beginning at the time that the patient first noted a departure from feeling well. The patient should be questioned concerning current and past medications, any allergic reactions or intolerance to foods or drugs, or exposure to contagious illnesses. It is important to determine if other members of the household or coworkers have similar symptoms. It is also useful to obtain information from previous examinations or diagnostic tests. For instance, a previously negative tuberculin skin test is important if tuberculosis is suspected. Elements of the personal, occupational, and social history should be included in the present illness if they are directly pertinent to the patient's current symptoms.

A systematic review of the symptoms of respiratory illnesses and their character and duration should be reported. Nonrespiratory symptoms should also be reviewed, because they may be related to the respiratory disease. Patients with carcinoma of the lung may present with complaints of headaches or seizures related to cerebral metastases; ankle swelling or a history of injury to the lower extremities is important if the patient has a suspected pulmonary embolism. Ascites and edema of the legs may be secondary to heart failure, cor pulmonale, or liver disease, all of which may cause abnormalities on the chest film, whereas joint pain may be caused by hypertrophic pulmonary osteoarthropathy. It is important to determine if a patient's complaints are seasonal, especially in patients with hay fever, sinusitis, postnasal drip, or asthma.

Previous illnesses and operations should be recorded, because they may be related to the present illness. For instance, childhood measles or pertussis may be the origin of bronchiectasis, and asthma during childhood that disappeared at puberty may return at a later age. Patients with reactivation tuberculosis often relate a history of household contact during their childhood years. Previous operations and biopsies may be the source of pathologic specimens that might be useful for re-examination. If previous chest films are available, they should be obtained for comparison with recent ones.

Occupational and Exposure History

Cigarette smoking is the most common preventable cause of death in the United States today (1). A smoking history is especially important in patients with respiratory complaints. Passive exposure to cigarette smoke in home or workplace is an increasingly recognized cause of respiratory symptoms in children whose parents smoke, and passive smoking has been shown to increase the incidence of respiratory infections (2).

The occupational history is especially important in patients with lung problems, because the lungs are constantly in contact with the environment. The patient should be encouraged to relate his or her job history in chronologic order. Occupational exposure may have occurred many years ago; exposure to asbestos may result in the development of a pleural mesothelioma 25 years or more after the exposure has ceased. It is important to ask the patient if he or she was advised to wear a mask at work or whether his or her fellow workers did so. The type of mask worn and the air source should be identified. Construction workers who are not directly involved in hazardous activities may work in closed areas containing toxic materials; for instance, carpenters, plumbers, and welders often work in areas where sandblasting is occurring. Although the sandblaster may have extensive protection, the workers nearby may be exposed.

Some symptoms of toxic reactions are not related to the lungs. Patients working with galvanized metal (zinc fumes) may complain of nausea, vomiting, and other systemic symptoms. Allergic alveolitis owing to thermophilic actinomycetes in workers exposed to moldy hay (farmer's lung) or sugar cane residue (bagassosis) is associated with fever, malaise, and headache in addition to nonproductive cough. The patient should be questioned about particularly irritating odors or upper respiratory symptoms, because toxic fumes usually affect the eyes, nose, and throat and this serves as an early sign of chemical exposure. Upper respiratory symptoms are common in toxic smoke inhalation.

Workers may not be aware of exposures to toxic materials. For instance, office workers have developed allergic alveolitis from air conditioners and humidifiers that were contaminated with fungal spores (3).

The family history is often useful. Cystic fibrosis and the immotile cilia syndromes are inherited, as are the hemoglobinopathies and α_1-antitrypsin deficiency. Patients with asthma often have a family history of allergic rhinitis, asthma, or other allergic symptoms. In addition, family members may have similar exposure. Tuberculosis is often spread by household contact, and viral respiratory diseases often affect several family members. Families may be exposed to the oxides of nitrogen (silo filler's disease) or moldy hay while working together on a farm.

SYMPTOMS OF RESPIRATORY DISEASES

Upper Respiratory Tract Symptoms

Rhinorrhea, conjunctivitis, and sneezing are common in patients with allergic rhinitis (hay fever), who may also have asthma; the two syndromes often coincide. Postnasal drip occurs in patients with upper respiratory disease and is manifested during the daytime by frequent clearing of the throat rather than by actual coughing. A postnasal drip is often a problem at night, and may produce a morning cough caused by chronic irritation of the upper airways.

Nosebleeds (epistaxis) may be a symptom of sinusitis or may be produced by trauma, foreign bodies, or tumors of the nose and nasopharynx. Systemic diseases such as hypertension, polycythemia, and bleeding disorders can also lead to bouts of epistaxis. Wegener's granulomatosis causes necrotizing granulomas of the upper respiratory tract as well as of the lungs. Blood from the nose and nasopharynx sometimes accumulates in the oropharynx and is coughed up; therefore, the patient thinks that it is coming from the lungs. A history of epistaxis and the finding of blood clots in the nose or nasopharynx are clues that the expectorated blood may be coming from the upper respiratory tract. Hoarseness may result from lesions of the recurrent laryngeal nerve (surgical trauma, mediastinal tumors, or infections) or from diseases of the larynx (tuberculosis, tumors, or allergy).

Patients who present with anaerobic infections of the lungs and pleura (lung abscess, empyema) often have upper respiratory abnormalities leading to aspiration of oral secretions. The patient should be questioned concerning recent mouth or dental surgery, anesthesia, aspiration of a foreign body, neurologic abnormalities, periods of unconsciousness, and seizures.

Chest Pain

Thoracic pain is an alarming symptom, because most people are aware of its association with cardiac disease, lung tumors, and other serious life-threatening diseases. There are two basic types of chest pain: that which arises in the chest wall structures and is conducted through the intercostal and phrenic nerves (lateral or chest wall pain) and that which arises in the internal organs and is conducted through the afferent fibers of the vagus nerve (central or visceral pain). These two types of chest pain are discussed separately.

Visceral chest pain occurs with neoplasms of the major bronchi or mediastinum; abnormalities of the heart, aorta, and pericardium; or diseases that cause esophageal pain, especially reflux esophagitis or tumors. Pain associated with acute bronchitis is usually central and is often accentuated by coughing.

Pain in the substernal area may indicate disease of the heart, pericardium, aorta, or esophagus. Angina pectoris is usually an effort-induced pain that is relieved by rest and vasodilators. It is often referred to the neck, shoulder, or arm. Pericardial pain is sometimes relieved by sitting up or leaning forward. Pain associated with a dissecting aortic aneurysm is frequently reported as severe and deep, and may be referred to the interscapular area of the back. Esophageal pain may mimic angina pectoris and may be relieved by sublingual nitroglycerin, which relaxes esophageal spasm. It is often related to meals and relieved by antacids. Patients with significant esophageal reflux are subject to aspiration, especially at night, and may present with recurrent bouts of acute bronchospasm and cough, mimicking asthma attacks.

Chest wall pain is sharp, often well localized, and is increased by deep breathing or coughing (pleuritic pain or pleurisy). Pleuritic pain is associated with any disease that causes inflammation of the parietal pleura such as infections (pneumonia, empyema, tuberculosis), trauma (pneumothorax, hemothorax, rib fracture), or tumors (cancer, lymphoma, mesothelioma). Older patients may suffer rib fractures following minor trauma or even severe coughing bouts. These fractures may not be visible on the initial chest film, but later callus formation around the fracture may make it apparent in retrospect. Irritation of the intercostal nerves (herpes zoster, spinal nerve root disease) may also lead to localized chest wall pain. Costochondritis of the second to fourth costosternal articulations (Tietze's syndrome) is common and may mimic the pain of myocardial ischemia or other serious diseases. The pain is clearly localized to the costal cartilage, and there is tenderness to pressure and often a palpable enlargement of the costosternal junction.

The peripheral innervation of the diaphragm is from the local intercostal nerves, and irritation of the peripheral diaphragm is referred to the adjacent chest wall. The central diaphragmatic pain fibers are conducted through the phrenic nerves, and pain in the central diaphragm is often felt in the ipsilateral trapezius region at the base of the neck and the shoulder, an area also supplied by the phrenic nerve.

Breathlessness

Breathlessness (dyspnea) is the sensation of difficulty in breathing, sometimes interpreted as the inability to take a deep breath. It is one of the most common reasons that patients with chest diseases consult a physician. Breathlessness is difficult to quantitate, because it is subjective and in certain situations (e.g., during and following exercise and at high altitudes) it is normal. Although exercise normally produces dyspnea, a rapid increase in breathlessness or a decrease in exercise tolerance is an important symptom. Breathlessness may occur intermittently, as with attacks of asthma, or it may be persistent, as with chronic obstructive pulmonary disease (COPD). It may be influenced by position, as in patients with left heart failure, who complain of orthopnea (dyspnea when lying flat). Orthopnea may also be seen in patients with asthma or chronic airway obstruction.

There are three basic causes of the sensation of breathlessness: an increased awareness of normal breathing, an increase in the work of breathing, and an abnormality of the ventilatory system itself. Increased awareness of normal breathing is usually a result of anxiety; in this situation the common complaint is that the patient cannot take a satisfactorily deep breath. The breathing pattern is often irregular, with frequent sighs. Severe psychogenic breathlessness is associated with rapid breathing, tingling of the hands and feet, circumoral numbness, respiratory alkalosis, and occasionally tetanic seizures. This *hyperventilation syndrome* is diagnosed only after organic causes, both respiratory and nonrespiratory, have been excluded and the respiratory mechanics and blood oxygen level have been determined to be normal.

The second cause of breathlessness is an increase in the work of breathing. This may be owing either to airways obstruction, in which case greater pressures are required to move air into and out of the lungs, or restriction of lung volumes and loss of compliance, in which case greater effort is required to expand the lungs and chest wall.

The third cause of breathlessness is an abnormality of the ventilatory apparatus. This involves dysfunction of the nerves, the respiratory muscles, or the thoracic cage itself. Neurologic abnormalities producing breathlessness include spinal cord injury, ascending polyneuritis, myasthenia gravis, amyotrophic lateral sclerosis, poliomyelitis, and exposure to paralytic agents or neurotoxins. Primary diseases of the respiratory muscles include polymyositis and muscular dystrophy, whereas examples of chest wall abnormalities include extreme obesity, kyphoscoliosis, large pleural effusions, and space-occupying lesions of the thorax.

Cough

Cough receptors are located in the large bronchi, trachea, and larynx and respond to respiratory secretions in the large airways. Irritation of the cough receptors may occur in the absence of abnormal secretions, as with inhalation of toxic fumes or a mild asthma attack. In such cases the nonproductive cough serves no useful purpose and may cause mechanical trauma, leading to more coughing. A nonproductive cough may also be a manifestation of anxiety. In such instances it may be useful to suppress the cough; however, in most cases coughing aids in airway clearance and suppression is not indicated.

A change in the character or frequency of cough is a common complaint in patients with pulmonary diseases. Most acute and self-limiting coughs are secondary to a viral respiratory infection (4), whereas chronic and persistent coughs are most often secondary to chronic bronchitis or postnasal drip. Patients who smoke cigarettes have a characteristic smoker's cough, a manifestation of chronic bronchitis, most noticeable in the morning on awakening. This cough may be productive of mucoid sputum and is often ignored by the chronic cigarette smoker.

Cough may be the sole complaint in patients with mild asthma (5). In such patients the cough may be relieved by a bronchodilator or the avoidance of inhaled allergens. If bronchospasm is not present at the time of examination, reversible airway obstruction may be demonstrated with the use of a nonspecific bronchial challenge such as methacholine (6). Cough (with or without bronchospasm) may occur as a side effect of β-adrenergic antagonists as well as the angiotensin converting enzyme (ACE) inhibiting drugs (7).

Sputum Expectoration

If the patient has a productive cough, the duration of sputum expectoration, the character of the sputum, and the presence or absence of blood should be determined. Cigarette smokers with chronic bronchitis have mucoid or occasionally purulent sputum without much change for months or years and without hemoptysis. The sputum is the result of chronic stimulation and hypertrophy of the bronchial glands as a defense mechanism (8).

In patients with COPD and chronic sputum production, it is important to examine grossly the character of an expectorated sputum sample (color, opacity, and consistency). The patient should be asked about any changes in the quantity, color, or opacity, which may indicate an acute infectious exacerbation requiring antibiotic therapy. It is useful to look at an unstained wet preparation of purulent-appearing sputum to identify neutrophils or eosinophils as the cause of the purulence, because therapy is with antibiotics in the case of neutrophils, and with antiinflammatory agents in the case of eosinophils (9). It is not usually necessary to obtain a Gram stain in cases of chronic bronchitis with acute exacerbation, and the results usually indicate a mixed flora with both Gram-positive and Gram-negative organisms. Likewise, a sputum culture and sensitivity are rarely indicated; antibiotic therapy is empiric, based on the usual causes of such exacerbations.

Viral infections of the lower respiratory tract are associated at first with scant mucoid sputum, which may contain a few streaks of blood. Later the sputum may become copious and purulent with or without bacterial superinfection. Patients recovering from influenza who begin to produce large volumes of purulent sputum associated with a febrile relapse most likely have a bacterial superinfection. Viral and mycoplasmal pneumonias are associated with relatively scant sputum production initially.

Patients with acute lower respiratory tract infections usually produce sputum containing neutrophils. A Gram stain of grossly purulent sputum may help to identify a predominant bacterial organism. In pneumococcal lobar pneumonia the sputum produced early is usually scanty and composed of mucus tinged with blood ("rusty"); later, sputum may become purulent. As opposed to the scant mucoid sputum in early lobar pneumonia, the sputum in patients with bronchopneumonia (frequently a complication of chronic bronchitis) is usually copious and purulent. The chronic production of purulent sputum with episodes of blood streaking is suggestive of severe bronchitis, bronchiectasis, a bronchogenic tumor, or the presence of an aspirated foreign body. Suppurative lung diseases—including bronchiectasis, lung abscess, or bronchopleural fistula with empyema—are associated with expectoration of large volumes of yellow or green sputum. The color is produced by pigments released from degenerating neutrophils. Approximately 60% of patients with lung abscess have foul-smelling sputum associated with bad breath, anorexia, and weight loss (10).

Asthmatics who are recovering from an acute attack usually produce sputum that is thick and tenacious and contains bronchial mucus plugs. The sputum may be purulent but, when examined, is found to contain predominantly eosinophils rather than neutrophils. A simple wet preparation or a Wright stain allows ready determination of the predominant cell type (9).

Lung tumors and tuberculosis are associated most often with the chronic production of mucoid sputum that may be associated with blood streaking. Hemoptysis is an important symptom in such patients; it is the appearance of bloody sputum that often brings the patient to the physician.

Sputum Induction

If the patient is unable to produce sputum, inhalation of a nebulized solution of 3 or 4 mL distilled water or 10% sodium chloride results in the induction of an adequate specimen for examination in over 90% of cases. Any type of nebulizer may be used; however, ultrasonic nebulizers, which produce a concentrated mist, are preferred. The patient should be placed in a private room or isolation booth if he or she is suspected of having a contagious disease. The patient inhales the nebulizer mist deeply and is encouraged to cough frequently, saving all material produced. Chest percussion and/or postural drainage may be used. The procedure is terminated when an adequate specimen is obtained, the nebulizer solution is exhausted, or after a maximum of 15 to 20 min. The procedure is most often used for patients suspected of having tuberculosis or a lung malignancy, and to search for *Pneumocystis carinii* infection in patients with acquired immunodeficiency syndrome (AIDS). Sputum induction has largely replaced gastric lavage to obtain specimens for mycobacteria or fungi because sputum induction results in higher yield and less patient discomfort (11).

Hemoptysis

The term hemoptysis means simply the coughing of blood; to say that a patient has hemoptysis is not enough. It is important to determine the duration of the hemoptysis and to note whether there is gross blood, blood-tinged sputum, or blood-streaked sputum. An attempt should be made to determine the amount of blood produced and to record whether it is bright red or dark and whether or not it contains blood clots.

Hematemesis, or vomiting of blood, may be confused with hemoptysis; however, hemoptysis tends to produce bloody sputum that is at least partly frothy, whereas hematemesis does not. Hematemesis more often produces dark red blood that is usually acid, whereas hemoptysis is alkaline. With hematemesis blood streaking of sputum is unusual, whereas with hemoptysis it is common. Vomited blood frequently contains food particles, whereas this is rare with hemoptysis.

The common causes of hemoptysis are shown in Table 4.1. Although the majority of episodes in earlier years were caused by bronchiectasis, tuberculosis, or unknown causes, in more recent reports (following the appearance of fiberoptic bronchoscopy), the most common causes are bronchitis and carcinoma (12,13). One-third of cases are still owing to unknown causes. Grossly bloody sputum is often seen in patients with tuberculosis, pulmonary infarction, bronchial adenoma, mitral stenosis, and lung abscess. A ruptured aortic aneurysm communicating with a bronchus usually results in exsanguination. Recurrent episodes of hemoptysis, sometimes massive, may occur in mycetomas that invade air spaces caused by inactive tuberculosis or sarcoidosis.

TABLE 4.1 INCIDENCE OF CAUSES OF HEMOPTYSIS

Cause	Percent of Cases
Bronchogenic carcinoma	13
Chronic bronchitis	53
Bronchiectasis	1
Tuberculosis	3
Other	30
Total cases	320

Data compiled from two published series (12, 13).

Bleeding may occur with tumors of the larynx; hoarseness is frequently present in this case. Problems in the nasopharynx and oropharynx are usually associated with obvious abnormalities of these areas on physical examination. Bleeding dyscrasias often cause hemoptysis, in which case there is usually evidence of hemorrhage elsewhere (e.g., in the skin or gastrointestinal tract).

PHYSICAL EXAMINATION

As in recording the medical history, it is important to develop an organized, systematic approach to examining the patient. Initially, the patient's general condition should be observed and his or her body habitus and state of nutrition noted. The presence of acute distress, such as pain, dyspnea, or mental confusion, should be recorded. Evidence of chronic illness, such as weight loss or debilitation, should also be noted. The patient's psychological attitude, awareness and appreciation of events, handicaps, and use of prosthetic devices should be noted. If the patient is receiving oxygen, the amount and method of administration should be recorded.

Inspection and Palpation

During the inspection and palpation of the head, neck, and chest, it is useful to have the chest radiograph handy. This is true during the entire examination of the chest because it allows correlation of physical and radiographic findings. In examining the chest, it is useful to recall the normal location of the five lobes of the lungs and their areas of contact with the chest wall (Fig. 4.1).

The nose, throat, and ears should be examined carefully, because lower respiratory diseases are often associated with upper respiratory tract abnormalities. Rhinorrhea and the presence of pale, edematous nasal mucosa occur with allergic rhinitis. Nasal polyps occur with respiratory allergies and may cause epistaxis. The frontal, ethmoid, and maxillary sinuses are often tender in the presence of sinusitis, which may produce postnasal drip or bleeding. A red, edematous throat may result from infection, toxic fume exposure, or chronic postnasal drip. Patients with pneumonia often have inflamed mucous membranes caused by associated viral or bacterial upper respiratory infections. Oropharyngeal candidiasis (thrush) may be associated with inhaled steroids or antibiotic therapy and is also common in immunosuppressed patients. Tumors, strictures, or inflammation of the oropharynx can cause upper airway obstruction leading to extreme breathlessness; sleep-related disorders of breathing may occur in the presence of lesions that obstruct the upper airway. Patients with lung abscess or empyema frequently have poor dental hygiene and foul-smelling breath, and may have problems with swallowing.

Sarcoidosis may involve the salivary and lacrimal glands,

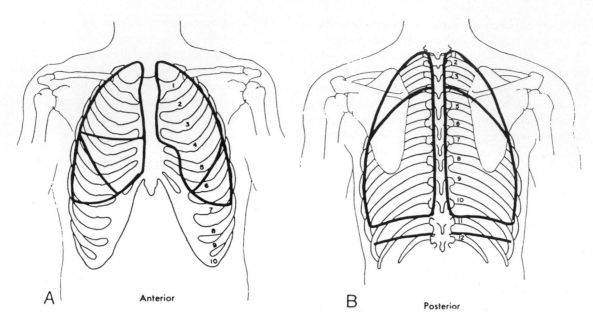

A Anterior B Posterior

FIGURE 4.1. A, Normal relationship of the lungs to the anterior chest wall. The upper part of the chest overlies the upper lobes. The middle lobe lies under the fourth and fifth interspaces to the right of the heart. The lower lateral chest wall lies over the anterior and lateral basal segments of the lower lobes. **B,** Normal relationship of the lungs to the posterior chest wall. The upper lobe areas are covered by the bones and muscles of the shoulder girdle and are therefore not readily accessible to percussion and auscultation. Most of the posterior chest wall overlies the lower lobes. Diaphragm positions at inspiration and expiration are shown. (Modified from Prior JA, Silberstein JS, Stang JM. *Physical Diagnosis, the History and Examination of the Patient,* ed 6. St. Louis, CV Mosby, 1981.)

with dryness of the oral mucosa and conjunctivae; involvement of the parotid gland may be associated with paralysis of the facial nerve (Bell's palsy). Inflammation of the uveal tract in sarcoidosis is detected by slit lamp examination. Drying of the oral mucous membranes may be associated with anticholinergic drug therapy or with rheumatoid disease (keratoconjunctivitis sicca), which may affect the lungs also.

The position and mobility of the trachea should be determined, because shift of the mediastinum is associated with shift of the trachea, whereas fixation of the mediastinum by carcinoma or mediastinal fibrosis is associated with decreased tracheal mobility. The position of the trachea is easily ascertained from the front by comparing the distance from the trachea to each clavicular head. Nodes and masses in the neck and supraclavicular areas are usually best palpated from the rear.

An examination of the neck veins is important in patients with lung diseases. Right heart failure and severe obstructive airway disease are associated with neck vein distention. With airway obstruction the veins usually collapse during inspiration unless elevated venous pressure is also present. With obstruction of the superior vena cava there is marked distention of neck veins, sometimes associated with edema of the neck, eyelids, and hands, and dilation of veins over the anterior chest wall.

The presence of tenderness, discoloration, bruises, or scars over the chest wall should be noted. If there is a history of recent trauma and if chest pain is present, an attempt should be made to palpate the chest wall for crepitus, indicating the presence of a rib fracture or subcutaneous emphysema. If scars from previous surgery are noted, the patient should be questioned about this. Examination of the spine for kyphoscoliosis may reveal the cause in patients with restrictive lung disease. Expansion of the chest wall should be evaluated both by inspection and palpation. In patients with severe hyperinflation of the chest owing to COPD or asthma, the chest is rounded and barrel-shaped, and because the diaphragm is low and flat there may be inward deflection of the lower chest with inspiration (Hoover's sign). In each step of the physical examination, advantage should be taken of the fact that the chest is a bilaterally symmetrical structure, and each side should be compared with the other as a control. For example, tension pneumothorax produces an ipsilateral hyperinflation of the chest, with hyperresonance and decreased breath sounds.

In patients with significant emphysema and air trapping, pneumothorax may occur spontaneously or with minor trauma, such as chest physical therapy. The presence of a pneumothorax may be difficult to detect on physical examination in such patients, because the findings are similar to those of the underlying COPD (increased thoracic diameter, hyperresonance, decreased breath sounds, decreased fremitus) (14). The pneumothorax may not be evident on inspiratory chest films because of the pulmonary hyperinflation; an expiratory film is useful in such cases.

Percussion

Percussion of the chest is useful because the chest contains structures of both air and fluid density; in the presence of disease their relationships may vary. With pleural effusions, consolidation, large intrathoracic masses, or atelectasis, the chest is dull to percussion. With pneumothorax or hyperinflation, the chest is hyperresonant. The generalized hyperresonance in patients with emphysema may cause the examiner to miss a small pneumothorax; in such patients, mediastinal shift may be limited because of air trapping on the opposite side (14).

Percussion over the area of the diaphragm during maximal inspiration and expiration allows the examiner to estimate the extent of diaphragm motion. This is one of the few objective measurements for assessing diaphragm movement. The diaphragm is low and flat and movement is minimal with emphysema.

Auscultation

The examiner should become familiar with the character of normal breath sounds. In the average resting person, inspiration involves approximately one-third of the respiratory cycle and expiration the remaining two-thirds. Breath sounds vary according to the site of auscultation. Bronchial breath sounds are a normal finding over the trachea.

Transmission of voice-generated sounds to the chest wall can be evaluated by either palpation or auscultation. Again, it is important to compare the two sides when listening for the conduction of voice sounds. A localized increase in the clarity of whispered or spoken sounds is associated with bronchial breathing and occurs with consolidation around open airways. Several words have been devised to describe this increased conduction of sound through fluid—bronchophony, egophony, and whispered pectoriloquy. Decreased conduction of whispered or spoken sounds occurs in the presence of obstructed bronchi, pneumothorax, or large collections of fluid or tissue between the lung and chest wall.

The terminology of adventitious sounds in the chest has been confusing in the past, and there are still differences in terminology in different countries. In an attempt to unify the terminology a series of symposia have been held in several countries. The recommendations of the International Lung Sounds Association are those used in this chapter (15).

Discontinuous Sounds

The word rale was originally devised by Laennec to signify a variety of abnormal chest sounds. Because of the confusion

TABLE 4.2 CLINICAL CONDITIONS AND TIMING OF CRACKLES

Early Crackles	Late Crackles
Chronic bronchitis	Diffuse interstitial fibrosis
Asthma	Airspace pneumonia
Emphysema	Pulmonary congestion and edema
"Atelectatic crackles"	Sarcoidosis
	Scleroderma
	Bronchopneumonia
	Rheumatoid lung
	Asbestosis

associated with this term, Robertson and Coope introduced the term crackles to describe the series of tiny explosions heard over the chest wall during inspiration (16). A number of qualifying adjectives have been used, such as crepitant, subcrepitant, dry, and wet. To avoid confusion only the terms coarse and fine should be used.

A careful analysis of chest physical findings with waveform analysis has revealed that the *timing* of crackles is important. Those that begin early in inspiration are likely to be associated with airway obstruction (Table 4.2). Early, fine crackles are usually caused by small airway closure at end-expiration and disappear after a few deep breaths. Coarse, early inspiratory crackles are usually associated with bronchitis or bronchopneumonia. Fine, superficial crackles that occur late in inspiration ("Velcro") are usually associated with diseases that cause a restrictive ventilatory defect, such as idiopathic diffuse interstitial fibrosis, asbestosis, and sarcoidosis.

Continuous Sounds

These sounds have a longer duration than crackles, usually lasting more than 250 msec. They have a musical quality that crackles do not have. Continuous breath sounds are either wheezes, which are high-pitched and arise in small airways, or rhonchi, which are low-pitched and occur in large airways (17). Wheezes generally occur in the presence of bronchospasm and are an important finding in asthma. Occasionally, a wheeze may begin with an audible pop as a small airway opens during inspiration. This crackle, followed by a high-pitched wheeze, has been called a sibilant crackle and has the same significance as a wheeze.

The word rhonchus means snore; rhonchi are common in severely ill patients whose secretions have collected in proximal airways. They occur in the presence of large-airway disease (stricture, foreign body, tumor, or mucus secretions), and those that clear with coughing are associated with sputum in larger airways. The presence of a localized wheeze or rhonchus that does not clear with coughing and does not change from one examination to another suggests an intrinsic defect in a large airway, such as a bronchogenic neoplasm. Because of the constricting nature of these lesions, the rhonchus usually occurs during both inspiration and expiration.

Other Adventitious Sounds

In the presence of air in the pericardium or mediastinum, a coarse, crackling sound called a mediastinal crunch may be heard that is synchronous with systole. This sound may be associated with a pericardial friction rub.

A pleural friction rub is a grating sound associated with breathing. Rapid tape recordings have demonstrated that pleural friction rubs are actually a series of tiny explosions, just as crackles are (17). Pleural friction rubs are generally loud and sound as if they are immediately under the stethoscope. They occur during both inspiration and expiration, generally at the end of inspiration and the beginning of expiration. If a patient has pleuritic chest pain, it is useful to ask him or her to point to the location of the pain and to listen over that area, because the rub will be loudest there. The rub often occurs simultaneously with the patient's chest pain.

Pericardial friction rubs are similar to pleural rubs except that they occur with atrial and ventricular systole and diastole. They are best heard at the left sternal border at about the third interspace. It is useful to have the patient stop breathing, at which time the pericardial friction rub should persist. Pericardial and pleural friction rubs may occur simultaneously.

Extrapulmonary Signs

A wide variety of physical findings outside the thorax may occur in patients with pulmonary diseases. Hypoxemia is associated with cyanosis if 5 g/dL or more of reduced hemoglobin is present in the capillary blood. Central cyanosis implies involvement of gas transfer in the lungs and affects the tongue as well as the extremities. Peripheral cyanosis without central cyanosis implies a circulatory problem (e.g., vascular spasm or shock).

Clubbing of the digits may or may not be associated with cyanosis. It is seen with many chest diseases, including neoplasms, bronchiectasis, and lung abscess. It may be inherited as a familial trait or may occur with diseases of other organs (e.g., the liver). The most reliable evidence of digital clubbing is an increase in the ratio of the diameter of the digit at the base of the nail to the diameter of the distal interphalangeal joint (Fig. 4.2). This ratio is always less than unity unless clubbing is present.

Patients who have pulmonary neoplasms may have one of several paraneoplastic syndromes, which are usually related to the production of hormones by tumor cells (Chapter 14, Lung Neoplasams). Horner's syndrome occurs when apical lung tumors invade outside the pleura and into the superior cervical ganglion. There is ipsilateral enoph-

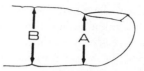

FIGURE 4.2. Clubbing of the fingers is best assessed by determining the ratio of the diameter at the base of the nail (**A**) to the diameter at the distal interphalangeal joint (**B**). This ratio is normally less than 1.

thalmos, loss of sweating, and meiosis. Invasion of the brachial plexus nerves by these tumors may produce pain, atrophy, and loss of function in the ipsilateral arm.

OFFICE AND HOME TESTING OF PATIENTS WITH RESPIRATORY DISEASE

Increasingly, the emphasis in medical care is shifting to the outpatient setting. Economic considerations and patient preference have resulted in a shift of diagnostic activity from the inpatient hospital setting to outpatient facilities, including the physician's office. This important trend has been facilitated by the development of technologically advanced, highly accurate, portable diagnostic equipment. Appropriate use of this equipment combined with a thorough history and physical examination may greatly enhance the speed and accuracy of the initial evaluation of the patient with suspected lung disease.

Office-based spirometry can be useful in several ways. Spirometry may be used to evaluate and characterize signs and symptoms of lung disease as well as to monitor disease progression (or regression) in patients with known lung disease. Therapeutic interventions by the physician may be more accurately quantitated using spirometry. Preoperative risk assessment can be facilitated with data obtained by spirometry. Prognostic information concerning the patient's disease may be obtained as well. On occasion, data obtained with spirometry may be useful in better defining occupational exposures causing or contributing to the observed pulmonary dysfunction. Degree of physical impairment based on lung function may be quantitated providing valuable information that may help the lung impaired patient find appropriate employment or gain appropriate disability benefits.

It is important to select the appropriate equipment for office spirometry. Volume-displacement spirometers may be the water-seal, rolling seal, or bellows type. The Stead-Wells water-seal type spirometer has been considered the gold standard for many years. Volume-displacement machines are highly accurate and frequently less costly than other types of spirometers; however, they tend to be bulky and less portable, and require manual calculations unless they are connected to computers. Flow-sensing spirometers are highly computerized and offer the advantage of small size and portability. They are probably the instrument of choice in most office settings. The pneumotachograph is the most common type of flow-sensing spirometer. Other types include machines that operate with thermistors, turbines, or vortex-sensing devices. Several companies manufacture spirometers. Not all of these machines are equally accurate, and the American Thoracic Society has established minimal standards for spirometers used for diagnostic and monitoring purposes (18). In addition, technician training is important and should not be neglected (19).

Peak flow meters are inexpensive and readily available. Although peak flow meters are less accurate than spirometry, they nonetheless may provide useful data regarding airflow, especially in asthmatic patients. Current expert panel guidelines recommend the measurement of peak flow, particularly in asthma patients with moderate to severe disease (20). Peak flow can be utilized as a formal part of an action plan for the patient to follow during exacerbations. Out-of-office phone consultations between patient and physician may be expedited if the patient can compare his or her current peak flow to his or her personal best. Patients with asthma that is difficult to control may benefit from recording peak flow in the morning and afternoon for several weeks. During an office visit, the physician and patient observe the variability in airflow patterns, which correlates with the degree of airway hyperresponsiveness.

Oximeters are an important addition to the office equipment of the pulmonologist. The ability to measure accurate oxygen saturation both at rest and with varying degrees of exertion is of great importance in the evaluation of lung disease. Because oxygen is the only therapeutic modality that has been demonstrated to prolong survival in COPD, it is important to identify those individuals who require supplemental oxygen. After a resting value is obtained, saturation values with exercise should also be measured. By use of a treadmill or simply by walking a known distance in the hallway, accurate oxygen saturation values with exercise may be obtained. Saturation values at rest and with exercise should be recorded in the chart for documentation purposes and to provide the basis for reimbursable oxygen prescriptions.

REFERENCES

1. U.S. Public Health Service. The health consequences of smoking—cardiovascular disease. A report of the Surgeon General. Washington, DC: US Government Printing Office, 1983.
2. Wall M, Brooks J, Holsclaw D, et al. Health effects of smoking on children. ATS Statement. *Am Rev Respir Dis* 1985;132:1137–1138.
3. Banaszak EF, Thiede WH, Fink JN. Hypersensitivity pneumonitis due to contamination of an air conditioner. *N Engl J Med* 1970;283:271–276.
4. Irwin RS, Rosen MJ, Braman SS. Cough, a comprehensive review. *Arch Intern Med* 1977;137:1186–1191.
5. Corrao WM, Braman SS, Irwin RS. Chronic cough as the sole presenting manifestation of bronchial asthma. *N Engl J Med* 1979;300:633–637.
6. Pratter MR, Irwin RS. The clinical value of pharmacologic bronchoprovocation challenge. *Chest* 1984;85:260–265.
7. Bucknall CE, Neilly JB, Carter R, et al. Bronchial hyperreactivity in patients who cough after receiving angiotensin converting enzyme inhibitors. *Br Med J* 1988;296:86–88.
8. Reid L. Measurement of the bronchial mucous gland layer: a diagnostic yardstick in chronic bronchitis. *Thorax* 1960;15:132–141.
9. Epstein RL. Constituents of sputum: a simple method. *Ann Intern Med* 1972;77:259–265.
10. Bartlett JG. Anaerobic infections of the lung. *Chest* 1987;91:901–909.
11. Elliott RC, Reichel J. The efficacy of sputum specimens obtained by nebulizer versus gastric aspirates in the bacteriologic diagnosis of pulmonary tuberculosis. *Am Rev Respir Dis* 1963;88:223–227.
12. Soll B, Selecky PA, Chang R, et al. The use of the fiberoptic bronchoscope in the evaluation of hemoptysis. *Am Rev Respir Dis* 1977;115:165–168.
13. Corey R, Hla KM. Major and massive hemoptysis: reassessment of conservative management. *Am J Med Sci* 1987;294:301–309.
14. George RB, Herbert SJ, Shames JM, Ellithorpe DB, Weill H, Ziskind MM. Pneumothorax complicating pulmonary emphysema. *JAMA* 1975;234:389–393.
15. Mikami R, Murao M, Cugell DW, et al. International symposium on lung sounds: synopsis of proceedings. *Chest* 1987;92:342–345.
16. Robertson AJ, Coope R. Rales, rhonchi, and Laennec. *Lancet* 1957;2:417–422.
17. Forgacs P. Crackles and wheezes. *Lancet* 1967;2:203–205.
18. American Thoracic Society. Standardization of spirometry: 1994 update. Am J Respir Crit Care Med 1995;152:1107–1136.
19. Wanger J, Irvin CG. Office spirometry: equipment selection and training of staff in the private practice setting. Journal of Asthma 1997;34:93–104.
20. National Heart, Lung, and Blood Institute. Expert Panel Report II: Guidelines for the diagnosis and management of asthma. Bethesda, MD: National Institutes of Health; [NIH publication no. 97–4051], 1997.

5

CHEST IMAGING

H. DIRK SOSTMAN
FRANK M. MELE
RICHARD A. MATTHAY

CONVENTIONAL CHEST RADIOGRAPHY
Radiographic Technique
Routine Projections
Portable Chest Radiographs
Observer Error

RADIOGRAPHIC ANATOMY OF THE AIRWAYS
The Trachea and Main Bronchi
The Lobar Bronchial Segments

RADIOGRAPHIC ANATOMY OF THE HILA AND PULMONARY VASCULAR SYSTEM

SPECIAL CHEST RADIOGRAPHIC VIEWS
Oblique Views
Lateral Decubitus Views
Lordotic View
Expiration Film

Other Views
Fluoroscopy

TOMOGRAPHY
Indications for Tomography
Conventional Tomography
Computed Tomography
Magnetic Resonance
Ultrasound

CONTRAST EXAMINATIONS
Barium Swallow
Bronchography
Pulmonary Angiography

VENTILATION-PERFUSION LUNG SCANNING

POSITRON EMISSION TOMOGRAPHY

The lungs are composed of a complex of tissues, each of which has a unique function, but all of which together perform the act of respiration (1). The morphologist examines each tissue and describes its normal or abnormal characteristics. The radiologist similarly can assess individual components of the lungs through application of special techniques such as bronchography and angiography. The most commonly and generally used examination is the plain chest film (taken without added contrast material) (Figs. 5.1 and 5.2). The plain radiograph is the cornerstone of chest radiographic diagnosis (1). All other radiographic procedures (e.g., fluoroscopy, tomography, and special contrast studies), are strictly ancillary. With few exceptions, establishing the presence of a disease process by plain radiography of the chest should constitute the first step; if this first examination does not show clearly the nature and extent of the lesion, additional studies can be performed to complement the plain chest radiograph.

Accordingly, in this chapter the normal chest radiograph and the normal radiographic anatomy of the airways and the pulmonary vasculature are discussed first; then special chest radiographic views, fluoroscopy, tomography, ultrasound, magnetic resonance imaging, contrast examinations, and ventilation-perfusion scans are reviewed. Radiographic manifestations of diseases of the lungs, mediastinum, diaphragm, chest wall, and pleura are discussed in subsequent chapters.

CONVENTIONAL CHEST RADIOGRAPHY

Radiographic Technique

The basic principles of radiographic technique are as follows: (a) positioning must be such that the x-ray beam is properly centered, the patient's body is not rotated, and the scapulae are rotated sufficiently anteriorly to be projected free of the lungs; (b) respiration must be fully suspended, preferably at total lung capacity; (c) exposure factors should be such that the resultant radiograph permits faint visualization of the thoracic spine and the intervertebral discs so that lung markings behind the heart are clearly visible (2).

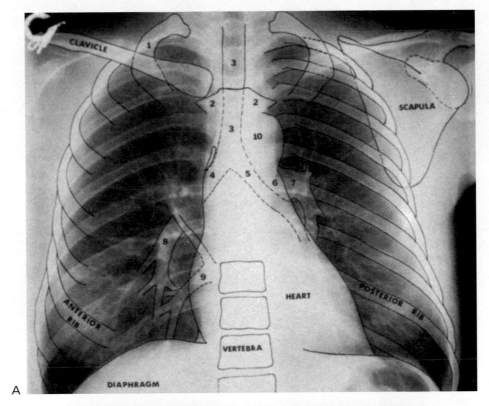

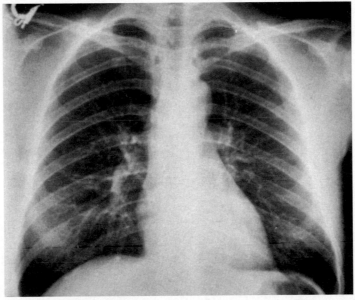

FIGURE 5.1. **A,** Posteroanterior (PA) chest radiograph with diagrammatic overlay. Various structures are identified by label or numbers. *1,* first rib; *2,* upper portion of manubrium; *3,* trachea; *4,* right main bronchus; *5,* left main bronchus; *6,* main pulmonary artery; *7,* left pulmonary artery; *8,* right interlobar pulmonary artery; *9,* right pulmonary vein; *10,* aortic arch. **B,** Chest radiograph of the same subject without diagrammatic overlay.

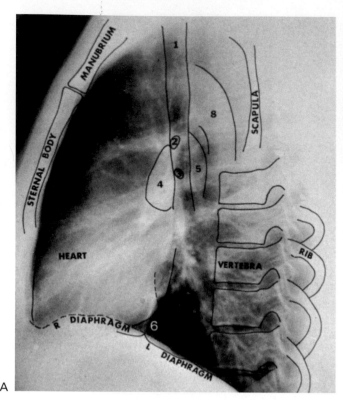
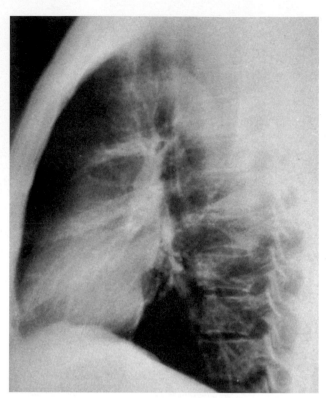

A   B

FIGURE 5.2. **A,** Lateral chest radiograph of the same patient as in Figure 5.1, with diagrammatic overlay. Structures are identified by labels or numbers. *1,* trachea; *2,* right upper lobe bronchus; *3,* left upper lobe bronchus; *4,* right pulmonary artery; *5,* left pulmonary artery; *6,* inferior vena cava; *7,* ascending aorta; *8,* descending aorta. **B,** Lateral chest radiograph without diagrammatic overlay.

Routine Projections

The normal chest radiograph in the posteroanterior (PA) and lateral projections is shown in Figures 5.1 and 5.2. A diagrammatic overlay shows the normal anatomic structures numbered or labeled in both projections. In young persons or in asymptomatic patients a PA projection alone is generally used as a screening procedure (3). From an analysis of over 100,000 chest radiographs of a hospital-based population, Sagel and coworkers concluded that routine screening examinations, obtained solely because of hospital admission or scheduled surgery, are not warranted in patients under 20, and that the lateral projection can be safely eliminated from routine screening examination in patients 20 to 39 years of age (4). A lateral film should be obtained whenever chest disease is suspected and in screening examination of patients 40 years of age or older.

For the PA film, the x-ray beam is projected from the back to the front of the patient, with the film cassette against the anterior thorax. Because the heart is in the front of the thorax, there is much less cardiac and mediastinal magnification on a PA than on an anteroposterior (AP) film (5).

The upright position is used because the diaphragms are lower and the lungs are larger in this position since the abdominal viscera do not push the diaphragms up as they do in the supine position. If pleural fluid is present, it is more easily identified on the upright film than on a supine film, because it gravitates to the dependent portion of the thorax, where small spaces (e.g., the costophrenic angles) are filled and altered in contour. Ultrasound is more sensitive than the chest radiograph for detecting small to moderate-size pleural effusions. Air-fluid levels, as seen in lung abscess and hydropneumothorax, are clearly visible on the upright chest film. If fluid must be identified and the patient cannot stand or sit upright, a lateral decubitus film should be obtained.

It is not always possible or advisable to take films upright or in the PA projection. The very sick patient must be recumbent, and infants and young children are usually radiographed in the supine position.

The lateral view adds valuable information about certain areas that are not seen well on the PA view (3). This is particularly true of the anterior part of the lung close to the mediastinum, which may be obscured by the overlying heart and aortic shadows, the mediastinum, and the vertebral column (Figs. 5.1 and 5.2). Moreover, a small pleural effusion is best seen, and often only seen, as blunting of a costophrenic sulcus posteriorly (3).

Portable Chest Radiographs

Portable x-ray films that are made in the intensive care unit, operating suite, or patient's room are generally of poorer quality than the erect PA x-ray or even recumbent films made in the radiology department. Positioning is difficult in a hospital bed; consequently, the patient's true position is often unknown, which causes difficulty in assessing the pulmonary vascularity or the presence of pleural fluid. The film focal distance is short, with resultant magnification of the heart and aorta and obscuration of part of the lung fields. Further, the x-ray generator used on portable equipment is not as powerful as stationary generators available in the x-ray department. Hence, it is preferable to obtain a film in the radiology department unless the patient absolutely cannot be moved without hazard. If a portable film must be taken, an upright portable film is preferable to a supine film. The position and distance from the beam generator to the film should be recorded on the film.

Recent advances in storage phosphor technology have made it possible to significantly improve the consistency and quality of portable radiographs and to produce them in a digital format so that they may be transmitted easily to video terminals (which might be located, for example, in the intensive care unit).

Observer Error

As Fraser and Paré have emphasized, radiologic diagnosis of chest disease begins with identification of an abnormality on a radiograph; what is not seen cannot be appreciated (1). Many studies of the accuracy of diagnostic procedures, notably those by Garland and coworkers, have revealed an astonishingly high incidence of both intraobserver and interobserver error among experienced radiologists (6–9). For example, in one series the interpreters missed almost one-third of radiographically positive minifilms and overread about 1% of negative films; in another series, based only on positive radiographs, interobserver error ranged from 9% to 24% and intraobserver error from 3% to 31% (6,7). Since these figures are derived from studies by competent, experienced observers, it is clear that no student of chest radiography should be lulled into a false sense of security concerning his or her competence to detect a lesion.

To minimize observer error, a radiograph can be inspected in two ways, each of which may be employed usefully in different situations. *Directed search* is a method by which a specified order of inspections is carried out (e.g., thoracic and extrathoracic scans), followed by examination of soft tissues, bony thorax, mediastinum, diaphragm, pleurae, and finally the lungs themselves (1). The lungs usually are analyzed by individual inspection and comparison of the zones of the two lungs from apex to base. Such a method *must* be used by those in training, because it is only through the exercise of this routine that the pattern of the normal chest can be recognized (1).

The alternative method of inspection is *free search,* in which the radiograph is scanned without a preconceived orderly pattern. This is the method employed by the majority of experienced radiologists. However, such free search must be followed by an orderly pattern of inspecting to avoid overlooking less obvious abnormalities.

It is important to view every chest radiograph from a distance of at least 6 to 8 feet or through diminishing lenses (1). There are two reasons: (a) the slight nuances of density variation between similar zones of the two lungs can be appreciated better at a distance, and (b) the visibility of shadows with ill-defined margins is improved significantly by minification (10).

As a further means of reducing the frequency of "missing" lesions radiographically, the practice of double viewing has been advocated (1,6,10). In one study, the dual interpretation by the same observer on two occasions or by two different observers decreased by at least one-third the number of positive films missed (6). Many physicians, particularly chest physicians and surgeons, become highly competent in radiograph interpretation as a result of many years of personal viewing; if their chest radiograph reading is done in consultation with the radiologist, the second look may reveal abnormalities missed on the first interpretation.

RADIOGRAPHIC ANATOMY OF THE AIRWAYS

The Trachea and Main Bronchi

The trachea is a midline structure; however, a slight deviation to the right after entering the thorax is a normal finding and should not be misinterpreted as evidence of displacement (Fig. 5.1) (1). The walls of the trachea are parallel except on the left side just above the bifurcation, where the aorta commonly impresses a smooth indentation; rarely, the azygos vein causes a smaller indentation at the tracheobronchial angle on the right side (1).

The trachea divides into the two major bronchi at the carina. The angle of bifurcation is varied and is most acute in asthenic persons (1). The course of the right main bronchus distally is more vertical than that of the left.

The transverse diameter of the right main bronchus at total lung capacity is greater than that of the left (average 15.3 mm versus 13.0 mm in adults), although its length before the origin of the upper lobe bronchus as measured at necropsy is shorter (average 2.2 cm compared with 5 cm on the left) (Fig. 5.3) (11–13).

The air column of the trachea, both major bronchi, and the intermediate bronchus should be visible on well-exposed

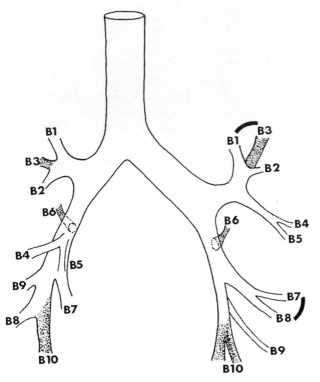

FIGURE 5.3. Diagram of the bronchopulmonary segments, following the Boyden classification. Segments that are relatively more posteriorly located are shaded; these areas are frequent sites of aspiration pneumonia. See Table 5.1 for correspondence of the Boyden system with the more frequently used Jackson-Huber classification. Note that the latter combines the segments connected with bars on the diagram into single segments.

TABLE 5.1 NOMENCLATURE OF BRONCHOPULMONARY ANATOMY

Jackson-Huber	Boyden
Right upper lobe	
Apical	B1
Anterior	B2
Posterior	B3
Right middle lobe	
Lateral	B4
Medial	B5
Right lower lobe	
Superior	B6
Medial basal	B7
Anterior basal	B8
Lateral basal	B9
Posterior basal	B10
Left upper lobe	
Upper division	
Apical-posterior	B1, B3
Anterior	B2
Lower (lingular) division	
Superior lingular	B4
Inferior lingular	B5
Left lower lobe	
Superior	B6
Anteromedial	B7, B8
Lateral basal	B9
Posterior basal	B10

Adapted from Fraser RG, Paré JAP, Paré PD, et al: *Diagnosis of Diseases of the Chest,* ed 3. Philadelphia, WB Saunders, 1988, vol 1, p 37.

standard radiographs of the chest in the frontal projection (Fig. 5.1). A thin vertical shadow is usually well visualized on lateral chest radiographs; it is formed by the posterior boundary of the tracheal air column (Fig. 5.2). This thin band is chiefly the posterior tracheal wall and is formed anteriorly by the junction of the tracheal air column and the tracheal wall and posteriorly by the junction of aerated lung in the right retrotracheal space with the external aspect of the tracheal wall and a thin layer of areolar tissue (14).

Pathologic processes within the mediastinum (e.g., carcinoma of the middle third of the esophagus) or in the medial portion of the right upper lobe can lead to deformity or obliteration of the posterior tracheal band, providing evidence for a pathologic process that otherwise might not be readily apparent (1).

The Lobar Bronchial Segments

The anatomic distribution of the bronchial segments is illustrated in Figure 5.3. Each of the lobes divides into segments, which have been classified by the nomenclature shown in Table 5.1 (1).

Of clinical significance is the fact that several segmental bronchi are located posteriorly, which renders them frequent recipients of aspirated material and likely sites for the development of aspiration pneumonia. The dorsally located segments that are frequent sites for aspiration include the posterior segment of the right upper lobe (B3); the posterior basal and superior segments of the right lower lobe (B10, B6); and the posterior basal and superior segments of the left lower lobe (B10, B6) see (Fig. 5.3).

Lobar consolidation of the lung is frequently associated with loss of volume (atelectasis). However, atelectasis of pulmonary segments occurs less often because collapse is prevented by collateral air drift; thus, most x-ray presentations of atelectasis are lobar (3). The patterns of atelectasis of various lobes are illustrated in Figures 5.4 through 5.8. It is important to recognize the patterns of atelectasis, because it is a common manifestation of bronchial obstruction by carcinoma of the lung. Atelectasis is common in the postoperative period, when it is owing in part to inadequate clearing of secretions, and it may be seen in other conditions, such as asthma, in which viscid mucus occludes bronchi. It may also occur secondary to aspiration of a foreign body.

X-RAY ANATOMY OF THE HILA AND PULMONARY VASCULAR SYSTEM

The major vascular structures in the thorax that are visible on the normal chest radiograph are the aorta, pulmonary

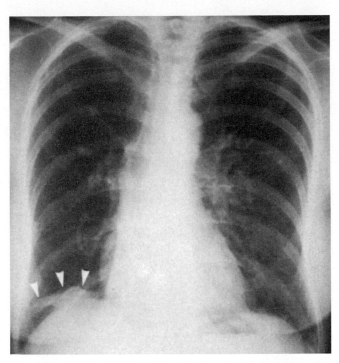

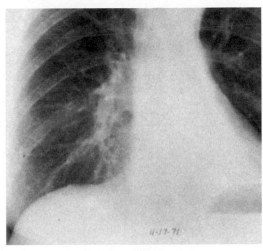

FIGURE 5.6. PA chest radiograph of another patient with left lower lobe atelectasis. Note the similarity to Figure 5.5**A**.

FIGURE 5.4. PA chest radiograph showing density in the right lung base behind the right portion of the cardiac silhouette obliterating the medial silhouette of the right hemidiaphragm. This is right lower lobe atelectasis. Note the relative paucity of vascular markings in the aerated portion of the right lung due to compensatory overaeration. Immediately above the right hemidiaphragm there is an area of linear atelectasis as well *(arrowheads)*.

arteries, and pulmonary veins (15). Each will be discussed individually; first the normal hila will be described.

The hila are composed of the pulmonary arteries and their main branches, the upper lobe pulmonary veins, the major bronchi, and the lymph nodes. The lower lobe pulmonary veins do not cross the hila and therefore do not contribute to the hilar shadows (15). The bronchi account for little of the hilar opacity, because they are filled with air, and normally lymph nodes are too small to add to the

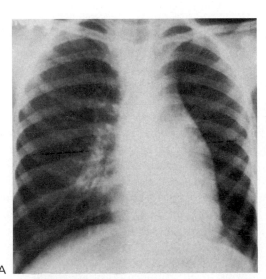

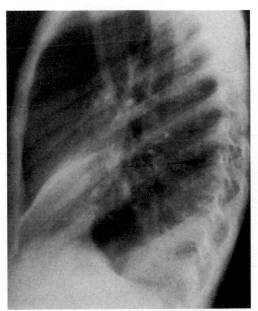

A

B

FIGURE 5.5. **A,** PA chest radiograph demonstrating middle lobe and left lower lobe atelectasis. The middle lobe atelectasis is seen as a triangular density obliterating the right cardiac silhouette. The left lower lobe atelectasis is demonstrated as a triangular-shaped area of increased density behind the left cardiac silhouette. Note that medial silhouette of the left hemidiaphragm is not visible. **B,** Lateral view of the same patient. The middle lobe atelectasis is more easily visible on this view, seen as a linear area of density overlying the heart silhouette. The left lower lobe atelectasis is seen as an area posteriorly and inferiorly, giving increased density to the vertebral bodies, which it overlies, and obliterating the silhouette of the left hemidiaphragm posteriorly.

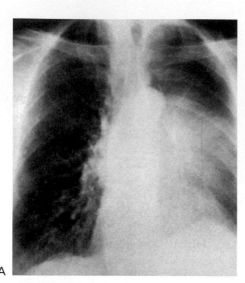

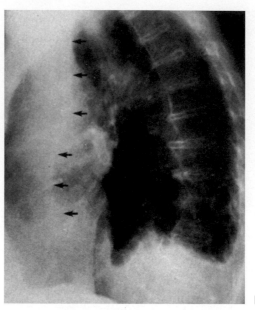

FIGURE 5.7. A, Chest radiograph of a patient with left upper lobe atelectasis. Note that the upper portion of the left heart border is not visible and there is a hazy density in the left upper lung field. There is evidence of volume loss in the left hemithorax (elevation of the left hemidiaphragm, shift of the heart and mediastinal structures to the left, and closer spacing of the left ribs than the right ribs). **B,** Lateral view of the same patient. The collapsed left upper lobe forms an anteriorly located density, which is outlined in the figure by *arrows.* This is because the left upper lobe collapsed upward and forward.

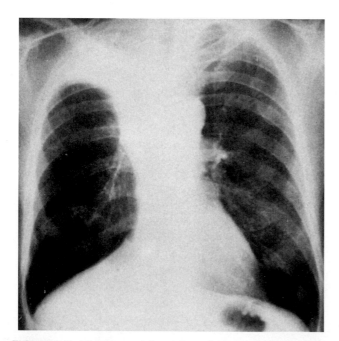

FIGURE 5.8. Right upper lobe atelectasis shown on the PA chest radiograph. Note the disparity in vascular markings between the right and left lungs. This is evidence of compensatory hyperinflation of the nonatelectatic portions of the right lung. Note that the right upper lobe collapse does not obliterate the cardiomediastinal silhouette as much as the left upper lobe collapse did. This is partly because the left upper lobe moves forward as well as upward as it collapses (see Fig. 5.7**A** and **B**), while the right upper lobe moves mostly upward, and partly because of differences in the mediastinal contour.

size or density. Therefore, normal hilar shadows consist mostly of the large pulmonary arteries and upper lobe veins (Figs. 5.9 and 5.10) (15).

The main pulmonary artery is 4 to 5 cm in length and about 3 cm in diameter in adults. It lies entirely within the pericardial sac, as does its bifurcation (15). The right pulmonary artery lies posterior to the aorta and the superior vena cava and anterior to the right main bronchus (Fig. 5.9 and 5.11). It remains within the pericardium until it gives off its first branch, and the artery continues as the descending or interlobar division to supply the middle lobe and right lower lobe. It accounts for the lower portion of the right hilum (15).

The left pulmonary artery lies within the pericardium for a short distance before entering the lung. This vessel divides within the left hilum after passing immediately anteriorly and laterally to the lower portion of the left main bronchus (Figs. 5.9 and 5.11) (1).

The component distribution pattern of pulmonary veins (Fig. 5.10) involves two large veins on each side entering the mediastinum slightly below the pulmonary arteries and anterior to them (Figs. 5.10 and 5.11). It may be difficult to distinguish arterial and venous trunks within the lungs owing to superimposition of artery and vein, especially in the upper lobes where their course is parallel; in the lower lung fields the veins run more horizontally than the arteries and can often be distinguished (1).

The caliber of the hilar pulmonary artery is important and should be assessed carefully. A significant sign is a

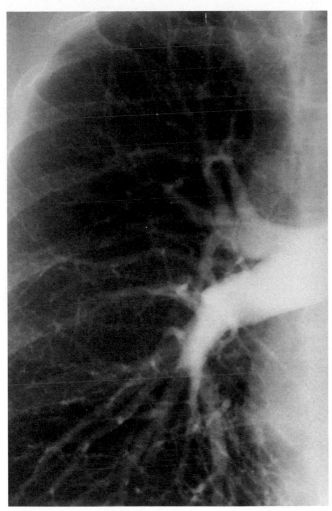

FIGURE 5.9. Normal pulmonary artery anatomy is shown on the arterial phase of a normal pulmonary arteriogram, obtained by injecting iodinated contrast material directly into the right main pulmonary artery.

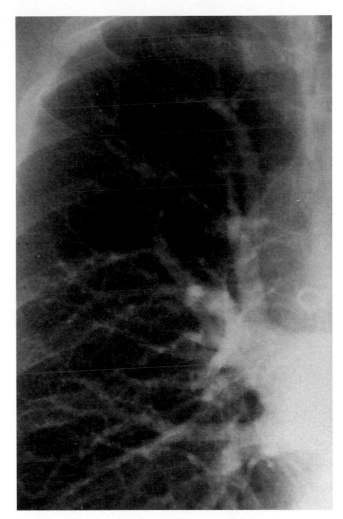

FIGURE 5.10. Levophase (venous and left heart phase) of the same pulmonary arteriogram shown in Figure 5.9. Note the differing course of the pulmonary veins as related to the pulmonary arteries.

change in caliber from one examination to another, particularly in relation to the diagnosis of pulmonary hypertension (1). Radiographic measurement of a segment of the pulmonary vascular tree may provide useful information (16). The width of the right descending pulmonary artery has been measured in over 1,000 normal adult subjects (16). The upper limit in inspiration was 16 mm in men and 15 mm in women; during expiration it was 1 to 3 mm greater. Pulmonary artery hypertension is generally associated with enlargement of the right descending pulmonary artery.

SPECIAL CHEST X-RAY VIEWS

Oblique Views

In addition to the PA and lateral views, other projections serve special purposes. Oblique views may be invaluable in delineating a pulmonary or mediastinal mass or pulmonary infiltrate from structures that overlie it on the PA and lateral view. A pleural effusion or mediastinal mass is often well demonstrated on oblique views (5). Oblique views are also useful for studying lesions that are visible in the PA view but not in the lateral view. They may help in determining the site of origin of an intrathoracic lesion. By observing the rotation of a lesion in relation to a rib or to the heart or aorta, it may be possible to ascertain how close the lesion is to that structure and thereby infer its site and sometimes even its point of origin (5). When there are bilateral lesions on the PA view, it may be difficult to decide from the lateral view which shadow belongs to which side. Oblique views usually resolve this dilemma (5). Some reports have emphasized the value of oblique chest radiographs in detecting pleural plaques caused by asbestosis. They are also helpful in the differential diagnosis of cardiac and great vessel enlargement, because the border-forming structures of the

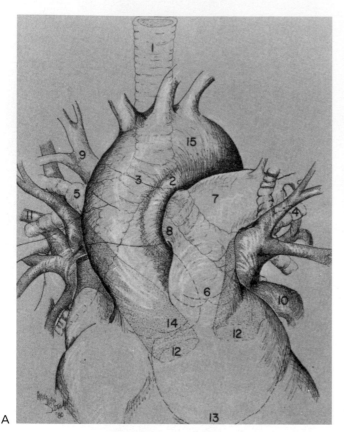
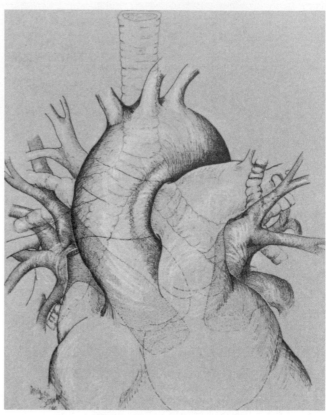

A

B

FIGURE 5.11. A, Depiction of the bronchial and vascular interrelationships in the mediastinum and hilum. Some of the individual structures are identified by numbers. *1,* trachea; *2,* left main bronchus; *3,* right main bronchus; *4,* segmental left upper lobe bronchus; *5,* right upper lobe bronchus; *6,* pulmonary valve; *7,* left main pulmonary artery; *8,* right main pulmonary artery; *9,* right upper lobe (truncus anterior) pulmonary artery; *10,* left lower lobe pulmonary vein; *11,* right upper lobe pulmonary vein; *12,* entrance of pulmonary vein to left atrium; *13,* left atrium; *14,* aortic valve; *15,* aortic arch. **B,** Depiction of the mediastinal, bronchial, and vascular structures without overlying identifying numbers.

cardiomediastinal silhouette are different in oblique projections than those in the frontal and lateral views.

Oblique positions are named according to which part of the chest is closest to the cassette: right anterior oblique (RAO) view, with the right front of the patient against the cassette, and left anterior oblique (LAO) view, with the left front of the patient against the cassette. The standard angles relative to the coronal plane are 45 degrees for the RAO and 60 degrees for the LAO (5).

Lateral Decubitus Views

The lateral decubitus film is useful for demonstrating a small amount of free pleural fluid or pneumothorax, the extent of a cavity or lung abscess, and the mobility of a mediastinal mass with gravity. As little as 25 to 50 mL of pleural fluid can be visualized (17). This view is particularly useful in determining if blunting of a costophrenic sulcus is owing to pleural effusion or to pleural thickening (3). Pleural thickening is usually a scar following organization of an

exudate or blood in the pleural space (3). The decubitus film may also be helpful in shifting free fluid out of the way to visualize the underlying lung (2,3,5). Bilateral decubitus films are usually necessary if the effusion is moderately sized or large.

A lateral decubitus view is taken with the patient on his or her side, the x-ray beam aimed parallel to the floor, and the area of interest closest to the film. Air rises and fluid falls; therefore, when right pneumothorax is suspected, for example, the patient should be placed on the left side with the film and x-ray beam centered over the uppermost part of the right chest. For right-sided pleural fluid, on the other hand, the patient should be lying on the right side, with centering over the dependent portion of the right chest (5).

Lordotic View

The original purpose of the lordotic view of the chest was to partially uncover the pulmonary areas from the bony grid

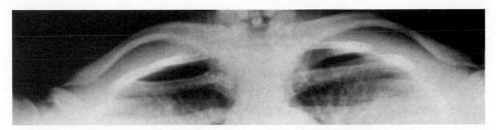

FIGURE 5.12. Normal apical lordotic view of the chest. Compare with Figure 5.1 to appreciate the difference in visualization of the lung apices.

created on the PA film by the ribs and clavicles. When the tube is angled upward, the shadows of the clavicles are projected above the thorax and the ribs become more horizontal (Fig. 5.12) (5). The anterior part of each rib is thereby superimposed on its posterior portion, reducing the number of obscuring bony structures. Thus, the lordotic projection enables evaluation of the apical portion of the lungs by displacing shadows of the first rib and the clavicle, which may be confusing on the PA projection (3). The lordotic view is also useful for recognizing collapse of the lingula or middle lobe when these areas become very thin and cast minimal shadows on the PA film (5). Lordotic and reverse lordotic views are often good for determining if a lesion is anterior or posterior. An anterior lesion is projected upward, as are other anterior structures (such as ribs and clavicles). The opposite is true for a posterior lesion. A reverse lordotic film produces exactly the opposite changes.

Expiration Film

Although chest radiographs are routinely taken at full inspiration, an expiratory film may be helpful under appropriate circumstances. For example, a small pneumothorax is often difficult or impossible to see on a routine inspiratory PA film. On expiration, the volume of the thorax and of the lungs within it is reduced, but the amount of air in the pleural sac remains essentially unchanged. The pneumothorax then occupies a larger percentage of the area of the thorax and is more easily visible. Also, when a film is taken in expiration, the lungs appear denser, because the blood-containing vessels are crowded into a smaller space. Because the blackness of the pneumothorax does not change, the density gradient between the pneumothorax and the lungs becomes larger and this also makes the pneumothorax easier to see.

Another indication of the expiratory film is to demonstrate air trapping. The bronchi increase in diameter with each inspiration and decrease with each expiration. With a foreign body or tumor in a main bronchus, a valve action may occur, with air bypassing the obstruction on inspiration and becoming trapped on expiration. With expiration, the normal lung is reduced in volume and becomes less radiolu-

cent. The obstructed portion of the lung retains its air, thereby retaining its radiolucency and forcing the mediastinum to shift toward the contralateral side. If a patient has a unilateral respiratory wheeze, air trapping is likely, and an expiratory film is mandatory (5).

Other Views

The *overpenetrated grid* radiograph is useful for evaluating densities that lie behind the heart or diaphragm and are seen poorly on routine radiographs. Stereoscopic views can be helpful in localizing any pulmonary lesion and are particularly useful with apical lesions, because they can separate pulmonary lesions from the overlying clavicle and first rib (3). *Magnification* radiographs are used occasionally in diffuse lung disease to clarify minute details of the pulmonary parenchyma (10). Double-exposed films in inspiration and expiration are sometimes helpful in evaluating motion of the diaphragms.

Fluoroscopy

Fluoroscopy of the chest is useful for examining the movement of pulmonary and cardiac structures and for localizing a pulmonary lesion that is only visible in one of the two conventional radiographic projections. It is particularly helpful for examining diaphragmatic motion (3,18). When searching for diaphragmatic paralysis, it is often best to use the lateral projection so that motion of both hemidiaphragms can be observed simultaneously (3). A paralyzed hemidiaphragm moves paradoxically. This paradoxical motion is often difficult to appreciate during quiet breathing but usually becomes readily apparent during a quick, short "sniff" (sniff test). Localized weakness in part of one hemidiaphragm (eventration) is often misinterpreted as diaphragmatic paralysis. This error can be avoided by fluoroscopy in the lateral projection; partial eventration is then manifested by paradoxical motion of one portion of the hemidiaphragm, whereas the other portion moves normally. Eventration of an entire hemidiaphragm is impossible to distinguish from paralysis, because in both instances the entire hemidiaphragm moves paradoxically (3).

Fluoroscopy of the heart is useful for demonstrating calcification in cardiac valves or coronary arteries. Fluoroscopy often helps to identify the nature of a mediastinal lesion. When fluoroscopy is combined with a barium swallow, lesions within the esophagus can be seen. Moreover, the pattern of displacement of the esophagus by a mass in the middle mediastinum helps to determine the nature of the mass (3,18). Respiratory maneuvers affect the size of large venous structures in the chest, which become smaller during a Valsalva maneuver and larger during a Müller maneuver. These maneuvers do not change the size of solid masses. Pulsation of a mediastinal mass suggests it is vascular. However, pulsation must be interpreted with care: masses that are adjacent to the aorta often transmit its pulsations and appear to be pulsating; in contrast, large aortic aneurysms often pulsate poorly (3).

Chest fluoroscopy also can be useful when trying to determine if a suspected pulmonary nodule on a chest radiograph (a) is real versus a superimposition of unrelated shadows, or (b) is intrapulmonary versus extrapulmonary.

In past years, fluoroscopy of the chest was used as a screening procedure for routine chest examination (2,3). This is no longer acceptable for at least three reasons: (a) the patient's exposure to x-rays is much greater during even a short fluoroscopic examination than during standard radiographs; (b) small lesions in the lung fields are overlooked at fluoroscopy; and (c) usually no permanent record of the fluoroscopic examination is available. However, fluoroscopy of the chest is warranted when specific information is being sought or when it is necessary to monitor "on line" the performance of a special procedure, such as needle aspiration of a pulmonary mass or transbronchial biopsy (3).

TOMOGRAPHY

Indications for Tomography

Tomography is useful when there is a need for precise knowledge of the morphologic characteristics of lesions visible on plain radiographs whose nature is obscured by superimposed images lying superficial or deep to them (2).

Tomography provides clearer visualization of shadows that on plain radiographs are indistinct because of image summation (e.g., the bronchi or the pulmonary interstitium) (2). Tomograms are widely used to determine the presence, size, number, and location of pulmonary nodules. Preoperative tomography is commonly used to detect pulmonary metastases and to determine if an apparently solitary lesion is in fact single. Further, within a solitary nodule, the detection of calcium is an important piece of data that is best obtained by tomography. Calcium usually denotes a benign rather than a neoplastic nodule, especially if there are multiple calcifications or if the calcium is centrally located, laminated, or homogeneous (18).

Conventional Tomography

If the x-ray tube and film are in motion during exposure, the resulting radiograph (called a *tomogram* or *laminagram*) will show a sharply focused plane or "cut" through the body with adjacent planes blurred (18). The thinness of the plane and successful blurring of the other planes are factors that can be controlled to some degree to determine the ultimate appearance of the film. Since the distance of the x-ray tube from the table determines the plane in focus, the films are usually made in a series of cuts so that each level through the lung is visualized sharply, without overlying shadows (Fig. 5.13) (18). Posterior oblique tomography at an angle of 55 degrees has been recommended for displaying a clearer outline of the anatomic components of the hila (19). Conventional tomography accurately detects calcification within pulmonary nodules and other thoracic lesions.

In most institutions, conventional tomography has been largely or completely superseded by computerized tomography (CT) in evaluating pulmonary nodules, the hila, the mediastinum, and the lung parenchyma. However, conventional tomography remains an accurate and useful technique (Fig. 5.14).

Computed Tomography

The development of CT brought diagnostic medical imaging into the modern age. It combined the basic phenomenon upon which the field of radiology was founded (differential x-ray attenuation by tissues) with the basis of subsequent developments (use of nonfilm x-ray detectors, digital computers, and video displays). Previous methods of forming x-ray images all used direct geometric projection of an x-ray shadowgraph of the patient's body on a piece of film by a large-area beam of x-ray photons. CT uses a series of planar projections made by a thin beam of x-ray photons. These planar projections are mathematically recombined by the *computer* to form a cross-sectional *tomographic* image of the patient that displays the attenuation values of the many small areas ("picture elements" or "pixels"). CT thus introduced into clinical practice an entirely new approach to diagnostic imaging, aspects of which have subsequently been utilized in digital radiography, fluoroscopy, ultrasound, and magnetic resonance imaging. The diagnostic advantages of CT are owing to its transaxial tomographic (slice-like) format and its high sensitivity to differences in electron density (and thus in x-ray attenuation) between different tissues. In addition, because the x-ray attenuation measurements are stored in the computer, the image can be enhanced or manipulated mathematically. Adjustments of the computer data (windowing) allow for differences in contrasts. For example, wider window (2200/ − 600 Hounsfield units [HU]) allows for better evaluation of the lung parenchyma and a narrower window (400/40

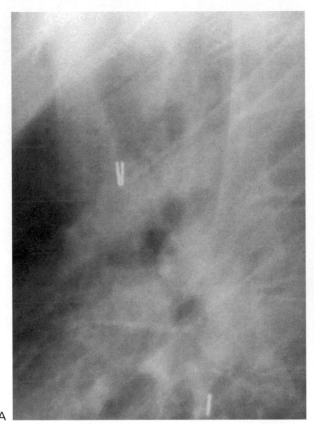
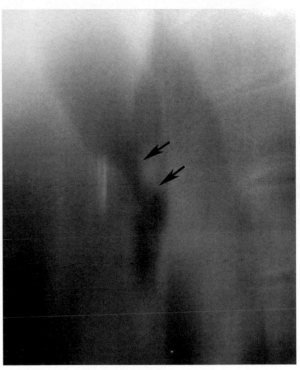

A   B

FIGURE 5.13. The value of plain tomography in evaluating pathology of the central airways. **A,** Lateral chest radiograph in a patient after resection of esophageal carcinoma who presented with wheezing. The lower portion of the tracheal air column is not well seen, but the presence of a lesion is not clear. **B,** Lateral tomogram through the trachea. Note that the overlying surgical clip that is seen clearly in **A** is blurred on the tomogram. This is the means by which tomography produces clearer visualization of selected planes. The tomogram clearly shows the presence of a constricting tumor recurrence narrowing the lower trachea *(arrows).*

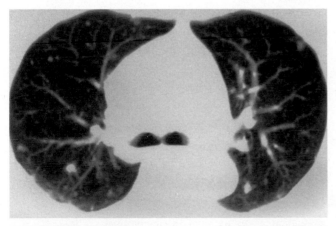

FIGURE 5.14. CT is the method of choice for detecting pulmonary metastases (as shown here in a patient with metastatic melanoma) and other kinds of pulmonary nodules.

HU) is better for assessing mediastinal structures (Figs. 5.15 and 5.16). The technique of high-resolution CT (HRCT), a valuable method of studying the lung parenchyma, combines very thin slices with mathematical filtering of the computer data to produce increased edge definition in the final image.

Thoracic CT has found widespread use in the assessment of masses and neoplasms, including primary lung cancer, hilar and mediastinal masses, and pulmonary nodules (Fig. 5.14; Fig. 5.17) (20–33). It is now the standard of care for patients with such conditions who require diagnostic imaging beyond the plain chest radiograph and its simple variants (e.g., fluoroscopy). High-resolution CT of the lung parenchyma has been developed in the last few years and has become widely used for evaluating interstitial lung disease and bronchial abnormalities (Fig. 5.18) (34–42). CT has application in vascular imaging in the thorax, most notably for suspected aortic dissection and superior vena cava obstruction (Fig. 5.19) (43,44). In addition, CT is unsurpassed in the detection and localization of pericardial and

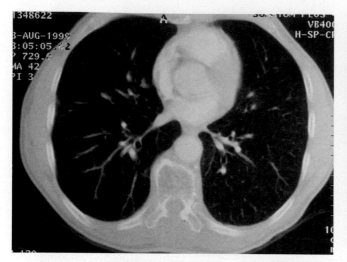
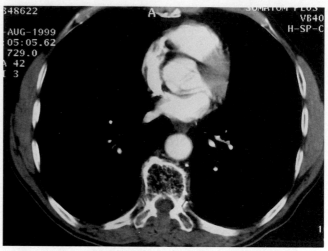

FIGURES 5.15 and 5.16. Images obtained of the chest at the level of the heart demonstrating differences in appearance owing to computer manipulations. The lungs (5.15) are well seen with the wider window while the heart and mediastinal structures (5.16) are better visualized with the narrow settings.

pleural fluid collections (Fig. 5.20) (45–48). Finally, CT may be used effectively to guide percutaneous biopsy and drainage of thoracic lesions (49,50). The patient is imaged to localize the lesion, and the skin entry site is identified with the aid of the CT scanner's positioning lights. A similar approach can be used to localize fluid collections or pneumothoraces that are not responding to blindly placed thora-

costomy tubes, and then to guide percutaneously placed drains into the refractory collections.

Helical CT

Over the past decade, CT has benefited from advance in technology with the advent of helical scanning (51). Con-

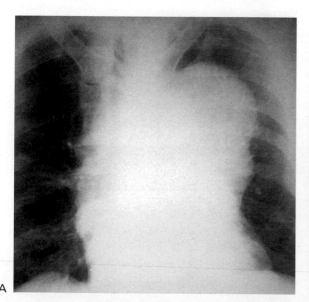
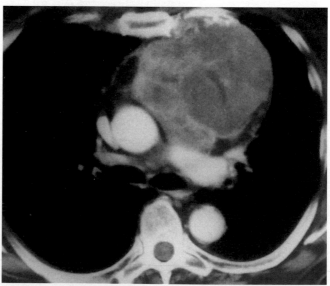

A   B

FIGURE 5.17. CT is the method of choice for detailed evaluation of most patients with mediastinal masses. **A,** The PA chest radiograph in this patient shows a large mass. **B,** The CT scan clearly delineates the anterior mediastinal location of the mass and separates it from the mediastinal vasculature, facilitating both the differential diagnosis and the surgical planning.

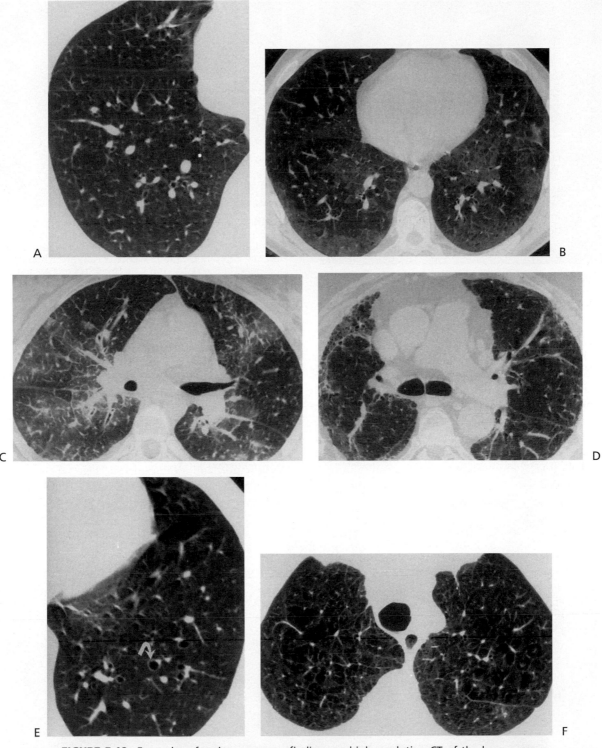

FIGURE 5.18. Examples of various common findings on high-resolution CT of the lung parenchyma. **A,** Normal lung. The vessels, bronchi, and fissures are seen clearly. **B,** Patient with alveolitis. There is multifocal faint opacification of the lungs, referred to as "ground-glass opacity." This usually, but not always, indicates the presence of an active, treatable process. **C,** Patient with lymphangitic carcinomatosis. Nodularity, bronchial wall thickening, and interlobular septal (interstitial) thickening are present. **D,** Patient with idiopathic pulmonary fibrosis. Characteristically subpleural changes of fibrosis and cyst formation ("honeycombing") are clearly visible on the HRCT image. **E,** Patient with focal bronchiectasis. Note the dilated bronchi compared with **A** and also compared with associated vessels in the same area, forming the so-called "signet-ring" *(arrow)* appearance. **F,** Patient with diffuse emphysema. Areas of destroyed lung tissue are apparent (due to their low density) as dark regions usually without definite walls.

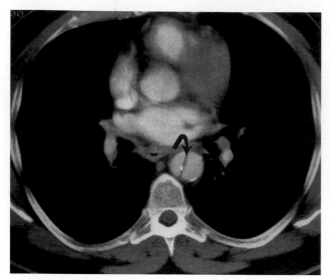

FIGURE 5.19. This contrast-enhanced CT section shows a Type B aortic dissection. The intimal flap, containing a fleck of calcium, is well seen *(arrow)*.

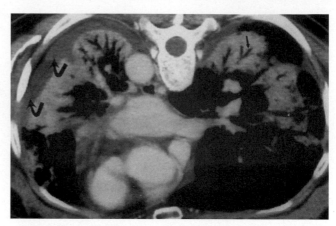

FIGURE 5.20. The left pleural effusion *(curved arrows)* is clearly visualized in this patient and easily distinguished from the adjacent lung consolidation. Note, in the consolidated areas of both left and right lungs, the presence of "air bronchograms" (one is indicated in the right lung by a small straight *arrow*).

ventional CT obtains images one section at a time as the x-ray tubes stop and rotate around the patient at each subsequent station. Conversely, with helical acquisition, the patient continuously moves as the x-ray tube rotates, resulting in a helical (spiral) pathway. Since all of the data are available from the entire acquisition, the images can be reconstructed at select levels and locations. A further benefit is the rapid speed of helical CT, which allows for acquisition during a single breathhold—an important feature in lung imaging to reduce respiratory motion artifacts.

CT pulmonary angiography utilizing helical CT is a less invasive method than conventional pulmonary angiography for evaluating patients with suspected pulmonary thromboembolism (PE) (52). In a prospective study by Remy-Jardin et al. of 75 patients helical CT angiography was highly sensitive (91%) and specific (78%) for detecting PE (51,52). Direct signs of PE on the CT pulmonary angiogram include vessel cutoff and a filling defect (Fig. 5.21). Indirect signs include low-attenuation in a segmental or subsegmental distribution (oligemia) or wedge-shaped infarct. Limitations

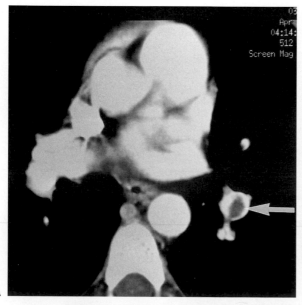

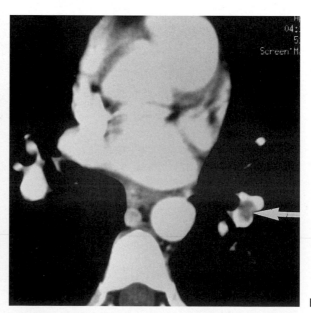

FIGURE 5.21 (A,B). Contrast enhanced CT scan of the mediastinum demonstrating a nonocclusive thrombus in the left lower lobar artery at its branch point consistent with an acute saddle embolus.

include respiratory motion artifact, observer inexperience, and inability to detect emboli in small peripheral pulmonary arteries. The CT pulmonary angiogram in the diagnostic algorithm for PE has yet to be defined, and a National Heart, Lung and Blood Institute (NHLBI) trial is underway to study this issue.

Contrast Helical CT for Assessing Solitary Pulmonary Nodules

The solitary pulmonary nodule is frequently encountered on the chest radiograph or chest CT scan. Although the detection of these nodules may be challenging, the diagnostic evaluation of these lesions can be even more challenging. Goals include minimizing removal of benign nodules, maximizing removal of malignant nodules at a curable stage, maximizing use of noninvasive studies, and maintaining cost effectiveness.

It has been recognized that malignant neoplasms have an abundant vascular supply (53). Applying this knowledge, Swensen et al. theorized that the degree of enhancement of a solitary pulmonary nodule on CT should be related to the amount of contrast entering that nodule, in turn related to the lesion's blood supply (54,55). These investigators imaged lung nodules using the helical technique with bolus IV contrast injection in 105 patients. Swensen found that malignant neoplasms enhanced significantly more than benign neoplasms (median 40 HU versus median 12 HU) and, with a threshold of 20 HU, sensitivity was 100% and specificity was 77%. No malignant nodule enhanced less than 20 HU; the authors concluded that the degree of enhancement is an indicator of malignancy.

Other Helical CT Applications

Other uses of helical CT include virtual bronchoscopy for evaluation of endobronchial abnormalities, three-dimensional reconstruction of mediastinal and vascular abnormalities and coronary artery evaluation (51,56,57). Evaluation of coronary arteries for calcification by chest CT is a noninvasive method to assess for hemodynamically significant stenoses, and may be used as a screening study in selected populations. By acquiring thin section helical images with cardiac gaiting, image quality is markedly improved and the amount of coronary artery calcification may be quantified. Recent studies have reported sensitivities and specificities of 88% to 91% and 52%, respectively (57,58).

Magnetic Resonance

MR imaging (MRI) is based on magnetization of the patient's tissue, generation of a weak electromagnetic signal by the application of a radiofrequency pulse, and spatially mapping that signal by manipulating its frequency and phase in a location-dependent manner using magnetic field gradients. Unlike CT, MRI does not require mechanical motions of the scanner; therefore, it can image directly in nontransaxial planes. However, like CT, it is a tomographic technique.

Although electromagnetic radiation is involved, the energy levels used in MRI are well below the levels needed to ionize molecules, and MR imaging appears to be remarkably free of significant bioeffects. However, the strong magnetic field is a major safety hazard, because the magnetic forces near a whole-body MR imager are strong enough to cause significant projectile hazards. For example, an oxygen cylinder brought into an MR examination room will fly into the bore of the magnet with a *terminal velocity of about 45 mph.* The possibility of displacements or torques on metallic implants within patients must also be considered. Finally, the magnetic field can operate reed relays in cardiac pacemakers and cause a change in the pacing mode. Accordingly, strict security around MR facilities is essential to prevent patients with certain types of metallic implants from entering the scanner and to prevent medical personnel from carrying objects that could become projectiles into the scan room.

MRI produces extremely high contrast between different types of soft tissue. This soft tissue contrast is based on intrinsic properties of the tissues and also on operator-selectable machine parameters. The tissue properties are: (a) the tissue concentration of protons available to produce an MR signal ("proton density"); (b) the presence of motion or blood flow; and (c) two tissue properties known as T1 and T2, time constants that describe how quickly an MR signal can be generated (T1) from a tissue and how quickly the MR signal, once generated, decays (T2). In general, pathologic tissues have long T1 times and appear dark on those MR images whose appearance is conditioned primarily by T1 effects ("T1-weighted images"). Usually, pathologic tissues also have long T2 times and appear bright on T2-weighted images. Flowing blood also can appear either bright or dark on MR images, depending on the examination technique that is used.

The usefulness of MRI in thoracic diseases is more limited than that of CT; for most patients who require further imaging beyond the plain chest radiograph, CT is the preferred initial choice because it is more effective, less expensive, and more widely available (59). In certain situations, however, MRI is useful to answer questions that remain after a CT examination has been performed. These situations include indeterminate mediastinal, chest wall, or vascular invasion by lung carcinoma and the evaluation of suspected hilar masses (20,23,25,26,59). In still other patients, MRI is the initial procedure of choice because the patient is allergic to contrast material that may be deemed necessary for a particular CT examination (60). The most common setting in which this occurs is suspected aortic dissection, but an allergy to contrast material can mandate the use of

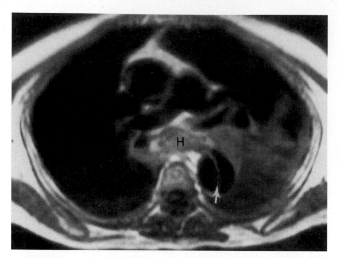

FIGURE 5.22. MRI was done in this patient with suspected aortic dissection who had renal dysfunction and thus was a poor candidate for intravenous contrast-enhanced CT. The intimal flap of a type B dissection is visible *(arrow)*, and a mediastinal hematoma *("H")* was found as well.

MRI for other vascular imaging problems as well (Fig. 5.22) (43,59,61–63). Finally, there are a few conditions in which MRI has a real diagnostic advantage over CT and should be used as the initial procedure of choice. These include upper-extremity deep venous thrombosis (DVT), brachial plexopathies and superior sulcus tumors, and cardiac and paracardiac masses (Fig. 5.23) (64–69).

Ultrasound

Like CT and MRI, ultrasound is a tomographic technique. Ultrasound has limited usefulness in evaluating the lungs, because the sound beam is transmitted poorly by the air-containing alveoli and airways. However, there are two situations in which ultrasound is very useful for evaluating chest diseases. First, ultrasound is widely used to evaluate disorders of the heart and aortic root. Areas in which the heart and mediastinal structures touch the chest wall without lung intervening are used as "acoustic windows" for transmission of the sound beam into the mediastinum.

Ultrasound is the procedure of choice to detect or exclude pericardial effusion. Unique information can also be obtained concerning valvular heart disease (e.g., mitral stenosis), the presence of vegetations or clots in the cardiac chambers, and global or segmental abnormalities of cardiac contraction. The second situation in which ultrasound is useful in the evaluation of chest pathology is in precisely localizing pleural effusions for aspiration or drainage (70,71). It should be emphasized that ultrasound should not be routinely used for this purpose, because most effusions can be safely and easily aspirated after localization by physical examination. Finally, ultrasound may be used to assess diaphragm motion analogous to the fluoroscopic

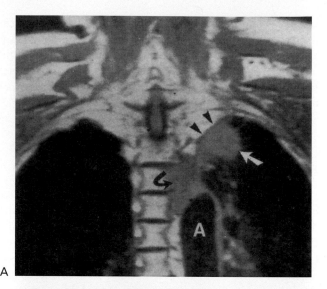

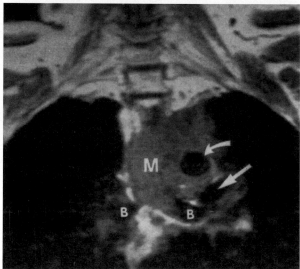

FIGURE 5.23. Magnetic resonance (MR) images of a 61-year-old man with a left superior sulcus (Pancoast) tumor, a squamous cell carcinoma. **A,** Coronal T1-weighted MR scan reveals a mass *(white arrow)* that is confined within the apical pleura. The subpleural fat, which has high signal intensity *(arrowheads),* is preserved. Medially, the mass is infiltrating the mediastinum *(black curved arrow)* and is contiguous with the thoracic aorta *(A).* **B,** Coronal MR scan 20 mm anterior to *top* demonstrates extension of the mass *(M)* into the mediastinum. The relationship of the mass to the aortic arch *(curved arrow),* main pulmonary artery *(straight arrow),* and bronchi *(B)* can be appreciated. (Reproduced with permission from Takasugi JE, Rapaport S, Shaw C: Superior sulcus tumors: the role of imaging. *J Thorac Imaging* 4:41–48, 1989.)

"sniff" test. This is particularly useful in ICU settings where the study can be done portably with ultrasound.

CONTRAST EXAMINATIONS

Air is the "natural" contrast material on which the diagnostic value of the plain chest film depends. Supplementary information is gained by introducing extraneous contrast material into different structural compartments of the thorax. "Positive" contrast material, (e.g., barium sulfate suspension), is commonly introduced into the esophagus, whereas other suitable media are used to visualize cardiac chambers, trachea and bronchi, pulmonary vessels, aorta, bronchial and mediastinal arteries, superior vena cava, and mediastinal veins. Intravenously administered contrast material has become commonly used in many CT and MRI examinations outside of the thorax. Iodinated contrast material is used for CT, whereas metal chelates are employed for MRI. In thoracic imaging with CT and MRI, the use of contrast is more selective and contrast is administered in a minority of examinations. To achieve "negative" contrast, air or other gases can be introduced, although this is no longer done in clinical practice.

Barium Swallow

Of all the contrast examinations, the barium swallow, which is usually performed under fluoroscopic guidance, is the simplest to perform. The esophageal lumen is outlined by radiopaque barium sulfate. Abnormalities of the esophagus itself, such as tumor or achalasia, can be seen (3). Formerly used to assess mediastinal masses and cardiac enlargement, the barium swallow has been replaced for these purposes by more specific tests (e.g., CT, MRI, and ultrasound).

Bronchography

The trachea and bronchi can be better defined by instillation of radiopaque contrast medium into the lumina of the trachea and bronchial tree (bronchography). It is mostly used for diagnosing bronchiectasis and mapping its location before surgical resection. In the past, prior to development of the flexible bronchoscope, bronchography was used to demonstrate an obstructing lesion that was inaccessible to the rigid bronchoscope. Today, bronchography is rarely performed. Bronchiectasis is infrequent and seldom requires surgical treatment (5). When present, it can be visualized accurately with the less hazardous CT examination. The advent of fiberoptic bronchoscopy has rendered fewer lesions inaccessible to direct vision, and bronchoscopic brush or forceps biopsy and transthoracic needle puncture are more precise methods of diagnosing a pulmonary lesion than bronchography. If bronchography is performed, it should be done in conjunction with fiberoptic bronchoscopy.

Pulmonary Angiography

Pulmonary angiography involves the rapid injection of a radiopaque dye into the pulmonary circulation via a catheter into the superior vena cava, right atrium, right ventricle, or main pulmonary artery; or by selective injection into the right or left pulmonary artery or branches of these (Figs. 5.9 and 5.10) (2,3). Direct injection into the pulmonary artery branches invariably produces the clearest opacification of the pulmonary vascular tree; this superior visualization usually outweighs any disadvantage inherent in the catheterization procedure (2).

Angiography is principally useful for investigating pulmonary thromboembolic disease. In recent years, the popularization of ventilation and perfusion scans of the lung ($\dot{V}/\dot{Q}$) using radioactive isotopes has relegated pulmonary angiography to a secondary role in most cases. The accuracy of ($\dot{V}/\dot{Q}$) scans for diagnosing pulmonary thromboemboli has recently been assessed and has been shown to be definitive in some circumstances but inaccurate in others (72). Angiography is almost always indicated when massive pulmonary embolus is suspected as the basis for circulatory collapse and immediate surgical intervention is contemplated. If surgical interruption of the inferior vena cava is planned because of failure of medical therapy or if thrombolytic therapy is planned, pulmonary angiography should usually be performed. Angiography is commonly used in a clinical setting in which anticoagulation is considered dangerous or in patients in whom $\dot{V}/\dot{Q}$ scan results are equivocal or the clinical and lung scan evaluations lead to markedly different conclusions.

Less common indications for angiography include: (a) suspected congenital abnormalities of the arterial system, such as agenesis or hypoplasia of a pulmonary artery; (b) suspected congenital abnormalities of the pulmonary venous circulation, such as anomalous pulmonary venous drainage and pulmonary varix; and (c) suspected pulmonary A-V malformations. In some instances, noninvasive techniques such as CT, ultrasound, and MRI provide diagnostic information in these settings.

The decision to perform pulmonary angiography should be made carefully, since the procedure is associated with slight morbidity and rare mortality. However, these risks are not great in experienced hands (73).

Before injection of contrast material into the pulmonary artery, the pulmonary artery pressure should always be measured since it is dangerous to perform angiography in a patient with severe pulmonary arterial hypertension. If physiologic measurements such as wedge pressure or oxygen saturations are needed, they should be obtained before contrast material is injected, because contrast material has numerous physiologic effects that may alter these parameters.

VENTILATION-PERFUSION LUNG SCANNING

There has been a rapid evolution of imaging devices and radiopharmaceuticals for the study of regional pulmonary function by inhalation and perfusion scintigraphy. Although the number of indications for lung scanning has increased, the major clinical application is in evaluation for pulmonary thromboembolism and performance of preoperative lung function studies (72,74–78). It is beyond the scope of this chapter to describe in detail the imaging techniques and methods of interpretation of lung scans. They are only summarized here, and the interested reader is referred to reviews of this subject (74–76).

Lung scans are obtained by measuring gamma radiation emitted from the chest after radiopharmaceuticals are injected into the bloodstream or inhaled into the air spaces. Ventilation-perfusion scintigraphy is performed with gamma cameras, which permit viewing a large area at once.

Interfacing the gamma camera with a computer allows quantification of pulmonary ventilation and perfusion scans and measurement of regional ventilation and perfusion ratios. Thus, prior to lung resection, the surgeon can discover the contribution to overall pulmonary function of the region of lung to be resected. Perfusion lung scans can be obtained for either particulate or gaseous radionuclides. For the particulate type, a standard quantity of particles (usually macroaggregates of human serum albumin) with a size of 10 to 60 mm is injected into a peripheral vein. Because the particles are larger than capillaries, they lodge in the first capillary bed encountered (74). Techniques for assessing pulmonary ventilation involve the inhalation of a radioactive gas or a nebulized aerosol of a radioactive material (such as albumin labeled with Technetium-99). For the latter, the particles must be small enough (less than 1 mm in diameter) to reach the alveoli.

As stressed previously, the major indication for lung scanning is the investigation of pulmonary thromboembolism. Perfusion studies are diagnostically valuable only when the scan image is normal or can be compared with a current chest radiograph and ventilation scan. The absence of perfusion in an area of lung is nonspecific. It can be owing to thromboembolic disease or to primary pulmonary vascular disease such as arteritis; it can be secondary to airway obstruction or other abnormalities of ventilation; or it can result from destruction of lung parenchyma, as in bullous emphysema. Only when the areas of perfusion abnormality correspond to pulmonary segments or subsegments (indicating a distribution comparable with the distribution of the pulmonary arteries) and ventilation in the analogous area is normal can pulmonary vascular disease be diagnosed with confidence. Pulmonary vascular disease is most commonly owing to pulmonary embolism, and thus the assumption is made that areas of normal ventilation and abnormal perfusion are owing to pulmonary embolism. The diagnostic scheme for evaluating perfusion defects with and without ventilation and chest x-ray abnormalities is presented in detailed reviews (74–77). A normal lung scan excludes pulmonary embolism for all practical purposes (Fig. 5.24). Multiple perfusion defects in areas of normal ventilation (Fig. 5.25 A,B) are characteristic of pulmonary embolism (Fig. 5.25 A,B). Intermediate patterns are more difficult to

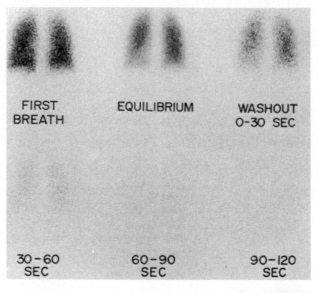

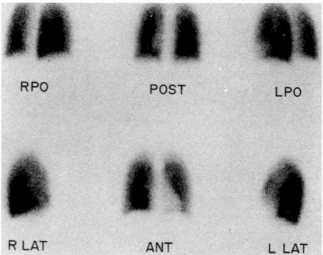

FIGURE 5.24. A, Ventilation phase of a ventilation-perfusion scan. Note that in the "first-breath" and "equilibrium" images there is homogeneous distribution of the radioactivity in both lungs. Note that in the "wash-out" phase (which is performed by serial imaging when the patient is no longer breathing in radioactive gas, so that the gas already in the lungs is imaged as it exits from the lungs) there is no evidence of abnormal retention of radioactive gas. **B,** Perfusion images of the same patient. It is important to obtain at least six views of the lungs. In this patient the perfusion is normal, with no focal defects seen in the images. The radioactive particles are injected with the patient lying supine. Note on the right and left lateral views that there is more perfusion in the posterior (dependent) portions of the lungs. This is a graphic demonstration of the effect of gravity on the pulmonary perfusion gradient.

interpret. In many of those cases, a pulmonary angiogram must be performed to make the diagnosis accurately (Fig. 5.25 C). Alternatively, evaluation of the deep venous system with ultrasound may be used as an ancillary study. If the ultrasound is diagnostic of clot in the deep venous system, pulmonary angiography may be avoided.

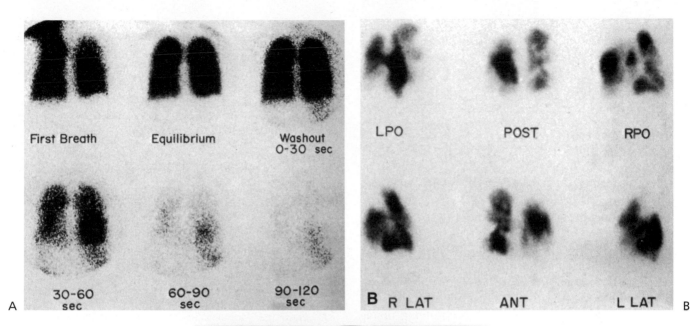

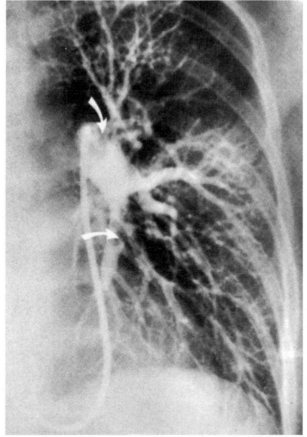

FIGURE 5.25. **A,** Ventilation scan in a patient with pulmonary embolism. There is no significant abnormality in ventilation. Focal activity in the later images is due to concentration of xenon in the liver. **B,** Perfusion scan in the same patient. Multiple perfusion defects that are wedge-shaped and bilateral are seen in the perfusion images. This is a classic appearance for pulmonary embolism. **C,** Selective pulmonary arteriogram on the same patient. Multiple filling defects in pulmonary arteries are demonstrated *(arrows)*. This is angiographic proof of pulmonary embolism.

An additional use of lung scanning has been in the preoperative evaluation of patients potentially undergoing lung resection (e.g., lobectomy or pneumonectomy) (78). By obtaining quantitative lung measurements of lung perfusion and ventilation, an estimation of the percentage of function that each lobe or lung contributes can be assessed.

POSITRON EMISSION TOMOGRAPHY

Positron emission tomography, or PET scanning, is an imaging technique based on annihilation of positrons (79,80). Photons from positron annihilation travel 180 degrees from each other, and when these photons strike the crystal detectors around the patient, the origin of the annihilation can be calculated. Only photons that strike the detectors 180 degrees apart within a very short interval are accepted for imaging improving sensitivity and resolution (i.e., photons detected by only detector or those not satisfying timing requirements are rejected for imaging).

PET uses physiologically and metabolically active radiopharmaceuticals labeled with positron emitters resulting in data that produce an image based on metabolic activity and not anatomy (as most of radiology does). PET originally was used in evaluation of cardiac and neurologic metabolism; however, PET now has oncological applications as well. The glucose analog fluorine-18 fluorodeoxyglucose (FDG) is currently used in the diagnosis and staging of cancer (79). The use of glucose analog is based on the increased glucose metabolism associated with malignant processes compared with normal tissues (80). However, glucose metabolism is affected in many disease states. This may result in potentially false-positive FDG PET studies in inflammatory or other nonneoplastic conditions (79). Clinical, radiographic, and functional data need to be incorporated in any given case to best assess any given abnormality.

As mentioned elsewhere in the text, lung cancer may present as a solitary pulmonary nodule (Chapter 14, Lung Neoplasms). Multiple studies have demonstrated the utility of FDG PET for pulmonary nodule evaluation (81–84). Sensitivities of 95% or higher and specificities of 78% or higher have been reported (79,81,83). The size of the nodule that can be detected depends on the instrument, but lesions less than 1 cm may be studied. Use of whole body PET imaging in pretherapy and posttherapy assessment of patients with lung cancer can allow for detection of local spread (e.g., mediastinal or hilar lymph nodes) and distant spread (e.g. adrenal, bone, brain) (79,85).

REFERENCES

1. Fraser RG, Paré JAP, Paré PD, et al. The normal chest. In Fraser RG, Paré JAP, Paré PD, et al, eds. *Diagnosis of diseases of the chest,* 3rd ed. Philadelphia: Saunders: 1988:1–291.
2. Fraser RG, Paré JAP, Paré PD, et al. Methods of roentgenologic and pathologic investigation. In Fraser RG, Paré JAP, et al, eds. *Diagnosis of diseases of the chest,* 3rd ed. Philadelphia: Saunders, 1988:315–387.
3. Miller TW. Radiographic evaluation of the chest. In Fishman AP, ed. *Pulmonary diseases and disorders,* 2nd ed. New York: McGraw-Hill, 1988:479–528.
4. Sagel SS, Evans RG, Forrest JV, et al. Efficiency of routine screening and lateral chest radiographs in a hospital based population. *N Engl J Med* 1974;291:1001–1004.
5. Felson B. The chest roentgenologic work up. *Basics of RD* 1980; 81:1–4.
6. Garland LH. Studies on the accuracy of diagnostic procedures. *AJR* 1959;82:25–38.
7. Garland LH. On the scientific evaluation of diagnostic procedures. *Radiology* 1949;52:309–327.
8. Garland LH, Cochrane AL. Results of international test in chest roentgenogram interpretation. *JAMA* 1952;149:631–634.
9. Felson B, Morgan W, Bristol VC, et al. Observations on the results of multiple readings of chest films on coal miners pneumoconiosis. *Radiology* 1973;109:19–23.
10. Tuddenham WJ. Problems of perception in chest roentgenology: facts and fallacies. *Radiol Clin NA* 1963;1:277–289.
11. Fraser RG. Measurements of the caliber of human bronchi in three phases of respiration by cinebronchography. *J Can Assoc Radiol* 1961;12:102–112.
12. Merendino KA, Kirilak LB. Human measurements involved in tracheobronchial resection and reconstruction procedures: report of case of bronchial adenoma. *Surgery* 1954;35:590–597.
13. Jesseph JE, Merendino KA. The dimensional interrelationships of the major components of the human tracheobronchial tree. *Surg Gynecol Obstet* 1957;105:210–214.
14. Bachman AL, Teixidor HS. The posterior tracheal band: a reflector of local superior mediastinal abnormality. *Br J Radiol* 1975; 48:352–359.
15. Felson B. *Chest roentgenology.* Philadelphia: Saunders, 1973.
16. Chang CH. The normal roentgenographic measurements of the right descending pulmonary artery in 1,085 cases. *AJR* 1962;87: 929–935.
17. Hesser I. Roentgen examination of pleural fluid. A study of the localization of free effusions, the potentialities of diagnosing minimal quantities of fluid and its existence under physiological conditions. *Acta Radiol Suppl (Stockh)* 1951;86:1–80.
18. Scanlon GT. Use of radiology in the diagnosis of lung disease. In Baum GL, ed. *Textbook of pulmonary diseases,* 2nd ed. Boston: Little, Brown, 1974:85–102.
19. Favez G, Willa C, Heinzer F. Posterior oblique tomography at an angle of 55 degrees in chest roentgenology. *AJR* 1974;120: 907–915.
20. Webb WR, Gatsonis C, Zerhouni EA, et al. CT and MR imaging in staging non-small cell bronchogenic carcinoma: report of the Radiologic Diagnostic Oncology Group. *Radiology* 1991;178: 705–713.
21. Patterson GA, Ginsberg RJ, Poon PY, et al. A prospective evaluation of magnetic resonance imaging, computed tomography, and mediastinoscopy in the preoperative assessment of mediastinal node status in bronchogenic carcinoma. *J Thorac Cardiovasc Surg* 1987;94:679–684.
22. Friedman PJ. Lung cancer staging: efficacy of CT. *Radiology* 1992;182:307–309.
23. Heelan RT, Demas BE, Caravelli JF, et al. Superior sulcus tumors: CT and MR imaging. *Radiology* 1989;170:637–641.
24. McLoud TC, Bourgouin PM, Greenberg RW, et al. Bronchogenic carcinoma: analysis of staging in the mediastinum with CT by correlative lymph node mapping and sampling. *Radiology* 1992;182:319–323.
25. Levitt RG, Glazer HS, Roper CL, et al. Magnetic resonance

imaging of mediastinal and hilar masses: comparison with CT. *AJR* 1985;145:9–14.

26. Glazer GM, Gross BH, Aisen AM, et al. Imaging of the pulmonary hilum: a prospective comparative study in patients with lung cancer. *AJR* 1985;145:245–248.

27. Khan A, Herman PG, Vorwerk P, et al. Solitary pulmonary nodules: comparison of classification with standard, thin-section and reference phantom CT. *Radiology* 1991;179:477–481.

28. Zwirewich CV, Vedal S, Miller RR, et al. Solitary pulmonary nodule: high resolution CT and radiologic-pathologic correlation. *Radiology* 1991;179:469–476.

29. Davis SD. CT evaluation for pulmonary metastases in patients with extrathoracic malignancy. *Radiology* 1991;180:1–12.

30. Chang AE, Schaner EG, Conkle DM, et al. Evaluation of computed tomography in the detection of pulmonary metastases: a prospective study. *Cancer* 1979;43:913–916.

31. Robertson PL, Boldt DW, DeCampo JF. Paediatric pulmonary nodules: a comparison of computed tomography, thoracotomy findings and histology. *Clin Radiol* 1988;39:607–610.

32. Costello P, Anderson W, Blume D: Pulmonary nodule: evaluation with spiral volumetric CT. *Radiology* 1991;179:875–876.

33. Feuerstein IM, Jicha DL, Pass HI, et al. Pulmonary metastases: MR imaging with surgical correlation—a prospective study. *Radiology* 1992;182:123–129.

34. Remy-Jardin M, Remy J, Deffontaines C, et al. Assessment of diffuse infiltrative lung disease: comparison of conventional CT and high-resolution CT. *Radiology* 1991;181:157–162.

35. Munk PL, Müller NL, Miller RR, et al. Pulmonary lymphangitic carcinomatosis: CT and pathologic findings. *Radiology* 1988;166:705–709.

36. Mathieson JR, Mayo JR, Staples CA, et al. Chronic diffuse infiltrative lung disease: comparison of diagnostic accuracy of CT and chest radiography. *Radiology* 1989;171:111–116.

37. Lee JS, Im J-G, Ahn JM, et al. Fibrosing alveolitis: prognostic implication of ground-glass attenuation at high-resolution CT. *Radiology* 1992;184:451–454.

38. Aberle DR, Gamsu G, Ray CS, et al. Asbestos-related pleural and parenchymal fibrosis: detection with high-resolution CT. *Radiology* 1988;166:729–734.

39. Munro NC, Cooke JC, Currie DC, et al. Comparison of thin section computed tomography with bronchography for identifying bronchiectatic segments in patients with chronic sputum production. *Thorax* 1990;45:135–139.

40. Silverman PM, Godwin JD. CT/bronchographic correlations in bronchiectasis. *J Comput Assist Tomogr* 1987;11:52–56.

41. Grenier P, Maurice F, Musset D, et al. Bronchiectasis: assessment by thin-section CT. *Radiology* 1986;161:95–99.

42. Naidich DP, Funt S, Ettenger NA, et al. Hemoptysis: CT-bronchoscopic correlations in 58 cases. *Radiology* 1990;177:357–362.

43. Petasnick JP. Radiologic evaluation of aortic dissection. *Radiology* 1991;180:297–305.

44. Godwin JD. Conventional CT of the aorta. *J Thorac Imaging* 1990;5(4):18–31.

45. McLoud TC, Flower CDR: Imaging the pleura: sonography, CT, and MR imaging. *AJR* 1991;156:1145–1153.

46. Waite RJ, Carbonneau RJ, Balikian JP, et al. Parietal pleural changes in empyema: appearances at CT. *Radiology* 1990;175:145–150.

47. Aberle DR, Balmes JR. Computed tomography of asbestos-related pulmonary parenchymal and pleural diseases. *Clin Chest Med* 1991;12:115–131.

48. Friedman AC, Fiel SB, Fisher MS, et al. Asbestos-related pleural disease and asbestosis: A comparison of CT and chest radiography. *AJR* 1988;150:268–275.

49. Fink I, Gamsu G, Harter LP. CT-guided aspiration biopsy of the thorax. *J Comput Assist Tomogr* 1982;6:958–962.

50. Lee KS, Im J-G, Kim YH, et al. Treatment of multiloculated empyemas with intracavitary urokinase: a prospective study. *Radiology* 1991;179:771–775.

51. Zeman RK, Baron RL, Jeffrey RB, et al. Helical body CT: evolution of scanning protocols. *AJR* 1998;170:1427–1438

52. Remy-Jardin M, Remy J, Deschildre F, et al. Diagnosis of pulmonary embolism with spiral CT: Comparison with pulmonary angiography and scintigraphy. *Radiology* 1996;200:699–706.

53. Viamonte M. Angiographic evaluation of lung neoplasms. *Radiol Clin NA* 1965;3:529–542.

54. Swensen SJ, Brown LR, Colby TV, et al. Pulmonary nodules: CT evaluation of enhancement with iodinated contrast material. *Radiology* 1995;194:393–398.

55. Swensen SJ, Brown LR, Colby TV, et al. Lung nodule enhancement at CT: prospective findings. *Radiology* 1996;201:447–455.

56. Nardich DP, Graden JF, McGuiness G, et al. Volumetric (helical spiral) CT (VCT) of the airways. *J Thorac Imag* 1997;12:11–28.

57. Broderick LS, Shemesh J, Wilensky RL, et al. Measurement of coronary artery calcium with duel-slice helical CT compared with coronary angiography: evaluation of CT scoring methods, interobserver variations and reproducibility. *AJR* 1996;167:439–444.

58. Shemesh J, Apter S, Rosenman J, et al. Calcification of coronary arteries: Detection and quantification with double-helix CT. *Radiology* 1995;197:779–783.

59. Webb WR, Sostman HD. MR imaging of thoracic disease: clinical uses. *Radiology* 1992;182:621–630.

60. Katayama H, Yamaguchi K, Kozuka T, et al. Adverse reactions to ionic and nonionic contrast media. *Radiology* 1990;175:621–628.

61. White RD, Dooms GC, Higgins CB. Advances in imaging thoracic aortic disease. *Invest Radiol* 1986;21:761–778.

62. Solomon SL, Brown JJ, Glazer HS, et al. Thoracic aortic dissection: pitfalls and artifacts in MR imaging. *Radiology* 1990;177:223–228.

63. Kersting-Sommerhoff BA, Higgins CB, White RD, et al. Aortic dissection: sensitivity and specificity of MR imaging. *Radiology* 1988;166:651–655.

64. Hansen ME, Spritzer CE, Sostman HD. Assessing the patency of mediastinal and thoracic inlet veins: value of MR imaging. *AJR* 1990;155:1177–1182.

65. Rapoport S, Blair DN, McCarthy SM, et al. Brachial plexus: correlation of MR imaging with CT and pathologic findings. *Radiology* 1988;167:161–165.

66. Castagno AA, Shuman WP. MR imaging in clinically suspected brachial plexus tumor. *AJR* 1987;149:1219–1222.

67. Gupta RK, Mehta VS, Banerji AK, et al. MR evaluation of brachial plexus injuries. *Neuroradiology* 1989;31:377–381.

68. Freedberg RS, Krozon I, Runnancik WM, et al. The contribution of magnetic resonance imaging to the evaluation of intracardiac tumors diagnosed by echo-cardiography. *Circulation* 1988;77:96–103.

69. Barakos JA, Brown JJ, Higgins CB. MR imaging of secondary cardiac and paracardiac lesions. *AJR* 1989;153:47–50.

70. Yan PC, Luh KT, Shen JC, et al. Ultrasonography and ultrasound guided aspiration biopsy. *Radiology* 1985;155:451–456.

71. Ammann AM, Brewer WH, Maull KI, et al. Traumatic rupture of the hemidiaphragm: Real-time sonographic diagnosis. *AJR* 1983;140:915–916.

72. The PIOPED Investigators. Value of the ventilation-perfusion scan in acute pulmonary embolism: results of the prospective investigation of pulmonary embolism diagnosis. *JAMA* 1990;263:2753–2759.

73. Nicod P, Peterson K, Levine M, et al. Pulmonary angiography in severe chronic pulmonary hypertension. *Ann Intern Med* 1987;107:565–568.

74. Anderson PO, Martin EC. Pulmonary embolism: diagnosis with multiple imaging modalities. *Radiology* 1987;164:297–312.

75. Gottschalk A, Juni J, Sostman HD, et al. Ventilation-perfusion scintigraphy in the PIOPED study. Part I: data collection and tabulation. *J Nucl Med* 1993;34:1109–1118.

76. Gottschalk A, Sostman HD, Juni J, et al. Ventilation-perfusion scintigraphy in the PIOPED study. Part II: evaluation of criteria and interpretations. *J Nucl Med* 1993;34:1119–1126.

77. Wernly JA, DeMeester TR, Kirchner PT, et al. Clinical value of quantitative ventilation-perfusion lung scans in the surgical management of bronchogenic carcinoma. *J Thorac Cardiovasc Surg* 1980;80:535–543.

78. Boysen PG, Block AJ, Olsen GN, et al. Prospective evaluation for pneumonectomy using the 99m-technetium quantitative perfusion lung scan. *Chest* 1977;72:422–425.

79. Scott WJ, Dewan NA. Use of positron emission tomograph to diagnose end stage lung cancer. *Clin Pulm Med* 1999;6:198–204.

80. Som P, Atkins HL, Bandoypadhyay D, et al. A fluorinated glucose analogue, 2-fluoro-2-deoxy-D-glucose (F-18): nontoxic tracer for rapid tumor detection. *J Nucl Med* 1980;21:670–675.

81. Dewan NA, Gupta NC, Redepenning LS, et al. Diagnostic efficacy of PET-FDG imaging in solitary pulmonary nodules. *Chest* 1993;104:997–1002

82. Gupta N, Chandramouli B, Reeb S, et al. Diagnostic evaluation of solitary pulmonary nodules using PET-FDG imaging. *J Nucl Med* 1994;35:76.

83. Gupta NC, Maloof J, Gunel E. Probability of malignancy in solitary pulmonary nodules using fluorine-18-FDG and PET. *J Nucl Med* 1996;37:943–948.

84. Rigo P, Paulus P, Kaschten B, et al. Oncological applications of positron emission tomography with fluorine-18 fluorodeoxyglucose. *Eur J Nucl Med* 1996;23:1641–1674.

85. Vansteenkiste JF, Stroobants SG, De Leyn PR, et al. Lymph node staging in non-small cell lung cancer with FDG-PET scan: a prospective study on 690 lymph node stations from 68 patients. *J Clin Oncol* 1998;16:2142–2149.

CLINICAL PULMONARY FUNCTION TESTING, EXERCISE TESTING, AND DISABILITY EVALUATION

RICHARD W. LIGHT

MEASUREMENTS OF VENTILATORY FUNCTION

Measurement of Expiratory Flow Rates
Measurement of Airway Hyperresponsiveness
Measurement of Lung Volumes
Airway and Pulmonary Tissue Mechanics
Distribution of Ventilation
Gas Transfer and Exchange

EXERCISE AND EXERCISE TESTING

Exercise Physiology and Pathophysiology
Measures of Work Capacity
Determinants of Work Capacity
Training
Aging and Exercise Performance
Performance of Exercise Testing
Use of Pulmonary Function and Exercise Tests

Pulmonary function testing consists of the performance of a set of maneuvers to detect and quantitate disorders of pulmonary ventilation and gas exchange. These tests provide objective evidence of the presence, type, and degree of abnormality. They allow for assessment of the course of a disease state over time, evaluation of the effectiveness of a therapeutic intervention, and determination of the risk of pulmonary complications of surgical procedures. In general, testing of the pulmonary system requires relatively little invasiveness or risk, enabling one to undergo repeated studies over relatively short intervals.

This chapter provides an overview of clinical pulmonary function testing as it exists today. The tests commonly performed in well-equipped clinical laboratories are discussed. The objective is not to detail the techniques but rather to emphasize the fundamental concepts.

The field of pulmonary function testing has acquired a system of nomenclature that may appear confusing to the student but has an underlying structure that is easily mastered. The American College of Chest Physicians and the American Thoracic Society Joint Committee on Pulmonary Nomenclature has provided a set of recommendations that are followed in this chapter (1). Where older terminology is commonplace, it is given as well.

MEASUREMENTS OF VENTILATORY FUNCTION

Measurement of Expiratory Flow Rates

Measurements of flow rates and cumulative exhaled volumes are the backbone of pulmonary function testing. The reader is referred to a recent monograph by the American Thoracic Society for guidance in the selection and calibration of equipment for this testing (2).

Simple Spirometry

With this test, the subject inhales maximally to total lung capacity (TLC) and then exhales as rapidly and forcefully as possible. The cumulative exhaled volume is recorded on the y-axis and time on the x-axis (Fig. 6.1). From the curve a series of timed volumes and flows are measured. The forced vital capacity (FVC) is the total volume exhaled. The $FEV_{0.5}$, FEV_1, and FEV_3 are the cumulative volumes exhaled after 0.5, 1.0, and 3.0 seconds, respectively. Although the $FEV_{0.5}$, FEV_1, and FEV_3 are volume measurements, they convey information on obstruction to flow because they are measured over a known period of time. They may be decreased by any process that inhibits expiratory flow, by a decrease in the TLC, or by lack of effort on the part of the subject.

A more sensitive means of evaluating obstruction is to express the forced expired volumes as a percentage of the vital capacity, abbreviated as FEV_t/FVC, with t representing time of measurement. The ratio is relatively independent of the patient's size. The FEV_1/FVC is a specific measure of airway obstruction with or without associated restriction of lung volumes. Normally it is 75% or greater. The FEV_3/FVC includes flows at relatively low lung volumes when flow rates are decreased relatively early in disease; thus, it may be abnormal in early airway obstruction. It is normally 95% or greater in adults.

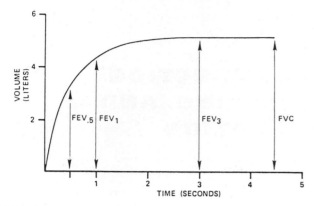

FIGURE 6.1. A typical forced expiratory spirogram showing the timed volumes obtained from the graph. $FEV_{0.5}$, FEV_1, and FEV_3 represent the forced expired volume at 0.5, 1, and 3 seconds, respectively. The forced vital capacity (FVC) is the maximum volume that can be forcefully exhaled.

Average flows can be graphically measured from the spirogram. Because flow is the change in volume with time, these forced expiratory flows (FEFs) may be determined graphically by dividing the volume change by the time required to make the change. Typically, the average flow between 25% and 75% of the vital capacity ($FEF_{25\%-75\%}$)—formerly called the maximal midexpiratory flow rate (MMF)—is recorded (Fig. 6.2). Other flows that are frequently reported include the flow between 75% and 85% of the vital capacity ($FEF_{75\%-85\%}$) and between 200 and 1200 mL of expired air ($FEF_{200-1200}$). These three average flow rates demonstrate marked variability in normal subjects (3). Accordingly, the 95% confidence limits for their normal values are so wide as to limit their utility in detecting disease in an individual subject.

Measures obtained from the FVC maneuver, whether recorded as spirograms or flow-volume loops, require the cooperation of the patient. It is recommended that a minimum of three acceptable FVC maneuvers be performed. If a subject has large variability between expiratory maneuvers, reproducibility criteria may require that up to eight acceptable maneuvers be performed. For the test results to be considered valid, the largest FVC and the second-largest FVC should not vary by more than 5% or 100 mL, whichever is greater. In addition, the largest FEV_1 and the second-largest FEV_1 should meet the same criteria. These reproducibility criteria are used as a guide to determine whether more than three FVC maneuvers are needed. The largest FVC and the largest FEV_1 should be recorded (2).

Flow-Volume Studies

The development of sophisticated electronic pulmonary function testing equipment has led to the popularity of the flow-volume curve. For this test, the subject makes a forced exhalation from TLC, as with the forced expiratory spirogram, followed by a forced inspiration. The recording device plots volume on the horizontal axis and flow on the vertical axis. Values of FEF are taken at volumes representing 25%, 50%, and 75% of the exhaled vital capacity and are recorded as $FEF_{x\%}$ ($\dot{V}max_{x\%}$), with x representing the exhaled fraction of the vital capacity (VC).

The flow-volume curve during forced exhalation has a characteristic appearance. The curve shows a rapid ascent to peak flow and a subsequently slow linear descent proportional to volume (Fig. 6.3). The initial portion of the curve depends at least in part on the effort of the patient. As a subject exerts increasing effort during exhalation, higher flow rates are generated. However, the latter two-thirds of the curve is relatively effort independent. For each point on the volume curve, a maximal flow exists that cannot be exceeded regardless of the effort of the patient (see discussion of isovolume pressure-flow curves in Chapter 3, Alveolar Ventilation, Gas Exchange, Oxygen Delivery). However, it must be emphasized that the maximal flow at a given lung volume will be achieved only if the patient generates sufficient intrathoracic pressure so that flow limitation is reached.

The flow-volume loop carries a great deal of information (4). Early in the development of obstructive airway disease, expiratory flow at low lung volumes is decreased but the volume exhaled is normal. This results in an expiratory curve that declines rapidly until the lung volume gets low, then persists at a low flow rate until the residual volume (RV) is reached (Fig. 6.4A). More severe obstructive disease results in an accentuation of upward concavity with a greatly decreased maximal flow (Fig. 6.4B) (5). Intrathoracic large airway obstruction, as in the trachea, results in decreased

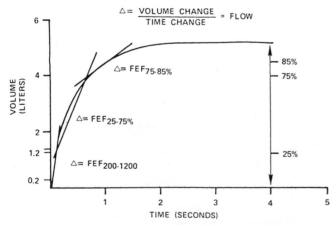

FIGURE 6.2. A typical forced expiratory spirogram showing the averaged flows obtained from the graph. The flow between 200 and 1200 mL of expired air ($FEF_{200-1200}$) is taken at high lung volume near TLC. The average flow between 25% and 75% of the expired vital capacity ($FEF_{25\%-75\%}$) measures flow in the midportion of the expired volume. The average flow between 75% and 85% of the expired vital capacity ($FEF_{75\%-85\%}$) measures flow at low lung volumes.

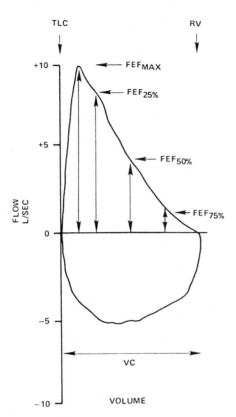

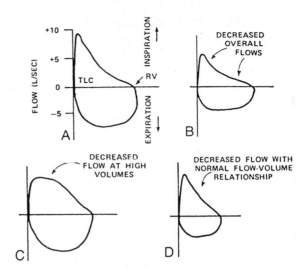

FIGURE 6.3. A typical flow-volume loop from a normal subject showing both expiratory *(upper)* and inspiratory *(lower)* portions. Instantaneous flows may be measured after 25% (FEF$_{25\%}$), 50% (FEF$_{50\%}$), and 75% (FEF$_{75\%}$) of the vital capacity has been exhaled. The peak flow is easily measured as the value of the peak of the graph.

FIGURE 6.4. Common examples of abnormal flow-volume loops. **A:** Mild obstructive airway disease characterized by decreased flow at low lung volume when elastic support is reduced. **B:** Significant obstructive airway disease characterized by decreased overall flows with a further decrease at low lung volumes. **C:** Variable intrathoracic large airway obstruction in which peak flow is decreased at higher lung volumes with preservation of normal flow-volume relationship at lower lung volumes. **D:** Restrictive pulmonary disease with decreased vital capacity and flows but preservation of normal flow-volume relationships.

flows at larger lung volumes, whereas the flows at low volumes are relatively unaffected. The result is a flattening of the flow-volume loop (Fig. 6.4C). The curve for patients with restrictive lung disease is one that has a decreased volume and peak flow but a normal relationship between the two (Fig. 6.4D).

There have been many studies comparing the flow-volume curves obtained when the subject is breathing air and breathing low-density gas mixtures such as 80% helium and 20% O_2. The clinical usefulness of these tests remains to be proved (6). The reader is referred to Chapter 2, Mechanics of Respiration, for a further discussion of these tests.

Peak Expiratory Flow Rate

The peak expiratory flow (PEF) is the highest flow rate that occurs during a forced exhalation from TLC. The PEF occurs very early in expiration, when the flow rates are effort dependent. A low value can result from slightly submaximal effort rather than from airway obstruction. In general, a relatively accurate prediction of the FEV$_1$ can be obtained from the PEF by multiplying the PEF (in liters per minute) by 9 to get the FEV$_1$ in milliliters (7).

The most common situation in which the PEF is used clinically is home monitoring. The availability of inexpensive, small, portable devices allows patients to objectively measure their degree of airway obstruction on an ambulatory basis. Essentially all published asthma practice guidelines recommend the use of PEF monitoring as an adjunct to asthma education in selected groups of patients (8,9). Groups most likely to benefit from home PEF monitoring are those who have labile asthma, and those who require repeated burst prednisone therapy, emergency room visits, and hospital admissions (9).

Maximal Voluntary Ventilation

The maximal voluntary ventilation (MVV) is the volume of air a subject can ventilate with maximal effort over a brief period. With this test, subjects are instructed to breathe rapidly and deeply for 12 to 15 seconds, and the cumulative expired volume is recorded. The results of the test are heavily dependent on subject cooperation and effort. Since the MVV can be predicted relatively accurately ($r = 0.94$) from the FEV$_1$ by multiplying the FEV$_1$ by 40, routine performance of this test is not recommended (10).

Measurement of Airway Hyperresponsiveness

Individuals with asthma have, by definition, hyperresponsive airways. At times when they are evaluated in the pulmonary function laboratory, their spirometry may be within normal limits. The diagnosis of asthma can still be established by demonstrating bronchial hyperreactivity to the inhalation of various agents. The two agents most commonly used to provoke bronchial responses are histamine and methacholine. Additional challenges that are used at times include distilled water, cold air, and exercise. With the typical procedure, the inhaled dose of the provocative agent is plotted on a logarithmic scale against the change in lung function, expressed as a percentage change from the normal value measured after an initial test dose of normal saline. Then the dose that produces a 20% fall in the FEV_1 is determined. Hyperresponsiveness is said to be present when the dose of histamine or methacholine that causes a 20% fall in the FEV_1 is 8.0 μmol or less. The lower the dose that induces the 20% decrease in FEV_1, the more hyperresponsive the individual. The primary uses of these tests are to establish the diagnosis of asthma in patients whose spirometry is normal and to quantitate the degree of hyperresponsiveness in known asthmatics (11).

One of the primary uses of bronchoprovocation tests is to exclude the diagnosis of asthma in patients with asthma-type symptoms or cough (11). A positive test in this situation is suggestive that the patient has asthma, but it should be remembered that 3% to 6% of asymptomatic individuals have airway hyperresponsiveness (12). A second primary use is to diagnose and follow subjects with occupational asthma. A third primary use is to document the severity of asthma and to assess the response to treatment (11). It should be noted that there is a high incidence of airway hyperresponsiveness in smokers with obstructive airway disease. In a recent study of 3,700 male and 2,200 female smokers with FEV_1/FVC less than 70%, 63% of the men and 87% of the women had a positive response to methacholine (13). It has also been shown that the presence of increased airway responsiveness is a significant predictor of subsequent accelerated decline in pulmonary function in adults (14).

Measurement of Lung Volumes

Spirometric Volume Determinations

The spirometric volume determinations are relatively simple to perform. The typical testing procedure consists of having a subject breathe several times with a normal, resting tidal pattern while recording the volume continuously. The subject is next instructed to inspire maximally, then exhale as completely as possible, but slowly, and then return to tidal breathing. A forceful expiration may induce air trapping and thus result in a lower volume measurement. A typical graph is given in Figure 6.5, from which the following measurements may be made:

Tidal volume (Vt): The average of the normal resting ventilatory excursions
Inspiratory reserve volume (IRV): The maximum volume that may be inhaled beyond a normal tidal breath

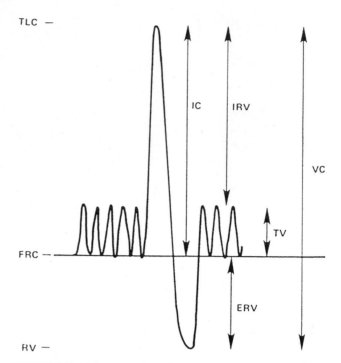

FIGURE 6.5. Volume tracing of a spirometer, showing the lung volumes and compartments measured from the tracing. The tracing is obtained by having the patient breathe quietly for a period of time, followed by a deep inspiration, and then a slow, complete expiration. The patient then returns to tidal breathing. The total lung capacity *(TLC)*, functional residual capacity *(FRC)*, and residual volume *(RV)* are shown for orientation. The measurements include the tidal volume *(TV)*, inspiratory reserve volume *(IRV)*, expiratory reserve volume *(ERV)*, inspiratory capacity *(IC)*, and vital capacity *(VC)*.

Expiratory reserve volume (ERV): The maximum volume that may be exhaled from a resting ventilatory level after a normal tidal expiration
Vital capacity (slow) (VC): The total volume of air that may be moved into or out of the lungs, including the inspiratory reserve, tidal, and expiratory reserve volumes
Inspiratory capacity (IC): The maximum volume of air that may be inhaled from a resting level, including the tidal volume and the inspiratory reserve volume

The main problem with the spirometrically determined lung volumes is that they do not provide any indication of the volume of air remaining after a maximal expiration, which is the residual volume (RV). Therefore, alternative methods must be used if one desires to measure the total lung capacity (TLC), which is the sum of the RV and VC. These alternative methods include gas dilution methods and body plethysmography.

Gas Dilution

The closed-circuit helium dilution method is performed by having the subject rebreathe a known volume of gas in a closed-circuit spirometer containing helium as a tracer (Fig.

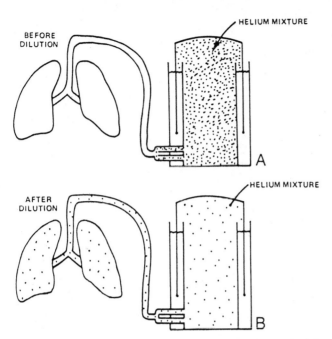

FIGURE 6.6. Diagram of the closed-circuit helium method for determination of the functional residual capacity. **A:** Prior to equilibration, the helium tracer is distributed in the spirometer circuit only. **B:** After equilibration with the patient's lungs by having him or her rebreathe the gas mixture the helium is diluted and distributed throughout the lungs and spirometer. Measurement of the spirometer gas volume and the amount of dilution of the helium tracer enables calculation of the total system volume. The FRC is calculated by subtracting the spirometer volume from the system volume.

6.6) (15). Helium is inert and does not readily diffuse across the alveolar-capillary membrane. The helium equilibrates throughout the volume of the entire patient-spirometer system. The carbon dioxide generated is removed and the oxygen lost is replenished with 100% oxygen to maintain a constant volume in the system. If the patient begins and ends the test at the end of a normal expiration, the functional residual capacity is determined. The residual volume is then obtained by subtracting the measured ERV from the calculated FRC. This method is sensitive to errors from leakage of gas and also fails to measure the volume of gas in lung bullae.

A second method is the open circuit or multibreath nitrogen washout technique (Fig. 6.7) (16). The nitrogen normally present in the lungs is used as the tracer gas. The subject begins breathing 100% oxygen at the end of a normal expiration (FRC). As the nitrogen is "washed out," the expired gas is collected and the concentration of nitrogen is continuously monitored. When the concentration in the expirate falls to a low level, the FRC may be determined by measuring the volume of gas exhaled and the nitrogen concentration of this gas in a manner similar to that used in the helium dilution method. This method has the advantage that it permits a simultaneous assessment of intrapulmonary gas mixing. This method is also sensitive to errors

from gas leakage and does not measure the volume of gas in poorly communicating air spaces such as bullae.

Two other measurements of lung volume can be obtained from the dilution of gases used in standard tests of pulmonary function. One involves the measurement of the mean concentration of nitrogen in the air exhaled after an inspiration of 100% oxygen with the single-breath nitrogen washout test. The other involves measuring the change in concentration of helium used as the inert tracer gas in the single-breath measurement of the diffusing capacity. However, because the time for dilution of the tracer gas is relatively short for both of these methods, the TLC is underestimated in patients with severe maldistribution of ventilation (17).

From the measurements obtained by spirometry and the gas dilution methods all of the lung volumes may be determined. All three techniques can give faulty results if the test begins and ends at a volume different from that to be measured, which is either the FRC or the RV. With the helium dilution method, gas leaks in the system can cause an overestimation of helium dilution and thus yield falsely elevated values.

Plethysmographic Volume Determinations

The technique of plethysmography is an alternate method used to measure the volume of the lungs (18). It is important to note that the results of these tests may differ from the results obtained by using gas dilution or washout methods. The gas dilution methods measure communicating FRC or RV, whereas the plethysmographic techniques measure both the communicating and noncommunicating compartments. Noncommunicating or poorly communicating air spaces are often present as a result of disease in which "air trapping" occurs. A pneumothorax is another example of a noncommunicating space. These gas compartments are compressible and therefore are included in the plethysmographic measurement but are not reflected in the gas dilution determination. The gas volume measured by a plethysmograph is known as the thoracic gas volume (V_{TG}) and in disease states is frequently higher than the value measured by gas dilution.

The measurement of V_{TG} via plethysmography is based on Boyle's law, which states that the product of the pressure times the volume of the gas in the thorax is constant if the temperature is unchanged. The subject is seated comfortably in the airtight plethysmograph and temperature equilibration is allowed to occur (Fig. 6.8). With the airway occluded, the subject makes inspiratory and expiratory efforts against the occluded airway. The lung volume can then be calculated, because changes in the volume of the thorax are reflected by changes in the pressure in the box and changes in the thoracic pressure are reflected by changes in the pressure recorded at the mouth.

The procedure described in the preceding is usually initiated at the end of a normal expiration, so the V_{TG} is equiva-

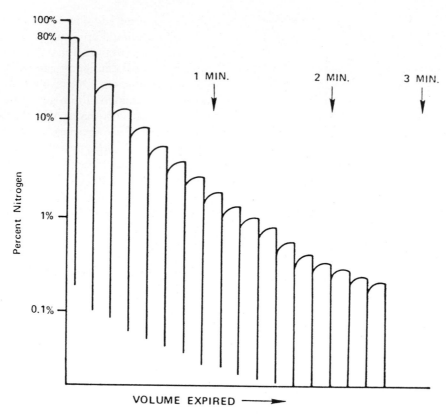

FIGURE 6.7. Graph of log nitrogen concentration versus volume exhaled in the multibreath nitrogen washout test used for determination of FRC and intrapulmonary gas mixing. The peak of the curve for each breath represents the end-tidal N_2 concentration. Analysis of the curve generated by the peak concentrations enables assessment of the homogeneity of gas distribution. On the log scale, mixing in the presence of ideal gas distribution would result in a curve that is nearly a straight line, with a rapid decrease in the concentration of N_2 to below 2.5%. By monitoring the volume exchanged, along with the N_2 concentration, the FRC may be calculated.

lent to FRC. By combining this measurement with spirometric measurements, one may determine all the lung volume compartments, as in the gas dilution methods. The volumes determined by plethysmography are subject to error if the test is performed at an inappropriate starting volume. The measurement reflects the actual volume in the thorax at the start and end of the test.

Airway and Pulmonary Tissue Mechanics

The tests discussed so far are affected by such extrapulmonary factors as thoracic and abdominal muscle function and the properties of the thoracic cage. It is possible to assess the mechanical properties of the lungs themselves by using tests that require more sophisticated equipment. These tests are discussed briefly in the paragraphs that follow.

Airway Resistance

Airway resistance (Raw) must be measured during air flow. By definition the airway resistance is the driving pressure

divided by the flow that results from the pressure differential. Resistance to flow in the airways may be measured through the use of body plethysmography (19). In measuring total airway resistance, the pressure differential is that between the alveoli and the atmosphere. It is not possible to measure alveolar pressure directly when air is flowing, but a body plethysmograph can be used to measure it indirectly. The flow at the mouth may be measured simultaneously to enable calculation of airway resistance. It is important to measure Raw at low flow rates (less than 0.5 L/sec) so that the measurement does not reflect dynamic compression of the airways (Chapter 3, Alveolar Ventilation, Gas Exchange, Oxygen Delivery).

Airway resistance changes with lung volume, so the Raw determination is made at a known volume, usually the FRC. The relationship is inverse: thus an increase in lung volume results in a decreased resistance. The inverse of airway resistance is *airway conductance* (Gaw), or flow per pressure change. Airway conductance is nearly linearly related to lung volume (Fig. 2.9B). The specific airway conductance (Gaw/VL or SGaw) is therefore independent of the lung volume and is the measurement that should be used in evaluating

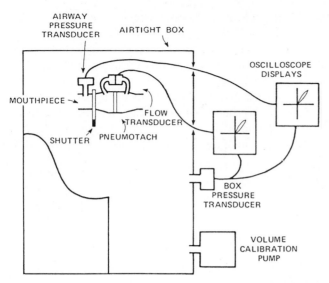

FIGURE 6.8. Body plethysmograph for the measurement of thoracic gas volume and airway resistance. The type shown is a pressure plethysmograph, which uses pressure changes in the box to estimate lung volume changes. Pressure transducers are used to monitor the box and mouth pressures. A flow transducer allows simultaneous recording of flow at the mouth. From these measurements, the thoracic gas volume and the airway resistance may be calculated using the techniques outlined in the text.

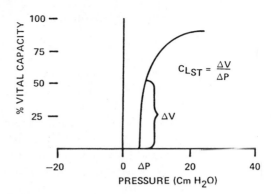

FIGURE 6.9. Volume-pressure graph obtained by measuring the pressure during static conditions at various lung volumes with the glottis closed. The test is usually performed by interrupting flow intermittently during an expiration from TLC while recording transpulmonary pressure and volume above FRC. The transpulmonary pressure is the alveolar pressure measured at the mouth minus the pleural pressure measured with an esophageal balloon. The pressure and volume points are plotted as a curve. The static compliance is measured as the slope of the curve at a given point, usually just above FRC.

changes in airway resistance with time in an individual patient or in comparing a given patient to normal values.

Lung Compliance

The distensibility of the lungs is assessed by measuring lung compliance, which is determined from the relationship between changes in *transpulmonary pressure* and changes in lung volume.

The measurement of static compliance is performed with a spirometer to measure volume change and with pressure transducers to measure pressures in the airway and esophagus. The pleural pressure is estimated from the pressure within a balloon placed in the esophagus. The subject inspires to TLC and begins a slow expiration. The air flow at the mouth is interrupted at small volume decrements of approximately 500 mL, during which time the volume and pressures are recorded. Since the airway pressure during occlusion of the airway is identical to alveolar pressure, the transpulmonary pressure is calculated as the difference between airway and esophageal pressures. The lung volumes and corresponding transpulmonary pressures are plotted to give a static lung compliance curve (Fig. 6.9). The slope of the curve ($\Delta V/\Delta P$) at any given volume represents the *static lung compliance* (C_{Lst}) at that volume. The portion of the curve 500 to 1,000 mL above the FRC is usually chosen for the measurement, because at higher lung volumes the relationship becomes highly nonlinear. The static compliance is often normalized to the absolute lung volume at which the measurement is made and is termed *specific compliance* (C_{Lst}/V_L). The reason for this is that compliance is directly related to absolute lung volume.

Static lung compliance reflects the elasticity of the lung parenchyma. It increases slightly with advancing age owing to changes in the elastic fibers of the lungs. It also increases in emphysema. A decreased compliance suggests interstitial disease or one with alveolar filling such as pulmonary edema.

During the measurement of static lung compliance, the transthoracic pressure (alveolar minus atmospheric) may be recorded in addition to the transpulmonary pressure to permit calculation of *total lung compliance* (C_{Tst}). This measurement includes pulmonary and chest wall factors. The difference between the transthoracic and transpulmonary pressures may be used to calculate the *chest wall compliance* (C_{Wst}).

Distribution of Ventilation

Tests of gas distribution are used to give a measure of the homogeneity of the distribution of inspired gas to the alveoli. In the normal lung, gas is transported along all airways and is distributed relatively equally to all areas of the lung, with more distribution to the lower regions of the lung in the upright subject. This is because alveoli in the upper zones are more distended than in the lower zones at FRC and are less able to expand. In certain disease states, especially those with destruction of pulmonary tissue, there is a variable degree of inhomogeneity that alters the intrapulmonary distribution of gas within each region. Several tests are available to detect this type of abnormality.

Single-Breath Nitrogen Elimination Test

The single-breath N_2 test may be used to assess the homogeneity of gas distribution (20). The results of the test give an index that reflects the overall mixing ability of the lungs, but no anatomic indication of areas of poor distribution is possible.

The test is performed with the subject seated after normal breathing of room air for a few moments. The subject exhales to residual volume, and then slowly inhales a breath of 100% oxygen to total lung capacity. During a slow expiration (under 1 L/sec), the concentration of nitrogen in the exhaled air is recorded continuously as a function of the volume exhaled. The resulting curve consists of four phases, which are depicted in Figure 6.10.

The shape of the curve can be explained on the basis of the underlying physiology. At RV the alveoli in the upper portions of the lungs are larger than those in the lower portions because of the more negative pleural pressure at the top part of the lung. At TLC all the alveoli are approximately the same size. Therefore, when an individual takes a breath of 100% O_2 from RV, the nitrogen concentration in the alveoli in the upper portion of the lungs will be greater at TLC than that in the lower portion of the lungs. On expiration, the dead space gas (100% oxygen) is exhaled first and is noted as phase I, in which the nitrogen concentration is zero. The nitrogen concentration rises abruptly (phase II) when alveolar gas with nitrogen begins to be exhaled. Phase III represents alveolar gas exhalation. If gas distribution were perfectly homogeneous, all alveoli would empty at an approximately equal rate and the phase III line would be horizontal. Nonhomogeneous emptying of the lungs results in different rates of nitrogen expiration, and there is normally a slight rise of the phase III line. In conditions of abnormal intrapulmonary mixing, the beginning of phase IV occurs when the small airways in the bases of the lungs begin to close, leaving only the upper zones, which have higher N_2 concentration, to empty, causing the abrupt increase in slope (21).

From the curve the following measurements are made:

Anatomic dead space (V_{Danat}): The volume of phase I and approximately half of phase II
Phase III slope: The change in nitrogen concentration over 1 L of the initial portion of phase III
Closing volume (CV): The volume above the RV, at which phase IV begins to occur, reported as percent of VC
Closing capacity (CC): The CV plus the RV, reported as percent of TLC

The phase III slope is an index of uniformity of gas distribution. Normally there is less than a 2% change in nitrogen concentration per liter during phase III. Increases in its value reflect relatively greater inhomogeneity than normal. Indeed, in one large study of over 2,500 adults, the slope of phase III was more strongly associated with mortality than was the FEV_1 (22). At one time the CV was proposed as a sensitive indicator of small airway disease and was thought to hold promise as a predictive test for the development of chronic obstructive pulmonary disease (23). However, subsequent studies designed to prove this contention were disappointing (24). At the present time, this test is rarely used in the clinical situation.

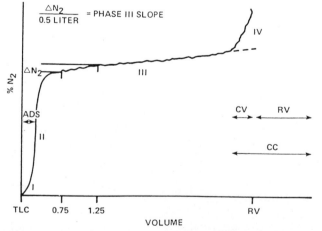

FIGURE 6.10. Graph of nitrogen concentration versus volume exhaled in the single-breath nitrogen test. Measurement of ΔN_2 is the change in nitrogen concentration over the curve from 750 to 1,250 mL. The phase III slope is the slope of the line over an initial portion of the curve, equal to the change in N_2 concentration over a 1-L portion of the curve. Measurements of closing volume and anatomic dead space are made directly from the graph.

Multibreath Nitrogen Washout

The use of this test to measure the FRC was described in a previous section (Fig. 6.7). It may also be used to assess the homogeneity of ventilation. The nitrogen concentration after 7 minutes is used as an index of the homogeneity of ventilation. Normally it is less than 2.5%. If uneven gas distribution exists owing to slower emptying of some lung compartments, the washout is prolonged and the nitrogen concentration after 7 minutes is greater than 2.5%. Occasionally, the multibreath nitrogen washout test may be abnormal when the single-breath nitrogen test is normal. This has been attributed to the exchange of gas with bullae or similar compartments, which is too slow to affect the single-breath test but is detectable by the washout method owing to the prolonged tidal breathing.

Radioactive Xenon Distribution

The two tests of distribution described in the preceding provide an index giving some overall indication of the degree of inhomogeneity. Visualization of the distribution of gas may be performed with the radioactive xenon test, in which the subject breathes a gas mixture containing ^{133}Xe while his or her chest is scanned with a gamma camera. The ^{133}Xe isotope may also be dissolved in saline and injected intravenously. Because the gas is poorly soluble in blood, it is almost completely eliminated in one passage through the lungs. Scanning over the chest wall immediately after injection yields an estimate of relative perfusion to various areas, and the rate of clearance from these areas indicates their relative ventilation.

Gas Transfer and Exchange

The ability of gases to transfer across the alveolar-capillary membrane is assessed by analyzing the concentration of respiratory gases on both sides of the membrane or by assessing the ease with which a foreign gas transfers from the alveoli to the blood. There are several factors that affect the process of gas exchange, including the total surface area available for gas exchange, the diffusion characteristics of the alveolar-capillary membrane, the perfusion of the capillaries with blood, and the matching of ventilation to perfusion. These tests, however, give an overall index of diffusion and do not allow an assessment of each of the factors involved.

Blood Gas and Acid-Base Analysis

The measurement of the pH and partial pressures of oxygen and carbon dioxide in the arterial and venous blood is fundamental to the diagnosis and management of patients with pulmonary disorders. These measurements are not only valuable in the management of critically ill patients but also enable one to determine a number of clinically useful indexes of cardiopulmonary function, including venous admixture (physiologic shunt fraction) and physiologic dead space fraction. They reflect the overall function of the cardiopulmonary system with respect to gas exchange. Detailed information on the use and interpretation of these measurements is presented in Chapter 3, Alveolar Ventilation, Gas Exchange, Oxygen Delivery.

Carbon Monoxide Diffusing Capacity

The diffusing capacity of the lungs (D_L) is a measure of the ability of gases to diffuse from the alveoli into the pulmonary capillary blood. Carbon monoxide is the usual test gas because it is not normally present in the lungs or blood and since it is much more soluble in blood than in lung tissues. When the diffusing capacity is measured with carbon monoxide, the test is called the carbon monoxide diffusing capacity (D_{LCO}).

To determine D_{LCO}, the amount of CO transferred per unit time and the average partial pressure difference of the gas across the alveolar-capillary membrane must be measured. The following equation represents this basic principle:

$$D_{LCO} = \dot{V}_{CO}/(P_{A_{CO}} - P_{c_{CO}}) \qquad (6.1)$$

where $\dot{V}_{CO}$ is the uptake of carbon monoxide and $P_{A_{CO}}$ and $P_{c_{CO}}$ are the partial pressures of carbon monoxide in the alveolar gas and capillary blood, respectively. The final result for D_{LCO} is expressed as milliliters of carbon monoxide transferred per minute per millimeter of mercury pressure gradient. Since the D_{LCO} is directly related to the alveolar volume, it is frequently normalized to this value (D_L/V_A), which allows for its interpretation in the presence of abnormal lung volumes.

Techniques

The most common manner by which the diffusing capacity is measured is the single-breath carbon monoxide test ($D_{LCO_{SB}}$) (25). With this method, the subject exhales to RV and then inhales a full breath of a gas mixture containing a low concentration of CO and a known concentration of an insoluble tracer gas, which is most commonly helium. The subject holds his or her breath for 10 seconds and then exhales completely (Fig. 6.11). The initial alveolar volume and alveolar concentration of carbon monoxide are derived from measurements of the concentrations of the tracer gas in the inspired and expired air and the carbon monoxide concentrations in the inspired gas. The final $P_{A_{CO}}$ is assumed to be the end-expiratory partial pressure of carbon monoxide. It is assumed that the $P_{A_{CO}}$ declines exponentially and that the capillary partial pressure is negligible. The D_{LCO} can then be easily computed from the following equation:

$$D_{LCO} = (V_A \times 60/(P_{bar} - 47) \times t) \times (\ln P_{A_{CO_i}}/P_{A_{CO_t}}) \qquad (6.2)$$

where V_A is the original lung volume, P_{bar} is the barometric pressure, t is the time of breath holding, and $P_{A_{CO_i}}$ and $P_{A_{CO_t}}$ are the initial and final partial alveolar pressures of

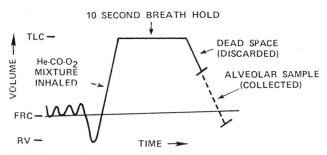

FIGURE 6.11. Kymograph tracing during the single-breath D_{LCO} maneuver. The patient first exhales to residual volume, then takes a full breath of a known mixture of oxygen, helium, and carbon monoxide. The breath is held at full inspiration for 10 seconds to allow gas transfer, then the subject exhales. After the initial dead space is exhaled, a sample of alveolar gas is collected and analyzed. The difference in gas concentration between the inhaled gas and the alveolar gas sample allows for calculation of the transfer of carbon monoxide from the lungs.

carbon monoxide (2). Recommendations for the standard technique for this measurement have been published (25).

A second technique is the steady-state method (DLCO$_{SS}$), of which there are several variations. With these methods, the subject rebreathes a gas with a known CO concentration until CO uptake reaches a steady-state, at which point several measurements are made for the calculation of the entities in Equation 6.1. The various methods differ in the way in which the mean PA$_{CO}$ and the capillary PC$_{CO}$ are calculated (26).

A less commonly used technique is the rebreathing method (DLCO$_{RB}$), in which a subject rebreathes a CO-He mixture for approximately 1 minute (27). The gas mixture and the measurement and calculations are nearly identical to those for the single-breath technique.

The choice of the technique used depends on several factors. The single-breath technique is the one most widely used, because it is simple and quick to perform. It is possible, however, that this technique does not give truly physiologic results, because breath holding does not provide proper conditions for complete gas distribution. It is also the method that is most sensitive to ventilation-perfusion abnormalities. It cannot be used for measurements during exercise. The steady-state and rebreathing methods can be applied to exercise testing and are less affected by ventilation-perfusion abnormalities but are more difficult and time-consuming to perform.

Factors Influencing the Diffusing Capacity

The resistance to the diffusion of carbon monoxide from the alveoli to the blood is determined primarily by two factors, the state of the alveolar-capillary membrane and the amount of hemoglobin in the pulmonary capillaries available for uptake of carbon monoxide (28). Mathematically, the following formula expresses this relationship:

$$1/D_L = 1/D_M + 1/\theta V_c \qquad (6.3)$$

where D$_L$ is the diffusing capacity of the lung, D$_M$ represents the membrane component, V$_c$ is the capillary blood volume, and the coefficient θ is the rate at which CO binds to intracellular oxyhemoglobin. Normally the two components on the right side of Equation 6.3 contribute approximately equally to the measured DLCO (29).

Both quantitative and qualitative abnormalities in the alveolar-capillary membrane may alter the measured DLCO. The measured DLCO will depend on the total surface area available for gas exchange. Therefore, large individuals will have a higher DLCO than small individuals. Also, the removal of a portion of the lung will reduce the DLCO. In areas of the lung that are poorly ventilated, carbon monoxide will not be transferred and a reduced diffusing capacity will result. In a given patient, a higher DLCO will be obtained with a higher lung volume (30).

The DLCO may also be reduced if there is increased resistance to diffusion across the alveolar membrane. Historically, qualitative abnormalities in the alveolar-capillary membrane have been considered to be primarily owing to an increased thickness of the membrane. However, the relative contribution of a "thick" membrane to loss of DLCO appears to have been overestimated. In diseases with interstitial thickening, other factors such as an alteration in the alveolar architecture with loss of surface area for gas exchange appear to play a greater role in producing the low DLCO (28).

The second major factor that influences the diffusing capacity, which is represented by the last term in Equation 6.3, is the ability of the blood to accept and bind carbon monoxide. Fundamentally, this is dependent on two factors: the pulmonary capillary blood volume and the level of hemoglobin in this capillary blood. The pulmonary capillary blood volume is obviously reduced in areas of the lung that are not perfused. Changes in position and alterations in intrathoracic pressure at the time of measurement can both alter pulmonary capillary blood volume.

Diffusing capacity measurements are usually made to determine the status of the lung. Since anemia can result in a decreased diffusing capacity in the presence of a normal lung, it is recommended that diffusing capacity measurements be corrected for the level of hemoglobin in the blood by using the following equations (31):
In men

$$\text{Adjusted } D_{LCO} = \text{observed } D_{LCO} + 1.40\,(14.6 - [Hb]) \qquad (6.4)$$

In women

$$\text{Adjusted } D_{LCO} = \text{observed } D_{LCO} + 1.40\,(13.4 - [Hb]) \qquad (6.5)$$

EXERCISE AND EXERCISE TESTING

In recent years exercise pathophysiology and exercise testing have received more and more attention. This is because an individual's capacity to function on a daily basis is more closely related to the maximal performance of his or her pulmonary and cardiovascular systems than to the performance of these organ systems at rest. If an individual is perfectly comfortable at rest but becomes very dyspneic with minimal exercise, he or she will be miserable. Life is a series of exercises that range from grooming oneself to feeding oneself to generating an income through work. Under normal conditions, one's ability to perform exercise depends on the capacity of the circulatory and respiratory systems to increase the transport of oxygen to the exercising muscles and on the status of the local factors that determine whether the increased quantity of oxygen reaches the cell interior, where it is used to produce energy for muscle fiber contraction. If a certain activity requires a greater oxygen consumption than can be generated by the individual, then that activity is closed to that individual.

There are at least eight reasons to study individuals while

they exercise. First, an exercise test can quantitate the degree of functional impairment. The maximal work load tolerated by the individual or the oxygen consumption during maximal exercise ($\dot{V}O_2$max) can be measured and compared with those predicted for individuals of the same age, size, and sex. Second, analysis of the results of the exercise test can help indicate whether the limiting factor is pulmonary, cardiac, or owing to lack of conditioning or to poor effort. Third, responses to various therapeutic interventions (e.g., vasodilator therapy for intractable heart failure) can be assessed with serial exercise tests. Fourth, the results of the exercise test can provide the basis for the development of a rational reconditioning program. Fifth, the results of exercise testing are sometimes useful in the preoperative assessment of patients with bronchogenic carcinoma (32). Sixth, the results of exercise tests are sometimes used to select patients for lung or heart transplantation. Seventh, exercise tests can be used to diagnose exercise-induced asthma (33). Eighth, exercise tests can be used to monitor disease progress, especially early interstitial lung disease.

This section briefly considers alterations in the respiratory and circulatory systems that occur during exercise. Excellent reviews are available that discuss the actual performance of exercise testing and the physiologic responses to exercise and training in more depth (33–37). In addition, the use of exercise testing in the differential diagnosis of work intolerance and disability evaluation is discussed.

Exercise Physiology and Pathophysiology

To exercise, an individual must generate more energy. Adenosine triphosphate (ATP) is the obligatory energetic intermediary in the transduction of ingested food energy into the mechanical energy of muscle contraction and work. ATP is generated primarily through the oxidation of carbohydrate and fat. When insufficient oxygen is present, ATP can also be generated via the anaerobic metabolism of carbohydrates to lactic acid. However, anaerobic metabolism is much less efficient than aerobic metabolism. To generate the same amount of energy with anaerobic as with aerobic metabolism, approximately 18 times as much glucose must be used. Accordingly, to all intents and purposes, an individual's ability to exercise is limited by his or her capacity to deliver oxygen to the exercising muscles and use the delivered oxygen (38).

The oxygen required to perform various tasks is shown in Table 6.1. Note that the oxygen requirements vary more than 15-fold, from 200 mL/min at rest to more than 3200 mL/min for carrying loads up stairs. Note also that eating and conversing require relatively low levels of oxygen consumption. Therefore, it becomes evident that if a patient is breathless during an interview or during eating, it will be very difficult for that patient to dress himself or herself, take a shower, drive a car, or do any housekeeping. The fact that propulsion of a wheelchair takes much less oxygen than does

TABLE 6.1 ENERGY REQUIREMENTS FOR AN AVERAGE-SIZED ADULT DURING VARIOUS ACTIVITIES

Activity	O_2 Consumption (ml/min)
Rest, supine	200
Sitting	240
Standing relaxed	280
Eating	280
Conversation	280
Typing	360
Dressing, undressing	460
Propulsion, wheelchair	480
Driving car	560
Peeling potatoes	580
Walking 2.5 mph	720
Making beds	780
Bricklaying	800
Showering	840
Swimming 20 yd/min	1000
Golfing	1000
Walking 3.75 mph	1120
Tennis	1420
Ambulation, braces and crutches	1600
Shoveling	1700
Ascending stairs, 22-lb load, 54 ft/min	3240

From Gordon EE: Energy costs of activities in health and disease. *Arch Intern Med* 101:702, 1958. Reproduced with permission of the author and publisher.

walking at 2.5 mph suggests that more people with severe exercise limitation might benefit from this device. If physicians keep in mind the oxygen requirements for the activities listed in Table 6.1, they can counsel their patients more rationally in what they should and should not do.

Measures of Work Capacity

As mentioned earlier, an individual's ability to perform muscular work is dependent on his or her capacity to transport oxygen from the atmosphere to the mitochondria of the cells in the exercising muscles. The best metabolic index of the work capacity in a given individual is the maximum O_2 consumption per unit time ($\dot{V}O_2$max) of the individual. Since the oxygen requirement to do a given task depends on the weight to the individual, the best indication of an individual's exercise capacity is the $\dot{V}O_2$max/kg. Prediction equations for the $\dot{V}O_2$max are given later in this chapter (Equations 6.9 to 6.16). The $\dot{V}O_2$max is determined by measuring oxygen consumption ($\dot{V}O_2$) at progressively higher work loads (35). Eventually a point is reached at which higher work loads do not result in higher $\dot{V}O_2$, and by definition the highest $\dot{V}O_2$ value attained is $\dot{V}O_2$max. The leveling off of $\dot{V}O_2$ provides objective evidence that the subject has attained maximal aerobic power. However, it is notable that one cannot demonstrate such a plateau in most individuals undergoing exercise testing (39). Since the energy for the additional work is provided by anaerobic metabolism, a demonstration that the blood lactate levels are substantial (8 mM/L or greater) also indicates that the subject has attained maximal aerobic power.

Since maximum exercise is at times uncomfortable to the subject, many exercise laboratories attempt to derive the $\dot{V}O_2$max from a $\dot{V}O_2$ measured at a submaximal load. This can be done because in most individuals there is a linear relationship between heart rate and $\dot{V}O_2$ after the $\dot{V}O_2$ reaches a certain level. The maximum heart rate for an individual can be estimated by subtracting the patient's age from 220. Therefore, if $\dot{V}O_2$ is measured at two submaximum exercise levels, $\dot{V}O_2$max can be estimated as demonstrated in Figure 6.12. This method of determining the $\dot{V}O_2$max by derivation from submaximal load is relatively accurate for normal subjects, deconditioned patients, and most patients with heart disease. However, it is usually not applicable to patients with moderate to severe pulmonary disease because their exercise is limited by their ventilatory abilities and they do not achieve their predicted maximum heart rate. Many patients with left ventricular failure also fall far short of reaching their predicted maximal heart rate (40).

Other indexes of work capacity frequently used are watts, kilopound meters (kpm) per minute, and multiples of resting O_2 consumption (metabolic equivalents, or METS). The relationship between these indexes of work capacity and the $\dot{V}O_2$ is shown in Table 6.2. Most bicycle ergometers are calibrated in watts or in kpm per minute; therefore, a reasonable estimate of the $\dot{V}O_2$ for bicycle ergometer exercise can be obtained from Table 6.2. When exercise is per-

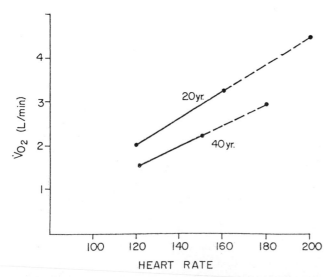

FIGURE 6.12. Predicting the $\dot{V}O_2$max from submaximal exercise levels. On the top line, a 20-year-old had a $\dot{V}O_2$ of 2,100 at a heart rate of 120 and a $\dot{V}O_2$ of 3,250 at a heart rate of 160. By extrapolating to a heart rate of 200 (220 − 20), we find an estimated $\dot{V}O_2$max of 4,500. In an analogous manner the 40-year-old represented by the bottom line was found to have an estimated $\dot{V}O_2$max of 3000 mL/min.

TABLE 6.2 RELATIONSHIP BETWEEN O_2 CONSUMPTION AND OTHER MEASURES OF WORK

O_2 Consumption (ml/min)	kpm/min	watts	METS
225	0	0	1
900	300	50	4
1500	600	100	7
2100	900	150	10
2800	1200	200	13
3500	1500	250	16
4200	1800	300	19
5000	2100	350	22

formed on a treadmill, the $\dot{V}O_2$ is dependent on the patient's weight, the speed of the treadmill, and the inclination of the treadmill. Nomograms are available for the prediction of an individual's $\dot{V}O_2$ from his or her weight and the speed and inclination of the treadmill (41). Therefore, relatively accurate estimates of $\dot{V}O_2$ can be obtained without the collection of expired gases. Such estimates do not take into consideration the contribution of anaerobic metabolism to the work performed. Moreover, with repeated testing, individuals tend to become more efficient on both the treadmill and the bicycle ergometer. Hence, these indirect estimates of the $\dot{V}O_2$max tend to overestimate actual improvements in the $\dot{V}O_2$max.

Determinants of Work Capacity ($\dot{V}O_2$max)

The oxygen consumption ($\dot{V}O_2$) of an individual is given by the following equation:

$$\dot{V}O_2 = \dot{Q} \times (CaO_2 - C\bar{v}O_2) \qquad (6.6)$$

where $\dot{Q}$ is the cardiac output, CaO_2 the oxygen content of arterial blood, and $C\bar{v}O_2$ the oxygen content of mixed venous blood. Since almost all the oxygen in the blood is bound to hemoglobin, Equation 6.6 can be rewritten as follows:

$$\dot{V}O_2 = \dot{Q} \times [Hb] \times (SaO_2 - S\bar{v}O_2) \times 1.34 \quad (6.7)$$

where Hb is the concentration of hemoglobin in the blood, SaO_2 is the hemoglobin saturation in arterial blood, $S\bar{v}O_2$ is the hemoglobin saturation of mixed venous blood, and 1.34 is the amount of oxygen it takes to fully saturate 1 g of hemoglobin. From Equation 6.7 one can readily appreciate that the $\dot{V}O_2$max is dependent on the cardiac output, the hemoglobin concentration, the arterial oxygen saturation, and the ability of the exercising muscles to extract oxygen from the blood during maximum exercise as reflected by the $S\bar{v}O_2$. We will discuss exercise physiology by examining the factors that influence the different terms in Equation 6.7.

Cardiac Output

The cardiac output is the limiting factor for $\dot{V}O_2$max in normal subjects (35). Attempts to go beyond maximal work capacity are associated with a further increase in ventilation but no further increase in the cardiac output or $\dot{V}O_2$max. The cardiac output during exercise increases linearly with increasing $\dot{V}O_2$. Although an increase in cardiac output can result from an increase in either heart rate or stroke volume or both, most of the increase in cardiac output during exercise is related to increases in the heart rate, and the increases in stroke volume are proportionately smaller.

The cardiac output at a given $\dot{V}O_2$ is essentially identical in trained and untrained subjects during arm and leg exercise and during running, bicycling, and swimming. Therefore, the $\dot{V}O_2$ provides an indirect measure of the cardiac output. The cardiac output is approximately 5 L plus the $\dot{V}O_2$ times 5. Therefore, the cardiac output with a $\dot{V}O_2$ of 1 L/min is approximately 10 L/min, whereas the cardiac output with a $\dot{V}O_2$ of 3 L/min is approximately 20 L/min.

The work capacity of patients with heart disease is also limited by their cardiac output. In general, cardiac patients generate the same maximal heart rates as do normal subjects, but because they have much lower stroke volumes than do normal individuals, the cardiac output at a given heart rate is reduced in proportion to the reduction in the stroke volume. In these patients the cardiac output can be improved by surgical correction of valvular defects, improvement of the perfusion of the myocardium by rehabilitative training or surgery, or administration of inotropic agents such as digitalis (40).

Hemoglobin Concentration

From Equation 6.7, it is obvious that Hb is a critical factor in determining $\dot{V}O_2$max. Either an abnormally high or a low Hb may be associated with a decreased work capacity. The explanation for the decrease in work capacity with a low Hb is obvious. Support for the relationship between the Hb and exercise tolerance is provided by a recent study of patients with kidney disease on chronic dialysis. When these patients were given erythropoietin such that their Hb increased from 7.3 to 10.8 g/dL, their exercise capacity increased from 108 to 130 watts (42).

The detrimental effects of a very high Hb on $\dot{V}O_2$max is not immediately apparent from Equation 6.6. Nevertheless, too high a hematocrit and Hb can result in increased viscosity of the blood, which in turn can decrease the maximum cardiac output. If the reduction in cardiac output is proportionately greater than the increase in Hb, $\dot{V}O_2$max is reduced. This appears to be the case for both the experimental animal and the COPD patient with polycythemia. In dogs the systemic oxygen transport during exercise is reduced when the animals are made polycythemic (43). In COPD patients, reduction of the hematocrit from above 60% to below 55% results in a marked improvement in exercise tolerance, which indicates that the increase in cardiac output is proportionately greater than the decrease in Hb (44).

In recent years, athletes have attempted to increase their performance by the administration of erythropoietin or transfusions; the practice is popularly called "blood doping." It appears that such practices do indeed result in a significant increase in the $\dot{V}O_2$max. One report summarized the results from 30 subjects who participated in four different investigations (45). These individuals exercised before and within 72 hours of reinfusing two 450-mL blood units. Overall erythrocyte reinfusion led to a mean increase in the $\dot{V}O_2$max of 0.357 L/min. In general, for every 1% increase in Hb there was a 1% increase in the $\dot{V}O_2$max, but there was marked interindividual variability in this relationship. At the present time the policing of blood doping via transfusion or the administration of erythropoietin is a major problem for sporting organizations (46).

Smoking can affect work capacity by transforming normal hemoglobin into carboxyhemoglobin (CO-Hb), which has no value in terms of O_2 transport. Smokers generally have CO-Hb values around 4% to 7%. In normal subjects it has been shown that $\dot{V}O_2$max decreases proportionately to the level of CO-Hb. A CO-Hb of 10% is associated with approximately a 10% decrease in the $\dot{V}O_2$max (1).

Peripheral O_2 Extraction ($S\bar{v}O_2$)

During exercise there is increased O_2 extraction by the exercising muscles, which results in a lowered mixed venous saturation ($S\bar{v}O_2$). The contribution of the decreased $S\bar{v}O_2$ to $\dot{V}O_2$ is obvious from Equation 6.7. Mixed venous blood is a mixture of the venous blood returning to the right heart from exercising muscles and from the remainder of the body. Blood returning from heavily exercising muscles is quite desaturated, with a $P\bar{v}O_2$ of 10 to 15 mm Hg and an $S\bar{v}O_2$ less than 10% (47). In superbly conditioned subjects at exhaustion, the mixed venous saturation averages about 10% (47).

Some authors have proposed that exercise is limited by the diffusion of oxygen from the capillaries to the mitochondria in the exercising muscles (38). In particular, there seems to be a "bottleneck" in the diffusion of oxygen from the capillary to the mitochondria as the oxygen enters the muscle cell before it combines with myoglobin (38). However, most maintain that the oxygen delivery to the muscles is the factor that limits exercise, because the hemoglobin is less than 10% saturated in blood emanating from a highly trained muscle.

During exercise the distribution of the systemic vascular resistance is altered so that a higher percentage of the blood is distributed to the exercising muscles. In unfit people this vasoregulation during exercise is suboptimal. They fail to adjust their regional peripheral vascular resistance, and so their exercising muscles receive less of the cardiac output. Therefore, their $S\bar{v}O_2$ at exhaustion is considerably higher than 25%. It follows from Equation 6.7 that their $\dot{V}O_2$ at a given level of cardiac output is lower than it is in the conditioned individual, since the $SaO_2 - S\bar{v}O_2$ is smaller (36). Other dysfunctions of the peripheral circulation can also result in a suboptimal distribution of cardiac output and a high $S\bar{v}O_2$ at maximal exercise.

Arterial Oxygen Saturation (SaO₂)

The SaO_2 depends on the alveolar O_2 tension (PAO_2) and the alveolar-arterial O_2 gradient ($PAO_2 - PaO_2$). The PAO_2 in turn is dependent on the partial pressure of the inspired O_2 (PIO_2), the $PaCO_2$, and the respiratory exchange ratio *(R)*, as shown by the alveolar air equation:

$$PAO_2 = PIO_2 - PaCO_2 \times [FIO_2 + (1 - FIO_2)/R]$$
$$(6.8)$$

where FIO_2 is the fractional concentration of O_2 in inspired gas. Note that an elevation of $PaCO_2$ will decrease the PAO_2. In normal subjects the $PaCO_2$ tends to remain constant or decrease with increasing levels of exercise to maintain a constant pH (48). Therefore the PAO_2 remains constant or increases. However, in some patients with COPD, the ventilatory reserve is insufficient to eliminate the additional CO_2 produced with exercise. Accordingly, the $PaCO_2$ increases and the PAO_2 decreases (49). For a given level of pulmonary dysfunction, patients in whom the $PaCO_2$ increases during exercise will have higher exercise tolerance, because they do not have to breathe as much to get rid of the same amount of CO_2 (49).

The $PAO_2 - PaO_2$ results from venous admixture ($\dot{Q}va/\dot{Q}t$), which is the fraction of the cardiac output that reaches arterial blood and acts as though it had not been exposed to alveolar gas. Venous admixture has three components: (a) that which results from the perfusion of units with low $\dot{V}/\dot{Q}$ ratios; (b) that which results from the failure of the capillary PO_2 and the alveolar PO_2 to reach equilibrium; and (c) that which results from true right-to-left shunts. In patients with lung disease, the majority of the $PAO_2 - PaO_2$ gradient is owing to inadequate ventilation of perfused alveoli. The amount of ventilation required to fully oxygenate the blood in a given alveolus is dependent on both the amount of perfusion and the degree of venous desaturation. West has shown that in a lung unit with a ventilation-perfusion ratio ($\dot{V}/\dot{Q}$) of unity the PaO_2 will fall from 100 to 42 mm Hg as PvO_2 falls from 100 to 10 mm Hg (50).

The best way to understand this phenomenon is to consider a numerical example. Table 6.3 lists the oxygen requirements to achieve full saturation of 100 mL blood at different $S\bar{v}O_2$ levels and the corresponding PAO_2 if this much oxygen is extracted from 100 mL of ventilated air. It can be seen that when the $S\bar{v}O_2$ falls below 55%, the resulting PAO_2 falls drastically, and accordingly the PaO_2

TABLE 6.3 INFLUENCE OF S$\dot{v}$O$_2$ ON PAO_2 ASSUMING R IS 0.8 AND HB 15 G/100 ML

S$\dot{v}$O$_2$ %	O$_2$ Required for SaO$_2$ = 100% ml	PAO_2 if SaO$_2$ = 100% $\dot{V}/\dot{Q}$ = 1	PAO_2 if SaO$_2$ = 100% $\dot{V}/\dot{Q}$ = 3
75	5	115	138
65	7	101	134
55	9	87	129
45	11	73	124
35	13	58	120
25	15	44	115

must fall. In the same example, if the $\dot{V}/\dot{Q}$ ratio had increased to 3, the PAO_2 would still be over 100 mm Hg when the $S\bar{v}O_2$ is 25%.

The preceding example illustrates that a $\dot{V}/\dot{Q}$ ratio of 1 is not ideal during exercise. If the $S\bar{v}O_2$ is substantially decreased, the $\dot{V}/\dot{Q}$ ratio must increase above 1, concomitantly, or arterial desaturation will result. The cardiac output of a normal subject at rest is about 5 L/min and increases fourfold to a level of 20 L/min on maximal exercise. The minute ventilation increases from 5 L/min at rest to 80 L/min during maximal exercise. Thus the overall $\dot{V}/\dot{Q}$ ratio increases from unity at rest to 4 to 1 during maximal exercise, and arterial desaturation does not normally result from the above mechanism.

Another factor that can increase the $PAO_2 - PaO_2$ is a reduced diffusing capacity of the lungs. If, at the end of the capillary, the PO_2 of the blood has not reached that of the alveolus, the $PAO_2 - PaO_2$ will be increased. Such an increase is said to be due to a diffusion abnormality. It is generally accepted that in normal individuals, complete equilibrium occurs between alveolar and capillary blood at most levels of exercise except when the individual is breathing low levels of oxygen. However, the SaO_2 is decreased in nearly 50% of elite cyclists and runners when they are performing maximally. A diffusion limitation is the most likely explanation for the desaturation in these athletes, but ventilation-perfusion imbalances could play a role (51).

It is thought that a reduced diffusing capacity does not contribute to the $PAO_2 - PaO_2$ at rest, even in patients with lung disease and markedly reduced diffusing capacities. However, when a patient with a reduced diffusing capacity exercises, equilibrium between the alveolar and capillary PO_2 may not occur, since the venous blood is more desaturated and the capillary transit time is shorter. Shepard, in a theoretical analysis, demonstrated that a reduced diffusing capacity can cause a substantial reduction in SaO_2 during exercise (52). Moreover, once the $PAO_2 - PaO_2$ is increased owing to diffusion limitations, slight increases in $\dot{V}O_2$ lead to dramatic reductions in SaO_2. For example, if the diffusing capacity is 16, the SaO_2 will start to fall when the $\dot{V}O_2$ reaches 1600 mL/min and will fall to less than 70% when the $\dot{V}O_2$ reaches 1800 mL/min, assuming that the $S\bar{v}O_2$ was

50%. In general, the higher the cardiac output, the more rapid the transit of blood in the pulmonary capillaries. Once the level is reached at which equilibrium between the alveoli and capillaries does not occur, further increases in the velocity of flow or decreases in $S\bar{v}O_2$ lead to large decreases in SaO_2.

The reduction in SaO_2 owing to a given fractional shunt ($\dot{Q}s/\dot{Q}t$) depends on the $S\bar{v}O_2$. For example, if the $\dot{Q}s/\dot{Q}t$ is 25%, the SaO_2 will be 94% if $S\bar{v}O_2$ is 75%, but will decrease to 81% if $S\bar{v}O_2$ is 25%. In view of the marked reduction in the $S\bar{v}O_2$ during strenuous exercise, one might expect that the SaO_2 would decrease substantially in many individuals during heavy exercise and that this reduction would limit their exercise capabilities. However, SaO_2 does not change in normal subjects even during exhaustive physical work. Most patients with lung disease have an increased $PAO_2 - PaO_2$ at rest, and the majority of this increase is owing to perfusion of units with low $\dot{V}/\dot{Q}$ ratios. As mentioned previously, patients with COPD increase their ventilation more than their cardiac output during exercise so that their PAO_2 does not decrease. This increase in total ventilation tends to improve the ventilation of units with low $\dot{V}/\dot{Q}$ ratios and decreases the fraction of the $\dot{Q}s/\dot{Q}t$ that is due to perfusion of poorly ventilated alveoli. The net effect of exercise on SaO_2 depends on whether the $\dot{Q}s/\dot{Q}t$ decreases enough to compensate for the decreased $S\bar{v}O_2$.

Ventilatory Limitation

As mentioned earlier, the cardiac output is the factor limiting exercise in normal subjects. At maximal exercise they have ventilatory reserve as manifested by their ability to increase their ventilation voluntarily. However, the exercise capacity of most individuals with moderate or severe lung disease is limited by their ventilatory abilities. Normal individuals are unable to maintain minute ventilations above 60% of their maximal voluntary ventilation (MVV). Patients with lung disease are also unable to sustain minute ventilations much above 60% of their MVV without developing dyspnea (53). Therefore, their exercise capabilities are limited by their ventilation even though their arterial blood gases frequently remain unchanged at exhaustion.

In addition to their reduced ventilatory reserves, patients with lung disease have increased ventilatory requirements for a given level of exercise. The ventilatory requirement is determined by the CO_2 production ($\dot{V}CO_2$), the $PaCO_2$, and the wasted ventilation fraction of each breath (VD/VT). In patients with lung disease, the VD/VT is much higher at rest (mean 0.45) than it is in normals (mean 0.28). Moreover, during exercise the VD/VT on the average does not change in patients with COPD, whereas it falls below 0.20 in normal individuals (49,54).

Therefore, the patient with lung disease needs more ventilation for a given work load. The ventilatory equivalent for CO_2 ($\dot{V}E/\dot{V}CO_2$) is a measure of the efficiency with which

additional CO_2 is eliminated. The normal $\dot{V}E/\dot{V}CO_2$ is about 30, but with COPD it can exceed 50 (55).

Anaerobic Metabolism

Exercise requires an increase in O_2 flow to the mitochondria of the exercising muscles. If the increase in O_2 flow is insufficient to generate the required ATP, anaerobic metabolism must be used to generate the ATP. The anaerobic threshold is the highest level of work that can be done without inducing a sustained metabolic acidosis. The anaerobic threshold normally occurs at between 50% and 60% of the $\dot{V}O_2$max.

Lactic acid is the end product of anaerobic metabolism. The metabolic acidosis that results from its accumulation produces the subjective feeling of fatigue that precludes extensive periods of anaerobic exercise. When lactic acid is produced it is immediately buffered, predominantly by the bicarbonate system:

$$H^+ \text{ lactate}^- + Na^+ HCO_3^-$$
$$\rightarrow Na^+ \text{lactate}^- + CO_2 + H_2O$$

The above reaction causes a reduction in the bicarbonate levels and an increase in the production of carbon dioxide gas. Until the anaerobic threshold is reached, the relationship between the work load or the $\dot{V}O_2$ and the $\dot{V}E$ is linear with progressive work loads. Above the anaerobic threshold $\dot{V}E$ increases more than $\dot{V}O_2$ for two reasons: (a) the increased carbon dioxide produced in the buffering of lactate must be eliminated, and (b) the metabolic acidosis produced in the buffering process acts as a respiratory stimulant so that $\dot{V}E$ increases more than the $\dot{V}CO_2$ and the $PaCO_2$ falls. In general, normal individuals and patients with cardiovascular or pulmonary disease attempt to regulate their ventilation such that the arterial pH remains stable (56).

The anaerobic threshold is best documented by demonstrating an increase in the blood lactate concentration. This is usually accompanied by a decrease in the plasma bicarbonate concentration. One can also try to identify the anaerobic threshold by examining the results of the expired gas analysis. One method is to plot $\dot{V}E$ versus the work load. The anaerobic threshold occurs when $\dot{V}E$ increases out of proportion to the work load (Fig. 6.13). A second method examines plots of the $\dot{V}E/\dot{V}O_2$ and the $\dot{V}E/\dot{V}CO_2$ versus the work load. The anaerobic threshold is the point where $\dot{V}E/\dot{V}O_2$ rises whereas $\dot{V}E/\dot{V}CO_2$ remains stable when plotted against work rate. A third method examines the relationship between the $\dot{V}O_2$ and the $\dot{V}CO_2$ and identifies the anaerobic threshold as the point where the $\dot{V}CO_2$ increases disproportionately to the $\dot{V}O_2$ (57). In general, noninvasive methods are relatively inaccurate in identifying the anaerobic threshold in patients with COPD (58). Moreover, the majority of patients with severe lung disease do not reach their anaerobic threshold (58).

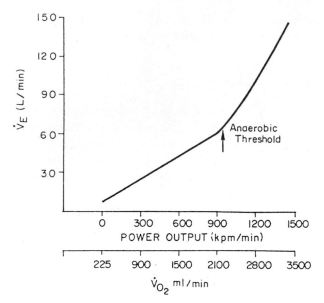

FIGURE 6.13. Determination of anaerobic threshold from plot of $\dot{V}_E$ versus work load or $\dot{V}_{O_2}$. The anaerobic threshold is identified as the work load at which the $\dot{V}_E$ starts to increase out of proportion to the $\dot{V}_{O_2}$ or the work load.

Training

It is widely recognized that it is possible to increase the maximum amount of exercise that a subject can perform by a period of physical training. By the same token, periods of inactivity will decrease the maximum amount of exercise that an individual can perform. In one study, $\dot{V}_{O_2}$max was measured in a group of elite Swedish swimmers at the height of their competitive swimming careers and then 4, 6, and 8 years after they had stopped swimming competitively (59). In these individuals the $\dot{V}_{O_2}$max decreased much more rapidly than would be expected from aging alone, and the rapid decrease persisted even between the sixth and eighth years. In another study, five adult males with varying degrees of physical fitness were studied before and after 21 days of bed rest and then periodically during 60 days of intensive reconditioning (Fig. 6.14) (60). During the 21 days of bed rest, $\dot{V}_{O_2}$max fell by over 25% in each of the five individuals. During the reconditioning period, $\dot{V}_{O_2}$max initially increased rapidly, then increased at a slower rate, and then appeared to level off after a mean of about 45 days. The $\dot{V}_{O_2}$max at the end of the training period had increased substantially more in the unfit than in the fit individuals.

In general, there are three different factors that should be considered in conditioning programs, namely, the intensity, the duration, and the frequency of the exercise (61). Of the three, the intensity is the most important. To increase $\dot{V}_{O_2}$max, the oxygen transport system must be challenged with exercise demanding at least 50% of the person's $\dot{V}_{O_2}$max. Moreover, the further above 50% of $\dot{V}_{O_2}$max is

the intensity of the exercise, the more rapid will be the improvement in $\dot{V}_{O_2}$max and the greater the eventual change. However, training should not be performed much above the anaerobic threshold. One can use the pulse to guide the intensity of exercise in that the anaerobic threshold is usually exceeded when the pulse is greater than 77% of the predicted maximal pulse (62). The exercise program should be performed at least twice a week, but every other day is preferable. The minimal duration of each training session should be 15 minutes, with 45 minutes optimal. The degree of improvement in $\dot{V}_{O_2}$max after 2 months of training is dependent on the initial level of fitness and the intensity of the exercise, as outlined in Table 6.4 (61).

The improvement in physical performance capacity that results from regularly performed, vigorous exercise involves multiple adaptive reactions occurring primarily in the circulatory system. The maximum cardiac output increases through an increase in the maximum stroke volume arising from two factors. First, the myocardial function improves, so that with a given peripheral vascular resistance the maximum cardiac output is increased. Second, local adaptive processes in the exercising muscle decrease the vascular resistance of the exercising muscles, so that the total vascular resistance is decreased and a higher fraction of the cardiac output is distributed to the exercising muscles. With conditioning, the improved myocardial function is a generalized process so that if nonconditioned muscles are exercised, the maximum cardiac output will still be increased. In contrast, the redistribution of the cardiac output is specific in that if nonconditioned muscles are exercised, the distribution of the cardiac output to them will not be facilitated.

An important byproduct of the redistribution of the cardiac output to the exercising muscles is its effect on $S\bar{v}_{O_2}$. When a larger fraction of the cardiac output goes to the exercising muscles, the $S\bar{v}_{O_2}$ decreases because of the very low $S\bar{v}_{O_2}$ of the larger fraction of the cardiac output returning from the exercising muscles. From Equation 6.7 it can be readily appreciated that this decrease in $S\bar{v}_{O_2}$ will increase $\dot{V}_{O_2}$max substantially.

Training also leads to changes in the muscle that has undergone training such that it can take up more oxygen (37). In particular, there is an increase in the oxidative capacity owing to an increase in mitochondrial volume and enhancement of the enzyme systems that promote the use of free fatty acids. These changes lead to a lower Sa_{O_2} at the end of the capillary. In addition, an increase in the vascular conductance owing to an increase in the capillary density increases oxygen extraction by increasing the surface area for oxygen movement.

It should be noted that the expected improvements outlined in Table 6.4 are those for normal individuals. Even though patients with COPD frequently have a very low $\dot{V}_{O_2}$max at the start of a physical training program, their $\dot{V}_{O_2}$max does not increase by as much as normals because

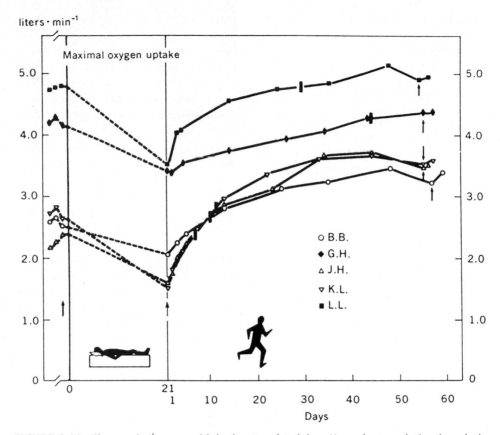

FIGURE 6.14. Changes in $\dot{V}o_2$max with bed rest and training. *Heavy bars* mark the time during the training period at which the maximal oxygen uptake had returned to the control value obtained before bed rest. Originally the top two patients were well conditioned, whereas the bottom three patients were poorly conditioned. (From Saltin B, Blomqvist G, Mitchell JH, et al. Response to exercise after bed rest and after training. A longitudinal study of adaptive changes in oxygen transport and body composition. *Circulation* 1968;38(Suppl 7):1. By permission of the American Heart Association, Inc.)

their ventilatory capabilities, which limit their exercise performance, do not increase significantly during a training program (63,64). In recent years there has been much interest in training the respiratory muscles of patients with lung disease. However, a recent meta-analysis of the results of respiratory muscle training concluded that there was little

evidence that patients with COPD clinically benefitted from respiratory muscle training (65).

Aging and Exercise Performance

As an individual ages, his or her capacity to exercise decreases. In untrained individuals there is an approximately 10% decrease per decade in the $\dot{V}o_2$max starting at age 25 (36). In trained individuals, the decrease in the $\dot{V}o_2$max is approximately 6% per decade (36). The initial $\dot{V}o_2$max is approximately 50% higher in the trained individual, but the absolute decrease in the $\dot{V}o_2$max is less in the trained individual. In the sedentary individual, most of the decline (72%) in the $\dot{V}o_2$max is due to a decreased cardiac output, whereas the remaining 28% is due to reduced peripheral oxygen extraction (36). Decreases in the stroke volume are more important than decreases in the maximal heart rate in producing the decrease in the $\dot{V}o_2$max (36). Interestingly, sedentary individuals above the age of 60 who embark on

TABLE 6.4 EXPECTED IMPROVEMENT IN $\dot{V}o_2$MAX AFTER TRAINING 3 TIMES A WEEK FOR 45 MINUTES FOR 2 MONTHS

Initial Status		Expected Improvement (%)		
Level of Fitness	$\dot{V}o_2$ max ml/kg/min	Exercise at 50–70% $\dot{V}o_2$max	Exercise at 70–90% $\dot{V}o_2$max	Exercise at 90–100% $\dot{V}o_2$max
Low	30	10	25	40
Medium	45	3	8	20
Excellent	60	0	0	5

a vigorous training program can improve their $\dot{V}O_2$max by approximately 25% (66). However, their exercise capabilities still remain far below those of individuals who remained trained throughout their lives (36,66).

Performance of Exercise Testing

Although the exercise test must in general be tailored to the individual patient, we believe that most exercise tests should be conducted along the following guidelines: The patient should be studied on a treadmill or bicycle ergometer at increasing work loads. The test should be performed in the presence of a physician and with constant cardiac monitoring. Resuscitation equipment, including a defibrillator, should be immediately at hand. The work load should be increased until the patient becomes physically exhausted.

However, it should be noted that the progressive ergometer test has little relevance to normal activities and may give no insight into the patient's difficulties in coping with daily living. Therefore, self-paced walking tests such as the 12-minute test or 6-minute test have been developed (67). These tests have the advantage of being a more natural test of exercise capacity. They are reproducible and simple. However, they give information only on overall exercise tolerance and they allow no physiologic measurements during the exercise. Self-paced walking tests have their greatest utility in evaluating the patient's response to a therapeutic intervention. In general, we prefer a 12-minute walking test because there is less variance (67).

An alternative to the 12-minute walk that has received attention lately is the shuttle walk. The patient walks in an oval with a largest diameter of 10 meters. The patient starts out walking slowly and each minute the walking speed is increased by 0.17 meters per second until the patient cannot keep up or is too short of breath to continue (68). Since this is a progressive test, its results correlate better with progressive exercise tests than do the 12-minute walk test. However, the 12-minute walk test probably is better correlated with the patient's activities of daily living.

The data collected during ergometer or treadmill exercise tests depend on the information desired from the test. In general, there are four stages of exercise testing (41). In stage 1 exercise testing, the patient is exercised at increasing work load until exhaustion, with monitoring of the heart rate and ventilation. An estimate of the $\dot{V}O_2$ can be obtained from nomograms that relate the power output or the treadmill grade and speed to the $\dot{V}O_2$ (41). Cardiovascular dysfunction is suggested by a stage 1 test demonstrating a heart rate that is high relative to the work load and an early onset of the anaerobic threshold as evidenced by nonlinear increases in ventilation. A ventilatory limitation is suggested when the maximum ventilation reaches 35 times the FEV_1 and the anaerobic threshold and the maximum predicted heart rates are not achieved.

In stage 2 exercise testing, mixed expired gases are also collected and analyzed. The additional information provided includes the $\dot{V}O_2$, the $\dot{V}CO_2$, the $\dot{V}E/\dot{V}O_2$, and the $\dot{V}E/\dot{V}CO_2$. Therefore, the aerobic capacity ($\dot{V}O_2$max) can be accurately determined. In addition, cardiac outputs and stroke volumes can be estimated if a rebreathing procedure is used to obtain the mixed venous PCO_2. These measurements are useful in further defining the factors limiting exercise but are unnecessary if the exercise capacity is normal. With stage 2 exercise testing, the end-tidal PCO_2 and PO_2 are usually also recorded. However, during exercise there is not a close correlation between the changes in the end-tidal PCO_2 and the arterial PCO_2 (69).

In stage 3 exercise testing, arterial blood gases are also collected. The additional data permit detection of hypoxemia, hypercapnia, and respiratory or metabolic acidosis during exercise. In addition, the VD/VT can be calculated. If the only reason for the measurement of arterial blood gases is to detect hypoxemia, a pulse oximeter is a possible noninvasive alternative. One study revealed that the when SaO_2 from the pulse oximetry was compared to SaO_2 as determined by cooximetry, the mean difference was 1.7% and the standard deviation of the difference was 2.9% (70).

In stage 4 exercise testing, a Swan-Ganz catheter is inserted into the pulmonary artery. The additional information provided includes the pressures in the lesser circulation, the mixed venous blood gases, and the cardiac output as calculated by the Fick method.

Predicted Values for $\dot{V}O_2$max

The following equations provide predicted values for the $\dot{V}O_2$max (71,72).

Males

$$\dot{V}O_2\text{max (L/min)} = 4.2 - 0.032 \times \text{age (SD} \pm 0.4) \tag{6.9}$$

$$\dot{V}O_2\text{max (mL/kg/min)} = 60 - 0.55 \times \text{age (SD} \pm 7.5) \tag{6.10}$$

Over the age of 55

$$\dot{V}O_2\text{max (L/min)} = 2.43 \text{ (SD} \pm 0.44) \tag{6.11}$$

$$\text{Work load (watts)} = 179 \text{ (SD} \pm 36) \tag{6.12}$$

Females

$$\dot{V}O_2\text{max (L/min)} = 2.6 - 0.014 \times \text{age (SD} \pm 0.4) \tag{6.13}$$

$$\dot{V}O_2\text{max (mL/kg/min)} = 48 - 0.37 \times \text{age (SD} \pm 7.0) \tag{6.14}$$

Over the age of 55

$$\dot{V}O_2\text{max (L/min)} = 1.49 \text{ (SD} \pm 0.31) \tag{6.15}$$

$$\text{Work load (watts)} = 104 \text{ (SD} \pm 25) \tag{6.16}$$

Use of Pulmonary Function and Exercise Tests

Pulmonary function tests and exercise tests can be used to answer many different questions. This section is organized according to the various questions that might be asked.

Does My Patient Have Lung Disease?

This is the question most frequently asked. The answer to this question is obtained primarily by comparing the results from a given individual to those obtained from a normal population. The predicted value of a test for a given patient represents the mean value of a group of normal individuals with similar characteristics. The characteristics involved depend on the test but usually include height, age, and sex. The predicted value is calculated from a prediction equation, usually an algebraic equation derived from multiple linear regression. Associated with each predicted value is a range representing the expected variation in the group of normal individuals. Conventionally this range has been defined as a somewhat arbitrary percentage of the predicted value. A better approach, which is gaining acceptance, is to use a range based on the standard error of the estimate obtained in the analysis of the normal group. In this manner, the range that includes 95% of the normal individuals can be calculated. A test result is labeled as abnormal only if it falls outside the range in which 95% of normals lie. This method takes into account intersubject variability. For specific equations, a number of references are available (73–80).

When a patient is initially evaluated, it is recommended that only spirometry be obtained. If the FVC, FEV_1, and FEV_1/FVC are all within normal limits, then one can assume that the patient does not have significant obstructive or restrictive ventilatory dysfunction (81). At times a diffusing capacity can be obtained in addition to the spirometry because patients with lung disease, especially pulmonary vascular disease, may have normal spirometry but an abnormal diffusing capacity. Usually there is no reason to obtain lung volume measurements or spirometry after the administration of bronchodilators in patients who have normal spirometry.

Inhalation challenge tests are useful at times in patients with normal spirometry. Asthma is an episodic disease and many patients have normal spirometry at least part of the time. Inhalational challenge tests can demonstrate airway hyperresponsiveness in such patients and suggest the diagnosis. In a similar manner, cough in some patients is due to airway hyperresponsiveness, and an inhalational challenge test may be necessary to demonstrate the airway hyperresponsiveness if the spirometry is within normal limits (11). It should be remembered that 3% to 6% of asymptomatic individuals do have airway hyperresponsiveness.

It should also be pointed out that the maximal exercise test is sometimes abnormal in patients with mild lung disease when the spirometry and diffusing capacity are normal. In one study of 30 patients with sarcoidosis, results from the maximal exercise tests were more sensitive than were spirometry or the diffusing capacity in identifying abnormalities. Excess ventilation and an increased V_D/V_T during exercise were the most common abnormality (82).

What Type of Lung Disease Does My Patient Have?

Once a patient has been found to have abnormal pulmonary function, the type and degree of dysfunction are sought. In general, abnormalities in pulmonary function can be classified as obstructive ventilatory dysfunction, restrictive ventilatory dysfunction, and mixed ventilatory dysfunction.

Obstructive Ventilatory Dysfunction
By definition, obstructive ventilatory dysfunction occurs when there are reduced expiratory flow rates with maximal effort owing to increased expiratory resistance. As discussed in Chapter 2, Mechanics of Respiration, the increased expiratory resistance can be due to either increased airway resistance or decreased elastic recoil of the lung.

In determining whether airway obstruction is present, one should look at the FEV_1/FVC and the FEV_3/FVC. In general, if the FEV_1/FVC is above 0.75 and the FEV_3/FVC is above 0.95 the patient does not have significant obstructive ventilatory dysfunction. The forced vital capacity is often reduced with moderate to severe airway obstruction as a result of air trapping. The peak expiratory flow and the forced expiratory flows at different lung volumes are also reduced.

The degree of obstructive ventilatory dysfunction can be quantitated as outlined in Table 6.5. The absolute value of the FEV_1 should be used only if the patient does not also have restrictive ventilatory dysfunction. The patient is classified according to the most severe criterion that he or she meets. For example, if the FEV_1/FVC is 0.35 and the FEV_1 is 1800 mL, the individual is classified as having severe obstructive ventilatory dysfunction.

Restrictive Ventilatory Dysfunction
By definition, restrictive pulmonary dysfunction indicates that the TLC is reduced. Most volume compartments are

TABLE 6.5 CRITERIA FOR QUANTITATING DEGREE OF OBSTRUCTION

Grade	FEV_1/FVC	FEV_1 (ml)
Very severe	<0.30	<600
Severe	0.3–0.4	600–1000
Moderate	0.4–0.6	1000–2000
Mild	0.6–0.7	2000–3000
Very mild	0.7–pred. value	>3000

affected, which results in decreases in VC, RV, and FRC as well as the total lung capacity. Frequently the residual volume is not reduced by as great a percentage as the other lung volumes. A diagnosis of restrictive impairment is made when the vital capacity falls below the predicted normal range and is associated with reductions in the other volume compartments. If the FVC is within normal limits, it is unlikely that the TLC will be abnormal and lung volume measurements are usually not indicated in this situation (81). If the patient has no obstructive ventilatory dysfunction, restrictive ventilatory dysfunction can be established from spirometry. However, if the patient has obstructive ventilatory dysfunction the FVC can be reduced due to the obstruction, and therefore the diagnosis of restrictive ventilatory dysfunction can only be established if lung volumes, including RV, are measured. In one recent study of 206 patients with obstructive ventilatory dysfunction and a reduced FVC, only 40 (19%) had restrictive pulmonary dysfunction when lung volume measurements were obtained (81). When both the FEV_1 and the FVC are reduced with spirometry, one can get some idea whether the individual has predominantly obstructive or restrictive ventilatory dysfunction by comparing the value for the FEV_1 and the FVC expressed as a percentage of the predicted value. If the individual has predominantly restrictive dysfunction, the FVC will be reduced proportionately more than the FEV_1. Alternatively, if the individual has predominantly obstructive dysfunction, the FEV_1 will be reduced proportionately more than the FVC.

The degree of restrictive ventilatory dysfunction can be quantitated as outlined in Table 6.6. Results of other ventilatory function tests—such as time forced expiratory volumes, expiratory flows, and MVV—are either normal or slightly reduced with restrictive impairment. Although the FEV_1 and FEV_3 expressed as a percentage of the predicted value are reduced in individuals with restrictive ventilatory dysfunction, the FEV_1/FVC and the FEV_3/FVC are normal or greater than predicted, which indicates an absence of airway obstruction.

Mixed Ventilatory Dysfunction

Some patients have both obstructive and restrictive ventilatory dysfunction. Lung volume measurements, including a determination of the residual volume, are necessary in such cases to quantitate the degree of dysfunction. Since the

TABLE 6.6 CRITERIA FOR QUANTITATING DEGREE OF RESTRICTION

Grade	VC % Predicted	TLC % Predicted
Very mild	>80	>90
Mild	60–80	70–90
Moderate	30–60	50–70
Severe	<30	<50

FEV_1 is reduced from the restrictive dysfunction, only the FEV_1/FVC should be used in quantitating the obstruction.

Does My Patient Have Predominantly Asthma, Chronic Bronchitis, or Emphysema?

The three main diseases that produce obstructive ventilatory dysfunction are asthma, chronic bronchitis, and emphysema. Some indication as to the pathogenesis of the obstruction can be obtained from the pulmonary function laboratory. However, it must be noted that in the older smoker the obstructive ventilatory dysfunction is usually due to a combination of all three diseases.

Measures of airway resistance are useful in separating the three entities. With pure emphysema, airway resistance is normal and the expiratory flow limitation is due to loss of lung elastic recoil. Therefore, an increased airway resistance indicates that the airways are abnormal and that the patient has a component of asthma or bronchitis. Emphysema results in destruction of pulmonary parenchyma and therefore loss of surface area for gas exchange. Accordingly, the DLco is reduced with emphysema, whereas it is normal with asthma or chronic bronchitis.

Bronchodilator Testing

By definition the obstructive ventilatory dysfunction with asthma is reversible. Therefore, many laboratories perform spirometry before and after administration of bronchodilators to distinguish asthma from chronic bronchitis and emphysema. A positive response is usually said to be present if the FEV_1 improves by at least 15% and 200 mL above baseline. However, it should be noted that most patients who appear to have chronic bronchitis or emphysema will have an improvement of 15% or more in their FEV_1 if they are repeatedly tested (83). It does appear that responses to bronchodilators are useful in predicting responses to oral corticosteroids in patients with COPD. Nisar and coworkers (84) administered 5 mg albuterol and 500 μg ipratropium bromide acutely to 100 patients with COPD (mean age 62 and mean $FEV_1 \sim 1,000$ mL). They reported that 33 responded to neither, 16 responded to albuterol only, 17 responded to ipratropium only, and 34 responded to both. Twenty-two patients improved after oral corticosteroid administration for 2 weeks, including 10 who improved after acute administration of both albuterol and ipratropium, five who improved only after acute administration of albuterol, two who improved only after acute administration of ipratropium, and three who did not improve after acute administration of either drug (84). Other studies have failed to demonstrate a relationship between the short-term response to bronchodilators and the long-term improvement with bronchodilators (85).

Large Airway Obstruction

A relatively uncommon cause of obstructive ventilatory dysfunction is upper or large airway obstruction. However, it is important not to overlook this possibility, because its presence is life-threatening. Upper airway obstruction is manifested as reduced flows early in expiration and normal flows during the latter part of the expiration (Fig. 6.4C). If the obstruction in the large airway is variable, its site inside or outside the thoracic inlet determines its effects on flow rates. Variable intrathoracic obstruction primarily affects forced expiratory flows, since positive pleural pressures cause further decrease in the size of the large airway. Variable extrathoracic obstruction affects forced inspiration, since the intratracheal negative pressure on inspiration tends to make the trachea collapse more. These changes are best demonstrated with the flow-volume loop as described above. The ratio of the FEV_1 to the $FEV_{0.5}$ is almost always greater than 1.5 except when obstruction of the large airways is present (86).

Is My Patient Going to Develop Lung Disease?

In the natural history of COPD, disease first develops in the small peripheral airways. Since only 10% to 20% of the total airway resistance is in these airways, the usual tests for obstructive ventilatory dysfunction, such as the FEV_1/FVC, are normal when significant disease is present (87). Accordingly, many different tests have been proposed, including the closing volume, the slope of phase III on the single-breath nitrogen washout test, comparison of flow-volume loops obtained with room air and a mixture of helium and oxygen, and sophisticated analyses of the forced expiratory spirogram. However, none of these has been shown to be very useful in predicting the development of significant COPD, and they are not recommended (24). A more cost-effective alternative is to ask the patient if he or she smokes. If the answer is affirmative, efforts should be expended to get him or her to stop smoking.

Is My Patient Responding to Therapy?

Once the diagnosis of pulmonary dysfunction is confirmed and therapy is undertaken, how should the response of the patient to therapy be monitored? The simplest way is to ask the patient how he or she feels. However, patients with lung disease are notoriously poor at assessing their pulmonary function. In one study of 82 asthmatics, more than 20% had an FEV_1 less than 70% of predicted when they were symptom free, and many did not become symptomatic when the FEV_1 fell to less than 50% of predicted after the inhalation of methacholine (88). Likewise, the physical examination of patients with COPD is less than ideal in quantitating the response to therapy. It has been shown that there is a very poor correlation between the auscultatory findings and the pulmonary function test results in patients with COPD (89).

Therefore, to evaluate the response to therapy, serial tests of pulmonary function should be obtained. Usually spirom-

etry is sufficient, and it is recommended that spirometry be performed each time a patient with pulmonary dysfunction is seen. The best indices for following patients with obstructive lung disease are the absolute values of the FEV_1 and the FVC, and not the FEV_1/FVC ratio, since the latter is very dependent on the duration of expiration. However, it should be noted that spirometry is not perfect for assessing the response to therapy. For the patient the most important consideration is whether his or her functional capabilities improve. However, significant improvements in spirometric results are not necessarily associated with increased exercise tolerance (90). Nevertheless, it is impractical to perform repeated exercise tests on most patients with pulmonary dysfunction.

Recent theories concerning the pathogenesis of chronic airway obstruction have focused on airway inflammation and airway hyperresponsiveness (11). Accordingly, serial inhalational challenge tests are being used more and more frequently to assess a patient's response to a therapeutic regimen. For example, a recent study documented that when aerosolized steroids were given to 16 mild asthmatics for 1 year, the hyperresponsiveness improved in 15 of the 16, and in five individuals the methacholine test became normal (91). Although at the present time such tests are used primarily in research situations, their use in the clinical setting will probably become more widespread in the future.

Why Is My Patient Short of Breath on Exertion?

Many patients complain of exercise intolerance. An explanation for the exercise intolerance is frequently lacking even after a careful history, physical examination, chest roentgenogram, electrocardiogram, and routine tests of pulmonary function. The performance of an exercise test frequently permits identification of the factor producing limitation in an individual patient. The characteristic profiles of exercise tests in patients limited by obstructive ventilatory dysfunction, exercise-induced asthma, restrictive ventilatory dysfunction, pulmonary hypertension, cardiovascular dysfunction, poor physical condition, and poor effort are described in the following section.

Obstructive Ventilatory Dysfunction

The exercise capacity of most patients with COPD is limited by their respiratory system. In general, this limitation is due to the facts that their ventilatory capacity is limited by their lung disease and that their ventilatory requirement for a given work load is increased since their wasted ventilation (V_D/V_T) is increased. The cardiovascular response to exercise in patients with COPD appears to be relatively normal, since the cardiac output for a given $\dot{V}O_2$ is normal (92).

The typical results of an exercise test of a patient with ventilatory limitation are as follows: (a) the patient stops exercising due to shortness of breath rather than leg fatigue (although even among those with FEV_1 below 40% of predicted, a sizable percentage stop on account of leg fatigue) (93); (b) the $\dot{V}O_2max$ is reduced, and $\dot{V}E$ at exhaustion is at least 35 times the FEV_1 or 70% of the MVV (93); (c) the VD/VT at rest is usually elevated and does not decrease with exercise, and the $\dot{V}CO_2/\dot{V}E$ is above 30; (d) for a given $\dot{V}O_2$ the heart rate is higher than normal, but the maximum heart rate is reduced because the $\dot{V}O_2max$ is so low (34); (e) the anaerobic threshold is frequently not reached due to the ventilatory limitation; (f) arterial blood gases during exercise may be unchanged from rest or may reveal an increased $PaCO_2$ or a decreased PaO_2.

Exercise-Induced Asthma

Exercise can precipitate bronchospasm in some individuals. If exercise-induced asthma is suspected, spirometry should be obtained before the exercise test and at 5-minute intervals after completion of the exercise test. The exercise should be for 6 to 8 minutes at an intensity of 85% to 90% of the predicted maximal heart rate. The diagnosis is established if the FEV_1 falls more than 10% after performance of the exercise test (94).

Restrictive Ventilatory Dysfunction

Restrictive lung disease encompasses a large and diverse group of disorders characterized by a diminished lung volume. In general, the functional disability in these patients is often out of proportion to the impairment in lung function and there is only a weak correlation ($r \sim 0.5$) between any resting measure of lung function and the exercise tolerance (95,96). Abnormal gas exchange is a major factor limiting exercise in patients with significant pulmonary interstitial disease. This is manifested during exercise by a decline in arterial oxygen saturation, a widened alveolar-arterial oxygen gradient and elevated VD/VT (95). The reduced FVC results in a relatively low maximal tidal volume, which necessitates a very high respiratory rate. This limitation, coupled with a decreased efficiency of gas exchange (increased VD/VT), leads to decreased exercise tolerance. Arterial blood gases during exercise usually reveal hypoxemia, and endurance exercise can be prolonged with supplemental oxygen (97).

Pulmonary Hypertension

The exercise tolerance as reflected by the $\dot{V}O_2max$ of patients with primary pulmonary hypertension is markedly reduced. The exercise capacity of these patients appears to be limited by a low cardiac output due to a decrease in the functional pulmonary vascular bed. The anaerobic threshold occurs at a relatively low work load, and the oxygen pulse is much lower than normal. The PaO_2 also tends to decrease in these patients with exercise. Although the ventilation at any given work load is higher in these patients than in normals (due to the increased VD/VT and the early onset of anaerobic metabolism), there is no evidence that these patients are

ventilatory limited (98). Exercise testing in patients with pulmonary hypertension carries a significant mortality risk and should not be performed when there is a history of arrhythmias or syncope, or clinical signs of right heart failure (33).

Cardiovascular Dysfunction

The exercise capacity of patients with cardiovascular dysfunction is limited by their cardiac output, as is that of normals. The main abnormality in such patients is a decreased stroke volume. Accordingly, their cardiac output at a given heart rate is less than normal. The maximum heart rate is also often reduced (40,99). Interestingly, there is a poor correlation between the left ventricular ejection fraction and the $\dot{V}O_2max$ (99). The $\dot{V}O_2max$ has been used to select patients for cardiac transplantation since a $\dot{V}O_2max$ of less than 12 mL/kg identifies a group of patients with a poor 1-year prognosis (99). When patients with cardiac dysfunction undergo maximal exercise tests, about 50% stop because of fatigue and about 50% stop because of dyspnea. The patients who stop due to dyspnea do not appear to have less ventilatory reserve than those who stop because of fatigue (100).

The typical results of an exercise test in a patient with cardiac dysfunction are as follows (55): (a) the $\dot{V}O_2max$ is reduced but the $\dot{V}E$ is less than 35 times the FEV_1 and less than 70% of the MVV; (b) the VD/VT is near normal and the $\dot{V}CO_2/\dot{V}E$ is below 30; (c) the heart rate is elevated relative to the $\dot{V}O_2$ (owing to the low stroke volume) and the anaerobic threshold is reached at a low $\dot{V}O_2$; (d) arterial blood gases reveal a normal PaO_2 but a reduced $PaCO_2$ and a metabolic acidosis.

Lack of Fitness

The results of exercise tests in an unfit individual are similar to those in a patient with cardiovascular disease. The anaerobic threshold will be reached at a low $\dot{V}O_2$ because of the poor distribution of the cardiac output. The maximum heart rate is normal and the $\dot{V}E$ is below 35 times the FEV_1. Arterial blood gases are similar to those of patients with cardiovascular dysfunction.

Malingering

Some individuals complain of exercise intolerance when their initial evaluation reveals no abnormalities that can explain such intolerance. Frequently the question arises as to whether they are actually impaired, particularly when litigation or disability compensation is involved. When subjected to a maximal exercise test, such individuals may not give maximum effort. Therefore, they have decreased $\dot{V}O_2max$. However, aside from this decrease, there is no evidence that they are limited by any of the above mechanisms. More specifically, their $\dot{V}E$ is less than 35 times their FEV_1; their maximal heart rate is reduced, but the $\dot{V}O_2$ for a given heart rate is normal; they fail to reach their anaerobic threshold and their blood lactate levels are less than 8 mM/L; and arterial blood gases do not demonstrate hypercapnia, hypoxia, or a metabolic acidosis.

If an individual appears not to give a maximum effort, a good approximation of their actual $\dot{V}O_2$max can be obtained by extrapolating the results of their exercise test to the maximal predicted heart rate, as shown in Figure 6.12. If their ventilatory reserve at exhaustion is less than their cardiac reserve percentagewise, then the extrapolation should be made with the ventilation rather than with the heart rate.

Is My Patient Physically Impaired from His or Her Lung Disease?

New and revised social legislation entitles an increasing number of Americans to compensation for disability. As a result, physicians are being asked more and more frequently to quantify impairment of health. The term impairment implies a physiologic, anatomic, or mental functional deficit, whereas the term disability implies an inability to perform or a limitation in the performance of tasks within a social environment. Rating of impairment falls within the sphere of the physician's expertise. In contrast, adjudication of disability requires consideration of additional factors, such as educational or cultural level and availability of suitable work, and is generally an administrative function outside the realm of the physician's practice (101). The following discussion concerns itself only with quantifying the degree of impairment. The recommendations are those of the American Thoracic Society (102,103).

Tests of Pulmonary Function

In the evaluation of respiratory impairment, the first step is to obtain pulmonary function testing. It is recommended that this initial testing include both forced spirometry measurements and testing for single-breath diffusing capacity. The results of these tests will allow the majority of subjects to be appropriately categorized as to their degree of impairment as follows:

Normal. FVC $\geq$80% of predicted, *and* FEV$_1$ $\geq$80% of predicted, and FEV$_1$/FVC $\geq$0.75, *and* DLCO $\geq$80% of predicted

Mildly impaired (usually not correlated with diminished ability to perform most jobs). FVC 60% to 79% predicted, *or* FEV$_1$ 60% to 79% predicted, *or* FEV$_1$/FVC 0.60 to 0.74, *or* DLCO 60% to 79% of predicted

Moderately impaired (progressively lower levels of lung function correlated with diminishing ability to meet the physical demands of many jobs). FVC 51% to 59% of predicted, *or* FEV$_1$ 41% to 59% of predicted, *or* FEV$_1$/FVC 0.41 to 0.59, *or* DLCO 41% to 59% of predicted

Severely impaired (unable to meet the physical demands of most jobs, including travel to work). FVC 50% or less of predicted, *or* FEV$_1$ 40% or less of predicted, *or* FEV$_1$/FVC less than 0.40, *or* DLCO 40% or less of predicted

Exercise Testing

Subjects found to have no impairment or mild impairment on the basis of their pulmonary function tests are usually able to perform all but the most unusually physically demanding of jobs. Patients with severe impairment usually are unable to perform almost all jobs, if for no other reason than that they are frequently unable to travel back and forth to their place of work.

Patients with mild or moderate impairment who complain of shortness of breath while working should be considered as possible candidates for exercise testing. Exercise testing is useful because there is not a close relationship between tests of pulmonary function and $\dot{V}O_2$max (Fig. 6.15). In such cases the exercise testing is performed for two reasons. First, to determine whether an individual is significantly impaired, and second, to determine whether the impairment is due to pulmonary dysfunction or some other cause. At a minimum, the testing should include measurement of ventilation ($\dot{V}E$), tidal volume, and frequency of breathing. Most testing should be done in laboratories that can also measure the composition of expired gas and arterial oxygen saturation.

The following rating of impairment is recommended:

1. If the $\dot{V}O_2$max is greater than 25 mL/kg per minute, then the subject will be capable of continuous heavy exertion throughout an 8-hour shift of all but the most physically demanding of jobs.
2. If the $\dot{V}O_2$ is between 15 and 25 mL/kg per minute and 40% of the observed $\dot{V}O_2$max is greater than the average metabolic work requirement of the subject's job, then the subject should be able to perform that job comfortably.
3. If the $\dot{V}O_2$max is less than 15 mL/kg per minute, then the subject will be unable to perform most jobs because he or she will be uncomfortable in traveling back and forth to the place of employment.

Impairment with Asthma

The determination of impairment in patients with asthma differs from that with other respiratory diseases because of the following factors: (a) in asthmatics the condition is much more variable; (b) the condition is associated with hyperresponsiveness to various agents such as dusts, fumes, and gases that the patient may encounter while working; (c) environmental or occupational exposures may increase airway inflammation, which on repeated exposures can become chronic and irreversible.

The American Thoracic Society has also developed guidelines for the evaluation of impairment in patients with

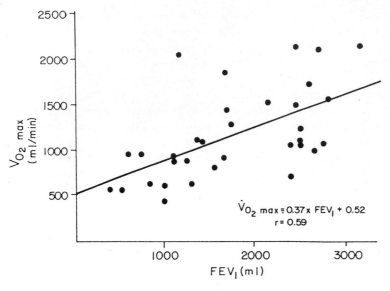

FIGURE 6.15. Relationship between the $\dot{V}_{O_2}$max and the FEV_1. Note how poorly the $\dot{V}_{O_2}$max correlates with the FEV_1. (Data courtesy VD Minh.)

asthma (103). In summary, these guidelines suggest the following three factors be considered in determining the level of impairment: (a) the postbronchodilator FEV_1; (b) the reversibility of the FEV_1 or the degree of airway hyperresponsiveness; and (c) the minimal amount of medication required by the patient. An asthmatic is severely impaired if the FEV_1 is less than 50% of predicted while taking at least 20 mg prednisone orally. The reader is referred to the recent ATS statement for further details about impairment in the asthmatic (103).

REFERENCES

1. Pulmonary terms and symbols: a report of the ACCP-ATS Joint Committee on Pulmonary Nomenclature. *Chest* 1975;67: 583–593.
2. Official statement of the American Thoracic Society. Standardization of spirometry—1994 update. *Am J Respir Crit Care Med* 1995;152:1107–1136.
3. Cochrane GM, Prieto F, Clark TJ. Intrasubject variability of maximal expiratory flow volume curve. *Thorax* 1977;32: 171–176.
4. Hyatt RE, Black LF. The flow volume curve: a current perspective. *Am Rev Respir Dis* 1973;107:191–199.
5. Kapp MC, Schachter EN, Beck GJ, et al. The shape of the maximum expiratory flow volume curve. *Chest* 1988;94: 799–806.
6. Meadows JA III, Rodarte JR, Hyatt RE. Density dependence of maximal expiratory flow in chronic obstructive pulmonary disease. *Am Rev Respir Dis* 1980;121:47–53.
7. Heaf PJD, Gillam PMS. Peak flow rates in normal and asthmatic children. *Br Med J* 1962;1:1595–1596.
8. National Heart, Lung, and Blood Institute. National Asthma Education Program: expert panel report 2: guidelines for the diagnosis and treatment of asthma. Bethesda, MD: National Institutes of Health; May 1997 (NIH publication No. 97-4051).
9. Jain P, Kavuru MS, Emerman CL, et al. Utility of peak expiratory flow monitoring. *Chest* 1998;114:861–876.
10. Campbell SC. A comparison of the maximum voluntary ventilation with the forced expiratory volume in one second: an assessment of subject cooperation. *J Occup Med* 1982;24:531–533.
11. Cockcroft DW, Hargreave FE. Airway hyperresponsiveness. Relevance of random population data to clinical usefulness. *Am Rev Respir Dis* 1990;142:497–500.
12. Rijcken B, Schouten JP, Mensinga TT, et al. Factors associated with bronchial responsiveness to histamine in a population sample of adults. *Am Rev Respir Dis* 1993;147:1447–1453.
13. Buist AS, Connett JE, Miller RD, et al. Chronic obstructive pulmonary disease early intervention trial (Lung Health Study). Baseline characteristics of randomized participants. *Chest* 1993; 103:1863–1872.
14. O'Connor GT, Sparrow D, Weiss ST. A prospective longitudinal study of methacholine airway responsiveness as a predictor of pulmonary function decline: the normative aging study. *Am J Respir Crit Care Med* 1995;152:87–92.
15. Meneely GR, Ball CO, Kory RC, et al. A simplified closed circuit helium dilution method for the determination of the residual volume of the lungs. *Am J Med* 1960;28:824–831.
16. Darling RC, Cournand A, Richards DW. Studies on the intrapulmonary mixing of gases. II. An open circuit method for measuring residual air. *J Clin Invest* 1940;19:609–618.
17. Burns CB, Scheinhorn DJ. Evaluation of single-breath helium dilution total lung capacity in obstructive lung disease. *Am Rev Respir Dis* 1984;130:580–583.
18. Dubois AB, Botelho SY, Bedell GN, et al. A rapid plethysmographic method for measuring thoracic gas volume: a comparison with a nitrogen washout method for measuring functional residual capacity in normal subjects. *J Clin Invest* 1956;35: 322–326.
19. Dubois AB, Botelho SY, Comroe JH Jr. A new method for measuring airway resistance in man using a body plethysmograph: values in normal subjects and in patients with respiratory disease. *J Clin Invest* 1956;35:327–335.
20. Comroe JH, Fowler WS. Lung function studies. IV. Detection of uneven alveolar ventilation during a single breath of oxygen: a new test of pulmonary disease. *Am J Med* 1951;10:408–413.
21. Buist AS, Ross BR. Quantitative analysis of the alveolar plateau in the diagnosis of early airway obstruction. *Am Rev Respir Dis* 1973;108:1078–1087.

22. Menkes HA, Beaty TH, Cohen BH, et al. Nitrogen washout and mortality. *Am Rev Respir Dis* 1985;132:115–119.

23. McCarthy DS, Spencer R, Greene R, et al. Measurements of "closing volume" as a simple and sensitive test for early detection of small airway disease. *Am J Med* 1972;52:747–753.

24. Buist AS, Vollmer WM, Johnson LR, et al. Does the single-breath N_2 test identify the smoker who will develop chronic airflow limitation? *Am Rev Respir Dis* 1988;127:293–301.

25. Crapo RO, Hankinson JL, Irvin C, et al. Single-breath carbon monoxide diffusing capacity (transfer factor). Recommendations for a standard Technique—1995 update. *Am J Respir Crit Care Med* 1995;152:2185–2198.

26. Lewis BM, Lin TH, Noe FE, et al. The measurement of pulmonary diffusing capacity for carbon monoxide by a rebreathing method. *J Clin Invest* 1959;38:2073–2086.

27. Official statement of the American Thoracic Society. Single breath carbon monoxide diffusing capacity (transfer factor). Recommendations for a standard technique. *Am Rev Respir Dis* 1987;136:1299–1307.

28. Weinberger SE, Johnson TS, Weiss ST. Use and interpretation of the single breath diffusing capacity. *Chest* 1980;78:483–488.

29. Bates DV, Varvis CJ, Donevan RE, et al. Variations in the pulmonary capillary blood volume and membrane diffusion component in health and disease. *J Clin Invest* 1960;39:1401–1412.

30. Ferris BG, ed. Epidemiology standardization project: recommended standardized procedures for pulmonary function testing. *Am Rev Respir Dis* 1978;118(pt 2):62–72.

31. Marrades RM, Diaz O, Roca J, et al. Adjustment of D_{LCO} for hemoglobin concentration. *Am J Respir Crit Care Med* 1997;155:236–241.

32. Larsen KR, Svendsen UG, Milman N, et al. Exercise testing in the preoperative evaluation of patients with bronchogenic carcinoma. *Eur Respir J* 1997;10:1559–1565.

33. Roca J, Whipp BJ, Agusti AGN, et al. Clinical exercise testing with reference to lung diseases: indications, standardization and interpretation strategies. *Eur Respir J* 1997;10:2662–2689.

34. Wasserman K, Hansen JE, Sue DY, et al. *Principles of exercise testing and interpretation.* Philadelphia: Lea & Febiger, 1994.

35. Sutton JR. Limitations to maximal oxygen uptake. *Sports Med* 1992;13:127–133.

36. Ogawa T, Spina RJ, Martin WH III, et al. Effects of aging, sex and physical training on cardiovascular responses to exercise. *Circulation* 1992;86:494–503.

37. Crawford MH. Physiologic consequences of systematic training. *Cardiol Clin* 1992;10:209–221.

38. Honig CR, Connett RJ, Gayeski TEJ. O_2 transport and its interaction with metabolism: a systems view of aerobic capacity. *Med Sci Sports Exerc* 1992;24:47–53.

39. Myers J, Walsh D, Buchanan N, et al. Can maximal cardiopulmonary capacity be recognized by a plateau in oxygen uptake? *Chest* 1989;96:1312–1316.

40. Arnold SB, Byrd RC, Meister W, et al. Long-term digitalis therapy improves left ventricular function in heart failure. *N Engl J Med* 1980;303:1443–1448.

41. Jones NL, Campbell EJM. *Clinical exercise testing,* 2nd ed. Philadelphia: Saunders, 1981.

42. Barany P, Freyschuss U, Pettersson E, et al. Treatment of anaemia in haemodialysis patients with erythropoietin: long-term effects on exercise capacity. *Clin Sci* 1993;84:441–447.

43. Weiss AB, Calton FM, Kuida H, et al. Hemodynamic effects of normovolemic polycythemia in dogs at rest and during exercise. *Am J Physiol* 1964;207:1361–1366.

44. Chetty KG, Light RW, Stansbury DW, et al. Exercise performance of polycythemic chronic obstructive pulmonary disease patients. Effect of phlebotomies. *Chest* 1990;98:1073–1077.

45. Sawka MN, Young AJ, Muza SR, et al. Erythrocytes reinfusion and maximal aerobic power. *JAMA* 1987;257:1496–1499.

46. Birkeland KI, Hemmersbach P. The future of doping control in athletes. Issues related to blood sampling. *Sports Med* 1999;28:25–33.

47. Astrand PO, Rodahl K. *Textbook of work physiology,* 2nd ed. New York: McGraw-Hill, 1977.

48. Oren A, Wasserman K, Davis JA, et al. Effect of CO_2 set point on ventilatory response to exercise. *J Appl Physiol* 1981;51:185–189.

49. Light RW, Mahutte CK, Brown SE. Etiology of CO_2 retention at rest and during exercise in chronic airflow obstruction. *Chest* 1988;94:61–67.

50. West JB. Ventilation-perfusion relationships. *Am Rev Respir Dis* 1977;116:919–943.

51. Powers SK, Martin D, Dodd S. Exercise-induced hypoxaemia in elite endurance athletes. Incidence, causes and impact on $\dot{V}_{O_2}$max. *Sports Med* 1993;16:14–22.

52. Shepard RH. Effect of pulmonary diffusion capacity on exercise tolerance. *J Appl Physiol* 1958;12:487–488.

53. Belman MJ, Mittman C. Ventilatory muscle training improves exercise capacity in chronic obstructive pulmonary disease patients. *Am Rev Respir Dis* 1981;121:273–280.

54. Jones NL. Normal values for pulmonary gas exchange during exercise. *Am Rev Respir Dis* 1984;129(Suppl):S44–S46.

55. Brown HV, Wasserman K. Exercise performance in chronic obstructive pulmonary diseases. *Med Clin NA* 1981;65:525–547.

56. Koike A, Hiroe M, Taniguchi K, et al. Respiratory control during exercise in patients with cardiovascular disease. *Am Rev Respir Dis* 1993;147:425–429.

57. Beaver WL, Wasserman K, Whipp BJ. A new method for detecting anaerobic threshold by gas exchange. *J Appl Physiol* 1986;60:2020–2027.

58. Belman MJ, Epstein LJ, Doornbos D, et al. Noninvasive determinations of the anaerobic threshold. Reliability and validity in patients with COPD. *Chest* 1992;102:1028–1034.

59. Eriksson BO, Engstrom I, Karlberg P, et al. A physiological analysis of former girl swimmers. *Acta Paediatr Scand* 1971;217(Suppl):68–72.

60. Saltin B, Blomqvist G, Mitchell JH, et al. Response to exercise after bed rest and after training. A longitudinal study of adaptive changes in oxygen transport and body composition. *Circulation* 1968;38(Suppl 7):1–78.

61. Knuttgen HG. Development of muscular strength and endurance. In Knuttgen HG, ed. *Neuromuscular mechanisms for therapeutic and conditioning exercise.* Baltimore: University Park Press, 1976:97.

62. Goldberg L, Elliot DL, Kuehl KS. Assessment of exercise intensity formulas by use of ventilatory threshold. *Chest* 1988;94:95–98.

63. Holle RHO, Williams DV, Vandree JC, et al. Increased muscle efficiency and sustained benefits in an outpatient community hospital-based pulmonary rehabilitation program. *Chest* 1988;94:1161–1168.

64. Sala E, Roca J, Marrades RM et al. Effects of endurance training on skeletal muscle bioenergetics in chronic obstructive pulmonary disease. *Am J Respir Crit Care Med* 1999;159:1726–1734.

65. Smith K, Cook D, Guyatt GH, et al. Respiratory muscle training in chronic airflow limitation: a meta-analysis. *Am Rev Respir Dis* 1992;145:533–539.

66. Kohrt WM, Malley MT, Coggan AR, et al. Effects of gender, age, and fitness level on response of $\dot{V}_{O_2}$max to training in 60 to 71 year olds. *J Appl Physiol* 1991;71:2004–2011.

67. Bernstein ML, Despars JA, Singh N, et al. Reanalysis of the 12-minute walk test in COPD patients. *Chest* 1994;105:163–167.

68. Singh SJ, Morgan M, Scott S, et al. Development of a shuttle walking test of disability in patients with chronic airway obstruction. *Thorax* 1992;47:1019–1024.

69. Liu Z, Vargas FS, Stansbury DW, et al. Comparison of the end-tidal arterial P_{CO_2} gradient during exercise in normal subjects and in patients with severe COPD. *Chest* 1995;107:1218–1224.

70. McGovern J, Sasse SA, Stansbury DW, et al. Comparison of oxygen saturation by pulse oximetry and co-oximetry during exercise testing in patients with COPD. *Chest* 1996;109:1151–1155.

71. Blackie SP, Fairbarn MS, McElvaney GN, et al. Prediction of maximal oxygen uptake and power during cycle ergometry in subjects older than 55 years of age. *Am Rev Respir Dis* 1989;139:1424–1429.

72. Jones NL, Makrides L, Hitchcock C, et al. Normal standards for an incremental progressive cycle ergometer test. *Am Rev Respir Dis* 1985;131:700–708.

73. American Thoracic Society. Lung function testing: selection of reference values and interpretative strategies. *Am Rev Respir Dis* 1999;144:1202–1218.

74. Morris AH, Kanner RE, Crapo RO, et al. *Clinical pulmonary function testing: a manual of uniform laboratory procedures,* 2nd ed. Salt Lake City: Intermountain Thoracic Society, 1984.

75. Clausen JL, Zarins LP, eds. *Pulmonary function testing—guidelines and controversies.* New York: Academic Press, 1982.

76. Knudson RJ, Lebowitz MD, Holberg CJ, et al. Changes in the normal maximal expiratory flow-volume curve with growth and aging. *Am Rev Respir Dis* 1983;127:725–734.

77. Morris JF, Koski A, Temple WP, et al. Fifteen-year interval spirometric evaluation of the Oregon predictive equations. *Chest* 1988;92:123–127.

78. Withers RT, Bourdon PC, Crockett A. Lung volume standards for healthy male lifetime nonsmokers. *Chest* 1988;92:91–97.

79. Crapo RO, Morris AH. Standardized single breath normal values for carbon monoxide diffusing capacity. *Am Rev Respir Dis* 1981;123:185–189.

80. Knudson RJ, Kaltenborn WT, Knudson DE, et al. The single-breath carbon monoxide diffusing capacity. Reference equations derived from a healthy nonsmoking population and effects of hematocrit. *Am Rev Respir Dis* 1987;135:805–811.

81. Aaron SD, Dales RE, Cardinal P. How accurate is spirometry at predicting restrictive pulmonary impairment. *Chest* 1999;115:869–873.

82. Miller A, Brown LK, Sloane MF, et al. Cardiorespiratory responses to incremental exercise in sarcoidosis patients with normal spirometry. *Chest* 1995;107:323–329.

83. Curtis JK, Liska AP, Rasmussen HK, et al. The bronchospastic component in patients with chronic bronchitis and emphysema. *JAMA* 1966;197:693–696.

84. Nisar M, Earis JE, Pearson MG, et al. Acute bronchodilator trials in chronic obstructive pulmonary disease. *Am Rev Respir Dis* 1992;146:555–559.

85. Guyatt GH, Townsend M, Nogradi S, et al. Acute response to bronchodilator. An imperfect guide for bronchodilator therapy in chronic airflow limitation. *Arch Intern Med* 1988;148:1949–1952.

86. Rotman HH, Liss HP, Weg JG. Diagnosis of upper airway obstruction by pulmonary function testing. *Chest* 1975;68:796–799.

87. Wright JL, Lawson LM, Pare PD, et al. The detection of small airways disease. *Am Rev Respir Dis* 1984;129:989–994.

88. Rubenfeld AR, Pain MC. Perception of asthma. *Lancet* 1976;1:882–884.

89. Marini JJ, Pierson JD, Hudson LD, et al. The significance of wheezing in chronic airflow obstruction. *Am Rev Respir Dis* 1979;120:1069–1072.

90. Tobin JM, Hughes JA, Hutchison DC. Effects of ipratropium bromide and fenoterol aerosols on exercise tolerance. *Eur J Respir Dis* 1984;65:441–446.

91. Juniper EF, Kline PA, Vanzieleghem MA, et al. Effect on long-term treatment with an inhaled corticosteroid (budesonide) on airway hyperresponsiveness and clinical asthma in nonsteroid-dependent asthmatics. *Am Rev Respir Dis* 1990;142:832–836.

92. Light RW, Mintz HM, Linden GS, et al. Hemodynamics of patients with severe chronic obstructive pulmonary disease (COPD) during progressive upright exercise. *Am Rev Respir Dis* 1984;130:391–395.

93. Killian KJ, Leblanc P, Martin DH, et al. Exercise capacity and ventilatory, circulatory, and symptom limitation in patients with chronic airflow limitation. *Am Rev Respir Dis* 1992;146:935–940.

94. Mahler DA. Exercise-induced asthma. *Med Sci Sports Exerc* 1993;25:554–561.

95. Hsia CCW. Cardiopulmonary limitations to exercise in restrictive lung disease. *Med Sci Sports Exerc* 1999;31:S28–S32.

96. LoRusso TJ, Belman MJ, Elashoff JD, et al. Prediction of maximal exercise capacity in obstructive and restrictive pulmonary disease. *Chest* 1993;104:1748–1754.

97. Bye PB, Anderson SD, Woolcock AJ, et al. Bicycle endurance performance of patients with interstitial lung disease breathing air and oxygen. *Am Rev Respir Dis* 1982;126:1005–1012.

98. D'Alonzo GE, Gianotti LA, Pohil RL, et al. Comparison of progressive exercise performance of normal subjects and patients with primary pulmonary hypertension. *Chest* 1987;92:57–62.

99. Piña IL, Fitzpatrick JT. Exercise and heart failure. A review. *Chest* 1996;110:1317–1327

100. Russell SD, McNeer FR, Higginbotham MB. Exertional dyspnea in heart failure: a symptom unrelated to pulmonary function at rest or during exercise. *Am Heart J* 1998;135:398–405.

101. Demeter SL. Disability evaluation. State of the Art Review. *Occupat Med* 1998;13:315–323.

102. Medical Section of the American Lung Association. Evaluation of impairment/disability secondary to respiratory disease. *Am Rev Respir Dis* 1986;133:1205–1209.

103. Medical Section of the American Lung Association. Guidelines for the evaluation of impairment/disability in patients with asthma. *Am Rev Respir Dis* 1993;147:1056–1061.

7

INVASIVE DIAGNOSTIC PROCEDURES

RICHARD W. LIGHT
R. MICHAEL RODRIGUEZ

THORACENTESIS AND PLEURAL FLUID EXAMINATION
Thoracentesis
Pleural Fluid Appearance
Separation of Transudates from Exudates
Pleural Fluid Cell Count and Differential
Pleural Fluid Chemistries
Pleural Fluid Bacteriology
Pleural Fluid Tests for Malignancy
Pleural Fluid Markers for Tuberculosis
Pleural Biopsy

BRONCHOSCOPY
Transbronchial Biopsy
Bronchoalveolar Lavage
Transbronchial Needle Aspiration
Bronchoscopic Ultrasonography

Complications of Bronchoscopy
Indications for Bronchoscopy

TRANSTHORACIC NEEDLE ASPIRATION

THORACOSCOPY
Pleural Effusions
Interstitial Lung Disease
Pulmonary Nodules
Mediastinal Disease
Miscellaneous Conditions
Complications of Thoracoscopy

MEDIASTINOSCOPY

ENDOSCOPIC ULTRASOUND-GUIDED FINE NEEDLE ASPIRATION

OPEN-LUNG BIOPSY

The majority of chest diseases can be diagnosed on the basis of the history, physical findings, pulmonary function tests, and chest radiographs including CT scans. When these basic procedures are not adequate to define a patient's illness, additional studies are available that allow the physician to define lung abnormalities with precision. These invasive tests, including the various biopsy procedures, not only carry increased risks, but are costly. In this time of fiscal responsibility the clinician must choose, from a battery of increasingly specialized diagnostic procedures, those that are most likely to yield the desired results while having the least risk and cost to the patient. This chapter discusses some of these specialized techniques: thoracentesis, pleural biopsy, bronchoscopy with specialized procedures including bronchoalveolar lavage, protected specimen brushing and transbronchial needle aspiration, transthoracic needle aspiration and biopsy, thoracoscopy, mediastinoscopy, and open lung biopsy. Other tests—such as arterial blood gases and oximetry, capnography, metabolic and nutritional evaluation, and various invasive and noninvasive tests for venous thrombosis—are discussed in the chapters devoted to the diseases for which they are most often used.

THORACENTESIS AND PLEURAL FLUID EXAMINATION

Pleural involvement often accompanies diseases of the lung parenchyma and is usually associated with abnormal amounts of fluid in the pleural space. The volume of pleural fluid present can be semiquantitated by obtaining a lateral decubitus chest radiograph with the suspected side down and measuring the thickness of the fluid between the inner border of the ribs and the lower part of the lung (Fig. 7.1). If the thickness of the fluid is greater than 10 mm, a sample of fluid can usually be obtained for diagnostic thoracentesis.

Thoracentesis

The site for insertion of the needle should be determined with care. It is best to make the insertion in the posterior thorax, where the ribs are easily palpable and to where the fluid gravitates. With the patient in the sitting position, the level is identified at which tactile fremitus is lost and the percussion note becomes dull. Thoracentesis should be attempted first in the interspace below this level. Ultrasound

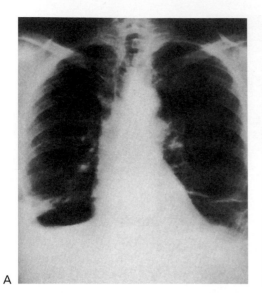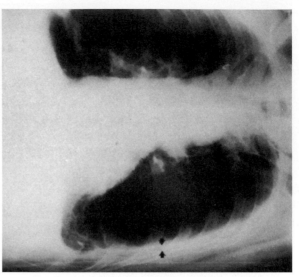

A

B

FIGURE 7.1. Lateral decubitus radiograph demonstrating pleural effusion. On the erect poster-oanterior radiograph **(A)**, both costophrenic angles are blunted. In the left lateral decubitus position **(B)**, there is a definite fluid line between the outer part of the lung and the inside of the chest wall. Since the distance between the *arrows* was greater than 10 mm, a diagnostic thoracentesis was performed.

should be used to guide the thoracentesis if there is only a small amount of pleural fluid, if loculation is suspected, or if the initial one or two attempts yield no pleural fluid (1).

The handling of the pleural fluid for the different tests is outlined in Table 7.1. For bacterial cultures, 5 mL of pleural fluid should be put into both aerobic and anaerobic culture media. For determination of pleural fluid pH, the sample should be sent to the laboratory on ice, in the original syringe.

TABLE 7.1 DISTRIBUTION OF PLEURAL FLUID OBTAINED WITH DIAGNOSTIC THORACENTESIS

Laboratory	Amount (mL)	Tests Ordered
Bacteriology	10	Aerobic and anerobic cultures Gram stain
Tuberculosis and mycology	5	Tuberculosis and fungal cultures
Cytology	10	Cytology
Hematology	5	Red cell count White cell count Wright stain
Chemistry	5	Glucose Amylase Lactic dehydrogenase Protein Marker for tuberculosis
Blood gas	5	pH

Pleural Fluid Appearance

The gross appearance of pleural fluid yields useful diagnostic information, and so the color, turbidity, viscosity, and odor of the pleural fluid should be recorded (2). Most transudative and many exudative effusions are clear, straw-colored, nonviscid, and odorless. A white milky appearance indicates chylothorax, a chyliform pleural effusion, or empyema. Pus in the pleural fluid can be distinguished from chylothorax and chyliform effusion, because after centrifugation there is a clear, yellowish, supernatant fluid in purulent effusions, while the fluid with a chylous or chyliform effusion remains cloudy after centrifugation. If the pleural fluid smells foul, the patient in all probability has an anaerobic pleuropulmonary infection.

Only 5,000 to 10,000 red blood cells per cubic millimeter are required to impart a red color to a pleural effusion. Thus, 1 mL of blood in a moderately sized effusion will result in blood-tinged pleural fluid. The diagnostic value of blood-tinged fluid is limited, since over 15% of transudates and over 40% of exudates are blood-tinged.[3] Grossly bloody effusions have red cell counts above 100,000 per mm³. This finding is suggestive of one of three disease processes: trauma, malignancy (including malignant mesothelioma and metastatic neoplasms), or, less commonly, pulmonary embolism (3). A hematocrit should be obtained on grossly bloody pleural fluid to determine whether or not a hemothorax is present. If the pleural fluid hematocrit is more than 50% that of the peripheral blood, a hemothorax is present (see Chapter 17, Diseases of the Pleura, Mediastinum, Chest Wall, and Diaphragm).

Separation of Transudates from Exudates

The first question that must be answered when a pleural effusion is discovered is whether the effusion is a transudate or an exudate. Transudates, by definition, are pleural effusions that result from imbalances of the hydrostatic and osmotic forces in the pulmonary or systemic circulation. Exudates are pleural effusions that result from increased permeability of the pulmonary or systemic circulation (4). If the effusion is a transudate, no further diagnostic procedures are necessary, and therapy is directed toward the underlying congestive heart failure, cirrhosis, or nephrosis. Alternatively, if the effusion proves to be an exudate, more extensive diagnostic procedures are needed to delineate the cause of the pleural disease.

Exudative pleural effusions can be separated effectively from transudative pleural effusions with the simultaneous use of protein and lactic acid dehydrogenase (LDH) levels in the pleural fluid and serum. Exudates meet at least *one* of the following three criteria, while transudates meet *none* (5).

1. The pleural fluid protein divided by the serum protein is greater than 0.5.
2. The pleural fluid LDH divided by the serum LDH is greater than 0.6.
3. The pleural fluid LDH is greater than two-thirds of the upper limit of normal for the serum LDH.

In the past decade several other tests—including the pleural fluid bilirubin level, the ratio of pleural fluid to serum bilirubin, the pleural fluid cholesterol, ratio of the pleural fluid to serum cholesterol, and the pleural fluid serum albumin gradient—have been suggested as being useful in the separation of transudates from exudates.[2] However, it appears that use of the protein and the LDH as described above (Light's criteria) is at least as effective as any of the newer criteria in making this differentiation (6).

The primary problem with Light's criteria is that they label some patients with transudative pleural effusions as having exudative pleural effusions. It is recommended that if a patient is thought to have a transudative effusion by clinical criteria, but the fluid is identified as exudative by Light's criteria, the difference between the serum and effusion albumin should be measured. If this is above 1.2 g per dL, the patient in all probability has a transudative effusion, and the exudative categorization by Light's criteria can be ignored (7).

Pleural Fluid Cell Count and Differential

The pleural fluid white blood cell count is of limited value in the differential diagnosis of pleural effusions. In general,

a white blood cell count (WBC) above 1,000 per mm^3 suggests an exudate. Parapneumonic effusions usually have white cell counts above 10,000 per mm^3; however, pleural fluid WBCs above 10,000 are also seen with pancreatitis, pulmonary infarction, collagen vascular diseases, malignancy, and tuberculosis (2,3).

The differential WBC should be obtained on all exudative pleural effusions. The cells in the pleural fluid can include neutrophils, small lymphocytes, mesothelial cells, other mononuclear cells and eosinophils. The presence of neutrophils suggests an acute inflammatory response. Pleural fluid neutrophilia is seen in effusions associated with pneumonia, pancreatitis, pulmonary embolism, and peritonitis. Occasionally, very early tuberculous effusions will have a predominance of neutrophils.

If the pleural fluid contains more than 50% lymphocytes, the patient probably has malignancy, tuberculosis, or a pleural effusion secondary to coronary artery bypass surgery (8). Mesothelial cells normally line the pleural cavity and are rarely present with tuberculous pleuritis or other processes in which the pleural surfaces are diffusely involved. The presence of pleural fluid eosinophilia is of little use in the differential diagnosis (2). Most effusions with eosinophil counts greater than 10% are either bloody or associated with a pneumothorax. Other etiologies for eosinophilic effusions include a drug reaction, paragonimiasis, asbestos exposure, the Churg-Strauss syndrome, or a resolving parapneumonic effusion.

Pleural Fluid Chemistries

It is recommended that all exudative pleural effusions be analyzed for protein, LDH, glucose, and amylase. As discussed above, the protein and LDH are used to separate transudative from exudative pleural effusions. The pleural fluid LDH should be measured each time a thoracentesis is performed, because it serves as an index of the degree of pleural inflammation (2). If the pleural fluid LDH increases with serial thoracenteses, the process responsible for the effusion is worsening and one should be more active in pursuing a diagnosis.

Pleural Fluid Glucose

Measurement of the pleural fluid glucose level is useful because a low pleural fluid glucose level (less than 60 mg per dL) indicates that the patient probably has one of four disorders, namely, a complicated parapneumonic effusion, a malignant pleural effusion, tuberculous pleuritis, or a rheumatoid effusion. Other rare causes of a low glucose pleural effusion include paragonimiasis, hemothorax, the Churg-Strauss syndrome, and occasionally lupus pleuritis (2).

Pleural Fluid Amylase

An elevated pleural fluid amylase (above the upper limit of normal for serum) indicates that the pleural effusion is due to pancreatic disease, esophageal rupture, or pleural malignancy. The incidence of pleural effusion with acute pancreatitis exceeds 50% (9). The pleural fluid amylase is usually markedly elevated in patients with chronic pancreatic pleural effusions which are due to a sinus tract leading from the pancreas into the mediastinum and then into the pleural space. The elevated amylase with esophageal rupture is due to saliva, with its high amylase content, entering the pleural space. The pleural fluid amylase level is elevated in approximately 10% of patients with malignant pleural effusions, and the primary tumor is usually not in the pancreas (10). Since the pleural fluid amylase with malignancy is the salivary type, determination of the pleural fluid amylase isoenzyme pattern can differentiate malignancy from pancreatic disease (10).

Pleural Fluid pH

The determination of pleural fluid pH is most useful in patients with parapneumonic effusions, because the lower the pH, the worse the prognosis. A pleural fluid pH below 7.00 suggests that the patient will require invasive procedures directed toward the effusion (11) (see Chapter 17, Diseases of the Pleura, Mediastinum, Chest Wall, and Diaphragm). The pleural fluid pH determination must be made with a blood gas machine because pH meters and pH indicator strips are not sufficiently accurate for clinical decision-making (12). Other types of effusions that may have a pleural fluid pH below 7.20 are malignant pleural effusion, tuberculous pleural effusion, and any other type of pleural effusion that has a low pleural fluid glucose (2).

Pleural Fluid Bacteriology

When a diagnostic thoracentesis is performed on a patient with an exudative effusion, the fluid should be cultured for both aerobic and anaerobic organisms. A Gram stain of the fluid should be examined to search for the presence of bacteria. Mycobacterial and fungal cultures should also be obtained if there is a possibility of tuberculosis or fungal infection.

Pleural Fluid Tests for Malignancy

Pleural Fluid Cytology

If a patient has malignancy, cytological examination of the pleural fluid is a fast, efficient, and minimally invasive means by which to establish the diagnosis. The percentage of malignant pleural effusions that are diagnosed with cytology has been reported to be anywhere between 40% and 87% (2). There are several factors that influence the diagnostic yield with cytology. If the patient has a malignancy but the pleural effusion has another etiology such as heart failure, pulmonary emboli, pneumonia, lymphatic obstruction, or hypoproteinemia, the cytology will be negative. The frequency of positive cytologic results also depends upon the tumor type. Almost all adenocarcinomas will be diagnosed with cytology, but the yield is less with squamous cell carcinoma, Hodgkin's disease and sarcomas. Obviously, the yield will also be dependent upon the skill of the cytologist. Overall, if three separate pleural fluid specimens are submitted to an experienced cytologist, one should expect a positive diagnosis in about 70% to 80% of patients.

Flow Cytometry

Flow cytometry can provide a rapid quantification of the nuclear DNA. The majority of malignancies are aneuploid and consequently have abnormal DNA levels. In contrast, the majority of benign effusions are diploid, with normal DNA levels. However, since some normals have abnormal DNA levels and some malignancies have normal DNA levels, the diagnosis of malignancy cannot be ruled either in or out with this test (13). Therefore, the routine use of flow cytometry is not recommended. It is, however, quite useful for demonstrating the homogeneity of a population of cells in patients with lymphoma (14).

Immunohistochemical Testing

Immunohistochemical staining using the monoclonal antibodies CEA, B72.3, and Leu-M1 is useful for distinguishing adenocarcinoma from mesothelioma (15). If the specimen stains positive for at least two of these antibodies, the patient in all probability has adenocarcinoma. Alternatively, if the specimen doesn't stain for any of the antibodies, the patient in all probability has mesothelioma (15). Immunohistochemical staining is not useful for distinguishing malignant mesothelioma cells from benign mesothelial cells.

Tumor Markers in the Pleural Fluid

There have been many publications evaluating the utility of tumor markers such as CEA, AFP, CA 15–3, CA 19–9, and enolase in the diagnosis of pleural malignancy. In general, the results with all have been disappointing, because there are false positives with all. Due to the poor prognosis with malignant pleural effusions, it is important not to make the diagnosis mistakenly. It is possible, however, that in the future better tumor markers will be developed.

Pleural Fluid Markers for Tuberculosis

Pleural Fluid Adenosine Deaminase Levels

Measurement of the adenosine deaminase (ADA) level in pleural fluid is diagnostically useful because ADA levels tend to be higher in tuberculous pleural effusions than in other exudates. In one recent study the ADA was above 47 U per L in 253 of 254 patients with tuberculous pleuritis (16). In a second report, only five of 173 patients (3%) with pleural effusions due to other etiologies, including 46 with malignancy and 30 with pneumonia, had ADA levels that exceeded 45 U/mL (17). The primary problem with using the pleural fluid ADA to establish the diagnosis of tuberculous pleuritis is that there are no commercial laboratories in the United States, to my knowledge, that reliably measure the ADA levels.

Pleural Fluid Gamma Interferon Levels

Pleural fluid gamma interferon levels are also elevated with tuberculous pleuritis. Pleural fluid gamma interferon levels are very efficient at separating tuberculous from nontuberculous pleural effusion. Using a cutoff level of 3.7 U per mL, Villena and coworkers demonstrated that this test resulted in a sensitivity of 0.99 and a specificity of 0.98 in a series of 388 pleural effusions, including 73 tuberculous effusions (18). Commercial laboratories in the United States do measure gamma interferon levels.

Pleural Fluid Polymerase Chain Reaction Tests

With polymerase chain reaction (PCR), one can demonstrate the presence of DNA from *Mycobacterium tuberculosis* in the pleural fluid, which should be diagnostic of tuberculous pleuritis. Querol and coworkers (19) performed PCR based on detecting a 123-bp DNA segment specific for *M. tuberculosis*. In their series of 21 patients with pleural tuberculosis and 86 controls, the sensitivity and specificity of PCR were very similar to those of ADA (19). Other series, however, have reported much poorer results with PCR (20). Since PCR test is more expensive and more technically difficult than either the ADA or the gamma interferon, it is not recommended.

Pleural Biopsy

The primary use of needle biopsy of the pleura over the past 40 years has been to diagnose tuberculous pleuritis. However, as outlined above, markers for tuberculosis obtained from the pleural fluid are very efficient at establishing this diagnosis. In recent years, with the emergence of multidrug-resistant tuberculosis, cultures for *M. tuberculosis* have become important in guiding the therapy of tuberculosis. Some have advocated performing a needle biopsy of the pleura so that a specimen of the pleura could be cultured. However, only about 33% of patients with tuberculous pleuritis will have a positive pleural biopsy culture and a negative pleural fluid culture (21). In addition, to my knowledge no patient has developed disseminated multidrug-resistant tuberculosis after presenting with a pleural

effusion and receiving a standard course of antituberculous drugs. In view of the above, pleural biopsy is usually not indicated for the diagnosis of tuberculous pleuritis.

Pleural biopsy can also establish the diagnosis of malignant pleural disease. However, in most series cytology of the pleural fluid is much more sensitive in establishing the diagnosis. If the cytology of the fluid is negative, the pleural biopsy is usually nondiagnostic. In one series, the pleural biopsy was positive in only 20 of 118 (17%) patients with pleural malignancy and negative cytology (22). Since thoracoscopy is diagnostic in more than 90% of patients with pleural malignancy and negative cytology, it is the preferred diagnostic procedure in the patient with a cytology negative pleural effusion who is suspected of having malignancy.

BRONCHOSCOPY

Bronchoscopy is the invasive procedure most commonly used in the diagnosis of pulmonary disease. With flexible bronchoscopes, the bronchoscopist can visualize up to 85% of the fifth-order subsegmental bronchi and 55% of the sixth-order bronchi. Directly visualized biopsies and bronchial washings are considered standard procedures with bronchoscopy. With advances in videochip technology, videobronchoscopy is being used more widely, contributing significantly to teaching and documentation of endocscopic images. Clinical studies have documented that image quality is far superior and allows for a more accurate and detailed evaluation of the tracheobronchial tree than does direct visualization through the older fiberoptic bronchoscopes (23). Over the last three decades, the diagnostic capabilities of bronchoscopy have been markedly increased due to the development of associated techniques such as transbronchial biopsy, transbronchial needle aspiration, and bronchoalveolar lavage. In this section, these various techniques will be briefly discussed. Subsequently, the primary indications for bronchoscopy as a diagnostic tool will be discussed.

Transbronchial Biopsy

Transbronchial lung biopsy (TBB) can be used to obtain tissue samples in patients with diffuse parenchymal disease or localized densities beyond direct endoscopic vision. With TBB, a biopsy forceps is passed through the channel of the scope and out into the lung parenchyma, usually using fluoroscopic guidance. In this manner, pieces of tissue of an average diameter of 3 mm can be obtained. In patients with diffuse lung disease, the forceps is engaged in a small peripheral airway, preferably in the lower lobe. If a focal lesion is present, fluoroscopy, CT scans, or bronchoscopic ultrasonography should be used to guide the biopsy. The main complications of TBB are pneumothorax and hemorrhage.

Bronchoalveolar Lavage

The basic premise which underlies bronchoalveolar lavage (BAL) is that the cells and noncellular material recovered after the endobronchial injection of saline reflect the constituents of the alveoli. Bronchoalveolar lavage is distinct from bronchial washing; in the latter instance, small amounts of saline are injected into the bronchi to obtain cells from the bronchi. With BAL, a total volume of 150 to 300 mL is infused, of which 40% to 60% is recovered while only a few milliliters of saline are used for bronchial washing. The first 20 to 30 mL returned with BAL is usually discarded because it may be contaminated with bronchial cells. Bronchoalveolar lavage is performed prior to transbronchial biopsies and brushings to avoid sampling errors and avoid contamination from bleeding. The bronchoscope is advanced into a peripheral fourth- or fifth-order bronchus that conforms to the area of abnormality. Once the bronchoscope is wedged into the bronchus, saline is infused through the bronchoscope and suctioned into a reservoir or trap. The recovered fluid may then be sent to the lab for cytologic (including cell count and differential), microbiologic, or biochemical analysis. There is no standard procedure for evaluation of the recovered BAL fluid, therefore, communication between the clinician and laboratory is important to avoid mishandling of the specimens.

The most common complication of BAL is hypoxemia. The incidence of fever ranges between 2% and 50% and this appears to depend on the volume of the infusate and the number of lobes washed (24). In addition, patients may develop bronchospasm or bleeding. Bleeding occurs in less than 0.7% of patients even in the presence of thrombocytopenia. BAL may be performed in patients with local anesthesia or in patients requiring mechanical ventilation. Relative contradictions include an uncooperative patient, hypercapnia, and cardiac instability (25).

Transbronchial Needle Aspiration

Transbronchial needle aspiration (TBNA) is a procedure in which a needle is inserted through a bronchial wall to sample a lesion that is not visible endobronchially. It is useful for establishing the diagnosis in patients with mediastinal or hilar adenopathy, extrinsic compression of the airway by a peribronchial process, and peripheral nodules. It is also useful in staging lung carcinomas in patients with mediastinal or hilar adenopathy. Its sensitivity is increased when it is used in conjunction with imaging techniques.

The complication rate of TBNA is low. Pneumothorax occurs in approximately 0.5% of patients. Significant bleeding is uncommon even if pulmonary and systemic blood vessels are inadvertently aspirated. Pneumomediastinum and mediastinitis are rare complications.

Bronchoscopic Ultrasonography

Use of endobronchial ultrasound was first described in 1990 (26). Normally the view of the bronchoscopist is limited to the visualization of the lumen and the inner surface of the airways. With endobronchial ultrasound, one can assess the depth of infiltration of the tumor into the bronchial wall or extrabronchial invasion (27). Endobronchial ultrasound can also be used to guide fine needle aspiration of mediastinal adenopathy (28), to demonstrate the length and diameter of bronchial stenoses, and to help obtain transbronchial biopsy specimens (26). It is anticipated that the use of endobronchial ultrasound will increase as bronchoscopists become more familiar with its use and as the technology improves.

Complications of Bronchoscopy

Flexible fiberoptic bronchoscopy is generally a well-tolerated procedure with few adverse effects. The commonly recognized complications include hypoxemia, bleeding, fever, cardiac arrhythmias, bronchospasm, pneumonia, and pneumothorax. The mortality rate is in the range of 0.01% and the rate of major complications is less than 1%. With bronchoscopy, the mean PaO_2 decreases by 15 to 20 mm Hg (29). Therefore, the oxygenation status of patients undergoing bronchoscopy should be monitored continuously and supplemental oxygen administered as required.

Bleeding is one of the most distressing and difficult management problems for the bronchoscopist. Minimal bleeding is defined as 50 mL of blood or less intermixed with saline lavage, and is not considered to be hazardous. The incidence of clinically significant bleeding varied from a low of 0.5% to a high of 1.3% in one study and appeared to be related to the types of procedures performed at bronchoscopy, including brushing and transbronchial biopsy (30). Risk factors associated with increased bleeding include an immunosuppressed host, platelet dysfunction and coagulopathies, drugs, organ failure, chest malignancy, and uremia (30). Uremia creates a major hazard of bleeding, and approximately 45% of uremic patients have significant hemorrhage after transbronchial biopsy. Pulmonary hypertension is also associated with a high incidence of bleeding and is frequently considered a contraindication to transbronchial biopsy.

Fever is another common complication of bronchoscopy and has been reported in as many as 16% of patients (31). Pereira and coworkers (31) reported pneumonia in 6% and death from rapidly progressive pneumonia in another 1%. Bacteremia following this procedure has not been demonstrated. Careful disinfection, cleaning, and sterilization of equipment are mandatory to prevent this complication (32).

Laryngospasm and bronchospasm are common airway complications, and patients with asthma are at especially high risk. The most severe airway obstruction occurs in patients with chronic obstructive pulmonary disease. In these patients, who may have borderline respiratory failure, endotracheal intubation and mechanical ventilation may be necessary during and after the procedure.

Indications for Bronchoscopy

Suspected Lung Cancer

Bronchoscopy is the procedure that is used most commonly to diagnose lung cancer. Approximately 170,000 new cases of lung cancer occur annually. Lung cancer may present as an endobronchial lesion, as a peripheral lesion, or as a hilar mass. Bronchoscopy is useful in establishing the diagnosis in each of these instances.

Endobronchial Lesions

The flexible bronchoscope is invaluable in examining the central airways to localize and diagnose endobronchial lesions. If an endobronchial lesion is *visible*, bronchoscopy will be diagnostic in more than 90% if bronchial brushing is combined with bronchial biopsy (33,34). With endobronchially visible lesions, three to five biopsies are usually sufficient (33). The diagnostic yield is increased when bronchial brushing is combined with biopsy (35,36). It is controversial whether the further addition of bronchial washing to bronchial biopsy and bronchial brushing increases the yield with endobronchially visible lesions (37).

Peripheral Lung Malignancies

Some lung carcinomas are located in the parenchyma of the lung and are not visible endoscopically. These lesions must be biopsied with a transbronchial biopsy. The diagnostic yield with these peripheral lesions depends upon their size and their distance from the hilum.[38] For all practical purposes, lesions that are over 2 cm in diameter or nodular or polypoid produce visible changes in the mucosa. Smaller lesions usually do not produce mucosal changes (39). The location of the lesion in the upper or lower lobes does not seem to influence the diagnostic yield, but the use of fluoroscopy or other imaging modalities is necessary when attempts are made to biopsy these lesions. It is recommended that at least six biopsy specimens be obtained when these peripheral lesions are approached (33). The diagnostic yield with peripheral lesions is lower than with central lesions and has been reported to be between 40% and 80% when biplane fluoroscopy is used and biopsy is combined with brushings and washings (38). Transbronchial needle aspiration (TBNA) is useful in the diagnosis of submucosal tumor (erythema, loss of bronchial markings, or a thickening of the mucosa) and tumors which extrinsically compress the bronchial lumen (40).

Solitary Pulmonary Nodules

Solitary pulmonary nodules (SPN) are defined as discrete lesions surrounded by aerated lung without associated lymphadenopathy, atelectasis, or pneumonitis. The physician's goal is to determine with the least morbidity whether the nodule is benign or malignant. Features that suggest malignancy are older age, prior tobacco use, growth on serial chest radiographs, lack of calcification, and a previous history of malignancy. Evaluation should include appropriate clinical history, review of previous radiographs (when available), routine laboratory data, and CT of the chest. High-resolution chest CT provides greater information regarding the characteristics of the nodule than does conventional CT (41).

The role of bronchoscopy in the management of SPN is limited (41). In general, if it is likely that the patient has a malignancy, it is best to proceed directly to thoracotomy since a negative bronchoscopy does not rule out malignancy. Bronchoscopy in this situation is performed for two reasons: to rule out synchronous endobronchial disease, and to establish a histologic diagnosis. In stage I disease, the likelihood of finding endobronchial disease is low. The size of the nodule is critical in determining the diagnostic yield from bronchoscopy. Nodules less than 2 cm in size are difficult to biopsy successfully and the yield is only 10% to 30%. The yield increases to 40% to 69% if the nodules are larger than 2 cm. When a "bronchus sign" is seen on a CT scan, there is an 80% chance of accurate diagnosis by transbronchial biopsy. This sign is defined as the finding of a bronchus leading directly to a peripheral pulmonary mass. In one recent study, bronchoscopy with bronchial washing, brushing, transbronchial needle aspiration, and transbronchial lung biopsy established the diagnosis in 40 of 49 patients (82%) with the CT bronchus sign and only 19 of 43 patients (44%) without the bronchus sign (42).

Staging

Once the diagnosis of lung cancer is established, staging of the disease becomes crucial not only to predict resectability but also to avoid unnecessary surgery and to provide the patient with prognostic information. One aspect of staging is to evaluate whether or not the mediastinum is involved. In general, histologic confirmation is necessary if imaging studies suggest mediastinal involvement by tumor. Sampling of the mediastinal nodes for the purpose of staging can be accomplished using TBNA, cervical mediastinoscopy, anterior mediastinoscopy, CT-guided transthoracic fine needle aspiration, or endoscopic ultrasound-guided fine needle aspiration. Of these procedures, TBNA is the least invasive since it involves aspiration of mediastinal nodes by aspirating through the tracheal wall at the time of bronchoscopy. This procedure is most useful in sampling paratracheal, hilar, and subcarinal nodes (43). The procedure has a reported yield of approximately 40% in patients with positive imaging studies of the mediastinum and a yield of approximately 10% in individuals with negative imaging studies (43). The yield can be increased if CT guidance is utilized to ascertain that the tip of the needle is exactly inside the node (44). False-positive results have been obtained with this procedure, but these are most likely due to faulty technique, with contamination of the sample with malignant cells from the airway (45).

Hemoptysis

Hemoptysis may be divided into two broad categories—massive and minimal—based on the volume of blood expectorated and/or the physiologic effects related to the loss of blood. In general, if the patient expectorates more than 150 mL/in 24 hours, the hemoptysis should be considered massive, because with this amount of hemoptysis the patient is in danger of drowning in his own blood. All patients with massive hemoptysis should undergo bronchoscopy, using a scope with a large suction channel; many prefer to use a rigid bronchoscope. If the hemoptysis is life-threatening, treatment options at the time of bronchoscopy include topical epinephrine, balloon tamponade, iced saline lavage, and insertion of a double-lumen endotracheal tube (46). The timing of bronchoscopy to localize the bleeding is controversial (47). Most clinicians, however, favor early bronchoscopy to localize the site in the event surgery is necessary.

The four primary causes of minimal hemoptysis are bronchiectasis, carcinoma of the lung, bronchitis, and infection (48). The primary reason to perform bronchoscopy in patients with minimal hemoptysis is to rule out endobronchial malignancy. There are certain clinical factors that should influence the decision whether or not to perform bronchoscopy. Patients who are less than 40 years of age, have a normal chest radiograph, have a bleeding duration of less than one week, have smoked for less than 40 pack years, or who expectorate less than 30 mL of blood daily are unlikely to have endobronchial carcinoma (49). The prognosis for patients with hemoptysis of undetermined origin (cryptogenic) with a negative bronchoscopy is generally good, usually with resolution of bleeding within six months of evaluation (50).

Diagnosis of Pulmonary Infections

The microbiologic diagnosis of pulmonary infections can be made by using specimens collected noninvasively or invasively. The bronchoscope allows direct access to the bronchi and pulmonary parenchyma. Transbronchial biopsy, bronchoalveolar lavage, and protected brush may be used independently or in combination in the diagnosis of pulmonary infections (35,51). When considering indications for bronchoscopy for the diagnosis of pulmonary infections, patients are generally subdivided into those with normal immune function and those who are immunocompromised.

Immunocompromised Patients

With the advent of AIDS, organ transplantation, and intensive chemotherapeutic regimens, the population of immunocompromised patients is increasing. Lung involvement by infectious and noninfectious agents is common in those who are immunocompromised. In patients with AIDS, the most common infectious agent is *Pneumocystis carinii*. This organism on occasion may be identified with induced sputum, but is usually diagnosed with bronchoscopy. Other diseases that affect the lungs of the immunocompromised include bacterial infections, tuberculosis, fungal infections, drug reactions, and neoplasms including Kaposi's sarcoma and lymphoma. The diagnosis of these other processes may be made using BAL and transbronchial biopsies (35).

The ability safely to obtain samples from infected alveoli using BAL has led to the widespread use of this modality in the immunocompromised host. Mycobacterial and fungal infections may be diagnosed using BAL. The presence of certain organisms found in the recovered fluid are diagnostic of infection, for instance, *P. carinii, Strongyloides, Histoplasma, Toxoplasma gondii, M. tuberculosis,* and *Mycoplasma* (25). Uses of semiquantitative cultures are necessary when infectious pathogens known to colonize the airway are recovered. At least 10^3 colony-forming units (cfu) should be present on a culture of a BAL specimen in order to consider the positive culture representative of the offending organism (52).

Immune-Competent Patients

Bronchoscopy is useful in identifying infectious agents in the immune-competent host also. Bronchoscopy is particularly useful at identifying chronic pulmonary infections such as fungal infections, actinomycosis, nocardiosis, and tuberculosis. When a chronic infection is suspected, BAL should be performed in conjunction with bronchoscopy. BAL is also useful in patients with community-acquired pneumonia in which the clinical course suggests progression of the infection despite appropriate antibiotic coverage (53). Furthermore, BAL may be a useful tool in the diagnosis of ventilator-associated pneumonia (54).

Protected Specimen Brushing

As the bronchoscope passes from the upper airway to the lower airways, it may become contaminated with nasal or endobronchial secretions which then result in false-positive cultures. Protected specimen brushings (PSB) are intended to avoid false-positive cultures. These catheters are designed with a plug over the distal end to avoid contact with the secretions encountered as the bronchoscope traverses the airways. When the catheter is advanced, the plug is extruded, the brush is allowed to come in contact with the infectious site, and material for cultures is then obtained. A positive diagnosis is made if there are more than 10^3 cfu. PSB is used most commonly in patients on respirators who develop infiltrates and in patients with community- or hospital-acquired pneumonia who are not responding to therapy.

Interstitial Lung Disease

There are many different diseases which cause interstitial lung disease. Some authors have advocated bronchoscopy with TBB for most patients with interstitial lung disease. In general, however, the only two common diagnoses that are easily established with TBB are lymphangitic carcinomatosis and sarcoidosis. The specimens obtained with TBB are usually too small to make the diagnosis of usual interstitial pneumonia or desquamative interstitial pneumonia. Accordingly, bronchoscopy with TBB is recommended only when the clinical picture is suggestive of lymphangitic carcinomatosis or sarcoidosis. In most cases, the preferred manner to get adequate tissue specimens is with thoracoscopy. The role of BAL in the diagnosis and management of patients with interstitial lung disease is controversial.

Cough

Chronic cough is a frequent presenting symptom in the outpatient setting. Cough is usually due to environmental exposure (especially cigarettes), postnasal drainage syndrome (PNDS) , gastroesophageal reflux disease (GERD), asthma, or medications (ACE inhibitors). Cough may also be the result of more serious pathology such as malignancy, tuberculosis, interstitial lung disease, congestive heart failure, aspiration, bronchiectasis, or other disorders affecting the upper or lower airway. Recently the American College of Chest Physicians published guidelines for the evaluation of chronic cough which suggested a very limited role for bronchoscopy. Bronchoscopy is indicated only in patients with radiographic abnormalities suggesting an underlying malignancy or other primary pulmonary process not explained by the initial noninvasive evaluation, which should include a history and physical, chest radiograph, and in certain instances pulmonary function testing, sinus films, and evaluation for GERD (55).

Undiagnosed Pleural Effusion

Bronchoscopy is useful in the diagnosis of pleural effusion only if one or more of the following three conditions are present (56): (a) There is a pulmonary infiltrate on the chest radiograph or the chest CT scan. In this situation, particular attention should be paid to the area that contains the infiltrate. (b) Hemoptysis is present. Hemoptysis in the presence of a pleural effusion is very suggestive of an endobronchial lesion. (c) The pleural effusion is massive, that is, it occupies more than three-fourths of the hemithorax. In patients with pleural effusions with positive cytology, but no hemoptysis or no parenchymal infiltrates, bronchoscopy will not identify the primary tumor (57).

Bronchoscopy in the Intensive Care Unit

Bronchoscopy is a useful tool in the intensive care unit. It may be used to facilitate intubation, evaluate the airway, change endotracheal tubes, and evaluate causes of stridor in the immediate postextubation period. Bronchoscopy may be used for diagnostic purposes in patients with persistent infiltrates or hemoptysis (58). Recent cardiac events are only a relative contraindication to bronchoscopy (59).

TRANSTHORACIC NEEDLE ASPIRATION

Percutaneous transthoracic needle aspiration (TTNA) is used most commonly to obtain tissue from patients who are suspected of having lung tumors, but it can also be used to establish the etiology of infections. Percutaneous needle aspiration is relatively good at establishing the diagnosis of lung malignancy, but it is not very good at establishing specific benign diagnoses. In one recent series of 130 patients who had undergone transthoracic needle aspiration, TTNA had a sensitivity of 74% for the detection of malignancy but established the diagnosis in only two of 28 (8%) of patients with benign disease (60). TTNA is more sensitive when the lesion is larger (60). In patients who are suspected of having lung cancer and who are operative candidates, TTNA should be performed only if the results of the aspiration will influence whether or not surgery will be performed. For example, if it is decided beforehand that surgery will be performed only if the aspiration is positive, TTNA should be performed. Also, if surgery will not be performed only if the TTNA is negative, then TTNA should also be performed. Visualization of the lesion for guidance of the procedure may be obtained with computed tomographic scanning, ultrasonography, or fluoroscopy (61).

The most common complication of TTNA is pneumothorax, which occurs in approximately 35% of patients undergoing the procedure (2). Indeed, TTNA is the most common cause of iatrogenic pneumothorax (2). Approximately 10% of the patients who develop a pneumothorax are treated with tube thoracostomy. Another complication is transient hemoptysis, which occurs in about 10%. Other rare complications include bacterial contamination of the pleural space, allergic anesthetic reactions, vasovagal reactions, soft tissue infection, cancer seeding at the insertion site, and air embolism (less than 0.1%) (61). Contraindications to the procedure include a bleeding diathesis, bullous lung disease in the area of the biopsy, local cutaneous lesions (e.g., pyoderma or herpes zoster), pulmonary hypertension, or a lesion abutting the mediastinum or hilum.

THORACOSCOPY

Although thoracoscopy has been a part of thoracic surgical practice for many years, the advent of video-assisted techniques has greatly expanded the indications and uses of this procedure. Whereas thoracoscopy was previously performed mainly for diagnostic purposes, video-assisted thoracic surgery (VATS) has now assumed a major role in the diagnosis and therapy of chest diseases. Indeed, in some institutions it is now the most commonly used operative approach for some general thoracic surgical practices (62). The primary advantage of VATS is that it produces less morbidity and mortality and shorter hospitalization times than does thoracotomy (63). The overall mortality with thoracoscopy is about 1%, while it is 1.5% in patients more than 70 years old and 2.1% in patients with an FEV_1 less than 1 L (63).

Two different techniques have emerged: video-assisted thoracoscopic surgery (VATS) and medical thoracoscopy. The former is performed in an operating room under general anesthesia with the patient selectively intubated to allow for single-lung ventilation. Multiple puncture sites are made in the chest wall through which the thoracoscope and surgical instruments are introduced. Medical thoracoscopy differs from VATS in that the patient may not be intubated and usually breathes spontaneously. The procedure is usually performed with conscious sedation and local anesthesia. Medical thoracoscopy primarily serves as a diagnostic tool rather than for intervention. Medical thoracoscopy is usually performed by pulmonologists, while VATS is performed by thoracic surgeons (64). For diagnostic purposes either VATS or medical thoracoscopy is appropriate and the choice of procedure depends primarily upon its availability at one's institution.

Pleural Effusions

In the diagnosis of pleural disease, thoracoscopic procedures should be used only when the less-invasive diagnostic methods, such as thoracentesis with cytology and markers for tuberculosis, have not yielded a diagnosis. In one series of 620 patients with pleural effusions, only 48 (8%) remained without a diagnosis and were subjected to thoracoscopy (65). If the patient has malignancy, thoracoscopy will establish the diagnosis more than 90% of the time, and the diagnosis of mesothelioma is probably best made with thoracoscopy. An advantage to thoracoscopy in the diagnosis of pleural disease is that pleurodesis can also be performed at the time of the procedure. It should be emphasized, however, that thoracoscopy rarely establishes the diagnosis of benign disease (66).

Interstitial Lung Disease

VATS procedures appear to be particularly useful for obtaining lung biopsies in patients with diffuse interstitial lung disease (67). Lung biopsy via VATS should not be attempted if the patient requires mechanical ventilation because he or she probably will not be able to tolerate one-lung ventilation. Patients with coagulation disorders or pulmonary hypertension should have an open-lung biopsy rather than a VATS procedure. With VATS, the visualization of the lung is better than it is with a limited thoracot-

omy, and more areas of the lung can be sampled. Most patients who previously needed an open-lung biopsy are currently best managed with VATS procedures (68).

Pulmonary Nodules

Pulmonary nodules may be safely removed via VATS procedures (62). If the nodule is benign, then no additional procedures need be done. If the patient is a good surgical candidate and has a primary lung cancer, then a lobectomy should probably be performed (62). If the patient is a poor surgical candidate, this wedge resection can serve as the definitive treatment. The primary advantage of using VATS is that for patients with benign disease, it is the definitive procedure and is associated with less discomfort and requires a shorter period of hospitalization. One problem with VATS for the removal of pulmonary nodules is that it is sometimes difficult to find the nodule. In one recent series, the nodule could not be localized in 46% of 92 patients (69). Nodules less than 10 mm in diameter and more than 10 mm deep to the pleura are particularly difficult to identify with VATS.

Mediastinal Disease

The role of thoracoscopy in the diagnosis of mediastinal masses is still controversial. Some surgeons recommend thoracoscopy only for lesions that are not within the reach of the mediastinoscope because the length of hospital stay and the complication rate are less with mediastinoscopy (70). In contrast, some surgeons now prefer VATS procedures to anterior mediastinotomy to approach mediastinal adenopathy located in the aortopulmonary window or the low periazygos area. The visibility of the entire mediastinal compartment afforded through the VATS approach is far superior to exploration through an anterior mediastinotomy. VATS procedures can also be used to resect benign posterior mediastinal neoplasms and carefully selected cases of early-stage thymoma (62).

Miscellaneous Conditions

VATS procedures have also been used for many other thoracic surgical procedures, including ligation of the thoracic duct, creation of a pericardial window, Zenker's diverticulum, lobectomy, lung volume reduction surgery, treatment of spontaneous pneumothorax with stapling of blebs and pleural abrasion, thoracic sympathectomy, benign esophageal tumors, removal of chest wall tumors, and removal of clotted blood with a hemothorax.

Complications of Thoracoscopy

Although there are less morbidity and mortality from VATS procedures than from thoracotomy, there are nonetheless significant complications. Kaiser and Bavaria (71) reviewed the complications of VATS encountered at the Hospital of the University of Pennsylvania between December 1991 and December 1992. They reported that 10% of the VATS procedures were associated with complications. The most common complication was prolonged (longer than seven days) air leak (3.7%) followed by superficial wound infection (1.9%), and bleeding significant enough to require either transfusion or reoperation (1.9%). In 4.1% of patients, they were unable successfully to complete the intended procedure thoracoscopically and resorted to an open procedure (71).

MEDIASTINOSCOPY

This endoscopic procedure is used to explore the mediastinum and to obtain biopsies of lymph nodes and other masses. General anesthesia is usually required, although a local anesthetic may be used safely in selected patients in a day surgery setting. All paratracheal nodes and the nodes in the tracheobronchial angle and proximally along the main bronchi are evaluable, as are the nodes in the anterior compartment of the subcarinal space. Lymph nodes in the aortopulmonary window as well as the left anterior mediastinum (usually along the phrenic nerve) cannot be reached by conventional mediastinoscopy, nor can the inferior posterior lymph nodes. In addition, nodes along the esophagus and in the inferior pulmonary ligament are not accessible (72).

A modified procedure has recently been developed involving extension of the conventional cervical mediastinoscopy incision using a parasternal approach as an alternative to left anterior mediastinotomy (73). This can aid in the evaluation of lymph nodes in the left hilar or left upper lobe areas. Complications from mediastinoscopy are uncommon, with no operative deaths reported in the series by Luke and coworkers[74] in 1986 from Toronto General Hospital. A complication rate of 2.3% was noted among the 1,000 patients described and included hemorrhage, pneumothorax, wound infection, and recurrent laryngeal nerve palsy (74).

Mediastinoscopy is recommended in patients with T2 or T3 primary cancerous lesions, as well as those with T1 lesions in whom the cell type is adenocarcinoma or large-cell carcinoma, even when the computed tomographic studies are negative. If nodes are identified, then cervical mediastinoscopy is performed. Patients with T2 or T3 lesions in the left upper lobe should undergo cervical mediastinoscopy with frozen section; if the other biopsy specimens are negative, a left anterior mediastinotomy through the second intercostal space should be performed (73). These procedures can be performed on an outpatient basis. A recent report of ambulatory mediastinoscopy and anterior mediastinotomy reveals that these procedures permitted a diagnosis to be made in 47 of 158 patients and confirmed unresectable malignant disease in 29 patients, thus barring unnecessary admission to the hospital in 48% of the patients reported (75). Mediastinoscopy may be omitted in patients with T1 squamous cell carcinoma and negative findings on CT. Patients with superior sulcus tumor or significant pleural effusion may be evaluated by mediastinal pleuroscopy on either side.[72,74]

Mediastinoscopy is also used for the diagnosis of other masses in the middle or anterior mediastinum. In one series of 21 such cases (76), definitive diagnoses were obtained in 67%. Since several of these patients had diseases for which the treatment of choice was not surgery, the procedure saved the patient from more extensive exploration. Carlens (77) reported that mediastinoscopy was positive in 96% of 123 cases of sarcoidosis. However, usually the diagnosis of sarcoidosis can be established by less-invasive means, such as peripheral lymph node biopsy or transbronchial lung biopsy.

ENDOSCOPIC ULTRASOUND-GUIDED FINE NEEDLE ASPIRATION

An alternative to mediastinoscopy in the diagnosis of mediastinal malignancy is endoscopic ultrasound-guided fine needle aspiration (EUS-FNA) (78). With this procedure, an echoendoscope is placed in the esophagus, and the lesion is localized with the echo. Once the lesion is localized, a needle is advanced through the esophageal wall incrementally under real-time endoscopic ultrasound guidance until the needle tip is visualized with the lesion. In one study, EUS-FNA established the diagnosis of mediastinal involvement in six of seven patients in whom cervical mediastinoscopy was positive (78).

OPEN-LUNG BIOPSY

To a large extent, thoracoscopic lung biopsy has replaced open-lung biopsy (68). The indications for either thoracoscopic lung biopsy or open-lung biopsy are as follows: (a) the patient with diffuse pulmonary infiltrates and progressive disease whose diagnosis is not apparent after a careful history, physical examination, sputum analysis, and bronchoscopy with transbronchial biopsy; (b) the patient with a progressive localized pulmonary infiltrate whose diagnosis is not apparent after a careful evaluation as described above, including bronchoscopy and transbronchial biopsy; (c) the immunocompromised host with pulmonary infiltrates but no specific diagnosis after bronchoscopy with transbronchial biopsy or percutaneous needle aspiration; and (d) the patient suspected of having pulmonary malignancy in whom the sputum cytologic examination, bronchoscopy, transbronchial biopsy, and needle aspiration are nondiagnostic. In general, thoracoscopy is preferred to open-lung biopsy if it is available because it is associated with less postoperative pain and requires a shorter hospitalization (68)

Open-lung biopsy via limited thoracotomy is a relatively safe procedure with little morbidity (19%) and approximately 0.5 to 0.6% mortality (79, 80). Biopsy specimens should be taken from at least two sites (an upper-lobe and a lower-lobe site) and should include both abnormal- and normal-appearing areas. Obtaining small subpleural samples (especially if pleuritis is present) in dependent segments of the right middle lobe or lingula may yield nonspecific findings. When the procedure is performed and the diagnosis of interstitial infiltrates with suspected fibrosis is found, the pathologist should quantitate both the extent and the severity of the inflammatory or exudative—as well as the fibrotic or reparative—tissue responses noted (79,80).

In patients with diffuse pulmonary infiltrates and acute respiratory failure, open-lung biopsy provided a specific etiologic diagnosis in 66% of patients in one series (79). Diagnosis influenced therapy in 70%; however, only 30% of the patients survived to hospital discharge, and only nine patients survived for more than one year. This study suggested that open-lung biopsy is helpful in yielding an etiologic diagnosis; however, this utility is limited by current shortcomings of therapy (79). Open lung-biopsy is also worthwhile in immunocompromised patients with pulmonary infiltrates. Cheson and coworkers (81) reviewed their results in 87 such patients and reported that a specific histologic diagnosis was obtained in 62 patients (71%), 33 of whom had infections. Specific therapy was available for 52 patients, and in 33 cases following the biopsy, a change in therapy was necessary for appropriate treatment. Forty-one patients received an adequate course of therapy, and 27 (66%) improved clinically, including those with infection, malignancies, and vasculitis. This report suggests that in immunocompromised patients in the pre-AIDS era (from 1971 to 1982), open-lung biopsy was safe and accurate in diagnosis, with clinical improvement following biopsy-directed patient management (81).

In contrast, in patients with AIDS, open-lung biopsy appears to have a limited role. In 42 patients reported by Fitzgerald and associates (82), 29 patients had a preceding nondiagnostic bronchoscopic procedure and nine had open-lung biopsy because of progressive deterioration despite treatment for diseases diagnosed bronchoscopically. Diagnoses of treatable diseases such as cryptococcosis, tuberculosis, and PCP were made in only five of the 42 patients subjected to open-lung biopsy in this study, and one of the procedures was a false negative. Based on this and other studies, many investigators suggest that open-lung biopsy in patients with AIDS should be reserved for highly selected patients and that a second bronchoscopic procedure or thoracoscopy should be considered because of the morbidity associated with open lung biopsy (83).

REFERENCES

1. Kohan JM, Poe RH, Israel RH, et al. Value of chest ultrasonography versus decubitus roentgenography for thoracentesis. *Am Rev Respir Dis* 1986;133:1124–1126.
2. Light RW. *Pleural Diseases*. 3rd Ed. Baltimore: Williams and Wilkins, 1995.
3. Light RW, Erozan YC, Ball WC Jr. Cells in pleural fluid: their value in differential diagnosis. *Arch Intern Med* 1973;132:854–860.
4. Broaddus VC, Light RW. What is the origin of pleural transudates and exudates? [Editorial]. *Chest* 1992;102:658.
5. Light RW, MacGregor MI, Luchsinger PC, et al. Pleural effusions: the diagnostic separation of transudates and exudates. *Ann Intern Med* 1972;77:507–513.
6. Romero S, Candela A, Martin C, et al. Evaluation of different criteria for the separation of pleural transudates from exudates. *Chest* 1993;104:399–404.
7. Burgess LJ, Maritz FJ, Taljaard FFJ. Comparative analysis of the biochemical parameters used to distinguish between pleural transudates and exudates. *Chest* 1995;107:1604–1609.
8. Light RW, Rogers JT, Cheng D-S, et al. Large pleural effusions occurring after coronary artery bypass grafting (CABG). *Ann Intern Med* 1999;130:891–896.
9. Lankisch PG, Groge M, Becher R. Pleural effusions: a new negative prognostic parameter for acute pancreatitis. *Am J Gastroenterol* 1994;89:1849–1851.
10. Kramer MR, Ceperao RJ, Pitchenik AE. High amylase in neoplasm-related pleural effusion. *Ann Intern Med* 1989;110:567–569.
11. Light RW, Girard WM, Jenkinson SG, et al. Parapneumonic effusions. *Am J Med* 1980;69:507–512.
12. Cheng D-S, Rodriguez RM, Rogers J, et al. Comparison of pleural fluid pH values obtained using blood gas machine, pH meter, and pH indicator strip. *Chest* 1998;114:1368–1372.
13. Rodriguez de Castro F, Molero T, Acosta O, et al. Value of DNA analysis in addition to cytological testing in the diagnosis of malignant pleural effusions. *Thorax* 1994;49:692–694.
14. Moriarty AT, Wiersema L, Snyder W, et al. Immunophenotyping of cytologic specimens by flow cytometry. *Diagn Cytopathol* 1993;9:252–258.
15. Brown RW, Clark GM, Tandon AK, et al. Multiple-marker immunohistochemical phenotypes distinguishing malignant pleural mesothelioma from pulmonary adenocarcinoma. *Human Pathol* 1993;24:347–354.
16. Valdes L, Alvarez D, San Jose E, et al. Tuberculous pleurisy: a study of 254 patients. *Arch Intern Med* 1998;158:2017–2021.
17. Ocana IM, Martinez-Vazquez JM, Seguna RM, et al. Adenosine deaminase in pleural fluids. *Chest* 1983;84:51–53.
18. Villena V, Lopez-Encuentra A, Echave-Sustaeta J, et al. Interferon-gamma in 388 immunocompromised and immunocompetent patients for diagnosing pleural tuberculosis. *Eur Respir J* 1996;9:2635–2639.
19. Querol JM, Minguez J, Garcia-Sanchez E, et al. Rapid diagnosis of pleural tuberculosis by polymerase chain reaction. *Am J Respir Crit Care Med* 1995;152;1977–1981.
20. Villena V, Rebollo MJ, Aguado JM, et al. Polymerase chain reaction for the diagnosis of pleural tuberculosis in immunocompromised and immunocompetent patients. *Clin Infect Dis* 1998;26:212–214.
21. Light RW. Closed needle biopsy of the pleura is a valuable diagnostic procedure. con closed needle biopsy. *J Bronchol* 1999;5:332–336.
22. Prakash URS, Reiman HM. Comparison of needle biopsy with cytologic analysis for the evaluation of pleural effusion: analysis of 414 cases. *Mayo Clin Proc* 1985;60:158–164.

23. Ahmad M, Dweik RA. Future of flexible bronchoscopy. *Clin Chest Med* 1999;20:1–17

24. Strumpf IJ, Feld MK, Cornelius MJ, et al. Safety of fiberoptic bronchoalveolar lavage in evaluation of interstitial lung disease. *Chest* 1981;80:268–271.

25. Goldstein RA, Rohatgi PK, Bergofsky EH, et al. Clinical role of bronchoalveolar lavage in adults with pulmonary disease. *Am Rev Respir Dis* 1990;142:481–486.

26. Steiner RM, Liu JB, Goldberg BB, et al. The value of ultrasound-guided fiberoptic bronchoscopy. *Clin Chest Med* 1995;16:519–534.

27. Kurimoto N, Murayama M, Yoshioka S, et al. Assessment of usefulness of endobronchial ultrasonography in determination of depth of tracheobronchial tumor invasion. *Chest* 1999;115:1500–1506.

28. Shannon JJ, Bude RO, Orens JB, et al. Endobronchial ultrasound-guided needle aspiration of mediastinal adenopathy. *Am J Respir Crit Care Med* 1996;153:1424–1430.

29. Ghows MB, Rosen MJ, Chuang MT, et al. Transcutaneous oxygen monitoring during fiberoptic bronchoscopy. *Chest* 1986;89:543–544.

30. Cordasco EM Jr, Mehta AC, Ahmed M. Bronchoscopically induced bleeding. *Chest* 1991;100:1141–1147.

31. Pereira W, Kovnat DM, Kahn MA, et al. Fever and pneumonia after flexible fiberoptic bronchoscopy. *Am Rev Respir Dis* 1975;112:59–64.

32. Prakash UBS. Does the bronchoscope propagate infection? *Chest* 1993;104:552–559.

33. Popovich J Jr, Kvale PA, Eichenhorn MS, et al. Diagnostic accuracy of multiple biopsies from flexible fiberoptic bronchoscopy: a comparison of central versus peripheral carcinoma. *Am Rev Respir Dis* 1982;125:521–523.

34. Dreisin RB, Albert RK, Talley PA, et al. Flexible fiberoptic bronchoscopy in the teaching hospital: yield and complications. *Chest* 1978;74:144–149.

35. Kavale PA. Bronchoscopic biopsies and bronchoalveolar lavage. *Chest Surg Clin N Am* 1996;6:205–222.

36. Man V, Johnston ID, Hassle MR, et al. Value of washings and brushings at fibreoptic bronchoscopy in the diagnosis of lung cancer. *Thorax* 1990;45:373–376.

37. Butcher G, Barbaric P, Delphian MS. Diagnostic, morphologic, and histopathologic correlates in bronchogenic carcinoma. A review of 1,045 bronchoscopic examinations. *Chest* 1991;99:809–814.

38. Zavala DC. Diagnostic fiberoptic bronchoscopy. Techniques and results of biopsy in 600 patients. *Chest* 1975;68:12–99.

39. Kato R, Sawafuji M, Kawamura M, et al. Massive hemoptysis successfully treated by modified bronchoscopic balloon tamponade technique. *Chest* 1996;109:842–843.

40. Witte MC, Opal SM, Gilbert JG, et al. Incidence of fever and bacteremia following transbronchial needle aspiration. *Chest* 1986;89:85–87.

41. Lillington GA, Caskey CI. Evaluation and management of solitary and multiple pulmonary nodules. *Clin Chest Med* 1993;14:111–119.

42. Bilaceroglu S, Kumcuoglu Z, Alper H, et al. CT bronchus sign-guided bronchoscopic multiple diagnostic procedures in carcinomatous solitary pulmonary nodules and masses. *Respiration* 1998;65:49–55.

43. Dasgupta A, Mehta AT. Transbronchial needle aspiration: an underused diagnostic technique. *Clin Chest Med* 1999;20:39–51.

44. Rong F, Cui B. CT scan directed transbronchial needle aspiration biopsy for mediastinal nodes. *Chest* 1998;114:36–39.

45. Schenk DA, Bryan CL, Bower JH, et al. Transbronchial needle aspiration in the diagnosis of bronchogenic carcinoma. *Chest* 1987;92:83–85.

46. Knott-Craig CJ, Oostuizen JG, Rossouw G, et al. Management and prognosis of massive hemoptysis. Recent experience with 120 patients. *J Thorac Cardiovasc Surg* 1993;105:394–397.

47. Dweik RA, Stoller JK. Role of bronchoscopy in massive hemoptysis. *Clin Chest Med* 1999;20:89–105.

48. Hirshberg B, Biran I, Glazer M, et al. Hemoptysis. etiology, evaluation, and outcome in a tertiary referral hospital. *Chest* 1997;112:440–444.

49. Haponik EF, Chin R. Hemoptysis: clinicians' perspectives. *Chest* 1990;97:469–475.

50. Adelman M, Haponik EF, Bleecker ER, et al. Cryptogenic hemoptysis. *Ann Intern Med* 1985;102:829–834.

51. Reynolds HY. Bronchoalveolar lavage. *Am Rev Respir Dis* 1987;135:250–263.

52. Marrie TJ. Community-acquired pneumonia: epidemiology, etiology, treatment. *Infect Dis Clin North Am* 1998;12:723–740.

53. Souweine B, Veber B, Bedos JP, et al. Diagnostic accuracy of protected specimen brush and bronchoalveolar lavage in nosocomial pneumonia: impact of previous antimicrobial treatments. *Crit Care Med* 1998;26:236–244.

54. Chastre J, Trouillet JL. Nosocomial pneumonia. *Curr Opin Pulm Med* 1995;1:194–201.

55. Irwin RS, Boudet LP, Cloutier MM, et al. Managing cough as a defense mechanism and as a symptom. A consensus panel report of the American College of Chest Physicians. *Chest* 1998;114[Suppl]:133S–181S.

56. Chang S-C, Perng RP. The role of fiberoptic bronchoscopy in evaluating the causes of pleural effusions. *Arch Intern Med* 1989;149:855–857.

57. Feinsilver SH, Barrows AA, Braman SS. Fiberoptic bronchoscopy and pleural effusion of unknown origin. *Chest* 1986;90:514–515.

58. Ovassapian A, Randel GI. The role of the fiberscope in the critically ill patient. *Crit Care Clin* 1995;11:29–51

59. Dunagan DP, Baker AM, Hurd DD, et al. Bronchoscopic evaluation of pulmonary infiltrates following bone marrow transplantation. *Chest* 1997;111:135–141.

60. Larscheid RC, Thorpe PE, Scott WJ. A percutaneous transthoracic needle aspiration biopsy. A comprehensive review of its current role in the diagnosis and treatment of lung tumors. *Chest* 1998;114:704–709.

61. Sokolowski JW, Burgher LW, Jones FL Jr, et al. American Thoracic Society Guidelines for percutaneous transthoracic needle biopsy. *Am Rev Respir Dis* 1989;140:255–256.

62. Landreneau RJ, Mack MJ, Hazelrigg SR, et al. The role of thoracoscopy in the management of intrathoracic neoplastic processes. *Semin Thorac Cardiovasc Surg* 1993;5:219–228.

63. DeCamp MM Jr, Jaklitsch MT, Mentzer SJ, et al. The safety and versatility of video-thoracoscopy: a prospective analysis of 895 consecutive cases. *J Am Coll Surg* 1995;181:113–120.

64. Loddenkemper R. Thoracoscopy—state of the art. *Eur Respir J* 1998;11:213–221.

65. Kendall SW, Bryan AJ, Large SR, et al. Pleural effusions: is thoracoscopy a reliable investigation? A retrospective review. *Respir Med* 1992;86:437–440.

66. Daniel TM. Diagnostic thoracoscopy for pleural disease. *Ann Thorac Surg* 1993;56:639–640.

67. Zegdi R, Azorin J, Tremblay B, et al. Videothoracoscopic lung biopsy in diffuse infiltrative lung diseases: A 5-year surgical experience. *Ann Thorac Surg* 1998;66:1170–1173.

68. Ravini M, Ferraro G, Barbieri B, et al. Changing strategies of lung biopsies in diffuse lung diseases: the impact of video-assisted thoracoscopy. *Eur Respir J* 1998;11:99–103.

69. Suzuki K, Nagai K, Yoshida J, et al. Video-assisted thoracoscopic surgery for small indeterminate pulmonary nodules. *Chest* 1999;115:563–568.

70. Gossot D, Toledo L, Fritsch S, et al. Mediastinoscopy vs thoracoscopy for mediastinal biopsy. *Chest* 1996;110:1328–1331.

71. Kaiser OR, Bavaria JE. Complications of thoracoscopy. *Ann Thorac Surg* 1993;56:796–798.

72. Pearson FG. Staging the mediastinum: role of mediastinoscopy and computed tomography. *Chest* 1993;103:346S–348S.

73. Ginsberg RJ, Rice TO, Goldbert M, et al. Extended cervical mediastinoscopy. *J Thorac Cardiovasc Surg* 1987;94:673–678.

74. Luke WP, Todd TRJ, Cooper SD. Prospective evaluation of mediastinoscopy for assessment of carcinoma of the lung. *J Thorac Cardiovasc Surg* 1986;91:53–56.

75. Vallieres E, Page A, Verdent A. Ambulatory mediastinoscopy and anterior mediastinotomy. *Ann Thorac Surg* 1991;52:1122–1126.

76. Widstrom A, Schnurer L. The value of mediastinoscopy—experience of 374 cases. *J Otolaryngol* 1978;7:103–109.

77. Carlens E. Mediastinoscopy. *Ann Otol Rhinol Laryngol* 1965;74:1102–1112.

78. Serna DL, Aryan HE, Chang KJ, et al. An early comparison between endoscopic ultrasound-guided fine-needle aspiration and mediastinoscopy for diagnosis of mediastinal malignancy. *Am Surg* 1998;64;1014–1018.

79. Warner DO, Warner MA, Divertie MB. Open lung biopsy in patients with diffuse pulmonary infiltrates and acute respiratory failure. *Am Rev Respir Dis* 1988;137:90–94.

80. Gaensler EA, Carrington CB. Open lung biopsy for chronic diffuse infiltrative lung disease: clinical, roentgenographic, and physiological correlations in 502 patients. *Ann Thorac Surg* 1980;30:411–426.

81. Cheson BD, Samlowski WE, Tang TT, et al. Value of open-lung biopsy in 87 immunocompromised patients with pulmonary infiltrates. *Cancer* 1985;55:453–459.

82. Fitzgerald W, Bevelagua FA, Garay SM, et al. The role of open lung biopsy in patients with acquired immunodeficiency syndrome. *Chest* 1987;91:659–661.

83. Vander Els NJ, Stover DE. Approach to the patient with pulmonary disease. *Clin Chest Med* 1996;17:767–785.

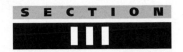

MANAGEMENT OF RESPIRATORY DISEASES

8

ASTHMA

MANI S. KAVURU
HERBERT P. WIEDEMANN

DEFINITION AND CLASSIFICATION

EPIDEMIOLOGY
Incidence, Prevalence, and Mortality
The β-agonist Controversy

NATURAL HISTORY

PATHOLOGY AND PATHOGENESIS

CLINICAL EVALUATION and assessment of severity
Diagnosis
Assessing Asthma Severity
Comorbid Conditions

GENERAL MANAGEMENT
Patient Education
Allergen Avoidance: Environmental Control Measures

PHARMACOTHERAPY FOR CHRONIC ASTHMA
Antileukotrienes

ACUTE ASTHMA

EXPERIMENTAL THERAPY

SUMMARY

Bronchial Asthma affects 3% to 5% of the U.S. population (approximately 14 to 15 million people), making it a frequently encountered clinical problem in both the pediatric and adult population. It is a major cause of morbidity in the United States and around the world. During the past decade, despite an increasing understanding of the pathogenesis of asthma, there has been an increase in the morbidity and mortality due to asthma. Although there are several potential hypotheses for the recent increases in asthma morbidity and mortality, attention has shifted away from excessive use of β-agonist aerosols as a significant cause. The National Asthma Education and Prevention Program (NAEPP) Expert Panel Report 2 (EPR-2) was published in 1997 (1). Since the publication of the first report in 1991, there has been a firmer scientific basis for the concept of antiinflammatory therapy for asthma. Also, several new drugs have been approved for asthma, including a new class of drugs (antileukotrienes).

Asthma is a heterogeneous disease, and multiple mechanisms are likely involved in the pathogenesis rather than a single unifying mechanism. The development of specific antagonists to the various mediators is accelerating our understanding of this disease. As a product of this understanding, it is to be hoped that additional therapeutic agents will emerge for subgroups of asthmatics. This chapter reviews recent trends in epidemiology, pathogenesis, and management principles of bronchial asthma.

DEFINITION AND CLASSIFICATION

Despite a number of formal attempts over a 30-year period, a universally accepted definition of asthma is unavailable (1–5). It is likely that asthma is not a specific disease but a syndrome that derives from multiple precipitating mechanisms and results in a common clinical complex involving reversible airflow obstruction (6). Important features of this syndrome include episodic occurrence of dyspnea and wheezing, airflow obstruction with a bronchodilator-reversible component, bronchial hyperresponsiveness to a variety of nonspecific and specific stimuli, and airway inflammation. All of these features need not be present. During the past 10 to 15 years, as a result of investigative bronchoscopic studies involving mild asthmatics, airway inflammation has become integral to the definition of asthma. Although there is some overlap in features between asthma and other chronic obstructive airflow disorders such as chronic bronchitis, emphysema, and cystic fibrosis, it is essential to make this distinction. Asthma typically occurs in younger individuals who are nonsmokers. In general, the baseline level of functioning, exercise tolerance, and spirometric parameters in asthmatics are much better preserved between acute exacerbations than in individuals with emphysema or chronic bronchitis. Patients with asthma exhibit a tremendous heterogeneity in the clinical features and the severity of disease. Asthma can range from being very mild, occurring perhaps only in relation to specific triggers such as pollen or exercise, to being a severe, unrelenting, and occasionally fatal disease without a definable external cause.

Asthma has traditionally been classified as either extrinsic or intrinsic. Patients with extrinsic asthma tend to have childhood onset, positive skin-test reactions to many allergens (atopy), a strong family history of atopy and asthma, and often a predictable seasonal variation of their asthma. Intrinsic asthma is not associated with any known immunologic reactions to external allergens, usually begins in adulthood, and exhibits little seasonal variation. However, this classification system is not particularly useful or relevant to the clinical management or treatment of most asthmatic patients, especially adults. Rather, current research to help further classify and characterize the asthma syndrome is focused on a variety of biologic markers of inflammation, including oxidation products, exhaled nitric oxide, bronchoalveolar lavage cellular and cytokine profiles, urinary leukotriene products, and various genetic markers. However, current knowledge does not permit these parameters to be used in the diagnosis, assessment of disease severity, prognosis, or likelihood to respond to specific therapies.

EPIDEMIOLOGY

Incidence, Prevalence, and Mortality

The true prevalence of asthma is difficult to ascertain due to the lack of a standard definition and the variations in epidemiologic methodology that have been used. In most surveys, asthma is found to be more common in children than in adults and slightly more frequent in males than in females. In the United States, a national survey by the Public Health Service in 1970 estimated that 3% of the population had asthma (7,8). In this survey, 60.3% of asthmatic individuals consulted a physician for asthma during the previous year and about 50% were using a medication or treatment for asthma. In a smaller study using better clinical documentation, performed in the Michigan town of Tecumseh, the 12-month prevalence of asthma was 4.0% in males and 3.4% in females (8,9). National Health and Nutritional Examination Surveys conducted five years apart, in 1975 and 1980, reported a significant increase in the prevalence of asthma from 4.8% to 7.6% among six- to 11-year-old children (10). The overall annual age-adjusted hospital discharge rate for asthma as the primary diagnosis decreased slightly from 18.4 per 10,000 population in 1982 to 17.9 per 10,000 in 1992 (11,12). From 1982 through 1992, the overall annual age-adjusted prevalence rate of self-reported asthma increased 42%, from 34.7 per thousand to 49.4

per thousand. For persons aged five to 34 years, the rate increased 52%, from 34.6 to 52.6 per thousand. The rate for women increased 82%, from 29.4 to 53.6 per thousand.

Skobeloff and coworkers conducted a retrospective review of all asthma admissions from southeastern Pennsylvania to define the role of age and sex as risk factors for asthma hospital admission. There were 33,269 patients admitted for asthma treatment over a four-year period that included 67 hospitals in five counties (13). In the 0- to 10-year-old age group, males were admitted nearly twice as often as age-identical females. In the 11- to 20-year-old age group, admissions for males and females were nearly identical. Between 20 and 50 years of age, the female-to-male ratio was nearly 3:1. Length of stay increased proportionally as the patient age increased, and the length of stay was greater for females than for males. Overall, the authors concluded that adult females are more severely affected by asthma than adult males.

Data from the National Center for Health Statistics disclosed gradual decreases in the number of deaths from asthma each year in the United States to a low of 1,674 in 1977 (11). From 1982 through 1991, however, the annual age-adjusted death rate for asthma as the underlying cause of death increased 40% from 13.4 per 1 million population (3,154 deaths) to 18.8 per 1 million (5,106 deaths). During this period, the death rate increased 59% for females (from 1.3 to 2.0 per 100,000) and 34% for males (from 1.3 to 1.6 per 100,000) (11). The annual asthma death rate was consistently higher for African Americans than for whites during this period. For African Americans the rate increased 52% (from 2.5 to 3.8 per 100,000), compared with a 45% increase (from 1.1 to 1.6 per 100,000) for whites. The increase in the death rate for black and white females was similar; however, the increase in the death rate for black males was more than twice that for white males and the mortality rate was three times the rate for whites. The increase in mortality rates has been even more dramatic in other countries, including Australia, England and Wales, West Germany, Japan, and Canada (14–16).

Several recent studies have critically reviewed whether the recent mortality trends are real or an epidemiologic artifact (17–19). Asthma mortality rates, determined from death certificate data, may underestimate actual asthma-related mortality. Data suggest that the recent increases in mortality due to asthma appear to be real and cannot be explained simply by false-positive reporting or a revision in the International Classification of Disease (ICD-9) coding. There are several potential causes for increased mortality due to asthma, including a change in the prevalence of asthma, change in the severity of disease, inadequate objective assessment of disease severity, toxicity of current therapy, or suboptimal usage of antiinflammatory therapy.

There are numerous retrospective studies that have examined the circumstances of asthma-related deaths (20–22).

Also, there are several case-controlled studies comparing matched survivors to patients who died of asthma (23,24). Review of these and other studies suggests that asthma deaths are of two types: type 1, slow onset–late arrival; and type 2, sudden onset (25). Consensus from these studies is that there are several risk factors that contribute to type 1 fatal asthma, including prior serious asthma requiring emergency room visits or mechanical ventilation. Factors that may interfere with compliance and access to medical care include socioeconomic factors, certain psychological features, and racial/cultural factors. Other factors include inadequate use of pulmonary function to assess objectively the severity of asthma. Inadequate treatment with either inhaled or systemic corticosteroids is also a frequently described finding. Therefore, underestimation of asthma severity and undertreatment are important contributing factors in type 1 asthma-related fatalities (26). A relatively small subset of patients with status asthmaticus have a predominantly hyperacute, bronchospastic component (27,28). Whether the fundamental mechanism in this type 2 subset is based on bronchospasm, smooth muscle contraction, neural mechanisms, or yet-unknown inflammatory mechanisms remains to be established (29).

Overall, data indicate upward trends in both the morbidity and mortality due to asthma. In 1990, the cost of illness related to asthma was estimated to be $6.2 billion, or nearly 1% of all U.S. health care cost (30,31). Inpatient hospital services represented the largest single direct medical expenditure for asthma, approaching $1.6 billion. Forty-three percent of the economic impact of asthma was associated with emergency room use and hospitalization. Nearly two-thirds of the visits for ambulatory care were to physicians in primary care specialties, including pediatrics, family medicine, general practice, and internal medicine.

The β-Agonist Controversy

There has been much controversy surrounding the potential role of β-agonist preparations in the increasing asthma mortality (32). The hypothesis is that excessive or regular use of β-adrenergic bronchodilators can actually worsen asthma, perhaps contributing to morbidity and mortality. Several studies from New Zealand suggested that the use of inhaled β-agonists increases the risk of death in severe asthma (15,33,34). Sears and coworkers conducted a placebo-controlled, crossover study in patients with mild stable asthma to evaluate the effects of regular versus on-demand inhaled fenoterol therapy for 24 weeks (35). In the 57 patients who did better with one of the two regimens, only 30% had better asthma control when receiving regularly administered bronchodilators, whereas 70% had better asthma control when they employed the bronchodilators only as needed.

Spitzer and coworkers conducted a matched, case-controlled study using a health insurance database from Saskatchewan, Canada, of a cohort of 12,301 patients for whom asthma medications had been prescribed (36). Data were based on matching 129 case patients who had fatal or nearly fatal asthma with 655 controls. The use of β-agonist administered by a meter dose inhaler (MDI) was associated with an increased risk of death from asthma, with an odds ratio of 5.4 per canister of fenoterol, 2.4 per canister of albuterol, and 1.0 for background risk (i.e., no fenoterol or albuterol). The primary limitation of this study, and indeed case-controlled studies in general, is concern regarding the comparability of the two groups in terms of the severity of the underlying disease (37).

More recently, a study by Drazen and coworkers randomly assigned 255 patients with mild asthma to inhaled albuterol either on a regular basis (two puffs four times per day) or only on an as-needed basis for 16 weeks (38). There were no significant differences between the two groups in a variety of outcomes, including morning peak expiratory flow, diurnal peak flow variability, forced expiratory volume in one second, number of puffs of supplemental as-needed albuterol, asthma symptoms, or airway reactivity to methacholine. Since neither benefit nor harm was seen, it was concluded that inhaled albuterol should be prescribed for patients with mild asthma on an as-needed basis.

Overall, the exact contribution of β-agonists to the recent mortality trend remains unknown, although it is unlikely to be a major contributor. If patients require increasing numbers of puffs of β-agonist aerosols, this is usually a marker for the need for more effective anti-inflammatory therapy. β-agonist aerosols remain a critical part of the regimen for acute emergency room management of bronchial asthma. For maintenance therapy, the ERP-2 guidelines recommend as-needed use of inhaled β-agonists (1). If a patient exceeds three to four puffs a day of a β-agonist, additional therapy should be considered.

NATURAL HISTORY

The natural history of asthma is complex and not well defined. In general, childhood asthma is frequently self-limited and carries a better prognosis than adult-onset asthma (8). In one large study, one-half of 449 children with onset of asthma before the age of 13 became symptom-free during 20-year follow-up (9,39). Another one-fourth had only minimal symptoms, which could be prevented by avoiding specific exacerbating factors such as dust or animals. The severity of asthma in childhood correlates with the persistence of asthma into adulthood and the severity of adult asthma in the childhood-onset group (40,41). There is increasing evidence to suggest that asthma alone can cause irreversible airflow obstruction (42–44). Recent studies indicate that the bulk of the "irreversible" loss of lung function may occur in the interval prior to the start of anti-inflammatory therapy (44,45). Data from Bronnimann and

Bronnimann and Burrows suggest that after the second decade, asthmatic subjects show a low rate of remission (46). Adults with a history of childhood asthma have a significant risk of future active asthma. In general, atopy is not useful in predicting remissions or relapses. Despite common belief, allergic rhinitis is not a harbinger of subsequent asthma. Although allergic rhinitis and asthma frequently coexist, if asthma does not occur within one year of the onset of allergic rhinitis, then there is only a 5% to 10% risk of asthma developing later (47). About 20% of asthmatics develop disease after the age of 65 (48).

PATHOLOGY AND PATHOGENESIS

Early pathologic observations have been made in patients who have succumbed to a severe exacerbation of asthma (49–51), although some information is available from asthmatic patients who died of other causes (52) and patients with symptom-free asthma (53). The pathologic findings in fatal asthma include (a) infiltration with eosinophils, (b) thickening of the basement membrane, (c) hypertrophy of the airway smooth muscle, (d) desquamation of the epithelium, (e) mucosal edema, and (f) mucus plugs containing shed epithelial cells and proteinaceous and cellular components of the inflammatory reaction (54).

Information from experimentally induced asthma as well as studies involving bronchoalveolar lavage (BAL) and endobronchial biopsy of milder, chronic, human asthma have contributed to the hypothesis that airway inflammation is a fundamental aspect of asthma (54–57). This concept underlies the growing clinical and investigational interest in the use of various antiinflammatory agents in the treatment of asthma. The relationship between airway inflammation and bronchial hyperreactivity remains unclear (58,59).

There are several well-described human models of experimentally induced asthma that form the basis of our current understanding of the pathogenesis of asthma (58,60). A well-known model involves an allergic asthmatic challenged with an inhaled allergen to which he is sensitive (61,62). This challenge results in a biphasic decline in respiratory function, an early asthmatic response (EAR) that occurs within minutes and resolves by two hours, and a late asthmatic response (LAR) that usually occurs within six to eight hours and may last 24 to 96 hours or longer (Fig 8.1) (54,63). The LAR, which appears to occur in 50% of adult asthmatics (64), is associated with increased airway reactivity to nonspecific stimuli (such as methacholine or histamine) and a cellular influx into airway lavage fluid. Pretreatment with β-agonists blocks only the EAR, whereas corticosteroids block only the LAR, and cromolyn sodium and nedocromil block both phases. In human studies, exposure to ozone results in LAR and influx of polymorphonuclear neutrophils in BAL (58). In the allergen and western red cedar (plicatic acid) model of asthma there again appears

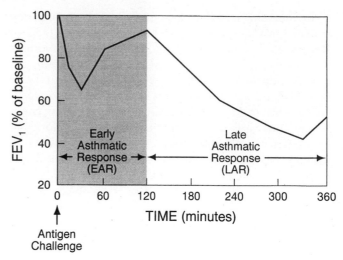

FIGURE 8.1. Biphasic decline in lung function as measured by forced expiratory volume in one second (FEV_1) in an allergic asthmatic after inhalation of an allergen (see text for details).

a LAR, but the lavage fluid has an influx of both polymorphonuclear cells and eosinophils. These and other studies suggest that the specificity of the stimulus affects the nature of the inflammatory process after exposure.

These observations in experimentally induced asthma have been extended to chronic stable asthma. Beasley and coworkers studied eight atopic stable asthmatics and four controls (57). Endobronchial biopsies of stable asthmatics showed extensive mucosal inflammation characterized by epithelial sloughing, eosinophil infiltration of the submucosa, and basement membrane thickening. Also, BAL studies in these stable asthmatics showed the presence of a fivefold increase in the shed epithelial cells and mast cells. Martin and coworkers analyzed BAL fluid in a group of asthmatics with nocturnal asthma and compared them to asthmatics without nocturnal asthma. BAL performed at 4:00 A.M. showed a significant increase in neutrophils, eosinophils, and lymphocytes in patients with symptomatic nocturnal asthma compared with asthmatics without nocturnal symptoms (65). These studies suggest that airway inflammation plays a significant role in both experimentally induced asthma and stable chronic human asthma. Numerous studies have suggested that the inflammation in asthma differs significantly from the inflammatory response seen in other airway or pulmonary parenchymal diseases by the distinct absence of bronchiolitis, fibrosis, and granulation tissue. The reasons for this remain unclear (54).

Numerous studies have recently advanced the notion that the T lymphocyte plays a pivotal role in the regulation and expression of local eosinophilia and IgE production in both asthma and allergic disease (66–68). Lavage fluid from patients with atopic asthma reveals expression of CD4-positive T helper cells. It appears that T helper cells can be further categorized as T_{H1} or T_{H2} cells based on the profile of cytokines these cells are capable of releasing (69). The T_{H1} cell produces interleukins 2 and 3 (IL-2, IL-3), granulocyte-macrophage colony-stimulating factor (GM-CSF), and interferon gamma (INF-γ), which leads to delayed hypersensitivity-type inflammatory response. On the other hand, T_{H2} lymphocytes mediate allergic inflammation in atopic asthmatics by a cytokine profile that involves interleukin-4 (which directs B lymphocytes to synthesize IgE), interleukin-5 (which is essential for the maturation of eosinophils), interleukin-3, and GM-CSF. Therefore, preliminary evidence suggests that atopic asthma is regulated by activation of a T_{H2}-like T-cell population (70).

Lipid mediators are products of arachidonic acid metabolism. They have been implicated in the airway inflammation of asthma and, therefore, have been the target for pharmacologic antagonism by a new class of agents: antileukotrienes (71–77). The prostaglandins are generated by the cyclooxygenation of arachidonic acid, and leukotrienes are generated by the lipoxygenation of arachidonic acid. The proinflammatory prostaglandins (PGD_2, PGF_2, TXB_2) cause bronchoconstriction, whereas other prostaglandins are considered protective and may elicit bronchodilation (PGE_2 and PGI_2 or prostacyclin). The cysteinyl leukotrienes (LTC_4, LTD_4 and LTE_4), formerly known as the slow-reacting substance of anaphylaxis (SRS-A), are formed by the lipoxygenation of arachidonic acid by the enzyme 5-lipoxygenase. These compounds, released by mast cells, eosinophils, and airway macrophages and epithelial cells, have a variety of potent effects, including bronchoconstriction, increased vascular permeability, and enhanced airway reactivity. Data over the past 10 years suggest that the leukotrienes are involved in the pathogenesis of experimentally induced asthma as well as spontaneously occurring chronic human asthma. Leukotrienes can be recovered from nasal secretions, bronchoalveolar lavage, and urine of patients with asthma at much higher levels than normal individuals (74,75). Leukotriene antagonists inhibit the asthmatic responses to a variety of triggers, including allergen, exercise, cold dry air, and aspirin (76–81). Three agents that antagonize the leukotriene pathway have been approved recently for use in asthma (82).

The paradigm of the asthma inflammatory cascade involves a complex interaction of resident airway cells, recruited inflammatory cells, a variety of cytokines, and a variety of proinflammatory chemical and neurogenic mediators (Fig. 8.2). The critical and rate-limiting steps in this process remain incompletely understood.

CLINICAL EVALUATION

The history and physical examination are important for several reasons: (a) to confirm a diagnosis of bronchial asthma and exclude asthma "mimics" such as upper airway obstruction (UAO), congestive heart failure, and so on; (b) to assess the severity of airflow obstruction and the need for hospitali-

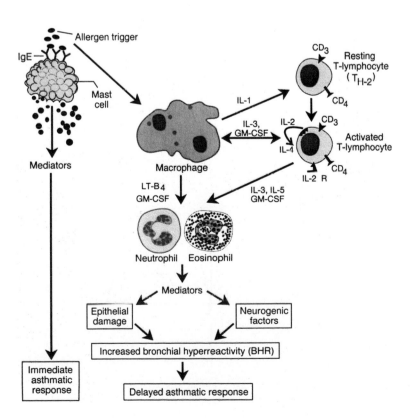

FIGURE 8.2. Asthma inflammatory cascade: summary of proposed mechanisms.

zation; (c) to identify factors that might place a patient at particular risk for poor outcome, including death; and (d) to identify comorbid diseases that may complicate the management of bronchial asthma, such as allergy to avoidable external triggers, sinusitis, or gastroesophageal reflux.

Diagnosis

In most instances, the diagnosis of asthma is not difficult. The typical patient exhibits dyspnea, and wheezes can be heard throughout the lung fields. It is essential to inquire specifically about nocturnal symptoms, since this is often missed (83). The clinician needs to remain alert both to possible atypical presentations of asthma and to conditions that may mimic asthma. Some individuals with symptomatic airway hyperresponsiveness exhibit a bothersome nonproductive cough rather than wheezing (84–88). Identification of the "cough variant" asthma syndrome may require the use of a bronchoprovocation test to document the presence of airway hyperreactivity. Such patients may achieve symptomatic relief with the use of inhaled bronchodilator medication (89). However, 29% of Irwin's patients in whom reactive airway disease was diagnosed as a cause of cough required prednisone to resolve their cough (90). No trials have compared the effectiveness of inhaled β-agonists with theophylline or inhaled corticosteroids.

The most important asthma mimic is upper-airway obstruction (UAO). Such obstruction can be caused by tumors, laryngeal spasm, aspirated foreign bodies, and tracheal stenosis, to name just a few potential causes. Patients with UAO may present with dyspnea and "wheezing" (stridor) that might be very difficult to distinguish from asthma on clinical inspection alone (although careful auscultation should reveal that the "wheeze" is located over the superior aspect of the thorax or neck). Some patients with chronic UAO have been misdiagnosed and treated for months or even years as having "refractory" asthma. Failure to diagnose and treat acute life-threatening UAO can have obvious consequences as well. Upper-airway obstruction can be detected through analysis of the flow-volume loops (expiratory and inspiratory) and confirmed by bronchoscopy.

The shape of the flow-volume loop may provide insight into the nature and location of airway obstruction. Figure 8.3 depicts several characteristic patterns of the loop that help to localize the site of obstruction and help distinguish asthma from asthma mimics such as UAO. Normally, there is a limitation of airflow at high lung volumes, which produces a sharp peak (peak expiratory flow, or PEF) in the expiratory limb of the flow-volume loop during periods of maximal flow. Both asthma and emphysema are examples of typical obstructive airway disorders characterized by a concavity of the expiratory limb of the flow-volume loop

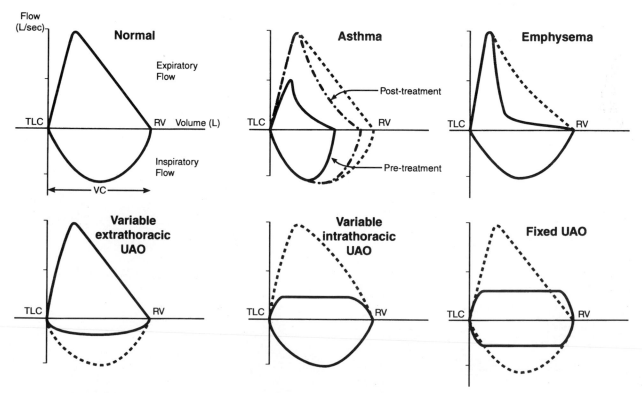

FIGURE 8.3. Representative flow-volume loops (see text for details). *RV,* residual volume; *TLC,* total lung capacity; *VC,* vital capacity; *UAO,* upper-airway obstruction.

with a fairly well preserved inspiratory limb. With UAO, the shape of the loop is related to the level of the obstruction (above or below the thoracic inlet) and the net effect of pressures acting on the extrathoracic or intrathoracic airway, which include the atmospheric pressure, intraluminal pressure, and intrapleural pressure. The flow-volume loop shows flattening of the inspiratory limb with variable extrathoracic UAO, likely due to a lesion involving the glottic or subglottic area. On the other hand, flattening limited to the expiratory limb of the flow-volume loop occurs with variable intrathoracic UAO, usually on the basis of an obstructing lesion of the mid or distal trachea. "Box-like" flattening of both the inspiratory and expiratory limbs of the flow-volume loop occurs with a fixed UAO due to any etiology.

Over the past decade, several reports have described patients with functional vocal cord disorders that mimic attacks of bronchial asthma ("factitious asthma") (91–94). The typical history involves episodes of wheezing and dyspnea that are refractory to standard therapy for asthma. These individuals may have wheezing that is often loudest over the neck, but the wheezing is often transmitted over both lung fields and may be misdiagnosed as bronchial asthma. During episodes of wheezing, the maximal expiratory and inspiratory flow-volume loop is consistent with variable extrathoracic UAO. The pathophysiology of factitious asthma, as noted by laryngoscopy, appears to be adduction of the true and false vocal cords throughout the respiratory cycle, including the inspiratory phase. During asymptomatic periods, both the flow-volume loop and the laryngoscopic examination are normal. Interestingly, methacholine or histamine provocation testing is usually negative for airway hyperreactivity. Christopher and coworkers described a variety of personality styles and psychiatric diagnoses in these individuals and suggested that factitious asthma is a form of conversion reaction (91). They described a dramatic response to speech therapy and psychotherapy in these patients. In general, factitious asthma should be included in the differential diagnosis of difficult-to-control asthma.

More recently, McFadden and coworkers described vocal cord dysfunction in elite athletes that presents as "choking" during exercise (95). This entity may be distinguished from typical exercise-induced asthma by several features (symptoms are maximal during, rather than after, exercise; absence of nocturnal symptoms; UAO pattern on flow-volume loops).

Assessing Asthma Severity

Assessing the severity of an asthmatic episode is important in determining the therapeutic approach. Although the magnitude of wheezing bears some relationship to the severity of airflow obstruction, use of auscultation alone is unreliable (96). In particular, wheezing may become weak or inaudible as airflow becomes significantly reduced. An early study by McFadden and coworkers evaluated the relationship between clinical and physiologic manifestations of acute bronchial asthma serially during initial therapy in the emergency room (97). Regardless of the initial presentation of the patients, when they became asymptomatic, the overall mechanical function of the lungs was only about 40% to 50% of predicted normal values. When they were without signs of asthma on examination, lung function was only 60% to 70% of predicted values. This study reinforces the need for objective measurement of airflow obstruction during acute asthma.

Patients may have a poor ability to perceive the presence and severity of airflow obstruction until it becomes quite severe (97–101). Some patients have remained asymptomatic even with an FEV_1 of 50% of predicted (102). Despite this, patients often have a better appreciation of the severity of airflow limitation than their physician, who is relying on the history and physical examination (103). It is true that physical findings such as pulsus paradoxus (inspiratory decline in systolic blood pressure greater than 12 mm Hg), accessory muscle use including sternocleidomastoid muscle retraction, respiratory rate greater than 30, and heart rate greater than 130 are generally associated with more severe airflow obstruction (104,105). However, none of these signs alone or in combination are specific or sensitive (106,107).

The importance of directly and objectively measuring airflow is underscored by the relative insensitivity of either arterial blood gases or subjective assessments for detecting anything less than severe obstruction. The measurements most frequently used for assessing air flow are the forced expiratory volume in one second (FEV_1) and peak expiratory flow (PEF). Both the FEV_1 and PEF yield comparable results (108–111). Severe airflow obstruction is indicated by a peak flow less than 120 L per minute or an FEV_1 less than 1 L.

Several attempts have been made to formulate a scoring index for the purpose of grading the severity of acute asthma and predicting the need for hospitalization (Table 8.1) (112–118). Fischl and coworkers described an index predicting relapse and the need for hospitalization in 205 patients with acute bronchial asthma (118). Of the 205 patients, 120 were successfully treated and discharged from the emergency room, 45 were hospitalized, and 40 were treated and discharged from the emergency room but had relapses within 10 days. A predictive index was developed based on awarding one point for each of a combination of seven factors on initial presentation, including tachycardia (heart rate above 120 per minute), tachypnea (respiratory rate above 30 per minute), pulsus paradoxus (18 mm Hg or above), and PEF (120 L per minute or less). Presence of four or more of the seven factors upon presentation to the emergency room (prior to therapy) was 95% accurate in predicting the risk of relapse and 96% accurate in predicting the need for hospitalization. However, two subsequent studies failed to support the clinical utility of this method

TABLE 8.1. PROPOSED SPIROMETRIC CRITERIA FOR ADMISSION

Basis	Indications for Admission	Reference No.
Initial presentation	• Fischl index	118
	• Inability to perform spirometry	113, 114
	• FEV_1 <0.61	114
Initial flow rate and response to first treatment	• Unresponsive to epinephrine and PEF <60 L/min	
	• Unresponsive to bronchodilators and <16% change in initial PEF value	113,115
	• <0.15 L increase in FEV_1 after subcutaneous administration of bronchodilator	114
	• PEF <100 L/min initially and <160 L/min after 0.25 mg terbutaline	116
	• FEV_1 <30% of predicted value; not improving to >40% of predicted value; >4 hours therapy needed	117
Initial flow rate and response to full treatment	• PEF <100 L/min and <300 L/min after full treatment	116
	• FEV_1 <0.61 and <1.6 L after full treatment	114
	• Change in FEV_1 <400 mL after bronchodilator administration	106
Other	• Deterioration of PEF by 15% after initial good response to bronchodilator therapy	115

Modified from Brenner AS. The acute asthmatic in the emergency department: the decision to admit or discharge. *Am J Emerg Med* 1985;3:74–77.

(119,120). Another early study indicated that the response to initial therapy could be a useful guide (106). Patients whose FEV_1 improved by more than 400 mL had an early relapse rate of only 29%, whereas those who failed to demonstrate such an improvement in FEV_1 had a 67% relapse rate.

The chest roentgenogram may be helpful to exclude other pathologic conditions (pneumonia, pneumothorax) but does not provide useful information to grade the severity of asthma. In fact, hyperinflation is the most common finding on the chest roentgenogram in patients with acute asthma. Clinical judgment should be used to decide which patients receive a chest roentgenogram (121).

Although life-threatening and severe hypoxemia can occur in asthma, it is relatively uncommon. Hypoxemia is secondary to ventilation/perfusion mismatch and readily responds to supplemental oxygen. Perhaps of more concern is the evaluation and correct interpretation of the arterial carbon dioxide tension ($PaCO_2$) (122,123). Mild and moderate degrees of airflow obstruction in asthma are usually accompanied by a hyperventilation response and a low $PaCO_2$. As airflow obstruction becomes more severe, $PaCO_2$ rises to about 40 mm Hg. The onset of hypercapnia usually begins when the FEV_1 declines below 750 mL or 25% of the predicted value (Fig. 8.4) (122,124). Thus the finding of a normal $PaCO_2$ in a patient with active asthma should be viewed with some concern, and increases in $PaCO_2$ above 40 mm Hg should be viewed with proportionately increasing alarm, since this heralds severe airflow obstruction and respiratory muscle fatigue. Nowak and coworkers prospectively compared arterial blood gas and pulmonary function measurements in 102 episodes of acute bronchial asthma initially seen in the emergency room (125). The PaO_2, $PaCO_2$, and pH were unable to distinguish patients requiring admission from those who could be discharged. All patients with $PaCO_2$ greater than 42 mm Hg and/or severe hypoxemia (PaO_2 less than 60 mm Hg) had a PEF below

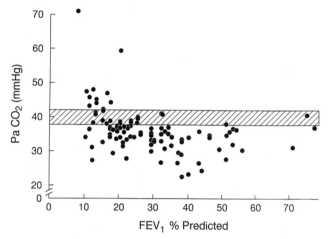

FIGURE 8.4. Correlation of the severity of acute airway obstruction with the arterial carbon dioxide tension in asthma. (From McFadden ER, Lyons HA. Arterial blood gas tension in asthma. Reprinted by permission of the *N Engl J Med*, 1968;278: 1027–1032.)

200 L per minute or an FEV_1 below 1 L. In general, in patients with an acute asthma exacerbation, arterial blood gas determination can be limited to patients who have evidence of severe airflow obstruction by a screening airflow measurement.

In the absence of completely reliable objective indicators, clinical judgment is necessary to help decide which patients with acute asthma require hospitalization.

Comorbid Conditions

Gastroesophageal Reflux

There is substantial literature that suggests a relationship between gastroesophageal reflux disease (GERD) and bronchial asthma (126). There are several possible associations between asthma and GERD: (a) these are two common diseases that coexist independently in some patients; (b) GERD either exacerbates or is causally related to the pathogenesis of asthma; or (c) bronchial asthma and/or anti-asthma medications exacerbate or induce gastroesophageal disease (127). It is likely that all three of these possibilities occur in subsets of patients with bronchial asthma. Some degree of reflux appears to be normal or "physiologic," especially for several hours in the postprandial period. The probable mechanisms for GERD-induced asthma are: (a) acid stimulation of sensory nerve fibers in the lower esophagus, with reflex vagal bronchoconstriction (128), and (b) micro-aspiration of acid into the trachea (129).

The magnitude of the association between GERD and asthma and its clinical significance remains unclear from the literature. GERD, with primary symptoms of heartburn and acid regurgitation, is common in the general population. A recent, random sample of 2,200 Olmstead County residents aged 25 to 74 years found that 20% of the respondants had reflux symptoms weekly and nearly 60% had either heartburn or acid regurgitation occurring in the past year (130). The prevalence of GERD in asthmatics is reported to range from 34% to 89% (126). Several reasons for this wide variability include the use of self-reported questionnaire data, comorbid confounding factors such as alcohol and cigarette smoking, and the variability of definition and choice of diagnostic techniques to establish GERD. Several methodologic limitations exist in the published literature relating GERD and asthma (126). The major limitation in all the published studies is the lack of attempts to optimize conventional, "standard" therapy for the underlying asthma. Inadequate use of inhaled corticosteroids is a major treatment shortcoming for many patients with poorly controlled asthma. All published trials on therapy for GERD-associated asthma involve asthmatics with symptoms of heartburn or acid regurgitation, therefore findings cannot be extended to asthmatics with so-called "silent GERD," where the reflux disease is diagnosed by a positive pH probe or endoscopic evidence of esophagitis in the absence of GERD symptoms. A practical approach to GERD in asthmatics could include aggressive empiric therapy for both GERD and asthma with judicious use of diagnostic studies. For patients with suboptimal control of asthma and symptomatic GERD, specific lifestyle changes along with empiric therapy with proton pump inhibitors (12-week trial at a dose of 20 mg twice a day with omeprazole or 30 mg twice a day with lansoprazole) should be adequate (126). The outcome of this intervention could fall into one of three groups. First, both GERD and asthma may be improved, which would suggest GERD as an important trigger. In this subset, the next challenge is long-term GERD management, possibly including gradual titration from proton pump inhibition to H_2-receptor antagonist and/or promotility drug, long-term proton pump inhibitor therapy, or evaluation for surgery. Alternatively, GERD may be improved, but asthma may remain unchanged, which would suggest that GERD is not an important trigger. And finally, if GERD is not improved with an empiric trial of proton pump inhibitor, further work-up should include specific diagnostic studies such as pH testing with manometry or endoscopy to ensure that acid reflux has been adequately controlled (126,131).

Drug-induced Asthma

A variety of over-the-counter and prescription medications may contribute to acute bronchospasm, either as an isolated response or as part of a generalized systemic anaphylaxis. The overall magnitude of drug-induced bronchospasm in the United States remains unknown. (132) Nonsteroidal anti-inflammatory drugs (NSAIDs) are by far the most common cause of drug-induced asthma. Reports indicate that 5% to 20% of adults with asthma will experience exacerbation of bronchoconstriction after ingestion of aspirin or other NSAIDs. An adverse reaction to aspirin or NSAIDs may occur at any time, often following many years of employing these drugs without difficulty. These reactions are not prevented by pretreatment with antihistamines, theophylline or cromolyn sodium. Corticosteroids do not prevent the bronchospasm unless given for an extended number of days. Other agents that have received a lot of attention in the literature include sulfites, β-adrenergic blocking agents, angiotensin converting enzyme (ACE) inhibitors, tartrazine, and a variety of miscellaneous agents (132–135). Drug-induced asthma should be suspected in all patients with difficult-to-control or steroid-dependent asthma. Careful history of all prescribed and over-the-counter medications should be obtained for all patients with asthma.

Allergic Bronchopulmonary Aspergillosis

The clinical course of an occasional patient with bronchial asthma may be complicated by pulmonary parenchymal infiltrates on the chest radiograph. The differential diagnosis for an infiltrate is extensive. However, specific entities to consider in an asthmatic include: (a) typical and atypical infections, (b) allergic bronchopulmonary aspergillosis (ABPA), (c) chronic eosinophilic pneumonia and other pulmonary infiltrate and eosinophilia (PIE) syndromes, and (d) allergic granulomatosis with angiitis (Churg-Strauss disease). Discussion here will be limited only to ABPA.

Allergic bronchopulmonary aspergillosis (ABPA) can be regarded as a complicated or special form of asthma in which immunologic reactions to *Aspergillus* species, usually *Aspergillus fumigatus,* play an important pathogenic role. Clinical syndromes analogous to ABPA have also been described in which noninvasive fungi other than *Aspergillus* appear to be the culprit. These related syndromes have been grouped under the term allergic bronchopulmonary fungoses (ABPF) (136).

Historical Aspects and Epidemiology

ABPA was first described in England in 1952 (137). In the United States, the first reported case did not appear until 1968 (138), and for several years ABPA was considered an extremely rare disease in this country. However, the relative paucity of reported cases may in part reflect underdiagnosis of this entity. In 1983, a survey of seven institutions in the United States with a known interest in ABPA identified a total of 352 patients with ABPA diagnosed since the late 1960s (139). The exact prevalence of the disease remains unknown. The vast majority of the reported cases in this country cluster in Illinois, Wisconsin, Minnesota, California, and Michigan (139). This geographic distribution likely reflects the diagnostic interest and knowledge of regional physicians, but a true difference in geographic incidence cannot be excluded as a possible explanation.

Diagnoses and Clinical Features

ABPA is an episodic and recurrent disorder with wheezing as an almost universal symptom (140). Mild or early cases resemble simple asthma and may resolve without therapy. More severe or chronic cases exhibit features of bronchiectasis with cough productive of purulent-appearing sputum that sometimes contains brownish sputum "plugs." A characteristic of advanced ABPA is proximal bronchiectasis (136).

The classic patient with ABPA has asthma, recurrent or fixed pulmonary infiltrates on the chest roentgenogram, proximal bronchiectasis, dual (immediate and late) skin test response to *A. fumigatus,* elevated total serum IgE level (above 1000 ng per mL), peripheral blood eosinophilia (above 1,000 per mm^3), and serum precipitins (specific IgG) to *A. fumigatus.* (136,141) *Aspergillus* species can frequently be identified or cultured from respiratory secretions.

Although recognition of the classic patient with ABPA should not be difficult, it is noteworthy that none of the individual diagnostic features listed in the preceding paragraph are completely specific or sensitive for the diagnosis of ABPA. Therefore, in patients who do not exhibit the full constellation of findings, differentiation of ABPA from other diseases may be difficult. In particular, it may be difficult to distinguish uncomplicated or typical asthma from ABPA. Many patients with asthma have an elevated serum IgE, peripheral eosinophilia, precipitins to *A. fumigatus* (about 10% of asthma patients), or positive skin-test reactivity. Furthermore, patients with asthma may at times exhibit an abnormal chest roentgenogram (atelectasis, pneumonia, etc.).

Patterson and colleagues have suggested that an index of elevated IgE and IgG serum antibodies *specific* against *A. fumigatus* is of value in separating ABPA patients from asthma patients who have cutaneous reactivity to *Aspergillus* species (142,143). Using this method, it was revealed that about 6% of asthma patients with cutaneous reactivity to *Aspergillus* species fulfill criteria for ABPA (144). However,

the quantitative assay for specific serum IgE or IgG is not widely available. Furthermore, it remains unclear whether ABPA needs to be rigorously excluded in all patients with chronic asthma, since the treatment for both is likely to include corticosteroids.

In patients with features suggestive of ABPA (asthma, lung infiltrates, elevated serum IgE, peripheral eosinophilia) but lacking evidence of specific immune sensitivity to *Aspergillus* species (absent precipitating antibodies, negative skin tests), the possibility of disease due to a different fungus should be considered. Such allergic bronchopulmonary fungoses (APBF) have been described (syndromes of candidiasis, curvulariosis, dreschleriosis, etc.) (136). In such cases, a diagnostic-therapeutic trial of prednisone may be warranted. If sera are obtained and stored before the initiation of therapy, subsequent assays (search for serum precipitins to specific fungal antigens) may provide insight to the specific cause (136).

It has been proposed that ABPA be described according to a five-stage classification system: acute (stage I), remission (stage II), exacerbation (stage III), corticosteroid-dependent asthma (stage IV), and fibrotic end stage (stage V) (145). Such a system may provide guidance in both the recognition and management of ABPA, although the natural history of ABPA still remains rather poorly defined and is probably quite variable.

Treatment

Prednisone is the drug of choice for treatment of ABPA. Patients who receive other therapy for asthma (cromolyn, inhaled bronchodilators, inhaled corticosteroids) without systemic corticosteroids appear to have an increased number of exacerbations and a greater likelihood of a progressive deterioration of lung function (136,146). When exacerbations of ABPA are treated with prednisone, it seems that most patients will maintain stable long-term lung function (136,147–150).

The suggested dosage of prednisone for stages I and III is 0.5 mg per kg daily for two weeks (or longer if lung infiltrates are slow to improve), followed by conversion to alternate-day therapy for another three months (136). Such therapy usually clears the patient's symptoms and chest roentgenogram. The total serum IgE is usually significantly reduced as well, but may not return to the normal level.

If clinical symptoms recur after cessation of prednisone therapy, resumption of therapy is indicated. However, monitoring of clinical status alone is insufficient, since asymptomatic pulmonary infiltrates can occur, presumably with the potential for progressive asymptomatic lung damage. The need for frequent chest roentgenograms, however, is obviated by the recognition that serum IgE levels are helpful in detecting asymptomatic relapses of ABPA (150).

During the first year off therapy, serum IgE measurements should be obtained frequently (perhaps every four to six weeks) to determine the patient's baseline value and to detect subsequent relapse. Once a patient's baseline is determined, a subsequent 100% rise in total IgE suggests a relapse. In many cases, the chest roentgenogram will indicate a new infiltrate. According to current concepts, even asymptomatic relapses of ABPA should be treated with a reinstitution of prednisone therapy.

GENERAL MANAGEMENT

The National Asthma Education Prevention Program (NAEPP) Expert Panel Report-2 provides an excellent algorithmic framework for the management of bronchial asthma (1). The general goals of asthma therapy include the following: (a) maintain normal activity levels, including exercise; (b) maintain nearly "normal" pulmonary function; (c) prevent chronic and troublesome symptoms and recurrent exacerbations of asthma; (d) avoid adverse effects from asthma medications and (e) meet patients' and family's expectation of care. Overall, asthma therapy has four key components according to EPR-2: (a) patient education; (b) lung function measurement, both initially and during periodic evaluation, including home PEF monitoring; (c) environmental control with avoidance of asthma triggers; and (d) pharmacologic therapy. Much effort has been expended to develop and disseminate asthma guidelines. Although the various guidelines represent the best collective experience and literature review by a group of experts, many of the recommendations are not based on rigorous prospective clinical trials (e.g., utility of PEF monitoring in chronic asthma), largely due to lack of head-to-head comparisons. Studies have shown that physican understanding and/or implementation of the guidelines is poor, even among specialists (151). The overall impact of NAEPP/EPR-2 remains largely unknown. It is best to view the guidelines as a dynamic process with the aim of improving outcomes.

Patient Education

Nonadherence or noncompliance with therapy is a major problem in the management of asthma. A recent study of patients with chronic asthma in a general practice setting found that only one in three patients used at least half of the prescribed amount of medication daily (152). Similarly, a number of studies have documented improper MDI technique in the majority of patients (153,154). Several studies have shown that only 40% of physicians correctly performed four or more of the seven steps in the recommended MDI inhalation maneuver (155–157). A provocative study of patients with Chronic obstructive pulmonary disease (COPD) participating in the lung health study (whose inhaler usage was monitored by self-reporting, canister weighing, and use of electronic recording devices) described a phenomenon of inhaler "dumping" (158). The investigators found that 87% of patients reported compliance with prescribed inhaler use (at least twice a day), and 85% compliance was observed if canister weights were used as measure of compliance. However, only 52% compliance was observed when the measure of compliance was the electronic monitoring device. Nearly 18% of patients who were uninformed about the function of the electronic recording device were found to have "dumped" their inhaler over a three-hour time period just prior to appointments. Reasons for nonadherence are complex and include patient-related factors (e.g., denial of disease, cultural perception of the use of medications, socioeconomic and educational status) as well as the complexity of care (e.g., need for regular maintenance therapy, use of MDIs with spacer rather than pills, etc.). Asthma education programs that are targeted (e.g., low income, ethnic minorities) may improve overall outcomes (159).

Asthma self-management education has received increasing attention in the literature recently (160,161). Several recent studies have highlighted the beneficial effects as well as the limitations of adult asthma education in clinical practice. At Bellevue Hospital, a randomized crossover trial was conducted to evaluate an outpatient educational program involving 104 adult asthmatics previously requiring multiple hospitalizations for asthma attacks (162). The program involved a combination of widely accepted modalities, including vigorous education about self-management skills, a written crisis plan, easy access to a nurse practitioner, home PEF monitoring, and proper MDI technique. The program enrollment resulted in a threefold reduction in readmission rate and a twofold reduction in hospital days. Notably, this study excluded patients with psychiatric disease, who have increased risk of asthma morbidity and mortality (162). Wilson and coworkers conducted a randomized controlled trial with one-year follow-up in a group of 323 adults with moderate-to-severe bronchial asthma (requiring three or more physician visits for asthma during a screening year) at a Kaiser Health Plan center (163). Patients were assigned to one of four treatment groups (small-group education, individual education, information workbook control group, or usual control group with no supplemental education). Both the small-group and individual asthma education programs improved patient understanding, control of asthma symptoms, and MDI technique. The small group was somewhat more effective. Additional controlled studies involving formal asthma education programs have documented their effectiveness in reducing the use of health services (164,165). Other studies have documented the cost-effectiveness of an adult asthma education program (166). However, attendance rates for formal asthma education programs have ranged from 31% to 66% (167,168). Yoon and colleagues reported that attenders at an asthma education program were more likely to be women, nonsmokers, and patients from a higher socioeconomic status (169). The EPR-2 recommends that patients, especially those with moderate-to-severe persistent asthma or a history of severe exacerbations, be given a written action plan based on signs and symptoms and/or PEF.

Peak expiratory flow (PEF) monitoring has been advocated as an objective measure of airflow obstruction in patients with chronic asthma. All published asthma practice guidelines uniformly recommend the use of PEF monitoring as an adjunct to asthma education in selected groups of patients. Unfortunately, even after nearly four decades of use, many aspects of PEF monitoring remain unclear. An important and largely unanswered question is whether PEF monitoring adds anything to a well-constructed, individualized asthma education program with management based on symptoms alone. Despite a sound theoretical rationale for PEF monitoring, evaluating the usefulness of PEF monitoring in ambulatory asthma patients shows conflicting results. Over the past decade, six out of 10 randomized trials failed to show an advantage for the addition of PEF monitoring above and beyond symptom-based intervention for the control group (110).

Although PEF monitoring is not an adequate substitute for office spirometry in the initial diagnosis, currently available inexpensive devices are acceptable for serial monitoring of airflow obstruction. Irrespective of the device used, regular PEF monitoring allows early detection of worsening airflow obstruction, which may be of particular value in "poor perceivers." Even though additional benefits above a well-constructed, symptom-based management plan have not been shown in patients with mild asthma, available data appear to support its role in moderate-to-severe asthma. PEF monitoring has some value in risk stratification in patients with asthma. Excessive diurnal variation and morning dip of PEF imply poor control and the need for careful reevaluation of the management plan. PEF alone is never appropriate; rather, PEF should be part of a comprehensive patient education program. Future studies to evaluate the usefulness of PEF should target patients who are at a higher risk for asthma-related morbidity and mortality. These are patients who are suspected to be poor perceivers. Future studies also need to identify the cutoff points or "action points" of high discriminatory value that can be easily applied by both patients and physicians in the primary care setting.

Aerosol delivery of the β-agonists can be achieved through the use of a handheld MDI in most patients. Proper instruction in the MDI technique is important to ensure effective use (153). It has been shown that increased deposition in the lung occurs when the actuator is held 2 to 4 cm from an open mouth position (170). Likewise, beginning inhalation at the end of normal expiration (functional residual capacity) is likely to optimize distribution of the inhaled aerosol (170). Optimal use of an MDI delivers only about 10% of the medication dose to the lung, whereas as much as 85% is deposited in the oropharynx (170). The use of a volume reservoir or spacer device is advantageous, especially in patients who are unable to learn or perform the unassisted MDI technique (171). Use of the volume reservoir may improve lung deposition to 15% of the dose and reduce oropharyngeal deposition to 5%, thereby potentially decreasing side effects as well (remaining 80% stays in the spacer device). Powered nebulizers have traditionally been used in patients with significant bronchospasm and in most hospital inpatients. However, recent studies suggest that properly supervised MDI aerosol delivery is as efficacious as powered nebulizer delivery, even in patients with acute or severe airflow obstruction (172–174). Data from non-ICU hospitalized patients suggests that use of MDIs rather than nebulizers results in substantial savings in direct costs (i.e., therapist's time) (175).

Allergen Avoidance: Environmental Control Measures

A variety of population and clinical studies have strongly suggested that exposure to aeroallergens in a susceptible host is associated with allergic sensitization in a subset of patients with both acute and chronic asthma (176–178). It is generally accepted that environmental control measures to reduce exposure to allergens should be considered in most asthmatics, and immunotherapy should be reserved for selected patients only (178–180). Broadly speaking, aeroallergens can be divided into outdoor allergens (pollen and molds) and indoor allergens (house dust mites, animal allergens, cockroach allergen, and indoor molds). Exposure to outdoor allergens is best reduced during the peak pollen season by remaining indoors as much as possible in an air-conditioned environment with the windows closed.

Much attention in the literature has recently focused on the composition of house dust and indoor allergens (181). It appears that house dust itself is not an allergen, but there are allergic components within house dust. Fecal pellets from two house dust mites, *Dermatophagoides farinae* and *Dermatophagoides pteronyssinus*, contain several well-characterized allergens (Der f I, Der f II, Der p I, and Der p II) (182). Similarly, allergens from cat dander (Fel d I) and cockroaches (Bla g I, Bla g II) have been well described. Data suggest that certain environmental conditions such as high temperature, high humidity, and perhaps closed urban surroundings can increase allergen burden from these sources. A variety of studies have quantitatively measured these allergens and have recommended "safe" levels (183). Specific recommendations have been published to help reduce indoor allergen burden (183). Overall, it seems clear that indoor allergens contribute to some morbidity related to asthma and that strategies to minimize allergen exposure are warranted in most patients with asthma.

PHARMACOTHERAPY FOR CHRONIC ASTHMA

Table 8.5 depicts the overview of therapy as outlined in the 1997 EPR-2 (1). The pharmacotherapy for asthma can be classified as symptomatic therapy with "relievers"/

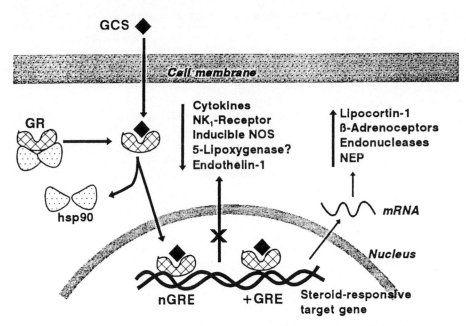

FIGURE 8.5. Molecular mechanism of glucocorticosteroid (*GCS*) action. GCS binds to a cytosolic glucocorticoid receptor (*GR*) that is normally bound to two molecules of heat shock protein (*hsp 90*). The activated GR translocates to the nucleus, where it binds to specific glucocorticoid receptor elements (GREs) in the upstream regulatory region of genes, which either inhibit (*nGRE*) or stimulate (+ *GRE*) transcription of steroid-responsive target genes (of which many are likely to be relevant in asthma therapy). (From Barnes PJ, Pedersen S. Efficacy and safety of inhaled corticosteroids in asthma. *Am Rev Respir Dis* 1993;148:S2, with permission.)

bronchodilators (β-agonists, theophylline) or "disease-modifying" therapy with "controllers"/antiinflammatory agents (corticosteroids, cromolyn, nedocromil or antileukotrienes). Medications commonly used in the treatment of asthma, along with possible routes and schedules of administration, are listed in Table 8.2. The ERP-2 guidelines target therapy based on the severity of asthma as assessed by frequency of symptoms or peak flow measurements (Table 8.3). The ERP-2 defines intermittent mild asthma as brief (less than one hour) wheezing, cough, dyspnea up to two times weekly, absence of symptoms between exacerbations, and nocturnal symptoms fewer than two times a month. Also, the FEV$_1$ or PEF are greater than 80% of the patient's personal best. For mild asthma as defined in this fashion, the guidelines recommend as-needed use of one to two puffs of a β$_2$-agonist and/or cromolyn prior to exposure to various triggers. Persistent asthma is classified as mild-persistent moderate-persistent, or severe-persistent. For persistent asthma, the guidelines recommend daily controller therapy (most often inhaled corticosteroids, alternatively cromolyn/ nedocromil or antileukotrienes). For breakthrough symptoms or nocturnal symptoms, additional therapy with salmeterol or sustained-release theophylline and/or higher doses of inhaled steroids are recommended. According to the EPR-2, severe asthma should be treated with a burst of oral corticosteroids at 40 mg a day for one week and then tapered for one week, in addition to the inhaled corticosteroids and as-needed inhaled β$_2$-agonists.

Bronchodilators: β-Adrenergic Agents

The β-adrenergic agonist drugs have structural similarities by virtue of a common catechol nucleus. The catecholamines (isoproterenol or isoetharine) are rapid-acting, potent, and relatively nonselective β$_1$ agonists (184). Resorcinols (metaproterenol, terbutaline, and fenoterol) and saligenins (albuterol and salmeterol) represent a modification of the central catechol nucleus, with resultant longer duration of action and greater β$_2$ airway selectivity. Stimulation of the β receptors activates adenyl cyclase, causing formation of intracellular cyclic AMP. This in turn provides energy for compartmental shifts in calcium, which results in bronchial smooth-muscle relaxation. The major therapeutic actions of β stimulation in the treatment of asthma include bronchodilation, facilitation of mucociliary clearance, and inhibition of acute mediator release from mast cells. β-agonists do not have an effect on cellular inflammation or the late asthmatic response.

In 1967, Lands and coworkers found that β receptors could be subclassified into β$_1$ and β$_2$ receptors (185). β$_2$ receptors mediate bronchodilation, whereas β$_1$ receptors increase heart rate and contractility. In the treatment of airflow obstruction, it is generally advantageous to use agents with a relatively selective β$_2$ effect such as metaproterenol, albuterol, terbutaline, and fenoterol to minimize side effects. Nevertheless, undesirable side effects occur even with selective agents, particularly when delivered orally. In

TABLE 8.2. PHARMACOLOGIC AGENTS FOR THE TREATMENT OF ASTHMA

Class	Generic Name	Brand Name (Manufacturer)	Delivery Route/Device	Suggested Dosage (Adults)	Comment
Anticholinergics	Atropine sulfate	Many	Solution 0.2% (1 mg/0.5 mL) 0.5% (2.5 mg/0.5 mL) (1.25 mg)	0.025 mg/kg diluted with 3–5 mL NS q 6–8 hr	Minimal side effects with ipratropium
	Ipratropium bromide	Atrovent (Boehringer)	MDI (18 μg/puff)	2–4 puffs qid; max = 12 puffs/day	
			Solution 0.02% (500-μg unit dose vial)	500 μg/tid, qid	
β-Adrenergic agents	Albuterol sulfate	Airet (Medeva)	Solution (0.083%)	2.5–10 mg q 6–8 hr	Inhaled agents have fewer systemic side effects; β_2-selective agents are albuterol, bitolterol, metaproterenol, pirbuterol, salmeterol, terbutaline
		Albuterol (various generic)	Solution (0.083%, 0.5%)	2.5–10 mg q 6–8 hr ml (0.5 mL)	
		Proventil (Schering)	MDI (90 μg/puff)	Acute: 2–4 puffs q 4–6 hr; max 16–20 puffs/day Prophylaxis: 2 puffs 15 min before exercise	
			Solution for nebulizer	2.5–10 mg a 6–8 hr (0.083%) (3 mL) or (0.5%) (0.5 mL)	
			Tablets (2, 4 mg)	2–4 mg q 6–8 hr; max: 32 mg/day	
		Proventil-HFA (Schering)	MDI (90 μg/puff)	2–4 puffs q 4–6 hr	
			Repetabs (sustained Release tablets), 4 mg	4 mg q 12 hr	
		Ventolin (Glaxo)	MDI (90 μg/puff)	Max: 16–30 puffs/day (200 puffs)	
			Rotohaler (200 μg/Rotacap)	00–400 μg q 6–8 hr; max dose = 2.4 mg/day	
			Solution for nebulizer (0.083%/3 mL, 0.5% 20 mL)	2.5–10 mg q 6–8 hr	
			Tablets (2, 4 mg)		
		Volmax (Muro)	Sustained-release tablets (4, 8 mg)	4–8 mg q 12 hr	
	Bitolterol mesylate	Tornalate (Sanofi Winthrop)	MDI (370 μg/puff)	2 puffs q 6 hr	
	Epinephrine	Medihaler-Epi (3M Pharm)	MDI (300 μg/puff)	2 puffs qid	
		Many	Solution for inhalation (15 mL)	nebulized q 2–3 hr	
		Adrenalin chloride (Parke-Davis)	SC injection 1:1000 (1 mg/mL)	0.2–0.5 mg SC (0.2–0.5 mL SC) q 20 min	
	Formoterol	Foradil (Novartis) (investigational in USA)	MDI DPI		
	Isoetharine HCl	Bronkometer (Sanofi Winthrop)	MDI (340 μg/puff)	1–2 puffs q 4 hr	
		Many	Solutions for Inhalation	0.25–1 mL nebulized with NS	
	Isoproterenol HCl	Medihaler-150 (3M Pharm)	MDI (800 μg/puff)	1–2 puff qid	
		Isuprel Mistometer (Sanofi Winthrop)	MDI (131 μg/puff)	1–2 puffs qid	
			Solution (0.5%, 1% 5%)	0.5 mL in 2.5 ml NS q 3–4 hr	
			Tablets (glossets 10, 15 mg)	10–20 mg q 4 hr	
	Levalbuterol	Xopenex (Sepracor)	Solution for nebulizer (0.63 mg)	0.63 mg q 6–8 hr	
	Metaproterenol	Alupent (Boehringer)	MDI (650 μg/puff)	2–3 puffs q 3–4 hr max = 12 puff/day	
			Solution (0.4%, 0.6%)	0.3 mL in 2.5 mL NS q 4–6 hr	
			Tablets (10, 20 mg)	10 mg q 6–8 hr, 10 mg up to 20 mg	
		Metaprel (Sandoz)	MDI (650 μg/puff)	2–3 puffs q 3–4 hr;max = 12	
			Solution (0.5%)	0.3 mL in 2.5 mL NS q 4–6 hr	
			Tablet (10, 20 mg)	10 mg q 6–8 hr, Up to 20 mg	
	Pirbuterol acetate	Maxair (3M Pharm)	MDI (200 μg/puff)	1–2 puffs q 4–6 hr hr;max = 12 puffs/day	
			AutoHaler	2 puffs q 6 hr	

(continued)

TABLE 8.2. *Continued.*

Class	Generic Name	Brand Name (Manufacturer)	Delivery Route/Device	Suggested Dosage (Adults)	Comment
	Salmeterol	Serevent (Glaxo)	MDI (46 μg/puff) Diskus (DPI 50 μg/puff)	2 puffs q 12 hr	
	Terbutaline sulfate	Brethaire (Geigy)	MDI (200 μg/puff) Solution for SC injection or nebulizer (1 mg/mL)	1–2 puffs q 4–6 hr 0.25 mg SC q 15–30 min; max = 0.50 mg/4 hr, 0.75–2.5 mg nebulized with NS	
			Tablet (2.5, 5 mg)	2.5–5 mg tid; max = 15 mg/24 hr	
		Bricanyl (Marion Merrell Dow)	MDI (200 μg/puff) Tablets (2.5, 5 mg)	1–2 puffs q 4–6 hr 2.4–5 mg tid; max = 15 mg/24 hr	
Cromoglycates	Cromolyn sodium	Intal (Fisons)	Spinhaler (20 mg capsules) MDI (800 μg/puffs) Solution (20 mg/2 ml ampule)	20 mg qid 2 puffs qid 1 ampule qid	Contraindication in acute asthma
	Nedocromil sodium	Tilade (Fisons)	MDI (1.75 mg/puff)	2 puffs bid, tid, qid	
Inhaled corticosteroids	Beclomethasone dipropionate	Beclovent (Allen & Hanburys)	MDI (42 μg/puff)	2 puffs tid-qid: max = 20 puffs/day	Need more than 400 μg/day to maintain off oral steroids, no adrenal suppression if <800–1200 μg/day
		HFA-BDP Qvar (3M)	MDI (50 μg/puff)	2–8 puffs bid	
		Vanceril (Schering) Vanceril DS	MDI (42 μg/puff) MDI (84 μg/puff)	2 puffs tid-qid; max = 20 puffs/day	
	Budesonide	Pulmicort (AstraZeneca)	Tubuhaler (200 μg/puff)	400–1600 μg in divided doses bid-qid	
	Flunisolide	AeroBid (Forest)	MDI (250 μg/puff)	2 puffs bid; max = 8 puffs/day	
	Fluticasone propionate	Flovent (Glaxo)	MDI (44, 110, 220, μg/puff) Diskus powder Inhaler (50, 100, 250 μg/puff)	100–800 μg/day	
	Mometasone furoate (investigational in US)	Asthmanex (Schering)	N/A	N/A	
	Triamcinolone acetonide	Azmacort (Rhone-Poulenc Rorer)	MDI (100 μg/puff)	2–4 puffs qid; max = 16 puffs/day	
Conbination products	Albuterol/ ipratropium	Combivent (Boehringer-Igelheim)	MDI (18 μg ipratropium/ 103 μg albuterol per puff)	2 puffs qid	
	Salmeterol/ fluticasone (investigational)	Advair (Glaxo)	Diskus (DPI)	50/100, 50/250, 50/500 (1 PUFF BID)	
	Formoterol/ budesonide (investigational)	Budoxis (AstraZeneca)	Turbuhaler	N/A	
Antileukotrienes	Montelukast	Singulair (Merck)	Tablet (5, 10 mg)	10 mg qd in the evening	Churg-Strauss
	Zafirlukast	Accolate (Zeneca)	Tablets (20 mg)	20 mg bid	Take on empty stomach; drug interactions
	Zileuton	Zyflo (Abbott)	Tablets (600 mg)	600 mg qid	Need to follow LFTs, drug interactions
Methylxanthines	Aminophylline	Various	IV	Load: if not on theophylline at home, 5–6 mg/kg over 20 min; if on theophylline, level pending, 3 mg/kg over 20 min; a bolus of 0.5 mg/kg will increase level by 2 in the average adult. Maintenance 0.5–0.9 mg/kg/hr 200–400 mq bid	Decreased clearance with cirrhosis, CHF, erythromycin, cimetidine, troleandomycin increased clearance with smoking, young age, and phenobarbital. Need to follow serum levels

(continued)

TABLE 8.2. *Continued.*

Class	Generic Name	Brand Name (Manufacturer)	Delivery Route/Device	Suggested Dosage (Adults)	Comment
	Theophylline	Anhydrous, immediate release (Slo-phyllin, Theolair, Quibron, Elixophyllin, etc.)	PO	qid	Normal dose range for an average adult is 300 to 1200 mg/day; immediate release preparation; dose should be given every 6 to 8 hr; sustained-release preparations: dose may be given every 12 to 24 hrs; this dose range is an approximate starting point; however, whenever possible, serum levels should be monitored, i.e., 8 hr after a dose after 5 to 6 consecutive doses
Systemic corticosteroids	Prednisone	Many	Tablets (1, 5, 10, 20, 50 mg)	10–50 mg/day	Long-term systemic side effects: cataracts, osteopenia, Cushingoid features, immune suppression, hypertension
	Methylprednisolone sodium succinate	Medrol (Upjohn) Solu-Medrol (Upjohn)	Tablets (2, 4, 8, 16, 24, 32 mg) IV (40, 125, 500, 1,000 mg)	4–48 mg/day 1–2 mg/kg q 4–6 hr	
	Hydrocortisone sodium succinate	Solu-Cortef (Upjohn)	IV (100, 250, 500, 1,000 mg)	4 mg/kg q 4–6 hr	

HFA, hydrofluoroalkane-134a; DPI, dry powder inhaler; MDI, pressurized metered dose inhaler; BDP, beclomethasone dipropionate; SC, subcutaneous; LFT, liver function tests; CHF, congestive heart failure; N/A, not available.

TABLE 8.3. CLASSIFICATION OF ASTHMA SEVERITY BY THE NATIONAL ASTHMA EDUCATION AND PREVENTION PROGRAM: EXPERT PANEL REPORT 2

	Clinical Features before Treatment*		
Classification	Symptoms†	Nighttime Symptoms	Lung Function
Mild Intermittent	■ Symptoms ≤2 times/week ■ Asymptomatic and normal PEF between exacerbations ■ Exacerbations brief (from a few hours to a few days); intensity may vary	≤2 times/month	■ FEV_1 or PEF ≥80% predicted ■ PEF variability 20%
Mild Persistent	■ Symptoms >2 times/week but <1 time/day ■ Exacerbations may affect activity	>2 times/month	■ FEV_1 or PEF ≥80% predicted ■ PEF variability 20%–30%
Moderate Persistent	■ Daily symptoms ■ Daily use of inhaled short-acting β_2-agonist ■ Exacerbations affect activity ■ Exacerbations ≥2 times/week; may last days	>1 time/week	■ FEV_1 or PEF > 60% to 80% predicted ■ PEF variability >30%
Severe Persistent	■ Continual symptoms ■ Limited physical activity ■ Frequent exacerbations	Frequent	■ FEV_1 or PEF ≤60% predicted ■ PEF variability >30%

* The presence of one of the features of severity is sufficient to place a patient in that category. An individual should be assigned to the most severe grade in which any feature occurs. The characteristics noted in this table are general and may overlap because asthma is highly variable. Furthermore, an individual's classification may change over time.
† Patients at any level of severity can have mild, moderate, or severe exacerbations. Some patients with intermittent asthma experience severe and life-threatening exacerbations separated by long periods of normal lung function and no symptoms.
PEF, peak expiratory flow; FEV_1, forced expiratory volume in 1 second.
National Heart, Lung, and Blood Institute. National Asthma Education and Prevention Program. Expert Panel Report 2. *Guidelines for the diagnosis and management of asthma.* Bethesda, MD: National Institutes of Health, 1997. Publication no. 97–4051, with permission.

particular, muscle tremor may occur due to stimulation of β_1 receptors in skeletal muscle. Vasodilation of peripheral vessels, another action of β_2 stimulation, may cause reflex tachycardia and palpitations. At higher doses, the selective agents may also directly stimulate myocardial β_1 receptors.

For several reasons, the use of oral β-adrenergic agonists has fallen into disfavor (1). Oral bioavailability of these agents is significantly confounded by patient-to-patient variability in bowel absorption and first-pass hepatic metabolism (1). Aerosol delivery provides a more rapid onset of action, a comparable sustained response, and a significantly decreased incidence of side effects (186). Aerosols have traditionally been administered through MDIs or dry powder inhalers (DPIs) for ambulatory care, while small-volume wet nebulizers have been used in emergency departments, on hospital wards and intensive care units, and for young children (187). Despite the fact that a large number of studies have found comparable bronchodilation for β-agonists administered by MDI or wet nebulization in patients with acute asthma (172–174), EPR-2 recommends delivery of aerosolized bronchodilators by wet nebulization for management of acute asthma in the emergency room (1). Nebulizer therapy continues to be widely prescribed for a number of reasons: (a) it is widely believed that acutely tachypneic patients are unable to use MDIs optimally, even with a spacer device; (b) patients are usually on MDI therapy at home, and an acute episode requiring emergency care typically represents a failure of home therapy, therefore patients expect alternative therapy; and (c) there is a widespread belief that nebulizer therapy is more effective than MDI usage in treating acute exacerbations of airway obstruction (188).

The environmental impact of chlorofluorocarbons (CFCs) used in pressurized metered dose inhalers has received much recent attention (189–193). Most currently used MDIs contain a blend of CFC propellants including CFC-12 (primary propellant), CFC-11 (primary solvent), and CFC-114 (moderates pressure and density). The CFCs (or Freons) used in MDIs represent 0.5% of the annual worldwide production of these compounds. CFCs are ideal propellants because of their stability and clinical safety. Several international conferences have been held that have resulted in an agreement to ban the use of CFCs after 1998 to 1999, including medical use (192,194). A number of pharmaceutical companies have responded to this challenge by developing new inhalers that do not use CFCs. One strategy is to utilize a non-CFC propellant such as hydrofluorocarbon-134a. CFC-free preparations are available for β-agonists as well as inhaled steroids. A second strategy is to use breath-actuated dry powder inhalers (DPIs). Examples of DPIs currently available (or under development) are the Spinhaler (Fisons), Rotahaler (Allen and Hanbury), Diskhaler (Allen and Hanbury), Turbuhaler (Astra), multidisk powder inhaler (Glaxo), and Aerolizer (Novartis). In addition to being environmentally safe, the breath-actuated

powder devices do not require the exact patient coordination and synchronization typically necessary for MDI use (195,196). Also, the powder preparations can be inhaled without the need for a spacer extension device. However, these devices do require a minimum inspiratory flow rate from a spontaneously breathing patient, and their use may sometimes cause throat irritation. Further studies demonstrating comparability and safety of these devices need to be conducted.

Salmeterol xinafoate is a long-acting β_2-agonist with a long lipophilic side chain, which confers a long duration of action (eight to 17 hours). It is available as a MDI and DPI. *In vitro* studies suggest that salmeterol is more potent than albuterol and has a slower onset (197). Short-term clinical trials have shown salmeterol to be more effective than albuterol (either with regular or on-demand doses), with a similar incidence of adverse reactions (198). A study by Castle and coworkers comparing the safety of salmeterol and albuterol in the United Kingdom noted fewer medical withdrawls due to asthma in patients taking salmeterol (199). This study found a small but nonsignificant excess mortality in the group taking salmeterol. The EPR-2 recommends that antiinflammatory therapy be initiated prior to long-acting β-agonists in patients with chronic asthma and does not recommend monotherapy with salmeterol. Numerous recent studies in mild-to-moderate asthmatics with inadequate symptom control despite low-to-moderate doses of inhaled steroids have found greater benefits with adding salmeterol than by increasing the inhaled steroid dose (200–203). Salmeterol is best suited for the following clinical situations: (a) predominantly nocturnal asthma symptoms; (b) exercise-induced asthma in patients who exercise regularly (may be preferred over short-acting β-agonists) (204); (c) as adjunctive therapy in patients with suboptimal asthma control while on low-to-moderate doses of inhaled steroids (as an alternative to increasing the dose of inhaled steroids).

It is important to educate patients that salmeterol is not to be used for short-term relief of acute asthma symptoms. All patients with symptomatic asthma should be prescribed and instructed on the proper use of a short-acting β-agonist. Several studies have confirmed the overall safety of daily use of salmeterol 100 mcg twice a day (total four puffs per day) when used in addition to inhaled steroids (201–203,205). Studies have also shown no tolerance to the bronchodilator effects of daily salmeterol therapy for months (206). Experimental studies do show a decrease in the bronchoprotective effect over time and the magnitude and significance of this finding remains unclear (207). Side effects of salmeterol may be additive with those of short acting β-agonists.

β_2-adrenergic agonists are derivatives of adrenaline and have been commercially available as racemates or as a racemic mixture of two enantiomers, levo-(R) and dextro-(S)-rotatory isomers (208). The R-isomer confers the racemate's pharmacologic bronchodilating activity, whereas the S-isomer is largely inactive, although it may be associated with inducing airway hyperreactivity in some models. Albuterol is a racemic mixture with a 1:1 ratio of the isomers R-albuterol (levalbuterol) and S-albuterol. Recently, levalbuterol has been approved as a nebulized solution for prevention and treatment of bronchospasm in asthmatics over the age of 12 (209). Although the early animal data with use of pure S-enantiomer aerosols was suggestive of an adverse effect, this has not been convincingly demonstrated in human clinical trials. A recent double-blind crossover study in mild-to-moderate asthmatics (N = 17) indicated that there was no adverse effect by S-albuterol compared with placebo (210). With the current data, there appears to be no advantage for levalbuterol compared to the widely used racemic albuterol (209).

Several mechanisms have been advanced to describe potential side effects related to regular administration of β agonists. These include paradoxical bronchoconstriction (211), downregulation of β_2-agonist receptors, tachyphylaxis as a result of depletion of norepinephrine stores, decreased protection against various stimuli, and an increase in bronchial hyperreactivity (211–215). A review of adverse reaction reports for inhaled β_2-adrenergic bronchodilators submitted to the U.S. Food and Drug Administration (FDA) between 1974 and 1988 identified 126 reports of paradoxical bronchoconstriction associated with the use of MDIs and 58 reports associated with nebulization solution (211). The denominator is difficult to ascertain, but approximately 78 million MDI canisters were distributed between 1985 and 1990. Several mechanisms have been postulated for paradoxical bronchoconstriction, including hypotonicity and acidity of the solution (216,217), and preservatives such as benzalkonium chloride (218), sorbitan, oleic acid, edetate disodium, sulfites (219,220), and alcohol. A recent report demonstrated paradoxical bronchoconstriction with nebulized albuterol but not with terbutaline, suggesting that this reaction could be specific to the drug preparation rather than a class effect (221). Overall, paradoxical bronchoconstriction is likely quite rare.

Bronchodilators: Methylxanthines

The naturally occurring methylxanthines caffeine and theobromine, found in coffee and tea respectively, have been used for hundreds of years in the treatment of bronchospasm (222). Currently, the most frequently prescribed methylxanthines are theophylline (used orally or intravenously) and aminophylline (the ethylenediamine salt of theophylline for intravenous use). Although the methylxanthines are proven bronchodilators, their mechanism of action remains unknown. Until recently, it was believed that relaxation of bronchial smooth muscle occurred through inhibition of the enzyme phosphodiesterase and the resulting intracellular accumulation of cyclic adenosine mono-

phosphate. However, it is now known that theophylline does not inhibit phosphodiesterase at the therapeutic concentrations used in patients (222). Another proposed mechanism, direct blockage of adenosine receptors, appears untenable since the xanthine derivative enprofylline has negligible adenosine antagonism and yet exhibits more potent bronchodilatory action than does theophylline (222,223). Several other mechanisms have been proposed, including translocation of intracellular calcium, prostaglandin antagonism, stimulation of endogenous catecholamine release, and direct β-agonist activity (224). However, in each case, it appears that the activity occurs at theophylline concentrations higher than those used clinically.

Although the mechanisms of action of theophylline are speculative, it is nevertheless clear that theophylline affects many different organs and its actions are not limited to bronchodilation. For example, several studies suggest that theophylline may improve diaphragm function, especially during fatigue of this muscle (225,226). Intravenous aminophylline improves right and left ventricular ejection fraction in patients with chronic obstructive lung disease (227). Oral therapy with theophylline produces a similar effect, which can be sustained for at least four months (228). Theophylline also stimulates the respiratory response to hypoxia but not hypercapnia (229). It is not clear which of these "alternative" actions of theophylline may play a therapeutic role in patients, but it is noteworthy that theophylline reduces dyspnea in some patients with chronic obstructive lung disease despite the absence of reversible airflow obstruction (230). The role of theophylline as an immunomodulator has recently received attention by the finding that slow-release theophylline increases suppressor T-cell counts in the peripheral blood of antigen-challenged asthmatics (231). Further studies are necessary to define the clinical importance of the nonbronchodilator effects of theophylline.

With the development of long-acting and potent inhaled β_2-agonists and inhaled corticosteroids, the use of theophylline now has a less central role in the chronic maintenance therapy of asthma. The reasons for this include the fact that theophylline has weak bronchodilating properties, modest and unclear antiinflammatory properties, and has the potential for side effects (numerous drug interactions, need to monitor serum levels, and a low therapeutic-to-toxicity ratio). However, although this medication is generally less effective as a single agent than aerosol β-agonists, at least some patients will achieve an enhanced benefit from combination therapy. Additionally, therapeutic advantages have been demonstrated when oral theophylline was combined with aerosolized metaproterenol (232), salbutamol (233), terbutaline (234), and oral terbutaline (235). Maintenance therapy with oral theophylline maybe beneficial in steroid-dependent asthmatics. In a placebo-controlled, randomized, and double-blind trial of steroid-dependent asthmatics, theophylline reduced the daily corticosteroid requirement

TABLE 8.4. FACTORS THAT ALTER THEOPHYLLINE CLEARANCE[a]

Decreased clearance	
Severe liver disease	⬇⬇⬇
Congestive heart failure	⬇⬇⬇
Cimetidine	⬇⬇
Troleandomycin	⬇⬇
Acute illness in ICU	⬇⬇
Fever	⬇
Erythromycin	⬇
Oral contraceptives	⬇
Old age	⬇
Viral infection	⬇
Increased clearance	
Smoking	
Phenytoin	
Young age	

Modified from Jeanne JW. Theophylline use in asthma. *Clin Chest Med* 1984;4:645–658, with permission.)
[a]⬇⬇⬇, Marked reduction (70%–90%); ⬇⬇, considerable reduction (50%); ⬇, mild to moderate reduction (25%–50%).

(235). The availability of sustained-release formulations provides theophylline with a role in the treatment of nocturnal asthma (236). Particularly useful in this regard are the "once-a-day" formulations (e.g., Theo-24 and Uniphyl) (237–240).

The potentially serious toxicity of theophylline mandates that the clinician be aware of certain pharmacokinetic features of the drug and the implication for dosing regimens. A recent retrospective chart audit evaluated 40 adult inpatients with theophylline toxicity (levels greater than 25 mg per L) to identify preventable factors (241). The study found that two-thirds (27 of 40 patients) of the inpatients became toxic because of inpatient or emergency department theophylline administration. A set of recurring management errors included a delay in taking action from the time toxic blood levels were drawn, inappropriately high dosing of patients with congestive heart failure, failure to recognize obvious symptoms of toxicity, emergency department treatment of already toxic patients, and overlapping of intravenous and oral therapy. The clearance of theophylline is affected by many different factors (Table 8.4) and exhibits significant variation among adults. The proper maintenance dose of theophylline should be given in accordance with the estimated clearance using guidelines provided. Aminophylline contains about 80% theophylline. Maintenance doses should be calculated using lean body weight. Serum theophylline levels need to be obtained to confirm the appropriateness of the chosen maintenance dose and to guide adjustments of the dose if necessary. Prior to initiation of the intravenous maintenance dose, a loading is required. The recommended loading dose of theophylline is 5.6 mg per kg (224). This will yield a serum level of approximately 10 to 12 μg per mL. The loading dose is not adjusted to account for expected variations in drug clearance, since this consideration affects only the maintenance dose. However, the loading dose recommendation assumes that the patient has an initial blood theophylline level of zero. In patients

TABLE 8.5. MANAGEMENT OF CHRONIC ASTHMA: OVERVIEW OF THERAPY

Severity	Therapy	Outcome/Goals
Mild Intermittent ■ Symptoms ≤2×/week ■ Asymptomatic, normal PEF between exacerbations	■ Inhaled β-MDI as required ■ No daily medication	■ Control symptoms ■ Maintain normal activity levels ■ Prevent exacerbations
Mild Persistent ■ Symptoms >2×/week <1×/day ■ May affect activity	■ One daily medication: — Low-dose inhaled corticosteroid or cromolyn/nedocromil — Sustained-release theophylline anti-leukotriene ■ Inhaled β-MDI as required	■ Normalize pulmonary function ■ Optimize pharmacotherapy with minimal side effects ■ Meet patient/family expectations of care
Moderate Persistent ■ Daily symptoms ■ Exacerbations ≥2×/week ■ Daily use of β-MDI	■ Daily medication ■ Medium-dose inhaled corticosteroid ± long-acting β-agonist	
Severe Persistent ■ Continual symptoms ■ Limited physical activity ■ Frequent exacerbations	■ Daily medication — High-dose inhaled corticosteroid + long-acting β-agonist — ? Prednisone	

PEF, peak expiratory flow; MDI, metered-dose inhaler.
Modified from National Heart, Lung, and Blood Institute. National Asthma Education and Prevention Program. Expert Panel Report 2. *Guidelines for the diagnosis and management of asthma.* Bethesda, MD: National Institutes of Health; 1997. Publication no. 97–4051.

who are currently taking methylxanthines, an appropriate reduction in the loading dose should be made.

Theophylline has a narrow therapeutic index. In fact, side effects and toxicity are sometimes noted at blood levels considered to be within the therapeutic range (10 to 20 μg per mL), making it impossible to disassociate adverse effects from therapeutic actions on all patients (222). The so-called minor side effects of theophylline include nausea, anorexia, diarrhea, insomnia, tachycardia, and tremor (224). Although these side effects become increasingly prominent at blood levels above the therapeutic range, they are not uncommon at therapeutic or even subtherapeutic levels and may necessitate the cessation of therapy. The major life-threatening side effects are seizures and ventricular arrhythmias. Although major toxicity is relatively rare at blood levels less than 35 μg per mL, it is important to realize that the major side effects can occur without warning signs. Thus the absence of minor side effects is not by itself adequate assurance that toxic blood levels are not present. Theophylline-induced seizures are relatively refractory to therapy and are reported to have a mortality of 50% (242). Life-threatening ventricular arrhythmias are usually responsive to lidocaine or other therapies (224,243). Of interest is that therapeutic concentrations of theophylline appear to have little, if any, significant adverse effects on cardiac rhythm, even in patients with underlying ventricular ectopy (244,245). Nevertheless, it is reasonable to exercise caution in the use of theophylline in patients with cardiac disease or rhythm disorders.

The presence of a dangerously high theophylline blood level (greater than 35 to 40 μg per mL), especially if accompanied by toxic side effects, requires urgent attention. In such emergent situations, theophylline blood levels can be rapidly lowered by instituting hemoperfusion with activated charcoal (246), or by the oral administration of activated charcoal (247). Of interest is that the orally administered charcoal is effective even when toxicity is due to intravenous aminophylline. Thus using oral activated charcoal should be considered while the hemoperfusion apparatus is being prepared (224). A recent study identified predictors of major toxicity in a series of 249 patients with theophylline levels greater than 30 mg per L (248). This study found that: (a) the risk of major toxicity in patients with acute theophylline intoxication is best predicted by the peak serum theophylline concentration; and (b) patients with chronic theophylline intoxication have a greater risk for major toxicity at lower serum theophylline concentrations than those with acute intoxication and that this risk cannot be predicted by the peak serum theophylline concentration. Age above 60 provides the best predictor of major toxicity in cases of chronic theophylline toxicity.

Anticholinergic Agents

For more than two centuries, naturally occurring anticholinergic substances (stramonium, found in the Datura plant, and atropine) have been used in the treatment of asthma. In general, these agents are less effective than β-agonists, and the systemic side effects after inhalation are considerable. However, the duration of action of the anticholinergic medications is often considerably longer than the β-agonists (249). However, the availability of a quaternary derivative of atropine, ipratropium bromide (Atrovent), which is topically active but poorly absorbed (and therefore has minimal side effects), stimulated renewed interest in using anticholinergic agents for both asthma and chronic obstructive pulmonary disease. Ipratropium bromide is available either in solution for use in a nebulizer or in a metered dose inhaler. When administered via metered dose inhaler, the recommended dose is two puffs (40 μg) four times daily. Of interest is that ipratropium bromide, in contrast to atropine, does not reduce mucociliary clearance in normal subjects or in patients with airway disease (250,251). An unpleasant, bitter taste appears to be the only significant unwanted feature of inhaled ipratropium.

The role of anticholinergic agents such as ipratropium (Atrovent) in the treatment of stable asthma is not yet clearly defined (252). When used as a single agent, ipratropium has been shown in some studies to be almost as effective as isoproterenol (253), albuterol (254), terbutaline (255), and metaproterenol (256). However, other clinical trials have indicated ipratropium to be less effective than either metaproterenol (257) or fenoterol (258). The discrepancy regarding the efficacy of ipratropium may be explained by patient selection; it is probable that there are "responders" and "non-responders" to ipratropium (256). It is difficult to predict which patients might respond to ipratropium, but patients with a "psychogenic" component to their asthma (in which vagal tone may play an important role) constitute a group that might be relatively responsive (259,260). Several studies indicate that combining ipratropium with a β-adrenergic agent is more effective in the treatment of chronic asthma than either drug alone (257,258,261).

Antiinflammatory Agents: Corticosteroids

The central role of airway inflammation in the pathogenesis of both acute and chronic asthma (both mild and severe) has been reviewed in detail. It is safe to say that there is a consensus that antiinflammatory treatment should represent a primary therapeutic approach for acute severe asthma in the emergency room setting (by use of parenteral or oral corticosteroids), in addition to repetitive dosing of inhaled β-agonists. For long-term maintenance therapy of patients with chronic asthma, treatment focus has shifted away from use of bronchodilator therapy alone and toward earlier use of inhaled antiinflammatory therapy.

Potential mechanisms of corticosteroid action include effects on leukocytes (T lymphocytes, polymorphonuclear

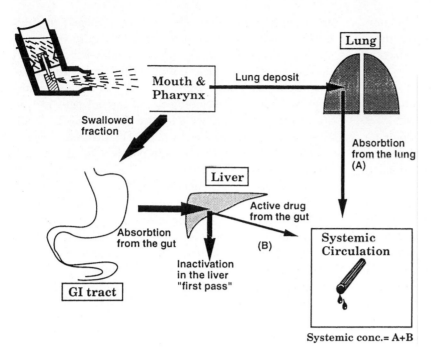

FIGURE 8.6. The fate of inhaled steroids. The amount of an inhaled glucocorticosteroid reaching the systemic circulation is the sum of the pulmonary and orally bioavailable fraction. The fraction deposited in the mouth will be swallowed, and the systemic availability will be determined by absorption from the gastrointestinal tract and degree of first-pass metabolism. The fraction deposited in the intrapulmonary airways is likely to be more or less completely absorbed in active form to the systemic circulation, as there is no evidence for any degree of metabolic inactivation in currently used inhaled steroids. The systemic concentration will be reduced by continuous recirculation and inactivation in the liver. (From Barnes PJ, Pedersen S. Efficacy and safety of inhaled corticosteroids in asthma. *Am Rev Respir Dis* 1993;148:S9, with permission.)

neutrophils), synthesis of regulator proteins, catecholamine receptors or function, eicosanoid synthesis and function, and vascular endothelial integrity (262). Although the precise mechanism of action of glucocorticoids is not known, recent advances in understanding the molecular mechanisms of the glucocorticoid receptor, steroid-responsive target-gene elements, and cytokine biology have provided insights (Fig. 8.6) (263–275). There is a single glucocorticoid receptor (GR) that is localized to the cytoplasm of target cells in airway epithelium and endothelium of bronchial vessels. After a glucocorticoid binds to a cytosolic GR, this complex translocates to the nucleus, where it binds to specific glucocorticoid response elements of genes, which either inhibit or stimulate transcription in steroid-responsive target genes. Steroids inhibit the transcription of several cytokines, including interleukin-1 (IL-1), tumor necrosis factor α (TNF-α), granulocyte-macrophage colony stimulating factor (GM-CSF), and interleukins 3, 4, 5, 6, and 8. The well-known eosinopenic effect of corticosteroids is believed to be due to the inhibitory effects on circulating IL-5 and GM-CSF (266). Steroids also increase the synthesis of lipocortin-1, which has an inhibitory effect on phospholipase A_2 and therefore inhibits the production of lipid mediators such as leukotrienes, prostaglandins, and platelet activating factor. Additional effects include inhibiting mucus secretion in airways and increasing the expression of β receptors by increasing gene transcription.

A variety of studies using bronchoscopy with lavage or biopsy have been performed in asthmatics of varying severity

to assess the antiinflammatory effect of inhaled and systemic steroid therapy (54,267–270). Limitations with these studies include small numbers of patients, usually with very mild asthma, with a short duration of follow-up. These studies have typically shown improvement in airway inflammation with three months' therapy, with more improvement in inflammation in endobronchial biopsy than on corresponding BAL cellular profile. Most studies have reported a marked posttreatment reduction in T lymphocytes, eosinophils, and mast cells in the lamina propria. Post-steroid-therapy biopsy has also shown a decrease in cells expressing mRNA for IL-4, IL-5, and GM-CSF along with an increase in cells expressing mRNA for IFN-γ. The reports on the effect of inhaled steroids on thickness of the epithelium and basement membrane have been inconclusive, with at least one study showing no improvement despite therapy for 10 years. Only one study has evaluated severe steroid-dependent asthmatics by the use of BAL and biopsy (271). Wenzel and colleagues studied 14 patients being treated with prednisone (mean dose 30 mg per day) in addition to inhaled steroids ranging between 800 and 4,000 mcg per day for a duration of more than five years (271). BAL from these patients continued to show elevated levels of LTB$_4$, LTE$_4$thromboxane, and histamine. Although there was no significant difference in the total number of BAL cells, the more severe asthmatics had greater numbers of neutrophils, whereas the milder asthmatics had more eosinophils. The same pattern of cellularity was also seen in biopsy specimens. There was no significant difference between endobronchial biopsy and transbronchial biopsy in this group. In summary, a large number of studies suggest that inhaled corticosteroids bring about a variety of antiinflammatory effects in the airway inflammation. There are conflicting data as to whether long-term therapy with inhaled corticosteroids reduces basement membrane thickening and substantially affects airway remodeling.

Additional studies have shown that inhaled steroids reduce airway responsiveness as measured by methacholine, histamine, or exercise challenge (272–275). This reduction in responsiveness (as assessed by an increase in PC_{20} for histamine or methacholine) occurs over several weeks to several months and usually ranges in the order of one or two doubling dilutions. Some had questioned whether these slight increases have clinical significance.

Numerous recent studies have shown that inhaled steroid therapy provides effective symptomatic control of chronic asthma (276–278). Haahtela and colleagues conducted a prospective parallel group trial involving 103 asthmatics over a two-year period randomly assigned to receive 600 μg of inhaled budesonide twice a day or 375 μg of inhaled terbutaline twice a day (276). Asthma in these patients had been newly diagnosed in the previous year and for the most part was mild. The group treated with budesonide showed a significant reduction in symptom scores and in use of rescue β_2-agonist and an improvement in morning and evening peak expiratory flow rates. This study is limited by the fact that the β-agonist was administered only on a twice-a-day basis and that a spacer device was not specified for either group. Kertjens and coworkers noted that inhaled beclomethasone at 800 μg per day improved symptoms and lung function over a 2.5-year period in patients with chronic asthma when given in addition to β-agonist inhaled therapy (277). Dompeling and coworkers, in a four-year prospective study, showed that therapy with beclomethasone at 400 μg two times daily slowed the deterioration of lung function of asthmatics, compared to bronchodilator therapy alone (278). Several studies have shown that higher doses of inhaled steroids reduces the need for maintenance oral steroids (279–285).

Inhaled corticosteroids have assumed the role of first line therapy for most patients with persistent asthma. Over the past five to 10 years, there have been several important trends in the way these agents have been used in clinical trials as well as in practice. One trend has been the use of higher doses of inhaled steroids, especially for the more severe asthmatics. This is predicated on the hypothesis that there is a dose-response effect for these agents. Although quite a number of studies support this hypothesis, there is continued debate (286). It is well documented that higher doses of corticosteroids facilitate a reduction in systemic corticosteroids in severe steroid-dependent asthma (284). A second trend has been the use of inhaled corticosteroids at

an earlier stage of asthma (45,278). Data suggest that this might improve the long-term forced expiratory volume in one second (FEV_1) by preventing subepithelial fibrosis. A third trend is less frequent dosing (i.e., either twice per day or once per day) (287–289). Limited data have suggested improved outcomes including cost of care for patients who are chronically treated with inhaled corticosteroids (290). Whether asthma controlled by inhaled corticosteroids translates to reduced mortality remains poorly defined. A fourth trend has been the increased use of topically more potent inhaled corticosteroids, including fluticasone and budesonide. Finally, the fifth trend involves the addition of another agent (e.g. salmeterol, theophylline, or an antileukotriene) to produce an inhaled steroid "sparing effect" (82,201–203,291). Currently there are five specific inhaled corticosteroids that are approved for maintenance therapy for asthma in the United States. Mometasone is undergoing late phase III clinical trials (292). The EPR-2 provides a table of inhaled steroids with comparative doses to achieve a similar clinical effect.

As discussed earlier, the conventional CFC-based metered dose inhalers are currently being reformulated with alternative propellants such as hydrofluoroalkanes (HFAs). Reformulation of beclomethasone with HFA-134a results in a solution that delivers an aerosol of extra-fine particles with a mass median aerodynamic diameter of 1 μm, compared to the CFC-based BDP, which has a MMAD of 4 to 5 μm. A recent randomized controlled-trial in patients with moderate asthma showed that 400 mcg HFA-134a BDP produced clinical effects equivalent to an 800 mcg dose of CFC-BDP in patients who had not been adequately controlled with 0 to 400 mcg per day of inhaled corticosteroids (194). There was no significant difference in the morning serum cortisol level. This preliminary study indicates that the extra-fine particles may deposit more peripherally in the lower airways and may be a more efficient method for delivery of steroid aerosols. Theoretically, this would mean increased clinical effectiveness with lower systemic absorption from more peripheral deposition using HFA-134a BDP.

Both the binding affinity to glucocorticoid receptor and the skin blanching test are *in vitro* parameters that are often used to compare relative potency of inhaled glucocorticoids (264,265,286) (Table 8.6). However, the pharmacokinetics of inhaled steroids and the subsequent clearance of these agents also determine both the efficacy and the side effects (Table 8.7). Long-term comparative clinical studies are needed before the clinician can rationally choose between the currently available inhaled glucocorticoids (265).

Side effects of inhaled corticosteroids are being increasingly recognized as a potential problem (293,294). The factors that may contribute to toxicity include the total dose, the dosing schedule, whether or not a spacer device is used, whether mouth rinsing is used, and the sensitivity of the pa-

TABLE 8.6. RELATIVE BINDING AFFINITY FOR HUMAN LUNG GLUCOCORTICOID RECEPTOR AND TOPICAL BLANCHING POTENCY IN HUMAN SKIN

Glucocorticosteroid	Binding Affinity	Blanching Potency
Dexamethasone	1.0	1
BDP/BMP	0.4/13.5	600/450
Budesonide	9.4	980
Flunisolide	1.8	330
Triamcinolone acetonide	3.6	330
Fluticasone propionate	18.0	1,200
	(Rat tissue)	

From Barnes PJ, Pedersen S. Efficacy and safety of inhaled corticosteroids in asthma. *Am Rev Respir Dis* 1993;148:57, with permission.
BDP, beclomethasone dipropionate; BMP, beclomethasone monopropionate.

rameter used to assess systemic toxicity (265,286). The adverse effects of inhaled corticosteroids can be broadly classified as topical or systemic (295). The three main topical side effects are cough, oral candidiasis, and dysphonia. Slow inhalation, use of a spacer device, and gargling reduce the incidence of these side effects (296). The systemic side effects may include suppression of the HPA axis, adverse effects on bone metabolism including osteoporosis, slowing of growth in children and adolescents, cataract formation, bruising and dermal thinning, and psychological changes (265,297–300). Many studies have suggested that doses of inhaled corticosteroids in excess of 800 μg per day in adults or 400 μg per day in children appear to result in dose-related suppression of the HPA axis, with substantial interindividual variability and response (286). Some studies suggest that beclomethasone may have a somewhat greater propensity to produce adrenal suppression in comparison with budesonide at higher doses, although the relevance of this is not clear. Inhaled corticosteroids with doses as low as 400 μg per day have been associated with the development of osteoporosis (299).

Studies have shown biochemical abnormalities with higher doses of inhaled steroids. These abnormalities may be viewed as markers for the absorption and systemic effects (toxicity) of the inhaled steroids. Parameters have included morning serum cortisol and 24-hour urinary-free cortisol excretion for HPA-axis suppression; serum osteocalcin, bone-specific serum alkaline phosphatase, urinary hydroxyproline/calcium excretion and bone densitometry for bone metabolism (bone formation and bone resorption); and slit lamp examination for cataract formation. The clinical significance of these subtle and sensitive markers of systemic effect and how they translate into clinical toxicity such as reduced bone growth, osteoporosis, or bone fractures remain poorly established. A variety of strategies may reduce the likelihood of systemic absorption and systemic side effects from inhaled steroids. These include: (a) use the lowest dose that is clinically necessary to achieve good asthma control (e.g., step down the number of puffs per day as control is achieved); (b) routinely use a spacer device with a MDI or use dry powder inhaler; (c) routinely use mouth rinsing; (d) twice-a-day dosing or dosing once a day at 4:00 P.M.; (e) for patients requiring higher doses of inhaled steroids, consider options for "inhaled steroid-sparing effect" with agents such as salmeteral, antileukotrienes, nedocromil, or theophylline (82,201–203,291).

Antiinflammatory Agents: Cromolyn Sodium and Nedocromil Sodium

Cromolyn sodium has been available in the United States since 1973 (301,302). This medication is poorly absorbed orally and therefore is effective only when inhaled. Initially, cromolyn was available only as a 20 mg capsule containing finely powdered cromolyn and lactose particles delivered by a turbo inhaler (Spinhaler). Its usefulness in this form was limited by oral pharyngeal irritation and cough. Subsequently, cromolyn was introduced as a nebulizer solution in 1982 and in a pressurized metered dose inhaler in 1986.

Cromolyn sodium administered prior to allergen exposure blocks both the early and late asthmatic response fol-

TABLE 8.7. PHARMACOKINETICS OF INHALED GLUCOCORTICOSTEROIDS

	Plasma Half-life (hr)	Volume of Distribution (L/kg)	Clearance (L/min)	First-Pass (%)
Triamcinolone acetonide	1.5	2.1	1.2	—
Beclomethasone dipropionate	—	—	—	—
Flunisolide	1.6	1.8	1.0	20
Budesonide	2.8	4.3	1.4	10
Fluticasone dipropionate	3.1	3.7[a]	0.87	—

From Barnes PJ, Pedersen S. Efficacy and safety of inhaled corticosteroids in asthma. *Am Rev Respir Dis* 1993;148:S7, with permission.
[a] Assuming a mean body weight of 70 kg.

lowing antigen inhalation (303). Cromolyn has not demonstrated smooth-muscle relaxant properties and therefore is not a bronchodilator. It has long been held that the primary mechanism of action appears to be inhibition of mediator release from mast cells. Although the exact mechanism by which cromolyn inhibits mast-cell mediator release is not known, it is believed to inhibit calcium influx by phosphorylation of a membrane protein. Other mechanisms of action of cromolyn include suppression of nonmyelinated vagal sensory nerve endings, inhibition of inflammatory cells other than mast cells, and reduction of airway permeability.

Many studies have documented the protective effect exerted by cromolyn against provocative stimuli such as allergen, cold air, SO_2, and exercise (303). The drug is most effective when administered before challenge. The protective effects against nonspecific agents such as methacholine and histamine have been less established. A number of studies have evaluated the effect of cromolyn on nonspecific bronchial hyperreactivity. Studies in which cromolyn was administered for longer than six weeks suggest an improvement in airway reactivity. Despite initial notions that cromolyn would be more effective in extrinsic than intrinsic asthma, most carefully designed studies do not support this concept. About 60% to 79% of asthmatics show a response to cromolyn. Studies comparing cromolyn and theophylline in the short-term management of chronic asthma suggest that both of these agents are equally effective, with perhaps greater side effects with theophylline. There are some data to show that there is an additive effect between these two agents. Toogood and coworkers did not find any advantage to adding cromolyn to an established regimen of beclomethasone (304).

Nedocromil sodium (Tilade) is structurally different from cromolyn, but it has very similar pharmacologic activities. Nedocromil was approved for use in the United States in MDIs in 1992. The mechanism of action of nedocromil appears to be quite similar to cromolyn. A number of *in vitro* and *in vivo* studies suggest that nedocromil blocks both the early and late asthmatic response (305,306). Nedocromil has antiinflammatory properties on a number of cells. There is some suggestion that nedocromil may be more potent in inhibiting bronchial C-fiber nerve endings.

A recent meta-analysis reviewed all known placebo-controlled, double-blind, randomized clinical trials involving nedocromil (a total of 4,723 patients from 127 centers) (305). This included both published and unpublished material. The authors compared the treatment effects of nedocromil and placebo using six efficacy variables, including symptom scores, peak flows, FEV_1, and inhaled bronchodilator use. The numerous studies were classified by trial design into five groups. Overall, nedocromil is more effective than placebo in treating asthma and is of most benefit to patients who are receiving monotherapy with bronchodilators (306–308). The aggregate data suggested that nedo-

cromil is less potent than inhaled corticosteroids, although some inhaled corticosteroid-sparing effects were noted. A recent nedocromil sodium workshop concluded that nedocromil could represent an alternative to cromolyn, although there was no clear advantage for nedocromil over inhaled steroids, and the costs are higher (309).

Overall, inhaled corticosteroids are preferred in the majority of patients for chronic asthma because of proven efficacy, greater potency than cromolyn or nedocromil, and effectiveness when administered twice a day as opposed to four times a day (310–314). Also, there are more data supporting improvement of inflammation as assessed by BAL and endobronchial biopsy in patients treated with inhaled corticosteroids (311). Additional studies directly comparing inhaled corticosteroids and nedocromil for newly diagnosed bronchial asthma are required.

Antileukotrienes

Since the 1970s, investigators have known of a link between leukotrienes and the airway inflammation typical of asthma. Several lines of evidence indicate that leukotrienes play an important role in asthma (315,316). First, leukotrienes stimulate airway smooth-muscle contraction, produce mucosal edema and mucus secretions, and attract a variety of cells including eosinophils and neutrophils. All of these features are important in asthma. Second, administering aerosolized leukotrienes can produce the typical physiologic and symptomatic changes characteristic of asthma. Third, antileukotrienes inhibit asthmatic responses to a variety of stimuli, including allergen, exercise, aspirin, and cold, dry air (76–81,317). Fourth, cysteinyl leukotrienes can be recovered from nasal secretions, bronchoalveolar lavage fluid, and urine of patients with asthma in increased concentrations compared to normal individuals. Fifth, recent placebo-controlled clinical trials have shown that leukotriene blockade has beneficial effects on chronic, spontaneously occurring asthma (i.e., without experimental provocation or challenge) in both adults and children (318–325).

Three antileukotriene agents have been approved in the United States for maintenance therapy for persistent asthma: zileuton, zafirlukast and montelukast (82). These agents have different mechanisms of action: zileuton blocks a critical step in leukotriene production involving 5-lipoxygenase enzyme, whereas zafirlukast and montelukast prevent leukotrienes from binding to the common leukotriene receptor. There are no published studies comparing the leukotriene synthesis inhibitors with the receptor antagonists, and the relative differences in efficacy remain unknown.

A number of randomized, placebo-controlled phase III clinical trials in patients with mild-to-moderate chronic asthma have been conducted with each of the three oral antileukotrienes and have demonstrated significant improvement compared to placebo in numerous parameters including symptoms, FEV_1, morning PEF, and need for rescue β-agonist use (318,320,325). These studies have varied in length from four weeks to six months and improvements in symptoms and FEV_1 were seen as quickly as the first or second day with peak responses by two weeks. These three agents are available as pills requiring dosing once a day for montelukast, twice a day for zafirlukast, and four times a day for zileuton. Montelukast is the only agent that is approved down to the age of six, whereas the other two agents have approval for children over the age of 12. Zafirlukast needs to be taken on an empty stomach (one hour before or two hours after meals) since food decreases absorption by as much as 40%. Studies suggest that there is a 5% incidence of liver function abnormalities with zileuton, and it is recommended that baseline alanine aminotransferase (ALT) be measured as well as follow-up monitoring approximately seven times during the first year. Many patients with liver function abnormalities may continue to take the drug. With zafirluast 20 mg twice a day, the risk of liver function abnormalities appears to be quite low and routine monitoring is unnecessary. However, there have been isolated reports of liver function abnormalities at the higher dose of 80 mg per day. There are no published reports of liver function abnormalities with montelukast. Both zafirlukast and zileuton have several drug interactions, especially agents which are metabolized with the cytochrome P-450 system. Clearance is reduced for coumadin, theophylline, phenytoin, and carbamazepine.

In the initial postmarketing experience with the antileukotrienes, a report described eight patients with steroid-dependent asthma who developed a Churg-Strauss vasculitis syndrome (allergic granulomatosis angiitis) while taking zafirlukast (326). All but one of these patients were receiving corticosteroids, and this syndrome occurred with tapering or discontinuation of systemic steroid therapy. Interestingly, all of these patients had an unusual cardiomyopathy as part of the vasculitis syndrome. Additional cases of Churg-Strauss syndrome have been reported with zafirlukast and more recently with montelukast as well (327). Whether this complication is related to zafirlukast and montelukast (either as an idiosyncratic drug reaction or by a class effect of cysteinyl leukotriene receptor blockade) or to tapering of systemic steroids and unmasking a *forme fruste* of Churg-Strauss syndrome remains unknown. There have been unpublished reports of Churg-Strauss-like syndrome in patients on high doses of inhaled corticosteroids during a taper.

A recent international clinical trial compared the clinical benefit of montelukast 10 mg once a day with inhaled beclomethasone administered 200 mcg twice a day versus placebo in a randomized, double-blind, double-dummy, parallel-group study (320). The study included 895 patients (2,253 patients were screened) with mild-to-moderate chronic asthma (FEV_1 50% to 85% predicted), aged 15 to 85. Over the 12-week treatment period, the average percentage in-

crease in FEV_1 from baseline was 13.1% with beclomethasone, 7.4% with montelukast, and 0.7% with placebo. Both active treatments had a $p < 0.001$ compared with placebo, and $p < 0.01$ for beclomethasone compared with montelukast. Patients receiving placebo, montelukast, and beclomethasone had asthma exacerbations on 26.1%, 15.2%, and 9.7% of days, respectively. After the end of the 12-week treatment period, a subset of patients was switched to placebo in a blinded manner and the remaining patients on active therapy were continued for a follow-up period of 100 weeks. During the blinded washout period, the FEV_1 for both of the active treatment arms returned to the same level as baseline with no evidence of rebound worsening. Interestingly, this study evaluated the FEV_1 response as a frequency distribution for montelukast and beclomethasone and noted for the montelukast group that 42% of the patients had an improvement in FEV_1 of at least 11% from baseline whereas 50% of beclomethasone recipients met that criteria. The proportion of patients who did not show an improvement in FEV_1 was 22% with beclomethasone and 34% with montelukast. Investigators concluded that the overall distribution of responses followed a similar, unimodal pattern with large overlap with both montelukast and beclomethasone. The authors concluded "these data do not support the hypothesis that response to antileukotrienes can be used to easily separate patients into responder and non-responder categories" (328). After the completion of the clinical trial, patients in both treatment groups were followed in a "real-world" setting without the mandates of a clinical trial. There was a notable decline in the FEV_1 response in the beclomethasone group, whereas the montelukast response was stable, and by 100 weeks there was no difference. These findings suggest that compliance with the inhaled steroid had declined over time (the compliance was greater than 95% during the 12 weeks of the clinical trial). There are few data to support an alternative explanation, which would imply a loss of response to inhaled steroid therapy over time. Overall, this study presents the best data to date, and in a head-to-head trial the magnitude of response over the 12 weeks is larger for the inhaled steroid. It is interesting to note that this difference was evident despite the fact that a very low dose of inhaled steroid was used, with no attempt at dose escalation or titration. Importantly, even though the antileukotriene appears to show less of an effect on the FEV_1 compared to the inhaled corticosteroid, the overall efficacy in a real-world situation at the end of 1.5 years was comparable, likely due to improved compliance with once-a-day oral therapy.

In another controlled trial, 226 stable asthmatics on high doses of inhaled corticosteroids were randomized to montelukast or placebo, with an attempt at steroid taper every two weeks over 12 weeks (319). Compared with placebo, montelukast allowed significant reduction in the inhaled corticosteroid dose (montelukast 47% versus placebo

30%). The clinical effectiveness of antileukotrienes has been noted whether patients were on inhaled steroids or not. Several other randomized clinical trials compared the antileukotrienes with other available antiasthma medications including theophylline and inhaled salmeterol (324,329). In these adult studies, theophylline was comparable to zileuton in steroid-naïve moderate asthmatics. Busse and colleagues published the results of a four-week treatment with inhaled salmeterol versus oral zafirlukast in patients with chronic persistent asthma, 80% of whom were on concurrent inhaled corticosteroids (324). This study found that salmeterol treatment resulted in significantly greater improvement from baseline for most efficacy measurements compared to zafirlukast. Finally, retrospective pooled data from a subgroup of 261 steroid-naïve patients from four randomized placebo controlled 13 week trials with zafirlukast were reviewed (321). This subset of patients had severe persistant asthma based on EPR-2 criteria but they received zafirlukast monotherapy. The authors noted a significant improvement in FEV_1, morning and evening PEF, daytime asthma symptoms and β-agonist usage.

The exact place for antileukotrienes in the chronic maintenance therapy for asthma remains to be established (82,315,316). EPR-2 indicates a possible role for these agents in the initial therapy for mild-persistent asthma as an alternative to inhaled corticosteroids, cromolyn, or nedocromil. Also, EPR-2 indicates a possible role for these agents as adjunctive therapy (in addition to inhaled steroids) for added asthma control at any level of severity for persistent asthma. These agents have effects on early and delayed asthma response; therefore, they act as a bronchodilator within one to three hours after administration as well as an antiinflammatory agent with a response over two to four weeks. The magnitude of increase in FEV_1 at four weeks is about 14% above the placebo. Data suggest that inhaled steroids have more potent effects compared to the antileukotrienes. A major cause for poor asthma outcome is patient nonadherence with prescribed inhaled steroid therapy. Once- or twice-a-day oral therapy with the antileukotrienes offers a significant compliance advantage. Whether the compliance advantage of prolonged once- or twice-per-day oral therapy balances the less potent effects compared to inhaled steroids seen in short-term controlled trials and thereby produces equal effectiveness in a real-world scenario remains to be confirmed. Montelukast represents a significant advance for pediatric patients, being approved as a 5 mg chewable tablet for use once a day for ages six to 14 (323). The antileukotrienes do facilitate a reduction in the need for β-agonist and inhaled steroids, thereby minimizing well-known side effects. Currently, the indications for antileukotrienes could be summarized as: (a) patients on moderate-to-high doses of inhaled steroids with break-through symptoms, as an alternative or adjunct to inhaled salmeterol, (b) maintenance therapy for aspirin-sensitive asthmatics, (c) initial therapy for mild or moderate persistent chronic asthma in settings where there is a particular problem with adherence (as an alternative to inhaled steroid therapy), (d) alternative therapy to salmeterol or short-acting β-agonist for children with exercise-induced asthma.

ACUTE ASTHMA

Status asthmaticus is an acute, severe exacerbation of asthma which requires care in a hospital setting. Recent epidemiologic data for acute asthma suggests there are about 500,000 hospitalizations per year in the United States, of which 65% occur in patients over 18 years of age (12). Acute asthma represents 4% of all emergency room (ER) visits involving about 1.8 million people. Between 15% to 25% of ER visits result in hospital admission. About 20% to 30% of patients initially managed and discharged from the ER have a relapse (330). The average length of stay for patients admitted to the hospital is about five days (30,31). Of all hospital admissions, about 4% require intensive care and of these 1% to 30% require mechanical ventilation (331–334). Patients typically come to the ER and/or hospital for acute asthma when the episode is severe and the tempo of illness is progressive and/or unresponsive to initial therapy. Acute asthma exacerbation often represents failure of outpatient maintenance therapy for several possible reasons: (a) lack of access to longitudinal medical care, (b) lack of objective monitoring of asthma, including home peak-flow monitoring, (c) poor self-management skills, including patient nonadherence, and (d) inadequate pharmacotherapy prescription by the physician, most often lack of inhaled corticosteroid maintenance therapy. For some patients, acute asthma exacerbation may be complicated by comorbid illness such as psychiatric illness, which makes outpatient management difficult.

The initial management of an acute asthmatic in any setting should include administration of aerosolized β-agonists on a repeated basis. β-agonist may be administered by metered dose inhaler (MDI) with a spacer device, intermittent bolus nebulization, or continuous nebulization (173,335). Comparable clinical effects can be achieved with all three delivery methods. Evidence suggest that patients with acute, severe airflow obstruction need higher doses of aerosolized β-agonist than patients with less severe, stable airflow obstruction (333). Selective β_2-agonists such as albuterol (2.5 mg per dose) or metaproterenol (15 mg per dose) are preferred over isoetharine (5 mg per dose). The potency ratio of a nebulizer to a MDI with spacer device is 7:1; therefore, one nebulization with 2.5 mg of albuterol is roughly equivalent to 4 to 12 puffs of albuterol MDI delivering 90 mcg per puff (equivalent dose range for the MDI is 0.36 to 1.08 mg). In an average adult, only 10%

of the MDI dose reaches the lower airway; in patients with airflow obstruction, about 6% reaches the lower airway, with 3% to the most distal airways (170). Use of a spacer device roughly doubles this amount.

Studies suggest that β-agonists may be effectively and safely administered continuously by a variety of nebulization devices for up to 72 to 96 hours in children with acute asthma (336,337). Two studies have extended these findings to adults with acute asthma (338,339). Colacone and associates randomly assigned 42 patients with acute, severe asthma to receive 5 mg albuterol by intermittent bolus nebulization at times 0 and 60 minutes or 0.2 mg/ml albuterol continuously by a calibrated nebulizer with an output of 25 mL per hour (338). Each patient received 10 mg of albuterol over two hours. The authors found that continuous and bolus nebulization were equally effective in the early management of asthma in the ER. Both modes of therapy were well tolerated. Interestingly, heart rate was significantly increased at 30 and 90 minutes in the bolus nebulization group. Olshaker and associates performed an open-label, prospective study of 76 adults with acute asthma exacerbation in the ER (339). The patients were given three continuous nebulizer treatments over 45 minutes; each dose was 2.5 mg albuterol in 3 mL of normal saline. All patients showed objective and subjective improvement, including an average improvement in baseline peak flow of 150%. This therapy was well tolerated with no significant tachyarrhythmia, despite the fact that the patients had underlying hypertension and coronary artery disease. In a study by Lin and colleagues, seven adults with asthma were given continuously nebulized albuterol at 0.4 mg per kg per hour delivered over four hours (340). Patients with a history of coronary artery disease were excluded. The mean patient age was 30.9 years. Patients showed a significant improvement in FEV_1. There was a mean increase in heart rate of 16.3%. One patient withdrew because of supraventricular tachycardia. In six of seven patients, serum albuterol levels at the end of treatment were greater than 25.0 mg per ml. The authors concluded that use of high-dose continuously nebulized albuterol can result in markedly elevated serum albuterol levels and potential cardiac stimulation in some patients with asthma.

Patients with acute airflow obstruction refractory to intermittent, frequently aerosolized β-agonist therapy may be candidates for continuously nebulized bronchodilator therapy until the effects of antiinflammatory therapy are achieved (341). Recommended regimens are albuterol, 2.5 to 15 mg per hour or terbutaline, 2 to 8 mg per hour. A variety of delivery methods for continuous nebulization have been described. Patients should receive continuous nebulization until they have improved enough to tolerate intermittent aerosol treatment every four hours. Extensive experience in children and the two reports in adults suggest

that this approach is safe, although further studies in adults with underlying coronary artery disease are required.

Subcutaneous injection of β-agonist is frequently used in the emergency treatment of acute asthma (342). In severe airflow obstruction, aerosol penetration into the bronchial tree may be suboptimal compared to systemically administered medication. Although epinephrine (0.3 to 0.5 mL of 1:1,000 aqueous solution) has long been used, terbutaline is available for subcutaneous administration as well. Epinephrine should be used extremely cautiously in patients with cardiac disease (especially if complicated by arrhythmias or severe hypertension) or hyperthyroidism (342). Despite theoretical expectations, subcutaneous terbutaline is not associated with a decreased incidence of cardiac side effects in comparison with subcutaneous epinephrine (342,343).

Intravenous administration of β-agonist has been used in the treatment of severe acute bronchospasm (344). The theoretical rationale for this approach is to overcome problems related to decreased drug penetration and decreased β-adrenergic receptor responsiveness, and thereby expose β-receptors to continuous and saturating levels of drug (345). Most of the experience with this therapy comes from Europe. In the United States, albuterol is not available for intravenous delivery. Albuterol might be preferable to isoproterenol, since the chronotropic effect is far less. However, it is not clear in which patients, if any, intravenous delivery is preferable over aerosol or subcutaneous administration. Available comparisons between intravenous albuterol and aerosol albuterol for the treatment of acute asthma provide conflicting conclusions (344–347).

The role of aminophylline in the treatment of acute, severe asthma remains controversial (348–349). The expert panel on the diagnosis and management of asthma has not recommended routine use of aminophylline in the treatment of asthma in the emergency department (4). However, both the expert panel and the British Thoracic Society recommend the routine use of intravenous theophylline in patients admitted to the hospital for an acute exacerbation of asthma (1,350). Early studies suggested that the addition of aminophylline to maximal therapy with inhaled β-agonists in the emergency room had little effect on pulmonary function parameters during three hours' observation (351–353). A recent meta-analysis of 13 controlled trials compared aminophylline therapy with a control regimen consisting of albuterol, epinephrine, or other sympathomimetic bronchodilators (354). Overall, the pooled data found no difference between the aminophylline-treated group and the control groups, with three studies favoring aminophylline, three favoring the control regimen, and seven showing no difference between the two.

More recently, several studies have evaluated the role of aminophylline in the treatment of acute exacerbation of asthma when used in addition to inhaled β-agonists and intravenous corticosteroids both in the emergency room and in the hospital for both adults and children (355–360). In a prospective study of 133 adult patients (356) maximally treated with intravenous corticosteroids and inhaled β-agonists, administration of aminophylline resulted in a three-fold decrease in the hospital admission rate for patients treated with aminophylline (6%) compared with placebo recipients (21%). Surprisingly, the reduction in admissions occurred despite an absence of improvement in pulmonary function as measured by spirometry. The admission decision was made by noninvestigator house staff by use of preexisting guidelines for admission. Huang and coworkers, in a placebo-controlled randomized trial of aminophylline infusion in addition to inhaled albuterol and intravenous methylprednisolone, found that the improvement in FEV_1 at three hours was greater in the aminophylline group (29% plus or minus 23% compared with 10% plus or minus 10%) and that the aminophylline-treated patients required fewer nebulizations of albuterol (358). A concern with this study is whether the patients received maximal inhaled β-agonist therapy. Also, it is unclear how the decision to administer "as-needed" albuterol therapy was made, since this was one of the endpoints of the study. In contrast, two recent studies in children did not find that intravenous theophylline added to the management of hospitalized pediatric asthmatics maximally treated with nebulized albuterol and intravenous corticosteroids (359,360).

The role of inhaled anticholinergic agents in the management of acute asthma is limited. The usefulness of atropine is limited by systemic side effects (361). Ipratropium is generally inferior to the β-agonists as sole therapy for acute asthma (362–365). Several studies have shown that the combination of high-dose ipratropium (500 μg) and the β-adrenergic agent is more efective than either drug used alone (366–368).

The efficacy of systemic corticosteroids (oral or intravenous) in acute severe asthma is quite well established in 15 clinical trials of acute asthma in adults (369). Fanta and colleagues demonstrated that in patients with acute severe episodes of asthma refractory to eight hours of conventional bronchodilator therapy, the subjects given intravenous corticosteroids had significantly greater resolution of airflow obstruction by the end of 24 hours (370). Littenberg and Gluck demonstrated that the prompt use of glucocorticoids in the emergency treatment of severe asthma can prevent significant morbidity, reduce the number of hospitalizations, and effect substantial savings in health care costs (371). In contrast, Stein and Cole, in a placebo-controlled trial of 81 adults with acute asthma in the ER, failed to show that early administration of intravenous corticosteroids reduces the hospital admission rate (18% for the steroid group and 13% for the control group) (372). However, the admitted patients did begin with lower PEFs and responded less at two hours to inhaled bronchodilators. It is likely that the severity of underlying airflow obstruction and

inflammation on initial presentation is what determines the need for admission (334). It is clear that the onset of action is delayed at least six to 12 hours following systemic administration of corticosteroids (373).

Much has been published about systemic corticosteroid therapy for patients with acute and chronic asthma as to the type of steroid preparation, route of administration (parenteral versus oral) (374), the ideal dosage (369,375), and the duration of taper (376,377). Although several studies have suggested that there are differences in penetration of different corticosteroid preparations in the lung, their clinical relevance is unclear (378,379). For parenteral use, methylprednisolone is preferred over hydrocortisone becase of more potent antiinflammatory properties and for being less expensive (369). For oral therapy, the available preparations appear to be fairly comparable, although cortisone and prednisone require hydroxylation before they become active. Since bioavailability after oral therapy is quite high for prednisone, some have recommended "noninvasive" therapy by the use of oral steroids in acute asthma exacerbation (380). Although the optimal dosage for systemic steroids has not been established, McFadden's review of the available studies suggest that hydrocortisone equivalent to 14 mg per kg per 24 hours is effective therapy for acutely ill asthmatic adults (369). It is common practice to administer 120 to 180 mg of methylprednisolone per day intravenously. As an alternative, oral therapy may be given in divided doses (150 to 225 mg of prednisone or 600 to 900 mg of hydrocortisone) (369). Likewise, the optimal schedule of steroid withdrawal following an acute exacerbation is not well established. In one study, Lederle and coworkers suggested that the relapse rate was not different between a steroid taper of one week compared to seven weeks, although the relapse rate was quite high in both groups (376).

Therefore, the conventional therapy for acute severe asthma exacerbation would include repeated aerosolized β-agonist, oxygen, and systemic corticosteroids. Forced hydration and antibiotics are usually not required. Reassessment at frequent intervals by physical examination and peak flow meter should be performed to determine whether the patient is improving, staying about the same, or deteriorating. Response to therapy is probably the single most important factor in helping to determine the need for hospital admission. It is true that patients showing improvements on this therapy and discharged home with oral corticosteroids do well without significant relapse. A practical duration of treatment in a typical ER setting is about four hours (334). If a patient requires further therapy after four hours, then the next decision is whether to admit the patient for prolonged inpatient care or continue therapy in the setting of an ER-based observation unit or holding room when these facilities are available. There are conflicting data on whether these observation units (typically consisting of care for 12 to 24 hours) lessen the need for hospital admission, reduce the total length of stay, or are cost-effective (381). For patients who are admitted to the hospital, the next decision is whether to manage them on a regular nursing floor or in the intensive care unit. Patients with severe airflow obstruction who are deteriorating despite conventional therapy (based on evidence of respiratory muscle fatigue and/or respiratory depression), should be managed in a closely monitored intensive care setting to assess serially the need for airway support and mechanical ventilation (344,382). For all other patients, therapy could be continued on a regular floor with frequent "every two to four hour" administration of aerosolized β-agonist and serial peak flow measurements.

Most patients with acute asthma respond to aggressive conventional therapy with aerosolized β-agonist and systemic corticosteroids. However, for the subset of patients with a delayed or inadequate response to initial therapy, a variety of unconventional therapies may be considered. These include the use of intravenous magnesium, mixture of helium-oxygen gas, non-invasive ventilation, ketamine, and inhalation anesthetics (333,344). Although there are published reports in support of each of these therapies, these therapies should be considered experimental and be reserved for patients who are not improving despite maximal conventional therapy. The rationale for the use of intravenous magnesium is based on the fact that magnesium inhibits calcium channels, reduces the acetylcholine release, and may improve respiratory function. In addition, serum level of magnesium may be low in 50% of patients with acute asthma exacerbation. Although there are several uncontrolled studies which have shown beneficial effects with intravenous magnesium, at least two recent randomized clinical trials have not shown a benefit compared to placebo (383,384). Heliox is a blend of helium and oxygen. When inhaled by an asthmatic, turbulent flow in narrowed airways may become laminar, thereby reducing the resistive work of breathing. Several prospective, uncontrolled studies have shown improvement in peak flows, respiratory muscle fatigue, and reversal of hypercapnia (385,386). It is important to recognize that the heliox mixture typically uses 50% to 80% helium; therefore patients who are severely hypoxemic are not appropriate candidates. Noninvasive positive-pressure ventilation has been used for patients with acute asthma with an inadequate initial response to therapy. Several uncontrolled small series and case reports suggest that continuous positive airway pressure therapy with 5 cm to 7.5 cm H_2O can help unload the inspiratory muscles and avoid intubation (387). The use of this modality is labor-intensive and should be reserved for a small number of carefully selected patients in the intensive care unit.

A small subset of patients may have such severe airflow obstruction and airway inflammation so as not to be able to maintain spontaneous ventilation despite aggressive initial therapy (344,382). These patients require intubation and mechanical ventilation in an intensive care setting. The in-

tubation itself may occur in the field, in an ER, on a regular nursing floor, or in the ICU. Technically, these patients are difficult to intubate because of dyspnea and respiratory distress. They do not tolerate lying flat and their airways are hyperreactive. Optimizing the conditions for intubation include using the most experienced operator and intubating in a controlled elective setting with the appropriate use of sedating agents. Good sedating agents to facilitate intubation include midazolam (a short-acting benzodiazepam), ketamine, or propofol. It is best to avoid morphine at the time of intubation, since it can produce hypotension, induce nausea and emesis, and contribute to bronchospasm by histamine release. Ketamine, a phencyclidine that inhibits the reuptake of catecholamines, is commonly used as an induction agent prior to administration of general anesthetics. It has a rapid onset, is short-acting, and has the advantage of being a bronchodilator, a vagolytic agent, and perhaps an antiinflammatory agent. A typical dose is 0.1 mg per kg to 0.2 mg per kg intravenous bolus followed by 0.5 mg per kg delivered by infusion over a three-hour period. Ketamine does have the potential to increase heart rate and blood pressure and lower the seizure threshold. A recent, prospective, randomized trial compared the addition of ketamine to acute asthmatics refractory to initial ER therapy with three doses of inhaled β-agonist and systemic steroids (388). Compared to placebo, ketamine did not show benefit.

Early studies of the use of mechanical ventilation in patients with status asthmaticus in the 1970s indicated significant mortality ranging from 9% to 39% as well as significant iatrogenic complications (331). However, over the past 20 years, the prognosis for ventilated acute asthmatics seems to have improved dramatically. More recent studies show a low death rate and a relatively low complication rate (389). The key principle that has evolved for mechanical ventilation of patients with status asthmaticus is controlled hypoventilation. The goal of mechanical ventilation in these patients is to support oxygenation, have an acceptable arterial pH, and avoid iatrogenic complications related to increased intrathoracic pressures. The complications of mechanical ventilation for status asthmaticus are due to incomplete emptying of the lungs, gas trapping, or auto-positive end expiratory pressure (auto-peep) (390). Normalization of the partial pressure of carbon dioxide should not be a goal, and "permissive hypercapnia" should be accepted with pH of 7.2 to 7.3. Occasionally, supplementation with intravenous bicarbonate is required. Specific ventilatory strategies to minimize airway pressure and auto-peep in this setting include reducing the minute ventilation by reducing the rate or tidal volume or both. Patients who are mechanically ventilated by this strategy will require heavy sedation with benzodiazepines or narcotics, and every effort should be made to avoid neuromuscular blockade. Patients with status asthmaticus are typically treated with systemic corticosteroids, and the combination of neuromuscular blockers and corticosteroids seem to be a significant risk factor for the development of prolonged paralysis (391). Therefore neuromuscular blockade should be reserved for patients who otherwise could not be ventilated. While patients are treated with nebulized β-agonist and systemic corticosteroids, and supported with mechanical ventilation, a number of heroic salvage therapies are available. These include the use of inhalational anesthetics and bronchoalveolar lavage. Anesthetic agents are felt to be effective because they potentiate β₂ receptors and they have direct bronchodilator properties (392,393). Anesthetics are effective in the presence of acidosis. However, these agents (including halothane and ether) have adverse effects including myocardial depression and irritability along with idiosyncratic reactions. Inhalation anesthetics should be reserved for the rarest situation where there is expertise in the use of these agents in the intensive care setting.

EXPERIMENTAL THERAPY

About 5% to 20% of patients continue to have troublesome asthma symptoms with frequent exacerbations requiring hospitalization despite maximal conventional therapy (1). The reversible factors that contribute to this subset of "steroid-dependent" asthma include patient noncompliance, poor self-management skills, inadequate control of allergen burden at home, inadequate inhaler technique, and suboptimal pharmacotherapy prescription by the physician. Data from the placebo arm of a number of studies have clearly shown that a compulsory conventional management plan, with frequent follow-up perhaps in an asthma center, can reduce the need for oral steroids by 16% to 40% in "steroid-dependent" asthmatics (394,395).

Carmichael and colleagues described 58 patients with chronic asthma who were clinically resistant to treatment with prednisolone (defined as absence of a 15% increase in FEV_1 after a seven-day course of at least 20 mg of prednisolone daily) (396). Dykewicz and colleagues studied the natural history of 40 randomly selected adult asthmatic patients refractory to inhaled beclomethasone and β-agonists and dependent on long-term prednisone therapy (mean duration 6.2 plus or minus 5 years) (397). Over a three- to five-year period, 24 patients (60%) had unchanged long-term prednisone requirement, 13 patients (32.5%) improved with a reduction in prednisone requirement, and three patients (7.5%) deteriorated with increased prednisone requirement. Unfortunately, this study did not report the maintenance dose of beclomethasone. Corrigan and co-workers evaluated the possible mechanism of glucocorticoid resistance in chronic asthma (398). Patients were defined as having glucocorticoid resistance if there was less than a 30% increase in FEV_1 after two weeks of daily prednisone, 20 mg for the first week and 40 mg for the second week. Glucocorticoid pharmacokinetics, receptor characteristics, and inhibition of peripheral blood T-cell proliferation by glucocorticoid were assayed. Overall, the investigators noted a relative insensitivity of T lymphocytes to glucocorticoid in patients with clinical glucocorticoid resistance compared to matched glucocorticoid-sensitive asthmatics. They noted that the resistance does not reflect abnormal glucocorticoid clearance. Additional studies by this group suggested that activated T lymphocytes may be the target, and perhaps an anti–T lymphocyte drug such as cyclosporine may be particularly useful in glucocorticoid-resistant asthmatic patients. Overall, the clinical relevance of glucocorticoid resistance in patients with chronic steroid-dependent asthma remains speculative and poorly understood (399).

The literature is replete with studies demonstrating the efficacy of alternative antiinflammatory therapies that provide a steroid-sparing effect in asthma (400–402). Discussion here will be limited to methotrexate, troleandomycin, and cyclosporine. Methotrexate has been evaluated in steroid-dependent asthma in 11 controlled clinical trials between 1988 and 1996. (394,403–407). The rationale for methotrexate trials in asthma is based on the long-standing experience with antiinflammatory properties of this drug in rheumatoid arthritis and psoriasis. Methotrexate is an inhibitor of dihydrofolate reductase, which appears to inhibit neutrophil-dependent inflammation. A meta-analysis attempted to combine the results of 11 published trials of methotrexate for steroid-dependent asthma (407). Overall, six of 11 studies concluded that methotrexate did not have a steroid-sparing effect. The average steroid dose at initiation of these studies was 18.4 mg per day and methotrexate treatment decreased steroid usage by 4.37 mg per day or 23.7% of initial dosage (p < 0.05). Subgroup analysis showed greatest steroid-sparing effects with methotrexate therapy greater than six months, low long-term steroid therapy (less than or equal to 20 mg per day), and a study design incorporating a run-in. In summary, based on the available studies, it is difficult to recommend therapy with methotrexate outside the setting of a clinical trial.

Both oral and parenteral gold preparations have been used in the therapy of steroid-dependent asthma (408–412). These studies have generally found that the addition of gold can decrease corticosteroid requirement, can improve symptoms, and perhaps can improve bronchial hyperreactivity as well. In addition to a number of methodologic limitations with these studies, overall patient tolerance has been poor and the incidence of side effects has been as high as 37%, including diarrhea, skin eruptions, and proteinuria. An eight-month controlled trial of 227 steroid-dependent asthmatics (prednisone 10 mg per day or more) randomized patients to oral gold (auranofin 4 mg twice daily) or placebo (412). Significant reduction in oral steroid dose (50% or more of baseline) was achieved in the auranofin group (60%) compared with the placebo group (32%) (p < 0.001). Gastrointestinal and cutaneous adverse effects were greater in the auranofin group. There are no data on long-term side effects or patient compliance with gold therapy for patients with bronchial asthma.

Another steroid-sparing approach in the treatment of chronic asthma has been the use of troleandomycin, a macrolide antibiotic. Several open-label studies have demonstrated a reduction in corticosteroid dose when troleandomycin is added to the medical regimen of patients with asthma (413–416). The principal effect of troleandomycin is the prolongation of the plasma half-life of corticosteroids through the inhibition of their elimination; in one study methylprednisolone half-life increased from 2.46 hours before troleandomycin therapy to 4.63 hours one week after troleandomycin therapy (414). Published protocols highlight the importance of using methylprednisolone rather than prednisone in conjunction with troleandomycin to have the steroid-sparing effect (416,417). A recent placebo-controlled parallel group study over a two-year period was performed in 75 steroid-dependent asthmatics comparing troleandomycin plus methylprednisolone versus methylprednisolone alone (418). Patients in both groups achieved alternate-day steroid therapy, and the reduction in methylprednisolone dose was not significantly different between the treatment groups. However, the patients in the troleandomycin group were observed to have significantly more steroid-related side effects as assessed by serum IgG, blood sugar, cholesterol, and osteoporosis. In summary, this was a well-designed study that strongly supports the notion that the steroid-sparing properties of troleandomycin are a pharmacologic phenomenon and do not translate into fewer long-term steroid-related side effects. Based on this study, further trials with troleandomycin are probably not indicated.

Cyclosporine is an immunosuppressive agent with a number of properties, including inhibition of mediator release from mast cells and basophils and inhibition of the synthesis of lymphokines, with the subsequent downregulation of CD4$^+$ T lymphocytes. Since recent data have implicated the T lymphocyte as playing a critical role in chronic asthma, several investigators have evaluated cyclosporine in steroid-dependent asthma (419–422). Most recently, Lock and colleagues conducted a 36-week placebo-controlled, randomized, double-blind trial using cyclosporine A (CsA) (5 mg per kg per day) in 39 steroid-dependent asthmatic patients (422). The 16 of 19 patients who completed CsA therapy achieved a significant reduction in prednisone dosage of 62% (10 mg reduced to 3.5 mg) compared with 25% (20 mg reduced to 7.5 mg) in the placebo group (p = 0.04). Side effects occurred more often in the CsA group, but these did not require withdrawal from the study. The well known side effects of CsA include hypertension, hypertrichosis, neurological disturbances, and nephrotoxicity.

SUMMARY

Asthma causes significant morbidity in the United States. In response to this need, several detailed practice guidelines have been put forth by expert panels and disseminated widely. A major challenge is the implementation of basic asthma management principles widely at the community level. Key issues include education of primary health care providers; establishment of programs for asthma education; use of longitudinal, outpatient, follow-up care with "easy access" to providers; and emphasis on chronic maintenance antiinflammatory therapy rather than acute episodic care.

Asthma is being aggressively targeted by a variety of research efforts. Whether asthma is a single disorder with a unique cause or a syndrome of multiple disorders with several etiologic mechanisms remains unclear. The critical and rate-limiting steps in the asthma inflammatory cascade remain to be established. The natural history of the disease is not well understood and the significance of airway hyperreactivity in asymptomatic individuals is unknown. The contribution of genetic factors, atopic status, environmental factors, and viral infections is not well understood. Future therapeutic strategies will in part be dependent on the answers to some of these unresolved issues.

REFERENCES

1. National Heart, Lung and Blood Institute. National Asthma Education and Prevention Program. Expert Panel Report 2. Guidelines for the diagnosis and management of asthma. Bethesda, MD. National Institutes of Health, 1997. Publication no. 97–4051.
2. Ciba Foundation Guest Symposium. Terminology, definitions and classification of chronic pulmonary emphysema and related conditions. *Thorax* 1959;14:286.
3. Scadding JG. The meaning of diagnostic terms in bronchopulmonary disease. *Br Med J* 1963;2:1423.
4. American Thoracic Society. Standards for the diagnosis and care of patients with chronic obstructive pulmonary disease (COPD) and asthma. *Am Rev Respir Dis* 1987;136:225–244.
5. International Consensus Report on Diagnosis and Management of Asthma. National Heart, Lung and Blood Institute, National Institutes of Health, Bethesda, MD. *Eur Respir J* 1992;5:601–641.
6. Snapper JR. Inflammation and airway function: the asthma syndrome [Editorial]. *Am Rev Respir Dis* 1990;141:531–533.
7. U.S. Department of Health. *Prevalence of Selected Chronic Respiratory Conditions—United States, 1970.* U.S. Department of Health, Education, and Welfare Series 10, No. 84, 1973.
8. Bonner JR. The epidemiology and natural history of asthma. *Clin Chest Med* 1984;5:557–565.
9. Broder I, Higgins MW, Mathews KD, et al. Epidemiology of asthma and allergic rhinitis in a total community, Tecumseh, Michigan. *J Allergy Clin Immunol* 1974;53:127–138.
10. Gergen PJ, Mullally DI, Evans R. National survey of prevalence of asthma among children in the U.S., 1976–1980. *Pediatrics* 1988;81:1–7.
11. Asthma mortality and hospitalization among children and young adults—United States, 1980–1993. *MMWR Morb Mortal Wkly Rep* 1996;45:350–353.
12. Mannino DM, Homa DM, Pertowski LA, et al. Surveillance for asthma—United States,1960–1995. *MMWR Morb Mortal Wkly Rep* 1998;47:1–27.
13. Skobeloff EM, Spivey WH, St. Clair SS, et al. The influence

of age and sex on asthma admissions. *JAMA* 1992;268: 3437–3440.

14. Jackson RT, Beaglehole R, Rea HH, et al. Mortality from asthma: a new epidemic in New Zealand. *Br Med J* 1982;285: 771–774.

15. Sears MR, Rea HH, Beaglehole R. Asthma mortality: a review of recent experience in New Zealand. *J Allergy Clin Immunol* 1987;80:319–325.

16. Wilson JD, Sutherland DC, Thomas AC. Has the change to beta-agonists combined with oral theophylline increased cases of total asthma? *Lancet* 1981;1:1235.

17. Sears MR. Epidemiological trends in bronchial asthma. In Kaliner MA, Barnes PJ, Persson CGA, eds. *Asthma, its pathology and treatment.* New York: Marcel Dekker, 1991:1–49.

18. Sly RM. Mortality from asthma. *J Allergy Clin Immunol* 1989; 84:421–434.

19. Buist AS, Sears MR, Reid LM, et al. Asthma mortality: trends and determinants. *Am Rev Respir Dis* 1987;135:1037–1039.

20. Rea HH, Sears MR, Beaglehole R, et al. Lessons from the national asthma mortality study: circumstances surrounding death. *N Z Med J* 1987;100:10–13.

21. Sly RM. Mortality from asthma, 1974–1984. *J Allergy Clin Immunol* 1988;82:705–717.

22. Benatar SR. Fatal asthma. *N Engl J Med* 1986;314:423–429.

23. Rea HH, Seragg R, Jackson R, et al. A case-control study of deaths from asthma. *Thorax* 1986;41:833–839.

24. Barger LW, Vollmer WM, Felt RW, et al. Further investigation into the recent increase in asthma death rates: a review of 41 asthma deaths in Oregon in 1982. *Ann Allergy* 1988;60:31–39.

25. Strunk RC. Death due to asthma. *Am Rev Respir Dis* 1993;148: 550–552.

26. Weiss KB, Wagener DK. Changing patterns of asthma mortality: identifying target populations at high risk. *JAMA* 1990;264: 1683–1687.

27. Molfino NA, Nannini LJ, Rebuck AS, et al. The fatality-prone asthmatic patient. *Chest* 1992;101:621–623.

28. Barriot P, Riou B. Prevention of fatal asthma. *Chest* 1987;92: 460–466.

29. Reid LM. The presence or absence of bronchial mucous in fatal asthma. *J Allergy Clin Immunol* 1987;80:415–416.

30. Weiss KB, Gergen PJ, Hodgson TA. An economic evaluation of asthma in the United States. *N Engl J Med* 1992;326:862–866.

31. Smith DH, Malone D, Lawson KA, et al. A national estimate of the economic costs of asthma. *Am J Respir Crit Care Med* 1997;156:787–793.

32. Nelson HS, Szeffler SJ, Martin RJ. Regular inhaled beta-adrenergic agonists in the treatment of bronchial asthma: beneficial or detrimental. *Am Rev Respir Dis* 1991;144:249–250.

33. Grant IWB. Asthma in New Zealand. *Br Med J* 1983;286:364.

34. Grainger J, Woodsman K, Pearce N, et al. Prescribed fenoterol and death from asthma in New Zealand, 1981–7: a further case-control study. *Thorax* 1991;46:105–111.

35. Sears MR, Taylor DR, Pring CG, et al. Regular inhaled beta-agonist treatment in bronchial asthma. *Lancet* 1990;336: 1391–1396.

36. Spitzer WO, Suissa S, Ernst P, et al. The use of B-agonists and the risk of death and near death from asthma. *N Engl J Med* 1992;326:501–506.

37. Ernst P, Habbick B, Suissa S, et al. Is the association between inhaled beta-agonist use and life-threatening asthma because of confounding by severity? *Am Rev Respir Dis* 1993;148:75–79.

38. Drazen JM, Israel E, Boushey HA, et al. Comparison of regularly scheduled with as-needed use of albuterol in mild asthma. Asthma Clinical Research Network. *N Engl J Med* 1996;335: 841–847.

39. Rackemann FM, Edwards MC. Asthma in children. *N Engl J Med* 1952;246:858–863.

40. Blair H. Natural history of childhood asthma. *Arch Dis Child* 1977;52:613–619.

41. Martin AJ, McLennan LA, Landau LI, et al. The natural history of childhood asthma to adult life. *Br Med J* 1980;1:1397–1400.

42. Brown PJ, Greville HW, Finvcane KE. Asthma and irreversible airflow obstruction. *Thorax* 1984;39:131–136.

43. Braman SS, Kaemmerlen JT, Davis SM. Asthma in the elderly: a comparison between patients with recently acquired and long-standing disease. *Am Rev Respir Dis* 1991;143:336–340.

44. Backman KS, Greenberger PA, Patterson R. Airways obstruction in patients with long-term asthma consistent with "irreversible asthma." *Chest* 1997;112:1234–1240.

45. Selroos O, Pietinalho A, Lofroos AB, et al. Effect of early vs late intervention with inhaled corticosteroids in asthma. *Chest* 1995;108:1228–1234.

46. Bronnimann S, Burrows B. A prospective study of the natural history of asthma. *Chest* 1986;90:480–484.

47. Broder I, Barlow PP, Horton RJM. The epidemiology of asthma and hay fever in a total community, Tecumseh, Michigan. *J Allergy* 1962;33:524–531.

48. Lee HY, Stretton TB. Asthma in the elderly. *Br Med J* 1972; 4:93–95.

49. Hogg JC. The pathology of asthma. *Clin Chest Med* 1984;5: 567–571.

50. Dunnill MS, Massarella GR, Anderson JA. A comparison of the quantitative anatomy of the bronchi in normal subjects, in status asthmaticus, in chronic bronchitis, and in emphysema. *Thorax* 1969;24:176–179.

51. MacDonald JB, MacDonald ET, Seaton A, et al. Asthma deaths in Cardiff 1963–74: fifty-three deaths in hospital. *Br Med J* 1976;2:721–723.

52. MacDonald JB, Seaton A, Williams DA. Asthma deaths in Cardiff 1963–74: ninety deaths outside hospital. *Br Med J* 1976; 1:1493–1495.

53. Laitinen LA, Heino M, Laitinen A, et al. Damage of the airway epithelium and bronchial reactivity in patients with asthma. *Am Rev Respir Dis* 1985;131:599–606.

54. Kavuru MS, Dweik RA, Thomassen MJ. Role of bronchoscopy in asthma research. *Clin Chest Med* 1999;10(1):153–189.

55. Smith DL, Deshazo RD. State of the art: bronchoalveolar lavage in asthma: an update and perspective. *Am Rev Respir Dis* 1993; 148:523–532.

56. Djukanovic R, Roche WR, Wilson JW, et al. Mucosal inflammation in asthma. *Am Rev Respir Dis* 1990;142:434–457.

57. Beasley R, Roche WR, Roberts JA, et al. Cellular events in the bronchi in mild asthma and after bronchial provocation. *Am Rev Respir Dis* 1989;139:806–817.

58. Sheppard D. Airway hyperresponsiveness: mechanisms in experimental models. *Chest* 1989;96:1165–1168.

59. O'Bryne PM, Hargreave FE, Kirby JG. Airway inflammation and hyperresponsiveness. *Am Rev Respir Dis* 1991;143: S35–S37.

60. Bigby TD, Nadel JA. Asthma. In: Gallin JI, Goldstein IM, Snyderman R, eds. *Inflammation: basic principles and clinical correlates,* ed 2. New York: Raven Press, 1992:889–906.

61. Herxheimer H. The late bronchial reaction in induced asthma. *Intl Arch Allergy Appl Immunol* 1952;3:323–328.

62. Cartier A, Thomson NC, Frith PA, et al. Allergen-induced increase in bronchial responsiveness to histamine: relationship to the late asthmatic response and change in airway caliber. *J Allergy Clin Immunol* 1982;70:170–177.

63. O'Bryne PM, Dolovich J, Hargreave FE. Late asthmatic responses. *Am Rev Respir Dis* 1987;136:740–751.

64. Booij-Noord H, De Vries K, Sluiter HJ, et al. Late bronchial

obstructive reaction to experimental inhalation of house dust extract. *Clin Allergy* 1972;2:43–61.

65. Martin RJ, Cicutto LC, Smith HR, et al. Airway inflammation in nocturnal asthma. *Am Rev Respir Dis* 1991;143:351–357.

66. Robinson DS, Hamid Q, Ying S, et al. Predominant T_{H2}-like bronchoalveolar T-lymphocyte population in atopic asthma. *N Engl J Med* 1992;326:298–304.

67. Rochester CL, Rankin JA. Is asthma T-cell mediated? *Am Rev Respir Dis* 1992;144:1005–1007.

68. Kay AB. Helper (CD4) T cells and eosinophils in allergy and asthma. *Am Rev Respir Dis* 1992;14:S22–S26.

69. Kay AB. Origin of type 2 helper T cells. *N Engl J Med* 1994; 330:567–568.

70. Wilson JW, Djukanovic R, Howarth PH, et al. Lymphocyte activation in bronchoalveolar lavage and peripheral blood in atopic asthma. *Am Rev Respir Dis* 1992;145:958–960.

71. Samuelsson B, Dahlen SE, Lindgren JA, et al. Leukotrienes and lipoxins: structures, biosynthesis, and biological effects. *Science* 1987;237:1171–1176.

72. Drazen JM, Austen KF. Leukotrienes and airway responses. *Am Rev Respir Dis* 1987;136:985–998.

73. Drazen JM. Inhalation challenge with sulfidopeptide leukotrienes in human subjects. *Chest* 1986;89:414–419.

74. Drazen JM, O'Brien JB, Sparrow D, et al. Recovery of leukotriene E_4 from the urine of patients with airway obstruction. *Am Rev Respir Dis* 1992;146:104–108.

75. Smith CM, Hawksworth FCK, Thien PE, et al. Urinary leukotriene E_4 in bronchial asthma. *Eur Respir J* 1992;5:693–699.

76. Busse WW, Gaddy JN. The role of leukotriene antagonists and inhibitors in the treatment of airway disease. *Am Rev Respir Dis* 1991;143:S103–S107.

77. Cloud ML, Enas GC, Kemp J, et al. A specific LTD4/LTE4-receptor antagonist improves pulmonary function in patients with mild, chronic asthma. *Am Rev Respir Dis* 1989;140: 1336–1339.

78. Taylor IK, O'Shaughnessy KM, Fuller Rw, et al. Effect of cysteinyl-leukotriene receptor antagonist ICI 204.219 on allergen-induced bronchoconstriction and airway hyperreactivity in atopic subjects. *Lancet* 1991;337:690–694.

79. Manning PJ, Watson RM, Margolskee DJ. Inhibition of exercise-induced bronchoconstriction by MK-571, a potent leukotriene D4-receptor antagonist. *N Engl J Med* 1990;2323: 1736–1739.

80. Israel E, Dermarkarian R, Rosenberg M, et al. The effects of 5-lipoxygenase inhibitor on asthma induced by cold, dry air. *N Engl J Med* 1990;323:1740–1744.

81. Dahlen B, Kumlin M, Margolskee DJ, et al. The leukotriene-receptor antagonist MK-0679 blocks airway obstruction induced by inhaled lysine-aspirin in aspirin-sensitive asthmatics. *Eur Respir J* 1993;6:1018–1026.

82. Kavuru MS, Subramony R, Vann AR. Antileukotrienes and asthma; alternative or adjunct to inhaled steroids? *Cleve Clin J Med* 1998;65:519–523.

83. Turner-Warwick M. Epidemiology of nocturnal asthma. *Am J Med* 1998;85:6–8.

84. Glauser FL. Variant asthma. *Ann Allergy* 1972;30:457.

85. McFadden ER. Exertional dyspnea and cough as preludes to acute attacks of bronchial asthma. *N Engl J Med* 1975;292: 555–559.

86. Corrao WM, Braman SS, Irwin RS. Chronic cough as the sole manifestation of bronchial asthma. *N Engl J Med* 1979;300: 633–637.

87. Hannaway PJ, Hopper GDK. Cough variant asthma in children. *JAMA* 1982;247:206–208.

88. Johnson D, Osborn LM. Cough variant asthma: a review of the clinical literature. *J Asthma* 1991:28(2):85–90.

89. Ellul-Micallef R. Effect of terbutaline sulphate in chronic "allergic" cough. *Br Med J* 1983;287:940.

90. Irwin RS, Corrao WM, Pratter MR. Chronic persistent cough in the adult: the spectrum and frequency of causes and successful outcome of specific therapy. *Am Rev Respir Dis* 1981;123: 413–417.

91. Christopher KL, Wood RP, Eckert RC, et al. Vocal-cord dysfunction presenting as asthma. *N Engl J Med* 1983;308: 1566–1570.

92. Downing ET, Braman SS, Fox MJ, et al. Factitious asthma: physiological approach to diagnosis. *JAMA* 1982;248: 2878–2881.

93. Miller RD, Hyatt RE. Evaluation of obstructing lesions of the trachea and larynx by flow-volume loops. *Am Rev Respir Dis* 1973;108:475–481.

94. Kavuru MS, Eliachar I, Sivak ED. Management of the upper airway in the critically ill patient. In: Sivak ED, Higgins T, Seiver A, eds. *The high risk patient: management of the critically ill.* Baltimore: Williams & Wilkins, 1995;189–211.

95. McFadden ER Jr, Zawadski DK. Vocal cord dysfunction masquerading as exercise-induced asthma. a physiologic cause for "choking" during athletic activities. *Am J Respir Crit Care Med* 1996;153:942–947.

96. Shim CS, Williams MH Jr. Relationship of wheezing to the severity of obstruction in asthma. *Arch Intern Med* 1983;143: 890–893.

97. McFadden ER, Kiser R, DeGroot WJ. Acute bronchial asthma: relations between clinical and physiologic manifestations. *N Engl J Med* 1973;288:221–225.

98. Veen J, Smits H, Ravensberg A, et al. Impaired perception of dyspnea in patients with severe asthma. *Am J Respir Crit Care Med* 1998;158:1134–1141.

99. Guidelines for the evaluation of impairment/disability in patients with asthma. *Am Rev Respir Dis* 1993;147:1056–1061.

100. Toren K, Brisman J, Jarvholm B. Asthma and asthma-like symptoms in adults assessed by questionnaires: a literature review. *Chest* 1993;104:600–608.

101. Juniper EF, Guyatt GH, Ferrie PJ, et al. Measuring quality of life in asthma. *Am Rev Respir Dis* 1993;147:832–838.

102. McFadden ER Jr. Clinical-physiologic correlates in asthma. *J Allergy Clin Immunol* 1986;77:1–5.

103. Shim CS, William MH. Evaluation of the severity of asthma: patients versus physicians. *Am J Med* 1980;68:11–13.

104. Knowles GK, Clark TJH. Pulsus paradoxus as a valuable sign indicating severity of asthma. *Lancet* 1973;11:1356–1359.

105. Rebuck AS, Pergelly LD. Development of pulsus paradoxus in the presence of airways obstruction. *N Engl J Med* 1973;288: 66–69.

106. Kelsen SG, Kelsen DP, Fleegler BF, et al. Emergency room assessment and treatment of patients with acute asthma: adequacy of the conventional approach. *Am J Med* 1978;64: 622–628.

107. Carden DL, Nowak RM, Sarkar D, et al. Vital signs including pulsus paradoxus in the assessment of acute bronchial asthma. *Ann Emerg Med* 1983;12:80–83.

108. Wright BM, McKerrow CB. Maximum forced expiratory flow rate as a measure of ventilatory capacity: with a description of a new portable instrument for measuring it. *Br Med J* 1959;2: 1041–1047.

109. Berube D, Cartier A, L'Archeveque J, et al. Comparison of peak expiratory flow rate and FEV_1 in assessing bronchomotor tone after challenges with occupational sensitizers. *Chest* 1991;99: 831–836.

110. Jain P, Kavuru MS, Emerman CL, et al. Utility of peak expiratory monitoring. *Chest* 1998;114:861–876.

111. Clark NM, Evans D, Mellins RB. Patient use of peak flow monitoring. *Am Rev Respir Dis* 1992;145:722–725.

112. Brenner BE. The acute asthmatic in the emergency department: the decision to admit or discharge. *Am J Emerg Med* 1985;3:74–77.

113. Banner AS, Shah RS, Addington WW. Rapid prediction of need for hospitalization in acute asthma. *JAMA* 1976;235:1337–1338.

114. Nowak RM, Gordon KR, Wroblewski DA, et al. Spirometric evaluation of acute bronchial asthma. *JACEP* 1979;8:9–12.

115. Lulla S, Newcomb RW. Emergency management of asthma in children. *Pediatrics* 1980;97:346–350.

116. Nowak RM, Pensier MI, Sarkar DD, et al. Comparison of peak expiratory flow and FEV$_1$ admission criteria for acute bronchial asthma. *Ann Emerg Med* 1982;11:64–69.

117. Fanta CH, Rossing TH, McFadden ER Jr. Emergency room treatment of acute asthma: Relationships among therapeutic combinations, severity of obstruction, and time course of response. *Am J Med* 1982;72:416–422.

118. Fischl MA, Pitchenik A, Gardner LB. An index predicting relapse and need for hospitalization in patients with acute bronchial asthma. *N Engl J Med* 1981;305:783–789.

119. Rose CC, Murphy JG, Schwartz JS. Performance of an index predicting the response of patients with acute bronchial asthma to intensive emergency department treatment. *N Engl J Med* 1984;310:573–576.

120. Centor RM, Yarbrough B, Wood JP. Inability to predict relapse in acute asthma. *N Engl J Med* 1984;310:577–580.

121. Gershel JC, Goldman HS, Stein REK, et al. The usefulness of chest radiographs in first asthma attacks. *N Engl J Med* 1983;309:336–339.

122. McFadden ER Jr, Lyons HA. Arterial blood gas tension in asthma. *N Engl J Med* 1968;278:1027–1032.

123. Jackson LK. Functional aspects of asthma. *Clin Chest Med* 1984;5:573–587.

124. Hopewell PC, Miller RT. Pathophysiology and management of severe asthma. *Clin Chest Med* 1984;5:623–634.

125. Nowak RM, Tomlanovich MC, Sarkar DD, et al. Arterial blood gases and pulmonary function testing in acute bronchial asthma. *JAMA* 1983;249:2043–2046.

126. Kavuru MS, Richter JE. Medical treatment of gastroesophageal reflux disease and airway disease. In: Stein MR, ed. *GERD and airway disease*. Lung Biology in Health and Disease Series. New York: Marcell Dekker, Inc., 1999:179–207.

127. Hubert D, Gaudric M, Guerre J, et al. Effect of theophylline on gastroesophageal reflux in patients with asthma. *J Allergy Clin Immunol* 1988;81:1168–1174.

128. Ing AJ, Ngu MC, Breslin ABX. Pathogenesis of chronic persistent cough associated with gastroesophageal reflux. *Am J Respir Crit Care Med* 1994;149:160–167.

129. Schan CA, Harding SM, Haile JM, et al. Gastroesophageal reflux-induced bronchoconstriction: an intraesophageal acid infusion study using state-of-the-art technology. *Chest* 1994;106:731–737.

130. Locke GR, Talley NJ, Fett SL, et al. Prevalence and clinical spectrum of gastroesophageal reflux: a population based study in Olmstead County, Minnesota. *Gastroenterology* 1997;112:1448–1456.

131. Mattox HE, Richter JE. Prolonged ambulatory esophageal reflux pH monitoring in the evaluation of gastroesophageal reflux disease. *Am J Med* 1990;89:345–356.

132. Meeker DP, Wiedemann HP. Drug-induced bronchospasm. *Clin Chest Med* 1990;11(1):163–175.

133. Hannaway PJ, Hopper GDK. Severe anaphylaxis and drug-induced beta-blockade. *N Engl J Med* 1983;308:1536.

134. Lois M, Honig EG. β-blockade post-MI: safe for patients with asthma or COPD. *J Respir Dis* 1997;18:568–591.

135. Moser M. Angiotensin-converting enzyme inhibitors, angiotensin II receptor antagonists and calcium channel blocking agents. a review of potential benefits and possible adverse reactions. *J Am Coll Cardiol* 1997;29:1414–1421.

136. Greenberger PA. Allergic bronchopulmonary aspergillosis and fungoses. *Clin Chest Med* 1988;9:599–608.

137. Hinson KFW, Moon AJ, Plummer NS. Bronchopulmonary aspergillosis. *Thorax* 1952;7:317–333.

138. Patterson R, Golbert TM. Hypersensitivity disease of the lung. *Univ Mich Med Cent J* 1968;34:8–11.

139. Akiyama K, Ricketti AJ, Greenberger PA, et al. Identification of allergic bronchopulmonary aspergillosis in the United States. *Immunol Allergy Prac* 1983;5:29–31.

140. Glimp RA, Bayer AS. Fungal pneumonias. Part 3: allergic bronchopulmonary aspergillosis. *Chest* 1981;80:85–94.

141. Rosenberg M, Patterson R, Mintzer R, et al. Clinical and immunologic criteria for the diagnosis of allergic bronchopulmonary aspergillosis. *Ann Intern Med* 1977;80:405–414.

142. Patterson R, Greenberger PA, Ricketti AJ, et al. A radioimmunoassay index for allergic bronchopulmonary aspergillosis. *Ann Intern Med* 1983;99:18–22.

143. Greenberger PA, Patterson R. Application of enzyme-linked immunosorbent assay (ELISA) in diagnosis of allergic bronchopulmonary aspergillosis. *J Lab Clin Med* 1982;99:288–293.

144. Greenberger PA, Patterson R. Allergic bronchopulmonary aspergillosis and the evaluation of the patient with asthma. *J Allergy Clin Immunol* 1988;81:646–650.

145. Patterson R, Greenberger PA, Radin RC, et al. Allergic bronchopulmonary aspergillosis: staging as an aid to management. *Ann Intern Med* 1982;96:286–291.

146. Safirstein BH, D'Souza MF, Simon G, et al. Five-year follow-up of allergic bronchopulmonary aspergillosis. *Am Rev Respir Dis* 1973;108:450–460.

147. Nichols D, Dopico GA, Braun S, et al. Acute and chronic pulmonary function changes in allergic bronchopulmonary aspergillosis. *Am J Med* 1979;67:631–637.

148. Patterson R, Greenberger PA, Halwig JM, et al. Allergic bronchopulmonary aspergillosis: natural history and classification of early disease by serologic and radiologic studies. *Arch Intern Med* 1986;146:916–918.

149. Patterson R, Greenberger PA, Lee TM, et al. Prolonged evaluation of patients with corticosteroid-dependent asthma stage of bronchopulmonary aspergillosis. *J Allergy Clin Immunol* 1987;80:663–668.

150. Ricketti AJ, Greenberger PA, Patterson R. Serum IgE as an important aid in management of allergic bronchopulmonary aspergillosis. *J Allergy Clin Immunol* 1984;74:68–71.

151. Doershug KC, Peterson MW, Dayton CS, et al. Asthma guidelines: an assessment of physician understanding and practice. *Am J Respir Crit Care Med* 1999;159:824–828.

152. Dekker FW, Dieleman FE, Kaptein AA, et al. Compliance with pulmonary medication in general practice. *Eur Respir J* 1993;6:886–890.

153. Shim C, Williams MH Jr. The adequacy of inhalation of aerosol from canister nebulizer. *Am J Med* 1980;69:891–894.

154. Epstein SW, Manning CPR, Ashley MK, et al. Survey of the clinical use of pressurized aerosol inhalers. *Can Med Assoc J* 1979;120:813–816.

155. Kelling JS, Strohl KP, Smith RL, et al. Physician knowledge in the use of canister nebulizers. *Chest* 1983;4:612–614.

156. Guidry CG, Brown WD, Stogner SW, et al. Incorrect use of metered dose inhalers by medical personnel. *Chest* 1992;101:31–33.

157. Hanania NA, Wittman R, Kesten S, et al. Medical personnel's

knowledge of and ability to use inhaling devices. *Chest* 1994;105:111–116.

158. Tashkin DP, Rand C, Nides M, et al A nebulizer chronolog to monitor compliance with inhaler use. *Am J Med* 91[Suppl 4A]1991;33S–36S.

159. Blixen CE, Havstad S, Tilley BC, et al. A comparison of asthma-related healthcare use between African-Americans and Caucasians belonging to a health maintenance organization (HMO). *J Asthma* 1999;36:199–204.

160. Clark NM. Asthma self-management education: research and implications for clinical practice. *Chest* 1989;95:1110–113.

161. Parker SR, Mellins RB, Sogn DD. Asthma education: a national strategy. *Am Rev Respir Dis* 1989;140:848–853.

162. Mayo PH, Richman J, Harris W. Results of a program to reduce admissions for adult asthma. *Ann Intern Med* 1990;112:864–871.

163. Wilson SR, Scamagas P, German DF, et al. A controlled trial of the two forms of self-management education for adults with asthma. *Am J Med* 1993;94:564–576.

164. Tougaard L, Krone T, Sorknaes A, et al. Economic benefits of teaching patients with chronic obstructive pulmonary disease about their illness. *Lancet* 1992;339:1617–1520.

165. Bailey WC, Richards JM, Brooks M, et al. A randomized trial to improve self-management practices of adults with asthma. *Arch Intern Med* 1990;150:1664–1668.

166. Bolton MB, Tilley BC, Kuder J, et al. The cost and effectiveness of an education program for adults who have asthma. *J Gen Intern Med* 1991;6:401–407.

167. Clark NM, Feldman CH, Evans D, et al. The impact of health education on frequency and cost of health care use by low income children with asthma. *J Allergy Clin Immunol* 1986;78:108–115.

168. Hilton S, Sibbald B, Anderson HR, et al. Controlled evaluation of the effects of patient education on asthma morbidity in general practice. *Lancet* 1986;1:26–29.

169. Yoon R, McKenzie DM, Miles DA, et al. Characteristics of attenders and non-attenders at an asthma education program. *Thorax* 1991;46:886–890.

170. Dolovich M, Ruffin RE, Roberts R, et al. Optimal delivery of aerosols from metered dose inhalers. *Chest* 1981;80[Suppl]:911–915.

171. Sackner MA, Kim CS. Auxillary MDI aerosol delivery systems. *Chest* 1985;99[Suppl]:161S–170S.

172. Shim CS, Williams MH Jr. Effect of bronchodilator administered by canister versus jet nebulizer. *J Allergy Clin Immunol* 1984;73:387–390.

173. Turner JR, Corkery KJ, Eckman D, et al. Equivalence of continuous flow nebulizer and metered dose inhaler with reservoir bag for treatment of acute air flow obstruction. *Chest* 1988;93:476–481.

174. Colacone A, Afilado M, Wolkove N, et al. A comparison of albuterol administered by metered dose inhaler (and holding chamber) or wet nebulizer in acute asthma. *Chest* 1993;104:835–841.

175. Orens DK, Kester L, Fergus LC, et al. Cost impact of metered dose inhalers vs small volume nebulizers in hospitalized patients: The Cleveland Clinic Experience. *Respir Care* 1991;36:1099–1104.

176. Sporik R, Holgate ST, Platts-Mills TAE, et al. Exposure to house-dust mite allergen (Der pI) and the development of asthma in childhood. *N Engl J Med* 1990;323:502–507.

177. Call RS, Smith TF, Morris E, et al. Risk factors for asthma in inner city children. *J Pediatr* 1992;121:862–866.

178. Gelber LE, Seltzer LH, Bouzoukis JK, et al. Sensitization and exposure to indoor allergens as risk factors for asthma among patients presenting to hospital. *Am Rev Respir Dis* 1993;147:573–578.

179. Creticos PS. Immunotherapy with allergens. *JAMA* 1992;268:2834–2839.

180. Platts-Mills TAE. Allergen-specific treatment for asthma. *Am Rev Respir Dis* 1993;148:553–555.

181. Platts-Mills TAE, de Week AL. Dust mite allergens and asthma—a worldwide problem. *J Allergy Clin Immunol* 1989;83:416–427.

182. Platts-Mills TAE, Pollart SM, Chapman MD, et al. Role of allergens in asthma and airway hyperresponsiveness: relevance to immunotherapy and allergen avoidance. In: Kaliner MA, Barnes PJ, Persson CGA, eds. *Asthma: its pathology and treatment.* New York: Marcel Dekker, 1991:595–631.

183. Hamilton RG, Chapman MD, Platts-Mills TAE, et al. House dust aeroallergen measurements in clinical practice: a guide to allergen-free home and work environments. *Immunol Allergy Pract* 1992;14:96–112.

184. Kaliner M, Lemanske R. Rhinitis and asthma. *JAMA* 1992;268:2807–2829.

185. Lands AM, Arnold A, McAuliff JP, et al. Differentiation of receptor systems activated by sympathomimetic amines. *Nature* 1967;214:597–598.

186. Popa VT. Clinical pharmacology of adrenergic drugs. *J Asthma* 1984;21:183–207.

187. Newhouse MT. Emergency department management of life-threatening asthma. *Chest* 1993;103:661–663.

188. Aerosol consensus statement. *Chest* 1991;100:1106–1109.

189. Newman SP. Metered dose pressurized aerosols and the ozone layer. *Eur Respir J* 1990;3:495–497.

190. Kerr RA. Ozone destruction worsens [News Report]. *Science* 1991;252:204.

191. Fisher DA, Hales CH, Wang WC, et al. Model calculations of the relative effects of CFCs and their replacement on global warming. *Nature* 1990;344:513–516.

192. Epstein SW. Is the MDI doomed to extinction? *Chest* 1993;103:1313.

193. Molina MJ, Rowland FS. Stratospheric risk for chlorofluoromethanes: chlorine atom-catalysed destruction of ozone. *Nature* 1974;249:810–812.

194. Gross G, Thompson PJ, Chervinsky P, et al. Hydrofluoroalkane-134a beclomethasone dipropionate, 400 μg, is as effective as chlorofluorocarbon beclomethasone dipropionate, 800 μg, for the teatment of moderate asthma. *Chest* 1999;115:343–351.

195. Brown PH, Lenny J, Armstrong S, et al. Breath-actuated inhalers in chronic asthma: comparison of Diskhaler and Turbohaler for delivery of beta-agonists. *Eur Respir J* 1992;5:1143–1145.

196. Newman SP, Weisz AWB, Talaee N, et al. Improvement of drug delivery with a breath activated pressurized aerosol for patients with poor inhaler technique. *Thorax* 1991;46:712–716.

197. Johnson M. The beta-adrenoceptor. *Am J Respir Crit Care Med* 1998;158(5 Pt 3):S146–153.

198. Verberne AA. An overview of nine clinical trials of salmeterol in an asthmatic population. *Respir Med* 1998;92(5):777–782.

199. Castle W, Fuller R, Hall J, et al. Screvent nationwide surveillance study: comparison of salmeterol with salbutamol in asthmatic patients who require regular bronchodilator treatment. *Br Med J* 1993;306:1034–1037.

200. Crompton GK, Ayres JG, Basran G, et al. Comparison of oral bambuterol and inhaled salmeterol in patients with symptomatic asthma and using inhaled corticosteroids. *Am J Respir Crit Care Med* 1999;159:824–828.

201. Greening AP, Ind PW, Northfield M, et al. Added salmeterol versus higher-dose corticosteroid in asthma patients with symp-

toms on existing inhaled corticosteroid. *Lancet* 1994;344: 219–224.

202. Woolcock A, Lundbash B, Ringdal OL, et al. Comparison of addition of salmeterol to inhaled steroids with doubling of the dose of inhaled steroids. *Am J Respir Crit Care Med* 1996;153: 1481–1488.

203. Verberne AA. Addition of salmeterol versus doubling the dose of beclomethasone in children with asthma. The Dutch Asthma Study Group. *Am J Respir Crit Care Med* 1998;158:213–219.

204. Leff JA, Busse WW, Pearlman D, et al. Montelukast, a leukotriene receptor antagonist, for the treatment of mild asthma and exercise bronchoconstriction. *N Engl J Med* 1998;339: 147–152.

205. Giannini D. Inhaled beclomethasone dipropionate reverts tolerance to the protective effect of salmeterol on allergen challenge. *Chest* 1999;115:629–634.

206. Boulet LP. Tolerance to the protective effects of salmeterol on methacholine-induced bronchoconstriction: influence of inhaled corticosteroids. *Eur Respir J* 1998;11:1091–1097.

207. January B. Salmeterol-induced desensitization, internalization and phosphorylation of the human β_2-adrenoceptor. *Br J Pharmacol* 1998;123:701–711.

208. Waldeck B. Enantiomers of bronchodilating β_2-adrenoceptor agonist: is there a cause for concern? *J Allergy Clin Immunol* 1999;103:742–748.

209. Levalbuterol for asthma. *Med Lett Drugs Ther* 1999;41(1054): 51–53.

210. Ramsey CM, Cowan JO, Flannery EM, et al. Broncho-protective and bronchodilator effects of single dose of the enantiomers of salbutamol [Abstract]. *Eur Respir J* 1998;12[Suppl 28]:324S.

211. Nicklas RA. Paradoxical bronchospasm associated with the use of inhaled beta-agonist. *J Allergy Clin Immunol* 1990;85: 959–964.

212. Galant SP, Durisetti L, Underwood S, et al. Decreased β-adrenergic receptors on polymorphonuclear leukocytes after adrenergic therapy. *N Engl J Med* 1978;299:933–936.

213. Cheung D, Timmers MC, Zwinderman AH, et al. Long-term effects of a long-acting β_2-adrenoceptor agonist, salmeterol, on airway hyperresponsiveness in patients with mild asthma. *N Engl J Med* 1992;327:1198–1203.

214. Pearlman DS, Chervinsky P, LaForce C, et al. A comparison of salmeterol with albuterol in the treatment of mild-to-moderate asthma. *N Engl J Med* 1992;327:1420–1425.

215. van Schayck CP, Graafsma SJ, Visch MB, et al. Increased bronchial hyperresponsiveness after inhaling salbutamol during one year is not caused by subsensitization to salbutamol. *J Allergy Clin Immunol* 1990;86:793–800.

216. O'Callaghan C, Milner AD, Swarbrick A. Paradoxical deterioration in lung function after nebulized salbutamol in wheezy infants. *Lancet* 1986;2:1424–1425.

217. Beasley R, Rafferty P, Holgate S. Paradoxical response to nebulized salbutamol in wheezy infants [Letter]. *Thorax* 1987;42: 702.

218. Zhang G, Wright WJ, Tam WK, et al. Effect of inhaled preservatives on asthmatic subjects: benzalkonium chloride. *Am Rev Respir Dis* 1990;141:1405–1408.

219. Koepke JW, Selner JC, Dunhill AL. Presence of sulfur dioxide in commonly used bronchodilator solutions. *J Allergy Clin Immunol* 1983;72:504–508.

220. Koepke JW, Christopher KL, Chai H, et al. Dose-dependent bronchospasm from sulfites in isoetharine. *JAMA* 1983;251: 2982–2983.

221. Finnerty JP, Howarth PH. Paradoxical bronchoconstriction with nebulized albuterol but not with terbutaline. *Am Rev Respir Dis* 1993;148:512–513.

222. Rossing TH. Methylxanthines in 1989. *Ann Intern Med* 1989; 110:502–504.

223. Lunell E, Andersson KE, Persson CG, et al. Intravenous enprofylline in asthma patients. *Eur J Respir Dis* 1984;65:28–34.

224. Bukowskyj M, Nakatsu K, Munt PW. Theophylline reassessed. *Ann Intern Med* 1984;101:63–73.

225. Aubier M, DeTroyer A, Sampson M, et al. Aminophylline improves diaphragm contractility. *N Engl J Med* 1981;305: 242–252.

226. Murciano D, Aubier M, Lecocguic Y, et al. Effects of theophylline on diaphragmatic strength and fatigue in patients with chronic obstructive pulmonary disease. *N Engl J Med* 1984;311: 349–353.

227. Matthay RA, Berger HJ, Loke J, et al. Effects of aminophylline upon right and left ventricular performances in chronic obstructive pulmonary disease: non-invasive assessment by radionuclide angiocardiography. *Am J Med* 1978;65:903–910.

228. Matthay RA, Berger HJ, Davis R, et al. Improvement in cardiac performance by oral long-acting theophylline in chronic obstructive pulmonary disease. *Am Heart J* 1982;104:1022–1026.

229. Lakshminarayan S, Sahn SA, Weil JV. The effect of aminophylline on ventilatory responses in normal man. *Am Rev Respir Dis* 1978;117:33–38.

230. Mahler D, Matthay RA, Snyder PE, et al. Sustained-release theophylline reduces dyspnea in nonreversible obstructive airway disease. *Am Rev Respir Dis* 1985;131:22–25.

231. Ward AJ, McKenniff M, Evans JM, et al. Theophylline: an immunomodulatory role in asthma? *Am Rev Respir Dis* 1993; 147:518–523.

232. Shim C, Williams MH Jr. Comparison of oral aminophylline and salbutamol in asthma: an in vivo study using dose-response curves. *J Int Med Res* 1979;7[Suppl 1]:52.

233. Smith JA, Weber RW, Nelson HS. Theophylline and aerosolized terbutaline in the treatment of bronchial asthma: double-blind comparison of optimal doses. *Chest* 1980;78:816–818.

234. Wolfe JD, Tashkin CP, Calvarese B, et al. Bronchodilator effects of terbutaline and aminophylline alone and in combination of asthmatic patients. *N Engl J Med* 1978;298:363–367.

235. Nassif EG, Weinberger M, Thompson R, et al. The value of maintenance theophylline in steroid-dependent asthma. *N Engl J Med* 1981;304:71–75.

236. Barnes PJ, Greening AP, Neville L, et al. Single-dose slow-release aminophylline at night prevents nocturnal asthma. *Lancet* 1982;1:299–301.

237. Arkinstall WW, Atkins ME, Harison D, et al. Once-daily sustained-release theophylline reduces diurnal variation in spirometry and symptomatology in adult asthmatics. *Am Rev Respir Dis* 1987;135:316–321.

238. Tilles DS, Hales CA. Comparison of 12-hour and 24-hour sustained-release theophylline in outpatient management of asthma. *Chest* 1987;91:370–375.

239. Mangura BT, Maniatis T, Abdel Rahman MS, et al. Bioavailability of a once daily-administered theophylline preparation: a comparison study. *Chest* 1986;90:566–570.

240. Helm SG. Diurnal stabilization of asthma with once-daily evening administration of controlled-release theophylline: a multi-investigator study. *Immunol Allergy Pract* 1987;9(11):414–419.

241. Schiff GD, Hegde HK, LaCloche L, et al. Inpatient theophylline toxicity: preventable factors. *Ann Intern Med* 1991;114: 748–753.

242. Zwillich CW, Sutton FD, Neff TA, et al. Theophylline-induced seizures in adults: correlation with serum concentrations. *Ann Intern Med* 1975;82:784–787.

243. Hendeles L, Bighley L, Richardson RH, et al. Frequent toxicity from IV aminophylline infusions in critically ill patients. *Drug Intell Clin Pharm* 1977;11:12–18.

244. Dutt AK, DeSoyza ND, Au WY, et al. The effect of aminophylline on cardiac rhythm in advanced chronic obstructive pulmonary disease: correlation with serum theophylline levels. *Eur J Respir Dis* 1983;64:264–270.

245. Banner AS, Sunderrajan EV, Agarwal MK, et al. Arrhythmogenic effects of orally administered bronchodilators. *Arch Intern Med* 1979;139:434–437.

246. Fleetham JA, Ginsburg JC, Nakatsu K, et al. Resin hemoperfusion as treatment for theophylline-induced seizures. *Chest* 1979; 75:741–742.

247. Berlinger WG, Spector R, Goldberg MJ, et al. Enhancement of theophylline clearance by oral activated charcoal. *Clin Pharmacol Ther* 1983;33:351–354.

248. Shannon M. Predictors of major toxicity after theophylline overdose. *Ann Intern Med* 1993;119:1161–1167.

249. Mann JS, Geroge CF. Anticholinergic drugs in the treatment of airways disease. *Br J Dis Chest* 1985;79:209–228.

250. Yeates DB, Aspin N, Levison H, et al. Mucociliary tracheal transport rates in man. *J Appl Physiol* 1975;39:487–495.

251. Pavia D, Bateman JRM, Sheahan NF, et al. Effects of ipratropium bromide on mucociliary clearance and pulmonary function in reversible airways obstruction. *Thorax* 1979;34:501–507.

252. Johns KA, Buse WW. Anticholinergic drugs: what role in asthma? *J Respir Dis* 1989;10:35–50.

253. Schleuter DP, Neumann JL. Double blind comparison of bronchial and ventilation perfusion changes to Atrovent and isoproterenol. *Chest* 1978;73:982–983.

254. Grandordy B, Thomas V, Marsac J. Compared bronchodilation after inhaled salbutamol and ipratropium bromide in asthma (abstract). *Am Rev Respir Dis* 1984;129[Part 2]:A91.

255. Jindal SR, Malif SR. Clinical experience with terbutaline sulfate and ipratropium bromide in bronchial asthma. *Indian J Chest Dis Allied Sci* 1979;21:130–133.

256. Storms WW, Bodman SF, Nathan RA, et al. Use of ipratropium bromide in asthma: results of a multi-clinic study. *Am J Med* 1986;81[Suppl 5A]:61–66.

257. Bruderman I, Cohen-Aronovski R, Smorzik J. A comparative study of various combinations of ipratropium bromide and metaproterenol in allergic asthmatic pateints. *Chest* 1983;83: 208–210.

258. Ruffin RE, McIntyre E, Crockett AJ, et al. Combination bronchodilator therapy in asthma. *J Allergy Clinic Immunol* 1982; 69:60–65.

259. McFadden ER Jr, Luparello T, Lyons H, et al. The mechanism of action of suggestion in the induction of acute asthma attacks. *Psychosom Med* 1969;31:134–143.

260. Neild JE, Cameron IR. Bronchoconstriction in response to suggestion: its prevention by an inhaled anticholinergic agent. *Br Med J* 1985;290:674.

261. Rebuck AS, Gent M, Chapman KR. Anticholinergic and sympathomimetic combination therapy of asthma. *J Allergy Clin Immunol* 1983;71:317–323.

262. Dunlap NE, Fulmer JD. Corticosteroid therapy in emphysema. *Clin Chest Med* 1984;5:669–683.

263. Morris HG. Pharmacology of corticosteroids in asthma. In: Middelton E, Reed CE, Ellis EF, eds. *Allergy: principles and practice.* St. Louis: CV Mosby, 1978.

264. Corticosteroids: their biologic mechanisms and application to the treatment of asthma. *Am Rev Respir Dis* 1990;141[Suppl]: 1–96.

265. Barnes PJ, Pederson S. Efficacy and safety of inhaled corticosteroids in asthma. *Am Rev Respir Dis* 1993;148:S1–S26.

266. Robinson D, Hamid Q, Ying S, et al. Prednisolone treatment in asthma is associated with modulation of bronchoalveolar lavage cell interlukin-4, interleukin-5, and interferon-γ cytokine expression. *Am Rev Respir Dis* 1993;148:401–406.

267. Laitinen LA, Laitinen A, Haahtela T. A comparative study of the effects of inhaled corticosteroid, budesonide, and a β_2-agonist, terbutaline on the airway inflammation in newly diagnosed asthma: a randomized double-blind, parallel-group controlled trial. *J Allergy Clin Immunol* 1992;90:32–42.

268. Djukanovic R, Wilson JW, Britten YM, et al. Effect of an inhaled corticosteroid on airway inflammation and symptoms of asthma. *Am Rev Respir Dis* 1992;145:699.

269. Jeffery PK, Godfrey RW, Adelroth E, et al. Effect of treatment on airway inflammation and thickening of basement membrane reticular collagen in asthma. *Am Rev Respir Dis* 1992;145: 890–899.

270. Lungren R, Soderberg M, Horstedt P, et al. Morphological studies on bronchial mucosal biopsies from asthmatics before and after ten years treatment with inhaled steroids. *Eur Respir J* 1988;1:883–889.

271. Wenzel SE, Szefler SJ, Leung DYM, et al. Bronchoscopic evaluation of severe asthma. Persistent inflammation associated with high-dose glucocorticoids. *Am J Respir Crit Care Med* 1997; 156:737–743.

272. Juniper EF, Kline AP, van Zieleshem MA, et al. Effect of long-term treatment with an inhaled corticosteroid (Budesonide) on airway hypcrresponsiveness and clinical asthma in non-steroid dependent asthmatics. *Am Rev Respir Dis* 1990;142:832–836.

273. Juniper EF, Kline PA, van Zieleshem MA, et al. Long-term effects of budesonide on airway responsiveness and clinical asthma severity in inhaled steroid-dependent asthmatics. *Eur Respir J* 1990;3:122–127.

274. Li JTC, Reed CE. Proper use of aerosol corticosteroids to control asthma. *Mayo Clin Proc* 1989;64:205–210.

275. Gedes DM. Inhaled corticosteroids: benefits and risks. *Thorax* 1992;47:404–407.

276. Haahtela T, Jarvinen M, Kava T, et al. Comparison of a β-agonist, terbutaline, with an inhaled corticosteroid, budesonide, in newly detected asthma. *N Engl J Med* 1991;325:388–392.

277. Kertjens HAM, Brand PLP, Hughes MD, et al. A comparison of bronchodilator therapy with or without inhaled corticosteroid therapy for obstructive airways disease. *N Engl J Med* 1992;327: 1413–1419.

278. Dompeling E, van Schayck CP, van Grunsven PM, et al. Slowing the deterioration of asthma and chronic obstructive pulmonary disease observed during bronchodilator therapy by adding inhaled corticosteroids. *Ann Intern Med* 1993;188:770–778.

279. Meltzer EO, Kemp JP, Orgel A, et al. Flunisolide aerosol for treatment of severe, chronic asthma in steroid-independent children. *Pediatrics* 1982;69:340–345.

280. Smith MJ, Hodson ME. High-dose beclomethasone inhaler in the treatment of asthma. *Lancet* 1983;1:265–269.

281. Toogood JH. High-dose inhaled steroid therapy for asthma. *J Allergy Clin Immunol* 1989;83:528–536.

282. Laursen LC, Taudorf E, Weeke B. High-dose inhaled budesonide in treatment of severe steroid-dependent asthma. *Eur J Respir Dis* 1986;68:19–28.

283. Tarlo SM, Broder I, Davies GM, et al. Six-month double-blind controlled trial of high dose, concentrated beclomethasone dipropionate in the treatment of severe chronic asthma. *Chest* 1988;93:998–1002.

284. Noonan M, Chervinsky P, Busse WW, et al. Fluticasone propionate reduces oral prednisone use while it improves asthma control and quality of life. *Am J Respir Crit Care Med* 1995; 152:1467–1473.

285. Pauwels RA, Lofdahl CG, Postma DS, et al. Effect of inhaled formoterol and budesonide on exacerbations of asthma. *N Engl J Med* 1997;337:1407–1411.

286. Lipworth BJ. Clinical pharmacology of corticosteroids in bronchial asthma. *Pharmacol Ther* 1993;58:173–209.

287. McFadden ER, Casale TB, Edwards TB, et al. Administration of budesonide once daily by means of turbuhaler to subjects with stable asthma. *J Allergy Clin Immunol* 1999;104:46–52.

288. Chisholm SL, Dekker FW, Knuistingh NA, et al. Once-daily budesonide in mild asthma. *Respir Med* 1998;92:421–425.

289. Weiner P, Weiner M, Azgad Y. Long-term clinical comparison of single versus twice daily administration of inhaled budesonide in moderate asthma. *Thorax* 1995;50:1270–1273.

290. Blais L, Ernest P, Boivin JF, et al. Inhaled corticosteroids and prevention of readmission to the hospital for asthma. *Am J Respir Crit Care Med* 1998;158:126–132.

291. Evans DJ, Taylor DA, Zetterstrom O, et al. A comparison of low-dose inhaled budesonide plus theophylline and high-dose inhaled budesonide for moderate asthma. *N Engl J Med* 1997;337:1412–1418.

292. Onrust SV, Lamb HM. Mometasone furoate: a review of its intranasal use in allergic rhinitis. *Drugs* 1998;56(4):725–745.

293. Toogood JH. Complications of topical steroid therapy for asthma. *Am Rev Respir Dis* 1990;141:S89–S96.

294. Lipworth BJ. Systemic adverse effects of inhaled corticosteroid therapy; a systemic review and meta-analysis. *Arch Intern Med* 1999;159:941–955.

295. Breslin ABX. New developments in anti-asthma drugs. *Med J Aust* 1993;158:779–782.

296. Newman SP, Moren F, Pavia D, et al. Deposition of pressurized suspension aerosols inhaled through extension devices. *Am Rev Respir Dis* 1981;124:317–320.

297. Allen DB, Mullen M, Mullen B. A meta-analysis of the effect of oral and inhaled corticosteroids on growth. *J Allergy Clin Immunol* 1994;93:967–976.

298. Silverstein MD, Yunginger JW, Reed CE, et al. Attained adult height after childhood asthma; effect of glucocorticoid therapy. *J Allergy Clin Immunol* 1997;99:466–474.

299. Luengo M, Picado C, Del Rio L, et al. Vertebral fractures in steroid dependent asthma and involutional osteoporosis: a comparative study. *Thorax* 1991;46:803–806.

300. Allen MB, Ray SG, Leitch AG, et al. Steroid aerosols and cataract formation. *Br Med J* 1989;299:432–433.

301. Patalano F, Ruggieri F. Sodium cromoglycate: a review. *Eur Respir J* 1989;2:556S–560S.

302. Kuzemko JA. Twenty years of sodium cromoglycate treatment: a short review. *Respir Med* 1989;83[Suppl]:11–16.

303. Murphy S, Kelly HW. Cromolyn sodium: a review of mechanisms and clinical use in asthma. *Drug Intell Clin Pharm* 1987;21:22–35.

304. Toogood JH, Jennings B, Lefcol NM. A clinical trial of combined cromolyn/beclomethasone treatment for chronic asthma. *J Pediatr* 1981;67:317–324.

305. Edwards AM, Stevens MT. The clinical efficacy of inhaled nedocromil sodium (Tilade) in the treatment of asthma. *Eur Respir J* 1993;6:35–41.

306. Callaghan B, Teo NC, Clancy L. Effects of the addition of nedocromil sodium to maintenance bronchodilator therapy in the management of chronic asthma. *Chest* 1992;101:787–792.

307. North American Tilade Study Group. A double-blind multicenter group comparative study of the efficacy and safety of nedocromil sodium in the management of asthma. *Chest* 1990;97:1299–1306.

308. De Jong JW, Deengs JP, Postma DS, et al. Nedocromil sodium versus albuterol in the management of allergic asthma. *Am J Respir Crit Care Med* 1994;149:91–97.

309. Geddes DM, Turner-Warwick M, Brewis RAL, et al. Nedocromil sodium workshop. *Respir Med* 1989;83:265–267.

310. O'Bryne RM. Is nedocromil sodium effective treatment for asthma? [Editorial] *Eur Respir J* 1993;6:5–6.

311. Bel EH, Timmers MC, Hermans J, et al. The long term effects of nedocromil sodium and beclomethasone dipropionate on bronchial responsiveness to methacholine in non-atopic asthmatic subjects. *Am Rev Respir Dis* 1990;141:21–28.

312. Svendsen UG, Jorgensen H. Inhaled nedocromil sodium as additional treatment to high dose inhaled corticosteroids in the management of bronchial asthma. *Eur Respir J* 1991;4:992–999.

313. Wong CS, Cooper S, Britton JR, et al. Steroid sparing effect of nedocromil sodium in asthmatic patients taking high dose of inhaled steroids. *Thorax* 1991;46:768–769.

314. Kemp JP. Approaches to asthma management. *Arch Intern Med* 1993;153:805–828.

315. Drazen JM, Israel E, O'Bryne PM. Treatment of asthma with drugs modifying the leukotriene pathway. *N Engl J Med* 1999;340:197–206.

316. Lipworth BJ. The emerging role of leukotriene antagonists in asthma therapy. *Chest* 1999;115:313–316.

317. Pearlman DS, Ostrom NK, Bronsky EA, et al. The leukotriene D$_4$ receptor antagonist zafirlukast attenuates exercise-induced bronchoconstriction in children. *J Pediatr* 1999;134:273–279.

318. Israel E, Rubin P, Kemp JB, et al. The effect of inhibition of 5-lipoxygenase by zileuton in mild-to-moderate asthma. *Ann Intern Med* 1993;119:1059–1066.

319. Lofdahl C, Reiss TF, Leff JA, et al. Randomized, placebo controlled trial of the effect of leukotriene receptor antagonist, montelukast, on tapering inhaled corticosteroids in asthmatic patients. *Br Med J* 1999;319:87–90.

320. Malmstrom K, Rodriguez-Gomez G, Guerra J, et al. Oral montelukast, inhaled beclomethasone and placebo for chronic asthma: a randomized controlled trial. *Ann Intern Med* 1999;130:487–495.

321. Kemp JP, Minkwitz MC, Bonuccelli CM, et al. Therapeutic effects of zafirlukast as monotherapy in steroid-naïve patients with severe persistent asthma. *Chest* 1999;115:336–342.

322. Lipworth BJ. Systemic adverse effects of inhaled salmeterol and oral zafirlukast in patients with asthma. *J Allergy Clin Immunol* 1999;103:1075–1080.

323. Knorr B, Matz J, Bernstein JA, et al. Montelukast for chronic asthma in 6- to 14-years old children. The Pediatric Montelukast Study Group. *JAMA* 1998;3279:1181–1186.

324. Busse W, Nelson H, Wolfe J, et al. Comparison of inhaled salmeterol and oral zafirlukast in patients with asthma. *J Allergy Clin Immunol* 1999;103:1075–1080.

325. Suissa S, Dennis R, Ernst P, et al. Effectiveness of the leukotriene receptor antagonist zafirlukast for mild-to-moderate asthma: a randomized double-blind placebo-controlled trial. *Ann Intern Med* 1997;126:177–183.

326. Wechsler ME, Garperstad E, Flier SR, et al. Pulmonary infiltrates, eosinophilia and cardiomyopathy following corticosteroid withdrawl in patients with asthma receiving zafirlukast. *JAMA* 1998;279:455–457.

327. Franco J, Artes MJ. Pulmonary eosinophilia associated with montelukast. *Thorax* 1999;54:558–560.

328. In KH, Asan K, Baeier D, et al. Naturally occurring mutations in the hum S-lipoxygenase gene promoter that modify transcription. *J Clin Invest* 1997;99:1130–1137.

329. Schwartz HJ, Petty T, Dube LM, et al. A randomized controlled trial comparing zileuton with theophylline in moderate asthma. *Arch Intern Med* 1998;158:141–148.

330. Emerman CL, Woodruff PG, Cydulka RK, et al. Prospective multicenter study of relapse following treatment for acute asthma among adults presenting to the emergency department. MARC investigators. Multicenter Asthma Research Collaboration. *Chest* 1999;115:919–927.

331. Braman SS, Kaemmerlen JT. Intensive care of status asthmaticus. A 10-year experience. *JAMA* 1990;264:366–368.

332. Brenner BE. The acute asthmatic in the emergency department: the decision to admit or discharge. *Am J Emerg Med* 1985;3: 74–77.

333. Corbridge TC, Hall JB. The assessment and management of adults with status asthmaticus. *Am J Respir Crit Care Med* 1995; 151:1296–1316.

334. Reed CE, Hung LW. The emergency visit and management of asthma. *Ann Intern Med* 1990;112:801–802.

335. Kavuru MS. Beta-agonist for acute asthma: which way to deliver? *J Respir Dis* 1994;15:312–314.

336. Moler FW, Hurquitz ME, Custer JR. Improvement in clinical asthma score and PacO$_2$ in children with severe asthma treated with continuously nebulized terbutaline. *J Allergy Clin Immunol* 1998;81:1101–1109.

337. Chipps BE, Blackney DA, Black LE, et al. Vortran high output extended aerosol respiratory therapy (HEART) for delivery of continuously nebulized terbutaline for the treatment of acute bronchospasm. *Pediatr Allergy Immunol* 1990;4(4):271–277.

338. Colacone A, Wolkove N, Stern E et al. Continuous nebulization of albuterol (salbutamol) in acute asthma. *Chest* 1990;97: 693–697.

339. Olshaker J, Jerrard D, Barish RA, et al. The efficacy and safety of a continuous albuterol protocol for the treatment of acute adult asthma attacks. *Am J Emerg Med* 1993;11:131–133.

340. Lin RY, Smith AJ, Hergenroder P. High serum albuterol levels and tachycardia in adult asthmatics treated with high-dose continuously aerosolized albuterol. *Chest* 1993;103:221–225.

341. Portnoy J, Nadel G, Amado M, et al. Continuous nebulization for status asthmaticus. *Ann Allergy* 1992;69:71–79.

342. Shim C. Adrenergic agonist and bronchodilator aerosol therapy in asthma. *Clin Chest Med* 1984;5:659–668.

343. Amory DW, Burham SC, Cheney FW Jr. Comparison of the cardiopulmonary effects of subcutaneously administered epinephrine and terbutaline in patients with reversible airway obstruction. *Chest* 1975;67:279–286.

344. Jederlinic RJ, Irwin RS. Status asthmaticus. *Intensive Care Med* 1989;4:166–184.

345. Parry WH, Martorano F, Colton EK. Management of life-threatening asthma with intravenous isoproterenol infusion. *Am J Dis Child* 1976;130:39–42.

346. Lawford P, Jones BJM, Milledge JS. Comparison of intravenous and nebulized salbutamol in initial treatment of severe asthma. *Br Med J* 1978;1:84.

347. Williams S, Seaton A. Intravenous or inhaled salbutamol in severe acute asthma? *Thorax* 1977;32:555–558.

348. Lam A, Newhouse MT. Management of asthma and chronic airflow limitation: are methylxanthines obsolete? *Chest* 1990; 98:44–52.

349. Milgrom H, Bender B. Current issues in the use of theophylline. *Am Rev Respir Dis* 1993;147:533–539.

350. British Thoracic Society. Guidelines for management of asthma in adults. *Br Med J* 1990;301:651–653.

351. Rossing TH, Fanta CH, Goldstein DH, et al. Emergency therapy of asthma: comparison of the acute effects of parenteral and inhaled sympathomimetics and infused aminophylline. *Am Rev Respir Dis* 1980;122:365–371.

352. Siegel D, Sheppard D, Gelb A, et al. Aminophylline increases the toxicity but not the efficacy of an inhaled β-adrenergic agonist in the treatment of acute exacerbations of asthma. *Am Rev Respir Dis* 1985;132:283–286.

353. Fanta CH, Rossing TH, McFadden ER Jr. Treatment of acute asthma—is combination therapy with sympathomimetics and methylxanthines indicated? *Am J Med* 1986;80:5–10.

354. Littenberg, B. Aminophylline treatment in severe, acute asthma: a meta-analysis. *JAMA* 1988;259:1678–1684.

355. Self TH, Abou-Shala N, Burns R, et al. Inhaler albuterol and oral prednisone theapy in hospitalized adult asthmatics. Does aminophylline add any benefit? *Chest* 1990;98:1317–1321.

356. Wrenn K, Solvis CM, Murphy F, et al. Aminophylline therapy for acute bronchospastic disease in the emergency room. *Ann Intern Med* 1991;115:241–247.

357. McFadden ER. Methylxanthines in treatment of asthma: the rise, the fall, and the possible rise again [Editorial]. *Ann Intern Med* 1991;115:323–324.

358. Huang D, O'Brien RG, Harman E, et al. Does aminophylline benefit adults admitted to the hospital for an acute exacerbation of asthma? *Ann Intern Med* 1993;119:1155–1160.

359. DiGiulio GA, Kercsmar CM, Krug SE, et al. Hospital treatment of asthma: lack of benefit from theophylline given in addition to nebulized albuterol and intravenously administered corticosteroid. *J Pediatr* 1993;122:470–476.

360. Carter E, Cruz M, Chesrown S, et al. Efficacy of intravenously administered theophylline in children hospitalized with severe asthma. *J Pediatr* 1993;122:470–476.

361. Karpel JP, Appel D, Briedbart D, et al. A comparison of atropine sulfate and metaproterenol sulfate in the emergency treatment of asthma. *Am Rev Respir Dis* 1986;133:727–729.

362. McFadden ER Jr, Elsanadi N, Strauss L, et al. The influence of parasympatholytic on the resolution of acute attacks of asthma. *Am J Med* 1997;102:7–13.

363. Qureshi F, Prestian J, Davis P, et al. Effect of nebulized ipratropium on the hospitalization rates for children with asthma. *N Engl J Med* 1998;339:1030–1035.

364. Bryant DH. Nebulized ipratropium bromide in the treatment of acute asthma. *Chest* 1985;88:24–29.

365. Ward MJ, McFarlane JT, Davies D, et al. A place for ipratropium bromide in the treatment of severe acute asthma. *Br J Dis Chest* 1985;79:374.

366. Lanes SF, Garrett JE, Wentworth CE, et al. The effect of adding ipratropium bromide to salbutamol in the treatment of acute asthma: a pooled analysis of three trials. *Chest* 1998;114: 365–372.

367. Rebuck As, Chapman KR, Abboud R, et al. Nebulized anticholinergic and sympathomimetic treatment of asthma and chronic obstructive airways disease in the emergency room. *Am J Med* 1987;82:59–64.

368. Weber EJ, Levitt MA, Covington JK, et al. Effect of continuously nebulized ipratropium bromide plus albuterol on emergency department length of stay and hospital admission rates in patients with acute bronchospasm: a randomized, controlled trial. *Chest* 1999;115:937–944.

369. McFadden ER. Dosages of corticosteroids in asthma. *Am Rev Respir Dis* 1993;147:1306–1310.

370. Fanta CH, Rossing TH, McFadden ER. Glucocorticoid in acute asthma: a critical controlled trial. *Am J Med* 1983;74:845–851.

371. Littenberg B, Gluck EH. A controlled trial of methylprednisolone in the emergency treatment of acute asthma. *N Engl J Med* 1986;314:150–152.

372. Stein LM, Cole RP. Early administration of corticosteroids in emergency room treatment of acute asthma. *Ann Intern Med* 1990;112:822–827.

373. McFadden ER, Kiser R, deGroot WJ, et al. A controlled study of the effects of single doses of hydrocortisone on the resolution of acute attacks of asthma. *Am J Med* 1976;60:52–59.

374. Ogirala RG, Aldrich TK, Prezant DF, et al. High-dose intramuscular triamcinolone in severe, chronic life-threatening asthma. *N Engl J Med* 1991;324:585–589.

375. Haskell RJ, Wong BM, Hansen JE. A double-blind, randomized clinical trial of methylprednisolone in status asthmaticus. *Arch Intern Med* 1983;143:1324–1327.

376. Lederle FA, Pluhar RE, Joseph AM, et al. Tapering of corticosteroid therapy following exacerbations of asthma. *Arch Intern Med* 1987;147:2201–2203.

377. Cydulka RK, Emerman CL. A pilot study of steroid therapy after emergency department treatment of acute asthma: is a taper needed? *J Emerg Med* 1998;16:15–19.

378. Vichyanond P, Irvin CG, Larsen GL, et al. Penetration of corticosteroids into the lung: evidence for a difference between methylprednisolone and prednisolone. *J Allergy Clin Immunol* 1989; 84:867–873.

379. Greos LS, Vichyanond P, Bloedow DC, et al. Methylprednisolone achieves greater concentrations in the lung than prednisolone. *Am Rev Respir Dis* 1991;144:586–592.

380. Aelony Y. Non-invasive oral treatment of asthma in the emergency room. *Am J Med* 1985;78:929–936.

381. McFadden ER Jr, Elsanadi N, Dixon L, et al. Protocol therapy for acute asthma: therapeutic benefits and cost savings. *Am J Med* 1995;99:651–661.

382. Manthous CA. Management of severe exacerbations of asthma. *Am J Med* 1995;99:298–308.

383. Tiffany R, Berk WA, Todd K, et al. Magnesium bolus or infusion fails to improve expiratory flow in acute asthma exacerbations. *Chest* 1993;104:831–834

384. Green SM, Rothrock SG. Intravenous magnesium for acute asthma: failure to decrease emergency treatment duration or need for hospitalization. *Ann Emerg Med* 1992;21:260–265.

385. Gluck EH, Onorato DJ, Castriotta R. Helium-oxygen mixtures in intubated patients with status asthmaticus and respiratory acidosis. *Chest* 1990;98:693–698.

386. Kudukis TM, Manthous CA, Schmidt GA, et al. Inhaled helium-oxygen revisited: effect of inhaled helium-oxygen during the treatment of status asthmaticus in children. *J Pediatr* 1997; 130:217–224.

387. Shivaram U, Miro AM, Cash ME, et al. Cardiopulmonary responses to continuous positive airway pressure in acute asthma. *J Crit Care* 1993;8:87–92.

388. Howton JC, Rose J, Duffy S, et al. Randomized, double-blind, placebo-controlled trial of intravenous ketamine in acute asthma. *Ann Emerg Med* 1996;27:170–175.

389. Marquette CH, Saulnier F, Leroy O, et al. Long-term prognosis of near-fatal asthma. A 6-year follow-up study of 145 asthmatic patients who underwent mechanical ventilation for a near-fatal attack of asthma. *Am Rev Respir Dis* 1992;146:76–81.

390. Tuxen DV. Detrimental effects of positive end-expiratory pressure during controlled mechanical ventilation of patients with severe airflow obstruction. *Am Rev Respir Dis* 1989;140:5–9.

391. Segredo V, Caldwell JE, Matthay MA, et al. Persistent paralysis in critically ill patients after long-term administration of vecuronium. *N Engl J Med* 1992;327:524–528.

392. Schwartz SH. Treatment of status asthmaticus with halothane. *JAMA* 1984;251:2688–2689.

393. Roy TM, Pruitt VL, Garner PA, et al. The potential role of anesthesia in status asthmaticus. *J Asthma* 1992;29:73–77.

394. Mullarkey MF, Blumenstein BA, Andrade WP, et al. Methotrexate in the treatment of corticosteroid dependent asthma. A double-blind crossover study. *N Engl J Med* 1988;318: 603–606.

395. Erzurum SC, Leff JA, Cochran JE, et al. Lack of benefit of methotrexate in severe steroid dependent asthma. *Ann Intern Med* 1991;114:353–360.

396. Carmichael J, Paterson IC, Diaz P, et al. Corticosteroid resistance in chronic asthma. *Br Med J* 1981;282:1419–1422.

397. Dykewicz MS, Greenberger PA, Patterson R, et al. Natural history of asthma in patients requiring long-term systemic corticosteroids. *Arch Intern Med* 1986;146:2369–2372.

398. Corrigan CJ, Brown PH, Barnes NC, et al. Glucocorticoid resistance in chronic asthma. *Am Rev Respir Dis* 1991;144: 1016–1032.

399. NIH Conference. Syndromes of glucocorticoid resistance. Moderator: Chrousos GP. *Ann Intern Med* 1994;119:1113–1124.

400. Lane DJ, Lane TV. Alternative and complementary medicine for asthma. *Thorax* 1991;46:787–797.

401. Schwartz YA, Kinity S, Ilfeld DN, et al. A Clinical and immunologic study of colchicine in asthma. *J Allergy Clin Immunol* 1990; 85:578–582.

402. Mazer BD, Gelfand EW. An open-label study of high-dose intravenous immunoglobulin in severe childhood asthma. *J Allergy Clin Immunol* 1991;87:976–983.

403. Mullarkey MF, Lammert JK, Blumenstein BA. Long-term methotrexate treatment in steroid dependent asthma. *Ann Intern Med* 1990;112:577–581.

404. Dyer P, Vaughan T, Weber R. Methotrexate in the treatment of steroid–dependent asthma. *J Allergy Clin Immunol* 1991;88: 208–212.

405. Shiner RJ, Nunn AJ, Chung KF, et al. Randomised, double-blind, placebo controlled trial of methotrexate in steroid dependent asthma. *Lancet* 1990;336:137–140.

406. Coffey MJ, Sanders G, Eschenbacher WL, et al. the role of methotrexate in the management of steroid-dependent asthma. *Chest* 1994;105:117–121.

407. Marin MG. Low-dose methotrexate spares steroid usage in steroid-dependent asthmatic patients: a meta-analysis. *Chest* 1997; 112:29–32.

408. Bernstein DI, Bernstein IL, Bodenheimer SS, et al. An open study of auranofin in the treatment of steroid dependent asthma. *J Allergy Clin Immunol* 1988;81:6–16.

409. Nierop G, Gijzel WP, Bel EH, et al. Auranofin in the treatment of steroid dependent asthma; a double-blind study. *Thorax* 1992;47:349–354.

410. Muranaka M, Myamoto T, Shida T, et al. Gold salts in the treatment of bronchial asthma: a double-blind study. *Ann Allergy* 1978;40:132–137.

411. Klaustermyer WB, Noritake DT, Kwong FK. Chrysotherapy in the treatment of corticosteroid dependent asthma. *J Allergy Clin Immunol* 1987;79:720–725.

412. Bernstein IL, Bernstein DI, Dubb JW, et al. A placebo-controlled multicenter study of auranofin in the treatment of patients with corticosteroid-dependent asthma. Auranofin Multicenter Drug Trial. *J Allergy Clin Immunol* 1996;98:317–324.

413. Spector SL, Katz, FH, Farr RS. Troleandomycin: effectiveness in steroid dependent asthma. *J Allergy Clin Immunol* 1974;54: 367–379.

414. Szefler SJ, Rose JQ, Elliott EF, et al. The effect of troleandomycin on methylprednisolone elimination. *J Allergy Clin Immunol* 1980;66:447–451.

415. Zeiger RS, Schatz M, Sperling W, et al. Efficacy of troleandomycin in outpatients with severe, corticosteroid-dependent asthma. *J Allergy Clin Immunol* 1988;66:438–446.

416. Wald JA, Friedman BF, Farr RS. An improved protocol for the use of troleandomycin in the treatment of steroid requiring asthma. *J Allergy Clin Immunol* 1986;78:36–43.

417. Kamada AK, Hill MR, Ikhe DN, et al. Efficacy and safety of low-dose troleandomycin therapy in children with severe, steroid-requiring asthma. *J Allergy Clin Immunol* 1993;91: 873–882.

418. Nelson HS, Hamilos DL, Corsello PR, et al. A double-blind study of troleandomycin and methylprednisolone in asthmatic subjects who require daily corticosteroids. *Am Rev Respir Dis* 1993;147:398–404.

419. Calderon E, Lockey RF, Bukantz SC, et al. Is there a role for cyclosporine in asthma? *J Allergy Clin Immunol* 1992;89: 629–636.

420. Finnerty NA, Sullivan TJ. Effect of cyclosporine on corticosteroid-dependent asthma [Abstract]. *J Allergy Clin Immunol* 1991; 87:297.

421. Alexander AG, Barnes NC, Kay AB. Trial of cyclosporin in corticosteroid dependent chronic severe asthma. *Lancet* 1992; 339:324–327.

422. Lock SH, Kay AB, Barnes NC. Double-blind, placebo-controlled study of cyclosporin A as a corticosteroid-sparing agent in corticosteroid-dependent asthma. *Am J Respir Crit Care Med* 1996;153:509–519.

9

CHRONIC OBSTRUCTIVE PULMONARY DISEASE, BRONCHIECTASIS, AND CYSTIC FIBROSIS

RONALD B. GEORGE
GERARDO S. SAN PEDRO
JAMES K. STOLLER

INTRODUCTION

CHRONIC OBSTRUCTIVE PULMONARY DISEASE
Definitions
Epidemiology
Pathophysiology
Clinical Assessment of Chronic Obstructive Pulmonary
    Disease
Prevention
Therapy of Chronic Obstructive Pulmonary
    Disease
Pulmonary Rehabilitation
Oxygen Therapy

Management of Acute Exacerbations
Prognosis in Chronic Obstructive Pulmonary Disease

BRONCHIECTASIS
Clinical Presentation
Evaluation
Treatment

CYSTIC FIBROSIS
Clinical Manifestations
Diagnosis
Atypical or Difficult Cases
Treatment
Complications

Chronic obstructive pulmonary disease (COPD) refers to a collection of clinical and pathologic findings which, individually, or in combination, produce chronic airflow obstruction, disability, and, sometimes, death. The American Thoracic Society defines COPD as a disorder characterized by abnormal tests of expiratory flow (on a structural or functional basis), that do not change markedly over periods of several months' observation (1). The diagnosis usually refers to the presence of chronic obstructive bronchitis associated with varying degrees of emphysema and bronchospasm (asthmatic bronchitis), but excludes specific causes of airflow obstruction such as bronchiectasis or cystic fibrosis.

COPD and allied obstructive lung diseases (asthma, bronchiectasis, cystic fibrosis, and hypersensitivity pneumonitis) rank as the fourth leading cause of death in the United States (2). This chapter seeks to focus on the epidemiology, pathophysiology, natural history, prevention, and treatment of COPD, with a brief discussion of bronchiectasis and cystic fibrosis. Asthma and hypersensitivity pneumonitis are considered in detail elsewhere.

CHRONIC OBSTRUCTIVE LUNG DISEASE

Definitions

A patient with COPD may have one or more of the following common conditions: chronic bronchitis, emphysema, and/or asthmatic bronchitis.

Chronic Bronchitis

Chronic bronchitis is a clinical diagnosis based on the symptoms of chronic cough and sputum production. The American Thoracic Society defines chronic bronchitis as the persistence of cough and excessive mucus secretion on most days over a three-month period for at least two successive years (1). The definition omits any specific pathologic feature, though mucous gland hypertrophy is the closest pathologic correlate. The Reid index, the ratio of the width of the mucous glands to the thickness of the bronchial walls, may be used to gauge the degree of hypertrophy. The definition excludes other clinical conditions that may have chronic cough and sputum production (3); for example, lung cancer, tuberculosis, and chronic congestive heart failure.

The majority of chronic bronchitis patients do not have airflow obstruction and hence do not have COPD. However, about 10% to 15% of cigarette smokers are susceptible to a more rapid decline in airflow than normal (4); understanding why this subpopulation is susceptible to lung injury from tobacco use remains incomplete. Patients who have chronic productive cough and normal airflow are diagnosed as having *simple chronic bronchitis;* those who demonstrate a progressive abnormal decline in airflow have *chronic obstructive bronchitis.* The latter group constitutes the majority of patients with COPD (4).

Emphysema

In contrast to chronic bronchitis, the diagnosis of *emphysema* is based on pathologic criteria. The American Thoracic Society defines emphysema as air space enlargement distal to the terminal bronchiole and destruction of the alveolar wall; later refinements of the definition include the requirements that the air space enlargement is permanent and that fibrosis is not a feature (1). Various subtypes of emphysema are identified based upon the pattern of destruction within the acinus. These subtypes include *centrilobular* (proximal), *panacinar,* and *paraseptal* (distal) emphysema. The three patterns of emphysema have somewhat different etiologies and clinical presentations. Correlation of clinical patterns with pathologic changes is frequently inaccurate, and much overlap exists among the three types.

Centrilobular emphysema is the classic form associated with cigarette smoking. Frequently, it involves the lung apices and peripheral areas of the lungs. Marked hyperinflation and airflow obstruction are observed.

Panacinar emphysema more often involves the lower lung zones; it is the pattern associated with deficiency of α_1-antitrypsin.

Paraseptal emphysema (distal emphysema) involves the periphery of the acinus and is a cause of spontaneous pneumothorax in young adults. Since proximal portions of the acinus are spared in paraseptal emphysema, airflow obstruction may not be prominent.

Asthmatic Bronchitis

Marked reversibility of airway obstruction over relatively brief periods is the pathophysiologic hallmark separating asthma from COPD. However, some patients with otherwise typical chronic obstructive bronchitis who are smokers or ex-smokers have significant changes in airflow following bronchodilator administration. Data from the Intermittent Positive Pressure Breathing Trial show that some patients with COPD have responses to inhaled bronchodilators that are comparable to those seen in patients with asthma (5).

Ten percent of patients in this trial demonstrated an improvement in FEV_1 of 25% or more following inhalation of a β-adrenergic agent.

Little agreement exists on the precise definition of *asthmatic bronchitis,* although it is clear that emphysema and asthmatic bronchitis represent opposite ends of the clinical spectrum of COPD. Patients with emphysema have lower values for gas transfer in the lungs (D_LCO), exhibit more fixed obstruction, and respond less well to bronchodilator administration. Those with asthmatic bronchitis have more significant bronchospasm and little alteration in gas transfer. In addition, patients with asthmatic bronchitis may have wheezing on physical examination and increased numbers of eosinophils in the blood and sputum; the patient or family members may be atopic. Although the disease has not been defined by consensus, a reasonable working definition of asthmatic bronchitis is the presence of significant reversibility of airway obstruction (i.e., an increase in FEV_1 of 20% or more following bronchodilator administration) in a current or former cigarette smoker who has other symptoms of chronic obstructive bronchitis.

Epidemiology

COPD affects over 14 million people in the United States (6% of the total population); it is the second leading cause of disability (behind back pain), and the fourth most common cause of death in adults (1,2). It is responsible for over 14 million office visits per year and over 500,000 hospitalizations per year, and is the third most frequent justification for home care services (2,6). Data from the 1991 National Health Interview Survey (NHIS) suggest that chronic bronchitis is the most prevalent cause of COPD (12.5 million Americans), followed by emphysema (1.6 million) (7).

Chronic obstructive pulmonary disease accounted for approximately 102,000 deaths in 1994; the age-adjusted mortality rate was 21.4 per 100,000 persons, representing a 46.6% increase since 1979 (2,8). The increase in age-adjusted mortality from COPD stands in contrast to declining mortality trends from other leading causes of death, for example, heart and cerebrovascular disease (9). Death rates from COPD rise sharply with advancing age to a peak rate of 26.6 per 100,000 for chronic bronchitis and 60.8 per 100,000 for emphysema among Americans older than 85 years (7). From 1979 to 1993, the overall age adjusted mortality rate increased 47.3%; mortality for men increased 17.1% from 96.3 to 112.8 per 100,000 while that for women increased an alarming 126.1% from 24.5 to 55.4 per 100,000 (10,11).

The NHIS data further clarify the demographic and geographic patterns of COPD in the United States. Chronic bronchitis and asthma are fairly evenly distributed across all ages. In contrast, emphysema is a disease of the elderly, with 59.6% of all cases occurring in patients over 65 and 96.2% of all cases occurring in patients over 45. Approximately 4% to 6 % of men and 1% to 3% of women have COPD, with a greater frequency of chronic bronchitis in women and greater prevalence of emphysema in men (7). Racial differences between chronic bronchitis and emphysema are less striking, with age-specific increases in both blacks and whites. Overall, both diseases are more common among white than black persons. Geographic patterns of occurrence also differ for chronic bronchitis and emphysema. Chronic bronchitis has the greatest prevalence in the Midwest (55.8 cases per 1,000 Americans), followed by the Northeast (52.8 per 1,000), the South (48.2 per 1,000), and finally the West (46.0 per 1,000). Emphysema is least common in the West (4.8 per 1,000) and most common in the southern United States (7.9 per 1,000) (7).

In addition to the substantial mortality and morbidity impact of these diseases, the economic impact of COPD in the United States is striking. The total 1986 cost of all lung diseases collectively was $40.9 billion, with COPD (23.5%) second only to lung cancer (26.4%) as the largest component (12). From 1993 to 1994 the total number of hospital discharges for COPD increased from 504,477 to 511,064 individuals, or an increase of 1.4% (13,14). This represents 1.48% of all hospital discharges for 1994.

Pathophysiology

COPD is primarily a disease of cigarette smokers. Tobacco smoke has adverse effects on the central airways, small airways (i.e., terminal bronchioles and beyond), and lung parenchyma resulting in mucus gland hyperplasia, respiratory bronchiolitis, and emphysema, respectively. Any or all of these lesions are present in smokers even in the absence of dyspnea. In those individuals that develop COPD, symptoms typically arise in the fourth or fifth decade of life after a cumulative cigarette exposure of twenty pack-years or more. The predominant symptoms are cough, sputum production, and dyspnea (1,15).

Risk Factors

Risk factors for the development of COPD include cigarette smoking, α_1-antitrypsin deficiency, occupational dust exposure, air pollution, "secondhand" smoke, airway hyperresponsiveness, gender, and infections. The predominant risk is inhalation of tobacco smoke, although only 10% to 15% of regular smokers develop COPD (1).

Pathogenesis

Cigarette Smoking
The relationship between cigarette smoking and the development of COPD is firmly established. Epidemiological studies attribute 80% to 90% of the deaths from COPD to smoking (16). There is a dose-response relationship between cumulative cigarettes smoked and rate of lung function decline (17,18). Smoking cessation may lead to improved lung function and will certainly reduce the accelerated rate of reduction in lung function seen in smokers (17,19).

Overall, the percentage of smokers in the adult population in the United States has dropped from more than 50% to approximately 25% in the last 30 years; the drop has been particularly dramatic among males (20). Accordingly, morbidity and mortality from COPD may decline in the years ahead, reflecting these favorable trends in smoking practices. However, COPD will continue to be a significant problem well into the future—3,000 people, mostly teenagers, take up the habit of smoking daily. In fact, smoking appears to be increasing among teenagers (21).

Airway Hyperresponsiveness
As only a minority of cigarette smokers develops COPD, investigators have speculated on host factors that may predispose the airways to injury. The "Dutch hypothesis" (so-named for the Dutch investigators who first proposed it) postulates that an "asthmatic constitution," defined as atopy, eosinophilia, and airway hyperresponsiveness (AHR), is a basic component in the development of chronic lung disease (1). The resulting chronic narrowing of the airways over years leads to remodeling and fixed airflow obstruction.

Several longitudinal studies provide persuasive evidence linking AHR to an accelerated decline in lung function in cigarette smokers (22–27). The Lung Health Study (LHS), a multicenter intervention trial in adult smokers with early COPD, defined AHR as a more than 20% reduction of FEV_1 after inhalation of less than 25 mg/mL methacholine. Approximately 85% of women and 60% of men included in the survey fit the definition of AHR. The higher prevalence of AHR in women was ascribed to their reduced airway caliber compared with their male cohorts (28). In both groups, the degree of impairment (expressed as the percentage of predicted FEV_1 at baseline) was strongly associated with the presence of AHR (29). Moreover, AHR was a strong predictor of change in FEV_1 over time, independent of baseline lung function. The patients with greater methacholine reactivity at study onset experienced the steepest decline in lung function (26). A similar association between AHR and accelerated FEV_1 deterioration has been reported in older and more severely obstructed patients (25,27). In fact, AHR may more closely approximate lung function decline than the baseline FEV_1 (26). A relationship between AHR and baseline lung volumes had been previously observed in smaller studies involving both nonsmokers (30–32) and smokers (32,33).

Many criticisms have been leveled against these studies. Unfortunately, asthmatics have been included in many cross-sectional study populations, making a firm determination of the relationship between AHR and COPD a difficult one. In addition, the association between lung volumes (as a marker of airway caliber) and AHR may simply reflect geometric factors. A slight decrease in airway diameter significantly increases airway resistance (since resistance $\approx 1/$ radius[4]). Thus the same degree of bronchoconstriction causes a proportionately greater increase in airflow resistance in narrower airways. Moreover, edema, cellular infiltration, fibrosis, smooth muscle hypertrophy, and secretions narrow COPD patients' bronchioles. Airway inflammation, characterized by these anatomic findings, may also lead to nonspecific reactivity to inhalational agents.

Pharmacological attempts to regulate AHR by reducing bronchomotor tone do not alter the course of COPD. Though an earlier study suggested that regular use of an inhaled bronchodilator reduced the yearly rate of decline of FEV_1 in smokers, this conclusion was not supported by the LHS (15,34). If AHR in COPD is due to airway inflammation (as it is in asthma), bronchodilators are unlikely to reduce airway reactivity. Thus the absence of an effect of bronchodilators in this model is to be expected.

Mucus Hypersecretion and Infection

Another postulated mechanism for the accelerated decline in lung function in cigarette smokers is referred to as the "British hypothesis." This theory proposes that airway irritants cause bronchitis, which results in an overproduction of mucus. The increase in mucus predisposes the individual to recurrent infections of the respiratory tract, which leads to airway inflammation and destruction; this ultimately results in chronic airflow obstruction. Several prospective studies fail to show a relationship between mucus hypersecretion or the number or severity of acute chest infections and the rate of decline of FEV_1, leading many to discount this theory (35,36). However, a role for childhood infection as a risk factor for the development of COPD remains credible (37,38).

Patients with COPD exacerbations present with increased sputum volume and purulence, which is thought to indicate an infection. In the majority of cases, however, the cause of the acute deterioration in lung function is unknown. It is not surprising then, that the efficacy of antibiotics in exacerbations of COPD has not been consistently demonstrated (39). In a double-blind, placebo-controlled trial to examine the efficacy of antibiotic therapy in COPD exacerbations, resolution was 1.2 times more likely in the treatment group; nonetheless, patients treated with placebo had a favorable outcome over half the time (40).

Proponents of a role for bacterial infection in COPD have recently advanced the "vicious circle" hypothesis (Figure 9.1). In this view, bacterial products and the host's response to them propagate, but do not initiate, lung disease (39). Specifically, bacterial infection or colonization stimulates an inflammatory response causing local proteolytic injury and progression of obstructive lung disease. Concomitantly, bacterial injury of the airway epithelium impairs host defenses, predisposing to further bacterial infection/colonization, establishing the "vicious circle" (39).

In summary, mucus hypersecretion does not accelerate the rate of decline of lung function in cigarette smokers

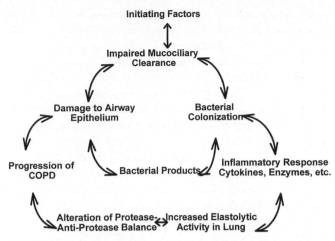

FIGURE 9.1. Diagram of the "vicious circle" hypothesis concerning the role of bacterial infections in the progression of COPD. (Reproduced with permission from: Murphy TF, Sethi S. Bacterial infection in chronic obstructive pulmonary disease. *Am Rev Respir Dis* 1992;146:1067–1083.)

with COPD. While childhood infection may lead to chronic airflow obstruction, there is no supporting evidence for a causal relationship between recurrent bronchitis in the adult and the development of COPD. Bacterial infections may, however, provoke acute exacerbations of COPD and ongoing lung injury.

Proteases and Oxidants

In 1963, Laurell and Eriksson (41) described families with a high prevalence of emphysema. Afflicted family members were found to have an absent alpha band on serum protein electrophoresis; the deficient protein was identified as α_1-antitrypsin, a protease inhibitor. Evaluation of other nonemphysematous family members revealed that α_1-antitrypsin levels fell into three groups: normal levels, 60% of normal, and less than 10% of normal, consistent with a genetic inheritance of this disorder (42). The deficiency appeared to predispose to the rapid development of panacinar emphysema. The disease develops rapidly in deficient smokers and leads to emphysema 10 to 15 years earlier than in nonaffected smokers (42–45).

These observations led to the "protease-antiprotease hypothesis" of emphysema (also referred to as the proteinase-antiproteinase or elastase-antielastase theory). This theory states that inhalation of microbes, particulate matter and other irritants initiates an inflammatory response in the lungs. This leads to an influx of alveolar macrophages and neutrophils, which release proteolytic enzymes to protect the lungs from these foreign agents. The delicate architecture of the lung parenchyma is protected from injury by a simultaneous release of antiproteolytic agents, the most important of which is α_1-antitrypsin (44). When the balance between proteolytic and antiproteolytic agents favors proteolysis, emphysema results (46–50).

α_1-antitrypsin is a 52,000 dalton (394 amino acid) glycoprotein that is synthesized in the liver and inhibits the actions of neutrophil elastase, cathepsin G, and other proteases in addition to trypsin; thus, it has also been called α_1-antiprotease (48,51). The gene for the protein is located on the long arm of chromosome 14; over 75 alleles have been identified, approximately 20% of which lead to a deficiency in active protein. α_1-antitrypsin deficiency is an autosomal recessive condition that involves a substitution or deletion mutation of a single amino acid codon (45). α_1-antitrypsin deficiency is one of the most common genetically linked lethal diseases among whites, affecting approximately one in every 3,000 Americans, or approximately 80,000 to 100,000 individuals (2% to 3% of all emphysema cases) (1,45).

The phenotypic variants of the α_1-protein are named to reflect the speed with which they migrate in an electric field at a pH between 4 and 5. For example, the normal M protein, which is present in at least 85% of individuals in most populations and at least 95% of those of northern European ancestry, migrates to an intermediate position, while the Z protein migrates slowest. The S form migrates to a position between the M and Z forms. Each allele at the α_1-antitrypsin locus is codominantly expressed in the offspring; therefore those heterozygous for the deficiency express intermediate levels of serum protein. Of the variants associated with decreased serum levels or protein activity, the S allele is most common, with a gene frequency of 3.4%, followed by the Z allele, which accounts for a gene frequency of 1.1%. However, the most common form of the deficiency is PiZZ (where there is the substitution of a lysine for a glutamic acid residue at position 342 of the molecule), which is present in over 95% of those significantly affected. A normal level of α_1-antiprotease (i.e., among P_iMM individuals) is 180 to 240 mg per dL (150 to 350 μmol per L); based on epidemiologic studies, a serum level of 80 mg per dL (or 11 μmol per L) of α_1-antitrypsin is deemed a "protective" threshold against emphysema. P_iZZ patients have serum levels that are approximately 15% of the normal PiMM state, approximately 35 mg per dL (150 to 350 μmol per L). Individuals with P_iSZ phenotypes (serum levels of 30 to 35% of normal) are considered to be at moderate risk for developing emphysema, and those with P_i Null-Null (in whom no α_1-antitrypsin is synthesized in the liver) are considered to be an even higher risk than P_iZZ individuals.

The primary clinical manifestations of severe α_1-antitrypsin deficiency involve the lung and the the liver. The major pulmonary manifestation is emphysema, although asthma and bronchiectasis have also been described (52). Two features of emphysema associated with severe α_1-antitrypsin deficiency are distinctive and should raise prompt suspicion of the diagnosis. Unlike "usual" emphysema, which characteristically presents in the sixth and seventh decades of life, the onset of emphysema in patients with severe α_1-antitrypsin deficiency occurs much earlier. The mean age of subjects in most large series of P_iZZ patients with fixed airflow obstruction is under 50 years (52). Second, the radiographic pattern of the emphysema associated with the disorder shows bullous changes that are more prominent at the bases of the lungs than at the apices. In the largest available series of radiographs in P_iZZ patients (n = 165), 99.8% had emphysematous changes that included the lung bases; 24% had those changes evident only at the bases (53). A smaller subgroup of deficient individuals develops liver injury during infancy and childhood; in fact, it is the most common genetic cause of chronic liver disease in children (54). Hepatic dysfunction typically presents as cholestasis in infancy but is usually not severe and generally remits by adolescence. Chronic liver disease develops infrequently; the risk for cirrhosis before the age of 20 is approximately 3%, but the risk for cirrhosis in deficient adults over the age of 50 years is at least 30% to 50% (55). Various theories have been put forth regarding the development of hepatic injury; intrahepatocyte endoplasmic reticulum aggregation of insoluble P_iZ protein is now widely considered to be the predominant cause of the liver damage (55).

The association of severe α_1-antitrypsin deficiency with emphysema is presented as strong support for the protease-antiprotease theory (56). The relationship between α_1-antitrypsin deficiency and lung function, however, is highly variable. Deficient individuals with normal spirometry and no respiratory symptoms have been well described (57,58). These findings suggest that other genetic or environmental factors (e.g., smoking, recurrent infections, AHR) may be required to unmask the risk of lung injury in patients with low levels of α_1-antitrypsin (58,59).

Since most patients with emphysema have normal serum levels of α_1-antitrypsin, several investigators sought to determine if tobacco smoke could influence the balance between proteases and antiproteases. In a series of animal experiments, tobacco smoke caused a 39% reduction in the elastase inhibitory capacity of lung α_1-antitrypsin collected by bronchopulmonary lavage. This effect could be reversed by treatment of the *(ex vivo)* bronchopulmonary lavage fluid with a reducing agent (60). These experiments suggested that tobacco smoke could induce oxidants that would inhibit α_1-antitrypsin activity. Unfortunately, supplementation with antioxidants does not improve symptoms in patients with COPD (61). In addition to inhibiting the actions of α_1-antitrypsin, tobacco smoke can tilt the balance of protease-antiproteases by augmenting the proteolytic burden in the lung. Cell suspensions, from bronchoalveolar lavage fluid and open-lung biopsies, reveal a significant increase in the absolute number and percent of neutrophils in smokers compared with nonsmokers (62). The elastase burden, defined as the elastase:α_1-protease inhibitor complex, has also been shown to correlate with the severity of emphysema (63).

Clinical Assessment of Chronic Obstructive Pulmonary Disease

Clinical Presentation and Physical Examination

Patients usually present because of progressively (over years) worsening dyspnea on exertion, decreasing exercise tolerance and persistent cough. Many individuals may actually hear wheezing respirations. Distinctions between chronic bronchitis and emphysema are summarized in Table 9.1. Chronic bronchitis, of course, typically features cough and mucoid phlegm production, which may become more copious and purulent during acute exacerbations. Hemoptysis may also accompany these exacerbations, although concerns about lung cancer are also appropriate.

In those patients with long-standing hypoxemia, symptoms of right heart failure may be prominent: pedal edema, liver enlargement and tenderness, and cyanosis. Digital clubbing is not a feature of chronic bronchitis or emphysema and should prompt consideration of other comorbid conditions such as bronchiectasis, lung cancer, interstitial disease, congenital heart disease, or inflammatory bowel disease.

Weight loss can be a presenting complaint; it occurs in about a third of the more severely impaired patients, but correlates only weakly with FEV_1. Notably, weight loss is an independent predictor of mortality in patients with COPD (64). The mechanism of weight loss appears to be a 10% to 20% increase in resting energy expenditure without a matched increase in dietary intake, although the total caloric intake may actually exceed the estimated daily requirements (64). This hypermetabolism can only partially be explained by increased work of breathing, and additional factors such as circulating catecholamines, cytokines, and drug therapy may contribute (65).

Hyperinflation of the lungs may result in a barrel chest, with percussion hyperresonance throughout. A characteristic posture is adopted by the patient using accessory muscles of respiration: the patient may lean forward with the elbows out and the neck extended ("tripod sign") to place the sternocleidomastoid and scalene muscles at maximum mechanical advantage for assisting inspiration. Inspection of the chest of hyperinflated patients may also show a paradoxic retraction or dimpling at the lower lateral chest wall during inspiration. Sometimes called "Hoover's sign," this finding reflects contraction of a flattened diaphragm, which pulls medially rather than moving caudally during contraction.

Auscultation of the chest may show diminished breath sounds when airflow obstruction is very severe or in areas with large bullae. With bronchitis and asthma, coarse inspiratory sounds (corresponding to large airway secretions) and wheezing may be prominent. Signs of cor pulmonale may include jugular venous distention, a right ventricular heave with a loud pulmonic valve component of the second heart sound, ascites, and sacral or pedal edema.

Laboratory assessment may show polycythemia in chronically hypoxemic individuals and metabolic alkalosis, which may reflect chronic diuretic use or compensation for hypercapnia of at least a day's duration. The electrocardiogram is an insensitive tool in detecting cor pulmonale, because electrocardiographic changes develop late. However, characteristic electrocardiographic features include evidence of a P pulmonale pattern (prominent P waves in inferior leads), right axis deviation, evidence of right ventricular hypertrophy (ratio of R to S wave in V_1 greater than 1), and an incomplete or complete right bundle branch block. Doppler flow echocardiography is a sensitive technique for detecting cor pulmonale, based on estimation of pulmonary artery pressures and the presence of right ventricular hypertrophy.

TABLE 9.1. CLINICAL FEATURES OF CHRONIC OBSTRUCTIVE PULMONARY DISEASE: DISTINCTIONS BETWEEN CHRONIC BRONCHITIS AND EMPHYSEMA

Features	Chronic Bronchitis	Emphysema
Symptoms, Signs		
Chronic cough, phlegm	Common	Less common
Cor pulmonale	Present (often with multiple exacerbations)	Present (but generally only in late disease stage)
Physiologic Function		
Airflow		
FEV_1	Decreased	Decreased
FEV_1/FVC	Decreased	Decreased
Lung volumes		
Residual volume	Normal	Increased, consistent with air trapping
Total lung capacity	Normal	Increased
Functional residual capacity	Mildly increased	Increased
Gas Exchange, Diffusion		
PaO_2	Often decreased	Often preserved until end stage
$PaCO_2$	Often decreased	Often preserved
Diffusing capacity	Normal	Decreased
Other		
Static compliance	Normal	Often increased

Pulmonary Function Tests

Bronchitic patients generally exhibit moderate airflow obstruction with mild degrees of hyperinflation (i.e., elevated residual volume and functional residual capacity), though less so than in patients with emphysema. In sharp contrast to patients with at least moderate emphysema, total lung capacity and diffusing capacity tend to be relatively normal in chronic bronchitis.

Emphysema results in abnormalities in airflow and lung volume measurements. The FEV_1 decrease reflects the progressive bronchiolar destruction. The loss of lung parenchyma results in a decrease in the radial traction on the airways, with consequent early airway closure. This decreased elastic recoil diminishes the lung's opposition to inspiratory muscle force, causing total lung capacity (TLC) to rise, although usually only slightly. Functional residual capacity (FRC—the amount of air in the lung after exhaling a normal tidal breath) is also increased as the elastic recoil of the lung falls. Lung forces opposing the tendency of the chest wall to expand at end-expiration are decreased, and FRC therefore increases. Residual volume (RV—the amount of air left in the lung after a maximal exhalation) is increased in emphysema as well. Vital capacity (VC—the difference between TLC and RV) is often decreased in emphysema, as the rise in RV usually exceeds the rise in TLC. Loss of elastic recoil also causes an increase in the static compliance of the lung, and static pressure-volume curves can distinguish patients with emphysema from those with normal lungs and from those with "pure" chronic bronchitis. However, because elasticity changes correlate poorly with the pathologic degree of emphysema and because these measurements require placement of an esophageal balloon, static pressure-volume curves have had limited clinical popularity.

As therapy of COPD is directed at maximizing available lung function, assessing the presence of reversible airflow obstruction (conventionally defined as a postbronchodilator increment of 15% and a rise in FEV_1 of 200 mL or more) has clinical appeal. While only a minority of patients with chronic obstructive pulmonary disease has reversible airflow obstruction as defined, the absence of reversibility during a single testing session does not discount its presence. For example, in a study of 985 patients with COPD, Anthonisen and coworkers (66) performed serial bronchodilator treatments and found that 68% of initially nonresponsive patients eventually satisfied criteria for air flow reversibility when tested up to seven times. In view of the insensitivity of a single bronchodilator trial for reversibility of airflow obstruction and the observation that bronchodilators may improve functional status in COPD patients without demonstrable reversibility (67,68), the absence of a rise in FEV_1 should not prevent a bronchodilator trial in such patients.

Resting hypoxia tends to develop late in the course of emphysema, though clinically significant desaturation may occur when the diffusing capacity for carbon monoxide (D_LCO) falls markedly (e.g., less than 55% of predicted). Preservation of gas exchange despite parenchymal loss in emphysema is best explained by the parallel loss of alveolo-capillary units, so ventilation-perfusion mismatch is not an early event.

Radiological Studies

The Plain Chest Radiograph

The plain chest radiographic features of emphysema include hyperinflation (e.g., depression and flattening of the diaphragms, blunting of the costophrenic angles, increased length of the lung, and increased size of the retrosternal air space) and features of vascular attenuation and hyperlucency (e.g., loss of lung parenchyma, bullous change, and disappearance of vascular markings, especially in the lung periphery) (Table 9.2). Less commonly recognized features include alteration of the tracheal shadow with development of "saber sheath" trachea, characterized by marked coronal narrowing associated with sagittal widening of the trachea (69). Finally, other vascular changes may reflect the development of pulmonary hypertension as a result of COPD. In a study of 1085 normal chest x-rays, Chang reported that the upper limit of the inspiratory diameter of the descending

---

TABLE 9.2. RADIOGRAPHIC SIGNS OF EMPHYSEMA

Signs in the posteroanterior chest radiograph
1. Peripheral vessels: a reduction in the caliber and number of the peripheral branches of the pulmonary artery in the outer half of the lung field when compared with the radiographs of normal persons.
2. Flattened diaphragm: depression and flattening of the diaphragm with blunting of the costophrenic angles. The actual level of the diaphragm is not as significant as the contour. The body build of the patient should also be considered. For example, in a short, stocky person, emphysema might be diagnosable even if the diaphragm were at the level of the tenth rib posteriorly.
3. Irregular radiolucency of lung fields: this manifestation is the result of the irregularity in distribution of the emphysematous tissue destruction. It is sometimes more clearly recognizable in laminograms.

Signs in the lateral chest radiograph
4. Abnormal retrosternal space: this is defined as a space showing increased radiolucency and measuring 2.5 cm or more from the sternum to the most anterior margin of the ascending aorta.
5. Flattened diaphragm: flattening of even concavity of diaphragmatic contour. A useful index of the change is the presence of a 90-degree or larger sternodiaphragmatic angle. In most patients with emphysema, this junction is more readily seen than in subjects with a normal chest.

From Nicklaus DW, Stowell DW, Christiansen WR, et al. The accuracy of the roentgenologic diagnosis of chronic pulmonary emphysema. *Am Rev Respir Dis* 1966;93:889–899, with permission.

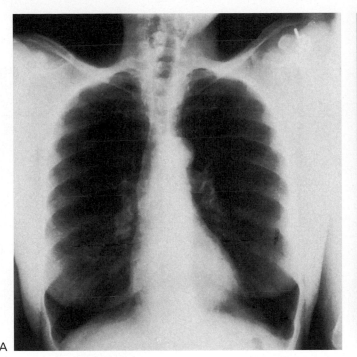
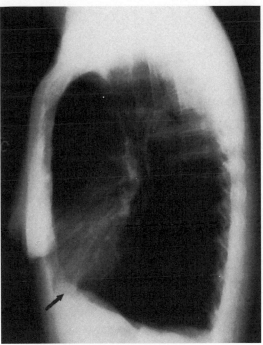

A   B

FIGURE 9.2. Chest radiograph (posteroanterior **A** and lateral **B** views) of a 62-year-old black female smoker with emphysema ($FEV_1 = 0.70$ L) and a normal α_1-antitrypsin level. Vascular attenuation, hyperlucency in the upper lung zones and diaphragm flattening (flattened costophrenic angles and an oblique sternocostal angle [**arrow**]) are demonstrated.

right pulmonary artery in normal males is 16 mm (70). Enlargement of the descending right pulmonary artery (width greater than 16 mm) is associated with elevation of the mean pulmonary artery pressure above 20 mm Hg (71) (Figure 9.2).

Because emphysema is a pathologic diagnosis, the most reliable studies of diagnostic criteria have assessed chest x-ray features in patients who subsequently come to necropsy (69). However, controversy still persists about the best single radiographic marker of emphysema. Proponents of using hyperinflation criteria (e.g., diaphragm flattening, increased retrosternal air space, etc.) suggest that hyperinflation is an early pathologic event in emphysema and that radiographic evidence of hyperinflation establishes emphysema even in the absence of airflow obstruction or symptoms (75). On the other hand, other observers use criteria for decreased vascularity and hyperlucency, arguing that these are sensitive in moderate to severe emphysema without falsely identifying patients with trivial emphysema (72,76). No consensus has emerged despite decades of study.

Radiographic criteria for chronic bronchitis have received less attention than emphysema, probably because chronic bronchitis is a clinical diagnosis and because the major role of the chest x-ray in chronic bronchitis is to exclude emphysema. Common chest x-ray features in chronic bronchitis (77) include hyperinflation; "tramlines," which are parallel-line shadows corresponding to thickened

bronchial walls seen in coronal section; and a diffuse increase in lung markings, especially at the bases, sometimes dubbed "dirty lungs." As with markers of emphysema, however, the reliability of these radiographic signs has been contested. For example, Fraser and Paré (77) suggest that tramlines more often indicate bronchiectasis than chronic bronchitis. Furthermore, attempts by these authors to identify other radiographic markers of chronic bronchitis (e.g., thickening of bronchial walls when seen "end on," or peribronchial cuffing) have not been successful to date (Figure 9.3).

Computed Tomography

Several studies have demonstrated the ability of computed tomography of the chest to diagnose emphysema, especially using high-resolution techniques. High-resolution computed tomography (HRCT) allows a display of fine anatomic details and is therefore particularly well suited to describe and quantitate the structural abnormalities of emphysema in living subjects (77–82). The accuracy of HRCT has been reported to rival direct pathologic examination, and may accurately diagnose emphysema in mild or even clinically silent emphysema (81,82). On the other hand, several investigators have shown that mild degrees of emphysema may be missed by computed tomography (78,79,82). For example, Gurney and colleagues observed that 20% of their patients with functional emphysema (de-

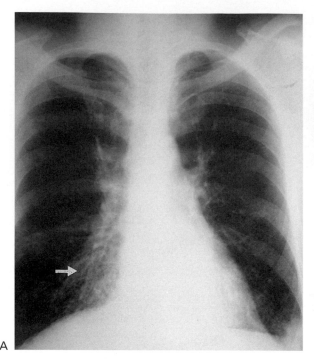

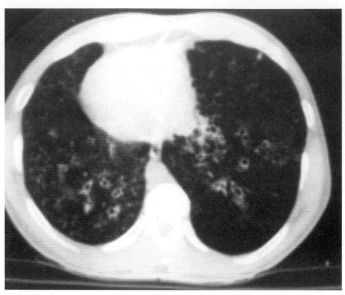

A

B

FIGURE 9.3. **(A)** Chest film from a man with severe chronic obstructive bronchitis who was seen during a bout of bronchopneumonia. The lungs are hyperinflated and the diaphragm is flattened and depressed. The heart is marginally enlarged and hilar vessel shadows are compressed toward the midline. Note the bilateral increase in interstitial nodular and linear shadows bilaterally ("dirty lung fields"), most marked at the bases. The parallel "tramlines" caused by thickened bronchial walls are most apparent in the right lower lung field (*arrow*). A small area of consolidation is present in the left costophrenic angle. **(B)** CT scan of the lower lung fields showing bilateral thickening of bronchial walls with peribronchial nodular changes, consistent with severe chronic bronchitis and early bronchiectasis.

fined as a diffusion capacity less than 75% of predicted and an FEV_1 less than 80% of predicted) had no subjective findings of emphysema on high-resolution computed tomography (82). Despite these limitations, HRCT of the chest is being advocated for the diagnosis of emphysema, particularly where intervention may have a clinical impact (e.g., smoking cessation in susceptible individuals, augmentation therapy for patients with emphysema associated with α_1-antitrypsin deficiency, lung volume reduction surgery in severe emphysema) (Figure 9.4).

Clinical Course

Among the most important contributions to our knowledge of the natural history of chronic bronchitis and emphysema is a study of transport workers in the London area conducted by Fletcher and colleagues (83). Nearly 800 working men, both smokers and nonsmokers, were studied over an eight-year period with serial recordings of the one-second forced expiratory volume (FEV_1). The rate of decline in FEV_1, which normally begins at the age of about 25 years, was markedly increased among the 10% to 15% of susceptible cigarette smokers. Clinical disability did not occur until late in the course of the disease, when the FEV_1 had declined by

about 70%. Typically, disability developed at approximately age 65 years, at which time smoking cessation prolonged life only slightly; disability persisted lifelong (Figure 9.5).

In order to improve longevity and quality of life, smoking cessation must occur at an early age, before disability is

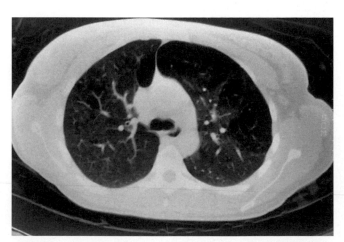

FIGURE 9.4. Computed tomographic section demonstrating extensive areas of lung destruction bilaterally consistent with the diagnosis of emphysema.

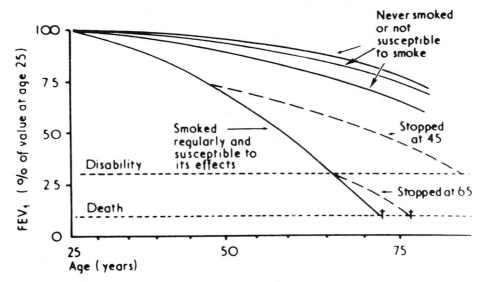

FIGURE 9.5. The effects of smoking and smoking cessation on the forced expiratory volume in one second (FEV_1) in men aged 25 years and older. The lower solid line represents a typical course in a smoker who is susceptible to developing COPD. Crosses indicate death due to respiratory failure. Disability usually occurs at about age 65 years, when airflow is already markedly decreased. At that time, smoking cessation will prolong life by a few years, but disability will persist. In order to effect a major improvement in life expectancy, smoking cessation must occur at an earlier age. (From Fletcher C, Peto R. The natural history of chronic airflow obstruction. *Br Med J* 1977;1: 1645–1648, with permission.)

evident. This underscores the importance of undertaking periodic evaluations of patients who smoke and vigorous attempts at breaking the smoking habit before disability occurs. As shown in Figure 9.5, smoking cessation will decrease the accelerated rate of decline in lung function to a normal rate, but pulmonary function will not return to the age-adjusted range for nonsmokers (1). Hence ex-smokers revert to a normal rate of decline in FEV_1, but they manifest a lower level of lung function at the time of smoking cessation.

The findings in Fletcher's study have been confirmed (19). The most recent confirmatory longitudinal study is the COPD Early Intervention Trial, or Lung Health Study, a multicenter, five-year study sponsored by the National Heart, Lung and Blood Institute (19); details of the study are discussed below. The Lung Health Study evaluated the effects of smoking cessation and use of bronchodilators in early, mild COPD. As expected, in this population of adults with mild disease, smoking cessation resulted in a significant delay in the expected decline in FEV_1 with age.

Late Stages of Chronic Obstructive Pulmonary Disease

The late stages of COPD are characterized by a marked decline in pulmonary function and a decrease in reversibility of obstruction following administration of inhaled bronchodilators. Initially, patients are dyspneic during exertion. However, as disease progresses, lower levels of routine activity result in dyspnea; finally dyspnea occurs at rest. Activities of daily living, such as bathing and dressing, become burdensome. During the very late stages of COPD, appetite is decreased and weight loss occurs. The weight loss is thought to be due to several factors, including decreased caloric intake and increased work of breathing; the latter is due to airway obstruction and a marked increase in physiologic dead space (wasted ventilation). As lung function declines, the alveolar-arterial gradient for oxygen increases due primarily to an increase in abnormal ventilation-perfusion relationships. Hypoxemia, pulmonary hypertension, and cor pulmonale develop. Psychologic effects of advanced COPD may be observed, including anxiety and depression.

Respiratory infections are common in patients with COPD. Late in the course of the disease, the infections are associated with episodes of severe hypoxemia, with or without hypercapnia. Acute exacerbations require intensive therapy, often in a hospital setting; and mechanical ventilation is sometimes necessary. During the final stages of the disease, weaning from mechanical ventilation becomes a major problem. The patient and family should be consulted in advance regarding their wishes on the use of mechanical ventilation to prolong life under these circumstances.

Prevention

The focus in prevention of COPD has been on smoking cessation and immunoprophylaxis with the use of pneumococcal and influenza vaccines.

Smoking Cessation

The major cause of chronic bronchitis is cigarette smoking; in fact, the United States Surgeon General has stated that tobacco use is the single most important preventable risk to human health in this country. Despite a significant decrease in cigarette smoking in the United States over the past 25 years, about 50 million Americans continue to smoke. While chronic bronchitis is rare among nonsmokers, the risk of COPD is increased up to 30-fold in smokers. Furthermore, a dose-response relationship exists between the number of cigarettes smoked and the rate of decline in airflow in patients with chronic obstructive bronchitis (4). In addition to the detrimental effects of active smoking, passive smoking among household members and workers exposed to cigarette smoke increases the normal rate of decline in pulmonary function with aging (84).

In the COPD Early Intervention Trial (begun in 1986), 5,887 adult smokers between 35 to 60 years of age who had mild airway obstruction (average FEV_1 of 75% of predicted) were studied over a five-year period. Subjects were entered randomly into three treatment groups: (a) a smoking intervention program and regular use of an inhaled bronchodilator (ipratropium bromide); (b) a smoking intervention program and administration of an inhaled placebo; and (c) usual care with no smoking intervention program. The smoking intervention program consisted of behavior modification, group therapy, and nicotine replacement. Subjects who quit smoking entered a maintenance program aimed at preventing recidivism. Initial results of the study, which was completed in 1994, have been reported (19). Consistent with results from previous investigations, smoking cessation resulted in a significant decrease in the age-related decline in FEV_1, even in patients with mild COPD (Figure 9.6).

Based on the studies cited, an organized approach to smoking cessation counseling should be considered an essential component of the management of all smokers, especially those with COPD. However, fewer than 50% of cigarette smokers are advised by their physicians to smoke less or to stop smoking (85). Intervention at an early age, when it is most effective, is rarely undertaken.

A simple, office-based smoking cessation program can effect success rates as high as 50% in highly motivated patients. Direct, unequivocal advice to stop smoking has, itself, been shown to result in abstinence in up to 10% of patients. A simple, useful tactic is to establish a quitting date when the patient's stress level is low, and to have the patient sign a one-sentence contract (e.g., "I, John Doe, agree to quit smoking on the following date: _____") written in the progress notes and witnessed by the physician. Most patients who quit smoking do so on their own, with advice and support from their physician and members of the office staff. The patient's efforts should be supported by visits to the office two weeks after quitting, one month later, and thereafter as necessary. Several self-help programs

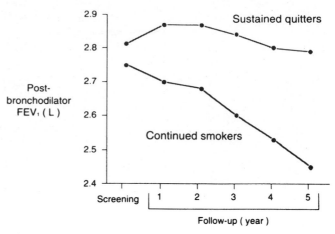

FIGURE 9.6. Mean postbronchial FEV_1 for participants in the Lung Health Study who were in the smoking intervention group; sustained quitters (open circles) and continued smokers (closed circles) are shown. The two curves diverge sharply from baseline. (From Anthonisen NR, Connett JE, Kiley JP, et al. Effects of smoking intervention and the use of an inhaled anticholinergic bronchodilator on the rate of decline of FEV_1. The Lung Health Study. *JAMA* 1994;272:1497–1505, with permission.)

are available at minimal cost from volunteer and government agencies, some of which are listed in Table 9.3. These programs assist the patient during the first few critical weeks of smoking withdrawal.

Commercial smoking cessation programs are available in most areas; however, they tend to be relatively expensive. Results from these programs are not superior to those of well-planned office-based programs. A variety of methods should be made available to patients, and patients should be encouraged to choose the plan that best suits their needs.

One cigarette delivers approximately 1 to 2 mg of nico-

TABLE 9.3. SOURCES FOR SELF-HELP GUIDES FOR SMOKING CESSATION

Title	Source
Smokers Self-Testing Kit	PHS Publication #1904 Office of Smoking and Health Department of Health and Human Services Atlanta, GA 30341
Freedom from Smoking in 20 Days, and A Lifetime of Freedom from Smoking	American Lung Association 1740 Broadway New York, NY 10019
Quit For Good	National Cancer Institute National Institutes of Health Bethesda, MD 20892
I Quit Kit	American Cancer Society 90 Park Avenue New York, NY 10016

tine to the lungs, which is rapidly absorbed into the bloodstream. Nicotine replacement will help reduce withdrawal symptoms (anxiety, irritability, anger, and difficulty concentrating) and will significantly improve the smoking cessation rate to approximately 25% at six months (85–89). Relative contraindications to nicotine replacement therapy include pregnancy and cardiovascular disease, though the risk appears to be minimal in the latter (90). Nicotine replacement therapy can be accomplished in several ways. Nicotine gum is available in 2 and 4 mg sizes. Nicotine patches are convenient and associated with improved compliance; a programmed series of decreasing doses allow gradual weaning of the patient off cigarettes. However, some patients may develop skin reactions that preclude their use. Nicotine spray can be used in the very addicted smoker. It is rapidly absorbed reaching peak blood levels within minutes after a 1 mg dose. Initial use may be associated with nasal, throat, and eye irritation, but these usually improve with continued use.

Smoking behavior during the initial stages of nicotine replacement has been shown to predict outcome: abstinence during the first two weeks of use of nicotine patches suggests success, while smoking during that interval is a good predictor of failure at six months. (91). Sustained-release bupropion hydrochloride (Zyban) has been shown to be as effective as nicotine replacement, with one-year quit rates of approximately 23% (92). The mechanism by which bupropion helps patients abstain from smoking is unknown; it is presumed that this action is mediated by the drug's noradrenergic or dopaminergic properties. In the recent guidelines for smoking cessation issued by the Agency for Health Care Policy Research, no conclusions were drawn regarding the effectiveness of acupuncture, hypnosis, and drug therapies such as clonidine, antidepressants, and anxiolytics/benzodiapines because of insufficient data or inconclusive evidence (85). Nicotine replacement therapy in conjunction with behavioral modification and motivational methods appears to double the likelihood of success. Unfortunately, the long-term relapse rate remains high, with less than 20% of smokers who quit remaining abstinent at one year (87). Repetitive reinforcement by the health care provider is necessary.

The importance of a "packaged approach" to smoking cessation has been emphasized, including counseling and follow-up visits (89). The "four As" approach includes: (a) *A*sking patients about their smoking status; (b) *A*dvising patients to quit; (c) *A*ssisting in setting a quit date; and (d) *A*rranging follow-up visits. Failure to adhere to a comprehensive program essentially guarantees failure, and patients should be encouraged not to depend on nicotine replacement therapies alone to stop smoking.

Pneumococcal and Influenza Vaccines

Secondary preventive measures in COPD include administration of influenza and pneumococcal vaccinations. COPD patients represent a group of individuals at high risk for development not only of these infections, but also of complications following these illnesses.

The pneumococcal polysaccharide vaccine is designed to elicit protective antibodies against *Steptococcus pneumoniae*. The current vaccine (licensed in 1983) covers 23 of the 83 capsular *S. pneumoniae* serotypes; these 23 serotypes are responsible for 88% of the invasive pneumococcal disease in the United States (93). The vaccine appears to be effective in preventing invasive disease (i.e., bacteremic pneumonia or meningitis), but with less protection against uncomplicated pneumococcal pneumonia (93). The Advisory Committee on Immunization Practices of the Centers for Disease Control and Prevention recommends that the vaccine be administered to: a) persons aged 65 years or over; (b) immunocompetent persons at risk for pneumococcal disease or its complications because of a chronic illness (diabetes mellitus, alcoholism, cirrhosis, chronic cardiopulmonary disease, cerebrospinal fluid leak); (c) immunocompromised persons at high risk for infection (including those with functional or anatomic asplenia). (93). In most healthy adults, titers persist for five or more years. Persons who have received the 14-valent vaccine (i.e., prior to 1983) need not be routinely revaccinated. However, persons at highest risk for pneumococcal infections (i.e., immunocompromised patients) should be revaccinated with the 23-valent vaccine if it has been more than 6 years since the previous dose. Patients with nephrotic syndrome, renal failure or transplants should be revaccinated every three to five years because of waning immunity. The most common side effects are erythema, localized pain, fever, and myalgias.

Influenza epidemics occur in the United States in the winter months every year and cause significant morbidity in all groups, but particularly among the very young, the aged, and debilitated patients. It is estimated that 20,000 deaths may be ascribed to influenza every year in the United States (94). During epidemics, deaths may occur directly from influenza and pneumonia or from complications of underlying chronic diseases. Influenza type A viruses may be classified on the basis of two surface antigens: hemagglutinin (which has three subtypes: H1, H2, and H3) and neuraminidase (which has two subtypes: N1 and N2). Influenza type A and type B viruses undergo almost annual antigenic variation, although the later has more antigenic stability. Immunity to the viral capsid antigens (especially influenza A hemagglutinin) reduces the chance of infection and the severity of disease if infection does occur. Every year, three influenza virus strains, usually two type A and one type B, are included in the influenza vaccine preparation. These represent the viruses that are anticipated to circulate in the United States during the influenza season. Influenza vaccine is strongly recommended for any person aged over six months who—because of age or underlying medical condition—is at increased risk for complications of influenza. In addition, health care workers and others (including household members) in close contact with persons in high-risk groups should be vaccinated to decrease the risk of transmitting infection to persons at high risk (94). The vaccine may also be administered to any person who wishes to reduce the chance of becoming infected with the virus (94). The inactivated virus may safely be administered to persons with HIV infection and to breast-feeding mothers. However, the vaccine should not be administered to persons known to have anaphylactic hypersensitivity to eggs or any other component of the vaccine preparation. Those with an acute febrile illness should not be vaccinated until their symptoms have abated. The optimal time to vaccinate high-risk persons is usually October to mid-November, as influenza activity in the United States generally peaks between late December and early March (95). The vaccine may be offered even after influenza virus activity is documented in a community. The vaccine contains killed virus and cannot cause influenza; respiratory disease after vaccination is coincidental and unrelated to vaccination. The most frequent (10% to 64% of patients) side effect of vaccination is soreness at the vaccination site that may last up to two days. Other reported adverse reactions include fever, malaise, and myalgias. In 1976, there was a reported increase in the frequency of Guillain-Barré syndrome (GBS) among persons receiving swine influenza vaccine (96). However, recent preparations have not been associated with increases in GBS (94). The incidence of vaccine-associated GBS appears to be occurring in greater frequency among those who have had a past history of GBS (97). Therefore it would be prudent to avoid influenza vaccination in persons who are not at high risk for severe influenza and who have had a previous bout of GBS. However, many experts believe that for most persons who have a history of GBS and who are at high risk for severe complications from influenza, the established benefits of influenza vaccination justify yearly vaccination (95).

We should be diligent in offering and administering these vaccines to patients who may benefit from them. Among national health objectives for the year 2000, the United States Public Health Service includes a goal to increase pneumococcal and influenza vaccination levels to over 60% for persons at high risk for complications from pneumococcal disease and influenza (98). In 1995, a random-digit-dialed telephone survey of adults (aged 18 years and over) showed that only 35% of persons aged over 65 years have ever received the pneumococcal vaccine; only 58% received the influenza vaccine in the 12 months immediately preceding the survey (99).

Other Measures

A general exercise plan and nutritional supplementation are also important adjunctive treatments for improving patients' functional status. These general measures are discussed further in the following sections on management of COPD.

Therapy of Stable Chronic Obstructive Pulmonary Disease

A suggested approach to the continuing outpatient care of the patient with COPD is illustrated in Figure 9.7 (1). The pharmacologic management of stable COPD is shown in Figure 9.8. Individual components are discussed in greater detail below. Surgical treatments for severe COPD (i.e., lung transplantation, reduction pneumoplasty for giant bullous emphysema, and lung volume reduction surgery) are discussed in greater detail in a following chapter.

Bronchodilators

Several classes of bronchodilator agents are used routinely in the management of COPD, including anticholinergic agents, β-adrenergic agonists, and methylxanthines.

Anticholinergic Agents
Anticholinergic agents are among the oldest drugs known and were some of the first drugs to be used to treat respiratory disorders. These agents inhibit the action of acetylcholine at parasympathetic cholinergic nerve endings by competing for acetylcholine receptors. As a result, intracellular guanosine 3′,5′-cyclic monophosphate (cGMP) levels are reduced, resulting in a decrease in bronchial smooth-muscle tone.

Atropine sulfate has long been available in aerosolized and oral forms; however, its use has been limited by exces-

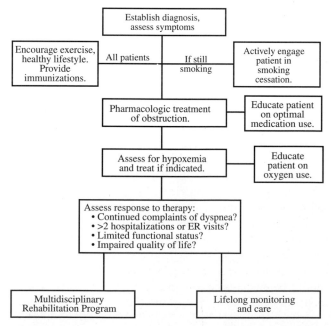

FIGURE 9.7. General outline for the outpatient management of stable COPD. (Adapted from Celli BR, Snider GL, Heffner J, et al. Standards for the diagnosis and care of patients with chronic obstructive pulmonary disease. *Am J Respir Crit Care Med* 1995; 152[Suppl]:S77–S120, with permission.)

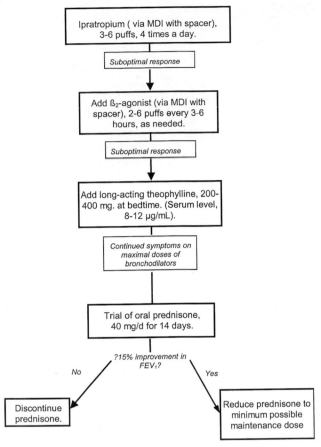

FIGURE 9.8. Proposed algorithm for the pharmacologic management of stable COPD. (Adapted from Ferguson GT, Cherniak RM. Management of chronic obstructive pulmonary disease. *N Engl J Med* 1993;328:1017–1022, with permission.)

sive side effects. Atropine is distributed rapidly in total body water and readily crosses the blood-brain barrier, making unpleasant side effects, including dry mouth, tachycardia, blurred vision, urinary retention, and mental status changes, common and dose-dependent. Atropine should not be given to patients with narrow-angle glaucoma or symptomatic prostatic hypertrophy.

New quaternary ammonium atropine derivatives have less mucosal absorption and fewer side effects. Currently, ipratropium bromide is the only such agent commercially available in the United States, though more agents are now undergoing clinical trials. Ipratropium bromide is available as a metered-dose inhaler and as a solution for nebulization. The drug has a relatively slow onset (60 to 90 minutes); however, it has a longer duration of bronchodilation (six to eight hours) than do most β-adrenergic agonists. Hence it is more suitable for use on a regular, rather than "as needed," basis. Submaximal bronchodilation has been demonstrated using the recommended dose of two puffs four times daily; consequently, the number of inhalations may be doubled or tripled without notable side effects (4). Ipra-

tropium bromide also reduces sputum volume without altering sputum viscosity.

In some studies, ipratropium bromide has been reported to produce greater bronchodilation in chronic bronchitis than do conventional doses of β-agonists (4). However, other investigations show that maximal doses of β-agonists produce the same degree of bronchodilation. A recent, large, multicenter, double-blind clinical trial compared the efficacy of the β-agonist albuterol with that of ipratropium and a combination of the two agents in 534 patients with severe COPD (100). The combination of drugs resulted in a greater change in FEV$_1$ from baseline than either drug alone; the benefit persisted over the 85 days of the study. The additive effects may derive from the agents' disparate mechanisms and sites of action, as well as their differing time courses for bronchodilation. The combination is now commercially available in the United States as a single metered-dose inhaler.

Other studies have demonstrated a prolonged benefit (over three months) of ipratropium bromide. The incidence of side effects is low, and the side effects are generally minor. No tachyphylaxis has been reported, even when ipratropium bromide has been used for as long as five years. Extended use of the agent does not appear to influence the long-term decline in FEV$_1$ (1). Given its effectiveness as a bronchodilator, prolonged duration of effect, wide therapeutic range, low incidence of side effects, and freedom from tachyphylaxis, ipratropium bromide has been recommended as a first-line agent for patients with COPD who have daily symptoms (4).

β-Adrenergic Agonists

β-adrenergic agonists have been the mainstay of treatment of obstructive lung disease. These agents increase cyclic adenosine monophosphate (cAMP) formation, which, in turn, results in a change in intracellular calcium ion concentration and a reduction of bronchomotor tone. Onset of action is more rapid than for inhaled ipratropium bromide, but duration of action is shorter. Characteristics of the available agents are presented in Table 9.4.

Several agonists are available in various forms; because of their high incidence of side effects, oral formulations generally are not used unless patients are unable to use the inhaled forms. The various agents provide similar bronchodilation in equivalent doses, and the choice of agent depends on such factors as patient preference, physician experience, availability, and cost. The drugs are best taken on an "as needed" basis; hence they may be used as primary therapy in patients who have dyspnea only intermittently. They may be added to regular doses of ipratropium when patients have daily symptoms. Excessive use of beta agonists may result in tachyphylaxis via a downregulation of beta-2 receptors, resulting in decreased bronchodilation. An algorithm for the proposed use of these and other therapeutic agents in patients with COPD is shown in Figure 9.8 (4).

TABLE 9.4. CHARACTERISTICS OF BETA-ADRENERGIC AGONISTS

Drug	Dose/Puff (mg)	Beta-receptor activity		Time of Effect (min)		
		β1	β2	Onset	Peak	Duration
Isoproterenol	0.08	+ + +	+ + +	3–5	5–10	60–90
Isoetharine	0.34	+ +	+ +	3–5	5–20	60–150
Metaproterenol	0.65	+	+ + +	5–15	10–60	60–180
Terbutaline	0.20	+	+ + + +	5–30	60–120	180–360
Albuterol	0.09	+	+ + + +	5–15	60–90	240–360
Bitolterol	0.37	+	+ + + +	5–10	60–90	300–480
Pirbuterol	0.20	+	+ + +	5–10	30–60	240–480
Salmeterol	0.025	+	+ + + +	10–20	~180	600–720

Adapted from Ferguson GT, Cherniak RM. Management of chronic obstructive pulmonary disease. *N Engl J Med* 1993;328(14):1018. Reprinted by permission of *The New England Journal of Medicine*, Copyright (1993), Massachusetts Medical Society.

The side effects of β-agonists are numerous, and most stem from activation of beta-1 receptors. Cardiovascular effects include tachycardia, dysrhythmias, exacerbation of myocardial ischemia, and hypo- or hypertension. Nervous system effects include tremor, agitation, and insomnia. Fortunately, tolerance to most subjective side effects develops within days without loss of bronchodilation. Hypokalemia has been noted in patients receiving large doses (4).

Reports on the incidence of serious adverse events during daily use of β-agonists by asthmatics have raised concerns regarding these drugs' safety. Asthma exacerbations, both fatal and near-fatal, have been linked to routine daily use of β-agonists; however there is no clear cause-and-effect relationship. The increased use of the agents may simply identify patients with more severe disease who have an increased likelihood of more frequent and severe exacerbations. No data exist on the association between β-agonist use and adverse events in COPD. At present, standard doses of the drugs are considered to be useful and safe in the management of patients with COPD.

Methylxanthines

Methylxanthines are drugs with a long tradition of use in respiratory disease. Despite this history, the exact mechanism of action for theophylline, the prototype methylxanthine, remains unclear. The drug relaxes bronchial smooth muscle (although only to relatively mild degrees) and increases diaphragmatic contractility and endurance. Theophylline also improves cardiac output, reduces pulmonary vascular resistance, and improves perfusion to ischemic myocardium (1). It has a narrow therapeutic window, with minimal improvement in lung function at serum levels less than 10 μg per mL; significant toxic effects are observed at levels greater than 20 μg per mL. It has multiple drug and food interactions that may result in altered drug levels (Table 9.5). Theophylline's unique multisystem effects, additive actions with other bronchodilators, and availability in sustained-release oral formulations provide a role for the agent in maintenance regimens for patients with COPD

(101). Nevertheless, the potential for serious side effects (nausea, vomiting, insomnia, agitation, seizures, cardiac dysrhythmias) mandates that serum levels be carefully monitored. This is especially true in the elderly and in patients with underlying medical disorders, including acute and chronic hepatic dysfunction, congestive heart failure, or febrile illnesses. In addition, several drugs commonly prescribed for patients with COPD (e.g., macrolide and quinolone antibiotics, H₂-blockers, propranolol) may prolong theophylline half-life, resulting in toxic side effects.

Corticosteroids

Several studies addressing use of systemic corticosteroids in patients with stable COPD have been conducted. Unfortunately, drug doses, routes of administration, duration of therapy, and endpoints have varied from one study to another. A meta-analysis of all English-language, placebo-controlled trials of oral corticosteroids in COPD published from 1966 to 1989 has been performed (102). Ten of the 15

TABLE 9.5. FACTORS THAT ALTER THEOPHYLLINE METABOLISM

Decreased half-life
  cigarette smoking
  marijuana
  high protein diet
  drugs (phenytoin, rifampin, isoniazid, phenobarbital, carbamazepine, aminoglutethimide, ketoconazole, isoproterenol)
  charbroiled food
Increased half-life
  liver disease
  congestive heart failure
  drugs (cimetidine, ciprofloxacin, allopurinol, erythromycin, propranolol, verapamil, nifedipine, tetracycline, hydrocortisone)
  viral illness
  influenza vaccine
  fever
  obesity

studies evaluated met all nine prospectively defined, explicit quality standards. Response to oral corticosteroids was defined as a 20% improvement in baseline FEV_1. Response rate was defined as the proportion of patients who responded to corticosteroid therapy minus the proportion who responded to placebo. Only 10% of patients fulfilled the criteria for response. No association was found between steroid responsiveness and clinical factors such as age or baseline FEV_1.

With only a limited number of patients demonstrating an objective response to corticosteroid therapy, is it possible to predict prospectively which patients will benefit from corticosteroids? Two measures that may be predictive are an increase in FEV_1 (by 15% or more) following administration of an inhaled β-agonist (103) and the presence of sputum eosinophilia (104).

The significant side effects associated with prolonged administration of systemic corticosteroids necessitate careful observation and documentation of the efficacy of therapy. If chronic oral therapy is required, alternate-day dosing, if possible, has been recommended (1); however, the efficacy of such a regimen has not been evaluated in patients with COPD. The recommended use of corticosteroids in patients with severe COPD is noted in Figure 9.8.

Inhaled corticosteroids are used in an attempt to further decrease systemic side effects, although their long-term efficacy in COPD is unclear. Nonetheless, their use has become accepted practice in the routine care of COPD; in one Canadian survey, as many as 43% of patients using inhaled corticosteroids had COPD (105). Recently, two large European studies challenged that long-standing practice. Vestbo and colleagues (106) identified 290 patients with fixed obstructive lung disease, defined as an FEV_1-to-FVC ratio of less than 70% and who did not exhibit reversibility (i.e., 15% or lower improvement from baseline FEV_1) after inhalation of terbutaline or 10 days of oral prednisolone. The patients were prospectively and randomly assigned into two groups: the first received inhaled budesonide (a potent long-acting corticosteroid) in addition to their usual regimen; the second received placebo from an identical inhaler. Rates of FEV_1 decline, number of exacerbations, and clinical symptoms were no different between the two groups after 36 months of close follow-up. Pauwels and colleagues (107) examined a similar group of 1,277 current smokers with mild COPD: prebronchodilator FEV_1-to-FVC ratio of less than 70%, postbronchodilator FEV_1 between 50% and 100% of predicted normal values, 10% or lower improvement from baseline FEV_1 after inhalation of terbutaline. The patients were randomly assigned to receive either budesonide or placebo from identical dry-powder inhalers. The patients who received the corticosteroid had a modest increase in their FEV_1 (approximating 17 mL per year) for the first six months of the study; those receiving placebo experienced a decline over the same period (approximating 81 mL per year, p < 0.001). However, from nine months to the end of the three years of follow-up, FEV_1 declined at similar rates in the two groups. Skin bruising occurred more often in those receiving the corticosteroid (10% versus 4%, p < 0.001); other adverse events were similar between the two groups. Therefore, the long-term use of inhaled corticosteroids can no longer be routinely recommended in COPD patients.

To date, use of nonsteroidal antiinflammatory agents, such as cromolyn and nedocromil, has not been evaluated in patients with severe COPD (1).

Other Therapeutic Agents

Chronic cough is the defining symptom in chronic bronchitis. However, cough may be a sign of associated diseases, such as cancer or acute respiratory infection. In most patients, the cause is readily identified. Therapy should be directed at the specific etiology, once identified. Antitussives and expectorants may be used to control the cough if it is a nuisance or results in other medical problems. Patients with ineffective, exhausting coughs can be trained to cough more effectively.

Mucolytics are of questionable benefit in the management of COPD. In one large, multicenter, randomized, placebo-controlled clinical trial of iodinated glycerol, subjective measures, such as cough frequency, cough severity, chest discomfort, ease of expectoration, and overall health status were improved in patients treated for eight weeks. However, objective evidence of benefit was considered insufficient, and the Food and Drug Administration mandated discontinuation of marketing of the drug. Other agents, including aerosolized water and acetylcysteine, have not been demonstrated to benefit patients with COPD (15).

Treatment of α_1-antitrypsin Deficiency

Treatment options for α_1-antitrypsin deficiency include liver transplantation, use of various drugs to augment hepatic synthesis (e.g., danazol, tamoxifen) (108–110), and, most recently, augmentation therapy by infusion of purified α_1-antitrypsin (111,112). While clearly effective, liver transplantation is a major intervention available to relatively few individuals, and drug therapy to promote protein synthesis has produced only modest increases in serum levels of α_1-antitrypsin (108–110). Replacement therapy with pooled human plasma purified α_1-antitrypsin has been available for limited use in the United States since 1988. The American Thoracic Society suggests augmentation therapy for patients older than 18 years with serum α_1-antitrypsin level less than 11 μM and severe obstructive lung disease (113,114). Wewers and colleagues have provided conclusive evidence that the antiprotease imbalance present in the lungs of individuals deficient in α_1-antitrypsin can be effectively corrected by regular infusions of the α_1-antitrypsin preparation (111,113). The ongoing National Heart, Lung and Blood Institute (NHLBI) Registry has enrolled more than 1,000 subjects in an observational study to assess the natural history of disease in these patients, whether or not they are receiving augmentation therapy. The experience of the registry will provide invaluable data on the beneficial effects of long-term α_1-antitrypsin augmentation.

Novel approaches include the administration of aerosolised α_1-antitrypsin, recombinant α_1-antitrypsin, and gene therapy. Preliminary studies (115,116) suggest that inhalation of a human recombinant DNA preparation of α_1-antitrypsin can augment serum and alveolar levels and activity, and this is a promising treatment strategy for which further investigation is needed. Recent exciting developments regarding "gene therapy" have involved the adenovirus-mediated transfer of a recombinant α_1-antitrypsin gene to the lung epithelium of rats, with subsequent detection of α_1-antitrypsin in epithelial lining fluid for at least one week (117). Also, the human gene has been introduced into rabbit lung, liver, and endothelium by means of a plasmid-liposome complex (118). Because augmentation therapy is already available, safety issues pertaining to the use of a viral transfer factor will need to be answered before gene therapy can be implemented as a treatment option for α_1-antitrypsin deficiency (119).

Finally, lung transplantation has become an option for patients with end-stage emphysema due to α_1-antitrypsin-deficiency. Although earlier observations raised concern that actuarial survival among α_1-antitrypsin deficient lung transplant recipients was lower than that of patients with centriacinar emphysema from smoking, more recent studies suggest similar survival rates following lung transplantation (120). The role of augmentation therapy to improve survival after lung transplantation has yet to be defined.

Pulmonary Rehabilitation

As the FEV_1 falls below 50% of predicted value in patients with COPD, essential activities of daily living become restricted. This limitation develops on a background of an already compromised quality of life due to shortness of breath and psychosocial disability. A vicious cycle ensues in which the patient performs less exercise and becomes more disabled and more depressed. Pulmonary rehabilitation is aimed at interrupting the cycle. The primary goal of rehabilitation is to restore the patient to the highest possible level of independent function. Rather than focusing solely on reversing the disease process, rehabilitation attempts to improve disability from disease.

Pulmonary rehabilitation is a broad therapeutic modality defined in a National Institutes of Health workshop (121) as:

> A multidisciplinary continuum of services directed to persons with pulmonary diseases and their families, usually by an interdisciplinary team of specialists, with the goal of achieving and maintaining the individual's maximum level of independence and functioning in the community.

Earlier studies failed to demonstrate any improvement in pulmonary function tests in patients completing rehabilitation measures, leading to conventional neglect of this modality. Recent work, however, provides evidence that pulmonary rehabilitation is an effective treatment option. Pulmonary rehabilitation is now recognized as an important component in the comprehensive management of patients with severe COPD. Guidelines for the conduct of such programs have been published (1,122–124).

Program Design

Selection of patients appropriate for pulmonary rehabilitation is an important element in the eventual success of any program. Patients with minimal functional limitations are not ideal candidates for rehabilitation as such patients may benefit little from programs designed to improve function. Furthermore, patients with mild disease may not justify the intense effort needed to maintain a viable program. Patients with the most severe degree of lung disease demonstrate significant psychologic improvement and increased exercise endurance after pulmonary rehabilitation. For instance, marked benefit is seen after intense rehabilitation efforts in patients awaiting lung transplantation and lung volume reduction surgery (124).

Patients with COPD who are on optimal medical therapy and who (a) continue to complain of dyspnea, (b) have had several emergency room visits or hospital admissions in the past year, (c) exhibit limited functional status, or (d) complain of impaired quality of life should be considered for a comprehensive rehabilitation program. Factors that may prevent the ultimate success of rehabilitation for the individual patient include the presence of disabling extrapulmonary diseases (i.e., severe heart failure, arthritis), very low educational level, lack of an emotional support system, and above all, poor motivation (124). The objectives of a pulmonary rehabilitation program are presented in Table 9.6.

TABLE 9.6. GOALS OF PULMONARY REHABILITATION

Reduce work of breathing
Improve pulmonary functions(?)
Normalize arterial blood gases
Alleviate dyspnea
Increase efficiency of energy utilization
Correct nutrition
Improve exercise performance and activities of daily living
Restore a positive outlook in patients
Improve emotional state
Decrease health-related costs
Improve survival

From Celli BR. Pulmonary rehabilitation for patients with advanced lung disease. *Clin Chest Med* 1997;18:521–534, with permission.

TABLE 9.7. RECOMMENDED COMPONENTS OF A CARDIOPULMONARY REHABILITATION PROGRAM

Patient and family education
Dyspnea assessment
Comprehensive exercise program
Nutritional assessment and support
Breathing retraining and expectoration techniques
Psychosocial support

From Lacasse Y, Guyatt GH, Goldstein RS. The components of a respiratory rehabilitation program: a systematic overview. *Chest* 1997;111(4):1077–1088, with permission.

Therapeutic Techniques

Because pulmonary rehabilitation is multimodal and multi-disciplinary, it is difficult to attribute improved global outcomes to the effects of individual components of a program. The basic elements of such a program include patient education, nutritional assessment, exercise training, breathing retraining, and psychosocial support (Table 9.7).

Patient Education

Education is a key factor in the routine care of the patient with advanced COPD. Many pulmonary patients have poor perceptions of their symptoms, lack understanding of their disease processes, and often practice inappropriate medication use (125). Instruction results in correct MDI use and even decreases the need for medications. Educational goals include having patients understand the basic pathophysiology of their disease, smoking cessation, and using medications properly. Patients who are educated about their disease generally demonstrate an increased ability to recognize and treat symptoms and develop practical ways of coping with disabling symptoms; they also manifest better adherence to the prescribed therapeutic regimen (1).

The educational program should be offered along with the other components of pulmonary rehabilitation, including physical reconditioning, nutritional assessment, and breathing retraining. Improvements in disease status, daily functional status, mental health, and quality of life in patients with COPD completing a relatively short (six to 12 hours) health education program cannot be demonstrated when other components of comprehensive care are not provided (126).

As part of patient education, the physician should explain the disease process and outline a management plan. The physician need not conduct the entire educational program, as studies have shown that nurses, respiratory therapists, physical therapists and other allied health personnel may be better than physicians at educating patients. These medical professionals often spend more time with the patient than does the physician.

Since adults vary in their learning styles, a variety of learning modalities should be made available, including printed materials (e.g., self-help programs for smoking cessation); videos, slides, or overheads for office and home use; didactic presentations; and group discussions. The patient should be encouraged to participate actively in the program, to maintain a healthy, active lifestyle, to obtain appropriate vaccines, and to avoid smoke and other irritants (1). Emotional support and encouragement are important, especially during periods of frustration and depression. The management team must accept the fact that some functional changes are irreversible; the goal is prevention rather than cure. In patients with advanced disease, the physical therapist or respiratory therapist may approach the patient about a living will or limited power of attorney. The physician must be available for advice about advance directives. Whenever possible, these issues should be discussed before the patient is hospitalized with acute respiratory failure.

Nutritional Assessment

About 25% of patients with COPD suffer from undernutrition (body weight less than 90% of ideal) (64). These patients have reduced respiratory muscle function and increased mortality. Even when receiving nutritional supplementation, many patients are unable to gain weight, perhaps related to underestimation of caloric needs or an inability to maintain adequate caloric intake. Dyspnea may play a role in limiting intake. In patients with chronic hypercapnia, excess production of carbon dioxide due to increased carbohydrate intake was once thought to increase P_aCO_2; however, recent studies have shown that this is not a problem unless the total caloric intake markedly exceeds caloric needs. Hypercapnic patients do not need to avoid carbohydrates, but should maintain a normal nutritious diet and optimum weight, eating foods they enjoy.

Exercise

Exercise is generally considered an important component of pulmonary rehabilitation programs. Reviews (123,127) of published studies of general exercise conditioning in chronic lung disease highlight consistent improvement in exercise endurance or maximum exercise tolerance. However, the optimal methods of training and the mechanisms underlying the improvements have not been clearly defined (122). Principles of exercise physiology derived from normal subjects or cardiac patients cannot be applied to patients with COPD due to the different limitations on exercise performance and coexisting problems of training in older patients.

The intensity of exercise training may be important, and recent reports suggest that high-intensity training in COPD is beneficial. In a study comparing the training response in patients with moderate COPD who performed high-intensity bicycle ergometry with a control group that trained at a lower intensity, the high-intensity group showed a greater decrease in lactate levels and heart rate at a given level of work and similar levels of oxygen consumption. The lower lactate levels resulted in less CO_2 generation from bicarbonate buffering and a lower ventilatory demand at any given workload (128).

Finally, it should be noted that exercise training is largely muscle-group-specific. Hence, it is unlikely that lower extremity bicycle or treadmill training will impact performance involving the arms. Indeed, a training program that involves both arm and leg exercise results in a greater improvement in activities of daily living than does a program limited to leg exercise (123). However, many studies have demonstrated benefit using arm training when compared to no training at all (124).

Breathing Retraining

Breathing retraining includes instruction in techniques of ventilatory muscle training, chest physiotherapy, diaphragmatic breathing, and pursed-lip breathing.

Respiratory muscle weakness from undernutrition, poor muscle mechanics, and chronic muscle stress is a common feature in advanced COPD. Ventilatory muscle training purports to enhance respiratory muscle function and potentially reduce the severity of breathlessness and perhaps improve exercise tolerance. One such attempt is the use of small, handheld devices that impose progressively increasing inspiratory resistance. However, reviews of such techniques have been unable to show clear benefit in the majority of patients (123,129). Unfortunately, only a minority of the studies actually imposed a sufficient training load (i.e., at least 30% of predicted maximal inspiratory pressure, or PI_{max}); in patients trained to 30% or more of PI_{max} measured clinical outcomes have shown some improvements in dyspnea and/or exercise tolerance (123). Therefore ventilatory muscle training may be considered in individual patients who remain symptomatic despite optimal therapy.

Many patients with COPD have abnormalities in lung clearance mechanisms that make them more susceptible to problems related to retained secretions (e.g., infection and atelectasis). Rehabilitation programs teach coughing and chest physiotherapy techniques for secretion control. However, the benefit of the individual techniques is difficult to determine, and many clinicians remain skeptical of their efficacy. Available evidence suggests that postural drainage and controlled coughing may be the most effective techniques (122), especially in patients who produce a large amount of sputum (over 30 mL per day). However, pulmonary function does not improve with any chest physical therapy maneuvers (124), so this modality is usually reserved for those patients with significant sputum production.

Diaphragmatic breathing is a maneuver in which the patient attempts to coordinate outward abdominal wall movement with inspiration and to slow expiration by pursed-lip breathing. Respiratory rate slows and, supposedly, tidal volume increases. In studies evaluating this technique, patients report subjective improvement, but objective results are mixed (122). In a recent study of patients with severe COPD studied before, during, and after diaphragmatic breathing training, no change in tidal volume or respiratory frequency was observed (130). Moreover, chest wall motion became discoordinated, mechanical efficiency of breathing declined, and the sensation of dyspnea increased.

In pursed-lip breathing, a technique often assumed naturally by some patients with COPD, the lips are tensed during expiration, resulting in prolongation of the expiratory phase. Pursed-lip breathing results in increased tidal volume, reduced respiratory rate, improved ventilation-perfusion matching, and increased arterial oxygen saturation as measured by pulse oximetry (122).

Psychosocial Support

Patients with COPD develop a variety of psychosocial symptoms that reflect their progressive feeling of hopelessness and their inability to cope with their disease. Depression is common. Successful pulmonary rehabilitation programs attend to the patient's psychosocial problems as well as physical ones. Patients who respond to rehabilitation, both early and long-term, have less severe psychologic symptoms (e.g., depression, anxiety, body preoccupation, fear of dyspnea) than do nonresponders (122). Family members and friends should be included in program activities so that they can understand and cope better with the patient's disease. Patients with severe psychological disorders may benefit from individual counseling and psychotherapy. Psychotropic drugs should be reserved for patients who have severe psychological dysfunction. As with education, psychosocial interventions alone (without the other components of rehabilitation) are insufficient (123).

Outcome Measures

One reason for the poor acceptance of pulmonary rehabilitation was the incomplete characterization of benefits achieved by such measures. Older studies reported little or no change in traditional measures such as FEV_1 or exercise capacity. However, new measuring tools have been developed that allow more insight into the gains acquired: disease-specific quality-of-life measures, validated questionnaires, health care resource cost studies, and the like. A recent meta-analysis of clinical trials of pulmonary rehabilitation in COPD examined results from 14 randomized controlled trials involving more than 400 patients (130). The study showed that rehabilitation, when compared to "usual care," improved health-related quality of life (as measured by specific instruments such as dyspnea indices, the St. George's respiratory questionnaire) and functional exercise capacity (measured by walking distances, dyspnea scores, patient-reported sense of well-being). Of interest were the findings that while quality-of-life indices were consistently improved in the rehabilitation group, exercise capacity results were rather heterogeneous, suggesting that the traditional methods of gauging improvement may not capture all benefits gained from rehabilitation (131). Unfortunately, many rehabilitation programs continue to rely solely on laboratory measures of exercise to grade efficacy of their efforts (132).

Older uncontrolled studies suggested that pulmonary rehabilitation decreased total hospital stay and recurrent hospitalization rates in COPD patients (133). However, results from more recent controlled studies have been less optimistic. More studies of the impact of rehabilitation on health care resource utilization are ongoing. One such trend is the great interest in delivering rehabilitation programs to patients in an outpatient setting or even at home (134,135).

Oxygen Therapy

In 1995, about 616,000 patients in the United States were treated with supplemental home oxygen at an estimated annual cost of $1.4 billion (136). The value of long-term supplemental oxygen therapy in hypoxemic patients with severe COPD has been demonstrated in major controlled trials. In the National Heart, Lung and Blood Institute's Nocturnal Oxygen Therapy Trial (NOTT) (137), patients with COPD and hypoxemia while breathing room air (P_aO_2 of less than 55 mm Hg) were randomly assigned to receive oxygen for either 12 hours a day (nocturnal group) or 24 hours a day (continuous group); all patients received oxygen during sleep. At 26 months, overall mortality in the continuous group (who actually received oxygen for an average of 19 hours a day) was approximately one-half that of the nocturnal group. In addition, morbidity in the continuous group was less than that of the nocturnal group. These findings, along with those reported in a study from the British Medical Research Council (138), serve as the basis for current recommendations regarding supplemental oxygen use in patients with COPD (see below).

Indications for Oxygen Therapy

Indications for long-term supplemental oxygen include a resting P_aO_2 of 55 mm Hg or less, or evidence of tissue hypoxia and organ damage, such as cor pulmonale, secondary polycythemia, edema from right heart failure, or impaired mental status. Evaluation of patients for nocturnal oxygen use should also be considered, since patients with COPD may have episodic arterial desaturation during sleep in the absence of daytime hypoxemia. These episodes are not always associated with sleep disturbances and may be related to abnormalities in gas exchange. In a study evaluating the long-term effects of nocturnal oxygen administration in patients with COPD who had nocturnal hypoxemia and a daytime P_aO_2 of 60 mm Hg or more, a group treated with nasal oxygen was compared with another receiving compressed air via nasal cannula (139). Over a three-year period, mean pulmonary artery pressure decreased by 3.7

mm Hg in patients receiving oxygen and increased by 3.9 mm Hg in those receiving compressed air ($p < 0.02$). Mortality was similar in the two groups. Finally, patients with COPD who are normoxemic at rest may become hypoxemic during exercise; exercise capacity and endurance may be improved with oxygen supplementation.

Techniques of Administration of Supplemental Oxygen

Home oxygen can be supplied using an oxygen concentrator, a compressed oxygen cylinder, or a source of liquid oxygen. The most cost-effective and reliable method is the oxygen concentrator, since it requires only an electrical source and periodic maintenance; backup sources of oxygen, such as a cylinder or liquid oxygen, should be available for extenuating circumstances, e.g., electrical power failure. Liquid oxygen and compressed oxygen cylinders permit patient mobility.

Oxygen is usually delivered by nasal cannula at continuous flows of 0.5 to 4 L per minute. Oxygen-conserving devices use reservoirs that allow delivery of a higher F_IO_2 at lower flows. The goal of oxygen therapy is to achieve a P_aO_2 of 60 mm Hg; using higher flows to achieve a significantly higher P_aO_2 will accomplish little clinically. The patient should be reevaluated with arterial blood gases after one, six, and 12 months; follow-up arterial blood gases are important, since about 20% of patients initially eligible for supplemental oxygen no longer need it following aggressive bronchodilator therapy (137).

Other techniques of oxygen administration have been developed in attempts to reduce supplemental oxygen requirements and improve cosmesis. Transtracheal oxygen delivery via a small-bore catheter offers several advantages over use of nasal cannula, including a 50% reduction in supplemental oxygen requirement, decreased dyspnea, improved exercise tolerance, and decreased rate of hospitalization (140). In a comparison of clinical outcomes in 20 stable patients with COPD who received oxygen for six months either by nasal cannula or transtracheal catheter, those treated with the transtracheal technique had reduced flow requirements, increased 12-minute walk distance, and decreased hospital days (141). Minor complications of the transtracheal technique include catheter displacement and mucus ball formation at the catheter tip.

A number of factors may be operative to account for the beneficial clinical and arterial blood gas effects achieved with transtracheal oxygen. For example, the oxygen "jet" may flush CO_2 from the upper airway; in addition, dead-space volume is reduced. Furthermore, the trachea acts as a reservoir, reducing the amount of supplemental oxygen wasted during expiration. Other potential benefits of the technique include better patient compliance and avoidance of hypoxemia during obstructive sleep disturbances, since the nose and glottis are bypassed. Since clothing can easily cover the device, patient satisfaction is increased.

Management of Acute Exacerbations

Acute decompensation of COPD is characterized by increased dyspnea, cough, and purulent sputum production. The decision to hospitalize a patient with an acute exacerbation is usually based upon the physician's subjective interpretation of clinical symptoms, including severity of dyspnea, short-term response to therapeutic efforts, and the presence of other conditions, such as bronchitis, pneumonia, or other comorbidities. Notably, up to 28% of patients with an acute exacerbation of COPD who are discharged from an Emergency Department (rather than admitted) have recurrent symptoms within 14 days (142); 17% of patients discharged after Emergency Department management will relapse and require hospitalization (1). The American Thoracic Society has devised guidelines for hospitalization (Table 9.8) and ICU admission of patients with an acute exacerbation of COPD (Table 9.9) (1).

Mortality rates for patients who require hospitalization are substantial. In one study of 590 patients, the mortality rate was 14.4%. Using multivariate, logistic regression analysis, the investigators identified several independent variables that predicted mortality: increased age, an alveolar-arterial oxygen gradient greater than 41 mm Hg, and presence of atrial fibrillation or ventricular dysrhythmias (143).

Pharmacologic therapy in an acute exacerbation of COPD centers on the use of β-agonists. Aerosol delivery is the most effective route of administration; delivery using

TABLE 9.8. INDICATIONS FOR HOSPITALIZATION OF PATIENTS WITH COPD

- Acute exacerbation (increased dyspnea, cough, or sputum production), plus one or more of the following:
  * Inadequate response to outpatient management
  * In a patient previously mobile, inability to ambulate due to dyspnea
  * Inability to eat or sleep due to dyspnea
  * Inadequate home care resources
  * Serious comorbid condition
  * Prolonged progressive symptoms before emergency visit
  * Altered mentation
  * Worsening hypoxemia
  * New or worsening hypercapnia
- New or worsening cor pulmonale unresponsive to outpatient management
- Planned invasive surgical or diagnostic procedure requiring analgesics or sedatives that may worsen pulmonary function
- Comorbid condition, e.g., severe steroid myopathy or acute vertebral compression fractures, that has worsened pulmonary function

Adapted from Celli BR, Snider GL, Heffner J, et al. Standards for the diagnosis and care of patients with chronic obstructive pulmonary disease. *Am J Respir Crit Care Med* 1995;152:S77–S120, with permission.

TABLE 9.9. INDICATIONS FOR ICU ADMISSION OF PATIENTS WITH ACUTE EXACERBATION OF COPD

- Severe dyspnea that responds inadequately to initial emergency therapy
- Confusion or lethargy
- Respiratory muscle fatigue (especially paradoxical diaphragmatic motion)
- Persistent or worsening hypoxemia despite supplemental oxygen or severe/worsening respiratory acidosis (pH under 7.30)
- Need for noninvasive or invasive assisted mechanical ventilation

Adapted from Celli BR, Snider GL, Heffner J, et al. Standards for the diagnosis and care of patients with chronic obstructive pulmonary disease. *Am J Respir Crit Care Med* 1995;152:S77–S120, with permission.

a metered dose inhaler (MDI) or nebulizer has been employed. Studies confirm the equal efficacy of two techniques (144). The safety and efficacy of continuous nebulization of β-agonists have not been established in COPD (1). The slow onset of action of ipratropium bromide has relegated this drug to a minor role in the acute setting; however, its apparent additive effects with β-agonists (100) should be considered. Ipratropium bromide is available in the United States in an MDI and as a solution for nebulization. High doses are generally well tolerated; an upper dosage limit has not been established. Ipratropium bromide may be combined with a β-agonist for nebulizer delivery.

In addition to β-agonists, theophylline has been used in the management of acute exacerbations of COPD. The efficacy of theophylline (or aminophylline) in this setting is uncertain (101). If used, theophylline levels should be monitored closely to avoid overdosage. Serum levels of eight to 12 μg per mL are appropriate for most patients, although some patients may tolerate higher levels (up to 18 to 20 μg per mL).

Corticosteroids

Controlled, double-blinded studies evaluating the effects of corticosteroids in the treatment of exacerbations of COPD have been relatively few in number; the results are conflicting (145). In a double-blind, randomized, placebo-controlled parallel study of 44 consecutive patients hospitalized for an exacerbation of COPD and acute respiratory insufficiency, patients received intravenous methylprednisolone (0.5 mg per kg every six hours for 72 hours) or placebo (146). All patients were given intravenous aminophylline, inhaled isoproterenol, supplemental oxygen, and antibiotics. The corticosteroid-treated group showed a statistically significant increase in postbronchodilator FEV_1 at every six to eight-hour time point from 12 to 72 hours; 12 of the 22 patients receiving methylprednisolone had a 40% or greater improvement in prebronchodilator FEV_1 by 72 hours, compared with only three of 21 receiving placebo ($p < 0.05$). No differences were noted in arterial blood gases. In a recent controlled study (147), no differences in FEV_1 and hospitalization rates were noted among 96 patients with COPD who were randomized to receive either 100 mg intravenous methylprednisolone or placebo during acute exacerbations. In the largest study to date (SSCOPE—Systemic Steroids in COPD Exacerbations), 271 patients from 25 Veterans Affairs medical centers were randomly enrolled in a double-blind, placebo-controlled trial examining the efficacy of systemic glucocorticoids (given for two or eight weeks) for acute COPD exacerbations (148). Corticosteroid-treated patients had a mild but statistically significant increase in FEV_1 (approximately 0.10 L, $p < 0.05$) within the first day, shorter hospital stays (8.5 days versus 9.7 days for placebo; $p = 0.03$) and at least 20% fewer treatment failures at 30 and 90 days. However, these benefits appeared to dissipate over time, so that no differences between patients treated with corticosteroids or placebo were evident. The eight-week corticosteroid regimen was not superior to the two-week regimen. Patients who received glucocorticoids were more likely to have hyperglycemia requiring therapy than did those receiving placebo (15% versus 4%, $p = 0.002$). This trial seems to argue for the use of intravenous corticosteroids in acute exacerbations severe enough to require hospitalization, followed by a short (two-week) course of oral prednisone.

Treatment of Infection

Bronchial infection is the most common precipitating factor for an acute exacerbation of COPD. *Streptococcus pneumoniae* and *Hemophilus influenzae* are the most common pathogenic bacteria isolated in the sputum of patients experiencing an acute exacerbation. However, the same bacteria can be isolated from stable patients. Thus there has been an ongoing debate over the efficacy of antibiotic therapy during acute flares. The most comprehensive study addressing this issue is a randomized, double-blinded, crossover trial in which 362 exacerbations in 173 outpatients were treated (149). Ten-day courses of trimethoprim-sulfamethoxazole (one double-strength tablet twice daily), amoxicillin (250 mg four times daily), or doxycycline (200 mg initially, followed by 100 mg twice daily) were administered. Patients treated with antibiotics had a higher clinical success rate—defined as resolution of all acute symptoms—within 21 days than those receiving placebo. Patients receiving placebo were two times more likely to experience deterioration of symptoms. There was no difference in efficacy among the three antibiotic regimens. Peak expiratory flow rates (measured on day 6 of the trial) were significantly more improved in antibiotic-treated patients. The incidence of side effects was similar in patients treated with antibiotics and those receiving placebo. Based on these findings, antibiotics appear to have a beneficial effect in patients experiencing an acute exacerbation of COPD. Indeed, a recent meta-analysis of the randomized trials of antibiotics in exacerbations of COPD published in the English literature from 1955 to 1994 confirms a small but statistically and clinically significant improvement with antibiotic therapy in this patient population—especially for those hospitalized with severe disease (manifested by low peak expiratory flow) (150). (Figure 9.9).

Other Measures

Supplemental oxygen should be administered to most patients with an exacerbation of COPD, since deterioration usually leads to increased ventilation-perfusion inequalities and worsening hypoxemia. Sputum may be tenacious and copious, so adequate hydration should be provided. Two to 3 liters of fluid daily should be supplied by mouth or parenterally, unless cardiac or renal insufficiency is of concern.

Prognosis in Severe Chronic Obstructive Pulmonary Disease

A number of factors are identified as associated with the clinical course and survival in patients with COPD (Table 9.10) (151–161). Unfortunately, few have evaluated the course and functional status of patients with severe COPD following hospitalization for an acute episode of COPD (162,163). Recently, Connors and fellow SUPPORT investigators reported on quality of life, functional status, and short- and long-term survival in 1,016 patients who were hospitalized for acute exacerbations of severe COPD (164). Their results indicate a rather grim prognosis in this population of patients following recovery from hypercapnic respiratory failure. While 89% of the patients recovered from the acute episode and were discharged from the hospital, half died within the two years posthospitalization. Furthermore, functional status was poor in the survivors, and six months posthospitalization, only 26% of the patients were able to report a good, very good, or excellent quality of life. Factors that affected survival following the episode of acute respiratory failure included severity of illness, body mass index, age, prior functional status, and the presence of congestive heart failure, low serum albumin, hypoxemia, or cor pulmonale.

Advance Directives

In view of the poor long-term survival in this group of patients with severe COPD, it is incumbent upon the physician, as well as the family and other caregivers, to discuss with the patient his or her wishes for acute and long-term care. This should be done early on, when the patient is alert and able to render rational decisions. Patients who survive an episode of mechanical ventilation have a substantial risk

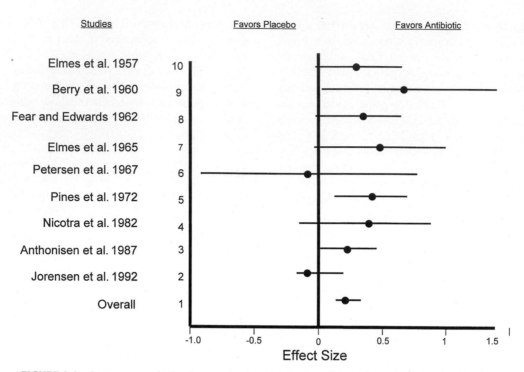

Studies | Favors Placebo | Favors Antibiotic

FIGURE 9.9. Outcome results in nine randomized trials of antibiotic therapy versus placebo therapy for patients with acute exacerbations of chronic bronchitis. An overall estimate of outcome results for all nine studies is shown at the bottom. Effect size indicates the differences between the mean outcome in the antibiotic and placebo groups divided by the pooled SD. Dots represent point estimates, while horizontal lines denote 95% confidence intervals. (Reproduced with permission from Saint S, Bent S, Vittinghoff E, et al. Antibiotics in chronic obstructive pulmonary disease exacerbations. A meta-analysis. *JAMA* 1995;273:957–960 based on the following studies: Elmes, PC, King TKC, Langlands JHM, et al. Value of ampicillin in the hospital treatment of exacerbations of chronic bronchitis. *Br Med J* 1965;2:904–908; Nicotra MB, Rivera M, Awe RJ. Antibiotic therapy of acute exacerbations of chronic bronchitis. *Ann Intern Med* 1982;97:18–21; Elmes PC, Fletcher CM, Dutton AAC. Prophylactic use of oxytetracycline for exacerbations of chronic bronchitis. *Br Med J* 1957;2:1272–1275; Fear EC, Edwards G. Antibiotic regimes in chronic bronchitis. *Br J Dis Chest* 1962;56:153–162; Anthonisen NR, Manfreda J, Warren CPW, et al. Antibiotic therapy in exacerbations of chronic obstructive pulmonary disease. *Ann Intern Med* 1987;106:196–204; Berry DG, Fry J, Hindley CP, et al. Exacerbations of chronic bronchitis treatment with oxytetracycline. *Lancet* 1960;1:137–139; Jorgensen AF, Coolidge J, Pedersen PA, et al. Amoxicillin in treatment of acute uncomplicated exacerbations of chronic bronchitis. *Scan J Prim Health Care* 1992;10:7–11; Petersen ES, Esmann V, Honcke P, et al. A controlled study of the effect of treatment on chronic bronchitis: an evaluation using pulmonary function tests. *Acta Med Scand* 1967;182:293–305; Pines A, Raafat H, Greenfield JSB, et al. Antibiotic regimens in moderately ill patients with purulent exacerbations of chronic bronchitis. *Br J Dis Chest* 1972;66:107–115.

of requiring care in a nursing home or other skilled care facility, and are subject to readmission to the hospital within the subsequent six months. They are likely to be dependent on others for activities of daily living, and may consider themselves a burden to their loved ones. The physician should discuss these facts with the patient and his or her family, and allow them to arrive at a carefully considered plan for future care. The determination of an advance directive is an important part of the care of the patient. A copy should be placed in the chart and should be made available to health providers when the patient is hospitalized.

TABLE 9.10. FACTORS ASSOCIATED WITH CLINICAL COURSE AND SURVIVAL IN PATIENTS WITH COPD

Cigarette smoking
Passive smoking exposure
Age
Rate of decline of FEV_1
Hypoxemia
Pulmonary artery pressure
Resting heart rate
Weight loss
Reversibility of airflow obstruction

BRONCHIECTASIS

Bronchiectasis is a condition anatomically defined by chronic, irreversible dilation and distortion of the bronchi caused by inflammatory destruction of the muscular and elastic components of the bronchial walls. Laennec described the postmortem appearance of bronchiectasis in 1826; his descriptions were incorporated over a century later into a contemporary classification system of bronchiectasis introduced by Reid in 1950 (165). This scheme divides bronchiectasis into cylindrical, varicose, and saccular (or cystic) varieties. Although this classification is helpful in roentgenographic and pathologic descriptions of the disorder, there appear to be very few, if any, epidemiologic, prognostic, or therapeutic distinctions among the various anatomic forms of bronchiectasis. The clinical utility of such classification systems is therefore minimal at best.

Bronchiectasis is best classified according to the underlying cause or predisposing factor. Bronchiectasis is not a discrete disease entity, but rather represents the possible result of several different diseases or insults. Some conditions associated with the development of bronchiectasis are listed in Table 9.11. The clinical features of a case of bronchiectasis such as the severity, distribution (localized versus diffuse), prognosis, and therapeutic potential are determined by the underlying cause. Another specific cause of bronchiecta-

TABLE 9.11. CONDITIONS ASSOCIATED WITH THE DEVELOPMENT OF BRONCHIECTASIS

Proximal airway obstruction
  Foreign body aspiration
  Middle lobe syndrome
  Benign airway tumors
Diffuse airway injury
  Inhalation of noxious gases (e.g., anhydrous ammonia, sulfur dioxide)
  Aspiration
Postinfection
  Bacterial pneumonia
  Tuberculosis
  Pertussis
  Measles
  Influenza
Genetic disorders
  Cystic fibrosis
  α_1-Antitrypsin deficiency (?)
Abnormal host defense
  Ciliary dyskinesia (e.g., Kartagener's syndrome)
  Humoral immunodeficiency
Other conditions
  Allergic bronchopulmonary aspergillosis
  Yellow nail syndrome
  Congenital cartilage deficiency (Williams-Campbell's syndrome)
  Tracheobronchomegaly (Mounier-Kuhn's syndrome)
Idiopathic

sis—cystic fibrosis—is discussed in this chapter, whereas allergic bronchopulmonary aspergillosis is discussed elsewhere.

Clinical Presentation

The hallmark of bronchiectasis is the production of large quantities of purulent and often foul-smelling sputum. The quantification of daily sputum production may serve as a helpful indicator of disease exacerbations or response to therapy. Ellis and colleagues (166) categorized less than 10 mL of sputum daily as indicating mild bronchiectasis, 10 to 150 mL as indicating moderate bronchiectasis, and greater than 150 mL as indicating severe bronchiectasis. Systemic manifestations of persistent infection—including fever, weight loss, and digital clubbing—may occur as well, but are now much less frequently observed in the antibiotic era.

Bronchiectasis is not always associated with sputum production, however. So-called "dry bronchiectasis" (to distinguish it from the more typical "wet" variety) may occur, especially when the involved area of the lung is limited to the upper lobes (such as with prior tuberculosis infection), presumably due to the beneficial effect of dependent drainage.

Hemoptysis is frequent in bronchiectasis and occurs more commonly in the dry variety than in the wet variety (167). Although hemoptysis is usually relatively mild, occurring most commonly as blood streaking of purulent sputum, the possibility of massive hemoptysis from dilated bronchial arteries or bronchial-pulmonary anastomoses under systemic pressure is ever present. In the preantibiotic era, hemoptysis accounted for about 7% of deaths (168) but was not the cause of a single fatality among 62 deaths analyzed in 1969 (169).

With modern treatment approaches, the average age at death is about 55 years (169). Most patients with bronchiectasis succumb to cor pulmonale, the underlying disease, or an incidental cause, rather than infectious complications.

Evaluation

Roentgenographic Studies

The plain chest film is unreliable in detecting and determining the anatomic distribution of bronchiectasis (170). Although patients with bronchiectasis rarely have an entirely normal chest radiograph, the typical findings (increase in size and number of bronchovascular markings) are quite nonspecific. In more severe forms of the disease, cystic spaces can be found and raise the suspicion that bronchiectasis is present. Bronchography is the traditional "gold standard" technique for assessing bronchiectasis. This method can be easily and safely performed via fiber-optic bronchoscopy using oily contrast agents. However, the advent of high-resolution CT techniques and discontinued production of some bronchography contrast agents has hampered the use of bronchography in the last decade. For example, in one large referral center, only one to five bronchograms are performed annually to evaluate or diagnose bronchiectasis (171). Bronchography has no role in the routine diagnosis or evaluation of bronchiectasis, because there is usually no impact on therapeutic approach. Computed tomography using thin contiguous sections (2 to 4 mm sections at 5 mm intervals) has a very high sensitivity and specificity in the diagnosis of bronchiectasis (170).

Bronchoscopy

Bronchoscopy is helpful in evaluating the proximal airways for lesions (obstructing tumors, foreign bodies, etc.) and for assessing the cause and localizing the source of hemoptysis.

Ancillary Evaluation

With the decrease in pyogenic infections of the lungs, bronchiectasis is now more commonly due to abnormal host defenses such as is seen with cystic fibrosis, immunoglobulin deficiency states, and dyskinetic cilia syndromes (172). Cystic fibrosis is reviewed elsewhere in this chapter.

Congenital or acquired humoral immunodeficiency has long been recognized as a cause of recurrent sinopulmonary infections and bronchiectasis. The most common humoral immunodeficient state associated with bronchiectasis is panhypogammaglobulinemia, which can be detected easily by measurement of serum immunoglobulin levels. Identification of patients with such a deficiency is important, because replacement therapy may be effective in reducing the frequency and severity of infectious episodes and their sequelae. Recently, it has become apparent that patients with selective immunoglobulin deficiencies may be at risk for bronchiectasis. In particular, abnormalities in IgG subclasses may be significant. Absence of IgG_4, even with no abnormalities in other IgG subclasses or other immunoglobulins, is associated with bronchiectasis (173,174). Reductions of IgG_2 and IgG_3, with or without IgA deficiency, are also associated with recurrent sinopulmonary infections (175,176). It is not entirely clear whether a selective deficiency of IgA is an independent risk factor for bronchiectasis. One large series of IgA-deficient patients made no mention of bronchiectasis (177). Because IgA deficiency is relatively common (about 1 in 700 individuals), it is unlikely that this condition confers a major risk for bronchiectasis.

In the 1930s, Kartagener reported patients with a triad of *situs inversus,* recurrent sinusitis, and bronchiectasis. It is now apparent that such patients, as well as many others who do not have *situs inversus,* share a defect in ciliary structure that renders the cilia nonfunctional. This defect has been termed the immotile cilia syndrome (178). In addition to sinopulmonary infections, male infertility due to immotile sperm is an important clinical hallmark. It is likely that variations of this syndrome will be identified; the term dyskinetic cilia syndrome is gaining favor with the increasing recognition that in many patients the cilia are in fact motile, albeit with abnormal motions. Of interest is that syndromes of male infertility (due to obstructive azoospermia) and recurrent respiratory infection have been identified that appear to be distinct from both cystic fibrosis and the dyskinetic cilia syndromes (179,180). Diagnosis of the various syndromes associated with bronchiectasis, sinusitis, and male infertility may require evaluation of biopsies of the testis and the mucosa of the bronchi or nasopharynx. Electron microscopy may be needed to detect ultrastructural abnormalities. Generally, such a complete evaluation is not required in routine clinical practice.

Treatment

Medical Management

The general therapeutic approach to bronchiectasis includes antibiotics and chest physical therapy with postural drainage and chest clapping. Antibiotic therapy should be guided through the use of sputum Gram stain and cultures. Despite the early promise of recombinant DNAse, which may lyse the DNA that causes sputum to be viscous (180–182), recent clinical trials have shown disappointing results.

Surgical Therapy

Surgical therapy is indicated in bronchiectasis only when recurrent and refractory clinical symptoms are due to a focal area of disease involvement. Full-lung imaging, either by high-resolution CT or, less commonly, bilateral full bronchograms, should usually be performed prior to consideration of surgical resection to ensure that significant diffuse bronchiectasis does not exist. Massive hemoptysis is a clear indication for surgery, but bronchial artery angiography and selective embolization may be considered instead, especially in patients whose suitability for surgery is poor (183).

CYSTIC FIBROSIS

Cystic fibrosis (CF) is the most common fatal inherited disease in whites. In the white population, about 5% of individuals carry the gene, and the disease occurs about once in every 2,500 live births (184). Cystic fibrosis is inherited as a simple autosomal recessive trait. The main pathophysiologic abnormality in cystic fibrosis is a defect in electrolyte transport. Decreased secretion of chloride into the airway lumen and increased sodium reabsorption from the airway lumen lead to a decrease in water content and increased viscosity of airway secretions (185).

A milestone was reached in 1989 with the identification of the cystic fibrosis gene (186). The classic cystic fibrosis phenotype, characterized by diagnosis at childhood, pancreatic insufficiency, and meconium ileus, is due to a mutation resulting in the loss of a phenylalanine residue at codon 508, hence its designation as ΔF508 (184). This mutation is responsible for 70% of all CF mutations, and results in an alteration in the secondary and tertiary structure of the cystic fibrosis transmembrane conductance regulator (CFTR) protein, which is thought to represent a chloride channel (184). About 170 other mutations of the CFTR gene account for the remaining 30%. The discovery of the cystic fibrosis gene and the ability to detect the common CFTR mutations now allow the routine screening of 33 mutations and the detection of 95% of carriers, and open the avenue of genetic counseling for couples at risk (184). Another consequence of the discovery of the CF gene has been the development of the first animal model for cystic fibrosis (187).

Although cystic fibrosis is typically diagnosed in infancy or early childhood, a recent review of 142 patients found that 5% were diagnosed between 16 and 30 years of age (188). Less commonly, the diagnosis is made as late as 35 years of age (189,190). While the correlation of genotype with phenotype is often imprecise, this variability may be ascribed to mutations outside the common ΔF508 locus. Milder mutations appear to be dominant in defining the phenotype of a compound heterozygote (184), but the genotype cannot be used to predict the severity of pulmonary disease (191).

Among the patients diagnosed after childhood, respiratory symptoms are frequently the major manifestation of the disease. Therefore, it is clearly important for pulmonary physicians, in particular, to have an awareness of cystic fibrosis and to be facile in its diagnosis.

Clinical Manifestations

The clinical manifestations are protean and are variably expressed from patient to patient. All organ systems that have exocrine gland function may be affected, including the exocrine pancreas, the small intestine, the biliary tract, the paranasal sinuses, the uterine cervix, the salivary glands, and the male reproductive tract. In young children, gastrointestinal problems often predominate. Meconium ileus occurs in 5% to 10% of newborns with cystic fibrosis. Clinical evidence of pancreatic insufficiency, including steatorrhea and failure to thrive, occurs in 85% of affected children but is a lesser problem for adults. Table 9.12 lists some clinical findings that should raise the suspicion that cystic fibrosis is present in the adult patient.

TABLE 9.12. CLUES TO CYSTIC FIBROSIS IN ADULTS

Respiratory
  Atypical asthma or unexplained airflow obstruction
  Chronic bronchitis (cough and sputum)
  Mucoid *Pseudomonas aeruginosa* in sputum
  Pneumothorax
  Nasal polyps
  Sinusitis
  Bronchiectasis
Gastrointestinal
  Biliary cirrhosis
  Pancreatitis
  Cholelithiasis
  Fecal impaction or intussusception
Other
  Infertility (azoospermia in males)
  Clubbing

Pulmonary Manifestations

Pulmonary manifestations of cystic fibrosis include cough, sputum production, wheezing, and intermittent radiographic infiltrates. As the disease progresses, mucoid strains of *Pseudomonas aeruginosa* often appear in the sputum. Such a finding is an important clue to the underlying diagnosis, but it is not entirely specific because mucoid *Pseudomonas* is also found in patients with bronchiectasis not caused by cystic fibrosis (192). Upper respiratory tract manifestations include nasal polyps (45% of adults) and radiographic evidence of sinusitis (90% of adults) (190).

The chest roentgenogram is normal in only about 2% of adults with cystic fibrosis. Many patients show only hyperinflation or increased bronchovascular markings (193,194). More advanced disease reveals evidence of bronchiectasis, including ring shadows and cysts, and mucoid impaction, seen as branching, fingerlike shadows. Bronchiectatic changes tend to occur first in the right upper lobe, followed by the left upper lobe and the right middle lobe (190,195). The "end-stage" chest roentgenogram reveals bronchiectasis, large cystic lesions, fibrotic areas, and hyperinflation.

Pulmonary function tests almost always reveal an obstructive impairment (188). The tests of small-airway function are most sensitive to the early changes of cystic fibrosis, correlating with the pathologic findings showing that the initial lesion is in the peripheral airways. As the disease worsens, large-airway obstruction (including a decline in FEV_1), elevation of arterial P_{CO_2}, and cor pulmonale occur.

Diagnosis

Sweat Chloride Test

In most instances, the diagnosis of cystic fibrosis is readily made by the presence of an elevated sweat chloride concentration (greater than 60 mEq per L) in conjunction with a clinical picture of typical pulmonary and gastrointestinal manifestations (196). The sweat chloride test involves collection of sweat via pilocarpine iontophoresis. The use of a standardized methodology is important to avoid false-positive or false-negative results. Up to 40% of patients referred to cystic fibrosis centers may have had inaccurate previous testing (197). One cause of faulty values is failure to obtain an adequate sweat collection of at least 100 mg in 45 minutes.

Atypical or Difficult Cases

Clinicians need to be aware that an elevated sweat chloride level can occur in conditions other than cystic fibrosis, including hypothyroidism, hypoparathyroidism, adrenal insufficiency, nephrogenic diabetes insipidus, and glycogen storage diseases (197). Fortunately, these disorders are readily distinguished from cystic fibrosis on clinical grounds.

More problematic is the fact that a small number of patients with cystic fibrosis have sweat chloride concentrations less than 60 mEq per L, and a small number of adults without cystic fibrosis have sweat chloride concentrations above 60 mEq per L. It is estimated that 1% to 2% of cystic fibrosis patients have values between 50 and 60 mEq per L, and that one in 1,000 of such patients will have values less than 50 mEq per L (195,196,198). There has also been one recent report of siblings with a demonstrable mutation of the CFTR gene and mild disease with normal sweat electrolyte levels (199).

Boat has proposed criteria to help the clinician diagnose or exclude cystic fibrosis in the borderline or atypical situation (Table 9.13) (197). A DNA probe specific for the currently identified mutations of the CFTR gene can be used to clarify difficult diagnoses.

Treatment

The prognosis of cystic fibrosis patients improved dramatically between 1940, when the median survival was about two years (197), and 1992, when the median survival reached about 29 years (184,200). The projected survival by actuarial methods for a CF child born today is 40 years (184). Although enhanced diagnosis of mild or atypical cases probably accounts for a portion of this improvement, comprehensive and aggressive multidisciplinary management has undoubtedly contributed in a major way to the improved outlook. Nevertheless, most of the approaches currently used have not been tested in controlled trials. The major goals of treatment are to improve nutrition, control infection, promote clearing of mucus, and optimize psychosocial factors. The recent discovery of the cystic fibrosis gene and the abnormal CFTR product opens the prospects of gene therapy, studies of which are currently under way (184).

Gene Therapy

In April 1993, the NHLBI announced the start of the first gene therapy trials for treating cystic fibrosis. The gene therapy technique under study involves the instillation into the airway of an adenovirus containing the normal human gene for CFTR with the goal of transfecting the host CF patient's respiratory epithelial cells. Resultant expression of the normal gene is hoped to compensate for the abnormal gene. Periodic administration of the modified adenovirus may be necessary to maintain the benefit (119,184).

Correction of Abnormal Salt Transport

Amiloride (a potassium-sparing diuretic) can block the uptake of sodium from the airway by respiratory epithelium, resulting in an increased mucus water content and improved clearance of secretions. Aerosolized amiloride has been shown to slow the deterioration in pulmonary function in moderately affected CF patients (201).

Similarly, triphosphate nucleotides (ATP or uridine triphosphate) applied to the apical surface of respiratory epithelium result in a chloride efflux, perhaps mediated through the P2 nucleotide receptor. Clinical trials of aerosolized nucleotides are being designed (202).

Decrease Viscosity of Airway Mucus

The presence of polymerized DNA from degenerating leukocytes significantly increases the viscosity of airway secretions. The use of aerosolized recombinant DNAse has been

---

TABLE 9.13. CRITERIA FOR THE DIAGNOSIS OF CYSTIC FIBROSIS IN ATYPICAL CASES[a]

Major criteria
   Sweat chloride over 60 mEq/L before age 20 (over 80 mEq/L in adults)
   Chronic obstructive lung disease with *Pseudomonas* infection of airways
   Unexplained obstructive azoospermia (confirmed by scrotal exploration and testicular biopsy)
Minor criteria
   Sweat chloride over 40 mEq/L (over 60 mEq/L in adults)
   Family history of classic cystic fibrosis
   Exocrine pancreas insufficiency before age 20
   Unexplained chronic obstructive lung disease before age 20
   Unexplained azoospermia (without scrotal exploration and testicular biopsy)

[a] The diagnosis is established by the presence of two major criteria or by one major and one minor finding. The two criteria used in diagnosis must involve different organ systems.
From Stern RC, Boat TF, Doershuk CF. Obstructive azoospermia as a diagnostic criterion for the cystic fibrosis syndrome. *Lancet* 1982;1: 1401–1404, with permission.

shown to be well tolerated and to result in significant improvement in lung function (181,182).

Modulation of Airway Inflammation

A recent study has shown that aerosolized leukoprotease inhibitor results in a significant decrease in interleukin-8, neutrophil elastase levels, and neutrophil numbers on the respiratory epithelial lining fluid of cystic fibrosis patients. This may result in decreased damage to epithelial cells (203).

Alternate-day corticosteroid administration decreased hospitalizations due to exacerbations of lung disease over a four-year period in a double-blind controlled study (204). The routine use of corticosteroids cannot be advocated at the current time, however. The preliminary results of a multicenter trial currently under way suggest a significant risk of adverse side effects (glucose abnormalities, cataracts, and growth retardation), requiring discontinuation of the drug in 30% of patients receiving high-dose (2 mg per kg) alternate-day prednisone therapy (205).

Control of Infections

Four bacterial species predominate as causes of lung infection in cystic fibrosis patients: *Staphylococcus aureus, Haemophilus influenzae, Pseudomonas aeruginosa,* and *Pseudomonas cepacia* (206,207). Nontuberculous mycobacteria (208,209), and viral infections (210–213) have also been implicated in exacerbations of cystic fibrosis.

Several aspects of antibiotic therapy in cystic fibrosis patients remain controversial. Specifically, a firm consensus is lacking with regard to indications for antibiotic therapy, the type of antibiotics to be used, or the route of administration. The interested reader is referred to a comprehensive review of this topic (214). The choice of antibiotics ideally should be based on results of sputum culture and sensitivity testing (206). In most instances, appropriate antibiotic therapy for *S. aureus* and *H. influenzae* will eliminate the organism from the sputum, at least temporarily. Suggested drugs for treating *H. influenzae* include trimethoprim-sulfamethoxazole, chloramphenicol, ampicillin (207), ampicillin-sulbactam, and ticarcillin-clavulanate. If *S. aureus* is present, the choice may include a cephalosporin, clindamycin, chloramphenicol, or a semisynthetic penicillin. *Pseudomonas* species are never completely eradicated from the sputum once chronic colonization and infection are initiated. Treatment is therefore aimed more at controlling clinical evidence of deterioration as might be manifested by fever (although patients are typically afebrile), cough, increased sputum, and changes in the chest roentgenogram or pulmonary function tests. Also, improvements in lung function have been found to correlate with the reduction of sputum *P. aeruginosa* bacterial density (215). Intravenous multidrug antibiotic therapy using an aminoglycoside and another antipseudomonal antibiotic (e.g., penicillin derivative, β-lactone drug, or third-genera-

tion cephalosporin) is commonly employed. To shorten hospitalization, home intravenous therapy should be considered. The duration of therapy for exacerbations should be over 14 days, as shorter courses of five to seven days may result in rapid recurrence. Despite the earlier controversy surrounding the use of inhaled antibiotic therapy in cystic fibrosis (216,217), a recent study has established the efficacy and safety of high-dose aerosolized tobramycin in the treatment of *P. aeruginosa* infections (218). The development of an oral antipseudomonal antibiotic effective for cystic fibrosis patients has been a major advance. In this regard, ciprofloxacin offers some promise (219) and is now commonly used. Although resistance to ciprofloxacin often rapidly emerges, the clinical virulence of the resistant organism may be less. Clearly, future research is required to resolve several issues concerning antibiotic use in cystic fibrosis.

Chest Physiotherapy

Patients with a productive cough have traditionally received indoctrination in proper daily chest percussion and postural drainage techniques. Nevertheless, the short- and long-term efficacy of these procedures remains unclear (220,221), although most physicians treating CF patients think they are clearly useful. Vigorous self-directed cough sessions are potentially as useful as more complex and time-consuming methods (222,223), though newer methods of inducing secretion clearance (e.g., positive expiratory pressure [PEP] treatment, autogenic drainage, etc.) may provide patients more autonomy in managing secretions than traditional chest physiotherapy that requires assistance of a caregiver (224). Self-administration of high-frequency chest compression therapy has also been shown to be efficacious, and also offers the advantage of increased independence (225).

Other Treatment

Patients should be immunized against influenza virus infection yearly.

Most CF centers routinely use β-agonist inhalers for nonbronchodilating effects on mucociliary clearance.

Acetylcysteine (Mucomyst) is of questionable efficacy and is injurious to respiratory epithelium when used chronically. Inhalation of this substance should be used selectively and for short duration (197).

Promotion of adequate nutrition is extremely important. Many patients require the regular use of pancreatic enzyme preparations to aid digestion and nutrient absorption. Typically, supplementation of vitamins A, D, E, and K is also provided.

Double lung transplantation is an option for patients with cystic fibrosis. The overall survival is about the same as transplant recipients with idiopathic pulmonary fibrosis and primary pulmonary hypertension. Complications specific to this group of patients include an increased rate of bacterial infections and erratic absorption of cyclosporine with concomitant seizures (215).

Complications

Hemoptysis

Massive hemoptysis occurs in about 5% to 7% of cystic fibrosis patients and carries a mortality rate of about 11% (195,226). Surgical therapy with lung resection is often contraindicated in many patients due to poor lung function. Even in those with adequate lung function, surgery should nevertheless be used only as a last resort. Sparing of lung tissue is important in the view of the chronic progressive nature of cystic fibrosis and the known high incidence of recurrent hemoptysis in these patients. Fortunately, acute control of massive hemoptysis can usually be achieved with endobronchial Fogarty balloon tamponade or bronchial artery embolization (226).

Pneumothorax

Pneumothorax rarely occurs in cystic fibrosis patients who are less than 10 years of age but is reported in about 20% of patients over 14 years of age (190,227). Treatment of pneumothorax in cystic fibrosis is similar to spontaneous pneumothorax due to other conditions, except that the high incidence of recurrence (50%) in cystic fibrosis argues for pleurodesis or other definitive therapy following the first large pneumothorax (190,228). The occurrence of a pneumothorax in cystic fibrosis indicates severe underlying disease and heralds a poor prognosis. In one series, the mean survival after the initial pneumothorax was only 3.4 years (190). Pleurodesis in the management of a pneumothorax may complicate subsequent lung transplantation.

REFERENCES

1. American Thoracic Society. Standards for the diagnosis and care of patients with chronic obstructive pulmonary disease. *Am J Respir Crit Care Med* 1995;152[Suppl]:S77–S120.
2. National Center for Health Statistics. Advance report of final mortality statistics, 1994. *Monthly Vital Statistics Report* 1996; 45[Suppl]:23.
3. Fletcher CM, Pride NB. Definitions of emphysema, chronic bronchitis, asthma, and airflow obstruction: 25 years on from the CIBA Symposium [Editorial]. *Thorax* 1984;39:81–85.
4. Ferguson GT, Cherniak RM. Management of chronic obstructive pulmonary disease. *N Engl J Med* 1993;328:1017–1022.
5. Anthonisen NR, Wright EC, Hodgkin JE. Prognosis in chronic obstructive pulmonary disease. *Am Rev Respir Dis* 1986;133: 14–20.
6. National Heart, Lung and Blood Institute, National Institutes of Health. 1996 chartbook on cardiovascular, lung and blood diseases. *MMWR,* Centers for Disease Control, 1996.
7. National Center for Health Statistics. Current estimates from the National Health Interview Survey, 1993. *Vital and Health Statistics,* series 10, No. 190. USDHHS (PHS), 95–1518.
8. Massachusetts Medical Society. Mortality patterns—United States, 1993. *MMWR* 1996;45.161–164.
9. Higgins MW, Thom T. Incidence, prevalence and mortality. intra- and intercountry difference. In: Hensley MJ, Sauners NA, eds. *Clinical epidemiology of chronic obstructive pulmonary disease.* New York: Marcel Dekker, 1990:23–43.
10. Szekely LA, Oelberg DA, Wright C, et al. Preoperative predictors of operative morbidity and mortality in COPD patients undergoing bilateral lung volume reduction surgery. *Chest* 1997; 111:550–558.
11. Mannino DM, Brown C, Giovino GA. Obstructive lung disease deaths in the United States from 1979 through 1993. *Am J Respir Crit Care Med* 1997;156:814–818.
12. Statistical compendium on adult lung diseases. New York: American Lung Association, 1987.
13. Statistics from the HCUP-3 Nationwide Inpatient Sample for 1993. Diagnosis-Related Groups. http://www.ahcpr.gov/data/93drga.htm. Anonymous 1998;1–10.
14. Statistics From the HCUP-3 Nationwide Inpatient Sample for 1994. Diagnosis-Related Groups. http://www.ahcpr.gov/data/94drga.htm. Anonymous 1998;1–10.
15. Senior RM, Anthonisen NR. Chronic obstructive pulmonary disease (COPD). *Am J Respir Crit Care Med* 1998;157[Suppl]: S139–S147.
16. Davis RM, Novotny TE. The epidemiology of cigarette smoking and its impact on chronic obstructive pulmonary disease. *Am Rev Respir Dis* 1989;140:S82–S84.
17. Camilli AE, Burrows B, Knudson RJ, et al. Longitudinal changes in forced expiratory volume in one second in adults: effects of smoking and smoking cessation. *Am Rev Respir Dis* 1987;135:794–799.
18. Dockery DW, Speizer FE, Ferris BG Jr, et al. Cumulative and reversible effects of lifetime smoking on simple tests of lung function in adults. *Am Rev Respir Dis* 1988;137:286–292.
19. Anthonisen NR, Connett JE, Kiley JP, et al. Effects of smoking intervention and the use of an inhaled anticholinergic bronchodilator on the rate of decline of FEV_1: the Lung Health Study. *JAMA* 1994;272:1497–1505.
20. Bartecchi C, MacKenzie T, Schrier R. The human costs of tobacco use. *N Engl J Med* 1994;330:907–912.
21. Kessler D. Nicotine addiction in young people. *N Engl J Med* 1955;333:186–189.
22. Frew AJ, Kennedy SM, Chan-Yeung M. Methacholine responsiveness, smoking, and atopy as risk factors for accelerated FEV_1 decline in male working populations. *Am Rev Respir Dis* 1992; 146:878–883.
23. Rijcken B, Schouten JP, Xu X, et al. Airway hyperresponsiveness to histamine associated with accelerated decline in FEV_1. *Am J Respir Crit Care Med* 1995;151:1377–1382.
24. O'Connor GT, Sparrow D, Weiss ST. A prospective longitudinal study of methacholine airway responsiveness as a predictor of pulmonary-function decline: the Normative Aging Study. *Am J Respir Crit Care Med* 1995;152:87–92.
25. Postma DS, de Vries K, Koëter GH, et al. Independent influence of reversibility of air-flow obstruction and nonspecific hyperreactivity on the long-term course of lung function in chronic air-flow obstruction. *Am Rev Respir Dis* 1986;134:276–280.
26. Tashkin DP, Altose MD, Connett JE, et al. Methacholine reactivity predicts changes in lung function over time in smokers with early chronic obstructive pulmonary disease. *Am J Respir Crit Care Med* 1996;153:1802–1811.
27. Villar MTA, Dow L, Coggon D, et al. The influence of increased bronchial responsiveness, atopy, and serum IgE on de-

cline in FEV_1: a longitudinal study in the elderly. *Am J Respir Crit Care Med* 1995;151:656–662.

28. Kanner RE, Connett JE, Altose MD, et al. Gender difference in airway hyperresponsiveness in smokers with mild COPD: the Lung Health Study. *Am J Respir Crit Care Med* 1994;150: 956–96.

29. Tashkin DP, Altose MD, Bleecker ER, et al. and the Lung Health Study Research Group. The Lung Health Study: airway responsiveness to inhaled methacholine in smokers with mild to moderate airflow limitation. *Am Rev Respir Dis* 1992;145: 301–310.

30. Rijcken B, Schouten JP, Weiss ST, et al. The relationship between airway responsiveness to histamine and pulmonary function level in a random population sample. *Am Rev Respir Dis* 1988;137:826–832.

31. Malo J-L, Pineau L, Cartier A, et al. Reference values of the provocative concentrations of methacholine that cause 6% and 20% changes in forced expiratory volume in one second in a normal population. *Am Rev Respir Dis* 1983;128:8–11.

32. Sparrow D, O'Connor G, Colton T, et al. The relationship of nonspecific bronchial responsiveness to the occurrence of respiratory symptoms and decreased levels of pulmonary function: the Normative Aging Study. *Am Rev Respir Dis* 1987;135: 1255–1260.

33. Ramsdell JW, Nachtwey FJ, Moser KM. Bronchial hyperreactivity in chronic obstructive bronchitis. *Am Rev Respir Dis* 1982; 126:829–832.

34. Anthonisen NR, Wright EC, and the IPPB Trial Group. Bronchodilator response in chronic obstructive pulmonary disease. *Am Rev Respir Dis* 1986;133:814–819.

35. Peto R, Speizer FE, Cochrane AL, et al. The relevance in adults of air-flow obstruction, but not of mucus hypersecretion, to mortality from chronic lung disease: results from 20 years of prospective observation. *Am Rev Respir Dis* 1983;128:491–500.

36. Bates DV. The fate of the chronic bronchitic: a report of the ten-year follow-up in the Canadian Department of Veteran's Affairs Coordinated Study of Chronic Bronchitis. *Am Rev Respir Dis* 1973;108:1043–1065.

37. Samet JM, Tager IB, Speizer FE. The relationship between respiratory illness in childhood and chronic air-flow obstruction in adulthood. *Am Rev Respir Dis* 1983;127:508–523.

38. Gold DR, Tager IB, Weiss ST, et al. Acute lower respiratory illness in childhood as a predictor of lung function and chronic respiratory symptoms. *Am Rev Respir Dis* 1989;140:877–884.

39. Murphy TF, Sethi S. Bacterial infection in chronic obstructive pulmonary disease. *Am Rev Respir Dis* 1992;146:1067–1083.

40. Anthonisen NR, Manfreda J, Warren CPW, et al. Antibiotic therapy in exacerbations of chronic obstructive pulmonary disease. *Ann Intern Med* 1987;106:196–204.

41. Laurell CB, Eriksson S. The electrophoretic alpha1 globulin pattern of serum in alpha1 antitrypsin deficiency. *Scand J Clin Lab Invest* 1963;15:132–140.

42. Eriksson S. Pulmonary emphysema and alpha1-antitrypsin deficiency. *Acta Med Scand* 1964;175:197–205.

43. Gross P, Babyak MA, Tolker E, et al. Enzymatically produced pulmonary emphysema: a preliminary report. *J Occup Environ Med* 1964;6:481–484.

44. Stoller JK. Alpha1-antitrypsin deficiency and augmentation therapy in emphysema. *Clev Clin J Med* 1989;56:683–689.

45. Crystal RG, Brantly ML, Hubbard RC, et al. The alpha1-antitrypsin gene and its mutations: clinical consequences and strategies for therapy. *Chest* 1989;95:196–208.

46. Kao RC, Wehner NG, Skubitz KM, et al. Proteinase 3: a distinct human polymorphonuclear leukocyte proteinase that produces emphysema in hamsters. *J Clin Invest* 1988;82:1963–1973.

47. Hautamaki RD, Kobayashi DK, Senior RM, et al. Requirement

for macrophage elastase for cigarette smoke-induced emphysema in mice. *Science* 1997;277:2002–2004.

48. Gadek JE, Fells GA, Zimmerman RL, et al. Antielastases of the human alveolar structures: implications for the protease-antiprotease theory of emphysema. *J Clin Invest* 1981;68: 889–898.

49. Gadek JE, Pacht ER. The protease-antiprotease balance within the human lung: implications for the pathogenesis of emphysema. *Lung* 1990;168[Suppl]:552–564.

50. Shapiro SD, Endicott SK, Province MA, et al. Marked longevity of human lung parenchymal elastic fibers deduced from prevalence of D-aspartate and nuclear weapons–related radiocarbon. *J Clin Invest* 1991;87:1828–1834.

51. Brantly M, Nukiwa T, Crystal RG. Molecular basis of alpha 1-antitrypsin deficiency. *Am J Med* 1988;84[Suppl 6A]:13–31.

52. Stoller JK. Clinical features and natural history of severe α_1-antitrypsin deficiency. Roger S. Mitchell Lecture. *Chest* 1997; 111[Suppl 6]:123S–128S.

53. Gishen P, Suanders AJS, Tobin MJ, et al. Alpha1-antitrypsin deficiency: the radiological features of pulmonary emphysema in subjects of PI-type Z and PI-type SZ: a survey by the British Thoracic Association. *Clin Radiol* 1982;33:371–377.

54. Perlmutter DH. Alpha-1-antitrypsin deficiency: biochemistry and clinical manifestations. *Ann Med* 1996;28:385–394.

55. Eriksson S. A 30-year perspective on α1-antitrypsin deficiency. *Chest* 1996;110[Suppl 6]:237S–242S.

56. Brantly ML, Paul LD, Miller BH, et al. Clinical features and history of the destructive lung disease associated with alpha-1-antitrypsin deficiency of adults with pulmonary symptoms. *Am Rev Respir Dis* 1988;138:327–336.

57. Silverman EK, Miletich JP, Pierce JA, et al. Alpha-1-antitrypsin deficiency: high prevalence in the St. Louis area determined by direct population screening. *Am Rev Respir Dis* 1989;140: 961–966.

58. Silverman EK, Pierce JA, Province MA, et al. Variability of pulmonary function in alpha-1-antitrypsin deficiency: clinical correlates. *Ann Intern Med* 1989;111:982–991.

59. Silverman EK, Chapman HA, Drazen JM, et al. Genetic epidemiology of severe, early-onset chronic obstructive pulmonary disease: risk to relatives for airflow obstruction and chronic bronchitis. *Am J Respir Crit Care Med* 1998;157:1770–1778.

60. Janoff A, Carp H, Lee DK. Cigarette smoke inhalation decreases α1-antitrypsin activity in rat lung. *Science* 1979;206: 1313–1314.

61. Rautalahti M, Virtamo J, Haukka J, et al. The effect of alpha-tocopherol and beta-carotene supplementation on COPD symptoms. *Am J Respir Crit Care Med* 1997;156:1447–1452.

62. Hunninghake GW, Crystal RG. Cigarette smoking and lung destruction: accumulation of neutrophils in the lungs of cigarette smokers. *Am Rev Respir Dis* 1983;128:833–838.

63. Fujita J, Nelson NL, Daughton DM, et al. Evaluation of elastase and antielastase balance in patients with chronic bronchitis and pulmonary emphysema. *Am Rev Respir Dis* 1990;142:57–62.

64. Wilson DO, Rogers RM, Wright EC, et al. Body weight in chronic obstructive pulmonary disease. National Institutes of Health IPPB Trial. *Am Rev Respir Dis* 1989;139:1435–1438.

65. Muers MF, Green JH. Weight loss in chronic obstructive pulmonary disease. *Eur Respir J* 1993;6:729–734.

66. Anthonisen NR, Wright EC, the IPPB Trial Group. Response to inhaled bronchodilators in COPD. *Chest* 1987;91:36S–39S.

67. Guyatt GH, Townsend M, Pugsley SO, et al. Bronchodilators in chronic air-flow limitation: effects on airway function, exercise capacity, and quality of life. *Am Rev Respir Dis* 1987;135: 1069–1074.

68. Berger R, Smith D. Effect of inhaled metaproterenol and exer-

cise performance in patients with stable "fixed" airway obstruction. *Am Rev Respir Dis* 1988;138:624–629.

69. Greene R. "Saber-sheath" trachea: relation to chronic obstructive pulmonary disease. *AJR* 1978;130:441–445.

70. Chang CH. The normal roentgenographic measurement of the right descending pulmonary artery in 1085 cases. *AJR* 1962; 87:929–935.

71. Matthay RA, Schwarz MI, Ellis JH, et al. Pulmonary artery hypertension in chronic obstructive pulmonary disease: determination by chest radiography. *Invest Radiol* 1981;16:95–100.

72. Thurlbeck WM, Simon G. Radiographic appearance of the chest in emphysema. *AJR* 1978;130:429–440.

73. Sutinen S, Christoforidis AJ, Klugh GA, et al. Roentgenologic criteria for the recognition of nonsymptomatic pulmonary emphysema. *Am Rev Respir Dis* 1965;91:69–76.

74. Palmer WH, Gee JB, Mills JBL, et al. The accuracy of the roentgenologic diagnosis of chronic pulmonary emphysema. *Am Rev Respir Dis* 1966;93:889–894.

75. Pratt PC. Role of conventional chest radiography in diagnosis and exclusion of emphysema. *Am J Med* 1987;82:998–1006.

76. Nicklaus DW, Stowell DW, Christiansen WR, et al. The accuracy of the roentgenologic diagnosis of chronic pulmonary emphysema. *Am Rev Respir Dis* 1966;93:889–899.

77. Fraser RG, Paré JAP. Roentgenologic signs in the diagnosis of chest disease. In: *Diagnosis of diseases of the chest,* 2nd ed. Philadelphia: WB Saunders, 1977:518–523.

78. Miller RR, Mueller NL, Morrison NJ, et al. Limitations of computed tomography in the assessment of emphysema. *Am Rev Respir Dis* 1989;139:980–983.

79. Kinsella M, Müller NL, Abboud RT, et al. Quantitation of emphysema by computed tomography using a "density mask" program and correlation with pulmonary function tests. *Chest* 1990;97:315–321.

80. Rienmüller RK, Behr J, Kalender WA, et al. Standardized quantitative high resolution CT in lung diseases. *J Comput Assist Tomogr* 1991;15:742–749.

81. Kuwano K, Matsuba K, Ikeda T, et al. The diagnosis of mild emphysema. Correlation of computed tomography and pathology score. *Am Rev Respir Dis* 1990;141:169–178.

82. Gurney JW, Jines KK, Robbins RA, et al. Regional distribution of emphysema: correlation of high-resolution CT with pulmonary function tests in unselected smokers. *Radiology* 1992;18(3): 457–463.

83. Fletcher C, Peto R, Tinker C, et al. *The natural history of chronic bronchitis and emphysema: an eight-year study of early chronic obstructive lung disease in working men in London.* New York: Oxford University Press, 1976.

84. US Department of Health and Human Services. *The health consequences of involuntary smoking: a report of the Surgeon General.* Rockville, MD: Office on Smoking and Health, 1986.

85. *Smoking cessation: A guide for primary clinicians.* Washington, DC: AHCPR Publications Clearinghouse, 1997. P.O. Box 8547, Silver Spring, MD 2009–8547.

86. *Smoking cessation: quick reference guide for smoking cessation specialists.* Washington, DC: AHCPR Publications Clearinghouse, 1997. P.O. Box 8547, Silver Spring, MD 2009-8547.

87. Huber GL, Burke M, Nett L. Smoking cessation. *Semin Respir Med* 1986;8(2):147–157.

88. Transdermal Nicotine Study Group. Transdermal nicotine for smoking cessation. Six-month results from two multicenter controlled clinical trials. *JAMA* 1991;266:3133–3139.

89. Fiore MC, Jorenby DE, Baker TB, et al. Tobacco dependence and the nicotine patch: clinical guidelines for effective use. *JAMA* 1992;268:2687–2694.

90. Joseph AM, Norman SM, Ferry LH, et al. The safety of transdermal nicotine as an aid to smoking cessation in patients with cardiac disease. *N Engl J Med* 1996;335.1792–1798.

91. Kanford SL, Fiore MC, Jorendy DE, et al. Predicting smoking cessation: who will quit with and without the nicotine patch. *JAMA* 1994;271:589–594.

92. Hurt RD, Sachs DPL, Glover ED, et al. A comparison of sustained-release bupropion and placebo for smoking cessation. *N Engl J Med* 1997;337:1195–1202.

93. Centers for Disease Control and Prevention. Prevention of pneumococcal disease: recommendations of the Advisory Committee on Immunization Practices (ACIP). *MMWR* 1997; 46(RR–8):1–24.

94. Centers for Disease Control and Prevention. Prevention and control of influenza: recommendations of the Advisory Committee on Immunization Practices (ACIP). *MMWR* 1999; 48(RR–4):1–29.

95. Centers for Disease Control and Prevention: Update. Influenza activity—United States and Worldwide, 1998–99 season, and composition of the 1999–2000 influenza vaccine. *MMWR* 1999;48(18):374–378.

96. Safranek TJ, Lawrence DN, Kurland LT, et al. Reassessment of the association between Guillain-Barré syndrome and receipt of swine influenza vaccine in 1976–1977; results of a two-state study. Expert Neurology Group. *Am J Epidemiol* 1991;133: 940–951.

97. Barohn RJ, Saperstein DS. Guillain-Barré syndrome and chronic inflammatory demyelinating polyneuropathy. *Semin Neurol* 1998;18:49–61.

98. Public Health Service. *Health people 2000: National health promotion and disease prevention objectives* [Full report, with commentary]. Washington, DC: US Department of Health and Human Services, Public Health Service, 1991; DHHS publication no. (PHS)91–50212.

99. Centers for Disease Control and Prevention. Pneumococcal and influenza vaccination levels among adults aged >65 years—United States. *MMWR* 1997;46(39):913–919.

100. Combivent Inhalational Aerosol Study Group. In chronic obstructive pulmonary disease, a combination of ipratropium and albuterol is more effective than either agent alone: an 85-day multicenter study. *Chest* 1994;105:1411–1419.

101. Ramsdell J. Use of theophylline in the treatment of COPD. *Chest* 1995;107[Suppl]:206S–209S.

102. Callahan CM, Dittus RS, Katz BP. Oral corticosteroid therapy for patients with stable chronic obstructive pulmonary disease: a meta-analysis. *Ann Intern Med* 1991;114:216–223.

103. Mendella LA, Manfreda J, Warren CPW, et al. Steroid response in stable chronic obstructive pulmonary disease. *Ann Intern Med* 1982;96:17–21.

104. Lebowitz M, Postma DS, Burrows B. Adverse effects of eosinophilia and smoking on the natural history of newly-diagnosed chronic bronchitis. *Chest* 1995;108:55–62.

105. Jackevicius CA, Chapman KR. Prevalence of inhaled corticosteroid use among patients with chronic obstructive pulmonary disease: a survey. *Ann Pharmacother* 1997;31:160–164.

106. Vestbo J, Sørensen T, Lange P, et al. Long-term effect of inhaled budesonide in mild and moderate chronic obstructive pulmonary disease. a randomized controlled trial. *Lancet* 1999;353: 1819–1823.

107. Pauwels RA, Löfdahl CG, Laitinen LA, et al. The European Respiratory Society Study on Chronic Obstructive Pulmonary Disease. Long term treatment with inhaled budesonide in persons with mild chronic obstructive pulmonary disease who continue smoking. *N Engl J Med* 1999;340:1948–1953.

108. Wewers MD, Gadek JE, Keogh BA, et al. Evaluation of danazol therapy for patients with PiZZ alpha 1-antitrypsin deficiency. *Am Rev Respir Dis* 1986;134:476–480.

109. Wewers MD, Brantly ML, Casolaro MA, et al. Evaluation of tamoxifen as a therapy to augment alpha 1-antitrypsin concentrations in Z homozygous alpha 1-antitrypsin deficient subjects. *Am Rev Respir Dis* 1987;135:401–402.

110. Eriksson S. The effect of tamoxifen in intermediate alpha 1-antitrypsin deficiency associated with the phenotype PiSZ. *Ann Clin Res* 1983;15:95–98.

111. Wewers MD, Casolaro A, Sellers SE, et al. Replacement therapy for alpha1-antitrypsin deficiency associated with emphysema. *N Engl J Med* 1987;316:1055–1062.

112. Hubbard RC, Crystal RG. Alpha 1-antitrypsin augmentation therapy for alpha 1-antitrypsin deficiency. *Am J Med* 1988;84[Suppl 6A]:52–62.

113. Stoller JK. Alpha 1-antitrypsin deficiency and augmentation therapy in emphysema. *Cleve Clin J Med* 1989;56:683–689.

114. American Thoracic Society. Guidelines for the approach to the patient with severe hereditary alpha-1-antitrypsin deficiency. *Am Rev Respir Dis* 1989;140:1494–1497.

115. Hubbard RC, Casolaro MA, Mitchell M, et al. Fate of aerosolized recombinant DNA-produced alpha 1-antitrypsin: use of the epithelial surface of the lower respiratory tract to administer proteins of therapeutic importance. *Proc Natl Acad Sci U S A* 1989;86:680–684.

116. Hubbard RC, McElvaney NG, Sellers SE, et al. Recombinant DNA-produced α_1-antitrypsin administered by aerosol augments lower respiratory tract antineutrophil elastase defenses in individuals with α_1-antitrypsin deficiency. *J Clin Invest* 1989;84:1349–1354.

117. Rosenfeld MA, Siegfried W, Yoshimura K, et al. Adenovirus-mediated transfer of a recombinant α_1-antitrypsin gene to the lung epithelium in vivo. *Science* 1991;252:431–434.

118. Canonico AE, Conary JT, Meyrick BO, et al. Aerosol and intravenous transfection of human α_1-antitrypsin gene to lungs of rabbits. *Am J Respir Cell Mol Biol* 1994;10:24–29.

119. Crystal RG. Gene therapy strategies for pulmonary disease. *Am J Med* 1992;92[Suppl 6A]:44S–52S.

120. Trulock EP. Lung transplantation for alpha 1-antitrypsin deficiency emphysema. *Chest* 1996;110[6 Suppl]:284S–294S.

121. Fishman AP. Pulmonary rehabilitation research. NIH workshop summary. *Am Rev Respir Dis* 1994;149:825–833.

122. Ries AL. Position paper of the American Association of Cardiovascular and Pulmonary Rehabilitation: scientific basis of pulmonary rehabilitation. *J Cardpulm Rehabil* 1990;10:418–441.

123. Pulmonary rehabilitation. Joint ACCP/AACVPR evidence-based guidelines. *Chest* 1997;112:1363–1396.

124. Celli BR. Pulmonary rehabilitation for patients with advanced lung disease. *Clin Chest Med* 1997;18:521–534.

125. Folgering H, Rooyakkers J, Herwaarden C. Education and cost/benefit ratios in pulmonary patients. *Monaldi Arch Chest Dis* 1994;49:166–168.

126. Howland J, Nelson EC, Barlow PB, et al. Chronic obstructive pulmonary disease: Impact of health education. *Chest* 1986;90:233–238.

127. Casaburi R. Exercise training in chronic obstructive lung disease. In: Casaburi R, Petty TL, eds. *Principles and practice of pulmonary rehabilitation*. Philadelphia: WB Saunders, 1993:204–224.

128. Casaburi R, Patessio A, Joli F, et al. Reductions in exercise lactic acidosis and ventilation as a result of exercise training in patients with obstructive lung disease. *Am Rev Respir Dis* 1991;143:9–18.

129. Smith K, Cook D, Guyatt GH, et al. Respiratory muscle training in chronic airflow limitation: a meta-analysis. *Am Rev Respir Dis* 1992;145:533–539.

130. Gosselink RAAM, Wagenaar RC, Rijswijk H, et al. Diaphragmatic breathing reduces efficiency of breathing in patients with chronic obstructive pulmonary disease. *Am J Respir Crit Care Med* 1995;151:1136–1142.

131. Lacasse Y, Wong E, Guyatt GH, et al. Meta-analysis of respiratory rehabilitation in chronic obstructive pulmonary disease. *Lancet* 1996;348(9035):1115–1119.

132. Lacasse Y. Is there really a controversy surrounding the effectiveness of respiratory rehabilitation in COPD? *Chest* 1998;114:1–4.

133. Bickford LS, Hodgkin JE, McInturff SL. National Pulmonary Rehabilitation Survey update. *J Cardpulm Rehabil* 1995;15:406–411.

134. Celli BR. Pulmonary rehabilitation in patients with COPD. *Am J Respir Crit Care Med* 1995;152:861–864.

135. Strijbos JH, Postma DS, van Altena R, et al. A comparison between an outpatient hospital-based pulmonary rehabilitation program and a home-care pulmonary rehabilitation program in patients with COPD. A follow-up of 18 months. *Chest* 1996;109:366–372.

136. O'Donohue WJ Jr, Plummer AL. Magnitude of usage and cost of home oxygen therapy in the United States. *Chest* 1995;107:301–302.

137. Nocturnal Oxygen Therapy Trial Group. Continuous or nocturnal oxygen therapy in hypoxemic chronic obstructive lung disease: A clinical trial. *Ann Intern Med* 1980;93:391–398.

138. Medical Research Council Working Party. Long-term domiciliary oxygen therapy in chronic hypoxic cor pulmonale complicating chronic bronchitis and emphysema. *Lancet* 1981;1:681–686.

139. Fletcher EC, Luckett RA, Goodnight-White S, et al. A double-blind trial of nocturnal supplemental oxygen for sleep desaturation in patients with chronic obstructive pulmonary disease and daytime P_aO_2 above 60 mmHg. *Am Rev Respir Dis* 1992;145:1070–1076.

140. Heimlich HJ, Carr GC. The Micro-Trach: a seven-year experience with transtracheal oxygen therapy. *Chest* 1989;95:1008–1012.

141. Hoffman LA, Wesmiller SW, Sciurba FC, et al. Nasal cannula and transtracheal oxygen delivery. A comparison of patient response after 6 months of each technique. *Am Rev Respir Dis* 1992;145:827–831.

142. Murata GH, Gorby MS, Chick TW, et al. Use of emergency medical services by patients with decompensated obstructive lung disease. *Ann Emerg Med* 1989;18:501–506.

143. Fuso L, Incalzi RA, Pistelli R, et al. Predicting mortality of patients hospitalized for acutely exacerbated chronic obstructive pulmonary disease. *Am J Med* 1995;98:272–277.

144. Kuhl DA, Agiri OA, Mauro LS. Beta-agonists in the treatment of acute exacerbation of chronic obstructive pulmonary disease. *Ann Pharmacother* 1994;28:1379–1388.

145. Hudson LS, Monti CM. Rationale and use of corticosteroids in chronic obstructive pulmonary disease. *Med Clin North Am* 1990 :661–690.

146. Albert RK, Martin TR, Lewis SW. Controlled clinical trial of methylprednisolone in patients with chronic bronchitis and acute respiratory insufficiency. *Ann Intern Med* 1980;92:753–758.

147. Emerman CL, Connors AF, Lukens TW, et al. A randomized controlled trial of methylprednisolone in the emergency treatment of acute exacerbations of COPD. *Chest* 1989;95:563–567.

148. Niewoehner DE, Erbland ML, Deupree RH, et al. Effect of systemic glucocorticoids on exacerbations of chronic obstructive pulmonary disease. *N Engl J Med* 1999;340:1941–1947.

149. Anthonisen NR, Connett JE, Kiley JP, et al. Effects of smoking intervention and the use of an inhaled anticholinergic bronchodilator on the rate of decline of FEV1; the Lung Health Study. *JAMA* 1994;272:1497–1505.

150. Saint S, Bent S, Vittinghoff E, et al. Antibiotics in chronic obstructive pulmonary disease exacerbations. A meta-analysis. *JAMA* 1995;273(12):957–960.

151. Boushy SF, Thompson HK, North LB, et al. Prognosis in chronic obstructive pulmonary disease. *Am Rev Respir Dis* 1973; 108:1373–1383.

152. Traver GA, Cline MG, Burrows B. Predictors of mortality in chronic obstructive pulmonary disease. A 15-year follow-up study. *Am Rev Respir Dis* 1979;119:895–902.

153. Postma DS, Burema J, Gimeno F, et al. Prognosis in severe chronic obstructive pulmonary disease. *Am Rev Respir Dis* 1979; 119:357–367.

154. Fletcher C, Peto R. The natural history of chronic airflow obstruction. *Br Med J* 1977;1:1645–1648.

155. White JR, Froeb HF, Kulik JA. Respiratory illness in nonsmokers chronically exposed to tobacco smoke in the workplace. *Chest* 1991;100:39–43.

156. Kanner RE, Renzetti AD Jr, Stanish WM, et al. Predictors of survival in subjects with chronic airflow limitation. *Am J Med* 1983;74:249–255.

157. Franie AJ, Prescott RJ, Biernacki W, et al. Does right ventricular function predict survival in patients with chronic obstructive lung disease? *Thorax* 1988;43:621–626.

158. Oswald-Mammoser M, Weitzenblum E, Quoix E, et al. Prognostic factors in COPD patients receiving long-term oxygen therapy. Importance of pulmonary artery pressure. *Chest* 1995; 107:1193–1198.

159. Vollmer WM, Johnson LR, Buist AS. Relationship of response to a bronchodilator and decline in forced expiratory volume in one second in population studies. *Am Rev Respir Dis* 1985;132: 1186–1193.

160. Burrows B, Bloom JW, Traver GA, et al. The course and prognosis of different forms of chronic airways obstruction in a sample from the general population. *N Engl J Med* 1987;317: 1309–1314.

161. Dompeling E, Van Schayk CP, van Grusven PM, et al. Slowing the deterioration of asthma and chronic obstructive pulmonary disease observed during bronchitis therapy by adding inhaled corticosteroids: a four year prospective study. *Ann Intern Med* 1993;118:770–778.

162. Burk RH, George RB. Acute respiratory failure in chronic obstructive pulmonary disease. Immediate and long-term prognosis. *Arch Intern Med* 1973;132:865–868.

163. Meugies R, Gibbons W, Goldberg P. Determinants of weaning and survival in patients with COPD who require mechanical ventilation for acute respiratory failure. *Chest* 1989;95: 398–405.

164. Connors AF, Dawson NV, Thomas C, et al. Outcomes following acute exacerbation of severe chronic obstructive lung disease. *Am J Respir Crit Care Med* 1996;154:959–967.

165. Reid LM. Reduction in bronchial subdivision in bronchiectasis. *Thorax* 1950;5:233–247.

166. Ellis DA, Thornley PE, Wightman AF, et al. Present outlook in bronchiectasis: clinical and social study and review of factors influencing prognosis. *Thorax* 1981;36:659–664.

167. Moll HH. A clinical and pathological study of bronchiectasis. *Q J Med* 1932;25:457–469.

168. Bradshaw HH, Putrey FJ, Clerf CH, et al. The fate of patients with untreated bronchiectasis. *JAMA* 1941;116:2561–2563.

169. Konietzko NFJ, Carton RW, Leroy EP. Causes of death in patients with bronchiectasis. *Am Rev Respir Dis* 1969;100: 852–858.

170. Stanford W, Galvin JR. The diagnosis of bronchiectasis. *Clin Chest Med* 1988;9:691–699.

171. Swartz MN. Bronchiectasis. In: Fishman AP, ed. *Pulmonary diseases and disorders.* New York: McGraw-Hill, 1988: 1553–1581.

172. Barker AF, Bardana EJ Jr. Bronchiectasis: update of an orphan disease. *Am Rev Respir Dis* 1988;137:969–978.

173. Beck CS, Heiner DC. Selective immunoglobulin G4 deficiency and recurrent infections of respiratory tract. *Am Rev Respir Dis* 1981;124:94–96.

174. Heiner DC, Moyer AS, Beck AS. Deficiency of IgG4: a disorder associated with frequent infections and bronchiectasis that may be familial. *Clin Rev Allergy* 1983;1:259–266.

175. Umetsu DT, Ambrosino DM, Quinti I, et al. Infection and impaired antibody response to bacterial capsular polysaccharide antigen in children with selective IgG-subclass deficiency. *N Engl J Med* 1985;313:1247–1251.

176. Bjorkander B, Bake B, Oxelius V, et al. Impaired lung function in patients with IgA deficiency and low levels of IgG2 or IgG3. *N Engl J Med* 1985;313:720–724.

177. Ammann AJ, Hong RR. Selective IgA deficiency: presentation of 30 cases and a review of the literature. *Medicine* 1971;50: 223–236.

178. Eliasson R, Mossberg B, Camner P, et al. The immotile-cilia syndrome: a congenital ciliary abnormality as an etiologic factor in chronic airway infections and male sterility. *N Engl J Med* 1977;297:1–6.

179. Handelsman D, Conway A, Boylan L, et al. Young's syndrome: obstructive azoospermia and chronic sinopulmonary infections. *N Engl J Med* 1984;310:3–9.

180. Schanker HMJ, Rajfer F, Saxon A. Recurrent respiratory disease, azoospermia, and nasal polyposis. *Arch Intern Med* 1985;145: 2201–2203.

181. Fuchs HJ, Borowitz DS, Christiansen DH, et al. Effects of aerosolized recombinant human DNase on exacerbations of respiratory symptoms and on pulmonary function in patients with cystic fibrosis. *N Engl J Med* 1994;331:637–642.

182. Ramsey BW, Astley SJ, Aitken ML, et al. Efficacy and safety of short-term administration of aerosolized recombinant human deoxyribonuclease in patients with cystic fibrosis. *Am Rev Respir Dis* 1993;148:145–151.

183. Uflacker R, Kaemmerer A, Neves C, et al. Management of massive hemoptysis by bronchial artery embolization. *Radiology* 1983;146:627–634.

184. Collins FS. Cystic fibrosis: molecular biology and therapeutic implications. *Science* 1992;256:774–779.

185. Davis PB. Cystic fibrosis from bench to bedside. *N Engl J Med* 1991;325:575–577.

186. Rommens JM, Iannuzzi MC, Kerem B, et al. Identification of the cystic fibrosis gene: chromosome walking and jumping. *Science* 1989;245:1059–1065.

187. Snouwaert JN, Brigman KK, Latour AM, et al. An animal model for cystic fibrosis made by gene targeting. *Science* 1992;257: 1083–1088.

188. Huang NN, Schidlow DV, Szatrowski TH, et al. Clinical features, survival rate, and prognostic factors in young adults with cystic fibrosis. *Am J Med* 1987;82:871–879.

189. Stern RC, Boat TF, Doershuk CF, et al. Cystic fibrosis after age 13: twenty-five teenage and adult patients including three asymptomatic men. *Ann Intern Med* 1977;87:188–191.

190. Murphy S. Cystic fibrosis in adults: diagnosis and management. *Clin Chest Med* 1987;8:695–710.

191. The Cystic Fibrosis Genotype-Phenotype Consortium. Correlation between genotype and phenotype in patients with cystic fibrosis. *N Engl J Med* 1993;329:1308–1313.

192. Rivera M, Nicotra MB. Pseudomonas aeruginosa mucoid strain. Its significance in adult chest disease. *Am Rev Respir Dis* 1982; 126:833–836.

193. Brasfield S, Hicks G, Soong SJ, et al. The chest roentgenogram

in cystic fibrosis: a new scoring system. *Pediatrics* 1979;63: 24–29.

194. Friedman PJ, Harwood IR, Ellenbogen PH. Pulmonary cystic fibrosis in the adult: early and late radiologic findings with pathologic correlation. *AJR* 1981;136:1131–1144.

195. di Sant'Agnese PA, Davis PB. Cystic fibrosis in adults: 75 cases and a review of 232 cases in the literature. *Am J Med* 1979;66: 121–132.

196. Davis PB, di Sant'Agnese PA. Diagnosis and treatment of cystic fibrosis: an update. *Chest* 1984;84:802–809.

197. Boat TF. Cystic fibrosis. In: Murray JF, Nadel JA, eds. *Textbook of respiratory medicine.* Philadelphia: WB Saunders, 1988: 1126–1152.

198. Davis PB, Hubbard VS, di Sant'Agnese PA. Low sweat chloride electrolytes in a patient with cystic fibrosis. *Am J Med* 1980; 69:643–646.

199. Strong TV, Smit LS, Turpin SV, et al. Cystic fibrosis gene mutation in two sisters with mild disease and normal sweat electrolyte levels. *N Engl J Med* 1991;325:1630–1634.

200. FitzSimmons SC. The changing epidemiology of cystic fibrosis. *J Pediatr* 1993;122:1–9.

201. Knowles MR, Church NL, Waltner WE, et al. A pilot study of aerosolized amiloride for the treatment of lung disease in cystic fibrosis. *N Engl J Med* 1990;322:1189–1194.

202. Knowles MR, Clarke LL, Boucher RC. Activation by extracellular nucleotides of chloride secretion in the airway epithelia of patients with cystic fibrosis. *N Engl J Med* 1991;325:533–538.

203. McElvaney NG, Nakamura H, Birrer P, et al. Modulation of airway inflammation in cystic fibrosis. In vivo suppression of interleukin-8 levels on the respiratory epithelial surface by aerosolization of recombinant secretory leukoprotease inhibitor. *J Clin Invest* 1992;90:1296–1301.

204. Auerbach HS, Williams M, Kirkpatrick JA, et al. Alternate day prednisone reduces morbidity and improves pulmonary function in cystic fibrosis. *Lancet* 1985;2:686–688.

205. Rosenstein BJ, Eigen H. Risks of alternate-day prednisone in patients with cystic fibrosis. *Pediatrics* 1991;87:245–246.

206. Michel BC. Antibiotic therapy in cystic fibrosis: a review of the literature published between 1980 and February 1987. *Chest* 1988;94[Suppl]:129S–140S.

207. Thomassen MJ, Demko CA, Doershuk CF. Cystic fibrosis: a review of pulmonary infections and interventions. *Pediatr Pulmonol* 1987;3:334–351.

208. Hjelte L, Petrinin B, Kallenius G, et al. Perspective study of mycobacterial infections in patients with cystic fibrosis. *Thorax* 1990;45:397–400.

209. Aitken ML, Burke W, McDonald G, et al. Non-tuberculous mycobacterial disease in adult CF patients. *Chest* 1993;103: 1096–1099.

210. Wang EEL, Prober CG, Manson B, et al. Association of respiratory viral infections with pulmonary deterioration in patients with cystic fibrosis. *N Engl J Med* 1984;311:1653–1658.

211. Shale DJ. Viral infections: a role in the lung disease of cystic fibrosis? *Thorax* 1992;47:89.

212. Conway SP, Simmonds EJ, Littlewood JM. Acute severe deterioration in cystic fibrosis associated with influenza A virus infection. *Thorax* 1992;47:112–114.

213. Pribble CG, Black PG, Bosso JA, et al. Clinical manifestations of exacerbations of cystic fibrosis associated with nonbacterial infections. *J Pediatr* 1990;117:200–204.

214. Kerrebijn KF, ed. Pulmonary infection and antibiotic therapy in patients with cystic fibrosis. *Chest* 1988;94[Suppl]:97S–169S.

215. Regelmann WE, Elliott GR, Warwick WJ, et al. Reduction of sputum Pseudomonas aeruginosa density by antibiotics improves lung function in cystic fibrosis more than do bronchodilators and chest physiotherapy alone. *Am Rev Respir Dis* 1990; 141:914–921.

216. Hodson ME, Penketh ARL, Batten JC. Aerosol carbenicillin and gentamicin treatment of Pseudomonas aeruginosa infection in patients with cystic fibrosis. *Lancet* 1981;2:1137–1139.

217. Wall MA, Terry AB, Eisenberg J, et al. Inhaled antibiotics in cystic fibrosis. *Lancet* 1983;1:1325.

218. Ramsey BW, Dorkin HL, Eisenberg JD, et al. Efficacy of aerosolized tobramycin in patients with cystic fibrosis. *N Engl J Med* 1993;328:1740–1746.

219. Hodson ME, Butland RJA, Roberts CM, et al. Oral ciprofloxacin compared with conventional intravenous treatment for Pseudomonas aeruginosa in adults with cystic fibrosis. *Lancet* 1987;1:235–237.

220. Zapletal A, Stefanova J, Horak J, et al. Chest physiotherapy and airway obstruction in patients with cystic fibrosis—a negative report. *Eur J Respir Dis* 1983;64:426–433.

221. Desmond KJ, Schwenk F, Thomas E, et al. Immediate and long-term effects of chest physiotherapy in patients with cystic fibrosis. *J Pediatr* 1983;103:538–542.

222. Rossman CM, Waldes R, Sampson D, et al. Effect of chest physiotherapy on the removal of mucus in patients with cystic fibrosis. *Am Rev Respir Dis* 1982;126:131–135.

223. Zinman R. Cough versus chest physiotherapy: a comparison of the acute effects on pulmonary function in patients with cystic fibrosis. *Am Rev Respir Dis* 1984;129:182–184.

224. Hardy K. A review of airway clearance: new techniques, indications, and recommendations. *Respir Care* 1994;39:440–455.

225. Warwick WJ, Hansen LG. The long-term effect of high-frequency chest compression therapy on pulmonary complications of cystic fibrosis. *Pediatr Pulmonol* 1991;11:265–271.

226. Porter DK, Van Every MJ, Anthracite RF, et al. Massive hemoptysis in cystic fibrosis. *Arch Intern Med* 1983;143:287–290.

227. Penketh A, Knight RK, Hodson ME, et al. Management of pneumothorax in adults with cystic fibrosis. *Thorax* 1982;37: 850–853.

228. Stern RC. Cystic fibrosis: recent developments in diagnosis and treatment. *Pediatr Rev* 1986;7:276–286.

10

LUNG TRANSPLANTATION AND LUNG VOLUME REDUCTION SURGERY

STEPHANIE M. LEVINE
JAY I. PETERS
STEPHEN G. JENKINSON

INDICATIONS FOR SINGLE LUNG TRANSPLANTATION

INDICATIONS FOR BILATERAL LUNG TRANSPLANTATION

INDICATIONS FOR HEART-LUNG TRANSPLANTATION

GUIDELINES FOR RECIPIENT SELECTION
Age
Contraindications
Systemic or Multisystem Disease
Corticosteroids
Psychosocial Criteria
Skeletal Disease
Mechanical Ventilation
Nutritional Status
Substance Abuse
Absolute Contraindications

DISEASE-SPECIFIC GUIDELINES FOR TIMING OF TRANSPLANTATION
Chronic Obstructive Lung Disease
Idiopathic Pulmonary Fibrosis
Cystic Fibrosis
Primary Pulmonary Hypertension

EVALUATION

DONOR SELECTION

SURGICAL TECHNIQUE: SINGLE LUNG TRANSPLANTATION

THE POSTOPERATIVE PERIOD
General Postoperative Management
Postoperative Problems

MANAGEMENT AFTER THE POSTOPERATIVE PERIOD

OUTCOME

COMPLICATIONS FOLLOWING LUNG TRANSPLANTATION
Airway Complications
Graft Rejection
Hyperacute and Acute Rejection

OBLITERATIVE BRONCHIOLITIS

INFECTIOUS COMPLICATIONS

LYMPHOPROLIFERATIVE DISORDERS

IMMUNOSUPPRESSION

LUNG VOLUME REDUCTION SURGERY
Selection of Patients
Surgical Techniques
Other Effects on Patient Outcomes Following LVRS
Mechanisms of Decreased Obstruction and Improved Exercise Tolerance following LVRS
Changes in Pulmonary Function following Surgery
Conclusions

Since the 1980s, lung transplantation (LT) has been a therapeutic option for patients with end-stage pulmonary parenchymal or vascular disease. Although Hardy performed the first human lung transplant in 1963, the patient survived only 18 days (1). From 1963 until 1980, nearly 40 more lung transplants were attempted; however, the longest survival was only 10 months (2,3). Early attempts at lung transplantation were unsuccessful because of the development of rejection or infection in the transplant recipients (2,3).

Since that time, research has led to improved surgical techniques, markedly improved immunosuppressive therapy initially with the discovery of cyclosporine A (4), and standardization of selection criteria for transplant recipients. As a result, in 1997 over 1,300 LT procedures were performed worldwide, as reported to the International Society of Heart and Lung Transplantation (ISHLT) (5). Pulmonologists must understand the surgical procedures available to their patients, the selection criteria for transplantation, the immunosuppressive regimens, and the management of complications that commonly occur in transplant recipients. The first part of this chapter reviews each of these topics. The second part of this chapter reviews the more recently utilized surgical option for patients with end-stage obstructive lung disease: lung volume reduction surgery.

INDICATIONS FOR SINGLE LUNG TRANSPLANTATION

In 1983, the Toronto Group reported the first long-term survival of a single lung transplantation (SLT) in a patient with idiopathic pulmonary fibrosis (6). Restrictive parenchymal lung disease is ideal for SLT. The transplanted lung possesses normal compliance and vascular resistance and allows preferential ventilation and perfusion to the transplanted organ. SLTs have been performed for idiopathic and familial pulmonary fibrosis, drug- or toxin-induced lung disease, occupational lung disease, sarcoidosis, limited scleroderma, and other disorders resulting in end-stage fibrotic lung disease.

Initially, there was concern that patients with obstructive lung disease might develop severe ventilation-perfusion mismatch after SLT. These disorders are characterized by increased lung compliance and destruction of the vascular bed. Perfusion could be diverted to the transplanted lung while ventilation remained in the native emphysematous lung. Early attempts at SLTs in patients with emphysema resulted in hyperinflation of the native lung with compression of the transplanted lung (7). Fortunately, careful management of mechanical ventilation and control of postoperative infections and rejection have resulted in successful SLTs in patients with obstructive lung disease (8). Although the patients have continued airway obstruction on pulmonary function testing, there is no significant ventilation-perfusion mismatch. This has allowed SLTs to be performed in patients with chronic obstructive lung disease (COPD) and in patients with α_1-antitrypsin deficiency. The first successful SLT for COPD in the U.S. was performed in 1989 by Dr. J. Kent Trinkle in San Antonio, Texas (9). Currently, COPD comprises the most common indication for SLT reported to the registry of the ISHLT at 45% (5).

SLT has also been used successfully in patients with pulmonary vascular disease. A single lung allograft with normal pulmonary vasculature can accommodate the entire right ventricular output without elevation of pulmonary artery pressure (10). The right ventricle has been shown to be extremely resilient, and SLTs have been done in patients

with right ventricular ejection fractions below 20%. The right ventricle shows significant improvement in function postoperatively. Patients with Eisenmenger's syndrome (a cardiac abnormality resulting in pulmonary hypertension) and a repairable cardiac anomaly are also candidates for SLT.

The advantages of SLT include reduced surgical morbidity, shortened hospitalization, and often the avoidance of cardiopulmonary bypass. This procedure also optimizes the use of donor organs, which are in critical shortage.

INDICATIONS FOR BILATERAL LUNG TRANSPLANTATION

Patients with suppurative pulmonary lung disease, such as cystic fibrosis, are not candidates for SLTs. Once immunosuppressed, the native lung would infect the transplanted lung or lead to systemic infection. Initially, patients with cystic fibrosis or bronchiectasis underwent heart-lung transplantation. Double lung transplantation (DLT) avoids concurrent or asynchronous rejection of the heart and may avoid the accelerated coronary artery disease seen with heart transplantation. Initially, this procedure was performed with an anastomosis at the level of the trachea; however, the rate of ischemic airway complications was prohibitive. Now transplant surgeons perform bilateral lung transplantation (BLT) or sequential SLT, with anastomoses performed at each mainstem bronchus.

Some transplant centers perform BLT for severe obstructive lung disease. In young patients with emphysema and a longer posttransplant life expectancy or in patients with extensive bilateral bullae, BLT may be preferable. Similarly, patients with pulmonary hypertension with reduced right ventricular function are the most difficult to manage in the intraoperative and postoperative periods. Some centers, therefore, prefer BLT for pulmonary hypertension in an attempt to distribute blood flow equally to both lungs.

INDICATIONS FOR HEART-LUNG TRANSPLANTATION

Few centers are currently performing heart-lung transplantation (HLT). However heart-lung transplantation remains the primary procedure for patients with combined end-stage lung disease and heart disease (e.g., emphysema with cardiomyopathy or irreparable coronary artery disease). Patients with Eisenmenger's syndrome and irreparable cardiac lesions also require HLT. Most transplant centers require that patients be less than 55 years of age for HLT. There is an approximately 25% risk of major morbidity in the postoperative period with HLT (11). Opportunistic infections and bronchiolitis obliterans are major causes of mortality after this procedure. Despite the increased incidence of complica-

TABLE 10.1. TRANSPLANTATION PROCEDURES BY DISEASE STATE

Transplant Procedure	Disease State
Single lung	Restrictive fibrotic lung disease, COPD (emphysema, α_1-antitrypsin deficiency), pulmonary hypertension
Bilateral lung	Suppurative lung disease (cystic fibrosis, bronchiectasis), some patients with COPD, pulmonary hypertension
Heart-lung	End-stage cardiac and pulmonary disease

Modified from Official ATS Statement—June 1992. Lung transplantation: report of the ATS Workshop on Lung Transplantation. *Am Rev Respir Dis* 1993;147:772–776, with permission.

tions, HLT remains the only appropriate option for some patients with combined end-stage cardiac and pulmonary disease. A summary of transplantation procedures by disease state is outlined in Table 10.1.

GUIDELINES FOR RECIPIENT SELECTION

Any patient with end-stage pulmonary or cardiopulmonary disease with the capacity for rehabilitation can be considered for transplantation. Obviously, many patients will not be suitable candidates, and the patients most likely to survive the early postoperative transplant period are those who, although terminally ill, maintain an active lifestyle and an acceptable nutritional status. The patient should have untreatable end-stage pulmonary disease, no other significant medical illness, and a limited life expectancy. The candidate should be ambulatory with rehabilitation potential. Patients must be psychologically stable, committed to the idea of transplantation, and willing to comply with the rigorous medical protocols required for successful lung transplantation. These general guidelines have been accepted by the American Thoracic Society (12) and are outlined in Table 10.2.

TABLE 10.2. GENERAL RECIPIENT SELECTION GUIDELINES

Untreatable end-stage pulmonary disease of any etiology
No other significant medical diseases
Substantial limitation of daily activity
Limited life expectancy
Ambulatory with rehabilitation potential
Acceptable nutritional status
Satisfactory psychosocial profile and emotional support system

Modified from Official ATS Statement—June 1992. Lung transplantation: report of the ATS Workshop on Lung Transplantation. *Am Rev Respir Dis* 1993;147:772–776, with permission.

Age

Recent international guidelines for selection of transplant candidates suggested age limits of 55 years for HLT, 65 years for SLT, and 60 years for BLT procedures (13). Although this is somewhat arbitrary, numerous patients with end-stage pulmonary disease are young to middle-aged, and there is a relative lack of available donors.

Contraindications

The general relative and absolute contraindications to lung transplantation as identified by the 1998 international guidelines are listed in Table 10.3 (13).

Systemic or Multisystem Disease

Transplantation is not contraindicated in patients with systemic diseases limited to the lungs, such as scleroderma, systemic lupus erythematosus, polymyositis, and rheumatoid arthritis. These cases should be considered on an individual basis (14).

Patients with diabetes mellitus, poorly controlled hypertension, or neurologic disease should be evaluated carefully before being considered candidates for lung transplantation, and should be accepted only if their disease is well controlled and there is no end organ damage.

Patients with active sites of infection are not considered good transplant candidates. Treated tuberculosis and fungal disease pose a particular problem, but are not contraindications to lung transplantation. Many centers will not consider transplanting a patient who is chronically colonized with a resistant organism (*Burkholderia cepacia,* methicillin-resistant *Staphylococcus,* atypical *Mycobacterium,* or *Aspergil-*

TABLE 10.3. CONTRAINDICATIONS TO LUNG TRANSPLANTATION

Relative	Mechanical ventilation
	Symptomatic osteoporosis
	Ideal body weight below 70% or over 130%
	Substance addiction in prior six months (including tobacco use)
	Psychosocial problems
	Severe musculoskeletal disease
	Colonization with fungus or atypical mycobacteria
Absolute	Extrapulmonic disease, i.e., renal (Creatine clearance below 50 mg/mL/min)
	HIV infection
	Malignancy within prior two years
	Hepatitis B antigen positivity
	Hepatitis C biopsy proven liver disease

Adapted from Guidelines for the selection of lung transplant candidates. Joint Statement of the American Society for International Transplant Physicians/American Thoracic Society/European Respiratory Society/International Society for Heart and Lung Transplantation. *Am J Respir Crit Care Med* 1998; 158:335–339, with permission.

lus). Centers should try to eradicate these organisms in the pretransplant period and patients should be considered on an individual basis (15). These patients should not be considered for SLT procedures since the colonized remaining lung could pose a serious threat to the new graft.

Corticosteroids

Initial data implicated corticosteroids as a cause of tracheal or bronchial dehiscence (16–17). At most centers, patients were required to have completely discontinued corticosteroids. This eliminated a large number of patients with chronic obstructive lung disease and pulmonary fibrosis. More recently, low-dose pretransplant corticosteroid therapy has proved to be acceptable in patients who cannot have corticosteroids completely discontinued (9,17,18). Most transplant programs will consider patients who can be chronically maintained on 20 mg or less per day of prednisone, and may consider patients on higher doses.

Psychosocial Criteria

The patient must be well motivated and emotionally stable to withstand the extreme stress of the pretransplant and perioperative period. A history of noncompliance or a significant psychiatric illness is a relative contraindication, although many patients will present with reactive depression or anxiety in the terminal phase of their pulmonary illness. Prior to transplantation, a thorough psychiatric evaluation is required to exclude an underlying psychiatric diagnosis. The importance of a support system cannot be overemphasized.

Skeletal Disease

Osteoporosis has become a significant problem in the posttransplant period, and preexisting symptomatic osteoporosis has been identified as a relative contraindication to transplantation (19). Bone densitometry should be part of the pretransplant evaluation, and treatment initiated in those with evidence of osteoporosis, symptomatic or asymptomatic. Nonosteoporotic skeletal disease, such as kyphoscoliosis is also a relative contraindication to transplantation.

Mechanical Ventilation

Requirement for invasive mechanical ventilation is a strong relative contraindication to transplantation. Patients who are on noninvasive ventilatory support can be considered for transplantation.

Nutritional Status

In order to be considered for transplantation, patients should have an ideal body weight of over 70 or less than 130% of predicted. Cachectic patients may be too weak to withstand the surgical procedure, and patients who are obese make more difficult surgical candidates.

Substance Abuse

Drug abuse or alcoholism are considered contraindications to transplantation because these patients are at high risk for noncompliance. Patients who continue to smoke despite end-stage pulmonary disease are not candidates for lung transplantation. Most transplant centers require a patient to abstain from cigarette smoking, alcohol abuse, or narcotics for six months to two years before being considered for lung transplantation.

Absolute Contraindications

Recent international guidelines identify absolute contraindications to lung transplantation to include major organ dysfunction, that is, renal (creatinine clearance of less than 50 mg per mL per minute), HIV infection, hepatitis B antigen positivity, and hepatitis C with biopsy-documented liver disease (13). Active malignancy within the prior two years is also a contraindication to transplantation. For patients with a history of breast cancer beyond stage 2, colon cancer beyond Dukes A, renal carcinoma, or melanoma at or beyond level III, this waiting period should be at least five years. Patients with a prior malignancy should be restaged before they become transplant candidates.

DISEASE-SPECIFIC GUIDELINES FOR TIMING OF TRANSPLANTATION

Patients who meet all criteria for lung transplantation are usually placed on the active waiting list when their life expectancy is less than 18 to 24 months. This period of time has been referred to as the "transplant window," when the patient is ill enough to require transplantation and healthy enough to assure a reasonable chance for success (20). Data from the United Network for Organ Sharing (UNOS) show that the mean waiting period ranges from 12 to 24 months. Guidelines for the timing of transplantation are difficult to determine but must be based on the natural history of each disease process. The recent international guidelines outline disease-specific criteria for transplant referral (Table 10.4) (13).

Chronic Obstructive Lung Disease

The variability in the natural course of COPD makes it especially difficult to predict when patients should be referred for lung transplantation. The National Institutes of Health's Intermittent Positive-Pressure Breathing (IPPB) trial demonstrated that patients less than 65 years old with an FEV_1 below 30% of predicted had a three-year survival rate of 80% (21). This study excluded patients with hypoxemia. Nevertheless, this study confirmed prior reports that the postbronchodilator FEV_1 was the best predictor of survival. Another study reviewed two community-based popu-

TABLE 10.4. DISEASE SPECIFIC CRITERIA FOR LUNG TRANSPLANTATION

COPD	FEV_1 under 25% of predicted (nonreversible)
	$PaCO_2$ at or over 55 mm Hg
	Cor pulmonale
	O_2-dependent hypercapnic patients (refer early)
IPF	Symptomatic disease despite medical therapy
	Abnormal pulmonary function:
	VC 60% to 70% of predicted
	Diffusing capacity 50% to 60% of predicted
CF	FEV_1 at or under 30% of predicted
	Clinical deterioration with FEV_1 >30% of predicted
	$PaCO_2$ over 50 mm Hg
	PaO_2 on room air under 55 mm Hg
	Young, female patients (refer early)
PPH	NYHA III-IV despite vasodilator treatment
	Cardiac index under 2 L/min/m^2
	Right atrial pressure over 15 mm Hg
	Mean pulmonary artery pressure over 55 mm Hg

CF, cystic fibrosis; COPD, chronic obstructive pulmonary disease; IPF, idiopathic pulmonary fibrosis; PPH, primary pulmonary hypertension.
Adapted from Guidelines for the Selection of lung transplant candidates. Joint Statement of the American Society for International Transplant Physicians/American Thoracic Society/European Respiratory Society/International Society for Heart and Lung Transplantation. *Am J Respir Crit Care Med* 1998; 158:335–339, with permission.

lations with COPD during a seven- to 15-year study period (22). Again, the best predictor of survival was the percentage of predicted FEV_1 after the administration of bronchodilators. The presence or absence of cor pulmonale further improved the prediction of subsequent mortality. Cor pulmonale was clinically determined by history and physical examination, radiographic findings, and electrocardiogram. Poor nutritional status (assessed by serum albumin) and carbon monoxide diffusing capacity (D_{LCO}) also showed some statistical significance. This study showed an overall one-year survival of 65% when the postbronchodilator FEV_1 fell below 30% of predicted. Patients with cor pulmonale and an FEV_1 below 30% of predicted had a two-year survival of 50% and a three-year survival of only 20%.

Both studies showed wide individual variability in survival with COPD, and the decision to transplant these patients is frequently based on the progression of disease. Analysis of registry and UNOS data have shown that this group of patients may achieve significant improvement in quality of life without clear survival benefit with transplantation (23).

Based on the above data, the international guidelines (13) suggest that patients with COPD are in the transplant window if FEV_1 is less than 25% of predicted (nonreversible), and/or $PaCO_2$ is at or over 55 mm Hg and/or there is cor pulmonale. Those patients with hypercapnia and hy-

poxemia requiring oxygen supplementation should be given preference.

Idiopathic Pulmonary Fibrosis

Prospective longitudinal studies show that the mean survival in patients with usual interstitial pneumonia (idiopathic pulmonary fibrosis—IPF) is 5.6 years after diagnosis (24). Although 10% of patients respond to therapy and 15% remain stable, this pattern is seen with only mild or moderate disease (24). Most patients have a progressive downhill course despite therapy. In one prospective randomized trial comparing prednisolone alone with cyclophosphamide and prednisolone, only the initial total lung capacity (TLC) and forced vital capacity (FVC) were associated with time to "failure." Patients with a TLC below 60% of predicted did poorly regardless of the initial regimen and had a 50% one-year survival (25).

Based on these high mortality statistics and the fact that many patients with IPF die while awaiting transplantation, the international guidelines suggest that these patients should be referred for transplantation early. Criteria include patients with symptomatic disease who have failed immunosuppressive therapy and/or patients with abnormal pulmonary function even with minimal symptoms, that is, vital capacity at or under 60% to 70% predicted and/or diffusing capacity at or under 50% to 60% of predicted (13).

Cystic Fibrosis

Despite the improvement in life expectancy with cystic fibrosis, most patients still die from respiratory failure and cor pulmonale. A recent study followed almost 700 patients with cystic fibrosis over 12 years to determine whether the risk from respiratory failure could be predicted one or two years in advance (26). The study concluded that patients with an FEV_1 less than 30% predicted, a partial pressure of oxygen below 55 mm Hg, or a partial pressure of carbon dioxide above 50 mm Hg had a two-year mortality of 50%.

The international guidelines (13) suggest that the following criteria should be used to define the transplant window for CF patients: an FEV_1 at or under 30%, or an FEV_1 over 30% with progressive deterioration (including increasing hospitalizations, rapid fall in FEV_1, cachexia, and massive hemoptysis), a PaO_2 under 55 mm Hg on room air and/or $PaCO_2$ over 50 mm Hg. Female patients and patients under the age of 18 years old had a more progressive course and should be considered for lung transplantation at an earlier stage.

Patients with CF are often colonized with multiple-resistant organisms (resistance to all agents in two of the following antibiotic classes: the beta-lactams, aminoglycosides, and/or quinolones) or panresistant organisms (resistant *in vitro* to all groups of antibiotics), particularly *Pseudomonas aeruginosa* and *Burkholderia cepacia*. Patients with multiple-resistant organisms can be successfully transplanted due to available synergistic use of antibiotics. However, panresistant organism colonization may be considered by some to be a strong relative contraindication. A recent study examined the outcome of CF patients with and without panresistant *P. aeruginosa* (n = 21) and *B. cepacia* (n = 6), versus those with sensitive organisms (n = 39) (15). Postoperative ventilator days, length of hospital stay, and antibiotic days were similar between groups. The incidences of bronchitis and pneumonia were also comparable between the groups. One-year survival was comparable at 81% and 83% respectively. However, when a subanalysis was performed, patients with *B. cepacia* had a lower one-year survival of 50% in comparison to resistant *P. aeruginosa* (90%). The authors concluded that CF patients with panresistant pseudomonas should not be excluded from transplantation based on that criteria alone.

Primary Pulmonary Hypertension

The natural median survival of patients with untreated primary pulmonary hypertension (PPH) is 2.8 years after diagnosis. The National Heart, Blood and Lung Patient Registry has followed approximately 200 patients for three to seven years to characterize variables associated with poor survival (27). Median survival decreased from 58.6 months (for patients in New York Heart Association [NYHA] class I or II) to 31.5 months (for patients in functional class III) to six months (for patients in functional class IV). An increase in mean pulmonary artery pressure from less than 55 mm Hg to more than 85 mm Hg was associated with a decrease in mean survival from 48 months to 12 months. A decrease in cardiac index of 4 L per minute per m² to 2 L per minute per m² was associated with a decrease in median survival from 43 months to 17 months. The presence of Raynaud's phenomena also predicted a poor prognosis, with a median survival of less than one year. Over 80% of patients were discharged on some drug therapy, usually a combination of vasodilators, anticoagulants, and diuretics.

The selection guidelines for transplantation suggested that PPH patients with NYHA III or IV who, despite optimal therapy, including vasodilators, that is, prostacyclin or calcium channel blockers, and those with significantly elevated pulmonary artery pressures (PA means above 55 mm Hg), depressed cardiac index (below 2 L per minute per m²), or right atrial pressure of over 15 mm Hg should be considered for transplantation. Others should be followed closely and reassessed for transplantation at six-month intervals. Referral to a transplant center is usually made when the patient reaches NYHA class III.

EVALUATION

Once a patient is a potential candidate for transplantation, a battery of studies is performed for further assessment.

Typically, these include pulmonary function tests (PFT) including lung volumes, spirometry and diffusing capacity, and a measure of exercise performance. Cardiac evaluation includes an electrocardiogram and an echocardiogram, in addition to some functional cardiac study such as dobutamine echocardiography and/or coronary angiography in patients over the age of 40. A high-resolution CT is usually obtained to look for bronchiectasis, which could indicate the necessity for a bilateral procedure, or to look for focal nodules not apparent on plain radiograph. Renal and liver functions are assessed by 24-hour creatinine clearance and liver function tests respectively.

DONOR SELECTION

The shortage of donor organs continues to be the rate-limiting factor for the number of LT procedures performed. Most potential donors are brain-dead as a result of head trauma or a primary noninfectious central nervous system event. Standard donor criteria are shown in Table 10.5. The ideal donor should be less than 65 years of age and have no history of lung disease and a low cumulative smoking history (under 30 pack-years). Serial chest radiographs should be grossly clear prior to consideration for lung donation. When donation is being considered for HLT or BLT, both lungs must meet criteria for donation. However, for SLT, unilateral lung injury secondary to trauma does not automatically exclude the contralateral lung from consideration for donation (28). The physiologic capacity of the potential donor graft is further accessed by gas exchange capability. Typically, a PaO_2 above 300 mm Hg on an FiO_2 of 1 and 5 cm H_2O of positive end–expiratory pressure (PEEP) is required. Oxygenation not meeting the above criterion could indicate potential ventilation/perfusion mismatch following surgery.

TABLE 10.5. GUIDELINES FOR DONOR SELECTION

Age under 65 years

No history of significant lung disease

Limited cumulative cigarette smoking history (under 30 pack-years)

Clear lung field on chest radiograph

Acceptable lung compliance (peak inspiratory pressure under 30 cm H_2O)[a]

Adequate oxygenation (PaO_2 above 300 mm Hg at F_iO_2 = 1.0 or PaO_2/FiO_2 above 250–300 mm Hg)[a]

Satisfactory gross appearance and bronchoscopic inspection

PaO_2 = arterial oxygen tension; F_iO_2, fraction of inspired oxygen.
[a]At PEEP = 5 cm H_2O.
Trulock EP. State of the art: lung transplantation. *Am J Respir Crit Care Med* 1997;155:789–818, with permission.

Most lung transplant centers require a Gram stain of a tracheal aspirate and/or bronchoscopy to be performed on all potential donor candidates to minimize the possibility of transmitting infectious agents from an infected donor organ. Fiber-optic bronchoscopy is often a routine part of the organ harvest to assess blood, purulent secretions, or foreign bodies in the tracheobronchial tree that are not apparent on chest radiograph. If bronchoscopic examination is abnormal, the organ should be excluded from consideration for donation.

The donor evaluation process is completed by obtaining serologic tests for HIV, hepatitis B, and cytomegalovirus (CMV). The patient is not a donor candidate if hepatitis B surface antigen or HIV antibody is present.

Certain donor-recipient compatibility tests should be met following availability of an acceptable donor organ. Unlike other solid-organ donations, SLT, HLT, and DLT are ABO blood groups matched only and not human leukocyte antigen (HLA) matched. Currently, lung graft preservation time is limited to approximately four to six hours, and this short time precludes HLA typing prior to transplantation. Furthermore, retrospective analysis of HLA compatibility of SLT donors and recipients does not appear to correlate with subsequent episodes of rejection or mortality (29). Two recent retrospective studies dispute this and suggest that HLA matching may result in a reduced incidence of posttransplant rejection (30,31).

Size matching of the donor and the recipient is not handled uniformly at all transplant centers. Some centers measure the chest circumference of the transplant recipient and match it to the corresponding donor chest wall circumference within 3 inches in either direction (9). Other groups estimate the size match by determining the lung capacities of the donor and recipient with a height and sex nomogram (32). Some institutions perform size matching by estimating chest wall size by plain radiograph or by using a combination of measurements of body weight and chest wall circumference plus horizontal thoracic length (33). Regardless of the method of size matching used, the donor lung size approximates that of the recipient soon after transplantation (32,34).

SURGICAL TECHNIQUE: SINGLE LUNG TRANSPLANTATION

The donor lung is usually removed at the time of cardiac harvest via a median sternotomy incision. The pulmonary veins with a residual 5 mm cuff of left atrium are detached from the heart. The pulmonary artery is transected from the main pulmonary trunk, and the mainstem bronchus is transected between two staple lines (9). The donor lung graft is preserved in Euro-Collins solution (a crystalloid solution with intracellular electrolyte composition) at 4°C during transportation to the recipient site and is usually stored in a partially inflated position.

The recipient surgery is performed through a posterolateral thoracotomy incision. Initially the donor pulmonary vein is anastomosed end to end to the recipient's left atrium. The technical details of the bronchial anastomosis vary among institutions. The lungs are the only solid organs that are transplanted without a complete vascular anastomosis (i.e., the bronchial circulation of the recipient and donor lungs are not anastomosed). Because of this lack of revascularization of the bronchial circulation, anastomotic complications including bronchial dehiscence, bronchial stenosis, and bronchial infection are major complications in lung transplantation. Some transplant centers perform an end-to-end anastomosis and wrap a piece of omentum with an intact vascular pedicle around the anastomosis to help in bronchial revascularization. Other institutions use the telescoping technique when performing the bronchial anastomosis. In the telescoping technique, the recipient and donor bronchi are overlapped by approximately one cartilaginous ring. This allows the intact bronchial circulation of the recipient better to supply the donor bronchus. The use of the telescoping technique has significantly reduced the incidence of anastomotic complications as reported in some series, but other centers have obtained fewer anastamotic complications with the end-to-end procedure (35). SLT surgery is completed by performing an end-to-end anastomosis of the donor and recipient pulmonary arteries.

An interesting issue to consider when performing SLT is which side to transplant. This choice is based on a number of factors. For example, if the recipient's pleural space has been previously invaded by open lung biopsy or pneumothorax requiring chemical or surgical pleurodesis, the contralateral hemithorax should be chosen. If preoperative quantitative ventilation and perfusion (V/Q) scanning shows one lung functioning significantly better than the other lung, the less-functional lung should be transplanted. Assuming that the lungs function equally and the recipient has had no prior surgery, the left side has traditionally been chosen for transplantation. Technically, the surgery is easier to perform on the left side, since it is easier to clamp the left atrium proximal to the left pulmonary vein and it is possible to leave a larger donor atrial cuff and longer recipient bronchus (9). When performing SLT for COPD, radiographically the transplanted left lung is apparently compressed by the native hyperinflated right lung. This compression is less dramatic when the transplant is placed on the right side. Despite the radiographic differences, the results of pulmonary function testing, exercise oximetry, and V/Q lung scanning do not support a functional difference between the right and left graft position for the treatment of obstructive lung diseases (36).

THE POSTOPERATIVE PERIOD

General Postoperative Management

Bilateral lung transplant procedures are usually performed through a transverse thoracosternotomy (clamshell incision) followed by sequential single lung procedures. Cardiopulmonary bypass may be required for cases of pulmonary hypertension. Following lung transplant surgery, patients remain intubated and require mechanical ventilation. Most patients are ventilated on a volume control mode, although some transplant centers have changed to pressure control ventilation in recent years. Airway pressures should be maintained as low as possible to avoid barotrauma and anastomotic dehiscence. Most institutions use routine pharmacologic sedation. Patients are generally maintained with tidal volumes of 6 to 10 mL per kg following surgery. At some institutions, a low level of PEEP is applied immediately after lung expansion in the operating room and continued following transplantation (9). Uncomplicated lung transplant recipients are extubated within the first 24 hours following transplantation. Both postural drainage and chest physiotherapy can be routinely employed without concern about mechanical complications at the anastomosis.

Certain patient populations require special ventilator management. In patients undergoing SLT for pulmonary hypertension, reperfusion pulmonary edema is often severe because nearly all perfusion is going to the newly implanted lung. Often prolonged sedation and pharmacologic paralysis for up to two to three days are required following surgery. This patient population should have aggressive diuresis, and they may require higher levels of PEEP for longer periods of time. Some transplant centers have recommended that patients with significant pulmonary hypertension be positioned for the first few days following surgery with the transplant side up to increase blood flow to the native lung, which is not as severely affected by the pulmonary reimplantation response.

In patients with obstructive lung disease, problems can be encountered if the delivered tidal volume or required levels of PEEP are high. Occasionally, significant hyperinflation of the native lung can result, which can compromise the newly transplanted lung. To reduce this problem, many transplant centers avoid PEEP when performing SLT for obstructive disease. Several reports have described the use of selective independent ventilation with a double-lumen tube to prevent this possible complication (37).

Since many patients are nutritionally depleted prior to transplantation because of their underlying disease, postoperative nutritional needs are important. Ideally, immediate nutritional alimentation should be begun.

Antibiotics are routinely administered for the first 48 to 72 hours following transplantation. Routine antibiotic regimens vary between centers but include a broad-spectrum Gram-negative agent. Several centers routinely use antifungal agents such as amphotericin B or itraconazole postoperatively. Empiric anaerobic coverage has been advocated by some centers. Gram stains and cultures of donor and recipient sputa may be used to choose appropriate antibiotics when available. Ganciclovir is administered for CMV prophylaxis in most transplant programs if either the patient or the donor is CMV-positive prior to surgery.

Induction immunosuppression is begun with cyclosporine and azathioprine preoperatively. Corticosteroids are administered as intravenous methylprednisolone 0.5 to 1 g in the operating room (usually given at the time of reperfusion), then 1 to 3 mg per kg per day for the subsequent three days, followed by 1 mg per kg per day, then converted to an equivalent oral dose. Many centers use lympholytic medications such as antilymphocyte globulin at 10 to 15 mg per kg per day intravenously or muromonab-CD3 (Orthoclone OKT3) 5 mg per day for the first five to 10 days following transplantation. Some programs are now using one or both of the newer immunosuppressive agents (tacrolimus and mycophenolate mofetil) *de novo*.

Postoperative Problems

Perhaps the most significant problem following lung transplantation is the development of the pulmonary reimplantation response (PRR) or primary graft failure (PGF). It is estimated that up to 80% of patients will experience some degree of reimplantation injury (37,38). To varying degrees, the PRR can persist for hours to days following lung transplant surgery. Clinically, the PRR is characterized by new radiographic alveolar and/or interstitial infiltrates, a decrease in pulmonary compliance, and disrupted gas exchange. Radiographic findings in these patients included a perihilar haze, patchy alveolar consolidations, and dense perihilar and basilar alveolar consolidations, with air bronchograms (Fig. 10.1). The PRR usually worsens or stabilizes over the subsequent two to four days and then begins to resolve.

Although the mechanism for the PRR has not been completely delineated, several contributing factors have been postulated, including the disruption of lymphatics, bronchial vasculature, and/or nerves, as well as lung injury occurring either during preservation of the graft or following reperfusion. The PRR is thought to be a form of membrane permeability edema that develops to various degrees in all lung transplant recipients in whom warm ischemia persists for more than 30 minutes or cold ischemia persists for more than two hours (39,40). Animal studies have suggested that the severity of the PRR is related to the ischemic time and may relate to the production of toxic oxygen-free radicals (39).

In general, the PRR appears in the immediate postoperative period, whereas rejection and infection are more common after the first 24 hours. However, since the timing of these disorders may vary, differentiation may be difficult. The PRR may be minimized by the avoidance of prolonged

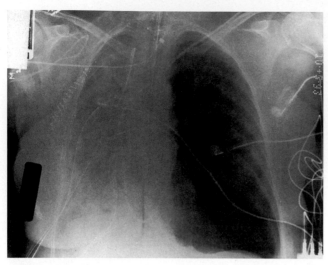

FIGURE 10.1. Anteroposterior portable chest radiograph of a 50-year-old woman with chronic obstructive lung disease taken six hours after a right single lung transplant procedure. Note the alveolar infiltrates caused by the pulmonary reimplantation response.

ischemic times, the optimization of organ preservation, the appropriate use of postoperative hemodynamic monitoring, and the timely use of diuretics, inotropic agents, and antibiotics or augmented immunosuppression if other diagnoses are suspected. There are reports of the use of inhaled nitric oxide and extracorporeal membrane oxygenation (ECMO) for severe early graft dysfunction (41,42).

A recent study examined the findings in 15 of 100 patients deemed by standard clinical criteria to have PGF (43). The study documented a 15% incidence of this complication with associated prolonged hospital course, prolonged mechanical ventilation, poor one-year survival (40% versus 69%) and compromised function among survivors. The authors found no clear risk factors for PGF, including with age, sex, underlying disease, pulmonary artery pressure, type of transplant, ischemic times, or use of cardiopulmonary bypass. In those patients with PGF, induction immunosuppressive therapy was used less frequently than those patients that did not develop this complication.

MANAGEMENT AFTER THE POSTOPERATIVE PERIOD

After discharge, follow-up is performed in the outpatient clinic. A sample follow-up schedule would be weekly for the first two months, biweekly for the next month, and monthly thereafter. After three months of uncomplicated posttransplant observation, patients often return home and resume follow-up with their referring pulmonologists.

Weekly studies include a cyclosporine or tacrolimus level, a CBC to monitor the leukocyte count on azathioprine or mycophenolate mofetil, blood chemistries to follow creati-

nine while on cyclosporine and to follow liver function tests, a chest radiograph, routine spirometry, and exercise oximetry. In addition, patients bring in their home spirometric measurements at each visit. Some institutions perform surveillance bronchoscopy on a routine schedule, while other institutions reserve this procedure for clinical deterioration.

The most efficient and effective way to monitor the patient following transplantation to detect early rejection, infection, or anastomotic complications remains controversial. Early in the transplant experience, quantitative ventilation and perfusion to the lung graft were examined as an indicator of graft rejection. Early acute rejection was often heralded by a decrease in perfusion to the lung graft (33). Subsequently, quantitative ventilation-perfusion lung scanning was found to be neither sensitive nor specific for graft complications.

Likewise, chest radiographs have been shown to be neither specific nor sensitive for early detection of infection or rejection (44,45–47). Seventy-four percent of cases of rejection or infection in HLT recipients were associated with abnormal chest radiographs in the first month following transplantation. However, after the first posttransplant month, only 23% of rejection episodes were associated with abnormal chest radiographs (46).

Close monitoring of pulmonary function has also been studied as a way of detecting graft complications (48,49). At most transplant centers, patients are given home spirometers and instructed to document their FEV_1 and FVC twice a day. Patients are instructed to notify their local physician or the transplant center if the FEV_1 or FVC declines by 10% to 15% on two subsequent measurements. If this decline is confirmed in the PFT laboratory, transbronchial biopsy is indicated, because this degree of deterioration in pulmonary function has been associated with either rejection or infection (48,49). A study of HLT recipients comparing pulmonary function, chest radiographs, and transbronchial biopsies found pulmonary function testing to have 86% sensitivity in detecting rejection in the first three months following transplantation and 75% sensitivity subsequently. The sensitivity for detecting infection was 75%. Although pulmonary function testing was not able to distinguish between rejection and infection, pulmonary function testing did have an 84% specificity for detecting complications in the lung graft. This study also reinforced prior data showing chest radiographs to be sensitive early following transplantation but subsequently having only 19% sensitivity for rejection (45). Desaturation of more than 4% or a drop below an absolute oxygen saturation of 90% on constant workload cycle exercise oximetry has also been suggested as an indicator of a complication in the lung graft (50).

Surveillance bronchoscopy has become a controversial issue in LT. Reports suggest that surveillance bronchoscopy may allow the early detection of asymptomatic complications such as acute rejection and could thus reduce future development of obliterative bronchiolitis (OB). A recent study using patients who had undergone surveillance bronchoscopy as historic controls did not support a difference in bronchiolitis obliterans syndrome (BOS) or survival in comparison to a group of transplant recipients who did not undergo surveillance bronchoscopy (51). However, a recent large survey of 57 transplant centers reported that 69% continue to perform surveillance bronschoscopy on a regular basis (52).

OUTCOME

Lung function gradually improves and reaches a plateau by three months following surgery. SLT for obstructive lung disease results in residual mild-to-moderate obstructive pulmonary dysfunction secondary to the remaining native lung (53). SLT recipients with underlying restrictive lung disease have a residual mild restrictive defect (54–57). SLT recipients with pulmonary vascular disease maintain their normal pulmonary function and develop normal hemodynamics following transplantation (58). BLT or HLT performed for any indication results in improved spirometry following surgery (59,60).

Most ventilation and perfusion go to the transplanted lung following SLT for obstructive or restrictive lung disease (59). SLT for pulmonary hypertension results in a nearly equal division of ventilation between the transplanted and native lung, with nearly all perfusion going to the new lung graft (58). This ventilation-perfusion imbalance results in normal gas exchange under baseline conditions but can pose a problem during episodes of graft complications (61). Following DLT, BLT, or HLT, ventilation and perfusion are divided between the lungs.

All of the different lung transplant procedures result in normal gas exchange following transplantation. Exercise testing uniformly results in reduced maximum exercise capacities with no evidence of ventilatory limitation or arterial oxygen desaturation. There is no significant difference in exercise capacities in patients undergoing SLT versus DLT, BLT, or HLT, despite the differences in spirometry for the SLT procedure (54–56,62). Proposed reasons for the reduced exercise capacity following transplantation include deconditioning, myopathy secondary to immunosuppressive medications, chronic anemia, and limited pulmonary vascular capacities in the case of SLT. Despite the reduced exercise capacities, all stable patients are able to carry out activities of daily living without compromise.

Although one-, two-, and three-year survival rates of lung transplant recipients are 72%, 62%, and 56%, respectively (5)—lower than those achieved with heart or liver transplantation—some improvement in survival has been made over the last 10 years. Some lung transplant recipients are surviving five to 10 years or more and maintaining a normal functional status. Mortality in the early postoperative period has been caused primarily by technical complications and primary graft failure. Mortality after the perioperative period (beyond 30 days) and up to one year is primarily due to infection. Mortality beyond the first year has been primarily related to bronchiolitis obliterans.

Quality-of-life (QOL) issues are a relatively recent area of research in lung transplantation. Several small studies have shown improvement in overall and health-related QOL (63–66). The large majority of patients have expressed satisfaction with their transplant decision. Even if survival advantage is in question, the improvement in QOL is worth the sacrifice to many patients.

COMPLICATIONS FOLLOWING LUNG TRANSPLANTATION

Airway Complications

Airway problems, a significant cause of morbidity and mortality following early attempts at lung transplantation, develope in 20% to 50% of transplant recipients (67–70). Airway complications can be divided into early and late time periods. Early complications typically develop in the first one to two months following transplantation and are characterized by anastomotic infection and/or partial or complete anastomotic dehiscence. Subsequently, anastomotic strictures and/or bronchomalacia can develop, which significantly compromise the function of the transplanted lung or lungs. Several theoretical causes of airway complications following lung transplantation have been postulated, including ischemia at the site of the anastomosis, infection of the anastomosis, poor organ preservation, pneumonia, graft rejection, early corticosteroid administration, and an excessively long donor bronchus. As stated previously, the lung is the only solid organ that is transplanted without complete revascularization of the systemic blood supply. Therefore oxygenation of the new lung graft or grafts depends upon collateral blood flow from the pulmonary to the bronchial circulation.

Airway complications have been reduced with the development of the omental wrap and the telescoping anastomotic technique (9). Experimental work in an animal model has been done on direct bronchial revascularization to decrease airway complications following transplantation (68,69). In contemporary series, airway complications have a prevalence of 10% to 20%, with a low mortality (35,71,72).

Clinically, bronchial stenosis can present with cough, shortness of breath, dyspnea on exertion, and worsening obstruction on pulmonary function testing. A characteristic flow volume loop with an inspiratory and expiratory concave pattern has been noted (73). Radiographically, bronchial strictures may be seen on posteroanterior chest radiographs and can be clearly visualized by CT and/or the definitive test, bronchoscopy. Partial or complete bronchial dehiscence can present with mediastinal emphysema on chest radiograph or air adjacent to the bronchial anastomosis on CT (47).

Many transplant centers advocate early routine surveillance bronchoscopy to evaluate the anastomosis and aid in early detection of complications. Anastomotic ischemia warrants close bronchoscopic observation. If an anastomotic infection is diagnosed, appropriate antibiotics should be initiated. There have been several cases described in HLT patients and more recently in SLT patients of *Aspergillus* tracheobronchitis involving the anastomosis (74). These have been successfully treated with amphotericin B followed by itraconazole.

Anastomotic strictures should be treated with balloon dilation, wire or silastic stent placement, laser, or surgery (72,75). Partial anastomotic dehiscence is managed conservatively. Complete dehiscence requires surgical revision of the anastomosis or retransplantation.

Graft Rejection

Any solid organ transplanted into a genetically nonidentical recipient is an allograft and provokes an immunologic response called rejection. Rejection results from the activation, differentiation, and proliferation of effector T cells directed against the donor organ cells. The transplanted organ is rejected primarily because of differences between the donor and the recipient cell-surface molecules that are encoded by genes in the major histocompatibility complex (MHC). The MHC molecules allow the immune system to discriminate between "self" and "nonself." The human MHC was discovered in the mid-1950s, when leukoagglutinating antibodies were found in the sera of multiparous women and were designated the human leukocyte antigen (HLA) complex.

Traditionally, graft rejection has been classified according to the time of onset and defined by the histopathologic pattern as hyperacute, acute, or chronic rejection.

Hyperacute and Acute Rejection

Hyperacute rejection occurs when preexisting alloantibodies bind to the vascular endothelium of the donor lung, activate complement, and cause widespread thrombosis of the vessels within the transplanted lung. Alloantibodies may be present in the donor's serum prior to transplantation through blood transfusions, pregnancy, or previous transplantation. Hyperacute rejection has been virtually eliminated by ABO blood group matching between the recipient and the donor and by pretransplantation screening of the recipients for panel-reactive antibodies (PRA). This panel uses a large group of antigens within the general donor population, and reactivity is measured between the panel and the serum of a prospective transplant recipient. Even though a recipient's serum shows no panel-reactive antibod-

ies, antibodies against donor alloantigens not represented in the screening panel could be present and cause hyperacute rejection. Fortunately, hyperacute rejection is uncommon, and only one pathologically proven case has been documented following lung transplantation (70,76).

Acute rejection is a common immunologic response that affects the majority of LT recipients and usually occurs between 10 and 50 days after lung transplantation. Many patients experience two to three episodes within the first few months. Acute rejection is usually not seen as frequently after the first year posttransplantation (77). The risk factors for acute rejection remain poorly defined, but a recent study found that HLA-DR and HLA-B loci mismatches have a correlation with high-grade rejection episodes (30).

The clinical features of acute rejection include cough, dyspnea, malaise, fever, and adventitious lung sounds (rales, wheezes). The chest radiograph is usually abnormal during rejection in the first month posttransplantation but is abnormal in only one-fourth of cases after the first month (46,78). The most common radiographic pattern has been a perihilar or lower lobe infiltrate, often associated with a small pleural effusion (79).

Hypoxemia and a deterioration in pulmonary function studies frequently occur in the setting of acute rejection. Although pulmonary function abruptly improves in the early postoperative period, pulmonary function values continue to improve for three to six months. Once lung function has stabilized, the coefficient of variation for most PFT parameters remains below 5% (45). Thus a decline of 10% or more in FVC or FEV_1 and a 10% to 15% decline in $FEF_{25\%-75\%}$ are significant changes and may signal either acute rejection or infection or an alternate graft complication (45).

Clinical criteria alone cannot differentiate acute rejection from infection. Transbronchial biopsy (TBB) with bronchoalveolar lavage (BAL) has emerged as the primary procedure in separating these entities. TBB has a positive predictive value of 69% to 83% in lung transplant patients with clinical deterioration (80,81). The sensitivity for diagnosing rejection has ranged from 70% to 95% and the specificity from 90% to 100% (81–83). A minimum of five transbronchial specimens containing pulmonary parenchyma should be obtained for histologic evaluation; however, 10 to 18 biopsies may be required to reach the 95% confidence level for the detection of rejection (83).

Histologically, acute rejection is characterized by perivascular mononuclear infiltrates and may also have airway involvement, lymphocytic bronchitis, or bronchiolitis (84) (Fig. 10.2). As rejection progresses, the perivascular lymphocytic infiltrate surrounding the venules and arterioles becomes dense and extends into the perivascular and peribronchiolar alveolar septa. With severe rejection, this process spills into the alveolar space and is usually associated with parenchymal necrosis, hyaline membranes, and a necrotizing vasculitis. A histologic grading system for acute pulmonary rejection, initially defined in 1990 and revised in

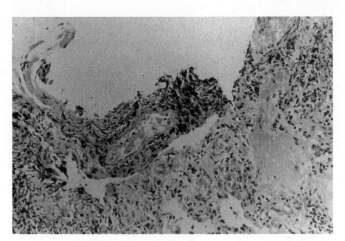

FIGURE 10.2. Transbronchial biopsy specimen revealing perivascular lymphocytic infiltration and necrosis around a small pulmonary artery, consistent with acute rejection.

1996, is outlined in Table 10.6 (84). Although rejection and infection frequently coexist, a definitive diagnosis of acute rejection is difficult to make in the setting of an active infection. Perivascular and interstitial infiltrates may occur with infections, particularly CMV and *Pneumocystis* pneumonia, as well as with acute rejection. Because of the problem in differentiating these disorders, the clinician may have to initiate antimicrobials as well as increase immunosuppression in some cases.

Currently, investigations are emerging examining exhaled nitric oxide as a marker of acute rejection (85).

Standard therapy for acute pulmonary rejection is high-dose corticosteroids. Methylprednisolone, 10 mg per kg per day for three days, is a common regimen and usually leads to a dramatic improvement in the patient's condition within 24 hours if the diagnosis is correct. The maintenance immunosuppressive regimen should also be optimized, and frequently the dose of azathioprine is increased to 1.5 to 2 mg per kg per day and the prednisone escalated to 1 mg per kg per day with a taper over several weeks. Some centers titrate azathioprine to maintain a total neutrophil count

TABLE 10.6. CLASSIFICATION AND GRADING OF ACUTE PULMONARY REJECTION

Grade A0	— None	
Grade A1	— Minimal	— Infrequent perivascular infiltrates
Grade A2	— Mild	— Frequent perivascular infiltrates
Grade A3	— Moderate	— Dense perivascular infiltrates with alveolar involvement
Grade A4	— Severe	— Diffuse perivascular and alveolar infiltrates with necrosis

Adapted from Yousem SA, Berry GJ, Cagle PT, et al. Revision of the 1990 working formulation for the classification of pulmonary allograft rejection: Lung Rejection Study Group. *J Heart Lung Transplant* 1996;15:1–15, with permission.

between 4,500 and 6,000 cells per mm³. Adjusting the immunosuppressive regimen is particularly important with severe episodes of rejection or when rejection occurs late in the posttransplant period (78). Conversion from a cyclosporine- to tacrolimus-based regimen may also result in improvement (decreased incidence and severity) of persistent or recurrent acute rejection (86). Lympholytic therapy, methotrexate, photophoresis, total lymphoid irradiation, and aerosolized cyclosporine have also been used for treatment of recurrent or persistent acute rejection (87–90).

Two recent studies have examined the newer immunosuppressant agent, mycophenolate mofetil (MMF) given *de novo* following LT. O'Hair and colleagues reported a decreased incidence of acute rejection in the first three posttransplant months in patients treated with MMF *de novo* in comparison to historic control groups treated with azathioprine. This difference did not persist after three months (91). Ross and colleagues reported a decreased incidence of acute rejection with a suggestion of decreased BOS in MMF-treated patients in comparison to concurrent azathioprine controls (92).

Obliterative Bronchiolitis

Obliterative bronchiolitis (OB) following transplantation is defined clinically by an obstructive pulmonary function defect and histologically by obliteration of terminal bronchioles (bronchiolitis obliterans). In the early HLT experience, 50% of recipients developed OB, a major cause of morbidity and mortality (93–95). With the use of increased immunosuppression, including corticosteroids and cyclosporine, and with the addition of azathioprine, the incidence of OB appeared to decrease (96). Furthermore, with augmented immunosuppression, the progression of disease has been slowed (93). Initially, it was thought that SLT and DLT procedures would result in a lower incidence of OB than HLT procedures; however, when followed over time, it is apparent that the incidence of OB in SLT and DLT recipients is comparable to that currently seen in HLT patients (97). Many large transplant centers are reporting a 25% to 50% incidence of OB in LT recipients (67,98,99). OB remains a major problem in lung transplantation and one of the leading causes of late mortality.

Although the etiology of OB remains unclear, several possible causes have been proposed, including uncontrolled acute rejection (94,100,101), CMV infection (102), HLA-A mismatches, total HLA mismatches, absence of donor antigen–specific hyporeactivity (101) bronchiolitis obliterans with organizing pneumonia (BOOP), and lymphocytic bronchiolitis (103,104). Acute rejection has been consistently identified as the most significant risk factor for BOS (105–108). Those patients with recurrent, high-grade, acute rejection had a higher incidence of BOS in the Pittsburgh series.

Clinically, OB has been reported any time following the third month posttransplantation, but the typical onset is 16 to 20 months after surgery (107,109). The onset of OB may he heralded by an upper respiratory tract infection and can be mistakenly treated as such. Other patients present without clinical symptoms but with a gradual obstructive dysfunction on pulmonary function testing (110). FEV_1 has been the standard spirometric parameter used, but midexpiratory flow rates may be a more sensitive parameter for early detection (111).

Typically, chest radiographs are not helpful in the diagnosis of OB, because most patients have radiographs that are unchanged from their baseline posttransplant film (110). Some investigators have described central bronchiectasis as an occasional radiographic finding suggesting a diagnosis of OB (112). High-resolution CT in OB may reveal peripheral bronchiectasis, patchy consolidation, decreased peripheral vascular markings, air trapping, and bronchial dilatation, which investigators feel may aid in the early diagnosis of OB (113–116). Air trapping on expiratory HRCT has been shown to be a sensitive (91%) and accurate (86%) radiologic indicator of OB in LT patients but may not be able to provide an early diagnosis of this disorder. Specificity of this finding is reported to be 80% (117).

TBB is used in the evaluation of suspected OB (Fig. 10.3). In addition to occasionally revealing histologic changes of OB, bronchoscopy is important in excluding other possible diagnoses such as acute rejection, infection, or airway complications as contributing causes of deteriorating pulmonary function. Unfortunately, it may be difficult to obtain diagnostic specimens of the terminal bronchioles by TBB. The sensitivity for detection of OB by TBB ranges from 15% to 87% (78,105,118–122). Since some patients are unable to tolerate open-lung biopsy, OB is sometimes a diagnosis of exclusion in a patient presenting with progres-

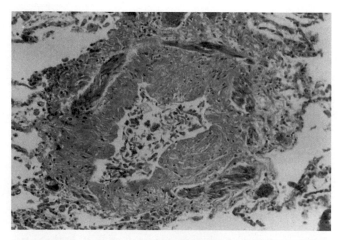

FIGURE 10.3. Transbronchial biopsy specimen revealing obliterative bronchiolitis.

TABLE 10.7. CLINICAL STAGING SYSTEM FOR OBLITERATIVE BRONCHIOLITIS

Stage[a]	FEV_1
0—No significant OB	at or over 80% of baseline
1—Mild OB	66% to 80% of baseline
2—Moderate OB	51% to 65% of baseline
3—Severe OB	at or under 50% of baseline

[a]Each stage is subdivided into *a* and *b*, where *a* is without histologic documentation of OB and *b* is with histologic documentation of OB. Adapted from International Society for Heart and Lung Transplantation staging system.
OB, obliterative bronchiolitis.
Adapted from Cooper JD, Billingham M, Egan T, et al. A working formulation for the standardization of nomenclature and for clinical staging of chronic dysfunction in lung allografts. *J Heart Lung Transplant* 1993;12:713–716, with permission.

sive obstruction on pulmonary function testing with an otherwise normal TBB.

Because of the variability in obtaining OB by transbronchial biopsy, the International Society of Heart Lung Transplantation has established a bronchiolitis obliterans syndrome (BOS) staging system (123). This staging is based on the reduction in FEV_1 in comparison to a posttransplant baseline FEV_1 with or without the pathologic documentation of OB (Table 10.7), and implies that other causes of the physiologic changes have been excluded by bronchoscopy, such as acute rejection, airway complications, and infection. Recent studies are examining the use of exhaled nitric oxide as a marker for BOS (124).

If OB has been diagnosed histologically or clinically by exclusion of alternate diagnoses, treatment is begun with high-dose methylprednisolone followed by a tapering course of oral corticosteroids. Lympholytic agents such as antilymphocyte globulin (ALG) or OKT3 can be considered if there is no clinical response to steroid treatment. Therapy may stabilize the pulmonary function but uncommonly results in significant improvement (124). The use of corticosteroids has been associated with a 65% response rate, while antilymphocytic agents resulted in a response in 81% of patients. Although relapses may be less likely with lympholytic therapy, relapses still occur in over 50% of patients (125).

Mycophenolate mofetil and tacrolimus have also been associated with stabilization of pulmonary function when used as salvage treatment for BOS (126–128). Methotrexate, total lymphoid irradiation, inhaled cyclosporine and newer immunosuppressive agents have been used in refractory cases of OB (129).

Unfortunately, infection frequently complicates intensive immunosuppression for OB and may result in death. Survival after diagnosis of OB were 74%, 50%, and 43% at one year, three years, and five years, respectively, in the Stanford series (130). Since most cases of OB can only be stabilized, strategies directed at prevention, early diagnosis, and treatment are necessary for preservation of lung function.

Infectious Complications

Infection is the leading cause of morbidity and mortality in recipients of lung or heart-lung transplantation (131,132). The act of surgically removing the donor lung, leaving it without a blood supply for several hours, and then reimplanting it without reestablishing the lymphatic drainage or nerve supply dramatically diminishes the defense mechanisms of the lung. Mucosal ischemia impairs mucociliary clearance, and the anastomosis impairs the movement of mucus up the trachea. These factors, along with immunosuppression, explain why 30% to 80% of transplant recipients develop major infections within the first four months following transplantation (133). Pneumonia accounts for 50% to 80% of infections and is the leading cause of death in these patients (131,132).

Bacterial, candidal, and herpes simplex viral infections occur in the first month after transplantation. More than 90% of the infections occurring in this time period are the usual nosocomial infections of the surgical wound, vascular-access, urinary tract, or lungs that occur in any postoperative patient.

Bacterial pneumonia is the most common life-threatening infection to occur in the early postoperative period. The risk of pneumonia in the first two postoperative weeks has been reported to be as high as 35% (134). *Pseudomonas aeruginosa* and *Staphylococcus* species have been the predominant pathogens. With the use of broad-spectrum antibiotic prophylaxis (usually an antipseudomonal cephalosporin and clindamycin) and routine culturing of the trachea of the donor and recipient at the time of surgery, the incidence of bacterial pneumonia has been significantly reduced to around 10%. If the cultures remain negative, prophylactic antibiotics are discontinued after three to four days.

The diagnosis of early bacterial pneumonia may be difficult because ischemic-reperfusion injury, pulmonary edema, rejection, and atelectasis may all present with similar clinical features. Gram-negative organisms are frequently found in the tracheal aspirate, and differentiating colonization from infection may require invasive procedures or semiquantitative bacterial cultures.

Atypical pneumonias, including *Pneumocystis carinii* pneumonia (PCP), *Legionella,* mycobacteria, and *Nocardia,* are uncommon in the first month and occur in 2% to 9% of lung and heart-lung transplant recipients (135,136). Other posttransplant infections include viral infections with herpes simplex virus and hepatitis B or C infections. Herpes simplex infections have almost been eliminated by the common use of acyclovir or gancyclovir, and the incidence of hepatitis B or C is minimal with better screening techniques of donors and blood products. Candidal infections are also seen in the early postoperative period, and the potential of this organism causing invasive disease should always be considered when isolated from cultures.

In transplant centers where trimethoprim-sulfamethoxazole prophylaxis is routinely used during the first year posttransplant and reinitiated when immunosuppression is augmented, the incidence of PCP is less than 1% (136–138). Nevertheless, lung transplant recipients have a fivefold higher prevalence of PCP than comparably immunosuppressed recipients of a cardiac allograft, and PCP must be considered in patients who are poorly compliant with their medications or intolerant to trimethoprim-sulfamethoxazole (138).

Most opportunistic infections occur one to six months after transplantation. The combination of sustained immunosuppression and the immunomodulating viruses, particularly CMV, predisposes the patient to opportunistic organisms including *Aspergillus, Mycobacterium, Nocardia, Listeria,* and geographically endemic fungi. During this time period, viral infections are a major cause of mortality and morbidity. CMV, a herpes virus, accounts for the majority of the viral infections in these patients.

CMV is the most common cause of infections in the interval between 30 to 150 days postoperatively (134). The overall prevalence of CMV illness (infection or disease) in lung transplant recipients has been around 50% (99). The risk of developing CMV disease is dependent on the serologic status of the donor and the recipient, as well as the use of high-intensity immunosuppressive therapy, especially cytolytic therapy (139). CMV positive recipients develop CMV disease approximately 25% to 35% of the time, while CMV-negative recipients have an 85% chance of developing disease when implanted with a CMV-positive lung (140). The case fatality rate for primary CMV disease (recipients that lack any intrinsic immunity) has been 20% to 25%.

CMV causes a wide spectrum of disease ranging from asymptomatic infection (shedding of virus in urine or bronchoalveolar secretions) to widespread dissemination. CMV infection in transplant patients is characterized by active replication and shedding of virus that can be associated with unexplained fever or constitutional symptoms as well as laboratory abnormalities including mild atypical lymphocytosis, leukopenia, or thrombocytopenia. CMV disease is established by cytologic or histologic changes in cell preparations or tissue. Although CMV disease can be manifested by hepatitis, gastroenteritis, or colitis, CMV pneumonia is the most common presentation after lung transplantation.

CMV pneumonia typically presents insidiously, with nonproductive cough, fever, malaise, hypoxemia, and a mild interstitial or alveolar infiltrate. Sputum smears and cultures are rarely diagnostic for CMV pneumonia. Fiber-optic bronchoscopy with TBB and BAL diagnoses 60% to 90% of patients with CMV pneumonia (133,136). A presumptive diagnosis is often made on the basis of a positive culture in a compatible clinical setting after other causes have been excluded.

The microscopic hallmark of CMV infection is the large (cytomegalic) 250 nm cell containing a large, central, baso-

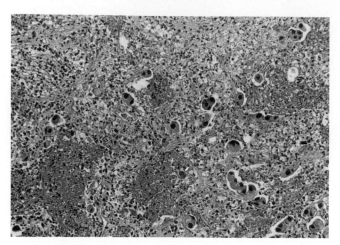

FIGURE 10.4. A photomicrograph revealing "owl's eye" intranuclear inclusions of cytomegalovirus in the lung graft.

philic intranuclear inclusion. The inclusion is referred to as an "owl's eye" because it is separated from the nuclear membrane by a halo. These inclusions are well seen on hematoxylin-eosin or Papanicolaou stain (Fig. 10.4). Cytologic identification of CMV inclusion cells is very specific (98%) but lacks sensitivity (21%) for the presence of infection (141). Biopsy specimens of the lung parenchyma contain CMV inclusion cells with a surrounding lymphocytic/mononuclear cell interstitial pneumonitis.

Ganciclovir, an acrylic guanine analogue, is currently the mainstay of therapy for invasive CMV disease. Initial doses of 5 mg per kg twice daily for two to four weeks reduce mortality from 60% to 80% to 15% to 20% in symptomatic CMV pneumonitis (141). If CMV relapses, ganciclovir at 5 mg per kg per day may be required for two to four months. Some patients develop bone marrow toxicity on ganciclovir and require therapy with foscarnet. Major toxic reactions associated with foscarnet include renal failure and severe electrolyte disturbances. CMV-specific IgG or polyclonal IgG in combination with ganciclovir is associated with an improved survival among bone marrow transplant recipients with CMV pneumonitis (142). Because of the cost of immunoglobulin and the lack of data in solid-organ transplant recipients, IgG preparations are often reserved for life-threatening episodes of CMV infection. With any severe CMV infection, a reduction in the level of immunosuppression is recommended.

Although there is no consensus about the optimal regimen for prevention of CMV disease, prophylaxis against CMV infection has become a major strategy in most transplant centers. The easiest way to reduce CMV infections is to match CMV-negative recipients with CMV-negative donors whenever possible. Limited studies suggest that CMV hyperimmune globulin may prevent or ameliorate serious CMV infections in high-risk patients after renal, liver, or heart transplantation (143,144).

Ganciclovir is very efficacious in preventing viral replication, and delays the onset of CMV infection. This delay in onset of the infection reduces the severity of the illness, since the patient's risk of morbidity and mortality is highest during the postoperative period and period of maximal immunosuppression.

A recent prospective study in liver transplant recipients demonstrated that a three-month regimen of oral ganciclovir significantly reduced the incidence of CMV infection and disease (145). At least one small, open, comparative study also showed efficacy of intravenous followed by oral ganciclovir in the lung transplant population (146). Widespread use of prolonged antiviral therapy has the potential to lead to ganciclovir resistance (147). A preemptive strategy is attractive since it treats only those patients at higher risk for developing CMV disease. Surveillance cultures using sensitive assays, such as CMV antigenemia or PCR, offer significant advantages over previous methods. CMV antigen has been detected at a mean of 28 days prior to the development of CMV disease in heart and lung transplant recipients, and should allow for sufficient time to initiate antiviral therapy and prevent disease (148–150). Standardization of quantitative antigenemia or PCR in blood or bronchoalveolar fluid may eliminate the need for universal prophylaxis for CMV in the near future.

Fungal infections are more common in lung and heart-lung transplant recipients than in those with other solid-organ transplants. The overall incidence of invasive fungal infections with lung or heart-lung transplantation ranges from 10% to 22% (151,152). Most fungal infections are caused by *Candida* or *Aspergillus* species, and over 80% of fungal infections occur within the first two months (152). The overall mortality of fungal infections in heart-lung and lung transplant recipients is reported to be between 40% and 70% (151,152).

Aspergillus species (*A. fumigatus, A. flavus, A. terreus,* and *A. niger*) may present as an indolent progressive pneumonia or as an acute fulminant infection that rapidly disseminates. *Aspergillus* exhibits a propensity to invade blood vessels and may present as an infarct or with hemoptysis. The radiographic features of pulmonary aspergillosis include focal lobar infiltrates, patchy bronchopneumonic infiltrates, single or multiple nodules with or without cavitation, thin-walled cavities, and opacification of the entire lung graft. High-resolution CT scan may reveal a halo sign felt to be pathognomonic for invasive aspergillosis (153). Prophylaxis with azoles or inhaled amphotericin has shown promise in decreasing the incidence of *Aspergillus* infections.

Definitive diagnosis of invasive aspergillosis requires identification of organisms within tissue. These organisms appear as septated hyphae that branch at acute angles and are visible on hematoxylin-eosin and methenamine-silver stains (Fig. 10.5). Even with documented cases of invasive aspergillosis, cultures are positive in less than 50% of cases (133,154). Another form of *Aspergillus* infection recently

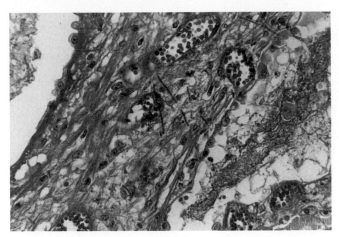

FIGURE 10.5. A photomicrograph revealing *Aspergillus* organisms in the lung graft.

recognized is *Aspergillus* tracheobronchitis (74,155). These patients develop ulcerative tracheobronchitis that usually starts distal to the anastomosis and may result in progressive narrowing of the airway.

Improved survival has been achieved with the early initiation of high-dose amphotericin (1 mg per kg per day) and the reduction of immunosuppressive therapy (156–158). Surgical resection as well as medical therapy may be required to maximize cure rates in patients with invasive aspergillosis, especially those with persistent signs of infections or necrotic tissue (154). Oral itraconazole (400 mg per day) compares favorably with amphotericin in uncontrolled studies (74,159). For life-threatening *Aspergillus* infections, amphotericin B remains the agent of choice. A lipid formulation of amphotericin B should be considered in the management of invasive fungal infections in patients who are intolerant of conventional amphotericin B and in patients with progressive fungal infection despite therapy with amphotericin-deoxycholate (153).

Candida species cause a variety of syndromes, including mucocutaneous disease, line sepsis, wound infections, and pulmonary involvement associated with widespread dissemination. A heavy growth of *Candida* in the donor tracheal culture has been associated with the occurrence of dissemination in the recipient (160). This has led to some programs initiating low-dose amphotericin (0.3 mg per kg per day) for the first 14 postoperative days (134); other centers have tried another azole, fluconazole (161). Although amphotericin B remains the therapy of choice for life-threatening invasive candidiasis, fluconazole has emerged as an effective alternative for infections caused by *C. albicans*. Fluconazole is less active against *C. glabrata* and inactive against *C. krusei*; therefore, amphotericin should be used in severe candidal infections until the species is identified (153).

Less common causes of fungal infections in lung transplant recipients include *Cryptococcus neoformans* and the dimorphic fungi (*Coccidioides, Histoplasma, Blastomyces*). Amphotericin B is the initial choice for therapy for serious infections with all these invasive mycoses. The dose, duration of therapy, and alternative therapy differ depending on the organism (158).

Mycobacterium tuberculosis (162), atypical mycobacteria (162–164), *Nocardia* (165–167), *Legionella* (135), and *Pneumocystis carinii* pneumonia (137,138) may all occur in lung transplant recipients, and the diagnosis and therapy of these organisms have recently been reviewed.

Lymphoproliferative Disorders

Posttransplant lymphoproliferative disorders (PTLDs) are reported more frequently following lung transplantation than in other solid-organ transplant recipients (99). Lymphomas comprise the majority (22%) of posttransplant malignancies. The PTLDs comprise a heterogenous group of lymphoid proliferation of variable clonality. The B-cell non-Hodgkin's lymphomas are the most frequent form of posttransplant lymphoma and have been associated with Epstein-Barr virus (EBV) activity, either serologically or by identification of viral DNA in tissue. No clear correlation has been made between episodes of rejection, specific immunosuppressive drugs, and development of PTLD. The incidence of PTLD following heart-lung and lung transplantation has been reported to be between 4.6% and 9.4% (47,168–174); however, patients who have negative EBV serology prior to transplantation may be at a significantly higher risk for developing PTLD (175). Clinical features of PTLD in LT recipients include development in the first posttransplant year, involvement of the allograft, and radiographic findings of solitary or multiple pulmonary nodules. Disseminated disease has also been reported. Treatment includes a reduction in immunosuppression as well as adjuvant treatment with radiation, chemotherapy, and/or surgery.

IMMUNOSUPPRESSION

One of the most important factors in the successful evolution of lung transplantation has been advances in the area of immunosuppression. Currently, most transplant centers use triple immunosuppression regimens including cyclosporine or tacrolimus, azathioprine or mycophenolate mofetil, and prednisone (See Table 10.8). Cytolytic agents such as antilymphocyte globulin (ALG) or OKT3 may be used for induction and/or treatment of refractory rejection (176). More recently, human monoclonal antibodies to activated T cells have been developed, since OKT3 may induce a capillary leak syndrome through cytokine release and ALG may induce serum sickness. Early studies have found human monoclonal anti T lymphocyte antibodies are effective as

TABLE 10.8. COMMON IMMUNOSUPPRESSIVE DRUGS IN LUNG TRANSPLANTATION

Drug	Dose[a]	Common Adverse Effects	Drug Interactions
Cylosporine and tacrolimus	For cyclosporine, the amount needed to achieve a whole-blood trough level of 250–350 ng/mL in the first six months after transplantation and a trough level of 150–250 ng/mL thereafter[b] For tacrolimus, the amount needed to achieve a whole-blood trough level of 8–20 ng/mL	Nephrotoxicity, hypertension neurotoxicity (tremor, seizures, white-matter disease, headache), hyperlipidemia, hyperkalemia, hypomagnesemia, GI disturbance. Hirsutism and gingival hyperplasia (with cyclosporine), hyperglycemia (with tacrolimus)	Blood levels are increased by azole antifungal agents, calcium channel blockers, cisapride, and macrolide antibiotics. Blood levels are decreased by anticonvulsant drugs, rifampin, or rifabutin
Azathioprine	1–2 mg/kg of body weight/day	Leukopenia. macrocytic anemia, thrombocytopenia, hepatotoxicity, pancreatitis, nausea	Enhanced bone marrow toxicity when given with allopurinol
Mycophenolate mofetil	1,000–1,500 mg twice daily	Diarrhea, abdominal pain, emesis, leukopenia, anemia	No clinically significant interactions
Prednisone	0.5 mg/kg/day for three months, followed by slow taper to 5 mg/day or 10–15 mg	Hyperglycemia, hypertension, hyperlipidemia, osteoporosis myopathy, insomnia, cataracts, weight gain	No clinically significant interactions

[a] Doses are based on the protocol used at the University of Texas Health Science Center at San Antonio; the regimens may differ at other transplantation centers.
[b] Cyclosporine levels are measured by immunoassay.

prophylaxis for rejection in solid-organ transplants, are well tolerated, and are easy to use because of prolonged half-life (177,178). There is no convincing evidence that induction therapy diminishes acute or chronic rejection in lung transplantation (179), and prospective studies are needed to establish its role in this setting.

A typical maintenance immunosuppression regimen consists of cyclosporine (3 to 5 mg per kg twice daily) or tacrolimus (0.1 mg per kg twice daily) adjusted to serum levels, azathioprine (1 to 2 mg per kg per day adjusted to maintain a leukocyte count above 4,500 per mm^3) or mycophenolate mofetil (1 to 1.5 gm twice daily), and prednisone (approximately 0.5 mg per kg per day for the first three months, tapered over the next three months to 15 mg per day, then to 5 mg per day or 10 to 15 mg on alternate days by the twelfth posttransplant month).

Cyclosporine and tacrolimus are the mainstays of immunosuppression. Each agent binds to intercellular proteins to create a complex that inhibits calcineuron (180). When calcineuron is inhibited, cytokine genes and other genes, such as the CD40 ligand, cannot be transcribed. Thus cyclosporine and tacrolimus functionally limit cytokine production and downstream lymphocyte proliferation (181,182). Tacrolimus is 50 to 100 times more potent than cyclosporine *in vitro* but its oral bioavailability is highly variable and ranges from 5% to 67% (183). The third-generation derivative of cyclosporine, cyclosporine microemulsion formulation, increases the absorption through the small bowel and reduces bile dependence and the effects of food on

absorption. Assessment of blood levels is critical to the use of tacrolimus and cyclosporine because of the narrow therapeutic index.

Unfortunately, immunosuppressive medications have numerous toxicities. The toxicities of tacrolimus and cyclosporine are similar (184). Nephrotoxicity is the major clinical toxic manifestation and occurs in 25% to 75% of patients receiving the drugs (185); the acute renal toxicity is usually dose-related and typically reversible. The drugs can decrease renal blood flow by causing afferent arteriolar vasoconstriction resulting in decreased glomerular filtration (186). Interstitial fibrosis, tubular changes, and vascular abnormalities can result with chronic use. Several other potentially nephrotoxic agents that can compound the nephrotoxicity include amphotericin B, aminoglycoside antibiotics, trimethoprim-sulfamethoxazole (even at low doses), and furosemide (187). The renal toxicity may resolve with a reduction in the dose or discontinuation of the drug, although this improvement is not universal. The concurrent administration of calcium channel blockers may diminish the vasoconstrictive effects of the agents (188).

A second serious complication of these agents is systemic hypertension, which develops in approximately 25% of lung transplant recipients. The most likely etiology of hypertension is a defect in renal sodium excretion (187). Many patients respond to sodium restriction and/or a reduction in cyclosporine dose, although approximately one-third of patients require antihypertensive medications to achieve adequate blood pressure control. Hypercholesterolemia is also commonly reported and can develop in up to 75% of transplant recipients. The incidence of posttransplant hypertension and hypercholesterolemia is lower with tacrolimus (184).

Numerous less common side effects of cyclosporine and tacrolimus can develop. The spectrum of neurologic toxicity includes tremors, parenthesis, headaches, confusion, depression, somnolence, and seizures. Neurotoxicity is more common with tacrolimus than cyclosporine. Posttransplant diabetes mellitus has been reported with both agents, but the incidence appears to be higher with tacrolimus. In some series, new-onset diabetes mellitus has been seen in up to 19% of patients on tacrolimus (188). Cosmetic changes that occur with cyclosporine, such as hirsutism and gingival hyperplasia, are uncommon with tacrolimus. Several electrolyte deficiencies have been reported with cyclosporine use, including hypomagnesemia in up to 50% of lung transplant patients (187) and hyperkalemia in 10% to 15% of transplant recipients. Cholestatic hepatotoxicity has also been reported (189).

Corticosteroids are the original drugs used in solid-organ transplantation (190). Corticosteroids bind to a cytoplasmic glucocorticoid receptor and undergo translocation into the nucleus, where they block the transcription of several genes. Corticosteroids exert inhibition of cytokine transcription (including IL-2), antigen presentation, eicosanoid production, and the expression of adherence molecules (191). The side effects seen in other patient populations on chronic corticosteroids occur in lung transplant recipients as well, including hyperglycemia, hypercholesterolemia, osteoporosis, cataracts, myopathy, exacerbation of peptic ulcer disease, Cushing's syndrome, and mood changes. Many of these side effects are improved with a reduction in corticosteroid dosage.

Azathioprine is metabolized to 6-mercaptopurine, which inhibits nucleic acid synthesis and suppresses mitosis and proliferation of lymphocytes (190). Bone marrow toxicity and suppression are the most common toxic effects of azathioprine, and it is important to adjust the dose to maintain a leukocyte count above 4,500 per mm^3. Miscellaneous side effects related to azathioprine include pancreatitis, hepatitis, cholestatic jaundice, and an increased risk of malignancy (192).

Mycophenolate mofetil, like azathioprine, is an inhibitor of purine synthesis. Mycophenolate acts on a lymphocyte-selective enzyme to inhibit *de novo* purine synthesis. Because lymphocytes have a unique requirement for *de novo* purine synthesis, this effect selectively suppresses lymphocyte clonal expansion (180). The results of pooled analysis indicate that mycophenolate reduces acute rejection and prolongs graft survival in solid-organ transplant recipients (193). Well-controlled studies with mycophenolate in lung transplantation are lacking. Mycophenolate lacks the marrow toxicity of azathioprine at a dose of 2 grams per day. Gastrointestinal symptoms of diarrhea and abdominal pain are the most common side effects of mycophenolate. The expense of mycophenolate and the inability to monitor drug levels are presently drawbacks to widespread use of this drug.

Ongoing research in the field of immunosuppressive therapy, as well as improvements in the prevention and treatment of infections and better graft preservation, has made lung transplantation a therapeutic option for the treatment of end-stage lung disease and has extended the life of these patients.

LUNG VOLUME REDUCTION SURGERY

Lung transplantation has provided a surgical option for patients with chronic obstructive pulmonary disease (COPD) who are relatively young and can find a donor match once they are listed as a possible recipient. Unfortunately, many people with emphysema are unable to qualify for lung transplantation or deteriorate during the time they have been listed as a possible lung transplant candidate with no donor available in the near future. For these types of patients, a second surgical option may be available. This option is known as lung volume reduction surgery (LVRS) or reduction pneumoplasty (194–197).

LVRS is actually a rediscovered surgical approach to emphysema that was first performed in the 1950s by Dr. Otto Brantigan (198). He removed areas of emphysematous lung in patients with severe emphysema in order to allow the remaining lung to hyperinflate, thereby increasing lung elastic recoil and increasing airflow conductance. Dr. Brantigan also hypothesized that by reducing the amount of lung in the hyperinflated emphysema patient, the diaphragm would be allowed to return to a more normal configuration and this could result in increased airflow due to increasing the efficiency of the muscle. LVRS was performed on a number of patients, but the complication rate of bronchopleural fistula was very high and the overall mortality rate from the surgery was unacceptable. For these reasons, the procedure was eventually abandoned (197).

In 1995, Dr. Joel Cooper and his colleagues described the use of LVRS in 20 patients with severe emphysema (199). No mortality from the surgery was reported, and the patients improved their FEV$_1$ by a mean of 82% over a six-month period. There was a significant increase in PaO$_2$ and a significant increase in exercise tolerance. The patients also reported an enhanced quality of life. During this same time period, several reports of laser LVRS were also published, and enthusiasm for this "reborn" procedure became heightened.

Initially, Medicare reimbursed for the surgery, but in late 1995 the Health Care Financing Administration (HCFA) released a national policy not to reimburse for LVRS until more data could be collected on the procedure's efficacy and safety (195). In order to obtain these data, the National Emphysema Treatment Trial (NETT) began in 1998. The primary goals of this study included answering the following questions:

   A. What are the benefits and risk of LVRS compared with good medical therapy alone?

   B. How long do any benefits last?

   C. Does LVRS benefit some patients more than others?

Selection of Patients

Patients who are candidates for LVRS should be experiencing end-stage emphysema with debilitation due to either severe dyspnea at rest or exercise intolerance. They should have evidence of hyperinflation with a total lung capacity of over 120% of predicted. The high-resolution chest CT and V/Q scans should reveal predominantly upper lobe heterogenous emphysema. Upper limits of age vary at different centers, but for the NETT study the patients must be younger than 75 years old. Their FEV_1 should be less than 35% of predicted. Alveolar hypoventilation is allowed, but the $PaCO_2$ should not exceed 50 mm Hg. All patients must undergo a six to 10-week rehabilitation program prior to surgery, during which they will receive maximum bronchodilator therapy, oxygen as needed, and a program of exercise and optimum breathing methods. Patients with significant comorbidity from nonrespiratory illnesses, especially cardiac disease, are excluded from LVRS treatment (Table 10.9).

Surgical Techniques

LVRS has been performed by both thoracoscopic and median sternotomy approaches. Laser ablation of pulmonary tissue is used much less than the above approaches because of an increase in postoperative complications, including delayed pneumothorax (197). The use of video-assisted thoracoscopy with stapling seems to have results similar to median sternotomy, both from operative mortality and functional outcome. This surgery is usually performed as a bilateral procedure but it can actually also be performed unilaterally. Simultaneous LVRS and resection of a sus-

pected bronchogenic carcinoma in an upper lobe are feasible and have been reported (200).

Other Effects on Patient Outcomes Following LVRS

Following LVRS, approximately 20% of the patients who required supplemental oxygen preoperatively were able to discontinue oxygen use postoperatively (199). In the report by Cooper and associates (201), 52% of patients (101 patients) had been using oxygen at rest preoperatively and 16% were using it postoperatively. Of that same group, 92% were using oxygen during exercise preoperatively and 44% were continuing to use oxygen during exercise postoperatively.

McKenna and associates (202) reported a 10% one-year mortality rate in 166 patients who received LVRS for emphysema. Cooper's report (201) on mortality in 150 patients receiving LVRS showed a one-year mortality of 7% and a two-year mortality of 8%. Persistent bronchopleural fistula (over seven days) is the most common postoperative complication and occurs in 30% to 50% of patients. Tracheostomy has been required in approximately 10% of patients during their postoperative course. Other significant complications include pneumonia and respiratory failure.

Mechanisms of Decreased Obstruction and Improved Exercise Tolerance following LVRS

Patients who undergo LVRS have decreased chest wall elastic recoil and increased lung elastic recoil following surgery, which increases airway conductance. Diaphragm function is also improved because the flattened diaphragm is able to assume a more normal configuration postoperatively as lung hyperinflation is decreased and the diaphragm ascends into the thorax (194). This allows the diaphragm to assume a resting position that is more favorably situated on the length-tension curve and thus permits the diaphragm to function more effectively as a pressure generator (196).

Improvement in exercise performance may occur due to improved lung mechanics. Patients are capable of longer six-minute walk distances and increased maximal oxygen uptake values. Ventilation/perfusion matching may also improve following LVRS because of the expansion of compressed atelectatic lung. Although the improved function and increase in FEV_1 are significant in patients with a good response to the procedure, one must remember that the increases are usually only a few hundred milliliters because these patients must have severe COPD in order to be candidates for the surgery.

Changes in Pulmonary Function following Surgery

Recent reports of changes in FEV_1 by Cooper and associates (201) in 150 patients reveal an increase of 51% in their

TABLE 10.9. INCLUSION CRITERIA

Age under 75 years
Severe emphysema—FEV_1 under 35% predicted
Maximum medical therapy
Ambulatory with rehabilitation capabilities
No present cigarette use
No severe comorbid illness
No severe cardiac disease
No severe pulmonary hypertension (mean PA pressure under 35 mm Hg)
No severe obesity or cachexia
$PaCO_2$ under 50 mm Hg
Perfusion to lower lung over 10% greater than perfusion to upper lung

FEV_1 at six months following surgery. Most patients experience subjective improvements in their exercise tolerance. Gelb and coworkers (203) reported a group of patients who received lung volume reduction by a video-assisted thoracoscopy, with stapling in 10 patients with one year of follow-up. The group's FEV_1 improved 68% at six months, but this declined to 34% by one year. Ingenito and colleagues (204) reported a two-year follow-up in nine patients receiving LVRS; their FEV_1 had declined by 19% at two years from their peak improvement, which occurred at six months following their surgery. All of these data suggest that maximum FEV_1 improvement occurs six months following the surgical procedure but there is increasing obstruction recurring over the following six-to-18-month period that exceeds rates reported in even continued smokers with severe COPD. Brenner and coworkers (205) reported an average loss of FEV_1 of 163 mL per year in 180 patients who had undergone a variety of LVRS procedures. The most rapid loss was 255 mL per year, which occurred in a group of patients who had undergone bilateral thoracoscopic LVRS, the procedure that produces the greatest improvement in function.

Conclusions

LVRS can drastically increase airflow in some patients with severe emphysema. The important questions concerning this new approach to emphysema include which patients are most likely to benefit from the surgery and how long the benefits will last. The cost-effectiveness of the procedure is also under intense scrutiny because of questions of long-term benefits and the large number of emphysema patients who could potentially be candidates for this surgery. The American Thoracic Society has stated that LVRS should be performed only at centers where experienced surgeons have demonstrated surgical expertise and where results can be studied in clinical trials. The National Emphysema Treatment Trial has the potential to answer many of the questions about LVRS, and the results of this trial will better define our approach and understanding of this surgical approach to emphysema.

REFERENCES

1. Hardy JD, Webb WR, Dalton ML, et al. Lung homotransplantation in man; report of the initial case. *JAMA* 1963;186:1065–1074.
2. Derom F, Barbier F, Ringoir S, et al. Ten-month survival after lung homotransplantation in man. *J Thorac Cardiovasc Surg* 1971;61:835–846.
3. Nelems JM, Rebuck AS, Cooper JD, et al. Human lung transplantation. *Chest* 1980;78:569–573.
4. Borel JF, Feurer C, Gubler HB, et al. Biological effect of cyclosporine A: a new antilymphocyte agent. *Agents Actions* 1976;6:465–475.
5. Hosenpud JD, Bennett LE, Keck BM, et al. The registry of the international society for heart and lung transplantation: Fifteenth official report—1998. *J Heart Lung Transplant* 1998;17:656–668.
6. Toronto Lung Transplant Group. Unilateral lung transplantation for pulmonary fibrosis. *N Engl J Med* 1986;314:1140–1145.
7. Stevens PM, Johnson PC, Bell RL, et al. Regional ventilation and perfusion after lung transplantation in patients with emphysema. *N Engl J Med* 1970;282(5):245–249.
8. Mal H, Andreassian B, Fabrice P, et al. Unilateral lung transplantation in end-stage pulmonary emphysema. *Am Rev Respir Dis* 1989;140:797–802.
9. Calhoon JH, Grover FL, Gibbons WJ, et al. Single lung transplantation—alternative indications and technique. *J Thorac Cardiovasc Surg* 1991;101(5):816–825.
10. Levine SM, Gibbons WJ, Bryan CL, et al. Single lung transplantation for primary pulmonary hypertension. *Chest* 1990;98:1107–1115.
11. Tuna I, Jamison SW. Human heart and lung transplantation. *Adv Surg* 1989;22:251–276.
12. Offical ATS Statement—June 1992. Lung transplantation. report of the ATS Workshop on Lung Transplantation. *Am Rev Respir Dis* 1993;147:772–776.
13. Guidelines for the Selection of lung transplant candidates. Joint Statement of the American Society for International Transplant Physicians/American Thoracic Society/European Respiratory Society/International Society for Heart and Lung Transplantation. *Am J Respir Crit Care Med* 1998;158:335–339.
14. Levine SM, Anzueto A, Peters JI, et al. Single lung transplantation in patients with systemic disease. *Chest* 1994;105:837–841.
15. Aris RM, Gilligan PH, Neuringer IP, et al. The effects of panresistant bacteria in cystic fibrosis patients on lung transplant outcome. *Am J Respir Crit Care Med* 1997;155:1699–1704.
16. Lima O, Cooper JD, Peters WJ, et al. Effects of methylprednisolone and azathioprine on bronchial healing following lung autotransplantation. *J Thorac Cardiovasc Surg* 1981;82:211–215.
17. Bryan CL, Anzueto A, Levine SM, et al. Corticosteroid therapy does not potentiate bronchial anastomotic complications in single lung transplantation (SLT) [Abstract]. *Am Rev Respir Dis* 1991;143(4):A461.
18. Shafers H-J, Wagner TOF, Dermertzis S, et al. Preoperative corticosteroids: a contraindication to lung transplantation? *Chest* 1992;102:1522–1525.
19. Aris RM, Neuringer IP, Weiner MA, et al. Severe osteoporosis before and after lung transplantation. *Chest* 1996;109:1176–1183.
20. Marshall SE, Kramer MR, Lewiston NJ, et al. Selection and evaluation of recipients for heart-lung transplantation. *Chest* 1990;98:1488–1494.
21. Anthonisen NR. Prognosis in chronic obstructive pulmonary disease: results from multicenter clinical trails. *Am Rev Respir Dis* 1989;140:S95–S99.
22. Traver GA, Cline MG, Burrows B. Predictors of mortality in chronic obstructive pulmonary disease. *Am Rev Respir Dis* 1979;119:895–902.
23. Hosenpud JD, Bennett LE, Keck BM, et al. Effect of diagnosis on survival benefit of lung transplantation for end-stage lung disease. *Lancet* 1998;351:24–27.
24. Carrington CB, Gaensler EA, Coutu RE, et al. Natural history and treated course of usual and desquamative interstitial pneumonia. *N Engl J Med* 1978;298:801–809.
25. Johnson MA, Kwan S, Snell NJC, et al. Randomised controlled trial comparing prednisolone alone with cyclophosphamide and low dose prednisolone in combination in cryptogenic fibrosing alveolitis. *Thorax* 1989;44:280–288.
26. Kerem E, Reisman J, Corey M, et al. Prediction of mortality

in patients with cystic fibrosis. *N Engl J Med* 1992;326: 1187–1191.

27. D'Alonzo GE, Barst RJ, Ayres SM, et al. Survival in patients with primary pulmonary hypertension. *Ann Intern Med* 1991; 115:343–349.

28. Puskas JD, Winton TL, Miller JD, et al. Unilateral donor lung dysfunction does not preclude successful contralateral single lung transplantation. *J Thorac Cardiovasc Surg* 1992;103(5): 1015–1017. Discussion 1992;1017–1018.

29. Mohar DE, Bryan CL, Jenkinson SG, et al. HLA matching as a predictor of OB or death in SLT [Abstract]. *Chest* 1993; 104(2):157S.

30. Schulman LL, Weinberg AD, McGregor C, et al. Mismatches at the HLA-DR and HLA-B loci are risk factors for acute rejection after lung transplantation. *Am J Respir Crit Care Med* 1998; 157:1833–1837.

31. Sundaresan S, Mohanakumar T, Smith MA, et al. HLA-A locus mismatches and development of antibodies to HLA after lung transplantation correlate with the development of bronchiolitis obliterans syndrome. *Transplantation* 1998;65:648–653.

32. Otulana BA, Mist BA, Scott JP, et al. The effect of recipient lung size on lung physiology after heart-lung transplantation. *Transplantation* 48(4):625, 1989.

33. The Toronto Lung Transplant Group. Experience with single-lung transplantation for pulmonary fibrosis. *JAMA* 1988; 259(15):2258.

34. Lloyd KS, Holland VA, Noon GP, et al. Pulmonary function after heart-lung transplantation using larger donor organs. *Am Rev Respir Dis* 1990;142:1026.

35. Date H, Trulock EP, Arcidi JM, et al. Improved airway healing after lung transplantation: an analysis of 348 bronchial anastomoses. *J Thorac Cardiovasc Surg* 1995;110:1424–1433.

36. Levine SM, Anzueto A, Gibbons WJ, et al. Graft position and pulmonary function after single lung transplantation for obstructive lung disease. *Chest* 1993;103(2):444–448.

37. Bierman MI, Stein KL, Stuart RS, et al. Critical care management of lung transplant recipients. *Intensive Care Med* 1991;6: 135.

38. Siegelman SS, Sinha SBP, Veith FT. Pulmonary reimplantation response. *Ann Surg* 1973;177:30.

39. Bryan CL, Cohen DJ, Gibbons WJ, et al. Lung transplantation: the reimplantation response. *Crit Care Rep* 1991;2:217.

40. Bryan CL, Cohen DJ, Dew JA, et al. Glutathione decreases the pulmonary reimplantation response in canine lung autotransplants. *Chest* 1991;100(6):1694–1702.

41. Glassman LR, Keenan RJ, Fabrizio MC, et al. Extracorporeal membrane oxygenation as an adjunct treatment for primary graft failure in adult lung transplant recipients. *J Thorac Cardiovasc Surg* 1995;110:723–727.

42. Date H, Triantafillou AN, Trulock EP, et al. Inhaled nitric oxide reduces human lung allograft dysfunction. *J Thorac Cardiovasc Surg* 1996;111:913–919.

43. Christie JD, Bavaria JE, Palevsky HI, et al. Primary graft failure following lung transplantation. *Chest* 1998;114:51–60.

44. Herman SJ, Rappaport DC, Weisbrod GL, et al. Single-lung transplantation: imaging features. *Radiology* 1989;170:89–93.

45. Otulana BA, Higenbottam T, Scott J, et al. Lung function associated with histologically diagnosed acute lung rejection and pulmonary infection in heart-lung transplant patients. *Am Rev Respir Dis* 1990;14:329.

46. Millet B, Higenbottam TW, Flower CDR, et al. The radiographic appearances of infection and acute rejection of the lung after heart-lung transplantation. *Am Rev Respir Dis* 1989;140: 62–67.

47. Herman SJ. Radiologic assessment after lung transplantation. *Clin Chest Med* 1990;11(2):333–347.

48. Otulana BA, Higenbottam TW, Scott JP, et al. Pulmonary function monitoring allows diagnosis of rejection in heart-lung transplant recipients. *Transplant Proc* 1989;21(1):2583.

49. Otulana BA, Higenbottam T, Ferrari L, et al. The use of home spirometry in detecting acute lung rejection and infection following heart-lung transplantation. *Chest* 1990;97(2):353.

50. Bryan CL, Levine SM, Anzueto A, et al. Exercise oximetry surveillance in single lung transplant recipients [Abstract]. *Am Rev Respir Dis* 1992;145(4):A702.

51. Tamm M, Sharples LD, Higenbottam TW, et al. Bronciolitis obliterans syndrome in heart-lung transplantation. *Am J Respir Crit Care Med* 1997;155:1705–1710.

52. Kukafka DS, O'Brien GM, Furukawa S, et al. Surveillance bronchoscopy in lung transplant recipients. *Chest* 1997;111: 377–381.

53. Levine SM, Anzueto A, Peters JI, et al. Medium term functional results of single lung transplantation for end-stage obstructive lung disease. *Am J Respir Crit Care Med* 1994;150:398–402.

54. Williams TJ, Patterson GA, McClean PA, et al. Maximal exercise testing in single and double lung transplant recipients. *Am Rev Respir Dis* 1992;145:101–105.

55. Miyoshi S, Trulock EP, Schaefers H-J, et al. Cardiopulmonary exercise testing after single and double lung transplantation. *Chest* 1990;97:1130–1136.

56. Gibbons SJ, Levine SM, Bryan CL, et al. Cardiopulmonary exercise responses after single lung transplantation for severe obstructive lung disease. *Chest* 1991;100:106–111.

57. Grossman RF, Frost A, Zamel N, et al. Results of single-lung transplantation for bilateral pulmonary fibrosis. *N Engl J Med* 1990;322:727–733.

58. Levine SM, Gibbons WJ, Bryan CL, et al. Single lung transplantation for primary pulmonary hypertension. *Chest* 1990;98: 1107–1115.

59. Patterson GA, Maurer JR, Williams TJ, et al. Comparison of outcomes of double and single lung transplantation for obstructive lung disease. *J Thorac Cardiovasc Surg* 1991;101:623–632.

60. Theodore J, Jamieson SW, Burke CM, et al. Physiologic aspects of human heart-lung transplantation. Pulmonary function status of the post-transplanted lung. *Chest* 1984;86(3):349–357.

61. Levine SM, Jenkinson SG, Bryan CL, et al. Ventilation-perfusion inequalities during graft rejection in patients undergoing single lung transplantation for primary pulmonary hypertension. *Chest* 1992;101:401–405.

62. Levy RD, Ernst P, Levine SM, et al. Exercise performance after lung transplantation. *J Heart Lung Transplant* 1993;12(1): 27–33.

63. Caine N, Sharples LD, Dennis C, et al. Measurement of health-related quality of life before and after heart-lung transplantation. *J Heart Lung Transplant* 1996;15:1047–58.

64. Dennis C, Caine N, Sharples L, et al. Heart-lung transplantation for end-stage respiratory disease in patients with cystic fibrosis at Papworth Hospital. *J Heart Lung Transplant* 1993;12: 893–902.

65. Gross CR, Savik K, Bolman RM III, et al. Long-term health status and quality of life outcomes of lung transplant recipients. *Chest* 1995;108:1587–1593.

66. Paris WP, Diercks M, Bright J, et al. Return to work after lung transplantation. *J Heart Lung Transplant* 1998;17:430–436.

67. de Hoyos AL, Patterson GA, Maurer JR, et al. Pulmonary transplantation: early and late results. *J Thorac Cardiovasc Surg* 1992; 103:295–306.

68. Laks H, Louie HW, Haas GS, et al. New technique of vascularization of the trachea and bronchus for lung transplantation. *J Heart Lung Transplant* 1991;10(2):280–287.

69. Nazari S, Prati U, Berti A, et al. Successful bronchial revasculari-

zation in experimental single lung transplantation. *Eur J Cardiothorac Surg* 1990;4:561–567.

70. de Hoyos A, Mauer JR. Complications following lung transplantation. *Semin Thorac Cardovasc Surg* 1992;4(2):132–146.

71. Kshettry VR, Kroshus TJ, Hertz MI, et al. Early and late airway complications after lung transplantation: incidence and management. *Ann Thorac Surg* 1997;63:1576–83.

72. Susanto I, Peters JI, Levine SM, et al. Use of balloon-expandable metallic stents in the management of bronchial stenosis and bronchomalacia after lung transplantation. *Chest* 1998;114:1330–1335.

73. Anzueto A, Levine SM, Tillis WP, et al. The use of the flow-volume loop in the diagnosis of bronchial stenosis after single lung transplantation. *Chest* 1994;105:934–936.

74. Kramer MR, Denning DW, Marshall SE, et al. Ulcerative tracheobronchitis after lung transplantation. *Am Rev Respir Dis* 1991;144:552–556.

75. Keller C, Frost A. Fiberoptic bronchoplasty. Description of a simple adjunct technique for the management of bronchial stenosis following lung transplantation. *Chest* 1992;102(4):995–998.

76. Frost AE, Jammal CT, Cagle PT. Hyperacute rejection following lung transplantation. *Chest* 1966;110:559–562.

77. Lawrence EC. Diagnosis and management of lung allograft rejection. *Clin Chest Med* 1990;11:269–277.

78. Trulock EP. Management of lung transplant rejection. *Chest* 1993;103:1566–1576.

79. Bergin CJ, Castellino RA, Blank N, et al. Acute lung rejection after heart-lung transplantation: correlation of findings on chest radiographs with lung biopsy results. *AJR* 1990;155:23–27.

80. Starnes VA, Theodore J, Oyer PE, et al. Pulmonary infiltrates after heart-lung transplantation: evaluation by serial transbronchial lung biopsies. *J Thorac Cardiovasc Surg* 1989;98:945–950.

81. Trulock EP, Ettinger NA, Brunt EM, et al. The role of transbronchial lung biopsy in the treatment of lung transplant recipients: an analysis of 200 consecutive procedures. *Chest* 1992;10:1049–1054.

82. Higenbottam T, Stewart S, Penketh A, et al. Transbronchial lung biopsy for the diagnosis of rejection in heart-lung transplant patients. *Transplantation* 1988;46:532–539.

83. Scott JP, Fradet G, Smyth RL, et al. Prospective study of transbronchial biopsies in the management of heart-lung and single lung transplant patients. *J Heart Lung Transplant* 1991;10:626–637.

84. Yousem SA, Berry GJ, Cagle PT, et al. Revision of the 1990 working formulation for the classification of pulmonary allograft rejection. Lung Rejection Study Group. *J Heart Lung Transplant* 1996;15:1–15.

85. Silkoff PE, Caramori M, Tremblay L, et al. Exhaled nitric oxide in human lung transplantation. *Am J Respir Crit Care Med* 1998;157:1822–1828.

86. Horning NR, Lynch JP, Sundaresan SR, et al. Tacrolimus therapy for persistent or recurrent acute rejection after lung transplantation. *J Heart Lung Transplant* 1998;17:761–767.

87. O'Riordan TG, Iacono A, Keenan RJ, et al. Delivery and distribution of aerosolized cyclosporine in lung allograft recipients. *Am J Respir Crit Care Med* 1995;151:516–521.

88. Iacono A, Zeevi A, Keenan R, et al. Treatment of refractory acute lung allograft rejection with aerosolized cyclosporine A: evidence for a dose response relationship [Abstract]. *J Heart Lung Transplant* 1996;15(1;Part 2):S102.

89. Valentine VG, Robbins RC, Wehner JH, et al. Total lymphoid irradiation for refractory acute rejection in heart-lung and lung allografts. *Chest* 1996;109:1184–1189.

90. Andreu G, Achkar A, Couetil JP, et al. Extracorporeal photochemotherapy treatment for acute lung rejection episode. *J Heart Lung Transplant* 1995;14:793–796.

91. O'Hair DP, Cantu E, McGregor C, et al. Preliminary experience with mycophenolate mofetil used after lung transplantation. *J Heart Lung Transplant* 1998;17:864–868.

92. Ross DJ, Waters PF, Levine M, et al. Mycophenolate mofetil versus azathioprine immunosuppressive regimens after lung transplantation: preliminary experience. *J Heart Lung Transplant* 1998;17:768–774.

93. Glanville AR, Baldwin JC, Burke CM, et al. Obliterative bronchiolitis after heart-lung transplantation: apparent arrest by augmented immunosuppression. *Ann Intern Med* 1987;107:300–304.

94. Burke CM, Glanville AR, Theodore J, et al. Lung immunogenicity, rejection, and obliterative bronchiolitis. *Chest* 1987;92(3):547–549.

95. McCarthy PM, Starnes VA, Theodore J, et al. Improved survival after heart-lung transplantation. *J Thorac Cardiovasc Surg* 1990;99:54–60.

96. Scott JP, Sharples L, Mullins, P, et al. Further studies on the natural history of obliterative bronchiolitis following heart-lung transplantation. *Transplant Proc* 1991;23(1):1201–1202.

97. LoCicero J III, Robinson PG, Fisher M. Chronic rejection in single-lung transplantation manifested by obliterative bronchiolitis. *J Thorac Cardiovasc Surg* 1990;99:1059–1062.

98. Maurer JR, Morrison D, Winton TL, et al. Late pulmonary complications of isolated lung transplantation. *Transplant Proc* 1991;23(1):1224–1225.

99. Trulock EP. State of the art: lung transplantation. *Am J Respir Crit Care Med* 1997;155:789–818.

100. Griffith BP, Paradis IL, Zeevi A, et al. Immunologically mediated disease of the airways after pulmonary transplantation. *Ann Surg* 1988;208(3):371–378.

101. Kroshus TJ, Kshettry VR, Savik K, et al. Risk factors for the development of bronchiolitis obliterans syndrome after lung transplantation. *J Thorac Cardiovasc Surg* 1997;114:195–202.

102. Kennan RJ, Lega ME, Drummer JS, et al. Cytomegalovirus: serologic status and postoperative infection correlated with risk of developing chronic rejection after pulmonary transplantation. *Transplantation* 1991;51(2):433–438.

103. Girgis RE, Tu I, Berry GJ, et al. Risk factors for the development of obliterative bronchiolitis after lung transplantation. *J Heart Lung Transplant* 1996;15:1200–1208.

104. Ross DJ, Marchevsky A, Kramer M, et al. "Refractoriness" of airflow obstruction associated with isolated lymphocytic bronchiolitis/bronchitis in pulmonary allografts. *J Heart Lung Transplant* 1997;16:832–838.

105. Bando K, Paradis IL, Similo S, et al. Obliterative bronchiolitis after lung and heart-lung transplantation: an analysis of risk factors and management. *J Thorac Cardiovasac Surg* 1995;110:4–14.

106. Scott JP, Higenbottam TW, Sharples L, et al. Risk factors for obliterative bronchiolitis in heart-lung transplant recipients. *Transplantation* 1991;51:813–817.

107. Keller CA, Cagle PT, Brown RW, et al. Bronchiolitis obliterans in recipients of single, double, and heart-lung transplantation. *Chest* 1995;107:973–980.

108. Sharples LD, Tamm M, McNeil K, et al. Development of bronchiolitis obliterans syndrome in recipients of heart-lung transplantation—early risk factors. *Transplantation* 1996;61:560–566.

109. Sundaresan RS, Trulock EP, Mohanakumar T, et al. Prevalence and outcome of bronchiolitis obliterans syndrome after lung transplantation. *Ann Thorac Surg* 1995;60:1341–1347.

110. Burke CM, Theodore J, Dawkins KD, et al. Post-transplant

obliterative bronchiolitis and other late lung sequelae in human heart-lung transplantation. *Chest* 1984;86(6):824–829.

111. Patterson GM, Wilson S, Whang JL, et al. Physiologic definitions of obliterative bronchiolitis in heart-lung and double lung transplantation: a comparison of the forced expiratory flow between 25% and 75% of the forced vital capacity and forced expiratory volume in one second. *J Heart Lung Transplant* 1996; 15:175–181.

112. Skeens JL, Fuhrman CR, Yousem SA. Bronchiolitis obliterans in heart-lung transplantation patients: radiologic findings in 11 patients. *AJR* 1989;153:253–256.

113. Halvorsen RA Jr, DuCret RP, Kuni CC, et al. Obliterative bronchiolitis following lung transplantation diagnostic utility of aerosol ventilation lung scanning and high resolution CT. *Clin Nucl Med* 1991;16(4):256–258.

114. Morrish WF, Herman SJ, Weisbrod GL, et al. Bronchiolitis obliterans after lung transplantation: findings at chest radiography and high-resolution CT. *Radiology* 1991;179:487–490.

115. Worthy SA, Park CS, Kim JS, et al. Bronchiolitis obliterans after lung transplantation: high-resolution CT findings in 15 patients. *Am J Roentgen* 1997;169:673–677.

116. Ikonen T, Kivisaari L, Tashinen E, et al. High-resolution CT in long-term follow-up after lung transplantation. *Chest* 1997; 11:370–376.

117. Leung AN, Fisher K, Valentine V, et al. Bronchiolitis obliterans after lung transplantation. *Chest* 1998;113:365–370.

118. Yousem SA, Paradis IL, Dauber JH, et al. Efficacy of transbronchial lung biopsy in the diagnosis of bronchiolitis obliterans in heart-lung transplant recipients. *Transplantation* 1989;47: 893–895.

119. Yousem SA, Ohori NP. Pathological classification of acute and chronic rejection of the lung. In: H Shennib, ed. *Immunology of the lung allograft.* Austin, TX: RG Landes Bioscience, 1989: 29–44.

120. Kramer MR, Stoehr C, Whang JL, et al. The diagnosis of obliterative bronchiolitis after heart-lung and lung transplantation: low yield of transbronchial lung biopsy. *J Heart Lung Transplant* 1993;12:675–681.

121. Chamberlain D, Maurer J, Chaparro C, et al. Evaluation of transbronchial lung biopsy specimens in the diagnosis of bronchiolitis obliterans after lung transplantation. *J Heart Lung Transplant* 1994;13:963–971.

122. Yousem SA, Paradis I, Griffith BP. Can transbronchial biopsy aid in the diagnosis of bronchiolitis obliterans in lung transplant recipients? *Transplantation* 1994;57:151–153.

123. Cooper JD, Billingham M, Egan T, et al. A working fomulation for the standardization of nomenclature and for clinical staging of chronic dysfunction in lung allografts. *J Heart Lung Transplant* 1993;12:713–716.

124. Date H, Lynch JP, Sundaresan S, et al. The impact of cytolytic therapy on bronchiolitis obliterans syndrome. *J Heart Lung Transplant* 1998;17:869–875.

125. Paradis IL, Duncan SR, Dauber JH, et al. Effect of augmented immunosuppression on human chronic lung allograft rejection [Abstract]. *Am Rev Respir Dis* 1992;145(4;pt2):A705.

126. Ross DJ, Lewis MI, Kramer M, et al. FK 506 "rescue" immunosuppression for obliterative bronchiolitis after lung transplantation. *Chest* 1997;112:1175–1179.

127. Kesten S, Chaparro C, Scavuzza M, et al. Tacrolimus as rescue therapy for bronchiolitis obliterans syndrome. *J Heart Lung Transplant* 1997;16:905–912.

128. Whyte RI, Rossi SJ, Mulligan MS, et al. Mycophenolate mofetil for obliterative bronchiolitis syndrome after lung transplantation. *Ann Thorac Surg* 1997;64:945–948.

129. Iacono AT, Keenan RJ, Duncan SR, et al. Aerosolized cyclospo-

130. rine in lung recipients with refractory chronic rejection. *Am J Respir Crit Care Med* 1996;153:1451–1455.

130. Valentine VG, Robbins RC, Berry GJ, et al. Actuarial survival of heart-lung and bilateral sequential lung transplant recipients with obliterative bronchiolitis. *J Heart Lung Transplant* 1996; 15:371–383.

131. Brooks RG, Hofflin JM, Jamieson SW, et al. Infectious complications in heart-lung transplant recipients. *Am J Med* 1985;79: 412.

132. Egan TM, Kaiser LR, Cooper JD. Lung transplantation. *Curr Probl Surg* 1989;26:675–751.

133. Lynch JP III, Chauncey JB III, Gyetko M. Pulmonary and infectious complications in organ transplant recipients. In: Tenholder MF, ed. *Approach to pulmonary infections in the immunocompromised host.* Mount Kisco, NY: Futura Publishing, 1991: 229–276.

134. Dauber JH, Paradis IL, Dummer JS. Infectious complications in pulmonary allograft recipients. *Clin Chest Med* 1990;11: 291–308.

135. Ampel NM, Wing EJ. *Legionella* infection in transplant patients. *Semin Respir Infect* 1990;5:30–37.

136. Ettinger NA, Trulock EP. Pulmonary considerations of organ transplantation. *Am Rev Respir Dis* 1991;143:1386–1405, 144: 213–223, 433–454.

137. Davey RT, Masur H. Recent advances in the diagnosis, treatment, and prevention of *Pneumocystis carinii* pneumonia. *Antimicrob Agents Chemother* 1990;34:499–504.

138. Dummer JS. *Pneumocystis carinii* infections in transplant recipients. *Semin Respir Infect* 1990;5:50–57.

139. Kirk AJB, Colquhoun IW, Dark JH. Lung preservation: a review of current practice and future directions. *Ann Thorac Surg* 1993;56:990–1000.

140. Paradis IL, William P. Infection after lung transplantation. *Semin Respir Infect* 1993;8:207–215.

141. Paradis H, Grgurick WF, Drummer JS, et al. Rapid detection of cytomegalovirus pneumonia by evaluation of bronchoalveolar cells. *Am Rev Respir Dis* 1988;138:697–702.

142. Snydman DR. Cytomegalovirus infection in solid organ transplantation. Prospects for prevention. *Transplant Rev* 1990;4: 59–67.

143. Saliba F, Arulnaden JL, Gugenheim J, et al. CMV hyperimmune prophylaxis after liver transplantation: a prospective randomized controlled study. *Transplant Proc* 1989;21: 2260–2262.

144. Havel M, Teufelsbauer H, Lackovics A, et al. Cytomegalovirus hyperimmunoglobulin prophylaxis in the prevention of cytomegalovirus infection in immunosuppressed heart transplant patients. *Transplant Proc* 1990;22:1805–1806.

145. Gane E, Saliba F, Valdecasas GJC, et al. Randomised trial of efficacy and safety of oral ganciclovir in the prevention of cytomegalovirus disease in liver transplant recipients. *Lancet* 1997; 350:1729–1733.

146. Speich R, Thurnheer R, Gaspert A, et al. Efficacy and cost effectiveness of oral ganciclovir in the prevention of cytomegalovirus disease after lung transplantation. *Transplantation* 1999; 67:315–320.

147. Singh N, Yu VL. Oral ganciclovir usage for cytomegalovirus prophylaxis in organ transplant recipients. *Dig Dis Sci* 1998; 43(6):1190–1192.

148. Singh N, Yu VL, Gayowski T, et al. Cytomegalovirus antigenemia guided preemptive therapy with oral versus intravenous ganciclovir for the prevention of cytomegalovirus disease in liver transplant recipients [Abstract H5]. 37th International Conference on Antimicrobial Agents and Chemotherapy, Toronto, Canada, 1997.

149. Schmidt CA, Oettle H, Peng R, et al. Comparison of polymer-

ase chain reaction from plasma and buffy coat with antigen detection and occurrence of immunoglobulin M for the demonstration of cytomegalovirus infection after liver transplantation. *Transplantation* 1995;59:1133–1138.

150. Egan JJ, Barber L, Lomax J, et al. Detection of human cytomegalovirus antigenaemia: A rapid diagnostic technique for predicting cytomegalovirus infection pneumonitis in lung and heart transplant recipients. *Thorax* 1995;50:9–13.

151. Peters JI, Levine SM, Anzueto A, et al. Infectious complications in single lung transplant recipients [Abstract]. *Am Rev Respir Dis* 1993;147(4):A601.

152. Paya CV. Fungal infections in solid-organ transplantation. *Clin Infect Dis* 1993;16:677–688.

153. Levine SM, Peters JI. Fungal infection in the lung transplant recipient. *Pulm Crit Care Update.* 1998;13(12):17.

154. Denning DW, Stevens DA. Antifungal and surgical treatment of invasive aspergillosis: review of 2,121 published cases. *Rev Infect Dis* 1990;12:1147–1201.

155. Levine SM, Peters JI, Anzueto A, et al. *Aspergillus* infection in single lung transplant recipients [Abstract]. *Am Rev Respir Dis* 1993;147(4):A599.

156. Saral R. *Candida* and *Aspergillus* infection in immunocompromised patients: an overview. *Rev Infect Dis* 1991;13:487–492.

157. Wajszczuk CP, Dummer JS, Ho M, et al. Fungal infections in liver transplant recipients. *Transplantation* 1985;40:347–353.

158. Zeluff BJ. Fungal pneumonia in transplant recipients. *Semin Respir Med* 1992;13:216–233.

159. Denning D, Tucker RM, Hanson LH, et al. Treatment of invasive aspergillosis with itraconazole. *Am J Med* 1989;86: 791–800.

160. Zenati M, Dowling RD, Dummer S, et al. Influence of the donor lung on development of early infections in lung transplant recipients. *J Heart Transplant* 1990;9:502–509.

161. Conti DJ, Tolkoff-Rubin NE, Baker GP, et al. Successful treatment of invasive fungal infection with fluconazole in organ transplant recipients. *Transplantation* 1989;48:692–695.

162. Sinnott JV IV, Emmanual PJ. Mycobacterial infections in the transplant patient. *Semin Respir Infect* 1990;5:65–73.

163. Novick RJ, Moreno-Cabral CE, Stinson EB, et al. Nontuberculous mycobacterial infections in heart transplant recipients: a seventeen-year experience. *J Heart Transplant* 1990;9:357–363.

164. Shelhamer JH, Toews GB, Masur H, et al. Respiratory disease in the immunosuppressed patient. *Ann Intern Med* 1992;117: 415–431.

165. Rolfe M, Strieter RM, Lynch JP III. Nocardiosis. *Semin Respir Med* 1992;13:216–233.

166. Wilson JP, Turner HR, Kirchner KA, et al. Nocardial infections in renal transplant recipients. *Medicine (Baltimore)* 1989;68: 38–57.

167. Lynch JP III, Rolfe MW. Today's approach to managing and preventing nocardiosis. *J Respir Dis* 1993;14:112–121.

168. Nalesnik MA, Makowka L, Starzl TE. The diagnosis and treatment of lymphoproliferative disorders. *Curr Probl Surg* 1988; 25:371–472.

169. Randhawa PS, Yousem SA, Paradis IL, et al. The clinical spectrum, pathology, and clonal analysis of Epstein-Barr virus-associated lymphoproliferative disorders in heart-lung transplant recipients. *Am J Clin Pathol* 1989;92:177–185.

170. Yousem SA, Randhawa P, Locker J, et al. Posttransplant lymphoproliferative disorders in heart-lung transplant recipients: primary presentation in the allograft. *Hum Pathol* 1989;20:361–369.

171. Armitage JM, Kormos RL, Stuart RS, et al. Posttransplant lymphoproliferative disease in thoracic organ transplant patients: ten years of cyclosporine-based immunosuppressiom. *J Heart Lung Transplant* 1991;10:877–887.

172. Walker RC, Paya CV, Marshall WF, et al. Pretransplantation

seronegative Epstein-Barr Virus status is the primary risk factor for posttransplantation lymphoproliferative disorder in adult heart, lung, and other solid organ transplantations. *J Heart Lung Transplant* 1995;14:214–221.

173. Marshall WF, Strickler JG, Wiesner RH, et al. Pretransplantation assessment of the risk of lymphoproliferative disorder. *Clin Infect Dis* 1995;20:1346–1353.

174. Leblond V, Sutton L, Dorent R, et al. Lymphoproliferative disorders after transplantation: a report of 24 cases observed in a single center. *J Clin Oncol* 1995;13:961–968.

175. Aris RM, Maia DM, Neuringer IP, et al. Post-transplantation lymphoproliferative disorder in the Epstein-Barr virus-naïve lung transplant recipient. *Am J Respir Crit Care Med* 1996; 154(6):1712–1717.

176. Goldstein G. An overview of Orthoclone OKT3. *Transplant Proc* 1986;18(4):927–930.

177. Knight RJ, Kurrle R, McClain J, et al. Clinical evaluation of induction of immunosuppression with a murine IgG$_{2b}$ monoclonal antibody (BMA 031) directed toward the human α/β-T cell receptor. *Transplantation* 1994;57:1581–1588.

178. Vicente F, Lantz M, Birnbaum J, et al. A phase I trial of humanized anti-interleukin 2 receptor antibody in renal transplantation. *Transplantation* 1997;63:33–38.

179. Kriett JM, Smith CM, Hayden Am, et al. Lung transplantation without the use of antilymphocyte antibody preparations. *J Heart Lung Transplant* 1993;12:915–922.

180. Halloran PF. Immunosuppressive agents in clinical trials in transplantation. *Am J Med Sci* 1997;313(5):283–288.

181. US Renal Data System. *USRDS 1995 Annual Data Report.* Bethesda, MD. National Institutes of Health, National Institute of Diabetes and Digestive and Kidney Diseases, 1995.

182. Hunsicker LG, Bennett LE. Design of trials of methods to reduce late renal allograft loss: the price of success. *Kidney Int.* 1995;48[Suppl]:S120–S123.

183. Briffa N, Morris RE. New immunosuppressive regimens in lung transplantation. *Eur Respir J* 1997;10:2630–2637.

184. Vasquez MA. New advances in immunosuppression therapy for renal transplantation. Southwestern Internal Medicine Conference, NM Kaplan, BF Palmer, eds. *Am J Med Sci* 1997;314: 415–435.

185. Vine W, Bowers LD. Cyclosporine: structure, pharmacokinetics, and therapeutic drug monitoring. *Crit Rev Clin Lab Sci* 1988;25:275–311.

186. Kaskel FJ, Devarajan P, Arbeit LA, et al. Effects of cyclosporine on renal hemodynamics and autoregulation in rats. *Transplant Proc* 1988;20(3):603–609.

187. Maurer JR. Therapeutic challenges following lung transplantation. *Clin Chest Med* 1990;11(2):279–291.

188. Mihatsch M, Thiel G, Ryffel B. Cyclosporin nephrotoxicity. *Adv Nephrol Necker Hosp* 1988;17:303.

188. *1996 Annual report of the U.S. scientific registry for transplant recipients and the organ procurement and transplantation network—transplant data. 1988–1995.* Rockville, MD: UNOS, Richmond, VA, and the Division of Transplantation, Bureau of Health Resources Development, Health Resources and Services Administration, U.S. Department of Health and Human Services, 1996.

189. Kahan BD. Cyclosporine. *Med Intell* 1989;321(25): 1725–1737.

190. Bach JF, Strom TB. *The mode of action of immunosuppressive drugs,* 8th ed. New York: Elsevier, 1985.

191. Lu CY, Sicher SC, Vasquez MA. Prevention and treatment of renal allograft rejection: new therapeutic approaches and new insights into established therapies. *J Am Soc Nephrol* 1993;4: 1239–1256.

192. Cameron DE, Traill TA. Complications of immunosuppressive

therapy. In: Baumgartner WA, Reitz BA, Achuff SC, eds. *Heart and heart-lung transplantation.* Philadelphia: WB Saunders, 1990:237–247.

193. The International MMF Renal Transplant Study Group. A pooled analysis of three randomized double-blind clinical studies in prevention of rejection with mycophenolate mofetil in renal allograft recipients. *Transplantation* 1997;63(1):39–47.

194. Fessler HE, Wise RA. Lung volume reduction surgery. Is less really more? *Am J Respir Crit Care Med* 1990;159:1031–1035.

195. Fein AM. Lung volume reduction surgery. Answering the crucial questions. *Chest* 1998;113:277S–282S.

196. Utz JP, Hubmayr RD, Deschamps C. Lung volume reduction surgery for emphysema: out on a limb without a NETT. *Mayo Clin Proc* 1998;73:552–566.

197. Payne DK, Markewitz BA, Owens MW. Surgical treatment of chronic obstructive pulmonary disease. *Am J Med Sci* 1993; 318(2):89–95.

198. Brantigan OC, Mueller E. Surgical treatment of pulmonary emphysema. *Am Surg* 1957;23:789–804.

199. Cooper JD, Trulock EP, Triantafillou AN, et al. Bilateral pneumectomy (volume reduction) for chronic obstructive pulmonary disease. *J Thorac Cardiovasc Surg* 1995;109:106–119.

200. Ojo TC, Martinez F, Paine R III, et al. Lung volume reduction surgery alters management of pulmonary nodules in patients with severe COPD. *Chest* 1997;112:1494–1500.

201. Cooper JD, Patters GA, Sundaresan RS, et al. Results of 150 consecutive bilateral lung volume reduction procedures in patients with severe emphysema. *J Thorac Cardiovasc Surg* 1996; 112:1319–1330.

202. McKenna RJ, Brennner M, Gelb AF, et al. A randomized prospective trial of stapled lung reduction versus laser bullectomy for diffuse emphysema. *J Thorac Cardiovasc Surg* 1996;111: 317–321.

203. Gelb AF, Brenner M, McKenna RJ, et al. Lung function 12 months following emphysema resection. *Chest* 1996;10: 1407–1415.

204. Ingenito EP, Evans RB, Loring SH, et al. Relation between preoperative inspiratory lung resistance and the outcome of lung volume reduction surgery for emphysema. *N Engl J Med* 1998; 338:1181–1185.

205. Brenner M, Kayaleh RA, Milne WN, et al. Thorascopic laser ablation of pulmonary bullae: radiographic selection and treatment response. *J Thorac Cardiovasc Surg* 1994;107:883–890.

11

PULMONARY THROMBOEMBOLISM AND OTHER PULMONARY VASCULAR DISEASES

ALEJANDRO C. ARROLIGA
MICHAEL A. MATTHAY
RICHARD A. MATTHAY

PULMONARY THROMBOEMBOLISM AND INFARCTION
Incidence

PATHOGENESIS
Pathology
Pathophysiology
Clinical Manifestations
Lung Scanning, Computerized Tomography, and
    Pulmonary Angiography
Differential Diagnosis
Prevention and Treatment
Chronic Thromboembolic Pulmonary Hypertension
Septic Thromboembolism
Pulmonary Emboli Other Than Thromboemboli

PULMONARY HYPERTENSION
Pathologic Characteristics
Pathogenesis
Precapillary Pulmonary Hypertension

Postcapillary Hypertension
Diagnosis of Pulmonary Hypertension
Hemodynamic Studies in Patients with Pulmonary
    Hypertension
Treatment of Pulmonary Hypertension

COR PULMONALE (PULMONARY HEART DISEASE)
Incidence
Symptoms and Signs
Electrocardiographic Abnormalities
The Chest Radiograph
Other Tests for Evaluating Patients with Cor Pulmonale
Therapy for Acutely Decompensated Cor Pulmonale
Long-Term Management of Cor Pulmonale

CONGENITAL PULMONARY VASCULAR DISORDERS AND ACQUIRED ANEURYSMS
Pulmonary Arteriovenous Malformations
Pulmonary Artery Aneurysms

NEOPLASIA OF THE PULMONARY VASCULAR BED

Abnormalities of the pulmonary vascular bed may be caused by various diseases, ranging from chronic obstructive lung disease to interstitial fibrosis (1,2). If the disease is extensive, pulmonary hypertension may ensue (1). Pulmonary hypertension is also a feature of many congenital and acquired heart diseases and such systemic disorders as scleroderma and systemic lupus erythematosus (1). This chapter reviews the disorders associated with pulmonary vascular disease, focusing on pulmonary thromboembolism and infarction, primary pulmonary hypertension, and pulmonary heart disease (cor pulmonale). Congenital and acquired pulmonary arteriovenous malformations and neo-

plasia of the pulmonary vascular bed are also discussed briefly.

PULMONARY THROMBOEMBOLISM AND INFARCTION

A crucial function of the pulmonary circulation is to act as a filter for particulate matter transported to the lung by venous blood (3). Particles that are too large to pass through the pulmonary capillary bed lodge in the lung as emboli, and smaller "sticky" materials (e.g., leukocytes or tumor cells) also may adhere to pulmonary vessels. The material most commonly filtered out by the lung is the bland thromboembolus transported from its origin by venous circulation (3).

Incidence

Pulmonary embolism is the most common acute pulmonary disorder among hospitalized patients in the United States, occurring in approximately 650,000 patients per year (4–8). It ranks third as a cause of death in this country, accounting for at least 50,000 to 100,000 deaths annually (5–7). The average annual incidence rate for pulmonary embolism is 69 per 100,000 (6).

Approximately one-third of the deaths from pulmonary embolism occur within 1 hour of the onset of symptoms, and the diagnosis is not even suspected in nearly 60% of the patients who die (7–9). Most of the deaths occur rapidly before the appropriate diagnosis and therapy are implemented; therefore, prevention is important (7). Patients in whom the diagnosis is made and therapy is instituted account for only about 7% of the deaths caused by thromboembolism; therefore, a simple, inexpensive screening test to detect asymptomatic deep venous thrombosis, the precursor of pulmonary embolism, would be invaluable (4).

In an autopsy studies major pulmonary embolism was seen in 13% of 2,356 autopsies. In 25% of autopsies, venous thromboembolism was found. Venous thromboembolism (pulmonary embolism and deep vein thrombosis) was significantly more common in patients who died in the hospital compared with nonhospital deaths (10). The prevalence of confirmed venous thromboembolism increases with age. The cumulative probability of suffering a first episode of venous thromboembolism is 10.7% by the age of 80 years (11). Multiple injuries, immobilization, and bed rest put patients, especially the elderly, at high risk for deep venous thrombosis (Tables 11.1 and 11.2) (10–12).

TABLE 11.1. FREQUENCY OF DEEP VENOUS THROMBOSIS IN VARIOUS HOSPITALIZED PATIENT GROUPS

Group	Frequency (%)
Orthopedic (fractured hip)	54–67
Urologic (prostatectomy)	25
Surgical patients over the age of 40	28
Gynecologic	18
Cardiovascular (acute myocardial infarction)	39
Obstetric	3

Source: Raskob GE, Hull RD. Diagnosis and management of pulmonary thromboembolism. *Quart J Med* 1990;76:787–797; Kudsk KA, Fabian TC, Baum S, et al. Silent deep vein thrombosis in immobilized multiple trauma patients. *Am J Surg* 1989; 158:515–519.

TABLE 11.2. CONDITIONS PREDISPOSING TO VENOUS THROMBOSIS AND PULMONARY THROMBOEMBOLISM

Advanced age
Postoperative status
Previous venous thrombosis
Trauma
Congestive heart failure
Cerebrovascular accidents
Thrombocytosis
Erythrocytosis
Homocystinuria
Sickle-cell anemia
Oral contraceptive use
Pregnancy
Prolonged bed rest
Long periods of travel
Carcinoma
Obesity
Antiphospholipid syndrome

Source: Raskob GE, Hull RD. Diagnosis and management of pulmonary thromboembolism. *Quart J Med* 1990;76:787–797; Kudsk KA, Fabian TC, Baum S, et al. Silent deep vein thrombosis in immobilized multiple trauma patients. *Am J Surg* 1989; 158:515–519.

PATHOGENESIS

Most pulmonary emboli arise from detached portions of venous thrombi that form in the deep veins of the lower extremities or the pelvis and in the right side of the heart (5,13,14). Thrombus formation is fostered by blood stasis, hypercoagulable states, and vessel wall abnormalities. Stasis may be caused by local pressure, venous obstruction, or immobilization after a fracture or surgery; stasis commonly occurs in patients with congestive heart failure, shock, hypovolemia, dehydration, and varicose veins. An enlarged fibrillating right atrium frequently contains blood clots.

Several conditions enhance the intravascular coagulability of blood (15–17). In polycythemia the blood viscosity increases, with resultant sluggish flow next to the vessel wall. In other hypercoagulable states, abnormalities of the platelets and dysfunction of the endothelium mediated by cytokine activation may be important (15). Activation of endothelium may lead to loss of its normal anticoagulant surface functions, resulting in a pro-inflammatory thrombogenic phenotype (15). Certain abnormalities of the coagulation or fibrinolytic system are associated with recurrent venous thromboembolism, including increased platelet adhesiveness and survival time, abnormalities of the coagulation cascade, such as high levels of factor V or factor VII or deficiency of antithrombin III, protein C, or protein S (15,16). The two most common thrombophilias are resistance to activated protein C (an anticoagulant protein) that is associated with an abnormal factor V gene (factor V Leiden), and a prothrombin gene variant (prothrombin 20210 A). The mutation in factor V gene makes it resistant to inactivation by activated protein C and the mutation in prothrombin gene increases the levels of plasma prothrombin (16). Other groups at risk for venous hypercoagulability are patients with primary or secondary antiphospholipid syndrome (15,17). The pathophysiologic mechanism in these patients is not fully understood, but inhibition of endothelial cell production of prostacyclin by autoantibodies and a block in endothelial-cell thrombomodulin-mediated protein C activation have been suggested (15). Severe hyperhomocysteinemia is known to be a risk factor for venous thromboembolism. In recent years, evidence has accumulated that even modest hyperhomocysteinemia is associated with a higher risk of developing venous thromboembolism (16).

Malignancy-associated phlebitis (Trousseau's syndrome) should be considered in patients 50 years of age or older without risk factors who develop deep venous thrombosis and/or pulmonary embolism or in whom thrombosis or embolism recurs during warfarin therapy (18). The pathophysiology in Trousseau's syndrome is not understood, but tumor cells interacting with thrombin and plasmin-generating systems can influence thrombus formation (15). Patients who present with deep venous thromboses and no known risk factors should have a minimal work-up for malignancy, including measurement of serum carcinoembryonic antigen as well as a test for fecal occult blood and measurement of prostate-specific antigen in men and mammography in women (15,18).

Local trauma or inflammation may damage a vessel wall. In instances of marked local phlebitis with tenderness, redness, warmth, and swelling, the thrombus may be more securely attached to the wall. When the thrombus fragment is released, it is carried into one of the pulmonary arteries (5). Large thrombi may become lodged in a large artery or break up and block several smaller vessels. Distribution is probably related to the normal regional blood flow in the upright position; the lower lobes are predominantly involved because of their higher blood flow (6).

Pathology

Autopsies reveal that fewer than 10% of pulmonary emboli cause a pulmonary infarction. Infection and left heart failure increase the likelihood of pulmonary infarction, as do poor premortem functional status, emboli in multiple lobes, and lung cancer (14,19).

In a pulmonary infarct, the necrotic tissue is hemorrhagic and the alveolar walls, bronchi, and vessels are necrotic. With time, the color of an infarct changes from dark red to brown when the hemosiderin pigment is ingested by alveolar macrophages. Finally, fibrosis occurs and a scar is formed (14).

Pathophysiology

Whatever the source of the embolic material, the acute pathophysiologic results of a sudden pulmonary arterial branch obstruction are similar and have been well defined (20). A total cessation of blood flow to the distal lung zone is the initial effect of embolic obstruction, and this leads to respiratory and hemodynamic consequences.

Respiratory Consequences

Embolic obstruction of a pulmonary artery is followed by three primary respiratory events: an increase in alveolar dead space, bronchoconstriction, and loss of alveolar surfactant (20). Alveolar dead space is ventilated but receives no blood flow. Because gas exchange cannot occur in a nonperfused zone, any ventilation to it is wasted. Adequate alveolar ventilation requires an increase in total ventilation, and this contributes to the patient's dyspnea (21). However, bronchoconstriction reduces the functional size of the ventilated, nonperfused lung zone. Because the terminal airways, including the alveolar zones, themselves are involved, the dead space is increased.

Among the factors contributing to the development of lung constriction is reduced carbon dioxide tension (P_{CO_2}) in the embolic zone. P_{CO_2} decreases in a lung zone that is ventilated with essentially CO_2-free inspired air and receives no pulmonary blood flow. It has been demonstrated that severely hypocapnic areas constrict; inhalation of air-containing carbon dioxide reverses this process, and inflation of the lungs overcomes the constriction temporarily (22). Additional studies have indicated that regional hypoxia is involved, because inhalation of oxygen can also reverse the constriction (23). It is also possible that humoral agents released from the lung or embolus itself (serotonin, histamine) promote constriction (24).

The activity of alveolar surfactant begins to decline shortly after pulmonary artery occlusion, resulting in alveolar collapse and regional atelectasis within 24 hours (25).

A secondary respiratory consequence of embolic obstruction is arterial hypoxemia (20). Not all patients with embolism have arterial hypoxemia, but a wide alveolar-arterial oxygen tension gradient and a reduced arterial oxygen tension are common, particularly in massive embolism. Ventilation-perfusion mismatch, intrapulmonary shunting of mixed venous blood (perfusion of nonventilated lung units caused by atelectasis), alveolar hypoventilation, and preexistent cardiopulmonary disease may contribute to hypoxemia (20). In massive embolic obstruction, hypoxemia may be aggravated by a reduction of cardiac output with a subsequent drop in mixed venous oxygen tension (20). Right ventricular failure accompanied by a patent foramen ovale in some patients may contribute to severe hypoxemia (20).

Hemodynamic Consequences

The main hemodynamic consequence of pulmonary embolism is a decrease in the functional cross-sectional area of the pulmonary arterial bed, causing increased resistance to blood flow. To maintain the same flow at a higher pressure, the right ventricle must work harder. Therefore, in patients with substantial occlusion of the pulmonary vascular bed caused by pulmonary embolism, there is an increase in pulmonary arterial resistance, pulmonary artery pressure, and right ventricular work (20).

Pulmonary vascular resistance and right ventricular work correlate directly with the extent of pulmonary vascular bed obstruction (20,26). The presence of right ventricular afterload stress is associated with a higher in-hospital and 1-year mortality (26). The substantial reserve capacity of the pulmonary vascular bed provides some protection to the right ventricle. When more than 50% of the pulmonary vascular bed is occluded, pulmonary arterial pressure rises, requiring additional right ventricular work to maintain cardiac output. In patients with acute pulmonary embolism, pulmonary arterial pressures rarely exceed a mean of 40 mm Hg (20,27,28). The thin-walled right ventricle is not designed to accept acute heavy pressure loads, which may result in right ventricular failure and cardiovascular collapse (20).

The role of reflex vasoconstriction in the pathogenesis of pulmonary hypertension associated with acute pulmonary embolism is uncertain (20). However, vasoactive amines such as the vasoconstrictors serotonin and thromboxane A_2 may play a role in the development of pulmonary hypertension after acute pulmonary embolism (20). Furthermore, experimental data suggest that administration of a serotonin antagonist (ketanserin) reduces mean pulmonary artery pressure (20,29,30).

Infarction

A rare consequence of embolism is ischemic death of the pulmonary parenchyma (i.e., pulmonary infarction) (19,20). Fewer than 10% of all pulmonary emboli result in the death of distal pulmonary parenchyma. The infrequency of infarction is because the lung obtains oxygen from the bronchial arterial system and the airways in addition to the pulmonary arterial system. At least two of the three oxygen sources must be compromised to promote infarction.

Infarction is most common in patients with preexisting left ventricular failure or pulmonary disease, because bronchial arterial flow, pulmonary venous outflow, and ventilation are most likely to be compromised in these patients (14,19,20). Pulmonary infarction occurs more commonly in patients with occluded small pulmonary arteries (20).

Resolution of Pulmonary Thromboembolism

Like venous thrombi, pulmonary emboli tend to resolve rapidly. Beyond the acute stage the most frequent course of thromboembolic obstruction is restoration of vascular patency (14,31–33). As with deep venous thrombosis, the removal of embolic material from the pulmonary vascular bed depends on thrombolysis, organization, and recanalization of the thrombus.

Emboli are lysed by the action of circulating fibrinolytic factors in the blood and fibrinolytic factors released by the intima of pulmonary arteries. Several factors influence the speed of fibrinolytic dissolution, and a thrombus that has aged or become organized before being released is less sensitive (or even completely resistant) to fibrinolytic attack (34).

Vascular patency is also restored by organization of thrombus, a slower process than fibrinolysis, requiring days to weeks for completion. Organization is a reparative response, with invasion of fibroblasts and neocapilarization of the embolus. After the embolus is converted to connective tissue, it shrinks and restores the original lumen (14).

The less thrombus that is removed through fibrinolysis, the more that remains for recanalization and organization and the more likely residual pulmonary artery obstruction becomes. Regardless of the mechanisms involved in the removal of embolic material, vascular patency is generally restored to normal (8,14). Studies in dogs have demonstrated substantial resolution of emboli within hours and established that administration of heparin can accelerate this rate (33,34). Perfusion lung scans and angiographic studies in humans have confirmed substantial resolution of emboli within a few days, with a progressive reduction in residual emboli within 4 to 6 weeks (31,32). Permanent residual emboli do occur, although the exact incidence is unknown (35,36). Fewer than 10% of patients appear to retain perfusion defects after 6 weeks (8). The rate and degree of resolution observed in humans are probably related to age, the composition and volume of the thrombus and individual differences in fibrinolytic activity. Even massive emboli are likely to resolve within days or weeks, particularly in young persons without coexisting cardiopulmonary disease.

Two groups of patients may develop late pulmonary hypertension: those with major "central" obstruction of main or lobar arteries, and those with obstruction of several more distal vessels. Their embolic events are not always recognized clinically, and incorrect diagnoses ranging from chronic lung disease to primary pulmonary hypertension are often made (3,36).

Clinical Manifestations

It is important to maintain a high index of suspicion for deep venous thrombosis and pulmonary thromboembolism, particularly in patients at risk (see Tables 11.1 and 11.2) (4,37). Clinical diagnosis of deep venous thrombosis can be difficult, but nearly all patients with deep venous thrombosis have pain or swelling in the affected leg. Physical findings include erythema and warmth in one-third of patients, and swelling and tenderness in three-fourths. The presence of Homan's sign or a palpable cord is variable. Moreover, proximal deep venous thrombosis is observed on venograms in only 42% of patients with two or more of the following

TABLE 11.3. SYMPTOMS IN 117 PATIENTS WITH PULMONARY EMBOLISM AND NO PREEXISTING CARDIAC OR PULMONARY DISEASE

Symptom	Frequency (%)
Dyspnea	73
Pleuritic pain	66
Cough	37
Leg swelling	28
Leg pain	26
Hemoptysis	13
Palpitations	10
Wheezing	9
Angina-like pain	4

Source: Stein PD, Terrin MC, Hales CA, et al. Clinical, laboratory, roentgenographic and electrocardiographic findings in patients with acute pulmonary embolism and preexisting cardiac or pulmonary disease. *Chest* 1991;100:598–608.

TABLE 11.4. SIGNS IN 117 PATIENTS WITH PULMONARY EMBOLISM AND NO PRE-EXISTING CARDIAC OR PULMONARY DISEASE

Sign	Frequency (%)
Tachypnea (respiration rate ≤20/min)	70
Rales (crackles)	51
Tachycardia (pulse >100/min)	30
Fourth heart sound	24
Increased pulmonary component of second sound	23
Deep venous thrombosis	11
Diaphoresis	11
Fever (temperature >38.5°C)	7
Wheezes	5
Homan's sign	4
Right ventricular lift	4
Pleural friction rub	3
Third heart sound	3
Cyanosis	1

Source: Stein PD, Terrin MC, Hales CA, et al. Clinical, laboratory, roentgenographic and electrocardiographic findings in patients with acute pulmonary embolism and preexisting cardiac or pulmonary disease. *Chest* 1991;100:598–608.

clinical findings: swelling above and below the knee, fever, and a history of immobility and cancer (38).

Dyspnea is the most common symptom of pulmonary embolism (Table 11.3) (8,39). It was present in 73% of patients with angiographically proven pulmonary embolism in a recent study of 117 patients (39). The severity of dyspnea is related to the extent of embolic obstruction of the pulmonary vasculature, resulting primarily from the sudden appearance of alveolar dead space in the lung and likely being a response to changes in lung mechanics caused by the emboli. Pulmonary embolism presents as transient episodes of dyspnea as well. Massive embolism can produce syncope and hemodynamic instability besides causing dyspnea (7).

Pleuritic chest pain and hemoptysis occur secondary to infarction or congestive atelectasis and develop after vascular occlusion. Massive embolism can cause severe chest pain, mimicking coronary insufficiency. Although these clinical findings are nonspecific and can occur in various cardiopulmonary disorders, the context in which they occur (e.g., in the postoperative period, after lower-extremity trauma, or in the postpartum period) may increase the likelihood that they are caused by pulmonary embolism (3).

Characteristic physical findings associated with embolism are few (Table 11.4) (8,37). Tachypnea and tachycardia may, like dyspnea, be transient. Sustained marked tachycardia and tachypnea occur in patients with extensive embolism (8,39). Fine crackles on lung examination arise from bronchoconstriction and atelectasis, but the lungs are usually clear to auscultation and percussion (3,39).

Additional physical findings may be present in up to 10% of patients in which congestive atelectasis or infarction occurs. These include pleural friction rub, pleural effusion, and fever (40). The friction rub generally is audible over the lung bases because embolism occurs most frequently in the lower lobes. Rarely is the effusion massive (39).

Patients with massive embolism may have cardiac findings suggestive of acute cor pulmonale (right heart disease), including large A waves in the jugular venous pulse, a "lift" palpable over the right ventricle, a right ventricular diastolic gallop (S_3), a scratchy systolic murmur in the pulmonary valve area, and an accentuated pulmonary valve closure sound (loud P_2). However, the intensity of the closure sound may not reflect the extent of embolism. In massive obstruction, the right ventricle may fail, pulmonary blood flow may decrease, pulmonary arterial pressure may fall to or below normal values, and the pulmonic closure sound may be barely audible (8).

Fixed splitting of the second heart sound is an ominous finding because it evolves only in patients with marked right ventricular compromise (41). Its development is controlled by two factors: premature closure of the aortic valve as the reduced volume of blood from the lungs rapidly flows out of the left ventricle, and delayed pulmonary valve closure as high resistance in the pulmonary vasculature delays the right ventricular ejection time (41).

Arterial Blood Gases

Most patients with acute pulmonary embolism have a respiratory alkalosis. Carbon dioxide retention is rare unless pulmonary embolism occurs in a comatose or paralyzed patient on assisted ventilation. The arterial oxygen tension (PaO_2) in patients with pulmonary embolism is uniformly 80 mm Hg or less; however, in 15% to 25% of patients the PaO_2 values may exceed 80 mmHg. A normal PaO_2 does not help to exclude the diagnosis of pulmonary embolism. The main utility of determination of PaO_2 is to document the severity of hypoxemia and direct oxygen therapy (42).

Byproducts of Thrombin and Plasmin

Until anticoagulation therapy is initiated for pulmonary embolism, clot formation associated with thrombin generation occurs simultaneously with clot lysis secondary to plasmin generation. Measurement of D-dimer, an epitope present after the stabilization of the fibrin network and subsequent lysis by plasmin, has been used to diagnose pulmonary embolism and deep venous thrombosis (43). Although the specificity of the test is only 39%, a value below 500 μg/L using ELISA has been shown to rule out deep venous thrombosis and pulmonary embolism in 98% of patients studied (43). A normal D-dimer test using a whole-blood assay has been found useful to exclude pulmonary embolism in patients with nondiagnostic lung scan or with a low clinical pretest probability (44).

Electrocardiogram

The electrocardiogram (ECG) can rule out other serious diagnoses, such as acute myocardial infarction or pericarditis, in patients with pulmonary embolism. Only 13% of ECG results are normal in such patients, but abnormalities are nonspecific in 70% to 75% of cases. The classic $S_1Q_3T_3$ occurs in only 15% of patients (45).

Chest Radiograph

The plain chest radiograph cannot be used by itself to diagnose or exclude pulmonary embolism, but it may rule out other potentially life-threatening conditions such as tension pneumothorax (46). In a dyspneic patient, however, a normal chest radiograph may be a clue to the presence of pulmonary embolism (46). A parenchymal density and even evidence of pleural reaction or effusion are often present in patients with pulmonary embolism who have infarction or atelectasis (39).

Subtle chest radiographic signs are more common than frank infiltration. Comparable vessels may be of unequal size (e.g., one main pulmonary artery may be enlarged, whereas the other is smaller or normal). A major pulmonary artery with a "rat tail" appearance is indicative of an organizing thrombus within it. Oligemia of the lung zone also suggests embolic obstruction, particularly in association with increased flow to other lung areas. The presence of a prominent central pulmonary artery or cardiomegaly (in the absence of previous cardiopulmonary disease) is suggestive of pulmonary hypertension (46).

Thoracentesis

Pulmonary embolism exhibits no diagnostic pleural fluid findings (47). Sixty-five percent of pleural effusions in patients with pulmonary embolism are sanguinous, and these are usually associated with infiltrates on the chest radio-graph. Total leukocyte count varies from 22,000 to 57,000/μL. Approximately half of the effusions are exudates, even in the absence of an infiltrate. Thoracentesis is used primarily to exclude empyema and to look for a grossly bloody pleural effusion, which occurs in up to 27% of patients with pulmonary embolism (47). Trauma, malignant neoplasms, and pulmonary embolism are the main causes of a grossly bloody pleural effusion, the presence of which is not a contraindication to therapy for pulmonary embolism.

Lung Scanning, Computerized Tomography, and Pulmonary Angiography

The mortality of patients with untreated pulmonary embolism is as high as 30%; patients appropriately diagnosed and treated have a mortality of 2.5% to 8%, substantiating the need for prompt and accurate diagnosis (48). Standard laboratory tests are of little help in the diagnosis, but the combination of history, physical examination, and the specific laboratory tests mentioned excludes many other possibilities, allowing therapy to be initiated (3,37,39). Although spiral computerized tomography of the chest has been used more frequently to diagnose pulmonary embolism, the ventilation-perfusion ($\dot{V}/\dot{Q}$) lung scan and pulmonary angiography are sensitive, and reliable in the diagnosis of pulmonary embolism. Because of the current emphasis on pulmonary embolism as the respiratory manifestation of venous thromboembolism, the diagnostic approach includes clinical evaluation, a combination of diagnostic modalities for pulmonary embolism ($\dot{V}/\dot{Q}$ scan and pulmonary angiogram) as well as noninvasive modalities for detecting deep venous thrombosis (impedance plethysmography and B-mode imaging ultrasound) (48–54).

The perfusion lung scan is performed after intravenous injection of 10- to 50-μm particles radiolabeled with a γ-emitting isotope, usually Technetium-99m macroaggregate of albumin (48). The particles are trapped in the pulmonary arteriolar capillary bed, their distribution representing pulmonary blood flow. Embolic obstruction is manifested as zones of reduced or absent blood flow or perfusion defects (Fig. 5.25). However, any process that destroys or constricts pulmonary arterial vessels (e.g., old or recent necrotizing infection or regional hypoventilation) can also cause perfusion defects (48). Therefore, although the scan is a sensitive detector of changes in regional blood flow, it lacks specificity; however, a normal scan essentially eliminates clinically significant thromboembolic obstruction (3,48,49). The specificity of an abnormal perfusion scan may be improved when it is combined with a ventilation scan. Most ventilation scans are done with Xenon-133, but Xenon-127, Krypton-181m, and Technetium-99m aerosols have been used (48). Embolism often causes regions of high or infinite $\dot{V}/\dot{Q}$ ratio—areas with reduced to absent blood flow but normal ventilation (Fig. 5.25) (48). In contrast, parenchymal disorders that cause perfusion defects are generally associated with decreased or absent ventilation in the same lung zones (48). Thus, embolism tends to cause a ventilation-perfusion "mismatch," whereas parenchymal diseases result in "matched" ventilation-perfusion abnormalities (48). Furthermore, if the V̇/Q̇ scan is abnormal, the result can be classified as high probability, intermediate or indeterminate probability, and low probability for pulmonary embolism based on the size of the defect and the degree of "mismatch" between the V̇/Q̇ scan and chest radiography abnormalities (Table 11.5) (48–54). Concomitant cardiopulmonary disease does not diminish the diagnostic utility of a V̇/Q̇ scan in acute pulmonary embolism (55).

In the Prospective Investigation of Pulmonary Embolism

TABLE 11.6. LIKELIHOOD OF IDENTIFYING PULMONARY EMBOLISM ON PULMONARY ANGIOGRAM BASED ON V̇/Q̇ LUNG SCAN READING AND CLINICAL PROBABILITY ASSESSMENT

Scan Interpretation	Probability of Pulmonary Embolism (%)		
	High Clinical Probability	Intermediate Clinical Probability	Low Clinical Probability
High probability	96	88	56
Intermediate probability	66	28	16
Low probability	40	16	4
Near normal/ normal	0	6	2

Source: The PIOPED investigators. Value of the ventilation/perfusion scan in acute pulmonary embolism. Results of the prospective investigation of pulmonary embolism diagnosis (PIOPED). *JAMA* 1990;263:2753–2759.

TABLE 11.5. REVISED PIOPED V̇/Q̇ SCAN INTERPRETATION CRITERIA

High probability: Two or more large (>75% of a segment) segmental perfusion defects without corresponding ventilation or abnormalities on chest radiograph

One large segmental perfusion defect and two or more moderate (25%–75% of a segment) segmental perfusion defects without corresponding ventilation or abnormalities on chest radiograph

Four or more moderate segmental perfusion defects without corresponding ventilation or abnormalities on chest radiograph

Intermediate probability: One moderate or up to two large segmental perfusion defects without corresponding ventilation defect or abnormalities on chest radiograph

Corresponding V̇/Q̇ defects and parenchymal opacity in lower lung zone on chest radiograph

Corresponding V̇/Q̇ defects and small pleural effusion

Single moderate matched V̇/Q̇ defects with normal findings on chest radiograph

Difficult to categorize as normal, low, or high probability

Low probability: Multiple matched V̇/Q̇ defects, regardless of size, with normal findings on chest radiograph

Corresponding V̇/Q̇ defects and parenchymal opacity in upper or middle lung zone on chest radiograph

Corresponding V̇/Q̇ defects and large pleural effusion

Any perfusion defects with substantially larger abnormality on chest radiograph

Defects surrounded by normally perfused lung (stripe sign)

Single or multiple small (<25% of a segment) segmental perfusion defects with a normal chest radiograph

Nonsegmental perfusion defects (cardiomegaly, aortic impression, enlarged hila)

Normal: No perfusion defects, and perfusion outlines the shape of the lung seen on chest radiograph

Source: Worsley DF, Alavi A, Palevsky JH. Role of radionuclide imaging in patients with suspected pulmonary embolism. *Radiol Clin NA* 1993;31:849–858.

Diagnosis (PIOPED) study, the usefulness of the V̇/Q̇ lung scan in the diagnosis of acute pulmonary embolism was assessed (56). The study protocol asked the clinicians to estimate the probability of pulmonary embolism before the lung scan was performed, and the clinical estimate was combined with the finding of the V̇/Q̇ scan to determine the probability of pulmonary embolism on the pulmonary angiogram. The V̇/Q̇ interpretive criteria are shown in Table 11.5. The likelihood of pulmonary embolism diagnosed by angiography as determined by the result of the scan and the clinical probability is shown in Table 11.6. Patients with a high-probability V̇/Q̇ scan and high clinical probability of pulmonary embolism had a 96% chance of having the embolism confirmed by pulmonary angiogram; on the other hand, patients with a normal or near normal scan, independent of the clinical probability, had a very low likelihood of having a pulmonary embolism. Patients with an intermediate- or low-probability scan still have a substantial probability of having pulmonary embolic disease, independent of the clinical probability, and pulmonary angiography was critical in establishing the diagnosis.

The study did not systematically evaluate the lower extremities for deep venous thrombosis. Other investigators have shown that combining the lung scan with impedance plethysmography, B-mode imaging ultrasound and D-dimers test is useful in patients suspected of having pulmonary embolism (44,51). (Figure 11.1 presents an algorithm for a combined diagnostic approach.) Impedance plethysmography and B-mode ultrasound have been shown to correlate positively with the leg venogram in 83% to 94% of cases in the diagnosis of proximal deep venous thrombosis (femoral and popliteal) (53,57–59). The correlation for distal (calf) venous thrombosis is less reliable (57). B-mode imaging has been used for the diagnosis of upper-extremity venous thrombosis, an increasing cause of pulmonary embo-

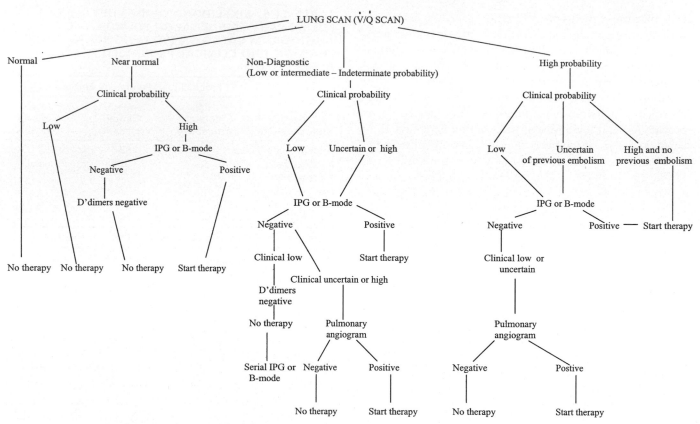

FIGURE 11.1. Strategy for diagnosis of pulmonary embolism in stable patients based on clinical suspicion, lung scan, pulmonary angiogram, and noninvasive tests for deep venous thrombosis. *IPG,* impedance plethysmography; *B-mode,* duplex, compression ultrasound. (Modified from Stein PD, Hull RS, Saltzman HA, Pineo G. Strategy for diagnosis of patients with suspected acute pulmonary embolism. *Chest* 1993;103:1553–1559).

lism; however, venography remains the most reliable technique (57).

Recent studies suggest that spiral computerized tomography of the chest may be a useful modality to diagnose pulmonary embolism (Fig 5.21) (50,52). A large multicenter, prospective study is underway in the United States to assess the potential role of spiral computerized tomography in the diagnosis of pulmonary embolism. Early studies showed that spiral computerized tomography is accurate and may be used in those patients in whom pulmonary embolism is suspected and the V̇/Q̇ scan is nondiagnostic (50,52).

The pulmonary angiogram is the definitive test for diagnosing pulmonary embolism (53,60). The false-negative rate is only 1% to 2% (53), the death rate from the procedure is 0.5%, and 1% of patients develop major complications (60). On the angiogram, the specific finding for pulmonary embolism is an abrupt cutoff of a major vessel caused by full embolic obstruction. However, the most common angiographic abnormality is a filling defect resulting from the flow of contrast medium around a partial obstruction (Fig. 5.25) (60). Additional angiographic signs that are less specific for pulmonary embolism include absent,

decreased, or delayed filling of a lung zone, delayed venous emptying, "pruning" (absence of small branches), and abnormal vessel tapering, as well as dilation of the right ventricle and great vessels (60).

When performed with a cardiac catheter inserted into the pulmonary artery, pulmonary angiography provides the opportunity to assess the hemodynamic status of the patient. Measurement of right heart pressures, pulmonary artery wedge pressure, and the assessment of cardiac output may provide information vital to therapeutic decisions (60). In those whose condition is unstable, segmental injection can be made into the abnormal area seen on perfusion scan (6,61).

The diagnostic approach to pregnant patients is generally similar; however, the perfusion scan is done with a low dose of radioisotope (1 to 2 mCi), and if impedance plethysmography of the lower extremities is positive, a venogram is obtained to rule out a false-positive result of the impedance study caused by the compression of the iliac vein by the gravid uterus, especially during the third trimester (62). During the performance of venography, the patient's abdomen is covered with a lead-lined apron.

Differential Diagnosis

The onset of an atrial arrhythmia in a patient with preexisting cardiac disease is commonly caused by pulmonary embolism, although the mechanisms involved are not clear. Sudden or progressive worsening of congestive heart failure also suggests embolic disease. Similarly, embolism may occur in a patient with chronic obstructive pulmonary disease (COPD) whose condition suddenly deteriorates or in a patient with worsening hypoxemia and dyspnea in the absence of infection or other obvious cause (8).

Attacks of syncope and dizziness in an apparently healthy person may indicate embolic phenomena, particularly in association with dyspnea (8), and recurrent attacks of hyperventilation should arouse suspicion. Moser observed patients with hyperventilation and fleeting episodes of chest discomfort who had recurrent embolization rather than psychological problems (3).

Bacterial or viral pneumonitis may mimic embolism in a clinical context that predisposes to pulmonary embolism. For example, in the postoperative period, a low-grade fever, dyspnea, and tachycardia may develop, and the chest radiograph may show a nonspecific infiltrate, possibly representing atelectasis, pneumonia, or pulmonary embolism (8).

Infarction secondary to embolism may be confused with any disorder capable of producing acute pleuritis, including collagen vascular diseases as well as infectious diseases. An exudative sanguineous pleural effusion with no organisms on Gram stain is typical of embolism but is not definitive (8).

Finally, patients with other acute cardiopulmonary disorders (e.g., myocardial infarction, dissecting aortic aneurysm, and pneumothorax) can present with substernal discomfort, dyspnea, tachycardia, and electrocardiographic abnormalities (8). Pulmonary thromboembolism should be included among the differential diagnoses in these contexts, because once the possibility of this diagnosis is considered, it can be confirmed.

Prevention and Treatment

Prophylaxis of Deep Venous Thrombosis

The frequency of proximal and distal deep venous thrombosis postoperatively ranges from 7% in general surgery patients to 80% in patients after hip and knee surgery (63). Patients with acute spinal cord injury (35%), myocardial infarction (24%), ischemic stroke (63%), and such other medical conditions as heart failure (20%) and pneumonia have an intermediate frequency (63). Despite the availability of agents that prevent deep venous thrombosis, up to 56% of patients who died of pulmonary embolism did not receive prophylaxis, despite having major risk factors and no obvious contraindication for prophylaxis (64).

It is clear that underutilization of prophylaxis is still common (65). There are two basic kinds of prophylaxis of deep venous thrombosis: mechanical and pharmacologic. The mechanical approaches, which reduce venous stasis, include early ambulation (desirable in all patients at risk for venous thrombosis), the use of elastic stockings, pneumatic calf compression, and electrical stimulation of calf muscles. The pharmacologic agents, which combat hypercoagulability of the blood, include warfarin, dextran, low-molecular weight heparin, heparinoids, and heparin (63). Standard heparin is the type of prophylaxis most commonly used in patients with medical conditions. Heparin is given in low doses or adjusted doses to maintain the activated partial thromboplastin time (aPTT) between 31 and 36 seconds 6 hours after therapy is administered. Low-molecular weight heparins are new pharmacologic agents recommended for prophylaxis. Low-molecular weight heparin, has restricted molecular weight distribution around 5000 daltons (66); heparinoids are a mixture of glycosaminoglycans, including heparin sulfate and dermatan sulfate (67). Table 11.7 summarizes the current recommendations for prophylaxis of deep venous thrombosis, as set forth by the Fifth Consensus Conference of the American College of Chest Physicians (63).

Treatment of Acute Deep Venous Thrombosis

Heparin is the drug of choice for acute deep venous thrombosis because of its immediate action, relative safety, and specific inhibitory effects on the coagulation system (68). Heparin catalyzes the effect of antithrombin III, a coagulation inhibitor that inactivates thrombin and factors Xa and IXa. Moreover, heparin inhibits the activation of factors V and VIII by thrombin (68). Heparin does not lyse existing clots, but prevents formation and propagation of further clots. Continuous intravenous therapy is generally preferred to intermittent intravenous bolus administration because is associated with fewer bleeding complications (68). If intravenous therapy is not possible, good alternatives are adjusted-dose subcutaneous therapy, usually starting at 17,500 units every 12 hours and adjusting the dose to give an aPTT of more than 1.5 time control within 1 hour of the next scheduled dose, or administration of low molecular weight heparin (63,68).

In patients with venous thromboembolic disease, heparin is frequently underdosed (68,69). The goal of heparin therapy is to maintain the aPTT at 55 to 60 seconds (70). Nomograms have been used to facilitate dosing, and three-fourths of patients treated according to a weight-based nomogram achieve therapeutic levels of heparin in a short period of time in three-fourths of patients with no major hemorrhagic complications (69,70).

In the first 24 to 36 hours of heparin therapy, when adequate anticoagulation is often difficult to achieve and

TABLE 11.7. PROPHYLAXIS OF DEEP VENOUS THROMBOSIS AND PULMONARY EMBOLISM

Type of Operation	Usual-Risk Patient	High-Risk Patient (e.g., prior DVT or PE)
General abdominothoracic surgery	<40 y/o, surgery <30 min; no risk factors, no prophylaxis, early ambulation All other patients: LDH, SCq 12 hr starting 2 hr preoperatively, *or* IPC or LMWH or ES	High-risk: LDH SCq 8 hr, LMWH and IPC Very high risk with multiple risk factors: LDH or LMW[b] or dextran plus IPC Alternative, consider perioperative Warfarin INR (2–3)
Orthopedic surgery[a] Hip replacement	Warfarin (INR 2–3) preoperatively or immediately after surgery *or* LMW (started 12–24 after surgery) or adjusted-dose heparin (aPTT 31–36 sec) started preoperatively	IVCF in selected patients with contraindications to anticoagulants
Hip fractures Knee operations	Warfarin (INR 2–3) or LMW IPC or LMW or warfarin or IPC	Consider LMWH or IPC and LMWH or IPC and LDH
Eye surgery Neurosurgery	IPC ± ES IPC ± ES	
Acute spinal cord injury with paralysis	LMWH or warfarin? *or* LOH, IPC ? ES, contraindications to acute coagulants	
Multiple trauma	LMWH or IPC	IVCF in selection of patients with contraindications to anticoagulants
General medical patient Myocardial infarction	LDH, IPC ? ES?	LDH or warfarin (INR 2–3) LMW ? IPC ? ES?
Ischemic stroke and lower-extremity paralysis	LDH or LMWH IPC ? ES ?	LMW or LDH Warfarin ? IPC ? ES?
Other medical condition (heart failure, pneumonia malignancy, etc.)	LDH or LMWH	
Long-term indwelling Catheter and malignancy	Warfarin 1 mg qd or LMWH	Warfarin 1 mg qd

[a] Consider maintaining prophylaxis for 24- to 35-day duration.
[b] LMWH should be used with caution if spinal tap is done or epidural catheter is used.
Source: Clagett GP, Anderson FA Jr, Geerts W, et al: Prevention of venous thrombi embolism. *Chest* 114:531S–560S, 1998.
Abbreviations: LDH, low-dose heparin 5000 units per dose; LMW, low-molecular weight heparin; ES, graduated compression elastic stockings; INR, international normalized ratio; IVCF, inferior vena cava filter; IPC, intermittent pneumatic compression; ?, probably indicated but insufficient data; DVT, deep venous thrombosis; PE, pulmonary embolism.

sustain, the aPTT should be determined every 4 hours, and the heparin dose should be adjusted according to the aPTT (Table 11.8).

Factors associated with an increased risk for bleeding complications are advanced age, uncontrolled hypertension, underlying coagulation abnormality, recent gastrointestinal hemorrhage, active vasculitis, chronic liver disease, uremia, and recent surgery or major arterial cannulation. In patients in which full-dose anticoagulation cannot be achieved (e.g., patients with intracranial bleeding), the insertion of a vena cava filter is indicated (68).

Heparin therapy should be initiated together with oral anticoagulation to reduce in-hospital days. Once anticoagulation has been achieved with the oral agent, heparin is discontinued when the prothrombin time (International Normalized Ratio, INR) is above 2 on 2 consecutive days (68). The minimal treatment with heparin is between 5 to 7 days.

TABLE 11.8. HEPARIN INFUSION NOMOGRAM: ADJUSTMENT TO INFUSION AFTER A BOLUS OF 5000 UNITS[a]

aPTT (sec)	Dose Change (U/hr)	Additional Action
≥45	↑240	Repeat aPTT in 4 hr
46–54	↑120	Repeat aPTT in 4 hr
55–850		None
86–110	↓120	Stop heparin for 1 hr, repeat aPTT in 4 hr after restarting heparin
>110	↓240	Stop heparin for 1 hr, repeat aPTT in 4 hr, after restarting heparin

[a]Concentration 20,000 U in 500 mL. Initial rate of 1240 U/hr (31 mL/hr) in patients with risk of bleeding and at 1680 U/hr in those without identified risk of bleeding.
Source: Elliott CG, Hiltunen SJ, Suchyta M, et al. Physician-guided treatment compared with a heparin protocol for deep vein thrombosis. *Arch Intern Med* 1994;154:999–1004.

Low-molecular weight heparin has been found to be safe and equivalent in efficacy to unfractionated heparin in the treatment of deep vein thrombosis and pulmonary embolism. Low-molecular weight heparin can be given as initial treatment and can be administered without laboratory monitoring, making management simple and in some patients allowing management in the outpatient setting (68,71). Recently, a randomized trial comparing subcutaneous low-molecular weight heparin (enoxaparin, 6,300 anti-Factor Xa units twice daily for patients weighing more than 60 kg and 4,200 units twice daily for patients between 45 kg and 60 kg) and intravenous unfractionated heparin, found that the fixed-dose low-molecular weight heparin is as effective and safe as unfractionated heparin in the treatment of venous thromboembolism (71).

The coumarin derivatives are orally administered drugs that inhibit vitamin K-dependent clotting proteins in the liver (factors II, VII, IX, and X); the most commonly used coumarin derivative is racemic warfarin sodium (68). These agents must be given for 6 to 7 consecutive days for a full antithrombotic effect (68). Coumarin derivatives are suitable for outpatient therapy and can provide long-term anticoagulation for patients with thrombotic problems. Early introduction of warfarin on day 1 in small loading doses of 5 mg can decrease the duration of heparin therapy to less than 7 days (68,72). An effective level of anticoagulation must be ensured reflected by an International Normalized Ratio of 2 to 3 (68). Coumarin therapy can be given to nursing mothers, but coumarin is contraindicated in pregnant patients. In those cases low-molecular weight heparin or unfractionated adjusted-dose heparin to prolong the aPTT to a level equal to a heparin level of 0.2 to 0.4 IU/mL is indicated (68).

The appropriate length of time for anticoagulation in patients with deep venous thrombosis is variable and depends on clinical circumstances. For example, patients developing deep venous thrombosis following transient immobilization or following a fracture in the lower extremity, should be treated for three months. Other patients who have risk factors that cannot be modified, for example, malignancy or patients with a hypercoagulable state and patients with recurrent venous thromboembolism, probably should be treated indefinitely (68,73).

Presenting a special problem are those patients with idiopathic venous thromboembolism. Aparently these patients are vulnerable to recurrent episodes, initiated by clinically obvious or occult stimuli (74). In patients with idiopathic venous thromboembolism, anticoagulant therapy should be given after a first episode for more than 3 months (75). The optimal duration is unknown, although in a recent analysis, patients with symptomatic pulmonary embolism or deep venous thrombosis treated with anticoagulant for 3 months had a low rate of fatal pulmonary embolism during and after the therapy was finished (76).

Thrombolytic Therapy in Deep Venous Thrombosis

The role of thrombolytic therapy in deep venous thrombosis is not defined, although streptokinase, urokinase, and tissue plasminogen activator have been used (68). Proximal, massive thrombi (iliofemoral veins) respond better than distal thrombi. Streptokinase is given in a dose of 250,000 units in 30 minutes, followed by 100,000 U/hr for 72 hours through an intravenous line. The thrombin time should be checked at 6 hours; if supratherapeutic, the infusion can be discontinued for a few hours and then reinitiated at a lower rate. In patients receiving streptokinase, the incidence of minor bleeding is increased; however, major bleeding episodes (requiring 2 or more units of blood) are apparently no more common than in patients receiving heparin only. Concomitant therapy with acetaminophen and intravenous corticosteroids is suggested to minimize allergic reaction (less than 5%) in patients receiving streptokinase therapy. After streptokinase therapy, heparin infusion (without a bolus) is needed. Heparin should not be infused together with streptokinase, urokinase, or tissue plasminogen activator (68,77). Direct infusion into a leg vein does not offer local benefit compared to systemic infusion into a peripheral vein. It has been suggested that thrombolytic therapy decreases pain and the incidence of postphlebitic syndrome; however, the risk–benefit ratio of thrombolytic therapy is not well established. Therefore, knowledge of patients' values and preferences should be used to guide therapy (68,78).

Treatment of Pulmonary Thromboembolism

The treatment plan for pulmonary embolism depends on the extent and sites of the obstruction and the hemodynamic condition of the patient. The first step is to stop the thrombotic process by instituting heparin therapy in a regimen similar to that established for deep venous thrombosis (68).

Additional supportive measures may be necessary. If arterial hypoxemia is present, supplemental oxygen should be administered. Mild analgesia may be required to alleviate pain. In patients with hypotension and shock, fluid therapy to increase right ventricular preload is the first line of treatment. Second, vasopressor support usually is needed, and norepinephrine is the vasopressor of choice in patients profoundly hypotensive to maintain systemic blood pressure, increase cardiac output, and maintain coronary perfusion of the right ventricle. Dobutamine can be used in those patients with moderate hypotension and a low cardiac output; however, it is important to follow the systemic blood pressure in patients in whom dobutamine is used because this agent can cause hypotension (79). Mechanical ventilation is often needed to support the patient because of the high work of breathing, increased dead-space fraction, and the metabolic acidosis that may be associated with a decline in cardiac output (8).

Streptokinase, urokinase, and tissue plasminogen activator can rapidly lyse pulmonary thromboemboli; these agents should be considered for patients with massive pulmonary embolism who are hemodynamically unstable and have no contraindication (e.g., bleeding) (68). These thrombolytic agents must not be administered concurrently with heparin (68). Thrombolytic therapy has been shown by angiography to result in early clot lysis, but it has not been shown to reduce the mortality from pulmonary embolism (68). In patients with submassive and massive life-threatening pulmonary emboli, streptokinase is administered in the same dose utilized for deep venous thrombosis for 24 hours (77). Therapy with urokinase, 4,400 U/kg over 30 minutes followed by 4,400 U/kg/hr for 24 hours, is an alternative and is the preferred agent in massive emboli because it produces more rapid thrombolysis. After thrombolysis, heparin should be given without a bolus to maintain the aPTT at 55 to 60 seconds.

Emergency surgical embolectomy is rarely done; it has a high mortality rate (50% to 94%), and good medical management may result in a lower mortality, especially with the availability of thrombolytic therapy to supplement other supportive treatment. Factors associated with enhanced mortality from submassive and massive pulmonary emboli include cardiac arrest, history of cardiopulmonary disease, and shock (68). Transvenous catheter extraction of emboli has a mortality rate of 27% and a success rate of 61%. Catheter thrombectomy for high-risk pulmonary embolism patients may be useful in a small group of patients in whom heparin therapy is insufficient and thrombolysis is contraindicated (68,80). Surgical embolectomy should be considered in otherwise healthy patients with large emboli who cannot receive thrombolytic therapy because of recent surgery or some other contraindication (68).

In patients with proximal leg deep venous thrombosis in whom anticoagulation is contraindicated, has failed, or has caused complications, inferior vena cava interruption is indicated. It is also indicated for chronic pulmonary embolism, in patients undergoing pulmonary embolectomy or pulmonary endarterectomy, and in patients developing recurrent pulmonary embolism in spite of adequate anticoagulation (68). In patients with a vena cava filter, the reported rate of pulmonary embolism is less than 2%, and insertion of a filter causes fatal complications in approximately 0.1% (81). Insertion of a vena cava filter has been suggested for prophylaxis of pulmonary embolism in patients at high risk of bleeding because of extensive trauma, cancer, or hip or knee surgery, and in paraplegic patients with spinal cord injury (81). In a prospective trial of patients considered to be at high risk for pulmonary embolism, patients were randomized to receive an inferior vena cava filter versus no filter. The patients who received a filter had less symptomatic and asymptomatic pulmonary embolism at day 12 compared with patients who received anticoagulation only (82). However, no difference in survival was detected, and, at 2 years, an increase in recurrent deep venous thrombosis was noted in the study group. Although patients with an inferior vena cava filter do not require anticoagulation, continuous warfarin therapy (if it is not contraindicated) is recommended to prevent the development and propagation of thrombi below the filter (68,82).

Chronic Thromboembolic Pulmonary Hypertension

Chronic thromboembolic pulmonary hypertension, a chronic disease of the pulmonary arteries, is the result of extensive obstruction of the pulmonary vasculature (83,84). It is a rare disorder, the prevalence being estimated at 0.1% (83). Up to 50% of affected patients have a history consistent with venous thrombosis or pulmonary embolism (84). When the pulmonary vessels become occluded, with extensive loss of cross-sectional area of the vascular bed, pulmonary hypertension develops at rest or with minimal exertion (83). Dyspnea on exertion is common, and other symptoms are conspicuously absent (83,84). In some patients the physical examination reveals only a systolic or continuous murmur heard over the lung fields (83). The murmur, which is caused by partial obstruction of major pulmonary arteries, is rare in other pulmonary vascular diseases and absent in primary pulmonary hypertension (83). Other physical findings late in the disease are suggestive of elevated right heart pressure (e.g., hepatomegaly, leg edema, loud P_2, murmur of tricuspid insufficiency) (83,84).

Laboratory tests are unremarkable in general. Fewer than 1% of affected patients have deficiencies of antithrombin III and protein C and S, and lupus anticoagulant is present in 10% (83). The chest radiograph may be normal, although such subtle findings as unequal central pulmonary vascular shadows and zones of avascularity are occasionally found (83). Right ventricular enlargement is a late finding (83). The electrocardiogram is normal early in the disease; later, right axis deviation, right ventricular hypertrophy, and T-wave inversion in the precordium may be present (83). Echocardiography shows an elevated pulmonary arterial systolic pressure and an increase in size of the right heart chambers (83). Pulmonary function tests are normal or show a restrictive ventilatory defect. The diffusing capacity for carbon monoxide (D_{LCO}) is normal or reduced (83). The arterial oxygen tension is normal at rest and declines during exercise (83). The most important noninvasive test in chronic thromboembolic pulmonary hypertension is the $\dot{V}/\dot{Q}$ lung scan (83). Affected patients have a segmental or larger perfusion-ventilation mismatch (83). In patients with primary pulmonary hypertension, the perfusion lung scan is normal or shows only patchy subsegmental defects (83). The pulmonary angiogram confirms the diagnosis; confirmatory findings include intraluminal bands, webs, intimal irregularities, vascular narrowing and obstruction, and "pouching defects" (occlusive thrombi that organize in a concave configuration) (83–86). The pulmonary arterial pressures are elevated with a normal wedge pressure.

The prognosis of chronic thromboembolic disease is related to the degree of pulmonary hypertension (84). The only successful therapy is thromboendarterectomy of the pulmonary arteries; the presence of comorbid conditions, such as coronary disease, increases the risk of this surgical procedure (85). The overall perioperative mortality is 6.4% in leading centers (85).

Septic Thromboembolism

Septic thromboembolism is encountered after gynecologic-obstetric procedures, as a complication of intravenous drug use and infective endocarditis (3,87). The classic inciting event in gynecologic-obstetric procedures is a septic abortion, but septic thromboembolism may occur after a normal delivery and after in-hospital sterile gynecologic procedures such as dilation and curettage. Additional potential sources of infected emboli are related to medical technology; for example, infection may develop from catheters placed in peripheral and central veins, ventriculoatrial shunt catheters, transvenous pacemakers, and catheters for hemodialysis. Patients with the acquired immunodeficiency syndrome (AIDS) and organ transplant recipients are at risk for pulmonary septic emboli (88).

In septic thromboembolism, a traumatized vein is invaded by microorganisms. In drug users, the vein is used for intravenous drug administration; in gynecologic-obstetric patients, the pelvic veins are involved; in patients with catheters, the cannulated vein is affected (3). The involved veins become occluded by mixtures of blood clot and bacteria, and small emboli are dislodged from such foci. The process may gradually resolve, with or without specific therapy, but if embolism develops, the already septic patient becomes more dyspneic; cough, sputum production, hemoptysis, and pleuritic chest pain often develop (3). The drug abuser often presents with severe sepsis and multiple pulmonary infiltrates (septic infiltrates) that tend to cavitate (88).

The chest radiograph characteristically shows multiple small, nodular densities, usually with fuzzy outlines (3). The number of these lesions may increase rapidly, and radiographs taken at 24-hour intervals often show striking changes that reflect the occurrence of repetitive, small infected emboli. There may be so many lesions that they become confluent. Cavitation usually appears within the nodules after hours or days and may lead to rapid development of thin-walled cavities. Computed tomographic scans may show multiple peripheral nodules of various sizes, predominantly basilar in distribution. These nodules may be cavitated and have air bronchograms (88). A blood vessel leading to a nodule (feeding vessel sign) is present in two-thirds of the patients (88). Wedge-shaped peripheral lesions abutting the pleura or extending into the pleural space are common.

Bacteremia is a common complication, sometimes resulting in endocarditis involving the tricuspid and, rarely, pulmonary valves (3). Echocardiography may be helpful in these cases. The friable valvular vegetations may subsequently embolize to the lungs and produce the clinical and radiographic features described in the preceding.

Both the infection and the thromboembolism must be treated with vigorous antibiotic therapy combined with heparinization. The value of adding heparin to the antibiotic regimen has been established (3). Because blood cultures may be negative, antibiotic selection must be made empirically; antibiotic coverage should include Gram-negative and Gram-positive organisms, including penicillinase-producing staphylococci (3). Any indwelling venous catheter should be removed immediately and cultured.

The use of heparin in patients with right-sided endocarditis is controversial because of the risk of hemorrhage. However, most evidence indicates that heparin plays a major role in the therapeutic regimen in these patients and that hemorrhagic risk is minor (3).

If antibiotic-heparin therapy fails to reverse the embolic process, surgical procedures to isolate drainage from the infected area should be considered (3). Ligation of the inferior vena cava and the left ovarian vein is necessary in septic pelvic thrombophlebitis. The source of the embolism determines the other sites of venous ligation. Combined antibiotic-heparin therapy usually precludes the necessity for ligation and other surgical procedures such as hysterectomy or extirpation of an infected valve (3).

Pulmonary Emboli Other Than Thromboemboli

Types of pulmonary emboli other than venous thromboemboli are shown in Table 11.9. This chapter briefly discusses certain of these entities; for a more detailed discussion the interested reader is referred to other reviews of the subject (3,89,90).

TABLE 11.9. PULMONARY EMBOLI OTHER THAN THROMBOEMBOLI

Fat emboli
Bone marrow emboli
Amniotic fluid emboli
Foreign body emboli
Air emboli
Tumor emboli
Trophoblast emboli
Brain emboli
Liver emboli
Bile thromboemboli
Plastic emboli (from intravenous tubing)
Cotton fiber emboli
Lymphangiographic (Ethiodol) emboli
Parasitic emboli (schistosomal flukes—*Schistosoma haematobium, S. mansoni, S. japonicum*)

Fat Emboli

Of the many types of tissue that obstruct the lungs, fat has received the most attention and is subject to some controversy (3,90). Fat cells and neutral fat are often found in the lungs of patients who have died after long-bone fractures and other types of severe trauma, burns, and surgery. In addition, intravenous infusion of large quantities of neutral fat can induce dyspnea, pulmonary hypertension, and gas exchange abnormalities in animals (3). However, the link between these facts and the fat embolism syndrome is open to question.

The typical case history involves a patient with long-bone fractures who, on admission, is alert, oriented, and in good condition with the exception of the traumatized areas. Within 12 to 36 hours, however, mental status changes occur and may progress to delirium and coma; high fever and marked dyspnea, tachypnea, and tachycardia may occur and a petechial rash may develop, particularly over the thorax and upper extremities. Inspiratory rales may fill the lungs, and the chest radiograph shows a diffuse alveolar filling-type pattern throughout both lung fields in 30% to 60% of patients. Arterial hypoxemia and hypocapnia develop; thrombocytopenia is common. Fat may be recovered from sputum and urine, a nonspecific finding that may occur in other conditions as well. Bronchoalveolar lavage specimens, when stained with oil red O, show fat droplets in 30% of the cells recovered from affected patients compared with less than 2% in patients who do not have fat embolism (91).

A mechanical theory of the pathogenesis of the syndrome proposes that bone marrow contents enter the venous system, lodge in the lungs, and may "cross" to the systemic circulation through the pulmonary capillaries or through a patent foramen ovale (90,92,93). A biochemical theory suggests that direct damage of pneumocytes by circulating free fatty acid causes the abnormalities of gas exchange (92). These two theories may not be mutually exclusive, but further studies are necessary (90). Treatment of suspected fat embolism is supportive, as with any form of adult respiratory distress syndrome. Infusion of heparin, ethanol, and low-molecular weight dextran seems to be ineffective, whereas corticosteroid therapy has been associated with ambiguous results (3,90).

Bone Marrow Emboli

Bone marrow is probably the most common tissue source of emboli. Marrow fragments sometimes lodge in the lungs after trauma to marrow-containing bones or after surgical procedures that involve bone transection or compression (thoracotomy, sternal splitting, total hip arthroplasty). Cardiac arrest during total hip arthroplasty occurs in 0.6% to 10% of patients (94). It has been suggested that a rise of intramedullary pressure caused by mechanical compression

of the femoral canal during the insertion of the stem, allows the intravasation of bone marrow, fat and debris into the venous system. The coagulation cascade is activated by the circulating bone marrow with occlusion of lung capillaries. The treatment is supportive care (3,94).

Amniotic Fluid Embolism

Amniotic fluid embolism usually occurs during or shortly after delivery. The exact incidence is unknown, but the mortality is high (80% to 90%), accounting for 10% to 20% of peripartum maternal deaths (90,95). Fifty percent of patients die within first hour of the presentation (90). The clinical presentation consists of sudden onset of dyspnea, restlessness, chills, and vomiting. Most patients are cyanotic, hypoxic, tachycardic, and hypotensive (95). Noncardiogenic pulmonary edema develops quickly, and mechanical ventilation is required. Grand mal seizures and disseminated intravascular coagulation occur in 10% to 15% of affected patients (95). All women in labor are at risk, but amniotic fluid embolism is more common in women with prolonged and tumultuous labor. Uterine stimulants have been used in 22% of cases (95). Other factors include multiparity, premature separation of membranes, increased maternal age, and large gestational size (90). In patients with suspected amniotic fluid embolism, cytologic examination of a specimen obtained from a pulmonary artery catheter in the wedge position supports the clinical diagnosis (90). The specimen reveals large numbers of fetal squames coated with neutrophils, and less frequently mucin and hair (95). The management of these patients is supportive, and most require mechanical ventilation and hemodynamic support with inotropes to treat the frequently present cardiac dysfunction (90). Corticosteroids, anticoagulants, and antibiotics have no role in the initial management (95).

Foreign Body Emboli

Various irritant agents used to "cut" heroin may enter the circulation and pulmonary arteries of narcotic addicts. Talcum powder is one of these agents; it has a marked effect on the pulmonary vessels, causing a granulomatous reaction in the lumina of small pulmonary arteries or causing an interstitial granulomatous reaction with few granulomas in the pulmonary arteries (89). These insults may be extensive enough to cause pulmonary hypertension. Perfusion lung scans and pulmonary function tests are often abnormal, and thrombi-obliterative changes are frequently seen at autopsy (3).

Air Emboli

Air can enter the pulmonary circuit after entering via the systemic veins or arteries (90). Small quantities of air are removed rapidly from blood and lungs without causing symptoms, although repeated small air injections have induced pulmonary vascular lesions and even acute noncardiogenic pulmonary edema experimentally (3,96). Rapid entry of a large bolus of air into the heart can obstruct pulmonary blood flow. Neurosurgical procedures, neck, and thorax wounds are particularly hazardous owing to the strong suction exerted during inspiration on veins in these areas. Air embolism may complicate cardiopulmonary bypass procedures and is always a possibility when intravenous catheters or needles are in place if the infusions are allowed to run out or if leaks in the tubing occur (3). Patients treated with mechanical ventilation for the adult respiratory distress syndrome (ARDS) may be at high risk of developing arterial air embolism as a form of barotrauma. In these patients, a high index of suspicion is necessary, particularly in the presence of livedo reticularis, angioedema of the face or neck, and cerebral and cardiac dysfunction (97). Venous air embolism must be treated promptly to prevent air entering into the heart. The patient must be placed immediately in the left lateral decubitus position to allow collection of air in the superiorly placed right atrium. Maintaining intravascular volume and β-adrenergic agents may be beneficial (90). If this is unsuccessful, compression in a hyperbaric chamber may be useful (3). However, prevention of air embolism is of paramount importance.

PULMONARY HYPERTENSION

Pulmonary hypertension may be defined as an increase in mean pulmonary artery pressure at rest or during exercise, as measured during catheterization (98,99). Pulmonary hypertension is present when the mean pulmonary artery pressure exceeds 25 mm Hg at rest and 30 mm Hg during exercise (98). A minor rise in pulmonary artery pressure usually causes no clinical, radiographic, or electrocardiographic changes (100).

Pulmonary hypertension could result from either increased pulmonary vascular resistance or increased pulmonary blood flow alone; however, even a large increase in pulmonary blood flow seldom leads to more than a mild elevation of the pressure as long as there are no pathologic vascular changes. Because of the elasticity of the pulmonary vasculature, the pulmonary vessels dilate in response to a large flow, causing the resistance to fall. The other factor explaining the low resistance of the pulmonary vessels is the capacity for recruitment of additional vessels (101). If flow increases, additional vessels open (usually in the upper lobes), decreasing pulmonary vascular resistance. Generally, pulmonary hypertension derives from either an increased resistance in the precapillary vessels or impedance to the pulmonary venous inflow. The resistance in the pulmonary arteries and arterioles may increase because of either functional changes (e.g., hypoxic vasoconstriction), organic

changes (e.g., thromboemboli) or destruction of the alveolar wall (e.g., emphysema).

Pathologic Characteristics

Pulmonary vessels undergo various pathologic changes in pulmonary hypertension; these changes depend on the cause of the hypertension and partially on the duration of exposure to high pressure (102). Both elastic and muscular pulmonary arteries are affected (103). In the elastic arteries, the muscular tunica media hypertrophies and the intimal connective tissue thickens. Medial hypertrophy may be followed by a form of mucoid degeneration, which, in conjunction with atrophy of the medial elastic tissue, may lead to aneurysmal dilation or even rupture. These conditions have been described in patent ductus arteriosus, mitral stenosis, and chronic pulmonary hypertension developing after corrective surgery for relief of tetralogy of Fallot (103). In addition to the medial changes, marked intimal atheromas usually develop, particularly at bifurcations. The atheroma may promote local thrombus formation, from which distal embolism may develop. Focal media aplasia is an additional feature resulting either from organization of mural thrombi or from healing of mural necrosis secondary to hypertensive pulmonary polyarteritis (103).

Although morphologic characteristics of the vessels may vary depending on the cause of hypertension, some changes develop regardless of the cause. These changes are most striking in arterioles and in arteries less than 500 μm in diameter. In the arterioles, changes consist of muscular thickening and intimal proliferation. Whereas arterioles normally have no tunica media, in mild to moderate pulmonary hypertension a distinct muscular tunica media develops, constituting up to 25% of the external diameter of the vessel and separated by internal and external elastic laminae. Later, intimal proliferation occurs, which is initially cellular but subsequently becomes fibrous. Finally, elastic tissue may develop and intimal proliferation may completely block the lumen. The tunica intima of the pulmonary trunk and the large elastic vessels become atherosclerotic, and muscular hyperplasia may thicken the tunica media (99,104).

Pathogenesis

The underlying process of pulmonary hypertension varies, and multiple factors are often responsible. The rise in pulmonary arterial pressure may be owing to vasoconstriction and thus should be reversible. In other cases, obstruction of the pulmonary vascular tree is largely or totally organic and thus irreversible (99). In Table 11.10, the causes of pulmonary hypertension are divided into three general groups, each with somewhat different clinical, physiologic, and radiologic characteristics: precapillary hypertension, postcapillary hypertension, and combined precapillary and postcapillary hypertension, a group in which the significant

TABLE 11.10. CLASSIFICATION OF PULMONARY HYPERTENSION

Precapillary pulmonary hypertension
  Primary vascular disease
    Increased flow (large left-to-right shunts)
    Decreased flow (tetralogy of Fallot)
    Primary pulmonary hypertension
    Connective tissue disease: scleroderma
    Pulmonary thromboembolic disease
      Thrombotic
      Metastatic neoplastic
      Parasitic
      Trophoblastic
      Foreign bodies; fat embolism; talc granulomatosis
      Sickle cell disease; myeloproliferative disorder
    Pulmonary arteritides
  Primary pleuropulmonary disease
    Emphysema
    Diffuse interstitial or air-space disease of the lungs
      Granulomatous
      Fibrotic
      Fibrotic
      Neoplastic: metastatic, bronchioalveolar
    Miscellaneous: alveolar microlithiasis, idiopathic hemosiderosis,
      Alveolar proteinosis, mucoviscidosis, bronchiectasis
      Preresection changes
      Postresection changes
    Pleural disease (fibrothorax)
    Chest deformity
      Thoracoplasty
      Kyphoscoliosis
    Alveolar hypoventilation
      Neuromuscular
      Obesity
      Idiopathic
      Chronic upper-airway obstruction in children
    High-altitude pulmonary hypertension
Postcapillary pulmonary hypertension
  Cardiac
    Left ventricular failure
    Mitral valvular disease
    Myxoma (or thrombus) of the left atrium
    Cor triatriatum
  Pulmonary venous
    Congenital stenosis of the origin of the pulmonary veins
    Mediastinal granulomas and neoplasms
    Idiopathic veno-occlusive disease
    Anomalous pulmonary venous return
Combined precapillary and postcapillary hypertension

Source: Modi, Parè JAP. Pulmonary hypertension and edema. In Fraser RG, Parè JAP, eds. *Diagnosis of disease of the chest*, 2nd ed. Philadelphia: Saunders, 1978:1201.

physiologic disturbance arises from vessels on both sides of the capillary bed. The capillaries may be involved to some extent in each case and may play a major role in the increase in vascular resistance. In emphysema or idiopathic pulmonary fibrosis, pressure rises as a result of obstruction of the capillary bed. In postcapillary venous hypertension, how-ever, edema surrounding the capillaries may become organized, thus limiting elasticity of the capillary bed.

Precapillary Pulmonary Hypertension

Increased Flow

Disorders classified in this group include congenital heart defects with left-to-right shunt such as atrial septal defect, ventricular septal defect, patent ductus arteriosus, aortopulmonary window, and partial anomalous pulmonary venous return. A substantial increase in pulmonary artery flow may be undetected for an extended period before increased resistance results in pulmonary artery hypertension. The heightened peripheral resistance is believed to result from an increase in vasomotor tone, with subsequent development of morphologic changes of increased flow and pulmonary hypertension. The major chest radiographic sign is enlarged pulmonary arteries throughout the lungs; the corresponding hemodynamic change is increased flow, and the main and hilar pulmonary arteries usually are distended. Normally invisible vascular markings in the peripheral 2 cm of the lungs may be seen. Fluoroscopic observation of greater pulsation amplitude of the enlarged pulmonary arteries (which usually is greatest in atrial septal defect and least in patent ductus arteriosus) and distention of individual cardiac chambers suggests the diagnosis of left-to-right shunt. The cardiac murmur may be distinctive, and specific signs may strongly suggest a particular anomaly, but accurate assessment often requires cardiac catheterization, with or without angiocardiography (104).

Primary Pulmonary Hypertension

Primary pulmonary hypertension is a disease or group of diseases clinically characterized by a mean pulmonary artery pressure greater than 25 mm Hg at rest and 30 mm Hg during exercise, with a normal pulmonary artery wedge pressure and absence of secondary causes (98,101). Three factors contribute to narrow the lumen of pulmonary artery and increase the pressure and the vascular resistance: vasoconstriction, vascular wall remodeling (medial hypertrophy) and thrombosis *in situ*. The pathogenesis of primary pulmonary hypertension is unknown, but the initial insult in a predisposed individual is probably at the pulmonary endothelium by shear forces, viruses, drugs, hypoxia, or autoimmune disorders (101). Damage to the endothelium probably alters the balance between vasoconstrictive mediators such as thromboxane and endothelin-1 and vasodilators such as nitric oxide and prostacyclin, the end result being vasoconstriction (98,101,105). Vasoconstriction may not be the primary event, but it is an important component in the pathophysiology of primary pulmonary hypertension (98).

Most of the structural changes are confined to the small pulmonary arterial branches and result in a progressive increase in pulmonary vascular resistance and thus pulmonary hypertension. Pharmacologic and pathologic evidence supports the view that functional and reversible vasoconstriction occurs in the early stages of primary pulmonary hypertension, with the development of irreversible vascular damage as the disease progresses.

Primary Thromboses

Thromboses are occasionally generated in the pulmonary arterial circulation itself. Decreased flow and increased blood viscosity typical of polycythemia and other myeloproliferative disorders probably contribute to their development (106). Pulmonary vascular changes caused by increased vasomotor tone, inflammation of the vessel wall, and sickling owing to hemoglobin SC and hemoglobin SS disease also are contributing factors (107). Pulmonary vasoconstriction owing to low PaO_2 and pH renders the lung vessels particularly susceptible to the increased viscosity caused by sickling, and various nonthrombotic emboli may occlude the vessels of the lungs and lead to pulmonary hypertension (Table 11.10).

Pulmonary Arteritides

Pulmonary arterial hypertension occurs in 6% to 60% of patients with scleroderma secondary to severe interstitial fibrosis (108). In a subgroup of patients with limited scleroderma, isolated pulmonary hypertension occurs independent of the degree of fibrosis (108). Occasionally, rheumatoid arthritis, systemic lupus erythematosus, and mixed connective tissue disease cause pulmonary hypertension. Pulmonary artery involvement in Takayasu's arteritis results in an uncommon and often unrecognized form of moderate pulmonary hypertension (109). Compression of the main pulmonary artery or its branches, sometimes as a result of an acquired mediastinal disorder, causes diffuse pulmonary oligemia of "central" origin (99). For example, a mediastinal mass exerting pressure on a pulmonary artery may compromise pulmonary artery flow. Dissecting aneurysms of the pulmonary artery or of the aorta, primary chondrosarcoma of the sternum, and fibrosing mediastinitis may have the same effect (99).

Primary Pleuropulmonary Disease

Numerous primary diseases of the lungs, pleura, chest wall, and respiratory control center may increase pulmonary arterial pressure and yet have no significant effect on pulmonary venous pressure (Table 11.10). Pulmonary artery pressures seldom reach the levels attained in cases of primary vascular disease. The hypertension may in fact be transient, reflecting pulmonary infection and associated hypoxia.

Hypoxemia, with or without respiratory acidosis, may be the most important cause of pulmonary artery hypertension in this group of conditions. Ventilation-perfusion inequality or generalized alveolar hypoventilation may be the source of reduced oxygen saturation. When arterial oxygen saturation is increased through treatment of pulmonary infections or the administration of oxygen, the pulmonary artery pressure usually falls significantly. Other contributory factors include hypervolemia and polycythemia, especially in cases of pulmonary emphysema and chronic bronchitis (110).

Pulmonary capillary destruction also may be associated with increased pulmonary artery pressure. The most common entities in this form of precapillary pulmonary hypertension include emphysema and chronic bronchitis and diffuse interstitial or air space disease of the lungs (102). Severe degrees of kyphoscoliosis or thoracoplasty may lead to pulmonary artery hypertension and cor pulmonale caused by a poorly ventilated but relatively well-perfused lung. Finally, there is a group of hypoventilation syndromes usually associated with sleep-disordered breathing that may be associated with severe arterial hypoxemia and hypercapnia. Patients with these disorders may present clinically in right-sided heart failure (111,112).

Pulmonary hypertension has been described in humans and animals living at high altitude and is known as chronic mountain sickness or Monge's disease (113). Affected individuals have a moderate degree of pulmonary hypertension (114). The symptoms and signs are similar to those of other causes of pulmonary hypertension caused by alveolar hypoventilation, although secondary polycythemia is more constant. Pulmonary hypertension is present as well in patients who develop high-attitude pulmonary edema. In those subjects prone to develop pulmonary edema, overactivation of sympathetic nerve activity has been described when the subjects are exposed to hypoxia (115).

Postcapillary Hypertension

There are two major forms of postcapillary hypertension: cardiac and pulmonary venous (Table 11.10). The most common causes of cardiac-induced postcapillary hypertension are failure of the left ventricle, mitral valve disease, myxoma (or thrombus) of the left atrium, and, rarely, cor triatriatum. The pulmonary venous causes of postcapillary hypertension include congenital stenosis at the origin of the pulmonary veins, mediastinal granulomas and neoplasms, idiopathic venoocclusive disease, and anomalous pulmonary venous return (116,117). Any condition that raises pulmonary venous pressure above a critical level can result in postcapillary hypertension. Mitral stenosis is the chief cause of this disorder (118).

Symptoms related to postcapillary hypertension usually are distinguished from those of precapillary origin. In left ventricular failure, perhaps the most common cause of pulmonary venous hypertension, symptoms and signs predominantly arise from acute or subacute pulmonary edema. Postcapillary hypertension causes orthopnea, dyspnea, and occasionally paroxysmal nocturnal dyspnea, reflecting interstitial and air space edema. In mitral stenosis, the pink frothy expectoration characteristic of acute cardiogenic pulmonary edema may be accompanied by bright red blood from hemorrhaging varicosities of the bronchial veins. Pulmonary vascular pressure remains steady until the mitral valve orifice shrinks to less than half its normal size (119). The symptoms and signs of pulmonary edema, the characteristic long opening snap of the first heart sound and the soft, low-pitched, rumbling diastolic murmur permit differentiation between this form of hypertension and primary pulmonary hypertension (120).

Pulmonary venous hypertension may occur from blockage of the left atrium by a myxoma or a thrombus. Episodes of pulmonary edema or syncope that can be relieved by a change in position are frequent. Left atrial myxomas may be the source of systemic embolization or may be associated with fever, weight loss, increased sedimentation rate, anemia, or elevated γ-globulin levels.

Diagnosis of Pulmonary Hypertension

Clinical Manifestations

Chronic, progressive pulmonary hypertension is generally characterized clinically by increasing exertional dyspnea, precordial discomfort, attacks of syncope, anginal pain, hoarseness, and occasional hemoptysis. Chest radiographs and electrocardiograms demonstrate enlargement of the right ventricle and subsequent evidence of right-sided heart failure.

Primary pulmonary hypertension is characterized by a slow, insidious onset of vague symptoms (101). On average the diagnosis is delayed for almost 2 years, and frequently patients have been misdiagnosed as having hyperventilation and depression (101). Primary pulmonary hypertension is rare and can occur at any age, although it is more common in the third and fourth decades. The female to male ratio is 1.7:1, and familial disease represents 6% of all cases. The disease may have a genetic basis, with dominant features and incomplete penetrance. Two recent studies identified an important locus in chromosome 2, region q 31–q 32 (121,122). The most common symptom is dyspnea, present in 60% of patients on initial presentation (98,101). Angina, probably as a result of underperfusion of the right ventricle or stretching of the large pulmonary arteries, is present in 47% of patients (101). Syncope is an early symptom in 8% of patients. Other symptoms include cough, hemoptysis, hoarseness resulting from compression of the recurrent la-

ryngeal nerve by the pulmonary vessels, and Raynaud's phenomenon in 10% of patients (98,101). Physical findings are similar in all patients with pulmonary hypertension. A loud second heart sound and right-sided fourth heart sounds are common (98). Other common signs are right ventricular heave, palpable systolic impulse of the pulmonary artery, pulmonary ejection murmur, and pulmonary tricuspid regurgitation murmur (101). Signs of right ventricular failure such as distended jugular veins, enlarged and pulsatile liver, ascites, and peripheral edema may be present (101). Cyanosis is present, owing to low cardiac output and right-to-left shunting across a patent foramen ovale. Clubbing does not occur in primary pulmonary hypertension (101).

Chest radiographic findings often include significant enlargement of the main and hilar pulmonary arteries, pruning of the peripheral arteries, and variable expansion of the right ventricle and atrium (98). Chest radiograph is normal in 6% of affected patients (101). Pleural effusions do not occur with right-sided heart failure alone (123).

In pulmonary veno-occlusive disease, a form of postcapillary hypertension, the signs and symptoms are similar (117). This form of primary pulmonary hypertension carries a poor prognosis (101). Radiographically, the main pulmonary artery and primary pulmonary branches are prominent, and there is evidence of increased bronchovascular markings and Kerley B lines (101). This contrasts with the radiolucent peripheral lung fields seen in classic pulmonary hypertension. In addition, there is no radiographic evidence of increased regional blood flow to the upper zones of the lungs such as that observed in pulmonary hypertension resulting from left atrial hypertension (e.g., mitral stenosis) (103). Electrocardiographic findings in both forms are right axis deviation with right ventricular hypertrophy and strain.

The physician must be aware of secondary forms of pulmonary hypertension, because mitral valve disease or other treatable lesions may be present (120). Patients with rheumatic mitral stenosis may present with severe pulmonary hypertension; subtle findings may indicate the presence of mitral valve obstruction. The symptoms, which suggest decreased cardiac output rather than mitral stenosis, reflect elevated pulmonary capillary pressure: severe exertional dyspnea, orthopnea, exertional cough, acute paroxysmal pulmonary edema, and hemoptysis. The murmur may not be evident at auscultation owing to low cardiac output and the rotation of the heart caused by right ventricular hypertrophy. The chest radiograph may show only a prominent main pulmonary artery and right-sided enlargement, with little evidence of left atrial enlargement. Cardiac catheterization may reveal only increased pulmonary artery pressure, low cardiac output, and limited increase in pulmonary artery wedge pressure, which on rare occasions may be within normal limits.

Radiographic studies, including fluoroscopy, may help detect underlying lesions. Even minor enlargement of the left atrium may suggest mitral stenosis; Kerley B lines, if present, are helpful, and the mitral valve area should be assessed for calcification, which if present generally confirms the presence of mitral valve disease until proved to result from other causes. P waves compatible with left atrial enlargement are an electrocardiographic abnormality suggestive of mitral valve disease. Echocardiography has largely replaced catheterization of the left side of the heart as a final study for detecting mitral stenosis.

Differential Diagnosis

Frequently, severe pulmonary hypertension secondary to increased vascular resistance is the obvious diagnosis. However, the specific cause may be difficult to define clinically. Symptoms developing after pregnancy, deep venous thrombosis, or a surgical operation likely represent thromboembolic obstructive hypertension. In patients with cirrhosis and portal hypertension significant pulmonary hypertension (porto-pulmonary hypertension) may be present in a small group of patients (124,125). Systemic lupus erythematosus, scleroderma, and schistosomiasis should be considered, and appropriate laboratory tests should be performed (126).

Excluding diseases of the pulmonary parenchyma requires careful assessment of the clinical picture and radiographic findings. Pulmonary function tests, particularly in the case of obstructive airways disease, may be helpful. High-resolution computed tomography may be useful in the group of patients with chronic interstitial lung disease and normal chest radiograph (127). A rise in pulmonary artery pressure, like that seen in patients with primary pulmonary hypertension, is rare in pulmonary parenchymal disease. Even moderate elevation in pulmonary artery pressure appears late in the course of the disease, well after the clinical picture has suggested primary pulmonary parenchymal disease. Primary pulmonary hypertension provides no clinical leads to diagnosis, and most laboratory tests are negative (98).

Hemodynamic Studies in Patients with Pulmonary Hypertension

Right and left cardiac catheterization are necessary to diagnose cardiac causes of pulmonary hypertension and, in the absence of secondary causes, make the diagnosis of primary pulmonary hypertension. Right heart catheterization is useful as well to determine the degree of pulmonary hypertension and prognosis and the response to vasodilators (98,128).

Patients with primary pulmonary hypertension and a high mean pulmonary arterial pressure and right atrial pressure and a low cardiac index (<2 L/min/m^2) have a very poor prognosis with a short survival (98,128).

Treatment of Pulmonary Hypertension

Primary pulmonary hypertension is progressive and often fatal (129). During the last decade, significant improvements have been made in the treatment of affected patients. The mainstay of treatment consists of supplemental oxygen, anticoagulation, and vasodilators (calcium channel blockers and epoprostenol). Supplemental oxygen must be given to patients who are hypoxemic at rest or during exercise. The arterial oxygen saturation needs to be maintained above 90% to attenuate hypoxic pulmonary vasoconstriction. Chronic warfarin therapy has been shown to improve survival in patients with primary pulmonary hypertension (98). The prothrombin time must be monitored to maintain the INR between 2 and 3.

Vasodilators have been advocated as a treatment of primary pulmonary hypertension for decades; several of them have been tested, with mixed results (101). The basis for vasodilator therapy in pulmonary hypertension is the assumption that reversible pulmonary vasoconstriction is present. The goal with vasodilator therapy is to reduce mean pulmonary artery pressure and pulmonary vascular resistance by at least 20%, with a concomitant rise in cardiac output, while not inducing systemic hypotension (98,101,129). Unfortunately, only 26% of patients have a therapeutic response to oral vasodilators (129). Calcium channel blockers are the oral vasodilators most frequently used, and nifedipine and diltiazem are preferred because they have fewer negative inotropic actions (101,129). Titration of nifedipine or diltiazem is done with hourly doses under close hemodynamic monitoring (pulmonary arterial catheter) until maximal effects or adverse effects are present. Patients who respond to calcium channel blocker therapy have a 5-year survival rate of 94% compared with 55% for nonresponders (129). The average daily dose of sustained-release nifedipine is 120 to 240 mg/day; diltiazem in doses up to 900 mg/day is an alternative in tachycardiac patients. Intravenous prostacyclin (epoprostenol), initially used as a screening agent for vasoreactivity, has been used in a continuous infusion with significant benefits in patients who failed to respond to calcium channel blockers(130–132). Long-term therapy with epoprostenol improves survival, functional class, and duration of exercise (130–132). Epoprostenol reduces pulmonary vascular resistance and pressures and increases the cardiac output (130,132). Patients receiving continuous prostacyclin need close monitoring, because tachyphylaxis occurs with chronic use. Other therapeutic agents used in pulmonary hypertension include digoxin and diuretics. Diuretics may be used in low doses to control hepatic congestion and leg edema.

Single or bilateral lung transplantation offers new hope for patients with primary pulmonary hypertension. Patients who need to be evaluated for transplantation include those with progressive disease despite optimal medical therapy (epoprostenol or calcium channel blockers) (133).

COR PULMONALE (PULMONARY HEART DISEASE)

The terms "cor pulmonale" and "pulmonary heart disease" refer to enlargement of the right ventricle (hypertrophy or dilation) secondary to disorders affecting lung structure or function (134). In general, the manifestations of cor pulmonale vary from initial adaptations of the right ventricle in response to the demands of increased pulmonary artery pressures to frank right ventricular failure. In cor pulmonale, the cause of the heart disease may be either intrinsic pulmonary disease (e.g., interstitial lung disease or COPD), inadequate function of the chest bellows (e.g., kyphoscoliosis), or insufficient ventilatory drive from the respiratory centers. Anatomic adaptation (dilation or hypertrophy) is confined predominantly to the right ventricle. The degree and duration of pulmonary arterial hypertension determine the relative effects of dilation or hypertrophy on right ventricular enlargement (135,136).

Incidence

Cor pulmonale is common, being closely associated with chronic bronchitis and emphysema, which are major causes of disability and death (135). In the United States, approximately 86,000 persons die of chronic bronchitis and emphysema each year (137). However, the incidence of cor pulmonale is difficult to determine because of unreliable reporting. In addition, anatomic hallmarks, particularly right ventricular hypertrophy, are often overlooked at autopsy. Of patients with COPD, approximately 50% of those older than 50 years develop pulmonary hypertension (135). In these patients, when pulmonary vascular resistance is more than 550 dynes-second-cm^{-5}, survival approximates that of patients with inoperable lung cancer (135). (Chronic bronchitis and pulmonary emphysema are discussed in detail in Chapter 9, Chronic Obstructive Pulmonary Disease, Bronchiectasis, and Cystic Fibrosis.)

Symptoms and Signs

Symptoms of cor pulmonale are nonspecific, although increases in pulmonary artery pressures frequently result in increasing dyspnea and easy fatigability. As the right ventricle loses its ability to meet mechanical work demands, symptoms related to fluid retention and weight gain may emerge. On physical examination, the patient is commonly cyanotic and dyspneic, often with audible wheezing and tachypnea (135). If considerable carbon dioxide is retained, the patient may be confused, somnolent, or even comatose. Hand flapping and tremors (asterixis) similar to those observed in hepatic decompensation are common. Examination of the ocular fundi occasionally reveals papilledema, a finding that is more likely if carbon dioxide retention has produced increased cerebral blood flow and increased intracranial pres-

sure. Except in patients with overt right ventricular failure—who have cyanosis, peripheral edema, and hepatomegaly—important physical findings may be limited to the cardiovascular system. The cardiac examination is frequently obscured by hyperinflated lungs or adventitious breath sounds. There may be a prominent left parasternal or epigastric lift owing to an enlarged right ventricle. The pulmonary second sound (P_2) may be palpable. Low-frequency diastolic gallops arising from the right heart may be heard to the left of the sternum; a presystolic or right atrial gallop sound (S_4) indicates increased right ventricular filling pressures and may coincide with prominent A waves in the jugular venous pulse. A protodiastolic gallop (S_3) is evidence of right ventricular failure and is usually accompanied by other signs of right heart failure. Less frequently, a diastolic decrescendo murmur of pulmonary insufficiency indicates dilation of the pulmonary valve ring caused by excessive pulmonary artery pressure (135).

In patients with severe right ventricular failure, the functional insufficiency of the valve owing to ventricular dilation gives rise to the holosystolic murmur of tricuspid regurgitation, a murmur that may increase with inspiration. Palpable pulsations in an enlarged, tender liver and prominent V waves in the jugular venous pulse are often seen as well (135).

Electrocardiographic Abnormalities

The diagnostic value of the electrocardiogram in cor pulmonale depends on the underlying pulmonary ventilatory disorder. Electrocardiographic findings are reliable if pulmonary artery hypertension is caused by primary pulmonary vascular or interstitial disease. However, characteristic electrocardiographic patterns of right ventricular enlargement are less common when cor pulmonale complicates chronic bronchitis and emphysema, caused by pulmonary hyperinflation with rotation and displacement of the heart, expanded distances between electrodes, or intrinsic cardiac disease and cardiac enlargement. However, the presence of electrocardiographic signs of cor pulmonale and hypoxemia in patients with chronic obstructive pulmonary disease is associated with a poor prognosis (138,139).

The Chest Radiograph

In patients with pulmonary heart disease, manifestations of the underlying disease may dominate the chest radiograph. Investigators have attempted to establish criteria for the radiographic diagnosis of pulmonary hypertension in severe COPD and have concluded that the chest radiograph is accurate (98%) in identifying pulmonary hypertension, although it cannot determine the severity of pulmonary hypertension. The most convincing evidence of the disorder is the combination of a large main pulmonary artery, a large right descending pulmonary artery (greater than 16 mm)

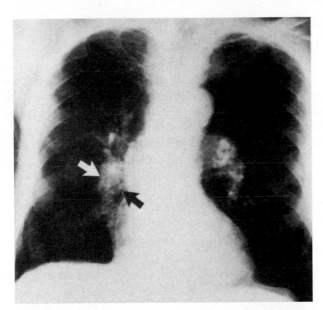

FIGURE 11.2. Enlarged right descending pulmonary artery (*arrows*) on posteroanterior chest radiograph in a patient with COPD. Note also the large left main pulmonary artery. The mean pulmonary artery pressure is 57 mm Hg (normal is 18 to 20 mm Hg). (Reproduced with permission from Matthay RA, Schwarz MI, Ellis JH Jr, et al. Pulmonary hypertension in obstructive pulmonary disease: determination by chest radiography. *Invest Radiol* 1981; 16:95–100.)

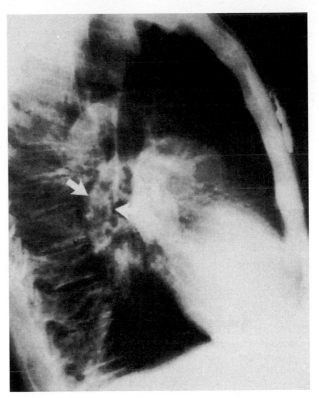

FIGURE 11.3. Enlarged left descending pulmonary artery (*arrows*) on left lateral chest radiograph in a patient with COPD and pulmonary artery hypertension. (Reproduced with permission from Matthay RA, Schwarz MI, Ellis JH Jr, et al. Pulmonary hypertension in chronic obstructive pulmonary disease: determination by chest radiography. *Invest Radiol* 1981;16:95–100.)

on the posteroanterior chest radiograph, and a large left descending pulmonary artery (greater than 18 mm) on the lateral chest radiograph (Figs. 11.2 and 11.3) (140,141). An additional clue is an enlarged right ventricular silhouette. Generally, cardiomegaly is more readily detected through serial chest films than a single examination. Computerized tomography and magnetic resonance imaging are accurate in the diagnosis of pulmonary hypertension. On computerized tomography the pulmonary artery cross-sectional area correlates well with mean pulmonary artery pressure (141).

Pleural effusions do not occur in the setting of cor pulmonale alone (123). The presence of pleural effusions should suggest left heart failure or a primary pleural process such as infection, malignancy, or pulmonary embolism.

Other Tests for Evaluating Patients with Cor Pulmonale

Patients with cor pulmonale have arterial hypoxemia with a resting P_{O_2} usually ranging from 40 to 60 mm Hg. In some patients the P_{O_2} falls further at night; therefore, the patient has periods of marked oxygen desaturation. The hypoxemia further aggravates the pulmonary hypertension, which then worsens the cor pulmonale. The arterial P_{CO_2} is usually in the range of 40 to 70 mm Hg. The degree of alveolar hypoventilation does not correlate well with the severity of airway obstruction. However, if the P_{CO_2} rises

at night, then the acidemia (associated with the increase in P_{CO_2}) can further potentiate the pulmonary hypertension and cor pulmonale (2).

Radionuclide ventriculography has been used to study the right and left ventricles in COPD. This method has provided reproducible values for right ventricular ejection fraction. The technique provides a noninvasive method for detection of right ventricular performance abnormalities secondary to pulmonary hypertension before they are manifested clinically in chronic bronchitis and cystic fibrosis (142). In patients with severe lung disease, the right ventricular ejection fraction is frequently reduced because of the increase of the right ventricle afterload.

Therapy for Acutely Decompensated Cor Pulmonale

The goal of therapy in cor pulmonale is to decrease the workload of the right ventricle by lowering pulmonary artery pressure. However, cor pulmonale caused by anatomic lesions such as primary pulmonary hypertension is not usually amenable to treatment. The disorders in which hypoxic pulmonary vasoconstriction is of primary importance are more responsive and include chronic bronchitis and emphysema.

Oxygen

The initial treatment for acutely decompensated cor pulmonale is supplemental oxygen therapy to restore arterial oxygen to acceptable levels (134). An endpoint of 90% arterial oxygen saturation (or an arterial P_{O_2} of 60 mm Hg that correspond to an arterial oxygen content of 18 vol%) is adequate in most settings (137). The coexistence of hypercapnia imposes constraint on administering oxygen; a practical approach consists of a cautious trial of a modestly enriched oxygen mixture (e.g., 25% to 30% oxygen), monitored by observance of the ventilation and sampling of arterial blood to detect an unacceptable rise in arterial P_{CO_2}. In the event of decreased ventilation with a rising arterial P_{CO_2}, mechanical ventilation may be necessary to improve oxygenation and avoid progressive respiratory acidosis. It should be remembered that it can take up to 30 minutes to achieve a steady-state after changing the oxygen concentration (137).

Diuretics

Oxygen is the best diuretic. As arterial P_{O_2} rises, pulmonary hypertension decreases and cardiac output rises, owing to a reduced right ventricular afterload. In some instances, diuretics are important in the management of cor pulmonale and heart failure. The lungs may share in accumulation of excess water in the body; this excess fluid may compromise pulmonary gas exchange and heighten pulmonary vascular resistance. In this setting, an initial diuresis can lower pulmonary artery pressure by decreasing total blood volume. Diuretics must be administered cautiously to avoid volume depletion and possible reduction in cardiac output (2). Another potential complication of diuretic therapy is a hypochloremic metabolic alkalosis, which can diminish the effect of the CO_2 stimulus on the respiratory centers and depress ventilatory drive. Therefore, serum electrolytes must be measured after diuretic administration or during periods of intensive salt and water retention. In some clinical circumstances, bed rest, modest salt restriction, and improved oxygenation alone may relieve significant water accumulation (2).

Digitalis

There is little proof that digitalis therapy is useful in patients with cor pulmonale. Digitalis therapy is considered appropriate only in the presence of coincident left heart failure or supraventricular arrhythmia (2,135,137). In patients with severe primary pulmonary hypertension, digoxin causes a modest increase in cardiac output (143).

Bronchodilators

Theophylline enhances biventricular performance in patients with COPD, particularly patients with cor pulmonale (137). Bronchodilators also alleviate reversible airway obstruction, and theophylline may improve diaphragmatic contractility and help prevent inspiratory muscle fatigue in acute respiratory failure in patients with COPD (144). Moreover, selective β-adrenergic bronchodilating agents, such as terbutaline, may reduce afterload on the right and left ventricles and thereby improve cardiac output. Therefore, these drugs should be given along with the theophylline preparation (145).

Antibiotics

Antibiotic therapy must be considered early in patients with acutely decompensated cor pulmonale and chronic bronchitis who have severe underlying disease or experience severe exacerbations (146). Sputum should be stained and cultured to identify the infecting organism and determine appropriate drug therapy. Therapy directed at *Moraxella catarrhalis, Haemophilus influenzae,* and *Streptococcus pneumoniae* should be considered in the previously nonhospitalized patient with purulent sputum, with or without pulmonary infiltrates, until culture results or clinical course indicate another pathogen or process (146).

Corticosteroids

Pulmonary function improves more rapidly in patients with acutely decompensated COPD if corticosteroids are given in addition to routinely used agents (147). However, it is important to avoid prolonged use of systemic corticosteroids in those patients who showed little or no clinical improvement (137).

Phlebotomy

Polycythemia impairs the vasodilatory response of the pulmonary artery in patients with severe chronic hypoxemic lung disease (110). The benefit of phlebotomy may be owing to a reduction in total blood volume, a change in viscosity, and a restoration of the normal vasodilatory response in the pulmonary arteries (110). In patients with severe erythrocytosis and stable cor pulmonale, reduction in hematocrit is accompanied by reduction in mean pulmonary artery pressure and pulmonary vascular resistance. However, in the setting of acute decompensation, the effect of phlebotomy is unknown. Accordingly, the procedure is best limited to patients with marked or refractory erythrocytosis (hematocrit greater than 65%) in whom supplemental oxygen has failed to reduce the hematocrit, or to patients in whom there is concern regarding thrombotic or central nervous system manifestations.

Long-Term Management of Cor Pulmonale

For many patients, reversing the acute precipitating factors of cor pulmonale restores satisfactory, or even normal, limits of pulmonary artery pressures and right ventricular function until additional causes of decompensation supervene or the underlying lung disease becomes more severe. However, in some patients qualitative disturbances of pulmonary vascular and myocardial function continue, although to a less marked degree. Persistent alveolar hypoxia sometimes contributes significantly to chronic elevation of pulmonary artery pressure; in these cases, continuous low-flow oxygen therapy is a useful tool. Long-term continuous administration of supplemental oxygen to carefully selected patients to relieve hypoxia can significantly decrease hematocrit and stabilize resting pulmonary artery pressure in spite of progression of airflow abnormalities and improve right ventricular performance (148,149). Such therapy has been shown to improve quality of life, reduce hospital admissions, and improve survival (149,150). Candidates for long-term oxygen therapy are patients with an arterial oxygen tension (PO_2) below 55 mm Hg or 88% arterial oxygen saturation. Patients with a PO_2 above 55 mm Hg but below 59 mm Hg or oxygen saturation below 89% in the presence of cor pulmonale, heart failure, or erythrocytosis (hematocrit above 55%) are candidates for supplemental oxygen therapy as well. The PO_2 must be re-evaluated at 1, 3, and 6 months to document the need for supplemental oxygen (137). The use of other agents to reduce the pulmonary hypertension in patients with chronic lung disease is not indicated at this time.

CONGENITAL PULMONARY VASCULAR DISORDERS AND ACQUIRED ANEURYSMS

A variety of congenital abnormalities are manifested in the pulmonary arteries and pulmonary veins (Table 11.11) (151).

Pulmonary Arteriovenous Malformations

Because arteries and veins develop from a common embryonic capillary plexus, persistent connections may develop even after birth (152). Shunts between large blood vessels and between chambers of the heart normally exist during fetal life. Trauma, chest surgery, infection, metastatic carcinomas, and hepatic cirrhosis are the chief causes of abnormal vascular shunts after birth (153). Multiple arteriovenous and other intervascular connections may also develop in the lungs as a result of chronic infection, such as bronchiectasis.

In certain pathologic disorders, a large volume of blood may be shunted from the pulmonary artery to the pulmo-

TABLE 11.11. CONGENITAL ABNORMALITIES OF THE PULMONARY ARTERIES AND PULMONARY VEINS

Pulmonary artery abnormalities
  Complete absence of the main trunk of the pulmonary artery
  Absence of one main pulmonary artery
  Hypoplasia of one or more pulmonary arteries or lobar divisions
  Postvalvular pulmonary stenosis of the pulmonary artery
  Aberrant pulmonary artery
Pulmonary vein abnormalities
  Failure of the stem of the common pulmonary vein to become incorporated into the atrium, resulting in cor triatriatum
  Failure of the pulmonary veins to join normally with the lung venous plexus or, in case of established union, subsequent atresia
  Drainage of the pulmonary veins or of a common pulmonary vein into the atrium of the heart
  Drainage of the right pulmonary vein into the superior vena cava, azygos vein, or right innominate vein
  Drainage of left pulmonary veins into a persistent left superior vena cava, coronary sinus, or anomalous pulmonary vein
  Persistent connections between the pulmonary veins and the adult portal vein (fetal vitelline-umbilical venous system, including the ductus venosus)
  Drainage of the pulmonary veins of the right lung into the inferior vena cava (scimitar syndrome)

Source: Spencer H. Congenital abnormalities of the lung, pulmonary vessels and lymphatici. In *Pathology of the lung,* 3rd ed. Oxford: Pergamon Press, 1977:71.

nary vein, resulting in considerable hypoxemia. Pulmonary arteriovenous malformation, a rare congenital lesion, is typical of true venous admixture. The shunt occurs from a pulmonary artery to a pulmonary vein. Such malformations may be single or multiple (153).

Pulmonary arteriovenous malformation may be isolated or, in 70% of cases, associated with hereditary hemorrhagic telangiectasia (HHT) (Osler-Weber-Rendu disease) (153). Approximately 15% to 35% of patients with HHT have pulmonary arteriovenous malformation.

The causes of HHT and pulmonary arteriovenous malformation are unknown. However, genetic mapping has found that HHT is linked to loci on chromosomes 3, 9, and 12. It has been suggested that changes in endoglin, a binding protein for transforming growth factor β, may result in an abnormal response of endothelial cells during vascular remodeling, resulting in formation of arteriovenous malformation (153). The exact pathogenesis of pulmonary arteriovenous malformation is unknown.

Women are more affected than men, in a ratio of 2:1; symptoms usually start between the fourth and sixth decades and are more frequent in patients with multiple lesions or when the lesion is greater than 2 cm (153). Epistaxis, dyspnea, and superficial telangiectasies are the most common findings in patients with HHT and pulmonary arteriovenous malformations. Dyspnea, platypnea, and hemoptysis are the most common symptoms in patients with pulmonary arteriovenous malformations. A bruit heard over the lung fields that increases with inspiration is present in almost half of the patients with pulmonary arteriovenous malformations. Clubbing and cyanosis are present in a third of patients (153).

Neurologic effects of pulmonary arteriovenous shunts are headaches, confusion, dizziness, seizure, syncope, paresthesia, diplopia, thick speech, and paresis, as well as cerebrovascular accidents. Such complications have been attributed to cerebral hypoxia, polycythemia, as well as to telangiectasia in the brain with or without associated cerebral thrombosis. Brain abscess owing to paradoxical emboli always needs to be considered as well (153).

The pulmonary arteriovenous malformation may be so small as to be barely discernible on chest radiograph, but a large pulmonary arteriovenous malformation can be seen on a routine posteroanterior chest radiograph. Typically, it is a lobulated or spherical opacity with smooth, discrete margins. It may be connected to the hilus by band-like linear or sinuous opacities, although the afferent and efferent vessels may not be visible. The aneurysm may involve any segment of either lung, although there appears to be a predilection for the lower and middle lobes. Fluoroscopic examination may demonstrate pulsations in the lobulated density as well as in the hilus. Ultrafast contrast enhanced chest computed tomography, three-dimensional helical computed tomography, contrast echocardiography, radionuclide perfusion lung scanning, and pulmonary angiography are important in the evaluation of patients with pulmonary arteriovenous malformations (153).

Physiologically, the presence of a true right-to-left shunt can be confirmed by the failure of the arterial P_{O_2} to rise above 500 mm Hg when a patient inhales 100% oxygen. Cardiac output is usually normal, although it may rise if

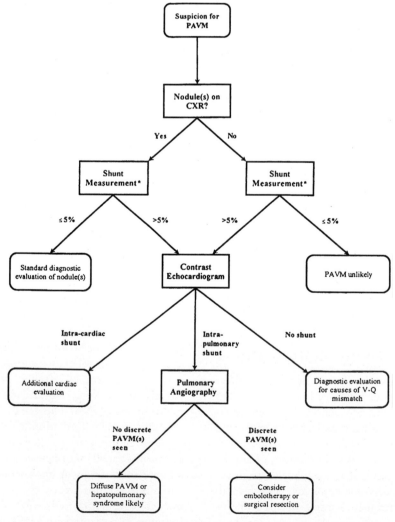

FIGURE 11.4. Algorithm for the evaluation of patients with pulmonary arteriovenous malformation. (Reproduced with permission from Gossage JR, Kanj G. Pulmonary arteriovenous malformations. *Am J Respir Crit Care Med* 1998:158:643–661.)

the oxygen tension is very low. Pulmonary hypertension is present in 1% of affected patients (153). The suggested work-up for a patient suspected to have a pulmonary arteriovenous malformation is shown in Figure 11.4.

Therapy can range from conservative management to surgical resection (153,154). Embolization of the malformation has been achieved with low morbidity and no mortality (153,154). Embolization reduces the shunting, alleviates dyspnea, and improves exercise capacity and gas exchange. Therapeutic embolization is now the modality of choice in patients with a single pulmonary arteriovenous malformation that is symptomatic, when the malformation is greater than 2 cm in diameter, in patients with multiple or bilateral malformations, or in patients who are poor surgical risk (153). It has been recommended as well to treat patients with small pulmonary arteriovenous malformations (less than 2 cm) when a feeding artery is greater than or equal to 3mm in diameter to reduce the risk of paradoxical embolization (153).

Pulmonary Artery Aneurysms

Pulmonary artery aneurysms are rare saccular dilatations of the walls of the pulmonary artery that are usually detectable on a chest radiograph (155). Risk factors for acquired aneurysms are infection (bacterial, fungal, tuberculosis, and syphilis); congenital and acquired cardiac abnormalities; abnormalities of the vessel walls, such as cystic medionecrosis and atherosclerosis; vasculitis; trauma; and other conditions, such as Hughes-Stovin syndrome, Behçet's syndrome, Takayasu arteritis, and primary pulmonary hypertension (155). The clinical presentation is nonspecific, but dyspnea, chest pain, cough, and hemoptysis may be present. Spiral computerized tomography and magnetic resonance imaging are helpful in the noninvasive diagnosis of these patients (156,157). Surgical resection of the aneurysm is the treatment of choice in most cases (155).

NEOPLASIA OF THE PULMONARY VASCULAR BED

True neoplasms of the pulmonary arteries, veins, and lymphatic vessels are rare. Sarcoma of the pulmonary arteries affect both sexes equally. The most common symptoms are dyspnea, chest pain, cough, and hemoptysis (158). On chest radiography the most common abnormalities are hilar and pulmonary artery enlargement, pulmonary nodules, enlargement of the heart shadow and decreased pulmonary vascularity. Computed tomography shows large filling defects in the pulmonary blood vessels (158). Pulmonary angiography usually shows intraluminal masses and perfusion abnormalities. Surgical resection is the treatment of choice and the survival is 31% at 1 year. Adjuvant radiation and chemotherapy may be helpful (158).

Metastatic lymphangitic carcinoma involves not only the lymphatic vessels of the lung, but also the pulmonary arteries (159,160). Lymphangitic cancer is usually a complication of adenocarcinoma; primary sites are the stomach, pancreas, breasts, prostate, ovaries, colon, and endometrium. In early reports, the most common primary tumor was carcinoma of the stomach, but now nearly 50% of metastatic lymphangitic carcinomas in North America arise from breast cancer (159). Lymphangitic carcinoma has been described as a complication of breast cancer in 24% of such patients (159).

Embolization of the tumor to the branches of the pulmonary artery with subsequent invasion of the arterial wall is regarded as the cause of lymphangitic cancer. Subsequent extension into the adjacent lymphatic vessels is followed by centripetal spread of the tumor. This theory is supported by the frequency with which tumor emboli are found in pulmonary arteries, 20 of 23 cases of one series (159). Further evidence of systemic hematogenous spread of tumor to other organs is often found in patients with lymphangitic carcinoma. The former belief that hilar lymph nodes were involved with retrograde spread of tumor has been disproved, and it is now apparent that hilar lymph nodes are free of tumor in as many as half of the patients (159).

REFERENCES

1. Gregoratos G, Karliner JS, Moser KM. Mechanisms of disease and methods of assessment. In Moser KM, ed. *Pulmonary vascular diseases.* New York: Marcel Dekker, 1979:279–339.
2. Fishman AP. Chronic cor pulmonale. *Am Rev Respir Dis* 1976; 224:775–794.
3. Moser KM. Pulmonary vascular obstruction due to embolism and thrombosis. In Moser KM, ed. *Pulmonary vascular disease.* New York: Marcel Dekker, 1979:341–386.
4. Mohr DN, Ryu JH, Litin SC, et al. Recent advances in the management of venous thromboembolism. *Mayo Clin Proc* 1988;63:281–290.
5. Raskob GE, Hull RD. Diagnosis and management of pulmonary thromboembolism. *Quart J Med* 1990;76:787–797.
6. Silverstein MD, Heit JA, Mohr DN, et al. Trends in the incidence of deep vein thrombosis and pulmonary embolism. *Arch Intern Med* 1998;158:585–593.
7. Hyers TM. Venous thromboembolism. *Am J Respir Crit Care Med* 1999;159:1–14.
8. Moser K. State of the art: venous thromboembolism. *Am Rev Respir Dis* 1990;141:235–249.
9. Wolfe WB, Sabiston DC Jr. Pulmonary embolism. *Major Probl Clin Surg* 1980;25:1–180.
10. Nordstrom M, Linbland B. Autopsy-verified venous thromboembolism within a defined urban population. The city of Malmo, Sweden. *APMIS* 1998;106:378–384.
11. Hansson PO, Welin L, Tibblin G, et al. Deep vein thrombosis and pulmonary embolism in the general population. *Arch Intern Med* 1997;157:1665–1670.
12. Kudsk KA, Fabian TC, Baum S, et al. Silent deep vein thrombosis in immobilized multiple trauma patients. *Am J Surg* 1989; 158:515–519.
13. Morpurgo M, Schmid C. The spectrum of pulmonary embolism. Clinicopathologic correlation. *Chest* 1995;107:18S–20S.

14. Wagenvoort CA. Pathology of pulmonary thromboembolism. *Chest* 1995;107:10S–17S.

15. Nachman RL, Silverstein R. Hypercoagulable states. *Ann Intern Med* 1993;119:819–827.

16. Murin S, Marelich GP, Arroliga AC, et al. Hereditary thrombophilia and venous thromboembolism. *Am J Respir Crit Care Med* 1998;158:1369–1373.

17. Ginsburg KS, Liang MH, Newcomer L, et al. Anticardiolipin antibodies and the risk for ischemic stroke and venous thrombosis. *Ann Intern Med* 1992;117:997–1002.

18. Sorensen HT, Mellemkjaer L, Steffensen FH, et al. The risk of diagnosis of cancer after primary deep venous thrombosis or pulmonary embolism. *N Engl J Med* 1998;338:1169–1173.

19. Schraufnagel DE, Tsao MS, Yao YT, et al. Factors associated with pulmonary infarction. A discriminant analysis. *Am J Clin Pathol* 1985;84:15–18.

20. Elliott CG. Pulmonary physiology during pulmonary embolism. *Chest* 1992;101:163S–171S.

21. Kakkar VV, Corrigan TP. Detection of deep venous thrombosis: survey and current status. *Prog Cardiovasc Dis* 1974;17:207–217.

22. Severinghaus JW, Swenson EW, Finley TN, et al. Unilateral hypoventilation produced in dogs by occluding one pulmonary artery. *J Appl Physiol* 1961;15:53–60.

23. Tisi GM, Wolfe WG, Fallat RJ, et al. Effects of O$_2$ on airway smooth muscle following pulmonary vascular occlusion. *J Appl Physiol* 1970;28:570–573.

24. Thomas D, Stein M, Tanabe G, et al. Mechanisms of bronchoconstriction produced by thromboemboli in dogs. *Am J Physiol* 1964;206:1207–1212.

25. Finley TN, Swenson EW, Clements JA, et al. Changes in mechanical properties, appearance and surface activity of extracts of one lung following occlusion of its pulmonary artery in the dog. *Physiologist* 1960;3:56.

26. Kasper W, Konstantinides S, Geibel A, et al. Prognostic significance of right ventricular afterload stress detected by echocardiography in patients with clinically suspected pulmonary embolism. *Heart* 1997;77:346–349.

27. Dexter L, Smith GT. Quantitative studies of pulmonary embolism. *Am J Med Sci* 1964;247:641–648.

28. Parmley LF Jr, North RL, Ott BS. Hemodynamic alterations of acute pulmonary thromboembolism. *Circ Res* 1962;11:450–465.

29. Huval WV, Mathieson MA, Stemp LJ, et al. Therapeutic benefits of 5-hydroxytryptamine inhibition following pulmonary embolism. *Ann Surg* 1983;197:3220–3225.

30. Huet Y, Brun-Buisson C, Lemaire F, et al. Cardiopulmonary effects of ketanserin infusion in human pulmonary embolism. *Am Rev Respir Dis* 1987;135:114–117.

31. Wessler S, Freeman DG, Ballon JS, et al. Experimental pulmonary embolism with serum induced thrombi. *Am J Pathol* 1961;38:89–101.

32. Fred HL, Axelrod MA, Lewis JM, et al. Rapid resolution of pulmonary thromboemboli in man. *JAMA* 1966;196:1137–1139.

33. Moser KM, Guisan M, Bartimmo EE, et al. In vivo and postmortem dissolution rates of pulmonary emboli and venous thrombi in the dog. *Circulation* 1973;48:170–178.

34. Freiman DG, Wessler S, Lertzman M. Experimental pulmonary embolism with serum-induced thrombi aged in vivo. *Am J Pathol* 1961;39:95–102.

35. Moser KM, Daily PO, Peterson K, et al. Thromboendarterectomy for chronic, major-vessel thromboembolic pulmonary hypertension. Immediate and long term results in 42 patients. *Ann Intern Med* 1987;107:560–565.

36. Rich S, Levitsky S, Brundage BH. Pulmonary hypertension from chronic pulmonary thromboembolism. *Ann Intern Med* 1988;108:425–434.

37. Fulkerson WJ, Coleman RE, Ravin CE, et al. Diagnosis of pulmonary embolism. *Arch Intern Med* 1986;146:961–967.

38. Landefeld CS, McGuire E, Cohen AM. Clinical findings associated with acute proximal deep vein thrombosis: a basis of quantifying clinical judgement. *Am J Med* 1990;88:382–388.

39. Stein PD, Terrin MC, Hales CA, et al. Clinical, laboratory, roentgenographic and electrocardiographic findings in patients with acute pulmonary embolism and preexisting cardiac or pulmonary disease. *Chest* 1991;100:598–608.

40. Hull RD, Raskob GE, Carter CJ, et al. Pulmonary embolism in outpatients with pleuritic chest pain. *Arch Intern Med* 1988;148:838–844.

41. Cobbs BW Jr, Logue RB, Dorney EG. The second heart sound in pulmonary embolism and pulmonary hypertension. *Am Heart J* 1966;71:843–844.

42. Stein PD, Goldhaber SZ, Henry JW. Alveolar-arterial oxygen gradient in the assessment of acute pulmonary embolism. *Chest* 1995;107:139–143.

43. Goldhaber SZ, Simons GR, Elliott CG, et al. Quantitative plasma D-dimer levels among patients undergoing pulmonary angiography for suspected pulmonary embolism. *JAMA* 1993;270:2819–2822.

44. Ginsberg JS, Wells PS, Kearon C, et al. Sensitivity and specificity of a rapid whole-blood assay for D-dimer in the diagnosis of pulmonary embolism. *Ann Intern Med* 1998;129:1006–1011.

45. Petruzzeli S, Palla A, Peeraccini F, et al. Routine electrocardiography in screening for pulmonary embolism. *Respiration* 1986;50:233–243.

46. Stein PD, Athanasoulis C, Greenspan RH, et al. Relation of plain chest radiographic findings to pulmonary arterial pressure and arterial blood oxygen levels in patients with acute pulmonary embolism. *Am J Cardiol* 1992;69:394–396.

47. Bynum LJ, Wilson JE III. Characteristics of pleural effusions associated with pulmonary embolism. *Arch Intern Med* 1976;136:159–162.

48. Worsley DF, Alavi A, Palevsky JH. Role of radionuclide imaging in patients with suspected pulmonary embolism. *Radiol Clin N Am* 1993;31:849–858.

49. Miniati M, Pistolesi M, Marini C, et al. Value of perfusion lung scan in the diagnosis of pulmonary embolism: Results of the prospective investigative study of acute pulmonary embolism diagnosis (PISA-PED). *Am J Respir Crit Care Med* 1996;154:1387–1391.

50. Mayo JR, Remy-Jardin M, Mueller NL, et al. Pulmonary embolism: prospective comparison of spiral CT with ventilation–perfusion scintigraphy. *Radiology* 1997;205:447–452.

51. Perrier A, Buswell L, Bounameaux H, et al. Cost-effectiveness of noninvasive diagnostic aids in suspected pulmonary embolism. *Arch Intern Med* 1997;157:2309–2316.

52. Ferretti GR, Bosson JL, Buffaz PD, et al. Acute pulmonary embolism: Role of helical CT in 164 patients with intermediate probability at ventilation-perfusion scintigraphy and normal results at Duplex US of the leg. *Radiology* 1997;205:453–458.

53. Stein PD, Hull RS, Saltzman HA, et al. Strategy for diagnosis of patients with suspected acute pulmonary embolism. *Chest* 1993;103:1553–1559.

54. Wells PS, Ginsberg JS, Anderson DR, et al. Use of a clinical model for safe management of patients with suspected pulmonary embolism. *Ann Intern Med* 1998;129:997–1005.

55. Stein PD, Coleman RE, Gottschalk A, et al. Diagnostic utility of ventilation/perfusion lung scans in acute pulmonary embolism is not diminished by preexisting cardiac or pulmonary disease. *Chest* 1991;100:604–606.

56. The PIOPED Investigators. Value of the ventilation/perfusion

scan in acute pulmonary embolism. Results of the prospective investigation of pulmonary embolism diagnosis (PIOPED). *JAMA* 1990;263:2753–2759.

57. Cronan JJ. Venous thromboembolic disease: the role of U.S. *Radiology* 1993;186:619–630.

58. Heijboer H, Buller HR, Lensing AWA, et al. A comparison of real-time compression ultrasonography with impedance plethysmography for the diagnosis of deep-vein thrombosis in symptomatic outpatients. *N Engl J Med* 1993;329:1365–1369.

59. Turkstra M, Pistolesi M, Marini C, et al. Diagnostic utility of ultrasonography of leg veins in patients suspected of having pulmonary embolism. *Ann Intern Med* 1997;126:775–780.

60. Stein PD, Athanasoulis C, Alavi A, et al. Complications and validity of pulmonary angiography in acute pulmonary embolism. *Circulation* 1992;85:462–468.

61. Quinn MF, Lundell CJ, Klotz TA, et al. Reliability of selective pulmonary arteriography in the diagnosis of pulmonary embolism. *AJR* 1987;149:469–471.

62. Lockshin MD. Venous thromboembolism during pregnancy. *N Engl J Med* 1996;335:108–114.

63. Clagett GP, Anderson FA Jr, Geerts W, et al. Prevention of venous thromboembolism. *Chest* 1998;114:531S–560S.

64. Gillies TE, Ruckley CV, Nixon SJ. Still missing the boat with fatal pulmonary embolism. *Br J Surg* 1996;83:1394–1395.

65. Bratzler DW, Raskob GE, Murray CK, et al. Underuse of venous thromboembolism prophylaxis for general surgery patients. *Arch Intern Med* 1998;158:1909–1912.

66. Weitz JI. Low-molecular-weight heparins. *N Engl J Med* 1997;337:688–698.

67. Salzman EW. Low-molecular-weight heparin and other new antithrombotic drugs (Editorial). *N Engl J Med* 1992;326:1017–1019.

68. Hyers TM, Agnelli G, Hull RD, et al. Antithrombotic therapy for venous thromboembolic disease. *Chest* 1998;114:561S–578S.

69. Raschke RA, Reilly BM, Guidry JR, et al. The weight-based heparin dosing nomogram compared with a "standard care" nomogram. A randomized controlled trial. *Ann Intern Med* 1993;119:874–881.

70. Elliott CG, Hiltunen SJ, Suchyta M, et al. Physician-guided treatment compared with a heparin protocol for deep vein thrombosis. *Arch Intern Med* 1994;154:999–1004.

71. The Columbus Investigators. Low-molecular-weight heparin in the treatment of patients with venous thromboembolism. *N Engl J Med* 1997;337:657–662.

72. Crowther MA, Ginsberg JB, Kearon C, et al. A randomized trial comparing 5 mg and 10 mg warfarin loading doses. *Arch Intern Med* 1999;159:46–48.

73. Schulman S, Granqvist S, Holmstrom M, et al. The duration of oral anticoagulant therapy after a second episode of venous thromboembolism. *N Engl J Med* 1997;336:393–398.

74. Schafer AI. Venous thrombosis as a chronic disease. (Editorial). *N Engl J Med* 1999;340:955–956.

75. Kearon C, Gent M, Hirsh J, et al. A comparison of three months of anticoagulation with extended anticoagulation for a first episode of idiopathic venous thromboembolism. *N Engl J Med* 1999;340:901–907.

76. Douketis JD, Kearon C, Bates S, et al. Risk of fatal pulmonary embolism in patients with treated venous thromboembolism. *JAMA* 1998;279:458–462.

77. Dalen JE, Alpert JS. Thrombolytic therapy for pulmonary embolism. Is it effective? Is it safe? When is it indicated? *Arch Intern Med* 1997;157:2550–2556.

78. O'Meara JJ, McNutt RA, Evans AT, et al. A decision analysis of streptokinase plus heparin as compared with heparin alone for deep vein thrombosis. *N Engl J Med* 1994;330:1864–1869.

79. Layish DT, Tapson VF. Pharmacologic hemodynamic support in massive pulmonary embolism. *Chest* 1997;111:218–224.

80. Goldhaber SZ. Integration of catheter thrombectomy into our armamentarium to treat acute pulmonary embolism. (Editorial). *Chest* 1998;114:1237–1238.

81. Becker DM, Philbrick JT, Selby JB. Inferior vena cava filters. Indications, safety, effectiveness. *Arch Intern Med* 1992;52:1985–1994.

82. Decousus H, Leizorovicz A, Parent F, et al. A clinical trial of vena caval filters in the prevention of pulmonary embolism in patients with proximal deep-vein thrombosis. *N Engl J Med* 1998;338:409–415.

83. Moser KM, Auger WR, Fedullo PF, et al. Chronic thromboembolic pulmonary hypertension: clinical picture and surgical treatment. *Eur Respir J* 1992;5:334–342.

84. Fedullo PF, Moser KM. Advances in acute pulmonary embolism and chronic pulmonary hypertension. *Adv Intern Med* 1997;42:67–104.

85. Jamieson SW. Pulmonary thromboendarterectommy. (Editorial). *Heart* 1998;79:118–120.

86. Auger WR, Fedullo PF, Moser KM, et al. Chronic major-vessel thromboembolic pulmonary artery obstruction: appearance at angiography. *Radiology* 1992;182:393–398.

87. Mansur AJ, Grinberg M, da Luz PL, et al. The complications of infective endocarditis. A reappraisal in the 1980's. *Arch Intern Med* 1992;152:2428–2432.

88. Kuhlman E, Fishman EK, Teigen C. Pulmonary septic emboli: diagnosis with CT. *Radiology* 1990;174:211–213.

89. Virmani R, Farb A, Burke AP, et al. Thromboembolic pulmonary hypertension, intravenous drug addiction, and rare forms of pulmonary embolization. In Saldana MJ (ed). *Pathology of pulmonary disease*. Philadelphia: Lippincott, 1994:225.

90. Dudney TM, Elliott CG. Pulmonary embolism from amniotic fluid, fat and air. *Prog Cardiovasc Dis* 1994;36:447–474.

91. Mimoz O, Edouard A, Beydon L, et al. Contribution of bronchoalveolar lavage to the diagnosis of posttraumatic pulmonary fat embolism. *Int Care Med* 1995;21:973–980.

92. Fabian TC. Unraveling the fat embolism syndrome (Editorial). *N Engl J Med* 1993;329:961–963.

93. Pell ACH, Hughes D, Keating J, et al. Brief report: fulminating fat embolism syndrome caused by paradoxical embolism through a patent foramen ovale. *N Engl J Med* 1993;329:926–929.

94. Pitto RP, Koessler M, Draenert K. Prophylaxis of fat and bone marrow embolism in cemented total hip arthroplasty. *Clin Orthop* 1998;355:23–34.

95. Masson RG. Amniotic fluid embolism. *Clin Chest Med* 1992;13:657–665.

96. Ohkuda K, Nakahara K, Binder A, et al. Venous air emboli in sheep: reversible increase in lung microvascular permeability. *J Appl Physiol* 1981;51:887–894.

97. Marini JJ, Culver BH. Systemic gas embolism complicating mechanical ventilation in the adult respiratory distress syndrome. *Ann Intern Med* 1989;110:699–703.

98. Rubin LJ. Primary pulmonary hypertension. *N Engl J Med* 1998;336:111–117.

99. Fraser RG, Parè JAP. Pulmonary hypertension and edema. In Fraser RG, Parè JAP, eds. *Diagnosis of diseases of the chest*, 3rd ed. Philadelphia: Saunders, 1988:

100. Sasamoto H, Hosono K, Viatayam K, et al. Electrocardiographic findings in patients with chronic cor pulmonale. *Respir Circ* 1961;9:55.

101. Olivari MT. Primary pulmonary hypertension. *Am J Med Sci* 1991;302:185–198.

102. Edwards WD. Pathology of pulmonary hypertension. *Cardiovasc Clin* 1988;18:321–359.

103. Crofton J, Douglas A. Pulmonary hypertension. In Crofton J, Douglas A. *Respiratory diseases,* 2nd ed. London: Blackwell Scientific Publications, 1975:360.

104. Foster E, Cheitlin MD. Recognition and management of adults with congenital heart disease. In Goldman L, Braunwald E, eds. *Primary cardiology,* Philadelphia: Saunders, 1998.

105. Kaneko FT, Arroliga AC, Dweik RA, et al. Biochemical reaction products of nitric oxide as quantitative markers of primary pulmonary hypertension. *Am J Respir Crit Care Med* 1998;158: 917–923.

106. Gruppo Italiano Studio Policitemia. Polycythemia vera: the natural history of 1213 patients followed for 20 years. *Ann Intern Med* 1995;123:656–664.

107. Sutton LL, Castro O, Cross DJ, et al. Pulmonary hypertension in sickle cell disease. *Am J Cardiol* 1994;74:626–628.

108. Minai OA, Dweik RA, Arroliga AC. Manifestations of scleroderma pulmonary disease. *Clin Chest Med* 1998;19:713–731.

109. Sullivan EJ, Hoffman GS. Pulmonary vasculitis. *Clin Chest Med* 1998;19:759–776.

110. Defouilloy C, Teiger E, Sediame S, et al. Polycythemia impairs vasodilator response to acetylcholine in patients with chronic hypoxemic lung disease. *Am J Respir Crit Care Med* 1998;157: 1452–1460.

111. Laks L, Lehrhaft B, Grunstein RR, et al. Pulmonary hypertension in obstructive sleep apnea. *Eur Respir J* 1995;8:537–541.

112. Laks L, Lehrhaft B, Grunstein RR, et al. Pulmonary artery pressure response to hypoxia in sleep apnea. *Am J Respir Crit Care Med* 1997;155:193–198.

113. Saldana MJ, Arias-Stella J. Pulmonary hypertension and pathology at high altitudes. In Saldana MJ, ed. *Pathology of pulmonary disease.* Philadelphia: Lippincott, 1994:247.

114. Naeije R. Pulmonary circulation at high altitudes. *Respiration* 1997;64:429–439.

115. Duplain H, Vollenweider L, Delabays A, et al. Augmented sympathetic activation during short-term hypoxia and high altitude exposure in subjects susceptible to high-altitude pulmonary edema. *Circulation* 1999;99:1713–1718.

116. Burke AP, Virmani R, Far B. Primary pulmonary hypertension and veno-occlusive disease. In Saldana MJ, ed. *Pathology of pulmonary disease.* Philadelphia: Lippincott, 1994:235.

117. Wagenvoort CA, Wagenvoort N, Takahashi T. Pulmonary veno-occlusive disease: involvement of pulmonary arteries and review of the literature. *Hum Pathol* 1985;16:1033–1041.

118. Farb A, Burke AP, Virmani R. Pulmonary hypertension caused by chronic left heart failure, obstruction of pulmonary venous return and parenchymal lung disease. In Saldana MJ, ed. *Pathology of pulmonary disease.* Philadelphia: Lippincott, 1994:203.

119. Gorlin R, Gorlin SG. Hydraulic formula for circulation of the area of the stenotic mitral valve, other cardiac valves, and central circulatory shunts. *Am Heart J* 1951;41:1–29.

120. Carabello BA. Recognition and management of patients with valvular heart disease. In Goldman L, Braunwald E, eds. *Primary cardiology.* Philadelphia: Saunders, 1998.

121. Nichols WC, Koller DL, Slovis B, et al. Localization of the gene for familial primary pulmonary hypertension to chromosome 2 q 31. *Nat Genet* 1997;15:277–280.

122. Morse JH, Jones AC, Barst RJ, et al. Mapping of familial primary pulmonary hypertension locus (PPH) to chromosone 2 q 31–32. *Circulation* 1997;95:2603–2606.

123. Wiener-Kronish JP, Goldstein R, Matthay RA, et al. Lack of association of pleural effusion with chronic pulmonary arterial and right atrial hypertension. *Chest* 1987;92:967–970.

124. Herve P, Lebrec D, Brenot F, et al. Pulmonary vascular disorders in portal hypertension. *Eur Respir J* 1998;11:1153–1166.

125. Kuo PC, Plotkin JS, Johnson LB, et al. Distinctive clinical features of portopulmonary hypertension. *Chest* 1997;112: 980–986.

126. Barbosa MM, Lamounier JA, Oliveira EC, et al. Pulmonary hypertension in schistosomiasis mansonii. *Tran R Soc Trop Med Hyg* 1996;90:663–665.

127. Mueller NL, Ostrow DN. High-resolution computed tomography of chronic interstitial lung disease. *Clin Chest Med* 1991; 12:97–114.

128. D'Alonzo GE, Barst RJ, Ayres SM, et al. Survival in patients with primary pulmonary hypertension. Results from a national prospective registry. *Ann Intern Med* 1991;115:343–349.

129. Rich S, Kaufmann E, Levy PS. The effect of high dose of calcium-channel blockers on survival in primary pulmonary hypertension. *N Engl J Med* 1992;327:76–81.

130. Barst RJ, Rubin LJ, Long WA, et al. A comparison of continuous intravenous epoprostenol (prostacyclin) with conventional therapy for primary pulmonary hypertension. *N Engl J Med* 1996;334:296–301.

131. Shapiro SM, Oudiz RJ, Caot, et al. Primary pulmonary hypertension: improved long-term effects and survival with continuous intravenous epoprostenol infusion. *J Am Coll Cardiol* 1997; 30:343–349.

132. McLaughlin VV, Genthner DE, Parella MM, et al. Reduction in pulmonary vascular resistance with long-term epoprostenol (prostacyclin) therapy in primary pulmonary hypertension. *N Engl J Med* 1998;338:273–277.

133. Maurer JR, Frost AE, Glanville AR, et al. International guidelines for the selection of lung transplant candidates. *Am J Respir Crit Care Med* 1998;158:335–339.

134. Wiedemann HP, Matthay RA. Cor pulmonale in chronic obstructive pulmonary disease: circulatory pathophysiology and new concepts of therapy. *Curr Pulmonol* 1987;8:127–162.

135. Salvaterra CG, Rubin LJ. Investigation and management of pulmonary hypertension in chronic obstructive pulmonary disease. *Am Rev Respir Dis* 1993;148:1414–1417.

136. Matthay RA, Arroliga AC, Wiedemann HP, et al. Right ventricular function at rest and during exercise in chronic obstructive pulmonary disease. *Chest* 1992;101:255S–262S.

137. Celli BR, Snider GL, Heffner J, et al. Standards for the diagnosis and care of patients with chronic destructive pulmonary disease. *Am J Respir Crit Care Med* 1995;152:S77–S120.

138. Behar JV, Howe CM, Wagner NB, et al. Performance of new criteria for right ventricular hypertrophy and myocardial infarction in patients with pulmonary hypertension due to cor pulmonale and mitral stenosis. *J Electrocardiol* 1991;24:231–237.

139. Incalzi RA, Fuso L, De Rosa M, et al. Electrocardiographic signs of chronic cor pulmonale. A negative prognostic finding in chronic obstructive pulmonary disease. *Circulation* 1999;99: 1600–1605.

140. Matthay RA, Schwarz MI, Ellis JH Jr, et al. Pulmonary hypertension in chronic obstructive pulmonary disease: determination by chest radiography. *Invest Radiol* 1981;16:95–100.

141. Takasugi JE, Godwin JD. Radiology of chronic obstructive pulmonary disease. *Radiol Clin NA* 1998;36:29–55.

142. Vizza CD, Lynch JP, Ochoa LL, et al. Right and left ventricular dysfunction in patients with severe pulmonary disease. *Chest* 1998;113:576–583.

143. Rich S, Seidlitz M, Dodin E, et al. The short-term effects of digoxin in patients with right ventricular dysfunction from pulmonary hypertension. *Chest* 1998;114:787–792.

144. Aubier M, Detroyer A, Sampson M, et al. Aminophylline improves diaphragmatic contractility. *N Engl J Med* 1981;305: 249–252.

145. Thomas P, Pugsley JA, Stewart JH. Theophylline and salbutamol improve pulmonary function in patients with irreversible chronic obstructive pulmonary disease. *Chest* 1992;101:160–165.

146. Murphy TF, Sethi S. Bacterial infections in chronic obstructive pulmonary disease. *Am Rev Respir Dis* 1992;146:1067–1083.

147. Albert RK, Martin TR, Lewis SW. Controlled clinical trial of methyl-prednisolone in patients with chronic bronchitis and acute respiratory insufficiency. *Ann Intern Med* 1980;92:753–758.

148. Zielinski J, Tobrasz M, Hawrylkiewicz I, et al. Effects of lonterm oxygen therapy on pulmonary hemodynamics in COPD patients. A 6-year prospective study. *Chest* 1998;113:65–70.

149. Nocturnal Oxygen Therapy Trial Group. Continuous or nocturnal oxygen therapy in hypoxemic chronic obstructive lung disease. *Ann Intern Med* 1980;93:391.

150. The Medical Research Council Working Party. Long-term domiciliary oxygen therapy in chronic hypoxic cor pulmonale complicating chronic bronchitis and emphysema. *Lancet* 1981;1:682–686.

151. Spencer H. *Pathology of the lung,* 3rd ed. Philadelphia: Saunders, 1978:71.

152. Perloff JK. *The clinical recognition of congenital heart disease,* 2nd ed. Philadelphia: Saunders, 1987.

153. Gossage JR, Kanj G. Pulmonary arteriovenous malformations. *Am J Respir Crit Care Med* 1998;158:643–661.

154. Haitgema TJ, Overtoom TThc, Westermann CJJ, et al. Embolisation of pulmonary arteriovenous malformations: results and followup in 32 patients. *Thorax* 1995;50:719–723.

155. Bartter T, Irwin RS, Nash G. Aneurysms of the pulmonary arteries. *Chest* 1988;94:1065–1075.

156. Rankin SC. Spiral CT: vascular applications. *Eur J Radiol* 1998;28:18–29.

157. Berkmen T. MR angiography of aneurysm in Behcet disease: a report of four cases. *J Comput Assist Tomogr* 1998;22:202–206.

158. Cox JE, Chiles C, Aquino SL, et al. Pulmonary artery sarcomas: a review of clinical and radiologic features. *J Comput Assist Tomogr* 1997;21:750–755.

159. Janower ML, Blennerhasset JB. Lymphangitic spread of metastatic cancer to the lungs. A radiologic-pathologic classification. *Radiology* 1971;101:267–273.

160. Filderman AE, Coppage L, Shaw C, et al. Pulmonary and pleural manifestations of extrathoracic malignancies. *Clin Chest Med* 1989;10:747–807.

12

DIFFUSE INTERSTITIAL AND ALVEOLAR INFLAMMATORY DISEASES

HERBERT Y. REYNOLDS
PAUL W. NOBLE
RICHARD A. MATTHAY

IDIOPATHIC PULMONARY FIBROSIS (CRYPTOGENIC FIBROSING ALVEOLITIS)
Clinical Presentation and Evaluation
Lung Histology and Staging Disease Activity
Immunopathogenic Concepts of IPF
Treatment and Prognosis

BRONCHIOLITIS OBLITERANS ORGANIZING PNEUMONIA

RESPIRATORY BRONCHIOLITIS

CONNECTIVE TISSUE (COLLAGEN VASCULAR) DISEASES
Systemic Lupus Erythematosus
Rheumatoid Arthritis
Progressive Systemic Sclerosis (Scleroderma)
Polymyositis-Dermatomyositis

SYSTEMIC GRANULOMATOUS VASCULITIDES
Wegener's Granulomatosis
Lymphomatoid Granulomatosis
Allergic Angiitis and Granulomatosis (Churg-Strauss Syndrome)

GOODPASTURE'S SYNDROME (ANTIGLOMERULAR BASEMENT MEMBRANE DISEASE)
Clinicopathologic Features
Chest Radiographic Findings
Pulmonary Function Abnormalities
Diagnosis and Pathologic Findings
Etiology and Pathogenesis
Therapy and Prognosis

IDIOPATHIC PULMONARY HEMOSIDEROSIS
Clinicopathologic Features

Chest Radiographic Findings
Diagnosis, Treatment, and Outcome

PULMONARY ALVEOLAR PROTEINOSIS
Clinicopathologic Features
Chest Radiographic Findings
Diagnosis
Course and Treatment

DRUG-INDUCED PULMONARY DISEASE
Cytotoxic Agents
Noncytotoxic Agents

SARCOIDOSIS
Clinical and Radiographic Presentations
Laboratory Findings in Blood and Lung
Immunologic Concepts
Disease Course and Therapy

HYPERSENSITIVITY PNEUMONITIS (EXTRINSIC ALLERGIC ALVEOLITIS)
Clinical Presentation
Laboratory and Immunologic Findings
Concepts of Immunopathogenesis
Therapy

LYMPHOID INTERSTITIAL PNEUMONITIS

EOSINOPHILIC SYNDROMES
Types of Eosinophilic Syndromes

EOSINOPHILIC GRANULOMA (LANGERHANS CELL GRANULOMATOSIS)

LYMPHANGIOLEIOMYOMATOSIS

The interstitial lung diseases are a diverse group of disorders characterized by inflammation and fibrosis involving the lung parenchyma or small airways (e.g., bronchioles). The interstitium of the lung includes the alveolar walls and lumens, pulmonary microvasculature, interstitial macrophages, fibroblasts, myofibroblasts, and extracellular matrix components such as collagen, elastin, and proteoglycans such as versican. The interstitium may extend to the terminal and respiratory bronchioles. Inflammation and fibrosis may involve both the conducting airways and the alveolar space (e.g., bronchiolitis obliterans with organizing pneumonia) or predominantly the lung parenchyma (idiopathic pulmonary fibrosis). The clinical presentation of ILDs has many common features, including similarity of patient symptoms, comparable appearance of chest radiographs, consistent derangements in pulmonary physiology, and typical histologic features (1,2). Although lung inflammation is a component of the disease, no known infectious agent is associated with the cause or onset of most of the various diseases. Exceptions include certain fungal and mycobacterial lung infections. For many of the diseases, the etiology is unknown.

The alveolar spaces, which are lined by type I epithelial cells, bring inspired air into close proximity with circulating blood contained in capillaries lined with endothelial cells, thus creating the air-exchange units of the lung (Fig. 12.1). Surrounding these units is the supporting tissue called the interstitium. This area is a potential space that can accumulate fluid and can contain such cells as fibroblasts, lymphocytes, dendritic cells, and monocytes that are undergoing maturation into macrophages; but few inflammatory cells are present in the normal interstitial space. In early phases of disease, inflammation is localized predominantly in the alveoli, and type II pneumocytes and alveolar macrophages may slough and accumulate in the air spaces (alveolitis). Other inflammatory cells, polymorphonuclear granulocytes (PMNs), and eosinophils also collect in the alveoli. In later stages of disease, interstitial abnormalities occur, of which

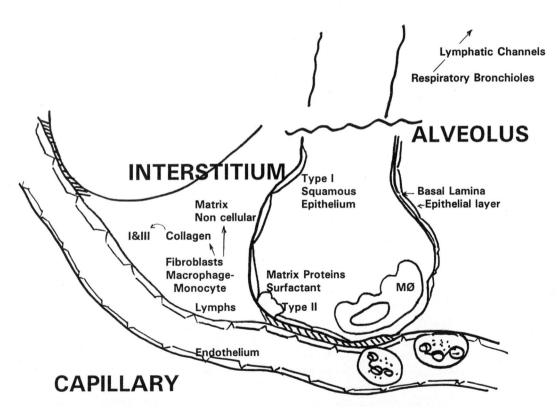

FIGURE 12.1. The diffuse interstitial lung diseases (DILDs) primarily involve the air exchange portion of the respiratory tract—the alveolar structures. Although there can be an element of bronchiolitis, this is not the site of inflammation or injury for most diseases. Bronchiolitis obliterans with organizing pneumonia is an exception. For DILD the initial process may involve the lining cells of the alveoli, after which inflammation spreads to the alveolar walls and their supporting structure, the interstitium, normally composed of fibroblasts capable of producing several forms of collagen and noncellular matrix glycoproteins and a few mononuclear cells, perhaps undergoing maturation before emerging as macrophages destined for the alveoli. Because of the proximity of the capillaries, the vascular component can be involved with inflammation as well. With chronicity the fibrotic reaction develops in which the discrete architecture of the alveolar unit becomes deranged and scarred or cytic changes result. In addition to inflammation, a granulomatous reaction may also occur concomitantly for many important diseases in the DILD group.

TABLE 12.1. MAJOR CATEGORIES OF DIFFUSE INTERSTITIAL AND ALVEOLAR INFLAMMATORY LUNG DISEASE

Lung Response	Unknown Cause	Known Cause
Interstitial inflammation and fibrosis without granuloma formation	Idiopathic pulmonary fibrosis[a]	Asbestos[b]
	Bronchiolitis obliterans pneumonia (BOOP)[a]	Fumes, gases[b]
	Collagen vascular diseases[a]	Drugs (antibiotics, chemotherapy drugs)[a]
	Pulmonary hemosiderosis[a]	Radiation
	Goodpasture's syndrome[a]	Neoplasia (lymphangitic)
	Pulmonary alveolar proteinosis[a]	Cardiac failure
	Ankylosing spondylitis	Aspiration (pneumonia)
	Lymphocytic Infiltration diseases	
	Eosinophilic lung syndromes[a]	
With granuloma also	Sarcoidosis[a]	
	Langerhans cell granulomatosis[a] (histiocytosis X or eosinophilic granuloma)	Hypersensitivity pneumonitis (organic dusts)[a]
		Beryllium[b]
		Silica[b]
	Granulomatous vasculitides[a]	Mycobacteria/fungi[c]
	• Wegener's granulomatosis	
	• Lymphomatoid granulomatosis	
	• Allergic granulomatosis of Churg-Strauss	

[a] Discussed in this chapter.
[b] Discussed in Chapter 14, Lung Neoplasms.
[c] Discussed in Chapter 16, Pulmonary Complications in the Immunosuppressed Patient.

derangement in the noncellular supporting structures, especially collagen, is most serious and causes fibrosis and distortion of lung architecture (3).

Although all the diffuse interstitial lung diseases share the common morphologic characteristic of an abnormal lung interstitium, a satisfactory classification of them has been difficult to construct. This is because approximately 150 individual diseases have a component of interstitial lung involvement, either as a primary disease or as a significant part of a multiorgan process, such as a collagen-vascular disease. This diversity precludes a tight and orderly classification. One reasonable approach broadly separates the interstitial lung diseases into two groups, those with known causes and those with unknown causes; each of these groups can be subclassified further according to the presence or absence of granuloma in interstitial or vascular areas as viewed in histologic specimens (Table 12.1) (2).

Interstitial lung diseases of known cause include several major subcategories. By far the largest group comprises occupational and environmental inhalant diseases; these include diseases owing to inhalation of inorganic dusts, organic dusts (hypersensitivity pneumonitis), gases, fumes, vapors, and aerosols (Chapter 13, Occupational and Environmental Lung Disease). Other categories include lung diseases caused by drugs, irradiation, poisons, neoplasia, and chronic cardiac failure. The number of diseases with an unknown cause is likewise very large. The major subgroups within this category are idiopathic pulmonary fibrosis (IPF) and connective tissue (collagen vascular) disorders with interstitial lung disease, including rheumatoid arthritis, systemic lupus erythematosus, progressive systemic sclerosis, polymyositis-dermatomyositis, and Sjögren's syndrome. Systemic vasculitides often have granulomas in tissue and

include a variant of polyarteritis nodosa called allergic granulomatosis, lymphomatoid granulomatosis, and hypersensitivity vasculitis (leukocytoclastic). A number of inherited disorders such as tuberous sclerosis, Hermansky-Pudlak syndrome and neurofibromatosis can have a component of interstitial lung disease. Forms of familial pulmonary fibrosis have been described, and amyloidosis can occasionally involve the lung (1,4).

Six major entities that are most frequently associated with diffuse interstitial lung disease are reviewed in this chapter: idiopathic pulmonary fibrosis, connective tissue (collagen vascular) diseases, systemic granulomatous vasculitis, sarcoidosis, hypersensitivity pneumonitis, and drug-related hypersensitivity disease, or fibrosis. In addition, bronchiolitis obliterans organizing pneumonia (BOOP), respiratory bronchiolitis, Goodpasture's syndrome, idiopathic pulmonary hemosiderosis, pulmonary alveolar proteinosis, and eosinophilic syndromes, representing diseases associated with both alveolar and interstitial abnormalities, will be discussed briefly.

IDIOPATHIC PULMONARY FIBROSIS (CRYPTOGENIC FIBROSING ALVEOLITIS)

Idiopathic pulmonary fibrosis (IPF) is an uncommon inflammatory/fibrotic interstitial lung disorder of unknown etiology. The clinical presentation is well characterized by cough, exertional breathlessness, bilateral predominantly lower zone infiltrates, and restrictive physiology with impaired diffusion. The original description of the disease is attributed to Hamman and Rich as a fulminant, fatal form of interstitial pneumonitis in which proliferating fibrotic tissue virtually occluded the peripheral airways (5). However, the typical presentation of IPF is of an insidious onset of exertional breathlessness. Clinicians have recognized a spectrum of disease, but progressive respiratory failure is typical within 3 to 5 years. Five-year mortality approaches 50%. Although the vast majority of patients succumb to respiratory failure, other causes of death include pulmonary emboli, cardiovascular disease, infections and cancer. Lung cancer complicates IPF in 10% of patients.

IPF is a syndrome of unknown etiology that is limited to the lungs. One of the most important aspects of initial evaluation is to determine if the lung disease is occurring in the context of a systemic disorder such as a connective tissue disease. Clinical features include symptoms of nonproductive cough, and breathlessness (dyspnea) increasing with exertion. Resting arterial hypoxemia is not usual except in advanced stages, but can frequently be elicited with exertion. However, 85% of patients have an elevated alveolar-arterial gradient (A-a O_2). Lung function tests reflect a pattern of restriction. In patients with a heavy smoking history, the restriction is less pronounced because of coexistent emphysema. This is usually reflected by an extremely reduced diffusing capacity. Chest radiographs are abnormal in 90% of patients with IPF. Radiographically, a pattern of alveolar filling may evolve into one of reticular (linear) or reticulonodular densities involving the peripheral (subpleural) and basilar regions of the lung producing a distinctive but nondiagnostic sequence of chest radiographs. Lung volumes are usually small. Pleural effusions and intrathoracic lymphadenopathy are not features of IPF. High-resolution thin section CT scans (HRCT) are superior to the conventional chest radiograph in evaluating IPF. Areas of ground-glass appearance, denoting inflammation and cellularity on lung histology, and of a reticular pattern correlating with fibrosis and cystic changes of traction bronchiectasis can be observed in subpleural portions of the lung. The HRCT findings can be highly distinctive for IPF, and under certain circumstances can obviate the need for lung biopsy (6). Cystic patterns 3 to 15 mm in diameter (termed honeycombing) connote irreversible fibrosis. Extensive honeycombing is associated with a poor prognosis.

Lung biopsies in IPF demonstrate varying degrees of fibrosis and inflammation within the interstitium. Recent attempts have been made to study the kinetics of the fibrosis process and to quantitate cellularity and fibrosis better in the biopsy specimen (7,8). Perhaps the most characteristic aspect of the IPF biopsy is the patchy nature of the abnormalities. Considerable distortion of lung architecture occurs, with thickening of alveolar septa and formation of cystic spaces in the parenchyma. Additional features of advanced disease include type II pneumocyte proliferation and hyperplasia, traction bronchiectasis, smooth muscle hypertrophy, and "muscularization" of pulmonary arteries. The pathologic term given to this constellation of findings is usual interstitial pnuemonitis (UIP). This is in distinction to the histological variant desquamitive interstitial pneumonitis (DIP), which is characterized by a homogenous pattern of alveolar filling with macrophages, preservation of alveolar architecture, absence of honeycombing, and ground glass opacities on HRCT. The relationship between UIP and DIP is debated. DIP appears to be more related to smoking and has a much better response to corticosteroids. The concept that DIP is an early form of UIP has been questioned. An additional histologic variant termed "nonspecific interstitial pneumonitis" (NSIP) has recently been described (9). NSIP is characterized by varying degrees of inflammation and fibrosis that appear to be temporally related. That is, the patchy nature of UIP with areas of extensive fibrosis abutting areas of inflammation is not as pronounced. Foci of bronchiolitis obliterans with organizing pneumonia denoting a tissue response to injury is observed more frequently than in UIP. There may be areas of overlap on biopsy. NSIP appears to have a more favorable response to corticosteroids than UIP. A challenge to the dogma that the early phases of UIP are characterized by inflammation that progresses to fibrosis has been issued by Katzenstein and Meyers (10). They have extolled the concept that true UIP is a fibrotic disease from the onset, rather than a consequence of persistent inflammation.

Clinical Presentation and Evaluation

At the inception of disease, the patient feels short of breath or notes a change in his or her tolerance to some prescribed or accustomed amount of exercise. A dry cough frequently occurs. Unless there are systemic symptoms or other organ involvement suggesting a generalized illness, the patient may do nothing more than try to adjust to the episodic dyspnea. The symptoms and physical signs can be very nebulous in the early phase of disease, leading to a delay in diagnosis. The most typical complaint from the patient is that they are "just getting older." Other respiratory signs, such as pleuritis, chest pain, wheezing, or hemoptysis, do not usually occur. Although sputum production is not present in many patients, about half may have mucus hypersecretion and expectoration. This occurrence has been correlated with glandular hypertrophy in the airway mucosa and accumulated mucus in the airways (11). Many patients have an occupational history that includes exposure to one or a variety of toxic inhalation products, and this may add uncertainty to the precise onset of symptoms and may suggest the contribution of several etiologic factors. A detailed work history, including each job dating back even to summer employment during school, is essential. Casual exposure to asbestos decades ago may provide a crucial link.

A surprising percentage of patients, perhaps 30%, can pinpoint their awareness of breathlessness as an aftermath of a respiratory infection that is usually described as a viral illness. Even minor upper respiratory tract infections (influenza A) cause acute small-airway changes, and these changes can take several months to clear completely, which emphasizes the widespread impact of even mild viral disease in the lungs (12). An association between IPF and serum antibodies to hepatitis C has been noted, but recently questioned (13,14). Months to several years (mean about 1 to 3 years) may elapse between the onset of dyspnea and its progression to the point of symptomatic breathlessness that is sufficient to bring the patient to the physician's attention. When dyspnea is noticeable and imposes physical limitation, other constitutional symptoms may be present, such as fatigue, poor appetite, and weight loss. Fever is infrequent. The incidence of IPF increases substantially with age. The prevalence among adults age 35 to 44 is three cases per 100,000. This increases to in excess of 175 cases per 100,000 in patients over the age of 75. Patients of all ages are affected and the disease has been described in infants (15). Factors associated with increased risk are male gender, smoking history, mining, residence in agricultural and polluted urban areas, and exposure to inhaled dusts, solvents and chemicals. Because several family clusters have been noted, it is likely that genetic factors can determine susceptibility to the disease.

Physical examination reveals crackles or rales on auscultation of chest in the majority of patients. Vivid adjectives have been used to describe these lung sounds—"Velcro," crackling or cellophane paper, or "close to the ear." Other findings may include tachypnea at rest (50% of patients), ability to speak only in phrases of a few words because of breathlessness, and finger clubbing (70%), without hypertrophic osteoarthropathy (2). Occasionally, cyanosis can be detected. In later stages, cardiac involvement is frequent, and signs pointing to pulmonary artery hypertension and right heart failure are noted in many (60% to 70%). An augmented pulmonic second heart sound, right-sided lift, and S(sub 3) gallop, in addition to peripheral signs of heart failure, signal the presence of pulmonary hypertension and cor pulmonale. Right ventricular ejection fraction by radionuclide scan is often depressed in the face of normal left ventricular performance. Except for clubbing and evidence of heart failure, physical signs are limited to the chest, and other organ systems are not prominently involved.

The chest radiograph is still important in establishing an initial diagnosis, for it usually reveals a pattern of diffuse reticular markings, prominent in the lower lung zones (Fig. 12.2). A most important consideration at this point is to retrieve any existing chest radiographs and compare them for prior changes. Again, for emphasis, it is important to investigate the patient's occupational and recreational history for evidence of a toxic environmental exposure. Not all patients with a chronic diffuse interstitial lung disease have an abnormal chest radiograph. In one series of 458 patients with biopsy-established forms of diffuse interstitial lung disease, about 10% had normal chest radiographs prior to a diagnostic lung biopsy (16). As stated, the HRCT represents a major diagnostic advance in the evaluation of ILD

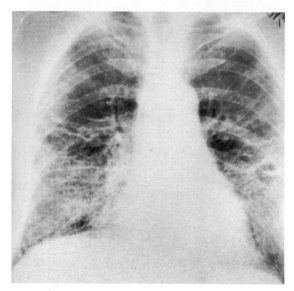

FIGURE 12.2. Idiopathic pulmonary fibrosis. Posterior-anterior (PA) chest radiograph of a 71-year-old man with end-stage pulmonary fibrosis. There are diffuse, bilateral interstitial infiltrates that form a honeycombing pattern.

and should be performed routinely. Characteristic findings, particularly in older patients can avoid a lung biopsy (Fig. 12.3). The HRCT may improve diagnostic accuracy from about one-third to about 46% for a form of diffuse interstitial lung disease when a group of pulmonary clinicians and radiologists compared both kinds of imaging studies (17).

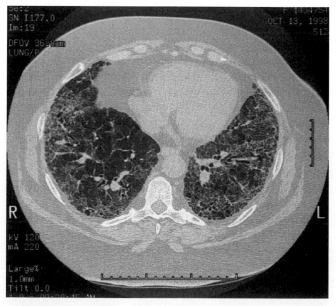

FIGURE 12.3. Idiopathic pulmonary fibrosis. High resolution chest CAT scan of a 58-year-old woman with end-stage disease. Subpleural honeycomb changes, traction bronchiectasis, and thickened interlobular septae are demonstrated.

Serologic and routine blood tests are indicated but may reveal few abnormalities of specific help. The erythrocyte sedimentation rate is elevated in most (90%), but does not exceed 100 Westergren units, circulating immune complex titers may be high, serum immunoglobulin levels are increased by 30% or so, and cryoimmunoglobulins may be found in a surprisingly high number (41%) (2,18). Serologic tests to screen for collagen-vascular diseases are necessary to exclude these diagnoses with confidence. In IPF, however, serum rheumatoid factor, lupus erythematosus cell preparations, low levels of complement activity, antinuclear antibodies, and autoimmune parameters can be detected (10% to 20%), but the titers are low and usually do not cause confusion with the collagen-vascular diseases, for which such serologic tests are much more important in establishing a diagnosis.

Use of ^{67}Ga gallium citrate isotope to scan the lungs has been touted to be helpful in assessing the overall inflammation in the lung parenchyma of many patients. In this disease, gallium uptake in lung was found to correlate with the presence of polymorphonuclear granulocytes in the airways and lung tissue (19). Initially, it was thought that lung scans might be a useful way to monitor treatment aimed at suppressing inflammation, but this has not developed (20). Recently, the proportional grading of the ground-glass and reticular patterns found in lung parenchyma by HRCT images has seemed to predict the long-term outcome of patients with IPF, which is notable but needs more substantiation in other series (6).

Lung function tests in virtually all patients with advanced disease reveal a reduction in total lung capacity and residual volume, indicating small, contracted lungs (21–23). Usually evidence of airway obstruction is minimal and the FEV-(sub 1)/FVC ratio is within normal limits. The restrictive respiratory function pattern is characteristic of stiff, noncompliant lungs. The diffusing capacity, assessed by a single-breath carbon monoxide method (DLco), is often reduced by 50% to 75% and is relied on heavily to support the diagnosis. The effect of cigarette smoking has to be factored into the lung function results, and this can produce obstructive changes. Thus, smoking introduces variability into these tests for lung volumes, pressure-volume characteristics and respiratory rate (24,25). There is usually resting arterial hypoxemia, but the carbon dioxide tension is not elevated.

Exercise performance to measure the alveolar-arterial oxygen gradient is a sensitive indicator of disease and can be useful in monitoring the course of disease and in assessing the effectiveness of various forms of treatment. Direct investigation of the airways by fiberoptic bronchoscopy is usually part of the evaluation, and transbronchial biopsy is an established means of obtaining samples of lung tissue for diagnosis. Bronchoalveolar lavage can be part of this procedure (26–34). Biopsies obtained through the bronchoscope are insufficient size to establish a diagnosis of IPF. However,

it is very effective for diagnosing diffuse, granulomatous interstitial diseases, such as sarcoidosis. Moreover, bronchoscopy allows one to do a lung lavage, which gives helpful information about cells and proteins in the airways that seem to correlate with histologic changes present in the interstitial and alveolar areas (28–35). Unfortunately, the early enthusiasm for being able to predict disease response based on bronchoalveolar lavage cell counts has not been borne out, with the exception that increased lymphocytes in the BAL does correlate with response to corticosteroids. If a transbronchial biopsy does not yield sufficient tissue for a confident diagnosis, the decision to proceed with an open biopsy must be weighed (35). Video-assisted thoracoscopic (VATS) lung biopsies are preferred to establish the diagnosis and represent an important advance over the traditional open lung biopsy (36). At least two biopsies from upper and lower lobes should be obtained to avoid "sampling error." The main reason to perform the biopsy is to establish a definitive diagnosis. The necessity of a definitive diagnosis must be individualized to each patient.

Lung Histology and Staging Disease Activity

Although general characteristics of lung pathologic changes are presented for each of the interstitial diseases discussed, a detailed description such as may be found in a pathology textbook is not given. For an excellent review of histologic changes in ILD, the article by Fulmer and Katzenstein is recommended (37). Presented here are a few concepts that correlate the patient's clinical status with findings present in lung tissue in an attempt to integrate pathophysiology and histology. The concepts include staging and activity of lung disease, characterizing inflammatory and immune effector cells in airways and lung parenchyma, and monitoring these immunologic parameters in a dynamic way that allow the natural progression of the disease to be assessed or the effects of immunosuppressive or cytotoxic therapy to be evaluated in an objective way (38).

Usually patients with very early forms of IPF are not extensively evaluated because of the mild or possibly confusing complex of signs and symptoms. Tissue histology is rarely available. Most undergo definitive work-up in the midperiod of disease. Thus, staging or assessing the activity of the cellular inflammatory reaction in the lungs becomes paramount because cellular forms of the disease usually respond best to therapy or have a higher rate of spontaneous regression (38–40). More advanced, acellular forms of disease in which excessive collagen deposition and fibrotic distortion of alveolar and interstitial architecture are pronounced are minimally responsive to therapy, as might be anticipated. Thus, the patient's clinical prognosis is determined largely by the histologic characteristics of lung tissue. Other factors that give the patient a better chance of response include younger age, recent onset of disease, female

TABLE 12.2. IDIOPATHIC PULMONARY FIBROSIS—CELLULAR AND IMMUNOLOGIC CHANGES IN BLOOD, BRONCHOALVEOLAR LAVAGE FLUID, AND LUNG TISSUE

Blood	Bronchoalveolar Fluid	Lung Tissue

Ig (IgG$_{1,3}$)
Immune complexes
Cryoglobulins
Serologic titers (low)
T-lymphs (sensitized to type I collagen)
	Alveolitis (characterized by more macrophages and increased percentage of PMNs [20%] and eosinophils [2–4%], but lymphs can be increased also [20%])
	Alveolar macrophages (active with numerous secretory components)
	  Chemotaxins to attract PMN (II-8 and LTB4) and smooth muscle cells
	  Plasminogen activator
	  Fibroblast growth factor
	  Fibronectin
	  Platelet-derived growth factor
	  Steroid receptors increased
	  Mitosis index increased
	Collagenase (PMN origin)
	IgG G$_3$, G$_1$ subclasses
	Immune complexes
	IgG-releasing cells
	Histamine elevated
	Abnormal content of surfactant Protein A
	N-Terminal type III procollagen peptides
		Interstitial inflammation
		  Plasma cells
		  Fibroblasts
		    Collagen synthesis (type 11 > 1)
		Fibrosis but no granulomas
		Bronchiolitis obliterans can develop

sex, finding of inflammatory cells in lung lavage analysis, and, especially, a relative increase in lymphocytes (20).

Three histologic features seem important. First is the degree of cellularity. Does the lung sample contain an abundance of inflammatory or reactive cells that suggest initial phases of disease, or is fibrosis already extensive? Second, what is the pattern or distribution of the cellular reaction? Collections of cells primarily in the alveolar spaces consisting of macrophages, type II pneumocytes, and inflammatory cells (polymorphonuclear granulocytes [PMNs] and eosinophils) suggest an alveolitis phase (3,33,41–43).

Third, the type of inflammatory or immune effector cells that are prevalent in the lung tissue is important and once again will give insight into the proposed efficacy of therapy. Biopsies that contain many PMNs, eosinophils, and especially lymphocytes often correlate with a response to corticosteroid therapy (30,34). This third feature is usually synonymous with that found in the previously described cellular lung specimen. Perhaps the most important aspect of the biopsy is to ascertain whether the classical UIP pattern of subpleural honeycombing is present, or whether there are atypical or more inflammatory changes as described. For example, biopsies with areas of bronchiolitis obliterans with organizing pneumonia (BOOP) portend a better response to treatment. The finding of areas of diffuse alveolar damage, BOOP as well as interstitial fibrosis, should lead one to consider an occult connective tissue disease such as the antisynthetase syndromes (polymysositis and ILD).

For assessing the immune reactivity of lung tissue, sampling the peripheral airways and alveoli by bronchoalveolar lavage (BAL) is a helpful method for assessing airway inflammation and the accumulation of immune effector cells and proteins in the alveoli and has greatly increased our understanding of the pathogenesis of IPF (44–47). BAL has led to the identification of a number of cytokines, growth factors and other inflammatory mediators that may be important in the pathogenesis of IPF (Table 12.2). Despite its value in research, BAL has marginal clinical value. BAL neutrophilia is observed in greater than 80% of patients but has no prognostic value. BAL eosinophilia (as high as 50%) has been associated with a worse prognosis in some studies but not others. BAL lymphocytosis (greater than 20%) does correlate with a cellular biopsy and better response to corticosteroids, but is uncommon (less than 20% of patients). High levels of lymphocytes should raise the concern for chronic hypersensitivity pneumonitis. BAL is most helpful in excluding an infectious etiology for ILD, but does not offer much value for staging or follow up of IPF.

Immunopathogenic Concepts of IPF

Idiopathic pulmonary fibrosis seems to be an immunologically mediated disease set in motion after an initial acute injury or infection and driven or perpetuated in a chronic phase by activated or poorly regulated macrophages. Increasing evidence has suggested a critical role for the fibroblast and the myofibroblast. The traditional concept has been that the fibroblast function is directed by activated macrophages, and although this may be true, the generally poor response to antiinflammatory therapy has suggested perhaps a primary dysfunction in the fibroblasts. The inciting antigen still remains unknown, but it might be a viral protein or some residual of a viral respiratory infection or hepatitis, because the association between a viral infection and the onset of symptoms that culminate in the IPF syndrome is quite clear in some patients. IgG in airway secretions and in blood, often in the form of immune complexes, is increased in most patients; specific antibody reactivity in the IgG fraction has not been identified (18). IgG-secreting plasma cells can be recovered in increased numbers in bronchoalveolar lavage. The intervening steps between immune complex formation and their localization in lung tissue and the influx of such cells as PMNs and eosinophils into alveoli and interstitial spaces are still incompletely known (47).

Referring to Table 12.2, the combination of airway cells retrieved by BAL reflects an alveolitis characterized by an abundance of macrophages and a mixture of PMNs and eosinophils; increased lymphocytes are unusual unless the IPF is associated with a collagen vascular disorder. The macrophages are activated cells and are capable of producing a number of mediators that may contribute to the inflammatory and fibrotic process. What activates the macrophages is not certain; but, should it be an IgG-containing immune complex on their cellular membranes, this would be a potent stimulus for the secretion of chemotaxins such as interleukin-8 and perhaps of the other fibrogenic factors, such as platelet-derived growth factor, transforming growth factor-β, and insulin-like growth factor-1 (47–56). Chemotaxins could attract PMNs into the alveoli, and subsequent elastolytic injury to the epithelial lining might develop. Likewise, substances like platelet-derived growth factor could attract smooth muscle cells and mesenchymal cells such as fibroblasts (57). Fibroblast proliferation, occurring either in the interstitial areas of the alveolar units or in the intraluminal alveolar spaces as buds that form from rents in the type I cell epithelial lining, is the essence of the fibrotic process (58). Transforming growth factor-β has been implicated as a critical mediator of fibrogenesis by stimulating collagen production and inhibiting the mechanisms responsible for breaking down and eliminating collagen (59). What is intriguing now is the possibility that other alveolar and interstitial-located cells may be participating in attracting and stimulating fibroblasts; therefore, a new role for epithelial cells, type II pneumocytes, and myofibroblasts is evolving in addition to the one of the macrophage (60–62). More recently, intriguing evidence has been provided that there may be activation of the cell death pathway, known as apoptosis in epethelial cells, may be a critical determinant of fibrosis (63). The potential link between apoptosis and fibrosis is an area of active research.

Treatment and Prognosis

Plans and expectations that the physician and the patient develop and share about the response of IPF to therapy are predicated on how well some of the foregoing information has been collected and analyzed. An accurate diagnosis based on good histologic conclusions, attempted staging of the disease, assembly of good baseline physiologic and immunologic parameters to compare with later values for objectively assessing "improvement," and a perspective of the natural history of the disease are all essential before therapy is undertaken. A decision not to pursue an adequate lung tissue biopsy because it entails the unpleasantness of chest surgery or thoracoscopic biopsy and instead just to give the patient an empiric trial of corticosteroid therapy may not be advantageous to the patient in the long run. It is important to keep in mind that if one is entertaining a diagnosis of IPF it carries a 5-year mortality of approximately 50%. In most circumstances, it is helpful for the patient and the physician to be certain of the diagnosis. If definitive tissue must then be obtained after failure of treatment, or if proper staging and baseline data have not been established, the clinician may have no basis for discontinuing treatment should significant side effects from corticosteroids or cytotoxic drugs develop. In general, cellular stages of IPF respond best, but such histologic findings suggest an early phase of disease and are often noted in the young patient, both being circumstances that improve prospects for suppressing or arresting the disease. In addition, therapy for a disease of still-undiscovered etiology is nonspecific by definition; therefore, the current strategy is directed at interrupting some step in the host's tissue response to the inciting agent and attacking the perceived injurious sequence. The drugs currently in use are far from specific in this respect.

Corticosteroids have been the mainstay of therapy for IPF, but increasing evidence is accumulating that they are ineffective as the sole therapeutic agent over the long run. Because the natural history of IPF is an inexorable deterioration, most patients should be offered a trial of therapy. What is unknown in each individual patient, is what the rate of deterioration will be. Prevention of deterioration is a reasonable goal in most patients. The response to existing therapies is poor and toxicities can be considerable; therefore, therapy must be individualized. Corticosteroids have been associated with a favorable response in only 10% to 30% of patients. High doses of corticosteroids have been advocated, but adequate studies to assess efficacy versus toxicity have not been performed. Recent studies have suggested no advantage of high doses versus medium level doses of corticosteroids. A reasonable approach is to institute prednisone at 40 to 60 mg daily for 2 to 3 months. Objective assessment of response to therapy should then be undertaken, although patients that are responding know it. The best methods for assessing response to therapy has not been definitively established but pulmonary function testing, especially exercise tests with measurement of arterial oxygen desaturation and diffusing capacity for carbon monoxide (D$_{LCO}$), and changes in the HRCT scan images apear to be the most useful. The prednisone should then be tapered by 2.5 to 5 mg every 2 weeks until a dose of 15 to 30 mg is reached. These doses should be continued for an additional 6 months. A critical unanswered question is whether a second immunosuppressive agent should be introduced or whether patients should show deterioration on prednisone before considering other potential therapies. The rationale for combination therapy is based on the potential mediators of fibrosis. A number of cytokines such as interleukin 8, tumor necrosis factor-α, and macrophage inflammatory protein-1β have been identified in BAL and lung tissue. The production of these mediators is sensitive to corticosteroids. However, the second major class of mediators, the growth factors such and platelet derived growth factor, transforming growth factor-β and insulin-like growth factor-1 are not sensitive to corticosteroids. Thus, it seems unlikely that corticosteroid therapy alone would be effective. After a total of 1 year of corticosteroid therapy, a careful decision should be made about weaning or continuing therapy. Some flexibility can be exercised in tailoring the maintenance therapy, and an alternate-day dose may be used if corticosteroid side effects are a significant management problem.

For patients who do not seem to be controlled with or responsive to corticosteroids, additional immunosuppressive therapy needs consideration (64). Cyclophosphamide, an alkylating drug, is a potent immunosuppressant and seems to be effective in some patients who are not controlled with corticosteroids (20,65). Some information substantiates the use of cyclophosphamide as the preferred treatment for IPF; hence, it has been tried as the initial treatment instead of corticosteroids. The drug is taken orally in graduated amounts (50 mg/day initially, with 50-mg dose increments at approximately biweekly intervals until a dose of 150 to 200 mg/day is reached for most patients) until a controlled and stable degree of peripheral blood lymphopenia is achieved. Ideally, a dose that suppresses the total lymphocyte count by half its baseline amount, yet preserves a circulating polymorphonuclear granulocyte count of 500/ mm^3 or more to prevent bacterial infection, should be the goal. With frequent patient follow-up for side effects and blood counts, reasonably tight control can be maintained with cyclophosphamide. If improvement in the lung disease is documented after 3 months of this therapy, it should be continued for a 12-month interval. Alternatively, an intermittent schedule every month using intravenous administration beginning with a 750 mg/m^2 dosage seems to be a reasonable alternative to daily oral therapy (65). However, significant toxicities have been reported in patients receiving cyclophosphamide for periods greater that 1 year; therefore, caution is advised.

Azathioprine has been used as an alternative to cyclophosphamide. No direct studies have been performed comparing the two agents. Penicillamine has been used in some patients in preliminary trials, with the rationale that it might prevent the cross-linking of abnormal collagen being synthesized in the interstitium and prevent or retard fibrosis (66). Patients who seem to show improvement with penicillamine tend to be those with earlier stages of disease, which suggests that this therapy is valuable in arresting disease rather than in improving established fibrosis. Patients with connective tissue diseases and interstitial fibrosis seem to show more improvement with penicillamine than those with IPF. Colchicine has been used and an antifibrotic agent and in a recent study, compared favorably to prednisone for some patients with IPF (67). A recent study suggested a possible role for the antifibrotic agent perfenidone in patients with advanced IPF, but more studies are required to assess the efficacy of this new approach (68). Single lung transplantation (SLT) is the most definitive option for patients failing medical therapy. Two-year survival following SLT approaches 70% and 5-year survival 50% (69–71). Survival is improved in younger patients and SLT is not an option for patients over 65 (72–75).

In addition to suppressing the patient's alveolitis and stabilizing the inflammatory process, several other measures may help respiratory function. It is imperative that these patients stop cigarette smoking. Although patients can have relatively normal oxygen saturation at rest, with exercise there is frequently a marked drop in arterial oxygen tension (Pao(sub 2)). Therefore, exercise tolerance may be significantly improved with supplemental oxygen therapy. When oxygen requirements are high (more than 4 L/min flow), direct administration of oxygen in the trachea may be preferred. Several modes of transtracheal catheter oxygen delivery are available (76). In addition to attaining a high local concentration of oxygen in the lungs, the cosmetic effect of not wearing obvious nasal prongs can be important. As the pulmonary vascular bed is impaired by progressive fibrosis, pulmonary hypertension and cor pulmonale can develop; right-sided congestive heart failure can be difficult to control. Judicious use of diuretics is advised, for a significant decrease in intravascular volume may be deleterious for lung perfusion. Digitalis or antiarrhythmic drugs might be required, although adequate oxygenation is probably the best treatment for heart failure. Some patients may also develop obstruction to air flow and be troubled with wheezing and coughing that may respond to bronchodilators. As infection may occur during immunosuppressive therapy, it is important to maintain a high index of suspicion and to treat infection aggressively. Prophylactic use of pneumococcal and influenza vaccines is encouraged.

In summary, the long-term prognosis of IPF is variable, and some patients may live 5 to 10 years with the disease. The stage at which the diagnosis is established and the degree of fibrosis are important features (77). Having a certain diagnosis based on an adequate specimen of lung tissue is important and may prevent some of the pitfalls of management and complications from inappropriate immunosuppression.

The identification of cellular mediators in the affected lung tissue and improved concepts of how these may injure tissue and promote fibrosis lead to different forms of specific antimediator therapy in the future. For a selected few, lung transplantation may be a hope for improved health. The smoldering fibrotic disease continues to create health problems chronically. Terminal problems experienced by patients include increasing dyspnea, severe hypoxemia requiring supplemental home oxygen therapy, right heart failure, and complications from prolonged immunosuppressive therapy. Approximately 10% of patients develop lung cancer, which means that patients with IPF have approximately a six-fold (women) or 14-fold (men) increased risk of cancer.

BRONCHIOLITIS OBLITERANS ORGANIZING PNEUMONIA

In 1985, Epler and coworkers reported 94 patients with bronchiolitis obliterans, of whom 50 had patchy organizing pneumonia and no apparent cause or associated disease (78). Histologic characteristics of this bronchiolitis obliterans with organizing pneumonia (BOOP) included polypoid masses of granulation tissue in lumens of small airways, alveolar ducts, and some alveoli. Clinically, patients had a cough or flu-like illness for 4 to 10 weeks, and crackles were heard in the lungs of 68% of the patients. Chest radiographs showed an unusual pattern of patchy densities with a "ground-glass" appearance in 81%. There was a restrictive ventilatory defect in 72% and an abnormal diffusing capacity in 86%. Only cigarette smokers had evidence of airway obstruction on pulmonary function tests. Corticosteroid treatment was efficacious, and over a mean follow-up period of 4 years, complete clinical and physiologic recovery occurred in 65% of patients; only two died of progressive disease. BOOP is most often confused with idiopathic pulmonary fibrosis, which generally has a poorer prognosis and does not respond in most cases to corticosteroids (78–82). Moreover, IPF has a more insidious onset and the chest radiograph shows bilateral interstitial opacities, whereas localized air space densities are a feature in BOOP (81). It is important to keep in mind that BOOP is a pathologic diagnosis that can be seen in a number of clinical settings including connective tissue disease, bone marrow and solid organ transplantation, following toxic fume exposure, in the setting of chemotherapy, or infections such as Legionella. The pathologic identification of BOOP must be placed in the appropriate clinical setting. When there is no apparent cause identified it is termed idiopathic BOOP or cryptogenic organizing pneumonia (COP) (83).

That classic presentation is that of a community acquired pneumonia failing to respond to antibiotics. The course is usually subacute, developing over 2 weeks to 6 months. Physical examination is notable for crackles on auscultation of the chest in over 50% of patients with a distinctive late inspiratory squeak heard in about 40%. Laboratory testing is nonspecific with an elevated white blood cell count and erythrocyte sedimentation rate in most patients. The chest radiograph can have a variety of manifestions, but the most frequent findings are patchy, hazy, peripheral infiltrates without evident air bronchograms. Involvement may be unilateral or bilateral. Infiltrates may be fleeting and resolve spontaneously or in the setting of antibiotics, but without corticosteroids they typically recur. However, one of the reasons that BOOP can be confused with IPF is that 20% to 30% of patients can present with bilateral lower lung zone reticulonodular infiltrates. Pleural effusions are not characteristic of idiopathic BOOP. The HRCT can be very helpful in the evaluation of the infiltrates when a peripheral pattern with air bronchograms is observed (84). Pulmonary function shows a restrictive pattern. This should not be confused with bronchiolitis obliterans, which has more recently been termed constrictive bronchiolitis, which is a pure obstructive ventilatory defect.

A tissue diagnosis should be obtained and transbronchial biopsies may provide adequate tissue to secure the diagnosis. The findings are an exuberant inflammatory response involving the terminal and respiratory bronchioles with extension of the tissue reaction into adjacent alveolar ducts. The so-called "Masson bodies" of granulation tissue without fibrosis. Recent studies have demonstrated the presence of inflammatory mediators such as interleukin-8 in BAL from patients with BOOP. One of the fascinating biological questions is why BOOP generally resolves with corticosteroids, whereas IPF does not. If transbronchial biopsies are insufficient, VATS is the indicated procedure.

The majority of patients respond to oral corticosteroids, but there are several caveats to successful treatment. Therapy should be initiated with prednisone at 1 mg/kg per day or at least 2 weeks. Patients usually note improvement within the first week. The rate of tapering the prednisone needs to be dictated by the radiographic response in accord with toxicities. Patients that are tapered too rapidly often relapse. As long as the radiograph or HRCT is improving the taper can continue. Treatment is usually required for at least 6 months and frequently 12 to 18 months. Again, the caveat is that as long as there is persistent infiltrate, therapy should be continued until it is clear the further reduction in dose does not precipitate recurrence. A minority of patients (3% to 10%) may progress despite corticosteroids and may have a fulminant course (85). Cytotoxic therapy should be considered early if there is a failure to respond to corticosteroids.

RESPIRATORY BRONCHIOLITIS

Respiratory bronchiolitis (RB) is a relatively recently recognized clinical and pathologic entity that can be confused with IPF (86). RB occurs exclusively in heavy cigarette smokers and can present with exertional breathlessness and dry cough. Constitutional symptoms are not typically seen with RB. Approximately 50% of patients have bibasilar crackles. The chest radiograph demonstrates bibasilar reticulonodular infiltrates, although it may be normal. The

HRCT is helpful in the distiction from IPF. The findings are fine peribronchiolar nodules (2 to 3 mm) and patchy ground glass infiltrates. The subpleural honeycombing and traction bronchiectasis of IPF are not seen. Pulmonary function tests reveal a restrictive pattern with reduced diffusion. Hypoxemia is not typically present. Lung biopsy is required for a definite diagnosis and shows pigmented macrophages filling the terminal and respiratory bronchioles. Recent studies have suggested that RB and DIP may represent a spectrum of smoking related illness (87). The prognosis is good in patients that cease smoking (unlike IPF). The role of corticosteroids is unclear but generally employed in patients with persistent symptoms despite cessation of smoking.

CONNECTIVE TISSUE (COLLAGEN VASCULAR) DISEASES

Connective tissue is an extracellular material composed of a physiologically active ground substance containing fibrils of elastin, collagen, and reticulin. Alteration in the chemical composition and physical constitution of the ground substance leads to edema, fibrinoid degeneration, and vascular lesions characteristic of the connective tissue diseases (88,89). The lungs may be the first organ involved in these diseases. In this section, the pulmonary manifestations of four connective tissue diseases are reviewed: systemic lupus erythematosus, rheumatoid arthritis, diffuse progressive systemic sclerosis (scleroderma), and polymyositis-dermatomyositis). Sjögren's syndrome and mixed connective tissue disease also have pleuropulmonary manifestations (90–98).

Systemic Lupus Erythematosus

Systemic lupus erythematosus (SLE) is a disease of unknown etiology that most often affects young women (99,100). Connective tissues of any organ in the body can be involved, but the vascular system, the epidermis, and the serous and synovial membranes are most common. Pulmonary illness, however, may be the presenting manifestation of SLE (88,101–112). Pleuropulmonary manifestations of SLE are summarized in Table 12.3 (92). The lungs and pleura are

TABLE 12.3. PLEUROPULMONARY MANIFESTATIONS OF SYSTEMIC LUPUS ERYTHEMATOSUS

Pleurisy with or without effusion
Diaphragmatic dysfunction with reduced lung volume
Acute lupus pneumonitis
Diffuse alveolar hemorrhage
Diffuse interstitial disease
Pulmonary hypertension
Pulmonary thromboembolism

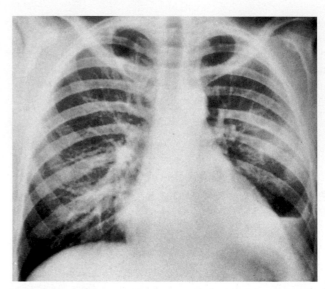

FIGURE 12.4. Systemic lupus erythematosus. PA chest radiograph of a 19-year-old man with an established diagnosis of systemic lupus erythematosus who developed fever and shortness of breath acutely. Note the left pleural effusion and enlarged cardiac silhouette. An echocardiogram revealed pericardial fluid. Corticosteroid therapy was instituted, and the chest radiograph returned to normal within 5 days.

frequently affected in SLE, with involvement occurring in 50% to 70% of SLE patients (92,101). Respiratory muscle dysfunction, including diaphragmatic muscle weakness, has been described in patients with SLE (113,114). This may in part explain the well-described basilar atelectasis and so-called vanishing lung syndrome noted in patients with this disease. Chest radiographic changes in patients with SLE include cardiac enlargement, pericardial effusion, pleuritis with or without effusion, and pulmonary infiltrates (Figs. 12.4 and 12.5) (88,92,101,106,115–117). The lung bases are most frequently involved with patchy areas of increased density, focal atelectasis with diaphragmatic elevation, and acute acinar or chronic interstitial infiltrates. The pulmonary infiltration tends to be recurrent and migratory in nature.

Pleural effusions, usually small but sometimes massive, are frequently bilateral (88,92,110,116,118–120). Winslow and coworkers emphasized the importance of pleuritis as an early manifestation of SLE (116). Pleural effusion occurred in 42 (81%) of their 57 patients; in three it was an isolated first sign, and in 16 others it was associated with only minor antecedent symptoms. Such pleural effusions are inflammatory exudates, containing both mononuclear and polymorphonuclear cells. The glucose concentration and pH of the pleural fluid are within normal range. The finding of LE cells in the fluid is diagnostic. Moreover, a high pleural fluid antinuclear antibody (ANA) titer (1:160 or greater) and a pleural fluid to serum ANA titer ratio of greater than 1 strongly support the diagnosis (119). Low

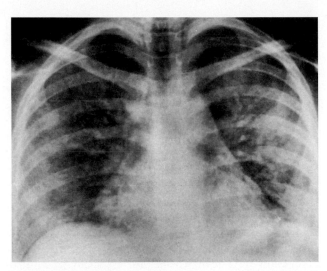

FIGURE 12.5. Systemic lupus erythematosus. PA chest radiograph of an 18-year-old woman with acute lupus pneumonitis. Note the bilateral alveolar filling process. Two weeks after corticosteroid and azathioprine therapy was instituted the chest radiograph had cleared markedly.

total and individual complement components are also characteristic of pleural effusion in SLE (98). Owing to the excellent response to corticosteroids, pleural fibrosis and resultant pleural entrapment and restrictive lung disease are uncommon sequelae (98).

Although many patients develop pulmonary infiltrates unrelated to infection, infection still appears to be the most frequent cause of pulmonary infiltrates in SLE (88,101,115,117). Some cases with pulmonary infiltrates not caused by infection have an acute onset; others are chronic. Acute lupus pneumonitis (ALP) is characterized by severe dyspnea, a cough productive of scant sputum, fever (100°F to 104°F), negative sputum and blood cultures, hypoxemia, and a bilateral alveolar filling process on the chest radiograph (Fig. 12.5) (101). Associated findings include cardiomegaly and pleuritis, with or without effusion. Clearing of the pulmonary infiltrates in response to corticosteroids is frequently rapid. Azathioprine has been administered with success to a small group of patients who did not respond to corticosteroids alone (101). ALP can develop during the course of the illness or can be the initial manifestation of SLE in 50% of cases with this complication (98,102). In half of the patients surviving the acute illness, the chest radiograph clears completely. In the other half, the disease progresses to chronic interstitial pneumonitis, with hypocapnia, restrictive pulmonary function, and decreased DLCO (102).

Diffuse alveolar hemorrhage owing to capillaritis, which can be confused with ALP, is characterized by the acute onset of fever, cough, dyspnea, and hemoptysis (98,118,121). The concomitant occurrence of a fall in hematocrit and a diffuse alveolar filling pattern on the chest radiograph support the diagnosis (118). Unlike ALP, diffuse alveolar hemorrhage is not associated with pleural or pericardial disease and is not a presenting manifestation of SLE (118). The incidence of this complication is low, but may be rising (118). In spite of treatment with corticosteroids, immunosuppressives, and plasmapheresis, the mortality rate is high (98,118).

In 1973, Eisenberg and coworkers reported 18 patients and in 1990 Weinrib, Sharma, and Quismorio reported 14 patients with SLE and chronic diffuse interstitial lung disease (117,122). Pulmonary symptoms in these patients included dyspnea, a nonproductive cough, and pleuritic chest pain. Physical findings were poor diaphragmatic movement and basilar crackles, but clubbing was not a feature in these patients. Hypoxemia, a restrictive ventilatory defect, and reduced diffusing capacity were evident on pulmonary function tests. Huang and coworkers and Andonopoulos and coworkers noted that patients with SLE may demonstrate these abnormalities in the absence of clinical symptoms or abnormal chest radiographs (123,124). In fact, Andonopoulos and coworkers found normal function in only one-third of 70 nonsmoking patients with SLE, and an isolated reduction in DLCO was the most commonly detected functional abnormality (31% of patients) (124).

Pulmonary hypertension in SLE can be secondary to progressive interstitial pneumonitis with resultant lung destruction and hypoxia, or it can be caused by a primary fibroproliferative pulmonary vasculopathy (118). Fewer than 50 cases of the latter, primary form have been reported (118). This entity must be differentiated from recurrent pulmonary embolism. Raynaud's phenomenon is present in 75% of the cases, and women are affected in more than 90% of the cases (118). There is an associated glomerulonephritis in 63% of patients and cutaneous vasculitis in 33% (125).

Although most patients who die of SLE have severe pathologic changes in their lungs, there are no features that are considered unique (126–132). Gross and coworkers found a high frequency of interstitial pneumonitis (98%), interstitial fibrosis (70%), and chronic pleuritis (95%) in 44 autopsy specimens (132). Acute inflammation of small pulmonary arteries and arterioles was found in 19%. Other common but nonspecific changes in those who die of SLE include alveolar hyaline membranes, hemorrhage, and capillary thrombi (101,126–130). The pleural lesions often seen in this disease are usually manifested pathologically by a fibrinous pleuritis (132).

Treatment of SLE is usually directed at control of the systemic disease and preservation of renal function if the kidneys are seriously involved. Corticosteroids and cyclophosphamide are the main immunosuppressive drugs used, and in severe cases plasmapheresis is indicated (88,92,101). A general statement about therapy of lung disease can be made for SLE and other collagen-vascular diseases. When therapy is required because of pulmonary involvement, corticosteroids are usually tried first in doses similar to those used in IPF (i.e., 1 mg/kg). Scleroderma lung involvement is an exception, because it does not respond to corticosteroids; therefore, such therapy is not indicated.

An additional important complication in patients with SLE and a circulating lupus anticoagulant (antiphospholipid antibody) is venous thrombosis and pulmonary thromboembolism (98,125,133). A 25% incidence of pulmonary emboli has been reported in patients with SLE in whom a circulating anticoagulant is present (133).

Rheumatoid Arthritis

Rheumatoid arthritis is a disease that primarily affects the joints, but it also involves other organs and tissues, including the lungs and pleura (92,134–145). Pleuropulmonary disease is more common in patients with rheumatoid arthritis who have severe chronic articular disease, high titers of rheumatoid factor, subcutaneous nodules, and other systemic manifestations such as Felty's syndrome, cutaneous vasculitis, myopericarditis, and ocular inflammation (98,142). There are several pleuropulmonary abnormalities associated with the rheumatoid process (Table 12.4) (88,110,134, 135,146–153). Pleural involvement by the rheumatoid process is the most common thoracic complication of rheumatoid arthritis and accounts for attacks of pleurisy, with or without effusion. Such pleurisy has a remarkable predilection for men, despite the fact that rheumatoid arthritis occurs predominantly in women in a ratio of 2:1. It appears that pleural disease is one of the systemic manifestations of rheumatoid arthritis. Such pleural disease rarely causes complications except for the occasional case of fibrothorax and restrictive lung disease that necessitates decortication. However, all patients with rheumatoid arthritis who present with pleurisy and effusion should have appropriate studies to exclude empyema, tuberculosis, and malignancy.

The prevalence of chronic interstitial lung disease as detected by chest radiographic screening of rheumatoid patients is small. In one series of 516 cases, only eight patients (2%) had radiographic evidence of interstitial lung disease (139). A much higher prevalence is detected by pulmonary function tests (139,148). Restrictive ventilatory impairment and a reduction of the diffusing capacity have been found in as many as 41% of a group of patients with rheumatoid arthritis (139). High-resolution CT (HRCT) may also iden-

TABLE 12.4. PLEUROPULMONARY MANIFESTATIONS OF RHEUMATOID ARTHRITIS

Pleurisy with or without effusion
Interstitial lung disease
Pulmonary nodules
Bronchiolitis obliterans organizing pneumonia
Bronchiolitis obliterans
Pulmonary hypertension

tify clinically silent interstitial lung disease (98). A higher prevalence of interstitial lung disease occurs in men with rheumatoid arthritis than in women. Other risk factors include smoking, high titers of rheumatoid factor, α-1-antitrypsin variants, subcutaneous nodules, or prominent extraarticular manifestations.

No specific pattern of arthritis is associated with interstitial lung disease, although 50% of such patients have subcutaneous nodules. Interstitial pneumonitis and pleural disease may precede articular manifestations (98). Cough and dyspnea are often present, and clubbing is found in up to 75% of cases (149). The chest radiograph shows diffuse interstitial infiltrates, most marked in the lung bases, and in far-advanced disease, small cysts (honeycomb lung) appear accompanied by loss of lung volumes (98). Histopathologic examination of tissue may be helpful, especially when rheumatoid nodules are present in the lung interstitium in addition to the interstitial pneumonitis (88). Large amounts of rheumatoid factor in alveolar walls and pulmonary capillaries have been demonstrated by direct immunofluorescent staining of rheumatoid lung tissue. This suggests a possible immune mechanism for the development of pulmonary disease associated with rheumatoid arthritis (102). Moreover, recent studies suggest a pathogenic role of neutrophils and collagenase in rheumatoid interstitial lung disease (107, 108). In patients with rheumatoid arthritis and interstitial pneumonitis in whom a cellular lung biopsy is obtained, there is a positive objective response to corticosteroids or other immunosuppressive medications (98,134). The mean survival for all patients with rheumatoid arthritis and interstitial pneumonitis is 5 years (134).

The intrapulmonary rheumatoid or necrobiotic nodule, which is pathologically identical to the subcutaneous nodule in rheumatoid arthritis, is more common in men than women (88,134,135). On the chest radiograph, necrobiotic nodules appear as single lesions or as bilateral, multiple, varying-sized coin lesions, with a predilection for the upper lung zones (98). Because the nodular form of rheumatoid lung disease may precede the arthritic manifestations, it must be differentiated from other granulomatous diseases. In the case of a single nodule, it may correlate with the activity and treatment status of the disease, and it must be differentiated from malignancy. Nodules may coexist with rheumatoid pleural effusions; spontaneous pneumothorax may also occur.

Caplan has described a syndrome in coal miners with rheumatoid arthritis (141). This rheumatoid pneumoconiosis (Caplan's syndrome) is characterized by the appearance on chest radiograph of rounded densities that evolve rapidly and can undergo cavitation—in contrast to the massive fibrosis of coal workers' pneumoconiosis. A similar syndrome has been reported in rheumatoid arthritis patients who are sandblasters, asbestos workers, potters, boiler scalers, and brass and iron workers (88,134,135). The pneumoconiotic nodule consists of layers of partially necrotic collagen and dust. Occa-

sionally there are foci of tuberculosis. The pulmonary disease may precede or coincide with the onset of the arthritis.

Bronchiolitis obliterans organizing pneumonia (BOOP) has been reported in a few patients with rheumatoid arthritis, and its frequency in this disease remains unknown (98,143). Treatment with corticosteroids has been effective (98).

Bronchiolitis obliterans, a disease of the terminal airways characterized by progressive air flow limitation with preservation or increase of lung volumes, has been described in patients with rheumatoid arthritis (98,144,145). Patients complain of cough and dyspnea, and in most cases the chest radiograph is clear or shows hyperinflation (98). Chest examination reveals rhonchi with an inspiratory squeak or diminished breath sounds (98). An autoimmunopathogenesis has been suggested (98). Unfortunately, no effective therapy is available for this disorder, and survival is usually less than 2 years following diagnosis (144).

In rare cases, pulmonary vasculitis may cause pulmonary hypertension in rheumatoid arthritis; more commonly, pulmonary hypertension is the result of advancing fibrosing alveolitis. Raynaud's phenomenon has been present in a few reported cases of rheumatoid arthritis and pulmonary vasculitis (88,134,135).

Progressive Systemic Sclerosis (Scleroderma)

Scleroderma is an inflammatory-fibrotic disorder of connective tissue that results in fibrosis and vascular abnormalities (98,154). The skin, gastrointestinal tract, musculoskeletal system, kidneys, heart, and lungs are frequently involved (154–156). The majority of patients are affected in their fourth through sixth decades; the disease is three times more common in women than in men. Prognosis is unfavorable, and the cause of death is usually either renal, cardiovascular, or pulmonary.

Among the visceral organs involved in scleroderma, the lungs are second only to the esophagus (92,154,155, 157–164). Clinical or autopsy evidence of pulmonary involvement is found in at least 70% of cases (159,164). Chest radiographic abnormalities have been reported in up to 25% of cases. Pulmonary symptoms have been found at some time during the course of the illness in 50% of patients. One series using pulmonary function tests reported abnormalities in 21 of 22 patients (158). Postmortem studies on 196 cases revealed that only 18% were free of pleuropulmonary involvement (159). Pulmonary fibrosis was found in 77%, pulmonary vascular disease in 30%, and pleural disease in 32%. Two recent studies suggest an increased risk of malignancy, particularly lung cancer, in patients with scleroderma (165,166).

The most prominent respiratory symptoms are dyspnea and, less commonly, a cough, which may be slightly productive (159). The most frequent signs are fine basilar crackles and limited expansion of the chest. Signs of cor pulmonale

may appear as a result of pulmonary vascular and interstitial disease (162,163).

The most common abnormality on chest radiograph is an interstitial reticular pattern, particularly affecting the lung bases, reminiscent of IPF. As the disease progresses, the pulmonary infiltration becomes denser, with subsequent honeycombing and cyst formation (154). The cysts are most often subpleural in the basal and paravertebral areas and are usually bilateral. Although they tend to be small (5 mm or less in diameter), large cysts may form and rupture, resulting in a pneumothorax. Other findings include micronodulation, increased vascular markings, and pulmonary edema. Disseminated pulmonary calcification or calcification of the soft tissue of the thorax may be seen on the chest radiograph (88,155,157). The latter may also demonstrate the presence of pleural thickening, pleural effusion, and signs of pulmonary hypertension secondary to scleroderma lung disease. Disturbance of esophageal motility may result in retention of food and recurrent aspiration pneumonia. HRCT of the chest has been utilized to detect early interstitial lung disease and to distinguish patients with predominantly fibrotic lung disease from those with significant inflammation (6,167, 168). Moreover, HRCT has been successful in detecting mediastinal adenopathy and asymptomatic esophageal involvement in patients with scleroderma (169,170).

Pulmonary function abnormalities include a restrictive pattern with reduction of vital capacity and normal flow rates (154,155,157,164,166–174). The compliance of the lung is reduced. A reduced DLCO is frequently the earliest abnormality noted and may be present prior to recognized chest radiographic abnormalities (159,175). Owens and coworkers and Silver and coworkers found a significant correlation between bronchoalveolar lavage cellular recovery and the single-breath DLCO (176,177). Sackner and coworkers showed that scleroderma involvement of the chest wall does not interfere with pulmonary function (158).

Pathological changes in the lung occur frequently, with or without clinical or chest radiographic abnormalities (159,175). In an autopsy study, Weaver and coworkers found pulmonary abnormalities in all their 28 cases of scleroderma (159). A progressive, nonspecific, bilateral lower-lobe interstitial fibrosis with bronchiectasis and cyst formation was the most prominent finding. Marked intimal thickening by loose myxomatous connective tissue occurred in small pulmonary arteries and arterioles.

In reviews of vascular disease in scleroderma, Norton and Nardo and Shuck and coworkers point out that involvement of the arterioles and capillary bed in many tissues, particularly the lungs, is the basis of scleroderma (162,178). They conclude that scleroderma must be regarded as a vascular disease. It is clear that the pulmonary vascular lesions are not merely an extension of interstitial fibrosis, because many

scleroderma lungs have areas of severe interstitial fibrosis without arterial lesions, as well as areas of vascular changes without interstitial disease (163). Thus, there are two predominant lung lesions in scleroderma: interstitial and pulmonary vascular (154). Other pathological findings in patients with scleroderma include pleural thickening or effusion, cardiomegaly, vascular congestion, pulmonary edema, and pneumonitis.

The course of chronic interstitial lung disese in scleroderma is more indolent than IPF and recent studies have suggested the 5-year mortality to be in the range of 15% (179). In general, corticosteroids are not beneficial in treating pulmonary disease in scleroderma (154). However, two studies demonstrated improvement in Dlco following penicillamine therapy, and one study suggested this drug may arrest worsening of pulmonary dysfunction (180,182). Moreover, in a 12-month trial of recombinant α-interferon therapy in 14 patients, nine of whom completed the trial, significant improvement was observed in skin involvement and in arterial oxygen tension (183). More recently, patients with evidence of alveolitis by BAL treated with low-dose prednisone and cyclophosphamide demonstrated clinical improvement (184). Nifedipine may be useful for treating patients with early pulmonary vascular disease (154). The 5-year survival rate for patients with scleroderma following the detection of lung disease is less than 50% (171,184).

Polymyositis-Dermatomyositis

Polymyositis and dermatomyositis (PM-DM) include a group of diffuse inflammatory and degenerative disorders of striated muscle that cause symmetrical weakness and atrophy of proximal muscle groups (185–191). The disease is twice as common in women as in men. It shows two peak age incidences: the first decade and the fifth and sixth decades (89). Patients commonly present with erythematous skin lesions accompanied by weakness and pain of proximal muscle groups.

The pulmonary complications of PM-DM may precede, follow, or occur simultaneously with the muscle and skin parenchymal disease (98). There are three mechanisms for the development of pulmonary parenchymal disease in polymyositis: primary interstitial pneumonitis; aspiration pneumonia owing to a hypotonic esophagus; and hypostatic pneumonia secondary to chest wall involvement, with resultant hypoventilation (192).

Respiratory muscle dysfunction caused by the inflammatory myopathy of PM-DM can lead to respiratory failure (alveolar hypoventilation) in up to 10% of patients (98). Subclinical respiratory muscle dysfunction is more frequent (98). These latter patients have tachypnea and dyspnea with exercise, and may develop the aforementioned hypostatic pneumonia owing to failure to generate an adequate cough (98).

In contrast to the other connective tissue diseases, pleural disease is not common in polymyositis (98,193). In one review of polymyositis lung, a total of 31 well-documented cases of interstitial pneumonitis was found in the world's literature (193). The exact prevalence of interstitial pneumonitis in polymyositis lung is difficult to determine; however, in a series from the Mayo Clinic, primary interstitial pneumonitis was present in 5%, likely an underestimate, because HRCT was not utilized to detect disease not seen on the plain chest radiograph (194).

The clinical presentation of this form of lung disease is quite variable. It may present as an acute pneumonitis with a mixed alveolar-interstitial pneumonitis in association with skin and muscle manifestations or as an asymptomatic finding on the chest radiograph. The most common presentation is one of gradual onset of dyspnea and cough with development of diffuse pulmonary infiltrates most prominent at the lung bases. Diffuse soft tissue calcification may be present, a finding more often seen in children with PM-DM than in adults. Histopathology is similar to that described for idiopathic pulmonary fibrosis (193). BOOP, usual interstitial pneumonia (UIP), diffuse alveolar damage, and pulmonary arteriolitis may be present (193).

In approximately 40% of patients, the pulmonary disease precedes the skin and muscle manifestations by 1 to 24 months (193). Clubbing is not often present. In most cases, the lung disease is progressive, causing severe restrictive lung disease and cor pulmonale. Corticosteroids have caused remission, with either stabilization or improvement in the symptoms, chest films, and physiologic abnormalities in 50% of patients (193).

A subset of patients with PM present with ILD as the predominant manifestation with minimal muscle weakness. Raynoud's phenomenon is often seen as well as arthralgias. Circulating autoantibodies to the amino-acyl tRNA synthetases are present. Most patients also have a positive ANA. The most common of the antisynthetase autoantibodies is against the histidyl-tRNA-synthetase (anti-Jo-1), but others have been described as well (195,196). Corticosteroids alone are insufficient and cyclophosphamide should be added. Refractory cases should be considered for therapy with immunoglobulin, which has been shown to benefit some patients with classic PM (197).

SYSTEMIC GRANULOMATOUS VASCULITIDES

Wegener's Granulomatosis

Wegener's granulomatosis (WG) has a distinctive clinicopathologic triad of necrotizing granulomatous vasculitis of the upper and lower respiratory tracts; glomerulonephritis; and variable degrees of disseminated small vessel vasculitis affecting arterioles, venules, and capillaries (198–226). A localized form of WG limited primarily to the respiratory

tract has been reported, but probably represents an early stage that, if not treated, eventually would involve the kidney and become a generalized Wegener's granulomatosis (212). However, some patients may have a forme fruste of the disease that never disseminates.

Clinicopathologic Features

Fauci and his colleagues have described the clinical features of Wegener's granulomatosis (211). The mean age at diagnosis was 41, range 14 to 75 years. The disease occurs in men almost twice as frequently as in women (204,211,212). Initially, clinical presentations vary widely among patients but generally are related to the upper respiratory tract. Typical findings include sinusitis (67%), otitis media (29%), rhinitis or nasal symptoms (22%), epistaxis (11%), ulcers (6%), and hearing impairment (6%) (194). Although chest radiographic abnormalities are present in 71%, fewer than one-half of Fauci's patients had noticed respiratory symptoms (cough in 33%, hemoptysis in 18%, chest pain in 8%, dyspnea in 7%, and pleurisy in 5%) (211,226). In one series, 8% of 77 patients with Wegener's granulomatosis presented with diffuse hemorrhage (227). Pulmonary function studies show loss of lung volume with a restrictive ventilatory defect in association with significant parenchymal lesions (89). More than 50% of patients with WG also have an obstructive ventilatory abnormality that cannot be related to cigarette smoking (92). In patients with obstructive changes, granulomatous lesions that have blocked a major airway may be found during fiberoptic bronchoscopy, and the severity of airflow obstruction has been shown to correlate with the extent of endobronchial disease (226,228).

Renal disease is the sine qua non of generalized Wegener's granulomatosis. Prior to the use of cytotoxic agents as therapy in this disorder, most patients succumbed to renal disease, with a mean survival of 5 months from the onset of clinically evident renal involvement (201,206). The urinary findings in generalized WG are of acute glomerulonephritis with hematuria, red blood cell casts, and proteinuria. Any of the other organ systems involved in WG may also be the focus of initial complaints (Table 12.5) (200,201,211). Among systemic signs and symptoms at presentation are fever (34%), weight loss (16%), and anorexia or malaise (8%) (211). Extrathoracic organ involvement at presentation includes arthritis (44%), skin rash (13%), ocular inflammation (6%), and proptosis (7%) (211,226).

Wegener's granulomatosis presents a characteristic complex of laboratory findings (201,204,211). The mild anemia of subacute or chronic diseases is seen frequently, as is mild leukocytosis. Thrombocytosis (up to 1 million platelets per cubic millimeter) can be present and probably represents an acute reaction (201). The results of antinuclear antibody and lupus erythematosus (LE) cell preparation tests are uniformly negative. The total complement level is normal or mildly elevated. Mild hyperglobulinemia, particularly involving the serum IgA fraction, occurs commonly (213). Almost all patients have strikingly elevated erythrocyte sedimentation rates, usually 100 mm/hour or more (Westergren method) (201). The C-reactive protein is almost always elevated. In 1982, a serum IgG against cytoplasmic components of polymorphonuclear leukocytes was described in eight patients with necrotizing granulonephritis (229). Subsequent studies have established the specificity of this anti-neutrophilic cytoplasmic antibody (c-ANCA or ANCA-PR3) for WG (230,231). Among 277 patients with WG and 1,657 control patients the specificity of ANCA was 99% (231). However, sensitivity is dependent on disease activity; thus, when only limited disease is present the sensitivity drops to 67%, and in patients in remission the sensitivity is between 32% and 40% (231). There is a good correlation between disease activity and c-ANCA titer (232). However, c-ANCA titers may persist in up to 40% of patients even after complete clinical remissions have been achieved. The antigen for the Wegener's granulomatosis-

TABLE 12.5. CHARACTERISTIC FEATURES OF ORGAN SYSTEM INVOLVEMENT IN WEGENER'S GRANULOMATOSIS

Organ System	Approximate Frequency %	Typical Features
Nasopharynx	75	Necrotizing granulomas with ulceration, saddle nose deformity
Paranasal	90	Parasinusitis, necrotizing granulomas, secondary bacterial infection
Eyes	60	Keratoconjunctivitis, granulomatous sclerouveitis
Ears	35	Serous otitis media, secondary bacterial infection
Lungs	95	Multiple nodular cavitary infiltrates, necrotizing granulomatous vasculitis
Kidney	85	Focal and segmental glomerulitis, necrotizing glomerulonephritis (later in course)
Heart	15	Coronary vasculitis, pericarditis
Nervous system	20	Mononeuritis multiplex, cranial neuritis
Skin	40	Dermal vasculitis with secondary ulcerations
Joints	50	Polyarthralgias

Source: Wolff SM, Fauci AS, Horn RG, et al. Wegener's granulomatosis. *Ann Intern Med* 1974;81:513–525; and Fauci AS, Wolff SM. Wegener's granulomatosis and related diseases. *Dis Mon* 1977;23:1–36.

specific c-ANCA is a 29-kd molecule found in the azurophilic granules of human neutrophils (proteinase-3) (233). A second antibody, reacting to the myeloperoxidase, forms a perinuclear pattern (p-ANCA) by immunofluorescence. p-ANCA occurs in a wide range of necrotizing vasculitides such as Churg-Strauss syndrome, polyarteritis nodosa with visceral involvement, and crescentic glomerulonephritis (232).

The etiology of WG remains unknown, although antineutrophilic cytoplasmic antibodies (ANCAs) are thought to play a role in the pathogenesis of this disease (234). Many research groups are attempting to create an animal model of ANCA-induced disease that might resemble human autoimmune diseases such as WG (235).

Chest Radiographic Manifestations

The pulmonary infiltrates of Wegener's granulomatosis are heterogeneous and may be of any size, shape, or lobar location (92,198–203,211,212,215–223). The most characteristic patterns (although not the most common) are solitary or multiple nodular densities or infiltrates, either poorly defined or sharply circumscribed (Figs. 12.6 and 12.7) (198). These opacities vary in size from less than 1 cm to greater than 9 cm, and occasionally air-fluid levels are found (198,216,217). The infiltrates may be quite transient, with one disappearing in one lung field and another appearing in a different location (217).

Atypical radiographic manifestations of WG include focal areas of collapsed lung adjacent to infiltrates, and mediastinal lymph node enlargement (217,218). The combination of hilar and mediastinal adenopathy on the chest radiograph should suggest an alternative diagnosis. Other occasional signs include bronchopleural fistula; narrow areas

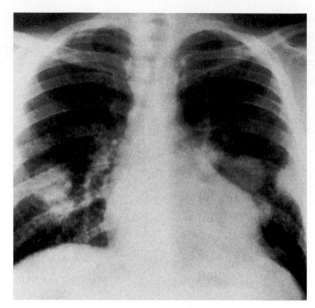

FIGURE 12.7. Wegener's granulomatosis. PA chest radiograph shows multiple large bilateral lung nodules. No cavitation, adenopathy, or pleural effusion is present.

in the larger airways, which may lead to lobar collapse; and pleural thickening and pleural effusions (92,216,219).

Diagnosis and Pathologic Findings

An important aspect of Wegener's granulomatosis is its pathologic and clinical similarity to a variety of other disorders characterized by granulomatous inflammation, vasculitis, or both (198,201,211). These include disorders such as polyarteritis nodosa; hypersensitivity vasculitis; the spectrum of connective tissue diseases; granulomatous diseases, such as sarcoidosis and midline granuloma; mixed granulomatous and vasculitis diseases, such as allergic granulomatosis; infectious granulomatous diseases, such as tuberculosis, leprosy, and fungal disease; Goodpasture's syndrome; and a variety of neoplasms accompanied by a granulomatous or vasculitic inflammatory response (201). The diagnosis of Wegener's granulomatosis is established when typical pathologic features accompany a characteristic clinical syndrome (226). The American College of Rheumatology criteria for WG include the presence of vasculitis (tissue or angiographically demonstrated) and any two of the following four findings: (*a*) painful or painless oral ulcers, or purulent or bloody nasal discharge; (*b*) chest radiograph showing the presence of nodules, fixed infiltrates, or cavities; (*c*) microhematuria (more than five red blood cells per high-power field) or red cell casts in urine sediment; (*d*) histologic changes showing granulomatous inflammation within the wall of an artery or in the perivascular or extravascular area (235). These criteria have an 88% sensitivity and 92% specificity in recognizing WG (235). Although c-ANCA was not used

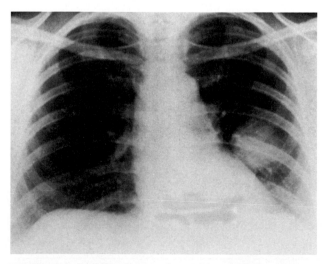

FIGURE 12.6. Wegener's granulomatosis. PA chest radiograph shows bibasilar lung nodules.

in developing these criteria, the presence of this highly specific, moderately sensitive marker of Wegener's granulomatosis may obviate the need for histologic confirmation (226,236).

Lung biopsy (open or thoracoscopic) is the procedure of choice for histologic confirmation of WG. This method has the added advantage of making specimens available to rule out infectious diseases. Transbronchial biopsies establish a diagnosis in less than 10% or cases owing to small sample size. The outstanding pathologic feature in all cases is the presence of inflammatory masses (0.5 to 5 cm) within the parenchyma of one or both lungs (224). Generally, the masses are few and sharply circumscribed on gross examination. Microscopically, they consist of necrotic areas surrounded by zones of granulation tissue. The earliest lesion in the kidney is a focal and segmental glomerulitis (201,225). If not treated properly, the lesions progress to a fulminant, necrotizing, and proliferative glomerulonephritis and eventually can lead to renal failure. At very early stages, glomerulitis may go undetected because the urinary sediment and renal function may be normal. Therefore, percutaneous renal biopsies are recommended when there is a high index of suspicion of WG, even when the urinary sediment is normal (201). Renal biopsies not only aid in establishing a diagnosis but also serve to monitor response to therapy as measured by subsequent biopsies.

Treatment and Prognosis

Untreated, Wegener's granulomatosis pursues a rapidly fatal course, with a mean survival time of 5 months in most cases (211,237,238). Eighty-two percent of patients die within 1 year and more than 90% within 2 years. Although corticosteroids increase mean survival to 12 months, the long-term prognosis is not significantly altered by this therapy, especially in patients with clinically apparent renal disease.

Although prospective, randomized trials have not been performed in treating Wegener's granulomatosis, oral cyclophosphamide plus corticosteroids is the mainstay of treatment (92,198,199,201,203,209,211,213,226). Fauci reported a complete remission in 79 of 85 patients (93%) using cyclophosphamide (211). The drug is administered orally or, in cases of rapidly progressive disease, intravenously. A clinical response is usually seen after 1 to 3 weeks of therapy. The dose of cyclophosphamide must be monitored continually and adjusted to keep the white blood cell count above 3000 cells/mm^3 (92,199,209,211). In patients who cannot tolerate cyclophosphamide because of severe leukopenia or hemorrhagic cystitis, or in young women who are not willing to accept the ovarian damage associated with cyclophosphamide, azathioprine and methotrexate are alternative agents (92,199). Recent evidence has suggested that milder cases or those limited to the lung involvement may be treated effectively with methotrexate (236). A recent study from the National Institutes of Health cited favorable responses in 35 of 42 patients with non–life-threatening WG treated with oral methotrexate (mean dose 20 mg/week) plus prednisone (1 mg/kg per day, with gradual taper) (239).

In 1985, De Remee et al. described improvement in 11 of 12 patients with WG treated with trimethoprim-sulfamethoxazole (T/S) (240). Since then the use of this agent in WG has been reported in additional patients, including 31 patients unresponsive to standard therapy (241). Twenty-six patients responded and five remained unresponsive to therapy. The role of this therapy for early limited disease, as an adjunct in generalized disease, or as maintenance therapy during remission for prevention of relapses, has yet to be elucidated (226). A recent study randomized patients with WG that had achieved complete remission with prednisone and cyclophosphamide to receive either (T/S) one double strength twice daily or placebo for 24 months in addition to their conventional therapy. Interestingly, there was an 18% relapse in the T/S group compared to 40% in the placebo (242).

Lymphomatoid Granulomatosis

Lymphomatoid granulomatosis (LYG) is a systemic disease characterized by an angiocentric, angiodestructive, and lymphoreticular granulomatous vasculitis, primarily of the lungs but also frequently involving the kidneys (45%), skin (45%), and central nervous system (20%) (92,205,209, 221,222,242,243). Although any organ system can be involved, the spleen, lymph nodes, and bone marrow usually are spared. This disorder resembles an indolent lymphoma, and in many instances it progresses to an atypical disseminated lymphoproliferative disease (92,221,242,243). LYG has been described as a late complication of Epstein-Barr viral infection (244,245). The cellular infiltrates are mixed, demonstrating normal as well as atypical lymphocytes, plasmacytoid cells, and cells apparently of reticuloendothelial origin (92,244).

Clinicopathologic Features

The male to female ratio is about 2:1, and most patients are in early middle age (221,243). Lung involvement is a sine qua non of LYG and is usually manifested as multiple pulmonary infiltrates of various sizes that tend to cavitate (92,203,221,242,243). Most patients present with chest symptoms (cough and shortness of breath) or systemic complaints (fever, weight loss, malaise) or both. Upper airway disease is uncommon in LYG (226). The skin and central nervous system are the two most common extrathoracic sites of involvement. Skin lesions occur in 30% to 50% of patients. A papular erythematous rash is typical, but painful and sometimes ulcerative nodules may develop. Central nervous system involvement occurs in 30% of patients and is usually manifested by signs and symptoms of a mass lesion (226–242).

There is no striking pattern of laboratory abnormalities. Most patients have a normal or only slightly reduced hematocrit. In the series of Katzenstein and coworkers, the presenting leukocyte count was normal in 50%, elevated in 30% (range, 9,000 to 38,000), and reduced in 20% (range, 1,200 to 3,900) (170). A relative lymphocytopenia was noted in 33% and lymphocytosis in 6%. Serum immunoglobulins were normal in 53% of cases, and nonspecific increases, usually in IgG or IgM, were seen in the remainder (242).

Chest Radiographic Manifestations

The chest radiographic manifestations of lymphomatoid granulomatosis depend in part on the duration of the disease. Lesions may appear and disappear without relation to therapy, as also occurs in Wegener's granulomatosis (92,199,203,221). The pulmonary lesions predominate in the lower lung fields peripherally and are usually bilateral (Fig. 12.8) (221). Typically, the early lesions present as multiple, bilateral, ill-defined densities (220). Later, they become better defined and resemble nodular metastases of various malignancies.

Diagnosis and Pathologic Findings

The definitive diagnosis of lymphomatoid granulomatosis is made histologically. Plasma cells, lymphocytic cells, and large "atypical" mononuclear cells in various stages of maturity infiltrating perivascular tissue are characteristic (246). Occlusion by infiltration of the vessels and subsequent tissue

necrosis are frequent findings. With peripheral nerve involvement, the infiltrate is seen surrounding the nerve, and spotty demyelination is present. When the skin is involved, small-vessel destruction with a lymphoreticular infiltrate is most often seen surrounding the dermal appendages.

This disorder is often confused clinically with Wegener's granulomatosis. However, granulomata are less copious and less distinct, and the vasculitis is remarkable in that it is not the characteristic leukocytoclastic or fibrinoid necrotic type seen in WG and other systemic vasculitides (205). In contrast, there is an angiotrophic invasion of blood vessels of various sizes with a bizarre cellular infiltrate. Blood supply through the involved vessels is compromised, and infarction and necrosis occur as in other vasculitides.

In addition to its characteristic histopathologic features, lymphomatoid granulomatosis differs from Wegener's granulomatosis in several other ways (209,210). As stated previously, sinus and upper airway involvement is unusual in lymphomatoid granulomatosis (201,221,225,243). In addition, renal involvement in lymphomatoid granulomatosis takes the form of a diffuse nodular infiltrate of the renal parenchyma with a characteristic cellular infiltrate, in contrast to the necrotizing glomerulonephritis seen in Wegener's granulomatosis. Leukopenia and anergy before therapy are rare in patients with WG but are seen frequently in lymphomatoid granulomatosis; the erythrocyte sedimentation rate may be normal or only mildly elevated in patients with active disease (198,199,213,226).

Etiology and Pathogenesis

The etiology of lymphomatoid granulomatosis is unknown. It may be an acquired abnormality of the lymphocyte in a

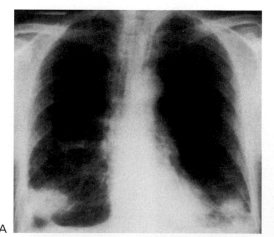 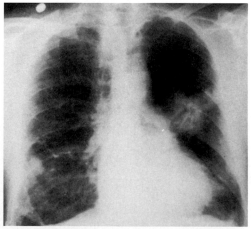

FIGURE 12.8. Lymphomatoid granulomatosis. **A:** PA chest radiograph shows bibasilar lung nodules. **B:** PA chest radiograph 2½ years later, after therapy with corticosteroids and chlorambucil, shows clearing of the bibasilar densities and appearance of at least two new lesions, one in the left midlung zone, the other in the lower third of the right lung. The left-sided lesion contains an air bronchogram. Open lung biopsy of the new, large left lung mass revealed lymphoma.

susceptible host, as is Sjögren's syndrome. Evidence for this includes absent delayed hypersensitivity, as demonstrated by nonreactivity to skin test antigens and the response of the lung lesions to corticosteroids (246). Like Sjögren's syndrome, lymphomatoid granulomatosis can terminate in a neoplastic disease (Fig. 12.8) (243,246). In fact, Colby and Carrington classified lymphomatoid granulomatosis as a malignant lymphoma (247).

Other diseases, such as lymphoma and mycosis fungoides, can have years of symptoms, with a biopsy showing nonspecific lymphoid and plasma cell infiltrates, before they assume the unusual features of neoplastic disease. Renal homotransplantation can be followed by lymphoreticular proliferation with involvement of the central nervous system (248–250). Antigenic exposure in an immunosuppressed host may alter the cell membrane and produce an autoimmune disease (243). Neoplastic disease may result with continued immunosuppression (251).

Therapy and Prognosis

Untreated, lymphomatoid granulomatosis is usually rapidly progressive and fatal (210). Death is often related to pulmonary or central nervous system complications (243). Preliminary reports indicate that a relatively high rate of long-term remissions (54%) can be achieved if patients are treated early with cyclophosphamide and corticosteroids in the same regimen used for Wegener's granulomatosis (199, 209,210,252).

Allergic Angiitis and Granulomatosis (Churg-Strauss Syndrome)

Churg and Strauss in 1951 and Rose and Spencer in 1957 described an uncommon granulomatous inflammation and vascular necrosis primarily involving the heart, lungs, skin, nervous system, and kidneys (205,209,210,253–255). This entity, commonly referred to as allergic angiitis and granulomatosis, occurs primarily in patients with an allergic background, often with asthma. Characteristically, high degrees of blood eosinophilia are found (255).

Clinicopathologic Features

In the 30 cases of the Churg-Strauss syndrome reported by Chumbley et al. 21 were men and nine were women (256). Ages ranged from 16 to 69 years; the average was 47 years. The mean duration of asthma was 8 years. It began at the same time as the manifestations of systemic vasculitis in six cases but preceded it in all others. Allergic rhinitis occurred in 21 of the 30 cases (70%). Most patients with Churg-Strauss syndrome have a fever at some point in their clinical course. Anemia and weight loss are common, as is leukocytosis. Both p-ANCA and c-ANCA may be positive. The elevation of the erythrocyte sedimentation rate and the degree of peripheral blood eosinophilia are good indicators of disease activity.

Chest Radiographic Manifestations

Chest radiographic abnormalities range from transient patchy densities to massive bilateral nodular infiltrates throughout the lung fields (257,258). New lesions may appear while older ones are disappearing; some remain stable after an initial period of improvement. Complete regression of a widespread active pulmonary process is sometimes seen with corticosteroids. Frequently, asthmatic symptoms recede as evidence of necrotizing vasculitis becomes prominent. The radiographic patterns are so varied that radiographic differential in this entity is not useful.

Diagnosis and Pathologic Findings

Histologically, the lung typically shows fibrinoid, necrotizing, and eosinophilic granulomatous lesions, which frequently involve the pulmonary arteries (258). In about half of their cases Churg and Strauss found parenchymal lesions in the form of an extensive pneumonic process involving septa and alveoli (253). In the acute stage, the exudate in the lungs had a predominance of eosinophilic leukocytes mixed with giant cells. Frequently, healing terminated in focal fibrosis. Histologic evidence of bronchial asthma (hyalinization of basement membrane, increased mucus secretion, and eosinophilic infiltration of the bronchial walls) was present in most cases but generally was not very marked (253).

Allergic granulomatosis (Churg-Strauss syndrome) strongly resembles classic polyarteritis nodosa, with some obviously distinguishing features (259). Churg-Strauss syndrome almost invariably is associated with an allergic diathesis, particularly severe asthma (199). Reports of the incidence of asthma with polyarteritis nodosa have ranged from 4% to as high as 54% (258). In general, unlike classic polyarteritis nodosa, in which pulmonary abnormalities are rare, lung involvement is invariable in Churg-Strauss syndrome. Also, this syndrome is characterized by high levels of peripheral eosinophilia (usually higher than $1500/mm^3$), eosinophilic tissue infiltration and granulomatous reactivity (254,256,257). In contrast, the predominant cellular infiltrate in polyarteritis nodosa is the polymorphonuclear leukocyte. In addition to the fibrinoid necrosis of small and medium-sized muscular arteries that is the hallmark of classic polyarteritis nodosa, a substantial degree of involvement of small vessels such as capillaries and venules is present in Churg-Strauss syndrome. Apart from these differences, the presentation, clinicopathologic manifestations, organ system involvement, and clinical course of these two syndromes are similar (199).

The "overlap" syndrome of the systemic vasculitides

combines many features that are characteristic of classic polyarteritis nodosa, other systemic vasculitides of the small- and medium-sized vessels, such as allergic angiitis and granulomatosis (Churg-Strauss syndrome), and the small-vessel hypersensitivity vasculitides (92,199,209,210). Large and small arteries, as well as capillaries and venules, may be involved in the vasculitic process. One patient may have features that would be considered characteristic or even pathognomonic of either classic polyarteritis nodosa or allergic granulomatosis. The overlap syndrome is a multisystem disease, with protean clinical manifestations. The same patient may have small-vessel involvement (arterioles, capillaries, and venules), as well as the classic small- and medium-sized muscular artery involvement with characteristic angiographic findings of small aneurysms. A history of allergy, peripheral eosinophilia, eosinophilic tissue infiltration, granulomatous reactions, and lung involvement described for Churg-Strauss syndrome may all be seen in the same patient, or one or more of these may be seen to the exclusion of the others (92,199). This syndrome is the most difficult to classify.

Recently, a Churg-Strauss-like disease process has been described in patients receiving leukotriene antagonists for the treatment of steroid-dependent asthma (260). It is controversial as to whether the disease process occurs because the steroid taper is allowing an underlying Churg-Strauss-like process to become exacerbated or as a consequence of the medication (260).

Therapy and Prognosis

Well-controlled experience with therapy for the Churg-Strauss syndrome is lacking. Chumbley and coworkers treated 27 of their 30 patients with prednisone; most received 40 to 60 mg daily, others 100 to 120 mg daily (256). Fifteen of these 30 patients died, three within a year after symptoms of vasculitis appeared. The interval from onset of signs and symptoms of vasculitis to death ranged from 6 months to 15 years; the average was 4.6 years. A recent prospective, randomized study failed to establish that plasma exchange adds to corticosteroids in preventing disease relapses (261). Cyclophosphamide and azathioprine therapy have theoretical rationale, because they are effective in treating another necrotizing vasculitis, Wegener's granulomatosis. Although experience with these agents is minimal, one prospective, randomized study showed that cyclophosphamide added to prednisone-plasma exchange therapy enhanced the relapse-free interval during long-term follow-up (262).

GOODPASTURE'S SYNDROME (ANTIGLOMERULAR BASEMENT MEMBRANE DISEASE)

Goodpasture's syndrome is characterized by pulmonary hemorrhage with hemoptysis, diffuse alveolar filling on the chest radiograph, anemia, and glomerulonephritis (often rapidly progressive) (263–271). Wilson and Dixon extended this definition to include the presence of antiglomerular basement membrane (anti-GBM) antibodies, which are found in most patients with Goodpasture's syndrome (265,266). Although the catalyst is unknown, production of these antibodies is usually self-limited, and the syndrome apparently is inactive when the antibody is not detected (266,269). Although the term Goodpasture's syndrome has gained wide popularity, to avoid confusion with a variety of other disorders (e.g., Wegener's granulomatosis and systemic lupus erythematosus) with similar clinical findings, Young has recommended using the term anti-GBM antibody disease (272). This latter term describes pulmonary hemorrhage, with or without associated glomerulonephritis, owing to circulating antibodies directed against basement membrane epitopes (272).

Clinicopathologic Features

Early reports on Goodpasture's syndrome indicated a marked male predominance of 9:1, but more recent studies describe lower male to female ratios of 3.5:1 and 2:1 (264). Seventy-five percent of patients are between the ages of 17 and 27 years at the onset of the illness, whereas the remainder range in age up to 75 years (264).

In most cases, the initial symptom is hemoptysis, which occurs at some point during the course of the disease in 99% of cases (206,207,263,264). Bouts of hemoptysis range in severity from slightly blood-streaked sputum to massive hemorrhage (263). In about one-fifth of the patients, upper respiratory tract infections of a nonspecific (viral) nature precede the appearance of the syndrome (263). Chills and fever occur acutely with pulmonary hemorrhage but are not otherwise prominent. Substernal chest pain occurs without relation to activity, although it can be aggravated by coughing.

Renal abnormalities may occur before pulmonary symptoms. Urinary findings, present on admission in over 80% of patients, include proteinuria, microscopic hematuria, and, less commonly, pyuria (263,264,266). In 26 (81%) of Wilson and Dixon's patients, renal failure requiring dialysis occurred within 1 to 14 months of onset (mean 3.5 months) (265).

Anemia is universally present early in the disease. The anemia is apparently not hemolytic, although a decreased erythrocyte life span has been demonstrated (263). Neither hemolysis nor jaundice is present.

Chest Radiographic Findings

The radiographic appearance of Goodpasture's syndrome is closely related to the distribution, volume, and temporal sequence of pulmonary hemorrhage. Both interstitial and alveolar involvement occur. Confluent densities are seen

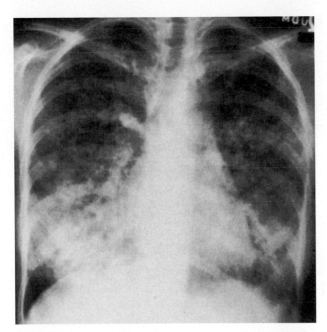

FIGURE 12.9. Goodpasture's syndrome. PA chest radiograph shows a characteristic alveolar filling pattern in a patient with hemoptysis and renal failure. The heart, pulmonary vascularity, and pleura are normal.

shortly after hemorrhage and may be indistinguishable from hypervolemia associated with azotemia or from noncardiogenic pulmonary edema of another origin (Fig. 12.9). All these conditions produce rapid alterations in the chest radiograph. Localized air space changes may progress to diffuse opacification within hours, whereas complete clearing may occur during remission. However, accentuated interstitial markings tend to persist in Goodpasture's syndrome after repeated episodes of bleeding owing to the presence of siderophages in the interstitium. If the bleeding is of sufficient duration, permanent reticulonodular infiltrates develop, resembling those seen in idiopathic pulmonary hemosiderosis. Generally these changes are diffuse, but they may be localized. The superimposition of fluffy alveolar densities on a reticulonodular background suggests recurrent pulmonary hemorrhage.

Goodpasture's syndrome demonstrates a predilection for perihilar involvement, whereas in contrast to the pulmonary venous congestion and edema of left ventricular failure, Kerley B lines, and pleural effusions are not characteristic.

Pulmonary Function Abnormalities

The diffusing capacity for carbon monoxide (D_{LCO}) may be useful in following the course of this disease (272,273). Because intraalveolar blood binds carbon monoxide, the D_{LCO} may be raised above baseline levels during lung hemorrhage (273). Thus, serial measurements of D_{LCO} may help

distinguish fresh pulmonary hemorrhage from other causes of radiographic opacities (e.g., infection) (272,273).

Diagnosis and Pathologic Findings

Diagnosis of Goodpasture's syndrome depends on the demonstration of circulating anti-GBM antibodies and/or the finding of linear deposits of immunoglobulin along glomerular or alveolar basement membranes (266,269,272,274). These findings are coupled with evidence of lung hemorrhage in a patient who typically presents with recurrent hemoptysis, dyspnea, and anemia (266,269). The erythrocyte sedimentation rate, although often slightly elevated, is usually not strikingly elevated as in most cases of systemic vasculitis (e.g., Wegener's granulomatosis) (272). The degree of renal injury is mirrored by elevations in serum creatinine and blood urea nitrogen, and active glomerulonephritis is almost always accompanied by proteinuria, hematuria (gross or microscopic), and red blood cell casts (272). Histologically, the renal abnormality in patients with Goodpasture's syndrome is an actively proliferating, often necrotizing, crescent-forming type of glomerulonephritis (266). This is accompanied by variable, probably secondary tubular alterations and interstitial infiltrative processes.

Etiology and Pathogenesis

The presence of antibodies is clearly involved in the glomerulonephritis and probably the pulmonary hemorrhage of Goodpasture's syndrome (206,209,266). The mechanism responsible for these antibodies, however, is not known, although environmental factors are thought to be instrumental in triggering their production (266,267). For example, antigens such as the influenza A2 virus might cause the production of antibodies that cross-react with the basement membrane structures (271). Many patients have a history of preceding viral syndromes, either of the upper respiratory tract or gastrointestinal tract. Infectious agents or chemical substances such as hydrocarbon solvents might uncover or alter some self-antigens so that they become immunogenic (265,275).

Therapy and Prognosis

The prognosis for Goodpasture's syndrome is generally poor (111,206,207,262,263,269,270). Patients die of either renal failure or lung hemorrhage. In Wilson and Dixon's study, in which the diagnosis was based on the presence of circulating anti-GBM antibodies, 28 of 32 patients developed renal failure and over half died within 1 year of diagnosis (265).

The most successful therapy includes plasmapheresis and treatment of the inflammatory response in tissues, and suppression of further antibody production through the use of corticosteroids and cyclophosphamide or azathioprine

(208,268,272,276–280). Because of the lack of controlled studies, the exact effects of this combined therapy are not clear. Because production of anti-GBM antibodies may be short-lived, plasma exchange should reduce damage to the glomerulus by lowering the levels of circulating anti-GBM antibody. Lockwood and coworkers reported on seven patients treated with plasma exchange, cytotoxic drugs, and corticosteroids (268). Renal function improved in three who were not already receiving dialysis at the initiation of therapy. Five patients had pulmonary hemorrhage that appeared to respond to therapy. These investigators reported that, although the fall in anti-GBM antibody titer was variable, there was also depletion of fibrinogen and complement. They believed that the reduction of the latter two substances could have been important therapeutically. Swainson and coworkers noted a rebound increase in anti-GBM antibody levels following periods of plasma exchange (279). They concluded that plasma exchange was only effective in substantially reducing the circulating amounts of complement or fibrinogen when performed on consecutive days. The rapid rise in concentrations after exchange reflects rapid turnover and distribution from extravascular pools. Plasma exchange is carried out every 1 to 3 days for 1 to 3 weeks, but the optimal frequency and duration have not been defined.

In general, plasma exchange may be useful in the early treatment of severe forms of Goodpasture's syndrome by controlling pulmonary hemorrhage and preventing irreversible renal damage from the high anti-GBM antibody levels. However, the removal of anti-GBM antibodies does not lead to recovery of renal function. Furthermore, there is considerable variation in the amount of reduction of anti-GBM levels in the serum produced by serial plasma exchange and immunosuppression.

IDIOPATHIC PULMONARY HEMOSIDEROSIS

Although it is likely that idiopathic pulmonary hemosiderosis (IPH) is a separate entity, its chest manifestations are identical to those of Goodpasture's syndrome. Both diseases are of unknown etiology and are characterized by repeated episodes of pulmonary hemorrhage, iron-deficiency anemia, and, in longstanding cases, pulmonary insufficiency. In contrast to IPH, Goodpasture's syndrome includes renal disease with circulating anti-GBM antibodies, in addition to the pulmonary manifestations (209,281–283).

IPH occurs most commonly in children, frequently below the age of 10 years; in this age group there is no sex predominance (283). When it develops in adults (and the incidence in adults appears to be increasing, especially in patients aged 40 years and more), it occurs twice as often in men as in women (282,284–287).

Clinicopathologic Features

The onset of IPH may be acute or insidious, with anemia, pallor, weakness, lethargy, and sometimes a dry cough; typical changes of air-space hemorrhage may be apparent radiographically without a clear-cut episode of hemoptysis (282). Rarely, patients present with unexplained iron-deficient hypochromic anemia without a history of hemoptysis. Fever may be present, possibly owing to elaboration of pyrogenic cytokines by pulmonary parenchymal cells (272).

Physical examination during an acute stage of pulmonary hemorrhage may reveal fine rales and dullness to percussion over the affected areas of lung. Liver, spleen, and lymph nodes are enlarged to palpation in 20% to 25% of cases.

Iron-deficiency anemia usually develops but may not be present when intrapulmonary hemorrhage is small, and it does not generally deplete the bone marrow iron stores. Serum iron and iron-binding capacity results are characteristic of iron-deficiency anemia, and it is generally agreed that hemolysis does not occur in this disease (282).

As in pulmonary hemorrhage of any cause, the DLCO may be increased (272). Other tests of pulmonary function may be normal initially, but may reveal a progressive restrictive ventilatory defect in chronic cases (272).

At the time of an acute episode of IPH, histologic material from the lungs reveals intraalveolar hemorrhage that may be extensive (288). Hemorrhage is typically confined to the peripheral air spaces; in fact, massive blood loss can occur into the lungs without hemoptysis, and the trachea and major bronchi may contain little or no blood. Sputum or lavage material may contain hemosiderin-laden macrophages. With repeated episodes of hemoptysis, interstitial fibrosis is present in most cases (283). The structural alteration of elastic fibers appears to be the consequence of intraalveolar bleeding rather than its cause; in fact, specimens of lung obtained by biopsy early in the course of the disease reveal morphologically normal elastic tissue (289). Alveolitis and alveolar necrosis are absent unless secondary pneumonia has been superimposed. In contrast to other syndromes considered to be immunologic, such as Wegener's granulomatosis, vasculitis is not an invariable pathologic feature of IPH and when present is usually minor (290,291).

IPH can be differentiated from Goodpasture's syndrome by the absence of renal disease, the absence of circulating anti-GBM antibodies, and the absence of an antigen-antibody reaction (i.e., the lack of antiglomerular basement membrane antibody on immunofluorescent staining of lung tissue) (292,293).

Chest Radiographic Findings

As mentioned, the changes apparent on the chest radiograph are identical in IPH and Goodpasture's syndrome. In the early stages, the pattern is one of diffuse mottled opacities characteristic of patchy air space consolidation throughout the lungs (282). An air bronchogram should be visualized in areas of major air space consolidation, and at this stage the radiographic pattern may simulate that of pulmonary edema.

During an acute episode, the fluffy deposits characteristic of acinar consolidation disappear within 2 to 3 days and are replaced by a reticular pattern whose distribution is identical to that of the air space disease (283,284). The appearance of the chest radiograph usually returns to normal about 10 to 12 days after the original acute episode (282).

With repeated similar episodes, increasing amounts of hemosiderin are deposited within interstitial tissue and there is progressive interstitial fibrosis. Thus, after subsequent fresh hemorrhage there is only partial clearing of the chest radiograph, which reveals a fine reticular pattern (282).

Diagnosis, Treatment, and Outcome

Although the diagnosis of IPH may be strongly suspected in young patients who manifest recurrent episodes of hemoptysis, iron-deficiency anemia, and the typical chest radiographic changes, definitive diagnosis may require lung biopsy. Examination of the sputum for hemosiderin-laden macrophages can provide supportive evidence. Lung biopsy specimens are obtained by transbronchial techniques or by limited thoracotomy.

The prognosis of IPH varies, with an interval from onset of symptoms until death of 2½ to 20 years (207,283,284). Remission can be permanent, with or without corticosteroid therapy and immunosuppressives such as azathioprine (272). To date, no therapy has been shown in a prospective, controlled trial to alter outcome.

PULMONARY ALVEOLAR PROTEINOSIS

Pulmonary alveolar proteinosis is a disease of unknown etiology characterized by accumulation of periodic acid-Schiff (PAS)-positive, lipid-rich, proteinaceous material in the distal air spaces of the lungs (294–304). Rosen, Castleman, and Liebow first described this entity in 1958 on the basis of human lung biopsies (304). Subsequent demonstrations that similar abnormalities could be produced in experimental animals by exposing them to a variety of dusts and fumes suggest that the disorder is a distinct but nonspecific response of pulmonary tissue to diverse inhaled injurious agents (296,305).

Clinicopathologic Features

Grossly, the lungs contain multiple, firm, yellow nodules ranging in size from several millimeters to 2 or 3 cm in diameter (297). Microscopically, large groups of alveoli and small distal bronchioles are filled with a granular, floccular

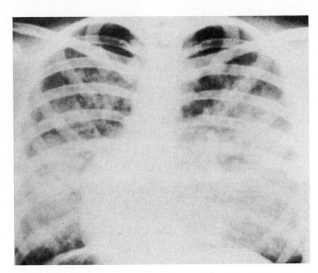

FIGURE 12.10. Pulmonary alveolar proteinosis. PA chest radiograph of a 21-year-old woman with a diffuse, bilateral alveolar filling process and a normal cardiac silhouette.

PAS-positive material (Figs. 12.10 and 12.11) (297,302). Generally, the alveolar walls are normal, but cellular infiltration and areas of fibrosis occur in the interstitial spaces of the lungs, particularly with longstanding disease (296–299). Electron microscopic examination of the proteinaceous material reveals alveolar macrophages that contain numerous lamellar osmiophilic inclusions within the cytoplasm. This lamellar material, rich in phospholipid, is found not only with macrophages but also lying free in amorphous debris in the alveolar spaces (296,297). The marked PAS positivity of this material is probably owing to the presence of large amounts of surfactant protein A, a heavily glycosylated surfactant constituent (306).

The age of onset is generally between 20 and 50 years,

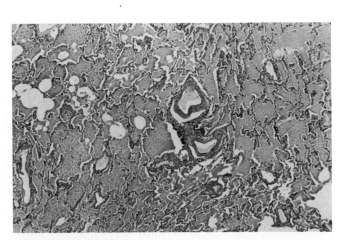

FIGURE 12.11. Pulmonary alveolar proteinosis. Open lung biopsy reveals diffuse alveolar flooding with a granular-like material that stained PAS positive. Note that the alveolar walls are relatively normal.

but the disorder also occurs in infants and the elderly (295,298,301–303,306). There is a male preponderance of greater than 3:1. Many, but not all, patients have been exposed to a variety of dusts and fumes, such as wood dust and silica (296). The onset is usually gradual and insidious, but occasionally the disorder follows an acute febrile illness. Dyspnea during exertion is characteristically the first manifestation, gradually evolving into a dyspnea at rest. Cough is common and is often associated with the production of a thick, white to yellow sputum. In those with extensive lung involvement, fatigability, and weight loss are common. Chest pain and hemoptysis are unusual.

Abnormal physical findings are few. The resonance of the percussion note over the thorax is diminished, and breath sounds have a coarse bronchovesicular quality; coarse crackles are audible over affected areas. Fingers and toes become clubbed in some patients (298).

There are no distinctive hematologic abnormalities associated with pulmonary alveolar proteinosis. Anemia does not occur; in fact, erythrocythemia may result if hypoxemia is severe. Leukocyte counts vary from normal to a brisk leukocytosis (i.e., to as high as 15,000 to 20,000 cells/mm³); this usually signifies the coexistence of an acute pulmonary infection. Hyperlipidemia, hyperglobulinemia, and elevated serum lactic dehydrogenase levels occur in some patients with pulmonary alveolar proteinosis (295,298,301–303).

Pulmonary function tests characteristically show a restrictive ventilatory pattern (224,226). The accumulation of the proteinaceous material in the air spaces reduces the number of functioning lung units, thereby altering the overall pressure–volume relationships of the lung and causing pulmonary compliance to decrease (296). The vital capacity, residual volume, and functional residual capacity are all proportionally reduced. Flow rates are usually normal during a forced expiratory maneuver (295).

Marked ventilation-perfusion ratio abnormalities occur in pulmonary alveolar proteinosis. Many areas of lung are perfused with mixed venous blood but receive little or no ventilation. As a result, the alveolar-arterial difference for oxygen widens, and arterial hypoxemia is prominent. Moreover, because abnormal material in the alveolar spaces effectively amputates some gas-exchange surface and interferes with gas transfer across the alveolar axillary membrane, the D$_{LCO}$ is reduced and a fall in arterial oxygen saturation can be demonstrated regularly during exercise (306). Moreover, in most cases a shunt fraction greater than 17% is demonstrated while the patient is breathing 100% oxygen (306).

Serum laboratory values are usually within normal limits except for an elevation in the serum lactic dehydrogenase (LDH) level (306,307). In fact, the combination of an elevated shunt fraction and an elevated serum LDH level suggests the diagnosis of pulmonary alveolar proteinosis (306). Of note, elevated serum LDH levels are also found in *Pneumocystis carinii* pneumonia.

Chest Radiographic Findings

The chest radiograph shows a diffuse alveolar filling process characterized by scattered patchy, confluent, nodular infiltrates (Fig. 12.10) (301–303). The pattern and distribution are similar to those of cardiogenic pulmonary edema, except that the cardiac silhouette is usually normal in alveolar proteinosis and the alveolar filling pattern resembles a bat wing (306). The involvement is usually bilateral and symmetrical, but asymmetrical or unilateral patterns are seen occasionally. Hilar adenopathy, Kerley's B lines, and pleural effusions do not occur (295,306).

Diagnosis

Based on clinical, functional, and chest radiographic findings (i.e., dyspnea, diffuse alveolar filling on chest radiograph, elevated serum LDH level, and arterial hypoxemia with an increased shunt fraction), a presumptive diagnosis can often be made (306). Bronchoalveolar lavage fluid demonstrates a thick opaque, milky effluent that sediments into multiple layers. However, definitive diagnosis is generally established by histologic examination of a lung biopsy obtained at bronchoscopy or thoracotomy (300,301). The diagnosis has also been made by the demonstration of PAS-positive material on light microscopic examination of sputum or lung washings. Electron microscopy of sputum or lung washings is also useful diagnostically by revealing granular material and lamellar bodies (308–311). Findings on light microscopy and the clinical presentation can be confused with those of *P. carinii* infection; a methenamine-silver stain is needed to exclude this possibility. Secondary PAP (pseudo-PAP) may complicate hematological malignancies and chronic infections.

Course and Treatment

Spontaneous recovery with complete resolution of clinical findings and chest radiographic changes occurs in about 25% of patients with pulmonary alveolar proteinosis (295,298,301–303,306). In others, the disorder is progressive, although the rate of progression is variable. In about 15% to 20% of patients, this disease runs a rapid, fulminant course with marked arterial hypoxemia, cor pulmonale, and respiratory failure. In others, progression is over months to years, and in some patients with longstanding disease, interstitial fibrosis develops.

Pulmonary infections with mycotic organisms are common in alveolar proteinosis, which suggests impaired lung defenses. In fact, the alveolar macrophage, the principal cellular defense against intracellular organisms, has been found to be defective in this disease (296,312,313). The most frequently encountered infections are nocardiosis, cryptococcosis, aspergillosis, and mucormycosis (301–303).

The management of pulmonary alveolar proteinosis is

made difficult by the fact that many patients improve spontaneously, which renders therapeutic intervention difficult to assess (314). Moreover, there have been no properly controlled studies of therapy in this disease. Corticosteroids are of no proven benefit. A few patients appear to improve following administration of agents that presumably thin or liquefy bronchial secretions (e.g., potassium iodide, aerosolized streptokinase-streptodornase, trypsin, and a combination of saline, heparin, and acetylcysteine delivered by intermittent positive-pressure breathing).

In patients with advanced disease and severe ventilatory compromise, lavage of an entire lung with large volumes of a saline solution has been proposed (306,315). The procedure is performed under general anesthesia. The airway is intubated with a double-lumen bronchospirometric tube, and mechanical ventilation is instituted with a high inspired oxygen concentration. The details of the procedure have been described at length (316). Usually amelioration of symptoms, with improvement in pulmonary function, begins within hours after lavage, and by 24 to 48 hours pulmonary function and arterial PO$_2$ exceed prelavage levels.

DRUG-INDUCED PULMONARY DISEASE

The development of antibiotics, cytotoxic antineoplastic agents, and various immunosuppressive drugs has had a remarkable impact on medical therapeutics and has made control of infection, cancer, collagen-vascular diseases, and organ transplant rejection everyday realities in medicine. One undesirable byproduct of drug therapy, albeit a rather minor one in the overall scheme, is related to iatrogenic and adverse complications of their use. Development of an allergy to drugs is common, and specific drug-induced pulmonary reactions occur frequently. In fact, almost every therapeutic agent used has (or may have) been noted to cause pulmonary disease; the lists compiled are impressive (317–330). A list of some of these drugs is provided in Table 12.6; the antineoplastic chemotherapy drugs and immunosuppressants are the most prominent offenders (331–340). Occasionally, lung toxicity results from a very commonly used drug such as hydrochlorothiazide or from an antibiotic such as nitrofurantoin, penicillin, or a sulfonamide drug (322,331).

The host reaction often seems to be a hypersensitivity one, for contact with the drug may eventually cause sensitization to occur. Subsequently, an immune response develops in the form of antibody or an exaggerated lymphocytic mitogenic response when the host is challenged with the offending drug antigen. However, the precise mechanisms are poorly understood, and for this reason experimental models have been difficult to develop, except for bleomycin, discussed in the following.

Most drugs are organic compounds of low molecular weight (less than 1,000). To become "antigenic" they must couple to larger carrier substances, which are usually serum proteins; in the process of drug-protein binding, the structure of the protein is denatured in that its tertiary molecular configuration is altered. The immune response that is elicited, however, is usually directed to the drug determinant, although a metabolite of the drug might be the actual antigen. Because the antigenic form is usually not known, this complicates selection of the correct metabolite to use in assaying the reaction *in vitro* or to use in an experimental model. Most of the drug reactions that affect the lung do not elicit IgE-antibody or cause a type 1 immediate hypersensitivity reaction as they do in other reactions, for example to penicillin, in which immediate or accelerated allergic reactions occur. Although asthmatic symptoms can be severe, it is the insidious onset of cough and dyspnea that characterizes most of the reactions caused by the drugs listed in Table 12.6.

Principal emphasis will be given to pulmonary disease caused by cytotoxic, immunosuppressive drugs, because the clinical setting of patients receiving them is complicated and the specific effect of drug toxicity is often difficult to factor out (318,321,332,333). Pulmonary infection (often with nosocomial or opportunistic microorganisms), radiation therapy to the thorax and lung, or progression of the disease under treatment can confuse and compound the issue of drug toxicity. For example, gold or penicillamine, both of which can cause interstitial lung injury, may be used to treat patients with rheumatoid arthritis, a disease with a 0 to 15% incidence of associated interstitial pulmonary fibrosis; whether disease progression or concomitant pulmonary drug toxicity is responsible may be difficult to decide (334,335). Moreover, a latent period may occur between the cessation of drug therapy and the onset of pulmonary symptoms that are in retrospect attributed to a toxic drug effect. A period of months to perhaps years, as noted with busulfan use, may elapse before the untoward drug reaction is evident (320,321,333).

Gradual development of shortness of breath and a nagging, dry, nonproductive cough are characteristic complaints of most patients with drug-related pulmonary disease (320,321). Tachypnea and lung crackles may be found on physical examination. The connection between the drug and the symptoms may be overlooked if the patient has progressive signs of the primary lung disease process or a systemic disease. Subtle development of congestive heart failure may occur from use of potentially myotoxic drugs such as adriamycin, now used frequently in multiple-agent chemotherapy protocols. Chest radiographic abnormalities are not usually noted until the patient experiences respiratory symptoms; then, diffuse linear densities and streaks occur, predominantly in the lower lung zones. The chest radiograph may have an appearance similar to those characteristic of the group of interstitial diseases (Table 12.1). However, certain drug-induced pulmonary reactions have

TABLE 12.6. DRUGS OR DRUG GROUPS THAT CAUSE PULMONARY REACTIONS

Drug	Syndrome(s)[a]	Frequency
CYTOTOXIC DRUGS		
Azathioprine	HP	<1%
Bleomycin	PF, NPE, HP, AP	3% to 25% (PF)
Busulfan	PF	<1%
Carmustine	PF, AP	10% to 30%
Cyclophosphamide	PF, NPE, HP	<1%
Cytosine arabinoside	NPE	<1%
Methotrexate	HP, NPE, PF, pleuritis	7% (HP)
Mitomycin	PF, AP	3% to 12%
Procarbazine	HP	<1%
Vinca alkaloids[b]	AP	20% to 40%
NONCYTOTOXIC DRUGS		
Amiodarone	PF, NPE, AP	6% to 15%
Aspirin	NPE,[c] bronchospasm	22%[c] (NPE)
β-Adrenergic blockers	Bronchospasm	Variable
Bromocriptine	PF, pleuritis	<1%
Captopril	Cough	10%
Carbachol	Bronchospasm	<1%
Carbamazepine	HP	<1%
Chlorambucil	PF	<1%
Chlordiazepoxide	NPE[c]	<1%
Dantrolene	Pleuritis	<1%
Diphenylhydantoin	HP	<1%
Enalapril	Cough	10% to 20%
Ethchlorvynol	NPE[c]	<1%
Gold salts	HP, PF, BO	<1%
Hydrochlorothiazide	NPE	<1%
Lidocaine	NPE	<1%
Methysergide	Pleuritis	<1%
Naloxone	NPE	<1%
Neuromuscular blocking agents	Bronchospasm	<1%
Nitrofurantoin	HP, PF	<1%
Nonsteroidal anti-inflammatory agents	Bronchospasm, HP	4% to 20%
Opiates	NPE	<1%
Penicillamine	BO, PRS, PF, HP	<1%
Protamine	NPE	<1%
Pyrimethamine-chloroquine	HP	<1%
Pyrimethamine-dapsone	HP	<1%
Sulfasalazine	PF, HP, BO	<1%
Tocolytic agents	NPE	<1%
Tocainide	PF, NPE	<1%

[a] PF, pulmonary fibrosis; HP, hypersensitivity pneumonitis; BO, bronchiolitis obliterans; NPE, noncardiogenic pulmonary edema; PRS, pulmonary renal syndrome; AP, acute pneumonitis.
[b] Not as single agent, in conjunction with mitomycin only.
[c] Overdose only.
Source: Cooper JA Jr. Drug-related pulmonary diseases. In Bone RC, Dantzker DR, George RB, et al. eds. *Pulmonary and critical care medicine,* vol 2. Chicago: Mosby-Year Book, 1993:1–9.

individual features that can heighten one's suspicion that they are causative or contributing to lung symptoms.

Cytotoxic Agents

Bleomycin, a mixture of glycopeptides isolated from *Strepto-myces verticillus,* is a versatile and effective drug used against squamous cell carcinoma, malignant lymphomas, and testicular tumors and is a popular drug to include in multiple-agent regimens (320,321). It is a rather predictable cause of interstitial pulmonary fibrosis, and for this reason it has provided one of the best experimental models of this disease. Toxicity correlates with the total dose of bleomycin given, for significant drug-related pulmonary illness is infrequent (less than 10%) if the cumulative dose is less than 150 to 200 mg; for doses of more than 300 to 500 mg, toxicity may approach 50% with approximately 10% mortality (336). Several factors seem to enhance pulmonary toxicity from bleomycin, and these should alert the physician to expect complications. Older people have more toxicity. Simultaneous administration of bleomycin and thoracic radiation increases the likelihood of toxicity, which also occurs at a lower cumulative dose of the drug. Prior use of radiation also increases the risk. Administration of high oxygen concentrations produces synergistic toxicity with bleomycin, and a fulminant form of interstitial pneumonitis and fibrosis can develop. Oxygen given during surgical procedures seems sufficient to trigger the response. Patients with esophageal carcinoma who have received radiation and bleomycin therapy and undergo subsequent surgery are at high risk to develop lung toxicity (337).

Whereas interstitial fibrosis is the usual manifestation of pulmonary toxicity, an apparent hypersensitivity form of toxicity can develop that is more amenable to improvement with corticosteroid therapy than the fibrotic form (338). Finally, the route of bleomycin administration accounts for a striking difference in lung susceptibility to injury. In experimental animals, a single intratracheal dose may cause a progressive form of pulmonary fibrosis to develop (339). In contrast, if the drug is given parenterally, much larger and repetitive doses can be tolerated; in fact, continuous intravenous administration of the drug in low doses may lower the incidence of toxicity somewhat. Pulmonary functional abnormalities generally include arterial hypoxemia and a restrictive ventilatory pattern with decreased lung volumes and a diminished diffusing capacity for carbon monoxide (320,321,336).

The lung response to the three cytotoxic agents busulfan, cyclophosphamide, and methotrexate shows similarities and is different from other forms of pulmonary toxicity. A considerable latent period may occur before pulmonary symptoms suggesting toxicity develop; often the patient is under treatment for a hematologic malignancy, and several years of rather stable drug usage may have elapsed before toxicity appears for inapparent reasons. Cough, dyspnea, and fever set in and the chest radiograph may show a combined alveolar filling and interstitial pattern and occasionally a pleural effusion. The troublesome differential is that of a drug reaction versus a leukemic infiltration of the lung, and an opportunistic infection may be present as well. The onset of illness in patients taking methotrexate can be quite variable, occurring within a few days of beginning therapy or after a latent period; the dosage of drug per week may be an important determinant of this illness (320). Bleomycin may also cause nodular lesions and the pathology in these circumstances can disclose BOOP. In all these drug reactions fever is an important part of the toxic syndrome. Sputum or bronchial washings may yield unusual-appearing type II pneumocytes that can be identified by cytology and are characteristic of these particular drug-induced toxic pulmonary reactions. Histopathologic features of cytotoxic lung disease include type II pneumocyte proliferation, macrophage infiltration of the interstitium, and fibrosis.

Mitomycin can cause chronic interstitial fibrosis in a pattern similar to bleomycin. Rarely, mitomycin C can cause a syndrome characterized by noncardiogenic pulmonary edema, vasculopathy, microangiopathic hemolytic anemia, and acute renal failure.

Noncytotoxic Agents

Amiodarone, a powerful antiarrhythmic agent, causes lung disease in between 4% and 27% of patients (326). Pulmonary fibrosis and hypersensitivity or acute pneumonitis can be induced by this drug. A major risk factor is a maintenance dose(s) of more than 400 mg/day. Diffuse reticular infiltrates are most commonly seen on the chest radiograph, although diffuse acinar infiltrates have also been described (326). HRCT scans demonstrate localized or diffuse areas of very high attenuation that can be highly characteristic of amiodarone toxicity (341). A restrictive ventilatory defect with a diffusion impairment is the most common physiologic abnormality (342). The D$_{LCO}$ is highly sensitive for amiodarone toxicity (320). Moreover, a D$_{LCO}$ greater than 80% of pretreatment level virtually excludes amiodarone toxicity (342). The major histologic is abundant, intraalveolar "foamy" macrophages. Amiodarone inhibits phospholipases leading to accumulation of lamellar inclusions that can be demonstrated by electron microscopy. However, foamy macrophages can be seen in patients without clinical evidence of lung disease; thus, their presence does not confirm toxicity. Discontinuation of the drug or reduction in drug dosage in conjunction with corticosteroid therapy can reduce the pulmonary disease. Recovery may be slow owing to the prolonged half-life (greater than 1 month) (326,342).

The antibiotic nitrofurantoin is one of the most widely recognized drugs causing pulmonary toxicity (317,320, 322,340). The acute onset of fever, chills, cough, and dyspnea can occur after a few days of therapy or within a few hours of the first dose in patients who have received the drug on previous occasions. Blood eosinophilia is likely and the symptom complex points to an allergic or hypersensitivity-type lung reaction, although the response has not been well characterized histologically. The pulmonary response seems to be one of pulmonary edema, with diffuse crackles heard in the lungs. A chest radiograph supports the impression of noncardiogenic pulmonary edema. Pleural effusion may be noted. The reaction clears within 48 hours after discontinuing the drug; the disease is self-limited without mortality. Episodes of recurrent pneumonia can occur if the patient resumes use of the drug. To conclusively prove the drug–disease relationship, a challenge dose will elicit the reaction. A chronic form of nitrofurantoin disease can occur that does not include fever, pleural effusion, and eosinophilia but rather an insidious onset of cough and dyspnea months after the drug has been taken on a regular basis, usually for suppression of chronic bacteriuria. In this form, the lung disease is virtually indistinguishable from interstitial pneumonitis and fibrosis. Discontinuance of the drug plus corticosteroid therapy will arrests the process.

Interstitial pulmonary fibrosis has been described following the treatment of prostate cancer with the antiestrogen medications leuprolide and nilutamide. Progressive disease can usually be avoided with cessation of therapy and institution of corticosteroids (343).

A variety of drugs are known to induce systemic lupus erythematosus; among the more than 20 drugs incriminated, procainamide, hydralazine, diphenylhydantoin, and sulfonamides are among the ones most frequently encountered (112,317,320,322). Drug-induced SLE differs from the spontaneous disease in that there is less kidney and skin involvement and more pleuropulmonary reaction. Antihistone antibodies are frequently positive. The lung reaction and the entire syndrome remit if the causative drug is discontinued.

SARCOIDOSIS

Sarcoidosis remains one of the most enigmatic diseases in the field of internal medicine. It occurs frequently, is variable in its severity, can affect multiple organs but has a propensity to involve the respiratory tract initially, and remains of unknown cause (344,345). Pulmonary sarcoidosis is often a clinical diagnosis made from the clinical presentation and compatible chest radiographic pattern; laboratory studies and tissue histology are obtained to confirm and support the diagnosis. It is also a diagnosis of exclusion after such diseases as lymphoma, bronchogenic carcinoma, beryllium exposure, tuberculosis, histoplasmosis, and coccidioidomycosis have been eliminated, because each may mimic the clinical picture and the tissue histology of sarcoidosis.

Sarcoidosis was once stereotyped as a disease that was considered to usually affect young African-American people, often women, who lived in rural parts of the southern United States. This is now recognized as a faulty categorization, for Caucasian-Americans frequently have the disease and geography is not specific. The hallmark of the host's immune response to the disease is activation of T cells and formation of tissue granuloma in affected organs. The peculiar noncaseating inflammation in the sarcoid granuloma, in contrast to those of tuberculosis, is not a specific histologic finding, contrary to the usual interpretation. However, sarcoidosis does feature many abnormalities in lymphocyte function, and these are described in detail.

Clinical and Radiographic Presentations

Sarcoidosis is protean in its clinical expression and at times can affect a variety of organs or begin with recurrent fever and vague constitutional symptoms. However, respiratory tract findings are by far the most common (Table 12.7) (346).

Sarcoidosis probably begins in the respiratory tract in response to some still-unknown inhaled substance or agent;

TABLE 12.7. MODE OF PRESENTATIONS OF SARCOIDOSIS

Presentation	Caucasian Patients (N = 105)	Black Patients (N = 103)
Respiratory symptoms	36	43
Routine chest film	25	6
Skin sarcoidosis	5	15
Arthralgia		
With erythema nodosum	5	2
Without erythema nodosum	8	5
Ocular symptoms	3	13
Fatigue, weight loss	8	5
Peripheral adenopathy	6	3
Fever	4	4
Cardiac symptoms	2	2
Neurologic symptoms	3	2
Hepatic symptoms	0	1
Nasal symptoms	1	0

Source: Israel H. Sarcoidosis. In Simmons DH, ed. *Current pulmonology.* New York: John Wiley & Sons, 1979:153.

certainly the lungs have a predilection to be involved with disease, although many other organs can be affected. The chest radiograph may provide the first clue, often in an asymptomatic person. Certain features of the disease vary between African-American and Caucasian patients, especially skin and ocular manifestations (347). After respiratory signs or symptoms, other findings are decidedly less frequent. Critical organ involvement may be striking and can confuse the diagnosis; when one is involved, this usually dictates prompt immunosuppressive therapy. Uveitis, cardiac arrhythmias, and neurologic signs—occasionally manifested as palsy of a single cranial nerve (the seventh with Bell's palsy)—and hypercalcemia are the major concerns (348–351). Although liver dysfunction is not a usual presentation, this organ is often involved and is the source of diagnostic tissue in many patients (352,353). Respiratory symptoms are not distinctive for sarcoidosis and are similar to those noted with other interstitial pulmonary diseases—breathlessness, often with minimal exertion, and nonproductive cough. Signs of pleural involvement or wheezing are unusual.

Sarcoidosis in the chest is suggested by a pattern of symmetrically enlarged bilateral hilar lymph nodes with ostensibly clear lung parenchyma on the chest radiograph (Fig. 12.12) (354). In such cases about half of the chest radiographs also reveal enlarged paratracheal nodes (usually right-sided and unilateral). In fact, sarcoidosis is one of the few chest diseases that commonly involves nodes in the lung (hilar) and mediastinum simultaneously. In some instances bilateral hilar adenopathy found on a routine chest radiograph may be the only manifestation of sarcoidosis (345,355). Approximately 5% to 9% of patients may present with only unilateral hilar adenopathy (356). In later stages of pulmonary sarcoidosis the lymph node response diminishes and progressive involvement of the lung parenchyma ensues; end stages of lung sarcoidosis may leave upper-zone cystic spaces and extensive linear streaking and infiltrates throughout, but reveal little residual adenopathy. Such disease progression has led to a still-applicable radiographic classification of sarcoidosis (357). Stage I disease features symmetrical, bilateral hilar adenopathy; stage II has hilar adenopathy and diffuse parenchymal changes; and stage III has diffuse pulmonary infiltrates without adenopathy (Figs. 12.12 and 12.13). This latter stage is often a burned-out, relatively stable period of disease in which extensive residual lung changes persist.

The classic chest radiographic sequence described in the preceding is not observed in every patient. When the hilar adenopathy stage is missed, clinicians often seem suspicious of the diagnosis of sarcoidosis and tend to think that the case is atypical. Dyspnea is roughly equated with higher radiographic stages of the disease that feature greater involvement of conducting airways and air-exchange tissue; however, some patients may not have respiratory symptoms despite obvious changes in the radiograph (357). The nonuniform, patchy distribution of sarcoid lesions in lung tissue can leave areas of parenchyma virtually normal, and this probably accounts for the preservation of good lung function and lack of symptoms in some patients. Unusual radio-

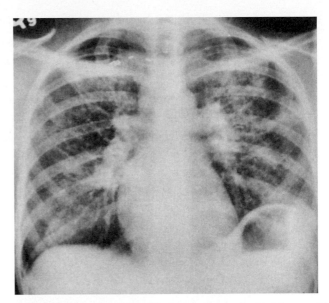

FIGURE 12.13. Sarcoidosis. PA chest radiograph of a 24-year-old woman with stage II sarcoidosis. Note the bilateral hilar adenopathy and interstitial infiltrates. (Clips from a previous surgical procedure are present in the right upper thorax.)

graphic patterns can be present, and one must be very alert to this possibility. Conglomerate infiltrates that give the appearance of pulmonary nodules or an alveolar filling pattern can occur, and evidence of pleural effusion may exist. In one series of 89 patients with an established tissue diagnosis of sarcoidosis, 15% had an atypical-appearing chest radiograph with one of the features listed in the preceding noted (356).

Laboratory Findings in Blood and Lung

For patients with overt lung tissue involvement and radiographic changes of the parenchyma, tests of pulmonary function usually reveal a restrictive pattern, small lung volumes, and diminished D_{LCO} as found with other forms of diffuse interstitial pulmonary fibrosis. Interestingly, the diminished D_{LCO} in sarcoid is more likely to correct for alveolar volume than in IPF (358). Patients with adenopathy and ostensibly clear lung fields may have normal lung function. As a rule, a decrement of at least 20% below a patient's predicted values for lung volumes and spirometric parameters must be present before any immunosuppressive therapy would be considered to control or arrest a decline in lung function. Other organs that require laboratory screening include the heart for possible arrhythmias, liver with a liver enzyme profile, and kidneys. Serum calcium should be monitored. Kveim antigen skin testing and subsequent biopsy of the skin papule for typical sarcoid histology has long been useful for confirming the diagnosis. Because of the general scarcity of a well-characterized and reliable

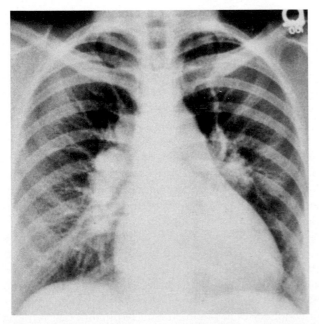

FIGURE 12.12. Sarcoidosis. PA chest radiograph of a 36-year-old woman with bilateral hilar and mediastinal adenopathy manifested by obliteration of the aortopulmonary window (ductus space). There is also right paratracheal adenopathy. The lung zones are normal; however, the cardiac silhouette is enlarged. The patient developed corticosteroid-responsive pulmonary infiltrates and cardiac arrhythmias, consistent with sarcoid cardiopulmonary involvement.

TABLE 12.8. CELLULAR AND IMMUNOLOGIC CHANGES IN SARCOIDOSIS

Blood	Bronchoalveolar Fluid	Lung Tissue
Skin test anergy	Lymphocytes increased (T cells, cells with T helper cell activity high)	Granulomas (giant epithelioid cells, few eosinophils)
Lymphopenia with low number of T cells but increased T suppressor cells	Lymphocytes with gamma or delta receptor increased	
	Peripolesis noted (lymphocytes clustering around a macrophage)	
	Secretion of interleukin-2 and spontaneous secretion of lymphokines (monocyte chemotactic factor, interferon gamma)	
Immune complexes	B lymphocytes and IgG secreting cells elevated	
IgG elevated	IgG increased	
Interferon gamma may be increased	Activated alveolar macrophages (can secrete interleukin-1 and angiotensin-converting enzyme)	
Angiotensin-converting enzyme and lysozyme elevated	Prostaglandin E_2	
	Tumor necrosis factor	
	PMNs in late stages of disease	

antigen, the Kveim test may be virtually impossible to perform nowadays.

Other changes in blood can be linked with the immunopathology occurring in affected organs such as the lung; Table 12.8 contrasts findings in blood and lung tissue (359).

Skin test anergy to common fungal and tuberculin antigens is a usual feature of active sarcoidosis; the cause of this faulty delayed hypersensitivity probably reflects the paucity of circulating T lymphocytes among the blood mononuclear cells. Leukopenia (total white cell count less than 4,000/mm^3) occurs in about 30% of patients (345). Patients with both active and chronic forms of disease can have fewer blood lymphocytes than normals, and the proportions of T and B cells are abnormal (360). The fraction of T cells is likely to be decreased and the mitogenic response to phytohemagglutinin is reduced in sarcoid patients. B cells, in contrast, especially those with immunoglobulin identified on their surface, are often increased in acute, active disease; this increase can be correlated with elevated serum γ-globulins in about half of the patients. In addition to the lymphocyte alterations, blood monocytes are activated and may show depressed chemotactic responses (361). Excessive activity of the subpopulation of T lymphocytes has been documented in sarcoid patients, and such activity may explain in part the skin anergy (362,363).

In serum, several enzyme and immunoglobulin changes can be documented. Serum globulin levels are increased in about half of patients with active disease and immune complexes can be identified (345,363,364). Two enzymes, lysozyme and angiotensin-converting enzyme (ACE) have been found to be elevated in patients with sarcoidosis and are used as diagnostic aids (365–368). ACE, which acts to convert serum angiotensin I to angiotensin II and helps metabolize bradykinin, is produced primarily by capillary endothelial cells; however, other cells such as fibroblasts and alveolar macrophages can also produce it at times (369,370). Whereas serum ACE is more helpful in the diagnosis of sarcoidosis because it is likely to be elevated in 60% or more of patients with active disease (an elevated value is greater

than 2 standard deviations above the normal mean), it is not specific for sarcoidosis. Other diseases that may have elevated levels are Gaucher's disease; leprosy; coccidioidomycosis; some cases of silicosis, asbestosis, berylliosis, and *Mycobacterium intracellulare* infection; osteoarthritis; diabetes mellitus with retinopathy; and miliary tuberculosis, primary biliary cirrhosis, or inflammatory bowel disease. Unfortunately, the list of diseases associated with elevated ACE levels is large, yet sarcoidosis continues to be the most common disease with high serum values. Several reports have indicated the usefulness of serial ACE values in monitoring sarcoid disease activity (371–375).

Bronchoscopy is indicated to inspect the airways for possible endobronchial sarcoid, often recognized by a cobblestone appearance of whitish plaques on the airway mucosa, and to obtain transbronchial biopsies that have a high yield of granulomatous tissue in this disease—up to 70% to 80% (376,377). Even though the chest radiograph may not show parenchymal evidence of disease, it is usually present, and parenchymal biopsies contain distinctive tissue changes.

The recovery of large numbers of lymphocytes in BAL fluid is a striking finding in many patients with active pulmonary sarcoidosis, and this is the important cellular feature that separates the diverse group of interstitial lung diseases into two general categories, granulomatous and nongranulomatous (Table 12.1) (27,378). As it is important to know the proportions of T lymphocyte subpopulations, a reference for normal cells is given in Table 12.9. For contrast with alveolar cells, in normal blood about 70% of the lymphocytes are T cells, and about the same ratio for T helper and T suppressor cells exists. Patients with active stages of pulmonary sarcoidosis usually have an increased percentage of lymphocytes in the mixture of respiratory cells retrieved by BAL (27,379–382). This percentage can be quite high and has been noted to be about 40% to 60% (normal is less than 10%). Moreover, the vast majority of lymphocytes can be identified as T cells, and these may constitute 90% of the total lymphocyte population (383). Concomitant blood T lymphocyte numbers are reduced. Smoking status

TABLE 12.9. PROFILE OF RESPIRATORY CELLS RECOVERED IN BAL FLUID (FOR NONSMOKER NORMALS FOLLOWING 100- to 300-ml LAVAGE)[a]

Cell Number Total	Viability	Macrophages	PMNs[b]	EOS/BASO[c]	Lymphocytes	Ciliated Cells	Erythrocytes
15×10^6	<90	85	1–2	<1	7–12	1–5	<5%
Lymphocytes T cells (% of total)	Subsets (%) T helper/inducer[d]	T suppressor/cytotoxic		T killer lymphs	B lymphs[e] (Plasma cells)	Untypable lymphs	
70	50[f]	30		7[g]	5–10	5	

[a] See references 41 and 42 for normal values.
[b] PMNs, polymorphonuclear granulocytes.
[c] EOS/BASO, Eosinophils/basophils.
[d] As percent of T cells. The T_H/T_s ratio is about 1.5:1.8.
[e] Amount plasma cells are immunoglobulin releasing cells with the following frequency: IgG = IgA > IgE (see reference 28).
[f] The T helper subset contains about 7% of cells with HLA DR + antigen, and these can preferentially produce interleukin-2 (see reference 371).
[g] Killer lymphocytes seem inactive when retrieved from a normal lung (see reference 374).
Source: Reynolds HY. Lung immunology and its contribution to the immunopathogenesis of certain diseases. *J Allergy Clin Immunol* 1986;78:833–847.

can influence the number of T cells and the CD4/CD8 ratio by decreasing them (384). In addition, the airway T cells are "activated" because they are capable of forming rosettes with sheep red blood cells at 37°C, instead of at 4°C as is the usual case, and they bear a surface receptor for IgG. Functionally, activated T cells spontaneously secrete a variety of lymphokines that affect other lymphocytes and monokines that interact with macrophages. Likewise, the macrophages are also activated and produce cytokines that modulate lymphocyte function. The sticking or clustering of lymphocytes around a macrophage (peripolesis) is complex and may reflect activity of the macrophage's membrane (385). These intraalveolar events probably mirror some of those ongoing in the tissue where the granuloma are formed. These cellular interactions are illustrated in Figure 12.14.

Immunologic Concepts

The inciting antigen or causative agent for sarcoidosis is still elusive, but evidence suggests that the T lymphocytes that accumulate in the lung have had surface antigen receptors stimulated (386). Whatever it is, it elicits a mononuclear cell lung response primarily of lymphocytes, especially of the T cell variety. Functionally these cells are activated, often adhere spontaneously to alveolar macrophages, forming rosettes, and secrete lymphokine substances (385). In examining Figure 12.14 and conceptually arranging the cell data for sarcoid immunopathogenesis, one might conclude that the alveolar macrophage may initiate the lung response.

Alveolar macrophages develop from circulating blood monocytes, which undergo further maturation or differentiation in the interstitial spaces before emerging on the alveolar surface. Vitamin D metabolites seem important in this process; lymphocytes are also affected (387). Although the first responsibility of the alveolar macrophage is to be a roving scavenger and phagocyte to clean debris from the alveolar surface, it is apparent that the macrophage, especially when activated as in sarcoidosis, can secrete a large array of cellular substances and mediators that affect the function of other cells (cytokines) (387a). As an example, macrophage chemotactic factors can attract other inflammatory cells to the alveoli, or fibroblast growth factors, such as platelet-derived growth factor and fibronectin, can influence fibroblast replication. Activated macrophages in sarcoidosis can secrete interleukin-1 (IL-1), which may attract lymphocytes into the alveoli (388). More recently, activated macrophages from patients with sarcoidosis have been shown to release interleukin-12 (IL-12) (389). IL-12 is a key mediator of the T helper 1 (T_h1) response (see the following). Such molecules as tumor necrosis factor and prostaglandin E_2 can have local effects that promote alveolitis, or they may diffuse into the systemic circulation as well (390). The list of enzymes, regulatory proteins, and inhibitors produced by macrophages continues to lengthen, as over 150 substances have been attributed to this heterogeneous cell population (391–393).

The macrophage also serves as an antigen presenting cell that can process an antigen, display it on its cell membrane where it is taken up by an appropriate T helper (T_H) lymphocyte and matched with respect to class II histocompatibility antigens. Antigen is received on the lymphocyte's membrane by a T cell antigen receptor that has an intricate structure composed of two (alpha and beta) chains. Whether or not the spontaneous lymphocyte-macrophage rosettes seen in sarcoidosis lung fluid represent an initial phase of antigen presentation to T cells is uncertain (385). Antigen presentation by macrophages is enhanced in sarcoidosis (393,394).

As noted, within the lumen of normal alveolar spaces, the majority of lymphocytes are T cells, and the T helper cells outnumber the suppressor cells by a ratio of about 1.5 to 1. A current paradigm in immunology is that the immune response to a given antigen is determined largely by the

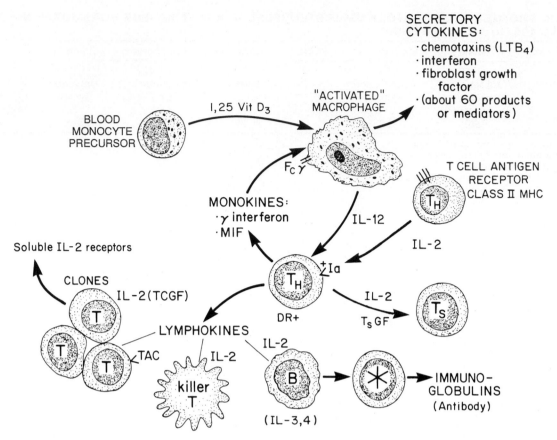

FIGURE 12.14. An interaction between the "activated" alveolar macrophage and subpopulations of T lymphocytes, especially T helper cells, occurs in sarcoid lung disease, and this creates the alveolitis. Details about macrophage effects on lymphocyte activity (secretion of cytokines and antigen presentation) and T lymphocyte action that feeds back to the macrophage or directs the function of other immune cells through lymphokine and monokine mediators are given in the text. (Adapted from Reynolds HY. Lung immunology and its contribution to the immunopathogenesis of certain diseases. *J Allergy Clin Immunol* 1986;78:833–847.)

pattern of cytokines produced by the activated $CD4^+$ (T helper) cells and the $CD8^+$ (T suppressor) cells. T helper 1 (T_h1) cells express γ interferon and IL-2, which are important in macrophage activation and delayed type hypersensitivity, respectively. T helper 2 (T_h2) cells express cytokines IL-4 and IL-5, which deactivate macrophage effector functions and mediate antibody responses and eosinophilia. IL-12 (produced by macrophages and dendritic cells) plays a critical role role in the development of the T_h1 response. It also directly stimulates T cells to produce γ interferon. Increased levels of IL-12 have been demonstrated in the BAL of patients with active sarcoidosis (389). Of the T helper cells, a small percentage (about 7% in normals) have an HLA-DR antigen; this subpopulation may increase when a lymphocytic alveolitis develops as in active sarcoidosis and is responsible for most of the interleukin-2 produced (395–397). Approximately 7% of the airway T cells are killer cells, but these seem dormant in normal subjects (398). In addition, about 5% of the lymphocytes are B cells or plasma cells. These cells can release various class-specific

immunoglobulins from their surface as already mentioned. In sarcoidosis, the expanded number of DR-positive T helper cells is responsible for producing the large amount of IL-2 that may cause expansion of clones of lymphocytes, activate the killer cells, and stimulate immunoglobulin production (IL-4 is needed as well). No defects in the function of lung sarcoid T suppressor cells have been noted, so lack of suppressor cell regulation is not the cause of the rather autonomous T helper cell function (399). In the activated T helper cell producing IL-2, increased expression of the IL-2 gene can be found (400). Thus, alveolar macrophages and lung T cells are selectively activated in the sarcoid lung (401).

In the other direction, the activated T_H cells can secrete a variety of monokines, such as gamma interferon (402) and migration inhibition factor (MIF), that modulate macrophage activity in turn. γ-Interferon in particular can energize or activate the macrophage. Having considered intraalveolar events in active sarcoidosis, a crucial intermediate step between the alveoli and development of granulomas in interstitial areas might involve hilar and mediastinal lymph nodes, which characteristically enlarge in early radiographic stages of disease and then subside as parenchymal tissue becomes more involved. The precise stimulus for the development of the complex tissue granulomas with epithelioid cell differentiation and concentric layers of surrounding T and B lymphocytes and fibroblasts remains unclear. However, soluble mediators, T helper cell activity, and macrophage-derived substances such as ACE may influence the kinetics of granuloma formation in the nodes and parenchymal tissue (403).

In advanced phases of sarcoid lung disease, an increased number of PMNs can be recovered in BAL fluid, and these inflammatory cells may contribute to the fibrotic stage of disease (404). Possibly, chemotactic factors produced by macrophages could have a role (405).

Thus, sarcoidosis involves complex cellular immune pathways; its pathogenesis is not simple. Peripheral blood findings do not reflect all the same changes noted in the airways; a compartmentalized immune response involving both macrophages and lymphocytes seems to occur. A relative excess of blood T suppressor cells probably contributes to the impaired cellular immunity often observed, whereas T helper cells are increased in the lungs of many patients with an active alveolar stage of disease. Finding evidence of numerous suppressor cells in the lung creating a CD8 alveolitis is unusual and may only be found in about 4% of patients when the diagnosis of sarcoidosis is made (406). In an early granulomatous stage some cases of sarcoidosis spontaneously resolve and granulomas regress. In others the disease may progress, causing considerable tissue destruction and lung fibrosis.

Disease Course and Therapy

Of 44 untreated, asymptomatic patients with symmetrical hilar adenopathy and no parenchymal infiltrates, spontaneous resolution of the radiographic disease occurred in most; 73% remitted and most did so in 6 to 17 months after diagnosis (354). Thus, advocacy of a particular form of therapy for patients in the earliest stages of disease must be tempered by the fact that spontaneous regression of the pulmonary process is frequent; this does not remove the lingering question about persistence of an inciting agent in a dormant stage. Prevention or environmental control is not possible because the cause of the disease is unknown.

For extrapulmonary sarcoidosis involving such critical organs as eyes, heart, or nervous system, corticosteroid therapy is indicated. For the lungs, the decision to treat is more difficult. To assess the effect of corticosteroid therapy on pulmonary dysfunction in sarcoidosis, a prospective study compared 6 months of moderate-dose prednisone therapy (60 mg/day for 1 month, then 20 mg/day for 5 months) with no treatment by monitoring pulmonary function for 1 to 2 years (407). Pulmonary dysfunction initially was rather modest in that mean D$_{LCO}$ was decreased 30% of predicted and mean arterial oxygen at rest was 80 mm Hg. Histologically, lung tissue had inflammatory changes and granulomas but was not severely distorted in most patients. In essence, treatment did nothing dramatic for these patients, for they neither improved nor worsened in pulmonary function when compared with the untreated control group.

If patients with pulmonary sarcoidosis, however, have troublesome respiratory symptoms and a 20% to 30% reduction in pulmonary function parameters (lung volumes, D$_{LCO}$, etc.), most clinicians institute a trial of corticosteroid therapy for approximately 6 months (408). Such therapy will generally improve symptoms, variably improve pulmonary function tests, and often improve the appearance of the chest radiograph. Long-term use of small doses of corticosteroid does seem beneficial for many patients, and relapse and exacerbation of symptoms occurs in some if the drug is tapered or withdrawn. However, the effectiveness of therapy for sarcoidosis remains controversial (407,409,410). Other cytotoxic and immunosuppressive drugs have been used to treat sarcoidosis but rarely in a controlled trial; therefore, none can be recommended as proven therapy for the disease. In the future, specific immunocytotoxic therapy that may obliterate certain hyperactive subsets of T cells, for example, may be developed and prove useful, or drug inhibitors or antibodies that neutralize enzymes such as ACE or that downregulate certain cell receptors may suppress the formation of granulomas (411). It is noteworthy that corticosteroids inhibit the secretion of IL-2 by T helper lymphocytes in active pulmonary sarcoidosis; therefore, the effect of this drug in suppressing cellular activity in this disease is now better understood (412). For the present, only corticosteroids are recommended for therapy. Corticosteroids can be envisioned to act on the alveolitis and interstitial inflammatory component of the disease by suppressing T lymphocytes that accumulate in affected tissue and perpetuate the disease.

As discussed for idiopathic pulmonary fibrosis, objective assessment that therapy is actually suppressing disease activity can be difficult given the subjective nature of symptoms and the insensitivity of chest radiographs in showing improvement. Pulmonary physiology may not suffice either. At present, the serial application of such tests as ACE measurement, gallium lung scans, and various cellular or immunologic components in bronchoalveolar lavage have no proven role, because they do not always correlate with disease activity nor predict response to therapy (413–418). Other more sensitive parameters need to be identified and are being sought (419). It remains important to find some mediator or cellular change that would identify the patient with sarcoidosis who may not have benign lung disease but will develop progressive fibrocystic debilitating lung changes. In this regard, IL-12 seems promising. In addition, subgrouping of patients based on immunologic parameters in BAL fluid needs more investigation (420,421).

For patients with established disease, the process eventually stabilizes and sarcoidosis seems to burn out. In this advanced stage, there is usually widespread cystic and fibrotic destruction of lung tissue, so the chest radiograph shows extensive honeycomb changes and diffuse interstitial markings. Pulmonary function is invariably impaired. In rare instances, successful lung transplantation has been performed in sarcoid patients with respiratory insufficiency. Interestingly, noncaseating granulomas have been described in the transplanted lung, but it is not apparent that the progressive disease recurs.

Sarcoidosis continues to be an enigmatic illness. Its cause remains elusive; it has a propensity to involve the respiratory tract, yet extrapulmonary disease can be severe and at times difficult to recognize; its course is unpredictable; and it is uncertain just how effective antiinflammatory therapy is. However, we are at an important juncture in understanding this disease. Continued investigation into ways of sampling the affected lung tissue will undoubtedly uncover more details of deranged immunology at the molecular and genetic levels in a related disease caused by beryllium, which in turn will produce more specific therapy (422,423). It may be that the association between sarcoidosis and another immunologic infectious disease, AIDS, will give further insight into the mechanisms of lymphocytic alveolitis that initiates the pulmonary phase (424).

HYPERSENSITIVITY PNEUMONITIS (EXTRINSIC ALLERGIC ALVEOLITIS)

Inhalation of a variety of organic dusts can cause hypersensitivity pneumonitis (425–428). Although many people are exposed to these environmental substances and many become sensitized and develop precipitating serum antibodies to the causative antigens, only a few develop overt lung disease. These dusts can be derived from animal dander and proteins; from saprophytic fungi that contaminate vegetables, wood bark, or water-reservoir vaporizers; and from dairy and grain products (Table 12.10) (426). Colorful, descriptive names for the diseases underscore the frequent occupational nature of exposure. Either the inhaled dust itself causes respiratory disease or a microbial contaminant passively carried with it may be incriminated. Usually a species of thermophilic actinomycetes is found; these ubiquitous bacteria thrive at high ambient temperatures (45°C to 60°C range) that are reached during the decomposition of vegetable matter. Perhaps about 10^9 mold spores per cubic millimeter of air must be inhaled on a daily basis for allergic alveolitis to develop, as was found for a group of Swedish farmers (429).

Some forms of occupational disease are easily recognized. When the clinical symptoms are temporally related to workplace exposure, the index of suspicion is high that an environmental or inhalation source is causing illness. However, subtle forms of exposure may occur among office personnel or individuals in the home (called sick building syndrome), and putting clinical symptoms together with unsuspected and episodic exposure or with a lower dose but constant exposure can be most difficult. A considerable amount of medical detective work may be required to find that a water-cooled air conditioning unit, a new down comforter or an infant's cold-mist vaporizer is the culprit or that an orchid grower is inhaling fungal spores from the bark chips he uses to mulch his flowers. The source may be obscure. In our experience, a mold growing on a kitchen wall provided a chronic exposure for a symptomatic homemaker (26). The list of potential antigens that can be inhaled and cause airway sensitization is increasing, and recognition of these diseases is becoming more prevalent.

TABLE 12.10. SOME ETIOLOGIC AGENTS IN HYPERSENSITIVITY PNEUMONITIS

Disease	Source of Exposure	Major Antigens or Microbe
Farmer's lung	Moldy hay	*Micropolyspora faeni* (also *Faenia rectivirgula*)
Grain handler's lung	Moldy grain	*Micropolyspora faeni, Thermoactinomyces vulgaris*
Bagassosis	Moldy sugar cane fiber	*Thermoactinomyces sacchari*
Summer type hypersensitivity	House dust or bird droppings	*Trichosporon cutaneum*
Humidifier or air-conditioner lung	Contaminated forced-air system, heated water reservoirs	*M. faeni, T. vulgaris,* occasionally amoebae are implicated
Maple bark stripper's lung	Moldy bark	*Cryptostroma corticale*
Malt workers' lung	Moldy malt	*Aspergillus clavatus*
Sequoiosis	Moldy redwood dust	*Aureobasidium pullulans* and *Graphium* spp.
Wheat weevil disease	Wheat weevil disease	*Sitophilus granarius*
Cheese worker's lung	Cheese mold	*Penicillium caseii*
Suberosis	Moldy cork dust	*Penicillium frequentans*
Bird breeder's lung	Pigeons, parakeets, fowl, rodents	Avian or animal proteins (in excreta)
Chemical workers lung	Manufacture of plastics, polyurethane foam, or rubber	Trimellitic anhydride, diisocyanate, methylene diisocyanate

Clinical Presentation

Sensitization to an organic dust is usually insidious, and the potential patient is unaware of the detrimental effects it can cause. In certain avocations such as bird handling, almost all people intimately involved in care of the birds develop serum-precipitating antibodies to some avian antigens, but this immune response is not associated with disease in most (430). Likewise, farm workers may have serum antibodies to certain thermophilic bacteria (431). The onset of respiratory symptoms may not occur at first but may appear only later after an exposure pattern is well established. In the acute form of disease, respiratory and systemic symptoms develop explosively within 4 to 6 hours after dust is inhaled and consist of dyspnea, cough, chills, fever, and malaise. The symptoms may persist for 12 hours or so and abate spontaneously; with each re-exposure the acute episode occurs again. When observed, the patient is acutely ill and dyspneic; inspiratory crackles can be heard prominently in the lower lung zones. Temperature may be alarmingly elevated and the peripheral blood leukocyte count can be in excess of 25,000/mm^3, with a left shift. The chest radiograph may appear normal but usually shows a fine, diffuse alveolar filling pattern and variable interstitial streaks.

Pulmonary function abnormalities, best measured in patients challenged with antigens in a pulmonary laboratory and followed with serial observations, appear in 4 to 6 hours when the clinical symptoms develop. A decrease in FVC and FEV$_{1.0}$ occurs; air trapping and hyperinflation may be documented; and the diffusing capacity for carbon monoxide is reduced. Also, pulmonary compliance decreases. These changes gradually return to normal as the clinical picture improves. Another pattern of pulmonary dysfunction may occur, involving a two-phase reaction. Initially, an immediate asthmatic-type reaction develops just after aerosol exposure to antigen that is characterized by air trapping and obstruction. This abates, to be followed in 4 to 6 hours by more restrictive and noncompliant lung function, as described.

Acute phases of the disease are seen infrequently, because a knowledgeable person will deduce the cause or make the connection between an airway exposure and subsequent respiratory symptoms. If the correlation is recognized, voluntary avoidance may solve the problem. On the other hand, if the exposure is continuous and protracted, a chronic form of disease may develop that does not include the acute exacerbations of respiratory symptoms (26,432). Instead, patients develop persistent symptoms of breathlessness, dyspnea with exertion, and cough that are indistinguishable from symptoms noted in other interstitial pulmonary diseases; fatigue, poor appetite, and weight loss can be significant in this disease. Symptoms and evidence of constitutional effects of disease may be evident for months and occasionally for years before the patient presents for evalua-

tion. Many patients with hypersensitivity pneumonitis are not diagnosed until this more advanced stage of disease is present. Chest radiographs are abnormal and appear like other IPF films. The HRCT scan can be helpful in the diagnosis. The most common findings are multiple fine nodules 2 to 4 mm in diameter with hazy, ground glass opacities. Pulmonary function is characterized by a restrictive ventilatory pattern and a deficit in diffusing capacity for carbon monoxide. Such patients with this chronic form of inhalational hypersensitivity disease are difficult to separate from those with IPF and a host of similar diseases unless the exposure history happens to be obvious (Table 12.1). A serum screen for hypersensitivity antigen precipitins will not establish a diagnosis but, if positive, might orient the clinician toward a possible environmental exposure. Physical examination does not provide any signs not found in other interstitial lung disease. Digital clubbing, initially considered an unusual occurrence, has been noted to develop in about half the patients in one series (426,427,433).

Laboratory and Immunologic Findings

Except for the consequences of weight loss and poor appetite, the disease is limited to the respiratory tract, and most laboratory abnormalities relate to that organ system. Blood parameters reflect the effects of chronic disease in patients with advanced illness but do not necessarily mirror immunologic events occurring in the airways. With the exception of acute episodes of pneumonitis, the white cell count is not elevated and eosinophilia is not usual. The erythrocyte sedimentation rate may be elevated, and serum immunoglobulins are often increased. The presence of precipitating antibodies (in IgM, IgA, and IgG classes) in serum to antigens causing hypersensitivity disease can give a helpful clue; because many people develop such antibodies, this finding is not diagnostic but only indicates that prior exposure and sensitization have occurred. Skin testing with hypersensitivity antigens is not well standardized and can provide confusing conclusions. *Aspergillus* antigens may be useful in patients with bronchopulmonary aspergillosis, but other fungal preparations are not. Peripheral blood lymphocytes can be stimulated with appropriate antigens to give mitogenic responses, but generally the lymphocytes, especially ones recovered from the alveoli by lavage, have not been studied in the same detail as those from patients with sarcoidosis.

Most of the details about immune responses in the lungs have come from patients with farmer's lung with chronic hypersensitivity pneumonitis and from patients with pigeon breeder's (bird fancier's) lung (427,434). These patients are evaluated with bronchoscopy like others with diffuse interstitial lung disease, and BAL and transbronchial biopsy help considerably to substantiate the diagnosis. Histologically, lung biopsy shows an infiltration with lymphocytes and inflammatory cells; granuloma formation and fibrosis are often evident as well. In patients with a chronic form of farmer's lung, the total recovery of cells from lung lavage was increased and reflected an increased number of lymphocytes. Of the respiratory cell population, 70% were lymphocytes, versus 8% customarily found in normal controls; most of the lymphocytes were T cells. On further analysis of subpopulations of T cells, a slight excess of T suppressor lymphocytes can be found (435–437). This is an interesting contrast to the striking increase in T helper cells that is characteristic of active sarcoidosis. There is a possibility that an elevated CD4-positive T-cell response is found with a more insidious onset of hypersensitivity pneumonitis, but this needs further study (438). Thus, there was an increase in the absolute number of lymphocytes found in bronchoalveolar lavage from patients with this form of chronic hypersensitivity pneumonitis. Moreover, lavage fluid from these patients contained high concentrations of immunoglobulin, especially IgG and IgM (439). The presence of IgM is unusual because this immunoglobulin class is rarely found in measurable amounts in normal lung fluid and is infrequently present in lavage fluid obtained in other lung diseases. Specific precipitating antibody to inciting antigens was found in most sera and in the BAL fluid from a number of these patients. Patients with acute forms of hypersensitivity disease have not been studied extensively by lung lavage and biopsy, because the illness is usually transient. One would expect that alveolitis and inflammation are present in the early phase. The reaction seems to be one of mononuclear cells and an acute but transient increase in polymorphonuclear granulocytes and virtually no eosinophils (440). In more chronic stages of organic dust inhalation, the lung response is rather similar to that in sarcoidosis, which is the prototype of a granulomatous cellular response. Finally, an intermediate stage of the disease, or more accurately a stage of exposure, is an asymptomatic form in which the subject has no special symptoms of respiratory illness but has a subclinical form as alveolitis (441–443). An increased percentage of lung lymphocytes can be found as well as specific precipitating antibody. In such subjects this form of benign alveolitis or lung inflammation is well tolerated for periods of at least 2 years without overt disease developing (442). It appears that a lymphocytic alveolitis as sampled in BAL fluid from an asymptomatic farmer does not have any long-term clinical significance (444,445).

Concepts of Immunopathogenesis

Immunologic data from lung lavage studies in patients in a chronic phase of hypersensitivity pneumonitis (HP) are summarized in Table 12.11 (446–448). It is satisfying to know the etiology of the hypersensitivity diseases so that a specific antigen can be inserted to initiate the reaction. The prominent lymphocyte accumulation in the alveoli is impressive, and T cells predominate, especially T suppressor cells. Less is known about lymphocyte function and subsets of T cells in HP than in sarcoidosis, and the mediators have not been as well described (as shown in Fig. 12.14). Tissue granulomas develop in chronic forms of the disease. A striking contrast between hypersensitivity pneumonitis and sarcoidosis, however, is the apparent lack of hilar and mediastinal lymph node enlargement and absence of splenomegaly. The striking increase in airway IgG and IgM in chronic hypersensitivity pneumonitis is notable. As the inciting antigen is known, specific antibodies can be identified and the ingredients for immune complex formation are present.

Therapy

If the environmental source of inhaled antigen is identified, simple avoidance is sufficient treatment. The acute form of

TABLE 12.11. IMMUNOLOGIC FEATURES OF THE BLOOD, BRONCHOALVEOLAR LAVAGE FLUID, AND LUNG TISSUE IN CHRONIC STAGES OF HYPERSENSITIVITY PNEUMONITIS

Blood	Bronchoalveolar Fluid	Lung Tissue
Normal blood cell counts Normal immunoglobulin levels, usually positive serum precipitins (IgG)	Lung cell recovery increase High lymphocyte percentages (50–70% of BAL cells) • T lymphocytes predominate • Possible to have an increased number of suppressor cells (slight reversal of T_H/T_S cell ratio) Large and foamy macrophages, a minimal number of eosinophils, and an increased number (up to 1% of all lavage cells) of basophils T-cell division high (RNA) Total protein increased • Elevated IgG and IgM levels • IgG and IgA antibodies present Abnormal surfactant composition Fibrogenic factors increased (hyaluronic acid, type III procollagen, fibronectin and fibroblast growth factors) Vitronectin Laminin P_1	Alveolitis • Lymphocytes, plasma cells, granulomas (intraalveolar septal distribution) and foamy histiocytes Bronchiolitis Fibrosis possible

disease abates without specific therapy. Preventing disease by avoiding the causative antigen is not always easy, however, especially if an occupational exposure is identified. A change of job or relocation within a factory to decrease exposure may not be a simple matter. With chronic forms of disease accompanied by respiratory symptoms and abnormal pulmonary function, a trial of corticosteroids can be given with modest expectations that this form of immunosuppression will be effective.

LYMPHOID INTERSTITIAL PNEUMONITIS

Lymphoid interstitial pneumonitis (LIP) is a rare form of interstitial lung disease characterized by the preferential accumulation of lymphocytic infiltrates in the interstitium and along lymphatics (449). Patients typically present with the subacute onset of exertional breathlessness and dry cough in the absence of constitutional symptoms. LIP can occur in the context of systemic diseases such as common variable immunodeficiency, dysproteinemias, monoclonal gammopathy, Sjögren's syndrome, primary biliary cirrhosis, and HIV infection. It may also occur in an idiopathic form. Chest radiographs demonstrate bilateral retinulonodular infiltrates in most cases, but mixed alveolar patterns can also be seen. Honeycomb changes are rare. The natural history of LIP is variable, but generally less progressive than IPF. Mortality exceeds 30% at 5 years. Corticosteroids are considered the first line of therapy even in HIV-related cases.

EOSINOPHILIC SYNDROMES

The presence of eosinophils in lung tissue is a common occurrence and indicates that these inflammatory cells are part of the host's cellular response to a variety of inciting agents and systemic immunologic diseases (449,450). Chemotactic factors released from degranulating mast cells attract eosinophils and localize them in sites of IgE-mediated reactions, whereupon eosinophils inactivate mediators and actually seem to control the extent of the reaction. Eosinophils are found in the airways and lung tissue of patients with idiopathic pulmonary fibrosis. In other interstitial diseases that seem to have an allergic component (such as hypersensitivity pneumonitis, drug-induced lung syndromes, and sarcoidosis), eosinophils are a minor component of the tissue reaction but can usually be identified in tissue sections. In contrast, eosinophils can be the most conspicuous inflammatory cell in certain primary lung or systemic diseases that have frequent lung involvement, and these are grouped together as eosinophilic syndromes. There is considerable overlapping among these syndromes, and precise separation is impossible because the etiology and pathogenesis are poorly understood. The classification developed by

Crofton and colleagues separated eosinophilic pneumonias into five groups: Loeffler's syndrome, prolonged pulmonary eosinophilia, pulmonary eosinophilia associated with asthma, tropical eosinophilia, and periarteritis nodosa (451). Although this classification is still useful, a more current modification has adapted this format to include: acute eosinophilic pneumonias, tropical pulmonary eosinophilia, chronic eosinophilic pneumonia, allergic bronchopulmonary aspergillosis, Churg-Strauss syndrome (discussed in the preceding), and idiopathic hypereosinophilic syndrome.

Types of Eosinophilic Syndromes

Acute Eosinophilic Pneumonias

Loeffler's Syndrome (Simple Pulmonary Eosinophilia)
This is usually a self-limited disease that features migratory, fleeting areas of infiltration in a peripheral pattern on the chest radiograph and is accompanied by minimal respiratory symptoms and blood eosinophilia (451,452). The disease seems to be an allergic response that can result from parasitic infection; the human parasite *Ascaris lumbricoides* and nonhuman ones such as dog and cat ascarids that produce visceral larva migrans, are known to be causative. Several other parasitic infections and exposure to numerous drugs such as sulfonamides have been implicated in a Loeffler's-like syndrome (483). The clinical presentation is that of a dry cough, fevers, and breathlessness. Peripheral eosinophilia can be striking and sputum frequently contains eosinophils. *Ascaris* larvae can be identified in sputum or gastric lavage during the period when pulmonary infiltrates are present. Tissue diagnosis is not usually required, but BAL can show a marked increase in eosinophils (453). When *Ascaris lumbricoides* is identified, mebendazole (100 mg twice daily for 3 days) is indicated to prevent the post-pneumonic GI manifestations.

Parasitic Infections

Numerous other parasitic infections can be associated with pulmonary infilatrates and peripheral eosinophilia (453). The more common offenders in the United States are *Strongylodes stercoralis*, *Toxocara canis (visceral larva migrans)*, and *Ancylostoma brasiliensis*. *Strongyloides* infection has been associated with the "hyperinfection syndrome" (453). This typically occurs in individuals with a previous exposure who develop defects in host defense, either in association with an illness such as HIV infection or malignancy, or when receiving systemic corticosteroids.

Drug-Induced Pulmonary Eosinophilic Syndromes

A variety of medications have been associated with pulmonary infiltrates and blood or pulmonary eosinophilia (454).

Patients typically present with acute or subacute symptoms of cough and dyspnea. Careful questioning is required because nonprescription medications may be the culprit. This was dramatically illustrated with L-Tryptophan-induced eosinophilia-myalgia syndrome (454). Symptoms usually abate with cessation of the drug, but corticosteroids are occasionally required. Resolution of the pulmonary infiltrates are typically very rapid (within 24 or 48 hours).

Idiopathic Acute Eosinophilic Pneumonia

Eosinophilic pneumonia can present as rapidly progressive respiratory failure with a clinical presentation compatible with the Adult Respiratory Distress Syndrome. This has been termed acute eosinophilic pneumonia (455,456). Patients present with fever, myalgias, dyspnea, and significant hypoxemia that may require mechanical ventilation. Importantly, peripheral eosinophilia is not usually present. BAL is critical in delineating the diagnosis. Demonstration of abundant eosinophils in BALF is diagnostic and is followed by systemic corticosteroids. There is typically a dramatic response to treatment with complete resolution of pulmonary infiltrates.

Tropical Pulmonary Eosinophilia

Respiratory symptoms of cough, dyspnea, and in some patients attacks of asthma may be present in those with filarial infection. Systemic symptoms of malaise, fatigue, weight loss, and fever also occur; peripheral blood eosinophilia and high levels of antibody to filarial antigens are characteristic of laboratory abnormalities. The chest radiograph may reveal areas of patchy consolidation or bilateral streaking and increased parenchymal linearities in the hilar and lower lung zones. Histologically, microfilaria can be identified in areas of tissue nodules showing necrotic debris and eosinophils (457–459,461). Recently, the inflammatory process in the lung has been characterized (459). A striking recovery of eosinophils in bronchoalveolar lavage fluid was found; after therapy with diethylcarbamazine, these cells decreased and lung function tests improved (460).

In the BAL fluid obtained from patients with TPE is an increase of filaria-specific antibody to *Brugia malayi,* especially in the IgE class, but also in IgG, IgM, and, to a lesser degree, IgA (461). After therapy for 1 to 2 weeks with diethylcarbamazine, the parasite-specific antibodies in lung fluids were found to decrease. However, lung inflammation can persist (462).

Chronic Eosinophilic Pneumonia

As suggested by its name, this disease differs from the simple form in that it is often chronic, and accompanying pulmonary and systemic symptoms can be severe. If this disease persists, it can lead to a form of interstitial pulmonary fibrosis that radiographically shows honeycombed lung changes and lung function abnormalities characteristic of other diseases in this group (Table 12.1).

Chronic eosinophilic pneumonia most commonly affects women and can present as a severe respiratory illness in which fever, night sweats, weight loss, and dyspnea are prominent symptoms (457,463,464). Presentation can be subacute or chronic. Blood eosinophilia is variable and often is not present. Extrapulmonary involvement does not occur. The disease is sometimes initially misdiagnosed as tuberculosis. A distinguishing feature in the first cases of eosinophilic pneumonia described was deterioration in the patient's condition despite a trial of antituberculosis therapy (457). However, one helpful clue is often evident in the chest radiograph. Dense alveolar infiltrates develop that have a peculiar location in the peripheral portions of the lung with a pronounced predilection for apical and axillary segments of the upper lobes. These peripheral infiltrates are not limited to a defined lobar or anatomical distribution but can extend across the usual anatomical barriers. Wheezing can be present or develop *de novo* in some patients. The clinical, laboratory and radiographic features are distinctive and an open or thoracoscopic biopsy is not usually required to establish the diagnosis. Fiberoptic bronchoscopy with transbronchial biopsy and BAL should be the first diagnostic test. Striking increases in BAL eosinophils (greater than 50%) are characteristic of chronic eosinophilic pneumonia (454). Infectious etiologies such as helminths need to be excluded. Once the diagnosis is established, treatment with corticosteroids causes a striking regression in the radiographic findings and in clinical symptoms; a chest film taken a few weeks later may appear normal. Although the response to corticosteroid therapy is usually impressive, the disease may exacerbate after therapy is discontinued, and relapse can occur in about half of the patients during a 10-year follow-up period (463). The infiltrates tend to recur in the same locations on the chest radiograph.

Pulmonary Eosinophilia with Asthma

Asthma is a frequent complaint in many forms of lung disease, including the eosinophilic syndromes; thus it is difficult to separate a single disease entity on this basis alone (465). Two diseases, allergic bronchopulmonary aspergillosis and allergic angiitis with granulomatosis, as described by Churg and Strauss, can fit this description (253,466). Since the eosinophilic component to the diseases seems incidental, it can be argued that these diseases are best discussed with respective asthma syndromes and systemic vasculitides affecting the lung, such as Churg-Strauss syndrome (see prior discussion in this chapter).

Idiopathic Hypereosinophilic Syndrome

Idiopathic hypereosinophilic syndrome (IHS) is a rare disorder characterized by severe peripheral eosinophilia with diffuse organ infiltration with eosinophils in which no underlying cause for the eosinophils can be identified (453,454). A variety of organs can be affected including the heart, CNS, bone marrow, visceral organs, GI tract, skin, and eyes. The cardiac manifestations can be life-threatening with CHF, intracardiac thrombi, mitral regurgitation and cardiomyopathy all described (453). Lung involvement is in about half the cases, with pulmonary infiltrates and cough the presenting manifestations. The disease was uniformly fatal prior to the advent of effective therapy with corticosteroids and hydroxyurea.

EOSINOPHILIC GRANULOMA (LANGERHANS CELL GRANULOMATOSIS)

The histiocytoses are a group of diseases that feature proliferation and activation of mononuclear phagocytic cells, especially macrophages (467). The term *histiocyte* is synonymous with *macrophage* and emphasizes the fact that tissue macrophages can exist in many forms as alveolar or peritoneal cells, dermal Langerhans cells, hepatic Kupffer cells, osteoclasts, and microglial brain cells. Thus, the range of diseases and the principal organs affected are very broad. Often a form of cell-mediated immunity is evident and a granulomatous tissue reaction is found. Both findings suggest an intimate macrophage-lymphocyte interaction, as discussed already for sarcoidosis. Eosinophils may be contained in the granulomatous reaction. Immune complexes in blood can contribute to the lung reaction and perhaps stimulate macrophages or histiocytes, but this too remains uncertain. The proliferation and accumulation of histiocytes in affected tissue, often producing a granulomatous lesion, are part of the disease process in the histiocytic disorders.

A comprehensive classification of the histiocytic diseases based on macrophage involvement presents obvious overlapping with other syndromes readily explained by etiology or easily recognized clinically (467). The spectrum includes (*a*) reactive histiocytic proliferation with a known microorganism (tuberculosis, fungal, or parasitic agents) or with inert particles; (*b*) reactive proliferation in which the inciting agent is unknown, which includes such diverse entities as eosinophilic granuloma, Wegener's and lymphomatoid granulomatosis of lung, and sarcoidosis; (*c*) lipid storage diseases, which include Gaucher's disease, Niemann-Pick disease, sea blue histiocytosis, and Fabry's disease; and (*d*) neoplastic disorders such as acute monocytic leukemia, chronic myelomonocytic leukemia, and histiocytic lymphoma. Eosinophilic granuloma is the only one that frequently affects the lungs, except for other granulomatous vasculitides and sarcoidosis.

Eosinophilic granuloma (EG) (or Langerhans cell granulomatosis) can be a multifocal disease involving bones of the skull, extremities, ribs, pelvis, vertebrae, and mandible with lytic lesions (468). The triad of lytic skull lesions, ex-

ophthalmos, and pituitary involvement producing diabetes insipidus is known as Hand-Schüller-Christian disease. A diffuse form of histocytosis of the Letterer-Siwe type is a fulminant disease generally unresponsive to therapy. A unifocal or local extraosseous form of EG involves the lungs and is a true cause of interstitial pulmonary fibrosis (467). Only the entity of EG is discussed here in detail (469,470).

EG is rare (estimated prevalence of two to five cases per million) and can affect all ages, but young adults, especially men, develop the disease most frequently. Symptoms may have an insidious onset, with cough and breathlessness with exertion as initial complaints. A spontaneous pneumothorax can be the presenting manifestation, although this is more likely to occur in advanced fibrotic stages of the disease when localized areas of airway obstruction lead to cyst formation and overdistention. Few constitutional symptoms may be present. Greater than 90% of cases occur in smokers. Blood eosinophilia is unusual, but circulating immune complexes can be measured in serum in many patients with active disease, and the titer reflects the degree of cellular reactivity in a lung biopsy (471). The chest radiograph usually reveals a diffuse micronodular and interstitial-appearing infiltrate, initially involving the middle and lower lung zones; later small cystic air spaces develop in the infiltrate, producing a honeycomb pattern (Fig. 12.15) (472). Adenopathy or pleural disease is unusual. The radiographic appearance differs from the one described for eosinophilic pneumonia, in which migratory infiltrates in the periphery of the lung are characteristic. Pneumothoraces occur in 10% to 30% of patients. The HRCT scan is highly distinctive, showing peribronchial cystic and nodular lesions predominantly in the mid- and upper lung zones. Numerous thin-walled cysts are observed with micronodules coexistent in most cases. Lung biopsies reveal a mixture of inflammatory, cystic, nodular and fibrotic abnormalities. Light microscopy shows a stellate pattern of fibrosis that is distinctive. The characteristic feature of EG is aggregates of Langerhans cells, which are large histiocytes derived from dendritic cells (473–475). They stain positively for S-100 protein or OKT6 antigen (476–479). Electron microscopy demonstrates the Birbeck granule (pentolaminar body), but is of marginal clinical utility because of expense. Diagnosis usually requires a thoracoscopic biopsy, the presence of more than 5% Langerhans cells in BAL fluid by S-100 or OKT6 strongly supports the diagnosis.

The course of EG is quite variable in adults, and the prognosis is generally better for focal disease limited to the lungs than for multifocal disease and bone involvement. A bone scan is advisable as part of the initial evaluation of a patient with focal EG and should certainly be made if bone symptoms occur later, because approximately 20% of patients eventually develop a lytic bone lesion. Rarely, diabetes insipidus occurs. The lung disease does have a significant rate of spontaneous remission. Regression of pulmonary symptoms and chest radiographic infiltrates may occur in

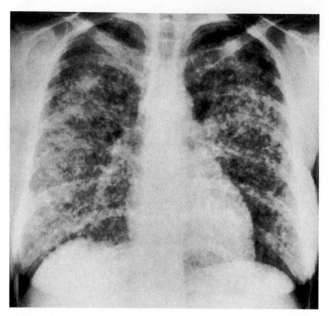

FIGURE 12.15. Eosinophilic granuloma of lung (Langerhans cell granulomatosis). A 31-year-old woman had a viral upper respiratory infection 3 months previously (a chest radiograph was not obtained), and a dry, nonproductive cough persisted. Dyspnea developed in the interim and shortness of breath limited her daily activities. Her chest radiograph shows extensive alveolar filling and interstitial infiltrates in all lung zones; also, small cystic spaces are evident. Tissue from an open lung biopsy revealed eosinophilic granuloma and evidence of cystic changes, suggesting that the disease process was chronic. Corticosteroid therapy improved the appearance of the chest radiograph and her symptoms. She also discontinued cigarette smoking, which is an essential part of the therapy.

10% to 25% of patients within several months of diagnosis, although the disease does not disappear entirely without some residual symptoms. As most patients are cigarette smokers, cessation of smoking greatly helps. Corticosteroid treatment is not especially effective overall in suppressing the disease, except for the initial boost in subjective well-being associated with the "steroid effect." In many cases, the lung disease stabilizes and in effect burns out, leaving the patient with moderate pulmonary symptoms (dyspnea on exertion), residual lung fibrosis, cystic spaces in the parenchyma, and a restrictive pattern of lung function (480). Therapy at this stage of disease is symptomatic. Some patients are troubled with persisting bronchitis, which is superimposed on the quiescent interstitial fibrosis. If wheezing or obstructive airway changes on pulmonary testing are noted, judicious use of antibiotics and bronchodilators can be effective.

As indicated, the precise kind of immune mechanisms involved in developing the histiocytic-eosinophilic granulomatous response in the EG lung is uncertain; failure to have an experimental animal model of the disease hampers investigative efforts. Because Hand-Schüller-Christian disease affects the head and airways, this form of disease is thought to be caused by some agent inhaled or concentrated in the nasooropharynx; multifocal osseous forms of the disease may reflect a different entry site (467). The disease does not seem to be a form of allergy, which seems important in the pathogenesis of certain eosinophilic lung syndromes, but instead features a granulomatous response and possibly an element of immune complex injury (Fig. 12.14) (471).

LYMPHANGIOLEIOMYOMATOSIS

Lymphangioleiomyomatosis (LAM) is a rare cystic lung disease causing progressive airflow obstruction in women of childbearing age. The histopathologic abnormality is a hamartomatous proliferation of atypical smooth muscle along lymphatics in a variety of organs but the most clinically evident are the lung and kidney (481,482). Patients typically present in the third or fourth decade of life with breathlessness. LAM is most frequently misdiagnosed as asthma or chronic bronchitis owing to the marked airflow limitation observed on pulmonary function testing. Pneumothoraces are common. Chylous effusions occur in 7% to 39% (482). Hemoptysis occurs approximately 25% of the time. In addition to severe airflow limitation without responsiveness to bronchodilators, the diffusing capacity is severely reduced. Lung volumes are typically normal or increased. Chest radiographs show cystic or reticulonodular infiltrates with hyperinflation. Abnormalities on HRCT are highly distinctive and given the clinical setting, virtually establish the diagnosis. Numerous thin-walled cysts are distributed throughout the lung fields. There is no predilection for the upper lobes. Unlike EG, the nodular component is not present. The cysts also are distinct from emphysematous changes. Angiomyolipomas are seen over one-third of patients and may cause severe hematuria. Positive staining for melanoma-related marker (HMB-45) in smooth muscle is highly specific for LAM. The natural history is variable, but most patients die of respiratory failure within 10 years of the onset of symptoms (482).

Major therapeutic approaches include oopherectomy or administration of antiestrogen regimens, but results have been disappointing. Medroxyprogesterone and/or oopherectomey are considered the major options for treatment. Lung transplantation has been performed in a few patients with a 2-year survival of approximately 60% (482).

REFERENCES

1. Keogh BA, Crystal RG. Chronic interstitial lung disease. In Simmons DH, ed. *Current pulmonology.* New York: John Wiley & Sons, 1981:237–340.
2. Crystal RG, Fulmer JD, Moss ML, et al. Idiopathic pulmonary fibrosis: clinical, histologic, radiographic, physiologic, scintigraphic, cytologic and biochemical aspects. *Ann Intern Med* 1976;85:769–788.

3. Crystal RG, Bitterman PR, Rennard SI, et al. Interstitial lung diseases of unknown cause: disorders characterized by chronic inflammation of the lower respiratory tract. *N Engl J Med* 1984; 310:154–166, 235–244.

4. Bitterman PB, Rennard SI, Keogh BA, et al. Familial idiopathic pulmonary fibrosis—evidence of lung inflammation in unaffected family members. *N Engl J Med* 1986;314:1343–1347.

5. Hamman L, Rich AR. Fulminating diffuse interstitial fibrosis of the lungs. *Trans Am Clin Climatol Assoc* 1935;51:154–163.

6. Wells AU, Hansell DM, Rubens MB, et al. The predictive value of appearance of thin section computed tomography in fibrosing alveolitis. *Am Rev Respir Dis* 1993;148:1076–1082.

7. Kuhn C III, Boldt J, King TE Jr, et al. An immunohistochemical study of architectural remodeling and connective tissue synthesis in pulmonary fibrosis. *Am Rev Respir Dis* 1989;140:1693–1703.

8. Hyde DM, King TE Jr, McDermott T, et al. Idiopathic pulmonary fibrosis. Quantitative assessment of lung pathology. *Am Rev Respir Dis* 1992;146:1042–1047.

9. Katzenstein AL, Fiorelli R. Nonspecific interstitial pneumonia/fibrosis. Histologic features and clinical significance. *Am J Surg Pathol* 18:136–147.

10. Katzenstein AL, Mcyers J. Idiopathic pulmonary fibrosis: clinical relevance of pathologic classification. *Am Rev Resp Crit Care Med* 1998;157:1301–1305.

11. Andoh Y, Aikawa T, Shimura S, et al. Morphometric analysis of airways in idiopathic pulmonary fibrosis patients with mucous hypersecretion. *Am Rev Respir Dis* 1992;145:175–179.

12. Little JW, Hall WJ, Douglas RG Jr, et al. Airway hyperreactivity and peripheral airway dysfunction in influenza A infection. *Am Rev Respir Dis* 1978;118:295–303.

13. Ueda T, Ohta K, Suzuki N, et al. Idiopathic pulmonary fibrosis and high prevalence of serum antibodies to hepatitis C. *Am Rev Respir Dis* 1992;146:266–268.

14. Irving W, Day S, Johnston I. Idiopathic pulmonary fibrosis and hepatitis C virus infection. *Am Rev Resp Dis* 1993;148:1683–1689.

15. Colin AA, Mark EJ. Lifelong progressive interstitial lung disease. Case records, Massachusetts General Hospital. *N Engl J Med* 1993;329:1797–1805.

16. Epler GR, McLoud TC, Gaensler EA, et al. Normal chest roentgenograms in chronic diffuse infiltrative lung disease. *N Engl J Med* 1978;298:934–939.

17. Nishimura K, Izumi T, Kitaichi M, et al. The diagnostic accuracy of high resolution computed tomography in diffuse interstitial lung diseases. *Chest* 1993;104:1149–1155.

18. Dreisin RB, Schwarz MI, Theofilopoulos AN, et al. Circulating immune complexes in the idiopathic interstitial pneumonias. *N Engl J Med* 1978;298:353–357.

19. Line BR, Fulmer JD, Reynolds HY, et al. Gallium-67 citrate scanning in the staging of idiopathic pulmonary fibrosis: correlation with physiologic and morphologic features and bronchoalveolar lavage. *Am Rev Respir Dis* 1978;118:355–365.

20. Turner-Warwick M, Haslam PL. The value of serial bronchoalveolar lavages in assessing the clinical progress of patients with cryptogenic fibrosing alveolitis. *Am Rev Respir Dis* 1987;135:26–34.

21. Fulmer JD, Roberts WC, von Gal ER, et al. Small airways and idiopathic pulmonary fibrosis. Comparison of morphologic and physiologic observations. *J Clin Invest* 1977;60:595–610.

22. Epler GR, Saber FA, Gaensler ET. Determination of severe impairment (disability) in interstitial lung disease. *Am Rev Respir Dis* 1980;121:647–659.

23. Keogh BA, Crystal RG. Pulmonary function testing in interstitial pulmonary disease. *Chest* 1980;78:856–865.

24. Schwartz DA, Merchant RK, Helmers RA, et al. The influence of cigarette smoking on lung function in patients with idiopathic pulmonary fibrosis. *Am Rev Respir Dis* 1991;144:504–506.

25. Hanley ME, King TE Jr, Schwarz MI, et al. The impact of smoking on mechanical properties of the lungs in idiopathic pulmonary fibrosis and sarcoidosis. *Am Rev Respir Dis* 1991; 144:1102–1106.

26. Reynolds HY, Fulmer JD, Kazmierowski JA, et al. Analysis of cellular and protein components of bronchoalveolar lavage fluid from patients with idiopathic pulmonary fibrosis and chronic hypersensitivity pneumonitis. *J Clin Invest* 1977;58:165–175.

27. Weinberger SE, Kelman JA, Elson NA, et al. Bronchoalveolar lavage in interstitial lung disease. *Ann Intern Med* 1978;89: 459–466.

28. David GS, Brody AR, Craighead JE. Analysis of airspace and interstitial mononuclear cell populations in human diffuse interstitial lung disease. *Am Rev Respir Dis* 1978;118:7–15.

29. Gadek JE, Kelman JA, Fells G, et al. Collagenase in the lower respiratory tract of patients with idiopathic pulmonary fibrosis. *N Engl J Med* 1979;301:737–742.

30. Rudd RM, Halslam PL, Turner-Warwick M. Cryptogenic fibrosing alveolitis: relationship of pulmonary physiology and bronchoalveolar lavage to response to treatment and prognosis. *Am Rev Respir Dis* 1981;124:1–8.

31. Lawrence EC, Martin RR, Blaese RM, et al. Increased bronchoalveolar IgG-secreting cells in interstitial lung diseases. *N Engl J Med* 1980;302:1186–1188.

32. Hunninghake GW, Kawanami O, Ferrans VJ, et al. Characterization of inflammatory and immune effector cells in the lung parenchyma of patients with interstitial lung disease. *Am Rev Respir Dis* 1981;123:407–412.

33. Reynolds HY. Idiopathic interstitial pulmonary fibrosis: contribution of bronchoalveolar lavage analysis. *Chest* 1986;89: 139–144.

34. Walters LC, Schwarz MI, Cherniack RM, et al. Idiopathic pulmonary fibrosis: pretreatment bronchoalveolar lavage cellular constituents and their relationships with lung histopathology and clinical response to therapy. *Am Rev Respir Dis* 1987;135: 696–704.

35. Reynolds HY. Idiopathic pulmonary fibrosis. In Lichtenstein LM, Fauci AS, eds. *Current therapy in allergy, immunology and rheumatology.* Toronto: Decker, 1988:214–220.

36. Bensard DD, McIntyre RC, Waring BJ, et al. Comparison of video thoracoscopic lung biopsy to open lung biopsy in the diagnosis of interstitial lung disease. *Chest* 1993;103:765–770.

37. Fulmer JD, Katzenstein AA. The interstitial lung diseases. In Bone R, Dantzker D, George R, et al, eds. *Pulmonary and critical care medicine.* St. Louis: Mosby Year Book, 1993:M1:1–15.

38. Reynolds HY. Classification, definition and correlation between clinical and histologic staging of interstitial lung diseases. *Semin Respir Med* 1984;6:1–19.

39. Liebow AA, Steer A, Billingsley JG. Desquamative interstitial pneumonia. *Am J Med* 1965;39:369–404.

40. Carrington CB, Gaensler EA, Coutu RD, et al. Natural history and treated course of usual and desquamative interstitial pneumonia. *N Engl J Med* 1978;298:801–809.

41. Haslam PL, Cromwell O, Dewar A, et al. Evidence of increased histamine levels in lung lavage fluids from patients with cryptogenic fibrosing alveolitis. *Clin Exp Immunol* 1981;44: 587–593.

42. Rankin JA, Kaliner M, Reynolds HY. Histamine levels in bronchoalveolar lavage fluids from patients with asthma, sarcoidosis and interstitial lung diseases. *J Allergy Clin Immunol* 1987;79: 371–377.

43. Reynolds HY. Bronchoalveolar lavage. *Am Rev Respir Dis* 1987; 135:250–263.

44. Cherniack RM (Coordinator) and other investigators. Bron-

choalveolar lavage constituents in healthy individuals, idiopathic pulmonary fibrosis and selective comparison groups. *Am Rev Respir Dis* 1990;141(Suppl):169–202.

45. Klech H, Hutter C, eds. Clinical guidelines and indications for bronchoalveolar lavage—report of the European Society of Pneumology Task Group on BAL. *Eur Respir J* 1990;3:937–974.

46. Robinson PC, Walters LC, King TE, et al. Idiopathic pulmonary fibrosis. Abnormalities in bronchoalveolar lavage fluid phospholipids. *Am Rev Respir Dis* 1988;137:585–591.

47. Hunninghake GW, Gadek JE, Lawley TJ, et al. Mechanisms of neutrophil accumulation in the lungs of patients with idiopathic pulmonary fibrosis. *J Clin Invest* 1981;68:259–269.

48. Lynch JP III, Standiford TJ, Rolfe MW, et al. Neutrophilic alveolitis in idiopathic pulmonary fibrosis. The role of interleukin-8. *Am Rev Respir Dis* 1992;145:1433–1439.

49. Ozaki T, Hayashi H, Tani K, et al. Neutrophil chemotactic factors in the respiratory tract of patients with chronic airway diseases or idiopathic pulmonary fibrosis. *Am Rev Respir Dis* 1992;145:85–91.

50. Carr PC, Mortenson RL, King TE Jr, et al. Increased expression of the interleukin-8 gene by alveolar macrophages in idiopathic pulmonary fibrosis. *J Clin Invest* 1991;88:1802–1810.

51. Merrill WW, Naegel GP, Matthay RA, et al. Alveolar macrophage-derived chemotactic factor—kinetics of in vitro production and partial characterization. *J Clin Invest* 1980;65:268–276.

52. Bitterman PB, Rennard SI, Hunninghake GW, et al. Human alveolar macrophage growth factor for fibroblasts: regulation and partial characterization. *J Clin Invest* 1982;70:806–822.

53. Martinet Y, Rom WN, Grotendorst GR, et al. Exaggerated spontaneous release of platelet derived growth factor by alveolar macrophages from patients with idiopathic pulmonary fibrosis. *Am Rev Respir Dis* 1988;137:572–578.

54. Cantin AM, Boileau R, Begin R. Increased procollagen III aminoterminal peptide-related antigens and fibroblast growth signals in the lungs of patients with idiopathic pulmonary fibrosis. *Am Rev Respir Dis* 1988;137:572–578.

55. McCormack FX, King TE Jr, Voelker DR, et al. Idiopathic pulmonary fibrosis. Abnormalities in the bronchoalveolar lavage content of surfactant protein A. *Am Rev Respir Dis* 1991;144:160–166.

56. Low RB, Giancola MS, King TE Jr, et al. Serum and bronchoalveolar lavage of N-terminal type III procollagen peptides in idiopathic pulmonary fibrosis. *Am Rev Respir Dis* 1992;146:701–706.

57. Shaw RJ, Benedict SH, Clark RAF, et al. Pathogenesis of pulmonary fibrosis in interstitial lung disease. Alveolar macrophage PDGF (B) gene activation and up-regulation by interferon gamma. *Am Rev Respir Dis* 1991;143:167–173.

58. Basset F, Ferrans VJ, Soler P, et al. Intraluminal fibrosis in interstitial lung disorders. *Am J Pathol* 1986;122:443–461.

59. Broekelman T, Limper A, Colby T, et al. Transforming growth factor beta 1 is present at sites of extracellular matrix gene expression in human pulmonary fibrosis. *Proc Natl Acad Sci USA* 1991;88:6642–6646.

60. Cherniack RM, Crystal RG, Kalica AR. Current concepts in idiopathic pulmonary fibrosis: a road map for the future. NHLBI Workshop Summary. *Am Rev Respir Dis* 1991;143:680–683.

61. Janson RW, King TE, Hance KR, et al. Enhanced production of Il-1 receptor antagonist by alveolar macrophages from patients with interstitial lung disease. *Am Rev Respir Dis* 1993;148:495–503.

62. Meyer KC, Powers C, Rosenthal N, et al. Alveolar macrophage surface carbohydrate expression is altered in interstitial lung disease as determined by lectin-binding profiles. *Am Rev Respir Dis* 1993;148:1325–1334.

63. Kuwano K, Hagimoto N, Kawasaki M, et al. Essential roles of the Fas-Fas ligand pathway in the development of pulmonary fibrosis. *J Clin Invest* 1999;104:13–19.

64. Dayton CA, Schwartz DA, Helmers RA, et al. Outcome of subjects with idiopathic pulmonary fibrosis who fail corticosteroid therapy. *Chest* 1993;103:69–73.

65. Baughman RP, Lower EE. Use of intermittent, intravenous cyclophosphamide for idiopathic pulmonary fibrosis. *Chest* 1992;102:1090–1094.

66. Turner-Warwick M. Evaluation and treatment of cryptogenic fibrosing alveolitis. *IM-Int Med Special* 1981;2:34.

67. Peters SG, McDougall JC, Douglas WW, et al. Colchicine in the treatment of pulmonary fibrosis. *Chest* 1993;103:101–104.

68. Raghu G, Johnson W, Lockhart D, et al. Treatment of idiopathic pulmonary fibrosis with a new antifibrotic agent, perfenidone: results of a prospective, open-label Phase II study. *Am J Respir Crit Care Med* 1999;159:1061–1069.

69. Venuta F, Rendina E, De Giacomo T, et al. Isolated lung transplantation for end-stage pulmonary disease. *Transplant Proc* 1998;30:1521–1529.

70. Chacon R, Corris P, Dark J, et al. Comparison of the functional results of single lung transplantation for pulmonary fibrosis and chronic airway obstruction. *Thorax* 1998;53:43–49.

71. Barbers R. Lung transplantation in interstitial lung disease. *Curr Opin Pulm Med* 1995;5:401–405.

72. Toronto Lung Transplant Group. Experience with single-lung transplantation for pulmonary fibrosis. *JAMA* 1988;259:2258–2262.

73. Grossman RF, Frost A, Zamel N, et al. Results of single-lung transplantation for bilateral pulmonary fibrosis. *N Engl J Med* 1990;322:727–733.

74. Trulock EP, Cooper JD, Kaiser LR, et al. The Washington University-Barnes Hospital experience with lung transplantation. *JAMA* 1991;266:1943–1946.

75. ATS Statement, lung transplantation. *Am Rev Respir Dis* 1993;147:772–776.

76. Hoffman LA, Wesmiller SW, Sciurba FC, et al. Nasal cannula and transtracheal oxygen delivery. *Am Rev Respir Dis* 1992;145:827–831.

77. Turner-Warwick M, Lebowitz M, Burrows B, et al. Cryptogenic fibrosing alveolitis: clinical features and their influence on survival. *Thorax* 1980;35:171–180.

78. Epler GR, Colby TV, McLoud TC, et al. Bronchiolitis obliterans organizing pneumonia. *N Engl J Med* 1985;312:152–158.

79. Guerry-Force ML, Muller NL, Wright JL, et al. A comparison of bronchiolitis pneumonia, and small airway diseases. *Am Rev Respir Dis* 1987;135:705–712.

80. Muller NL, Guerry-Force ML, Staples CA, et al. Differential bronchiolitis diagnosis of bronchiolitis obliterans with organizing pneumonia and usual interstitial pneumonia: clinical, functional, and radiologic findings. *Radiology* 1987;162:151–156.

81. Katzenstein AL, Myers JL, Prophet WD, et al. Bronchiolitis obliterans and usual interstitial pneumonia. A comparative clinicopathologic study. *Am J Surg Pathol* 1986;10:373–381.

82. Myers JL, Katzenstein AL. Ultrastructural evidence of alveolar epithelial injury in idiopathic bronchiolitis obliterans-organizing pneumonia. *Am J Pathol* 1988;132:102–109.

83. Alasaly K, Muller N, Ostrow D, et al. Cryptogenic organizing pneumonia. a report of 25 cases and a review of the literature. *Medicine (Balt)* 1995;74:201–211

84. Lee K, Kullnig P, Hatman T, et al. Cryptogenic organizing pneumonia. CT findings in 43 patients. *AJR* 1994;162:543–546.

85. Cohen A, King T, Downey G. Rapidly progressive bronchiolitis

obliterans with organizing pneumonia. *Am J Respir Crit Care Med* 1994;149:1670–1675.

86. Meyers J, Veal C, Shin M. Respiratory bronchiolitis causing interstitial lung disease. A clinicopathologic study of six cases. *Am Rev Resp Dis* 1987;135:880–884.

87. Yousem S, Colby T, Gaensler E. Respiratory bronchiolitis-associated interstitial lung disease and its relationship to desquamative interstitial pneumonia. *Mayo Clin Proc* 1989;64: 1373–1380.

88. Matthay RA, Schwartz MI, Petty TL. Pleuro-pulmonary manifestations of connective tissue diseases. *Clin Notes Respir Dis* 1977;16:3–9.

89. Boulware DW, Weissman DN, Doll NJ. Pulmonary manifestations of the rheumatic diseases. *Clin Rev Allergy* 1985;3: 249–267.

90. Constantopoulos SH, Drosos AA, Maddison PJ, et al. Xerotrachea and interstitial lung disease in primary Sjögren's syndrome. *Respiration* 1984;46:310–314.

91. Fairfax AJ, Haslam PL, Vavia D, et al. Pulmonary manifestations of Sjögren's syndrome. *Chest* 1976;70:354–361.

92. Hunninghake GW, Fauci AS. Pulmonary involvement in collagen vascular diseases. *Am Rev Respir Dis* 1979;119:471–503.

93. Sullivan WD, Hurst DJ, Harmon CE, et al. A prospective evaluation emphasizing pulmonary involvement in patients with mixed connective tissue disease. *Medicine* 1984;63:92–107.

94. Prakash UB, Luthra HS, Divertie MB. Intrathoracic manifestations in mixed connective tissue disease. *Mayo Clin Proc* 1985; 60:813–821.

95. Derderian SS, Tellis CJ, Abbrecht PH, et al. Pulmonary involvement in mixed connective tissue disease. *Chest* 1985;88:45–48.

96. Wiener-Kronish JP, Solinger AM, Warnock ML, et al. Severe pulmonary involvement in mixed connective tissue disease. *Am Rev Respir Dis* 1981;124:499–503.

97. Martyn JB, Wong MJ, Huang SH. Pulmonary and neuromuscular complications of mixed connective tissue disease: a report and review of the literature. *J Rheumatol* 1988;15:703–705.

98. Schwarz MI. Pulmonary manifestations of the collagen-vascular diseases. In Bone RA, Dantzker DR, George RB, et al, eds. *Pulmonary and critical care medicine.* St. Louis: CV Mosby, 1993:M4:1–16.

99. Steinberg AD, Gourley MF, Klinman DM, et al. NIH conference. Systemic lupus erythematosus. *Ann Intern Med* 1991;115: 548–559.

100. Tomer Y, Buskila D, Shoenfeld Y. Pathogenic significance and diagnostic value of lupus autoantibodies. *Int Arch Allergy Appl Immunol* 1993;100:293–306.

101. Matthay RA, Schwarz MI, Petty TL, et al. Pulmonary manifestations of systemic lupus erythematosus: review of 12 cases of acute lupus pneumonitis. *Medicine* 1975;54:397–409.

102. Brasington RD, Furst DE. Pulmonary disease in systemic lupus erythematosus. *Clin Exp Rheumatol* 1985;3:269–276.

103. Segal AM, Calabrese LH, Ahmad M, et al. The pulmonary manifestations of systemic lupus erythematosus. *Semin Arthritis Rheum* 1985;14:202–204.

104. Turner-Stokes L, Turner-Warwick M. Intrathoracic manifestations of SLE. *Clin Rheum Dis* 1982;8:229–242.

105. Schwartzberg M, Lieberman DH, Getzoff B, et al. Systemic lupus erythematosus and pulmonary vascular hypertension. *Arch Intern Med* 1984;144:605–607.

106. Ansari A, Larson PH, Bates HD. Cardiovascular manifestations of systemic lupus erythematosus: current perspective. *Prog Cardiovasc Dis* 1985;27:421–434.

107. Pines A, Kaplinsky N, Olchvsky D, et al. Pleuro-pulmonary manifestations of systemic lupus erythematosus: clinical features of its subgroups. Prognostic and therapeutic implications. *Chest* 1985;88:129–135.

108. Wohlegelertner D, Loke J, Matthay RA, et al. Systemic and discoid lupus erythematosus: analysis of pulmonary function. *Yale J Biol Med* 1978;51:57–164.

109. Perwz HD, Kramer N. Pulmonary hypertension in systemic lupus erythematosus: report of four cases and review of the literature. *Semin Arthritis Rheum* 1981;11:177–181.

110. Sahn SA. Immunologic disease of the pleura. *Clin Chest Med* 1985;6:83–102.

111. Leatherman SW, Davie SF, Hoidal JR. Alveolar hemorrhage syndromes: diffuse microvascular lung hemorrhage in immune and idiopathic disorders. *Medicine* 1984;63:343–361.

112. Cush JJ, Goldinas EA. Drug-induced lupus: clinical spectrum and pathogenesis. *Am J Med Sci* 1985;290:36–45.

113. Martens J, Demedts M, Vanmeenen MT, et al. Respiratory muscle dysfunction in systemic lupus erythematosus. *Chest* 1983;84:170–175.

114. Wilcox PG, Stein HB, Clarke SD, et al. Phrenic nerve function in patients with diaphragmatic weakness and systemic lupus erythematosus. *Chest* 1988;93:352–358.

115. Harvey AM, Shulman LE, Tumulty PA, et al. Systemic lupus erythematosus: review of the literature and clinical analysis of 138 cases. *Medicine* 1954;33:291–437.

116. Winslow WA, Ploss LN, Loitman B. Pleuritis in systemic lupus erythematosus: its importance as an early manifestation in diagnosis. *Ann Intern Med* 1958;49:70–88.

117. Eisenberg H, Dubois EL, Sherwin RP, et al. Diffuse interstitial lung disease in systemic lupus erythematosus. *Ann Intern Med* 1973;79:37–45.

118. Segal AM, Reardon EV. Systemic lupus erythematosus. In Cannon GW, Zimmerman G, eds. *The lung in rheumatic diseases.* New York: Marcel Dekker, 1990:261–278.

119. Good JT Jr, King TE, Antony VB, et al. Lupus pleuritis. Clinical features and pleural fluid antinuclear antibodies. *Chest* 1983; 84:714–718.

120. Bell R, Lawrence DS. Chronic pleurisy in systemic lupus erythematosus treated with pleurectomy. *Br J Dis Chest* 1979;73: 314–316.

121. Onomura K, Nakata H, Tanaka Y, et al. Pulmonary hemorrhage in patients with systemic lupus erythematosus. *J Thorac Imag* 1991;6:57–61.

122. Weinrib L, Sharma OP, Quismorio FP Jr. A long-term study of interstitial lung disease in systemic lupus erythematosus. *Semin Arthritis Rheum* 1990;20:48–56.

123. Huang CT, Hennigar GR, Lyons HA. Pulmonary dysfunction in systemic lupus erythematosus. *N Engl J Med* 1965;272: 288–293.

124. Andonopoulos AP, Constantopoulos SH, Galanopoulos V, et al. Pulmonary function of nonsmoking patient with systemic lupus erythematosus. *Chest* 1988;94:312–315.

125. Montes de Oca MA, Babron MC, Bletry O, et al. Thrombosis in systemic lupus erythematosus: a French collaborative study. *Arch Dis Child* 1991;66:713–717.

126. Haupt HM, Moore GW, Hutchins GM. The lung in systemic lupus erythematosus. Analysis of the pathologic changes in 120 patients. *Am J Med* 1981;71:791–798.

127. Abud-Mendoza C, Diaz-Jouanen E, Alarcon-Segovia D. Fatal pulmonary hemorrhage in systemic lupus erythematosus. Occurrence without hemoptysis. *J Rheumatol* 1985;12:558–561.

128. Desnoyers M, Bernstein S, Cooper AG, et al. Pulmonary hemorrhage in lupus erythematosus without evidence of an immunologic cause. *Arch Intern Med* 1984;144:1398–1400.

129. Myers JL, Katzenstein AA. Microangiitis in lupus induced pulmonary hemorrhage. *Am J Clin Pathol* 1986;85:552–556.

130. Carette S, Macher AM, Nussbaum A, et al. Severe, acute pulmonary disease in patients with systemic lupus erythematosus: ten

years of experience at the National Institutes of Health. *Semin Arthritis Rheum* 1984;14:52–59.

131. Miller LR, Greenberg SD, McLarty JW. Lupus lung. *Chest* 1985;88:265–269.

132. Gross M, Esterly JR, Earle RH. Pulmonary alterations in systemic lupus erythematosus. *Am Rev Respir Dis* 1972;105:572–577.

133. Petri M, Rheinschmidt M, Whiting-O'Keefe Q, et al. The frequency of lupus anticoagulant in systemic lupus erythematosus: a study of sixty consecutive patients by activated portal thromboplastin time, Russell viper venom time, and anticardiolipin antibody. *Ann Intern Med* 1987;106:524–531.

134. Walker WC, Wright V. Pulmonary lesions and rheumatoid arthritis. *Medicine* 1968;47:501–520.

135. Scadding JG. The lungs in rheumatoid arthritis. *Proc R Soc Lond (Med)* 1969;62:227–238.

136. Jones FL Jr, Blodgett RC Jr. Empyema in rheumatoid pleuropulmonary disease. *Ann Intern Med* 1971;74:655–671.

137. Hunder GG, McDuffie FC, Hepper NG. Pleural fluid complement in systemic lupus erythematosus and rheumatoid arthritis. *Ann Intern Med* 1972;76:357–363.

138. Turner-Warwick M, Haslam P. Antibodies in some chronic fibrosing lung disease. I. Non-organ specific autoantibodies. *Clin Allergy* 1971;1:83–95.

139. Frank ST, Weg JG, Harkleroad LE, et al. Pulmonary dysfunction in rheumatoid disease. *Chest* 1973;63:27–34.

140. DeHoratius RJ, Abruzzo JL, Williams RC Jr. Immunofluorescent and immunologic studies of rheumatoid lung. *Arch Intern Med* 1972;129:441–446.

141. Caplan A. Certain unusual radiological appearances in chest of coal miners suffering from rheumatoid arthritis. *Thorax* 1953;8:29–37.

142. King TE, Dunn TL. Connective tissue disease. In Schwarz MI, King TE, eds. *Interstitial lung disease.* Philadelphia: Decker, 1988:171–210.

143. Yousem SA, Colby TA, Carrington CB. Lung biopsy in rheumatoid arthritis. *Am Rev Respir Dis* 1985;131:770–777.

144. Geddes DM, Corrin B, Brewerton DA, et al. Progressive airway obliteration in adults and its association with rheumatoid disease. *Q J Med* 1977;46:427–444.

145. Herzog CA, Miller RA, Hoidal JR. Bronchiolitis and rheumatoid arthritis. *Am Rev Respir Dis* 1981;124:636–639.

146. Shiel WC Jr, Prete PE. Pleuropulmonary manifestations of rheumatoid arthritis. *Semin Arthritis Rheum* 1984;13:235–243.

147. Yousem SA, Colby TV, Carrington CB. Lung biopsy in rheumatoid arthritis. *Am Rev Respir Dis* 1985;131:770–777.

148. Hakala M. Poor prognosis in patients with rheumatoid arthritis hospitalized for interstitial lung fibrosis. *Chest* 1988;93:114–118.

149. Lee FI, Brain AT. Chronic diffuse interstitial fibrosis and rheumatoid arthritis. *Lancet* 1962;2:693–695.

150. Weiland JE, Garcia JG, Davis WB, et al. Neutrophil collagenase in rheumatoid interstitial lung disease. *J Appl Physiol* 1987;62:628–633.

151. Roschmann RA, Rothenberg RJ. Pulmonary fibrosis in rheumatoid arthritis: a review of clinical features and therapy. *Semin Arthritis Rheum* 1987;16:174–185.

152. Sassoon CS, McAlpine SW, Tashkin DP, et al. Small airways function in nonsmokers with rheumatoid arthritis. *Arthritis Rheum* 1984;27:1218–1226.

153. Garcia JG, James HL, Zinkgraf S, et al. Lower respiratory tract abnormalities in rheumatoid interstitial lung disease. *Am Rev Respir Dis* 1987;136:811–817.

154. Arroliga AC, Podell DN, Matthay RA. Pulmonary manifestations of scleroderma. *J Thorac Imag* 1992;7:30–45.

155. Barnett AJ. *Scleroderma.* Springfield, IL: Charles C Thomas, 1974.

156. Wilson RJ, Rodnan GP, Robin ED. An early pulmonary physiologic abnormality in progressive systemic sclerosis (diffuse scleroderma). *Am J Med* 1964;26:361–369.

157. Sackner MA. *Scleroderma.* New York: Grune & Stratton, 1966.

158. Sackner M, Akgun N, Kimbel P, et al. The pathophysiology of scleroderma involving the heart and respiratory system. *Ann Intern Med* 1964;60:611–630.

159. Weaver AL, Divertie MB, Titus JL. Pulmonary scleroderma. *Dis Chest* 1968;54:490–498.

160. Konig G, Luderschmidt C, Hammer C, et al. Lung involvement in scleroderma. *Chest* 1984;85:318–324.

161. Owens GR, Follansbee WP. Cardiopulmonary manifestations of systemic sclerosis. *Chest* 1987;91:118–127.

162. Norton WL, Nardo JM. Vascular disease in progressive systemic sclerosis (scleroderma). *Ann Intern Med* 1970;75:317–324.

163. Naeye RL. Pulmonary vascular lesions in systemic scleroderma. *Dis Chest* 1963;44:374–380.

164. Steen VO. Systemic sclerosis. In Cannon GW, Zimmerman G, eds. *The lung in rheumatic diseases.* New York: Marcel Dekker, 1990:279–302.

165. Rosenthal AK, McLaughlin JK, Linet MS, et al. Scleroderma and malignancy: an epidemiological study. *Ann Rheum Dis* 1993;52:531–533.

166. Abu-Shakra M, Guillemin F, Lee P. Cancer in systemic sclerosis. *Arthritis Rheum* 1993;36:460–464.

167. Pianone A, Matucii-Cerinic M, Lombardi A, et al. High resolution computed tomography in systemic sclerosis. Real diagnostic utilities in the assessment of pulmonary involvement and comparison with other modalities of lung investigation. *Clin Rheumatol* 1992;11:465–572.

168. Wells AU, Hansell DM, Corrin B, et al. High resolution computed tomography as a predictor of lung histology in systemic sclerosis. *Thorax* 1992;47:738–742.

169. Bhalla M, Silver RM, Shepard JA, et al. Chest CT in patients with scleroderma: prevalence of asymptomatic esophageal dilatation and mediastinal lymphadenopathy. *AJR* 1993;161:269–272.

170. Garber SJ, Wells AU, duBois RM, et al. Enlarged mediastinal lymph nodes in the fibrosing alveolitis of systemic sclerosis. *Br J Radiol* 1992;65:983–986.

171. Peters-Golden M, Wise RA, Hochberg MC, et al. Carbon monoxide diffusing capacity as predictor of outcome in systemic sclerosis. *Am J Med* 1984;77:1027–1034.

172. Greenwald GI, Tashkin DP, Gong H, et al. Longitudinal changes in lung function and respiratory symptoms in progressive systemic sclerosis. Prospective study. *Am J Med* 1987;83:305–312.

173. Owens GR, Fino GJ, Herbert DL, et al. Pulmonary function in progressive systemic sclerosis. Comparison of CREST syndrome variant with diffuse scleroderma. *Chest* 1983;84:546–550.

174. Peters-Golden M, Wise RA, Schneider P, et al. Clinical and demographic predictors of loss of pulmonary function in systemic sclerosis. *Medicine* 1984;63:221–231.

175. Harrison NK, Myers AR, Corrin B, et al. Structural features of interstitial lung disease in systemic sclerosis. *Am Rev Respir Dis* 1991;144:706–713.

176. Owens GR, Paradis IL, Gryzan S, et al. Role of inflammation in the lung disease of systemic sclerosis: comparison with idiopathic pulmonary fibrosis. *J Lab Clin Med* 1986;107:253–260.

177. Silver RM, Metcalf JF, Stanley JH, et al. Interstitial lung disease in scleroderma. Analysis by bronchoalveolar lavage. *Arthritis Rheum* 1984;27:1254–1262.

178. Shuck JW, Oetgen WJ, Tesar JT. Pulmonary vascular response

during Raynaud's phenomenon in progressive systemic sclerosis. *Am J Med* 1985;78:221–227.

179. Wells A, Cullinan P, Hansell D, et al. Fibrosing alveolitis associated with systemic sclerosis has a better prognosis than lone cryptogenic fibrosing alveolitis. *Am J Respir Crit Care Med* 1994;149:1583–1590.

180. Steen VD, Owens GR, Redmond C, et al. The effect of D-penicillamine on pulmonary findings in systemic sclerosis. *Arthritis Rheum* 1985;28:882–888.

181. DeClerck LS, Dequeker J, Francx L, et al. D-penicillamine therapy and interstitial lung disease in scleroderma. A long-term follow-up study. *Arthritis Rheum* 1987;30:643–650.

182. Akesson A, Blom-Bulow B, Scheja A, et al. Long-term evaluation of penicillamine or cyclofenil in systemic sclerosis. Results from a two-year randomized study. *Scand J Rheumatol* 1992;21:238–244.

183. Hein R, Behr J, Hundgen M, et al. Treatment of systemic sclerosis with gamma-interferon. *Br J Dermatol* 1992;126:496–501.

184. Silver R, Warrick J, Kinsella M, et al. Cyclophosphamide and low-dose prednisone therapy in patients with systemic sclerosis (scleroderma) with interstitial lung disease. *J Rheumatol* 1993;20:838–844.

185. Tuffanelli DL, Lavoie PE. Prognosis and therapy of polymyositis/dermatomyositis. *Clin Dermatol* 1988;6:93–104.

186. Kasner CS, White CL, Freeman RG. Pathology and immunopathology of polymyositis/dermatomyositis. *Clin Dermatol* 1988;6:64–75.

187. Sontheimer RD, Ziff M. Questions pertaining to the etiology and pathophysiology of polymyositis/dermatomyositis. *Clin Dermatol* 1988;6:105–119.

188. Benedek JG. Neoplastic associations of rheumatic diseases and rheumatic manifestations of cancer. *Clin Geriatr Med* 1988;4:333–355.

189. Callen JP. Dermatomyositis. *Dis Mon* 1987;33:237–305.

190. Hochberg MC, Feldman D, Stevens MD. Adult onset polymyositis/dermatomyositis: an analysis of clinical and laboratory features and survival in 76 patients with a review of the literature. *Semin Arthritis Rheum* 1986;15:168–178.

191. Dickey BF, Myers AR. Pulmonary disease in polymyositis/dermatomyositis. *Semin Arthritis Rheum* 1984;14:60–76.

192. Hepper NG, Ferguson RH, Howard FM Jr. Three types of pulmonary involvement in polymyositis. *Med Clin NA* 1964;48:1031–1042.

193. Schwarz MI, Matthay RA, Sahn SA, et al. Interstitial lung disease in polymyositis and dermatomyositis. Analysis of six cases and review of the literature. *Medicine* 1976;55:89–104.

194. Frazier AR, Miller RD. Interstitial pneumonitis in association with polymyositis and dermatomyositis. *Chest* 1974;65:403–407.

195. Hochberg M, Feldman D, Stevens M, et al. Antibody to Jo-1 in polymyositis/dermatomyositis: association with interstitial pulmonary disease. *J Rheumatol* 1984;5:663–665.

196. Kiely J, Donohoe P, Breshihan B, et al. Pulmonary fibrosis in polymyositis with the Jo-1 syndrome: an unusual mode of presentation. *Respir Med* 1998;92:1167–1169.

197. Moriguchi M, Suzuki T, Tateishi M, et al. Intravenous immunoglobulin therapy for refractory myositis. *Intern Med* 1996;35:663–667.

198. Fauci AS, Wolff SM. Wegener's granulomatosis: studies in 18 patients and a review of the literature. *Medicine* 1973;52:535–561.

199. Fauci AS, Haynes BF, Katz P. The spectrum of vasculitis: clinical, pathologic, immunologic, and therapeutic considerations. *Ann Intern Med* 1978;89:660–676.

200. Wolff SM, Fauci AS, Hom RG, et al. Wegener's granulomatosis. *Ann Intern Med* 1974;81:513–525.

201. Fauci AS, Wolff SM. Wegener's granulomatosis and related diseases. *Dis Mon* 1977;23:1–36.

202. Haworth SJ, Savage CO, Carr D. Pulmonary hemorrhage complicating Wegener's granulomatosis and microscopic polyarteritis. *Br Med J* 1985;290:1775–1778.

203. Wechsler RJ, Steiner RM, Israel HL, et al. Chest radiograph in lymphomatoid granulomatosis: comparison with Wegener granulomatosis. *AJR* 1984;142:79–83.

204. Littlejohn GO, Ryan PJ, Holdsworth SR. Wegener's granulomatosis: clinical features and outcome in seventeen patients. *Aust NZ J Med* 1985;15:241–245.

205. Churg A. Pulmonary angiitis and granulomatosis revisited. *Hum Pathol* 1983;14:868–883.

206. Salant DJ. Immunopathogenesis of crescentic glomerulonephritis and lung purpura. *Kidney Int* 1987;32:408–425.

207. Leatherman JW. Immune alveolar hemorrhage. *Chest* 1987;91:891–897.

208. Walker RG, Becker GJ, d'Apice AJ. Plasma exchange in the treatment of glomerulonephritis and other renal diseases. *Aust NZ J Med* 1986;16:828–838.

209. Leavitt RY, Fauci AJ. Pulmonary vasculitis. *Am Rev Respir Dis* 1986;134:149–166.

210. Chandler DB, Fulmer JD. Pulmonary vasculitis. *Lung* 1985;163:257–273.

211. Fauci AJ, Haynes BF, Katz P, et al. Wegener's granulomatosis: prospective clinical and therapeutic experience with 85 patients for 21 years. *Ann Intern Med* 1983;98:76–85.

212. Carrington CB, Liebow AA. Limited forms of angiitis and granulomatosis of Wegener's type. *Am J Med* 1966;41:497–527.

213. Fauci AS, Wolff SM, Johnson JS. Effect of cyclophosphamide upon the immune response in Wegener's granulomatosis. *N Engl J Med* 1971;285:1493–1496.

214. Howell SB, Epstein WV. Circulating immunoglobulin complexes in Wegener's granulomatosis. *Am J Med* 1976;60:259–268.

215. Flye MW, Mundinger GH, Fauci AS. Diagnostic and therapeutic aspects of the surgical approach to Wegener's granulomatosis. *J Thorac Cardiovasc Surg* 1979;77:331–337.

216. Felson B. Less familiar roentgen patterns of pulmonary granulomas. *AJR* 1959;81:211–223.

217. McGrego MB, Sandler G. Wegener's granulomatosis. A clinical and radiological survey. *Br J Radiol* 1964;37:430–439.

218. Kornblum D, Feinberg R. Roentgen manifestations of necrotizing granulomatosis and angiitis of lungs. *AJR* 1955;74:587–592.

219. Maguire R, Fauci AS, Doppman JL, et al. Unusual radiographic features of Wegener's granulomatosis. *AJR* 1979;130:233–238.

220. Landman S, Burgener F. Pulmonary manifestations of Wegener's granulomatosis. *AJR* 1974;122:750–757.

221. Liebow AA. The J Burns Amberson Lecture: pulmonary angiitis and granulomatosis. *Am Rev Respir Dis* 1973;108:1–18.

222. Gonzales L, Van Ordstrand HS. Wegener's granulomatosis: review of 11 cases. *Radiology* 1973;107:295–300.

223. Israel HL, Patchefsky AS. Wegener's granulomatosis of lung: diagnosis and treatment. Experience with 12 cases. *Ann Intern Med* 1971;74:881–891.

224. Godman GC, Churg J. Wegener's granulomatosis: pathology and review of the literature. *Arch Pathol* 1954;58:533–558.

225. Israel HL, Patchefsky AS, Saldama MJ. Wegener's granulomatosis, lymphoid granulomatosis, and benign lymphocytic angiitis and granulomatosis of lung. *Ann Intern Med* 1977;87:691–699.

226. Winterbauer RH. Wegener's granulomatosis and other pulmonary granulomatous vasculitides. In Bone RA, Dantzker DR,

George RB, et al, eds. *Pulmonary and critical care medicine.* St Louis: Mosby, 1993:M6:1–13.

227. Cordier JF, Valeyre D, Guillevin L, et al. Pulmonary Wegener's granulomatosis: a clinical and imaging study of 77 cases. *Chest* 1990;97:906–912.

228. Rosenberg DM, Weinberger SE, Fulmer JD, et al. Functional correlates of lung involvement of Wegener's granulomatosis. Use of pulmonary function tests in staging and follow-up. *Am J Med* 1980;69:387–394.

229. Davies DJ, Moran JE, Niall JF, et al. Segmental necrotizing glomerulonephritis with antineutrophil antibody. Possible arbor virus aetiology? *Br Med J* 1982;285:606.

230. Vander Woude FJ, Rasmussen N, Lobatto S, et al. Autoantibodies against neutrophils and monocytes: tool for diagnosis and marker of disease activity in Wegener's granulomatosis. *Lancet* 1985;1:425–429.

231. Nolle B, Specks U, Ludemann J, et al. Anticytoplasmic autoantibodies: their immunodiagnostic value in Wegener's granulomatosis. *Ann Intern Med* 1989;111:28–40.

232. Kallenberg CG, Mulder AH, Tervaert JW. Antineutrophil cytoplasmic antibodies: a still-growing class of autoantibodies in inflammatory disorders. *Am J Med* 1992;93:678–689.

233. Goldschmeding R, van der Schoot CE, ten Bokkel Huinink D, et al. Wegener's granulomatosis autoantibodies identify a novel diisopropylfluorophosphate-binding protein in the lysosomes of normal human neutrophils. *J Clin Invest* 1989;84:1577–1587.

234. Jeanette JC, Ewert BH, Falk RJ. Do antineutrophil cytoplasmic autoantibodies cause Wegener's granulomatosis and other forms of necrotizing vasculitis? *Rheum Dis Clin North Am* 1993;19:1–14.

235. Leavitt RY, Fauci AS, Bioch DA. The American College of Rheumatology 1990 criteria for the classification of Wegener's granulomatosis. *Arthritis Rheum* 1990;33:1101–1107.

236. Hoffman G, Kerr G, Leavitt R, et al. Wegener's granulomatosis. an analysis of 158 patients. *Ann Intern Med* 1992;116:488–498.

237. Walton EW. Giant-cell granuloma of the respiratory tract (Wegener's granulomatosis). *Br Med J* 1958;2:265–270.

238. Hollander D, Manning RT. The use of alkylating agents in the treatment of Wegener's granulomatosis. *Ann Intern Med* 1967;67:393–398.

239. Sneller M, Hoffman G, Talar-Williams C, et al. An analysis of forty-two Wegener's granulomatosis patients treated with methotrexate and prednisone. *Arthritis Rheum* 1995;38:608–613.

240. DeRemee RA, McDonald TJ, Weiland LH. Wegener's granulomatosis: observations on treatment with antimicrobial agents. *Mayo Clin Proc* 1985;60:27–32.

241. Specks U, De Remee RA. Granulomatous vasculitis. Wegener's granulomatosis and Churg-Strauss syndrome. *Rheum Dis Clin North Am* 1990;16:377–397.

242. de Groot K, Reinhold-Keller E, Tatsis E, et al. Therapy for the maintenance of remission in sixty-five patients with generalized Wegener's granulomatosis. Methotrexate versus trimethoprim/sulfamethoxazole. *Arthitis Rheum* 1996;39:2052–2061.

243. Liebow AA, Carrington CR, Friedman PJ. Lymphomatoid granulomatosis. *Hum Pathol* 1972;3:457–558.

244. Meyers JL. Lymphomatoid granulomatosis. Past, present, future? *Mayo Clin Proc* 1990;65:274–278.

245. Katzenstein AA, Peiper SC. Detection of Epstein-Barr virus genomes in lymphomatoid granulomatosis: analysis of 29 cases by the polymerase chain reaction technique. *Mod Pathol* 1990;3:435–441.

246. Bone RC, Vernon M, Sobonya RE, et al. Lymphomatoid granulomatosis: report of a case and review of the literature. *Am J Med* 1978;65:709–716.

247. Colby TV, Carrington CB. Pulmonary lymphomas: current concepts. *Hum Pathol* 1983;14:884–887.

248. Schnek SA, Penn I. Cerebral neoplasms associated with renal transplantation. *Arch Neurol* 1970;22:226–233.

249. Doak PB, Montgomerie JZ, North JDK, et al. Reticulum cell sarcoma after renal homotransplantation and azathioprine and prednisone therapy. *Br Med J* 1968;4:746–748.

250. Pierce JC, Madge GE, Lee HM, et al. Lymphoma: a complication of renal allotransplantation in man. *JAMA* 1972;219:1593–1597.

251. Fauci AS. Granulomatous vasculitides: distinct but related (editorial). *Ann Intern Med* 1977;87:782–783.

252. Fauci AS, Haynes BC, Costa J, et al. Lymphomatoid granulomatosis: prospective clinical and therapeutic experience with 85 patients for 21 years. *N Engl J Med* 1982;306:68–74.

253. Churg J, Strauss L. Allergic granulomatosis, allergic angiitis and periarteritis nodosa. *Am J Pathol* 1951;27:277–301.

254. Rose GA, Spencer H. Polyarteritis nodosa. *Q J Med* 1957;26:43–81.

255. Lanham JG, Elkon KB, Pusey CD, et al. Systemic vasculitis with asthma and eosinophilia: a clinical approach to the Churg-Strauss syndrome. *Medicine* 1984;63:65–81.

256. Chumbley LC, Harrison EG Jr, Remee RA. Allergic granulomatosis and angiitis (Churg-Strauss syndrome): report and analysis of 30 cases. *Mayo Clin Proc* 1977;52:477–484.

257. Levin DC. Pulmonary abnormalities in the necrotizing vasculitides and their rapid response to steroids. *Radiology* 1970;97:521–526.

258. Churg J. Allergic granulomatosis and granulomatous-vascular syndromes. *Ann Allergy* 1963;21:619–628.

259. Guillevin L, Lhote F, Gayraud, et al. Prognostic factors in polyarteritis nodosa and Churg-Strauss syndrome. *Medicine (Balt)* 1996;75:17–28.

260. Wechsler M, Garpestad, E, Flier S, et al. Pulmonary infiltrates, eosinophilia, and cardiomyopathy following corticosteroid withrawal in patients with asthma receiving zafirlukast. *JAMA* 1998;279:455–457.

261. Guillevin L, Fain O, Lhote F, et al. Lack of superiority of steroids plus plasma exchange to steroids alone in the treatment of polyarteritis nodosa and Churg-Strauss syndrome. A prospective, randomized trial in 78 patients. *Arthritis Rheum* 1992;35:208–215.

262. Guillevin L, Jarrousse B, Lok C, et al. Long term follow-up after treatment of polyarteritis nodosa and Churg-Strauss angiitis with comparison of steroids, plasma exchange and cyclophosphamide to steroids and plasma exchange. A prospective randomized trial of 71 patients. *J Rheumatol* 1991;18:567–574.

263. Teague CA, Doak PB, Simpson IJ, et al. Goodpasture's syndrome: an analysis of 29 cases. *Kidney Int* 1978;13:492–504.

264. Schwartz EF, Teplick JG, Onesti G, et al. Pulmonary hemorrhage in renal diseases: Goodpasture's syndrome and other causes. *Radiology* 1977;122:39–46.

265. Wilson CB, Dixon FJ. Anti-glomerular basement membrane antibody induced glomerulonephritis. *Kidney Int* 1973;3:74–89.

266. McPhaul JJ Jr, Dixon FJ. The presence of antiglomerular basement membrane antibodies in peripheral blood. *J Immunol* 1969;103:1168–1175.

267. Matthew TH, Hobbs JB, Kalowski S, et al. Goodpasture's syndrome: normal renal diagnostic findings. *Ann Intern Med* 1975;82:215–218.

268. Lockwood CM, Boulton-Jones JM, Lowenthal RM, et al. Recovery from Goodpasture's syndrome after immunosuppressive treatment and plasmapheresis. *Br Med J* 1975;2:252–254.

269. Whitworth JA, Lawrence JR, Meadows R. Goodpasture's syndrome: a review of nine cases and an evaluation of therapy. *Aust NZ J Med* 1974;4:167–177.

270. Klasa RJ, Abboud RT, Ballon HS, et al. Goodpasture's syn-

drome: recurrence after a five-year remission. Case report and review of the literature. *Am J Med* 1988;84:751–755.

271. Wilson CB, Smith RC. Goodpasture's syndrome associated with influenza A2 virus infection. *Ann Intern Med* 1972;76: 91–94.

272. Young KR. Pulmonary hemorrhage syndromes. In Bone RA, Dantzker DR, George RB, et al, eds. *Pulmonary and critical care medicine.* St. Louis: Mosby, 1993:M10:1–13.

273. Ewan PLO, Jones HA, Rhodes CG, et al. Detections of intrapulmonary hemorrhage with carbon monoxide uptake. Application in Goodpasture's syndrome. *N Engl J Med* 1976;295: 1391–1396.

274. Hudson BG, Kalluri R, Gunwar S, et al. Molecular characteristics of the Goodpasture autoantigen. *Kidney Int* 1993;43: 135–139.

275. Bombassei GJ, Kaplan AA. The association between hydrocarbon exposure and anti-glomerular basement membrane antibody-mediated disease (Goodpasture's syndrome). *Am J Ind Med* 1992;21:141–153.

276. Lang CH, Brown DC, Staley N, et al. Goodpasture's syndrome treated with immunosuppression and plasma exchange. *Arch Intern Med* 1977;137:1076–1078.

277. McLeish KR, Maxwell DR, Luft FC. Failure of plasma exchange and immunosuppression to improve renal function in Goodpasture's syndrome. *Clin Nephrol* 1978;10:71–73.

278. Cove-Smith JR, McLeod AA, Blamey RW, et al. Transplantation, immunosuppression and plasmapheresis in Goodpasture's syndrome. *Clin Nephrol* 1978;9:126–128.

279. Swainson CP, Robson JS, Urbaniak SJ, et al. Treatment of Goodpasture's disease by plasma exchange and immunosuppression. *Clin Exp Immunol* 1978;32:233–242.

280. Johnson JP, Whitman W, Briggs A, et al. Plasmapheresis and immunosuppressive agents in antibasement membrane antibody-induced Goodpasture's syndrome. *Am J Med* 1978;64: 354–359.

281. Fraser RG, Paré JAP. Diseases of altered immunologic activity. In *Diagnosis of diseases of the chest,* 3rd ed. Philadelphia: Saunders, 1988.

282. Soergel KH, Sommers SC. Idiopathic pulmonary hemosiderosis and related syndromes. *Am J Med* 1962;32:499–511.

283. Boyd DHA. Idiopathic pulmonary hemosiderosis in adults and adolescents. *Br J Dis Chest* 1959;53:41–51.

284. Bronson SM. Idiopathic pulmonary hemosiderosis in adults. Report of a case and review of the literature. *AJR* 1960;83: 260–273.

285. Ognibene AJ, Johnson DE. Idiopathic pulmonary hemosiderosis in adults. Report of a case and review of literature. *Arch Intern Med* 1963;111:503–510.

286. Cooper AS. Idiopathic pulmonary hemosiderosis. Report of a case in an adult treated with triamcinolone. *N Engl J Med* 1960; 263:1100–1103.

287. Smith WE, Fienberg R. Early nonrecurrent idiopathic hemosiderosis in an adult. Report of a case. *N Engl J Med* 1958;259: 808–811.

288. Hyatt RW, Adelstein ER, Halazum JF, et al. Ultrastructure of the lung in idiopathic pulmonary hemosiderosis. *Am J Med* 1972;52:822–829.

289. Soergel KH, Sommers SC. The alveolar epithelial lesion of idiopathic pulmonary hemosiderosis. *Am Rev Respir Dis* 1962;85: 540–552.

290. Overholt EL. Acute pulmonary-renal syndromes. *Dis Chest* 1965;48:68–77.

291. Irwin RS, Cottrell TS, Hsu KC, et al. Idiopathic pulmonary hemosiderosis. An electron microscopic and immunofluorescent study. *Chest* 1974;65:41–45.

292. Donlam CJ Jr, Srodes CH, Duffy FD. Idiopathic pulmonary

hemosiderosis—electron microscopic, immunofluorescent, and iron kinetic studies. *Chest* 1975;68:577–581.

293. Theros EG, Reeder MM, Eckert JF. An exercise in radiologic-pathologic correlation. *Radiology* 1968;90:784–791.

294. Rosen SH, Castleman B, Liebow AA. Pulmonary alveolar proteinosis. *N Engl J Med* 1975;258:1123–1146.

295. Claypool WD. Pulmonary alveolar proteinosis. In Fishman AP, ed. *Pulmonary diseases and disorders.* New York: McGraw-Hill, 1988:893–900.

296. Gehle DW, Territo M, Finley TN, et al. Defective lung macrophages in pulmonary alveolar proteinosis. *Ann Intern Med* 1976; 85:304–309.

297. Costello JF, Moriarty DC, Branthwaite MA, et al. Diagnosis and management of alveolar proteinosis: the role of electron microscopy. *Thorax* 1975;30:121–132.

298. Davidson JM, MacLeod WM. Pulmonary alveolar proteinosis. *Br J Dis Chest* 1969;63:13–28.

299. Hudson AR, Halprin GM, Miller JA, et al. Pulmonary interstitial fibrosis following alveolar proteinosis. *Chest* 1974;65: 700–702.

300. Rubinstein I, Muller JB, Hoffstein V. Morphologic diagnosis of idiopathic pulmonary alveolar lipoproteinosis—revisited. *Arch Intern Med* 1988;148:813–816.

301. DuBois RM, McAllister WA, Branthwaite MA. Alveolar proteinosis: diagnosis and treatment over a 10 year period. *Thorax* 1983;38:360–363.

302. Claypool WD, Rogers RM, Matuschak GM. Update on the clinical diagnosis, management and pathogenesis of pulmonary alveolar proteinosis (phospholipidosis). *Chest* 1984;85: 550–558.

303. Kariman K, Kylstra JA, Spock A. Pulmonary alveolar proteinosis: prospective clinical experience in 23 patients for 15 years. *Lung* 1984;162:223–231.

304. Rosen SH, Castleman B, Liebow AA. Pulmonary alveolar proteinosis. *N Engl J Med* 1958;258:1123–1142.

305. Abraham JL, McEuen DD. Inorganic particulates associated with pulmonary alveolar proteinosis: SEM and x-ray microanalysis results. *Appl Pathol* 1986;4:138–146.

306. Hoffman RM, Rogers RM. Pulmonary alveolar proteinosis. In Bone RC, Dantzker DD, George RB, et al. eds. *Pulmonary and critical care medicine.* St. Louis: Mosby Year Book, 1993:M12: 1–7.

307. Hoffman RM, Rogers RM. Serum and lavage lactate dehydrogenase isoenzymes in pulmonary alveolar proteinosis. *Am Rev Respir Dis* 1991;143:42–46.

308. Haslam PL, Hughes DA, Dewar A, et al. Lipoprotein macroaggregates in bronchoalveolar lavage fluid from patients with diffuse interstitial lung disease: comparison with idiopathic alveolar lipoproteinosis. *Thorax* 1988;43:140–146.

309. Takemura T, Fukuda Y, Harrison M, et al. Ultrastructural, histochemical, and freeze-fracture evaluation of multilamellated structures in human pulmonary alveolar proteinosis. *Am J Anat* 1987;179:258–268.

310. Hook GE, Gilmore LB, Talley FA. Dissolution and reassembly of tubular myelin-like multilamellated structures from the lungs of patients with pulmonary alveolar proteinosis. *Lab Invest* 1986;55:194–208.

311. Hook GE, Gilmore LB, Talley FA. Multilamellated structure from the lungs of patients with pulmonary alveolar proteinosis. *Lab Invest* 1984;50:711–725.

312. Nugent KM, Pesanti EL. Macrophage function in pulmonary alveolar proteinosis. *Am Rev Respir Dis* 1983;127:780–781.

313. Gonzalez-Rothi RJ, Harris JO. Pulmonary alveolar proteinosis. Further evaluation of abnormal alveolar macrophages. *Chest* 1986;90:656–661.

314. Wilson DO, Rogers RM. Prolonged spontaneous remission in

a patient with untreated pulmonary alveolar proteinosis. *Am J Med* 1987;82:1014–1016.

315. Ramirez RJ. Bronchopulmonary lavage: new techniques and observations. *Dis Chest* 1966;50:581–588.

316. Rogers RM, Szidon JP, Shelburne J, et al. Hemodynamic response of the pulmonary circulation to bronchopulmonary lavage in man. *N Engl J Med* 1972;286:1230–1233.

317. Rosenow EC. The spectrum of drug-induced pulmonary disease. *Ann Intern Med* 1972;77:977–991.

318. Cooper JA Jr, Zitnik RJ, Matthay RA. Mechanisms of drug-induced pulmonary disease. *Annu Rev Med* 1988;39:395–404.

319. Rosenow EC III. Drug-induced bronchopulmonary pleural disease. *J Allergy Clin Immunol* 1987;80:780–787.

320. Cooper JA Jr, Matthay RA. Drug-induced pulmonary disease. *Dis Mon* 1987;33:61–120.

321. Cooper JA Jr, White DA, Matthay RA. Drug-induced pulmonary disease. Part 1: cytotoxic drugs. *Am Rev Respir Dis* 1986;133:321–340.

322. Cooper JA Jr, White DA, Matthay RA. Drug-induced pulmonary disease. Part 2: noncytotoxic drugs. *Am Rev Respir Dis* 1986;133:488–505.

323. Rosenow EC III, Wilson WR, Cockerill FR III. Pulmonary disease in the immunocompromised host. *Mayo Clin Proc* 1985;60:473–487.

324. Adamson IY. Drug-induced pulmonary fibrosis. *Environ Health Perspect* 1984;55:25–36.

325. Gockerman JP. Drug-induced interstitial lung diseases. *Clin Chest Med* 1982;3:521–536.

326. Cooper JA Jr. Drug-related pulmonary diseases. In Bone RC, Dantzker DR, George RB, et al, eds. *Pulmonary and critical care medicine.* St. Louis: Mosby-Year Book, 1993:M8:1–9.

327. Rosenow EC 3d, Myers JL, Swensen SJ, et al. Drug-induced pulmonary disease. An update. *Chest* 1992;102:239–250.

328. Israel-Biet D, Labrune S, Huchon GJ. Drug-induced lung disease: 1990 review. *Eur Respir J* 1991;4:465–478.

329. Gregory SA, Grippi MA. The clinical diagnosis of drug-induced pulmonary disorders. *J Thorac Imaging* 1991;6:8–18.

330. Zitnik RJ, Cooper JA Jr. Pulmonary disease due to antirheumatic agents. *Clin Chest Med* 1990;11:139–150.

331. Beaudry C, Laplante L. Severe allergic pneumonitis from hydrochlorothiazide. *Ann Intern Med* 1973;78:251–253.

332. Sostman HD, Matthay RA, Putnam CE. Cytotoxic drug-induced lung disease. *Am J Med* 1977;62:608–615.

333. Weiss RB, Muggia FM. Cytotoxic drug-induced pulmonary disease—update 1980. *Am J Med* 1980;68:259–266.

334. Winterbauer RH, Wilske KR, Wheeis RF. Diffuse pulmonary injury associated with gold treatment. *N Engl J Med* 1976;294:919–921.

335. McCormick J, Cole S, Lahirir B, et al. Pneumonitis caused by gold salt therapy: evidence for the role of cell-mediated immunity in its pathogenesis. *Am Rev Respir Dis* 1980;122:145–152.

336. Pascual RS, Mosher MB, Sikand RS, et al. Effects of bleomycin on pulmonary function in man. *Am Rev Respir Dis* 1973;108:211–217.

337. Goldiner PL, Carlon GC, Cvitkovic E, et al. Factors influencing postoperative morbidity and mortality in patients treated with bleomycin. *Br Med J* 1978;1:1664–1667.

338. Holoye PY, Luna MA, Mackay B, et al. Bleomycin hypersensitivity pneumonitis. *Ann Intern Med* 1978;88:47–49.

339. McCullough B, Collins JF, Johanson WG Jr, et al. Bleomycin-induced diffuse interstitial pulmonary fibrosis in baboons. *J Clin Invest* 1978;61:79–88.

340. Hailey FJ, Glascock HW, Hewitt WF. Pleuropneumonic reactions to nitrofurantoin. *N Engl J Med* 1969;281:1087–1090.

341. Kuhlman J. The role of chest computed tomography in the diagnosis of drug-related reactions. *J Thorac Imaging* 1991;6:52–61.

342. Kennedy JI Jr. Clinical aspects of amiodarone pulmonary toxicity. *Clin Chest Med* 1990;11:119–130.

343. Wieder J, Soloway M. Interstitial pneumonitis associated with neoadjuvant leuprolide and nilutamide for prostate cancer. *J Urol* 1998;159:2099.

344. Mitchell DN, Scadding JG. Sarcoidosis (state of the art). *Am Rev Respir Dis* 1974;110:774–802.

345. Mayock RL, Bertrand P, Morrison CE, et al. Manifestations of sarcoidosis (analysis of 145 patients with review of nine series selected from the literature). *Am J Med* 1963;35:67–89.

346. Nolan JP, Klatskin G. The fever of sarcoidosis. *Ann Intern Med* 1964;61:455–461.

347. Israel H. Sarcoidosis. In Simmons DH, ed. *Current pulmonology.* Boston: Houghton Mifflin, 1979:163–182.

348. Roberts WC, McAllister HA, Ferrans VJ. Sarcoidosis of the heart (114 necropsy patients). *Am J Med* 1977;63:86–108.

349. Fleming HA. Sarcoid heart disease. *Br Heart J* 1974;36:54–68.

350. Delaney P. Neurologic manifestations in sarcoidosis. *Ann Intern Med* 1977;87:336–345.

351. Sharma OP, Sharma AM. Sarcoidosis of the nervous system—a clinical approach. *Arch Intern Med* 1991;151:1317–1321.

352. Klatskin G, Yesner R. Hepatic manifestations of sarcoidosis and other granulomatous diseases—a study based on histological examination of tissue obtained by needle biopsy of the liver. *Yale J Biol Med* 1950;23:207–248.

353. Israel HL, Goldstein RA. Hepatic granulomatosis and sarcoidosis. *Ann Intern Med* 1973;79:669–678.

354. Winterbauer PH, Belic N, Moores KD. A clinical interpretation of bilateral hilar adenopathy. *Ann Intern Med* 1973;78:65–71.

355. DeRemee RA, Andersen HA. Sarcoidosis—a correlation of dyspnea with roentgenographic stage and pulmonary function changes. *Mayo Clin Proc* 1974;49:742–745.

356. Littner MR, Schachter EN, Putnam CE, et al. The clinical assessment of roentgenographically atypical pulmonary sarcoidosis. *Am J Med* 1977;62:361–368.

357. Siltzbach LE, James DG, Neville E, et al. Course and prognosis of sarcoidosis around the world. *Am J Med* 1974;57:847–852.

358. Dunn T, Watters L, Hendrix C. Gas exchange at a given degree of volume restriction is different in sarcoidosis and idiopathic pulmonary fibrosis. *Am J Med* 1988;85:221–224.

359. Prior C, Haslam PL. Increased levels of serum interferon-gamma in pulmonary sarcoidosis and relationship with response to corticosteroid therapy. *Am Rev Respir Dis* 1991;143:53–60.

360. Daniele RP, Rowlands DT. Lymphocyte subpopulations in sarcoidosis. Correlation with disease activity and duration. *Ann Intern Med* 1976;85:593–600.

361. Manderazo EG, Ward PA, Woronick CL, et al. Leukotactic dysfunction in sarcoidosis. *Ann Intern Med* 1976;84:414–419.

362. Goodwin JS, DeHoratius R, Israel H, et al. Suppressor cell function in sarcoidosis. *Ann Intern Med* 1979;90:169–173.

363. Daniele RP, Dauber JH, Rossman MD. Immunologic abnormalities in sarcoidosis. *Ann Intern Med* 1980;92:406–416.

364. Daniele RP, McMillan LJ, Dauber JH, et al. Immune complexes in sarcoidosis—a correlation with activity and duration of disease. *Chest* 1978;74:261–264.

365. Pascual RA, Gee JBL, Finch SC. Usefulness of serum lysozyme measurement in diagnosis and evaluation of sarcoidosis. *N Engl J Med* 1973;289:1074–1076.

366. Lieberman J. Elevation of serum angiotensin converting enzyme level in sarcoidosis. *Am J Med* 1975;59:365–372.

367. Zorn SK, Stevens CA, Schachter EN, et al. The angiotensin converting enzyme in pulmonary sarcoidosis and the relative diagnostic value of serum lysozyme. *Lung* 1980;157:87–94.

368. Allen RK. A review of angiotensin converting enzyme in health and disease. *Sarcoidosis* 1991;8:95–100.

369. Gee JBL, Bodel PT, Zorn SK, et al. Sarcoidosis and mononuclear phagocytes. *Lung* 1978;155:243–253.

370. Hinman LM, Stevens C, Matthay RA, et al. Angiotensin convertase activities in human alveolar macrophages: effects of cigarette smoking and sarcoidosis. *Science* 1979;205:202–203.

371. Fanburg BL, Schoenberger MD, Bachus B, et al. Elevated serum angiotensin I converting enzyme in sarcoidosis. *Am Rev Respir Dis* 1976;114:525–528.

372. Silverstein E, Friedland J, Ackerman T. Elevation of granulomatous lymph-node and serum lysozyme in sarcoidosis and correlation and angiotensin-converting enzyme. *Am J Clin Pathol* 1977;68:219–224.

373. Lieberman J, Nosal A, Schlessner LA, et al. Serum angiotensin-converting enzyme for diagnosis and therapeutic evaluation of sarcoidosis. *Am Rev Respir Dis* 1979;120:329–335.

374. Nosal A, Schlessiner LA, Mishkin FS, et al. Angiotensin-I-converting enzyme and gallium scan in non-invasive evaluation of sarcoidosis. *Ann Intern Med* 1979;90:328–331.

375. DeRemee RA, Rohrbach MS. Serum angiotensin-converting enzyme activity in evaluating the clinical course of sarcoidosis. *Ann Intern Med* 1980;92:361–365.

376. Koontz CH, Joyner LR, Nelson RA. Transbronchial lung biopsy via the fiberoptic bronchoscope in sarcoidosis. *Ann Intern Med* 1976;85:64–66.

377. Wall CP, Gaensler EA, Carrington CB, et al. Comparison of transbronchial and open biopsies in chronic infiltrative lung diseases. *Am Rev Respir Dis* 1981;123:280–285.

378. Reynolds HY. The importance of lymphocytes in pulmonary health and disease. *Lung* 1978;155:225–242.

379. Hunninghake GW, Fulmer JD, Young RC Jr, et al. Localization of the immune response in sarcoidosis. *Am Rev Respir Dis* 1979; 120:49–57.

380. Daniele RP, Dauber JH, Rossman MD. Lymphocyte populations in the bronchoalveolar air spaces: recent observations in asymptomatic smokers and nonsmokers. In Biserte G, Chretien J, Voisin C, eds. *International Symposium on Bronchoalveolar Lavage in Man.* Paris: L'Institut National de la Sante et de la Recherche Medicale, 1979:193–209.

381. Hunninghake GW, Gadek JE, Young RC Jr, et al. Maintenance of granuloma formation in pulmonary sarcoidosis by T-lymphocytes within the lung. *N Engl J Med* 1980;302:594–598.

382. Hunninghake GW, Crystal RG. Mechanisms of hypergammaglobulinemia in pulmonary sarcoidosis. Site of increased antibody production and role of T-lymphocytes. *J Clin Invest* 1981; 67:86–92.

383. Hunninghake GW, Crystal RG. T-suppressor cells in sarcoidosis. *N Engl J Med* 1981;305:429–434.

384. Drent M, van Velzen-Blad H, Diamant M, et al. Relationship between presentation of sarcoidosis and T lymphocyte profile. A study in bronchoalveolar lavage fluid. *Chest* 1993;104:795–800.

385. Van Maarsseveen TC, deGroot J, Stam J, et al. Peripolesis in alveolar sarcoidosis. *Am Rev Respir Dis* 1993;147:1259–1263.

386. DuBois RM, Kirby M, Balbi B, et al. T-lymphocytes that accumulate in the lung in sarcoidosis have evidence of recent stimulation of the T-cell antigen receptor. *Am Rev Respir Dis* 1992; 145:1205–1211.

387. Biyoudi-Vouenze R, Cadranel J, Valeyre D, et al. Expression of 1,25(OH)$_2$D$_3$ receptors on alveolar lymphocytes from patients with pulmonary granulomatous diseases. *Am Rev Respir Dis* 1991;143:1376–1380.

387a. Reynolds HY. Cytokines: role in respiratory illnesses and potential control with immunomodulatory therapy. *Focus & Opinion: Int Med* 1994;1(6):1–10.

388. Hunninghake GW. Release of interleukin-I by alveolar macro-phages of patients with active pulmonary sarcoidosis. *Am Rev Respir Dis* 1984;129:569–572.

389. Moller D, Forman J, Liu M, et al. Enhanced expression of IL-12 associated Th1 cytokine profiles in active pulmonary sarcoidosis. *J Immunol* 1996;156:4952–4960.

390. Pueringer RJ, Schwartz DA, Dayton CS, et al. The relationship between alveolar macrophage TNF, I1–1, and PGE$_2$ release, alvcolitis, and disease severity in sarcoidosis. *Chest* 1993;103: 832–838.

391. Fels AOS, Cohn ZA. The alveolar macrophage. *J Appl Physiol* 1986;60:353–369.

392. Nathan CF. Secretory products of macrophages. *J Clin Invest* 1987;79:319–326.

393. Sibille Y, Reynolds HY. Macrophages and polymorphonuclear neutrophils in lung defense and injury. *Am Rev Respir Dis* 1990; 141:471–501.

394. Lem VW, Lipscomb MF, Weissler JC, et al. Bronchoalveolar cells from sarcoid patients demonstrate enhanced antigen presentation. *J Immunol* 1985;135:1766–1771.

395. Saltini C, Spurzem JR, Lee JJ, et al. Spontaneous release of interleukin 2 by lung T lymphocytes in active pulmonary sarcoidosis is primarily from the Leu + DR + T cell subset. *J Clin Invest* 1986;77:1962–1970.

396. Pinkston P, Bitterman PB, Crystal RG. Spontaneous release of interleukin-2 by lung T-lymphocytes in active pulmonary sarcoidosis. *N Engl J Med* 1983;308:783–800.

397. Hunninghake GW, Bedell BN, Zavala DC, et al. Role of interleukin 2 release by lung T-cells in active pulmonary sarcoidosis. *Am Rev Respir Dis* 1983;128:634–638.

398. Robinson BWS, Pinkston P, Crystal RG. Natural killer cells are present in the normal human lung but are functionally impotent. *J Clin Invest* 1984;74:942–950.

399. Saltini C, Spurzem JR, Kirby MR, et al. Sarcoidosis is not associated with a generalized defect in T cell suppressor function. *J Immunol* 1988;140:1854–1860.

400. Muller-Quernheim J, Saltini C, Sondermeyer P, et al. Compartmentalized activation of the interleukin-2 gene by lung T lymphocytes in active pulmonary sarcoidosis. *J Immunol* 1986;137: 3475–3483.

401. Muller-Quernheim J, Pfeifer S, Männel D, et al. Lung-restricted activation of the alveolar macrophage/monocyte system in pulmonary sarcoidosis. *Am Rev Respir Dis* 1992;145:187–192.

402. Robinson BWS, McLemore T, Crystal RG. Gamma interferon is spontaneously released by alveolar macrophages and lung T-lymphocytes in patients with pulmonary sarcoidosis. *J Clin Invest* 1985;75:1488–1495.

403. Gilbert S, Steinbrech DS, Landas SK, et al. Amounts of angiotensin-converting enzyme mRNA reflect the burden of granulomas in granulomatous lung disease. *Am Rev Respir Dis* 1993; 148:483–486.

404. Roth C, Huchon GJ, Arnoux A, et al. Bronchoalveolar cells in advanced pulmonary sarcoidosis. *Am Rev Respir Dis* 1981;124: 9–12.

405. Sibille Y, Naegel GP, Merrill WW, et al. Neutrophil chemotactic activity produced by normal and activated human bronchoalveolar lavage cells. *J Lab Clin Med* 1987;110:624–633.

406. Agostini C, Trentin L, Zambello R, et al. CD8 alveolitis in sarcoidosis: incidence, phenotypic characteristics, and clinical features. *Am J Med* 1993;95:466–472.

407. Young RL, Harkleroad LE, Lordon RE, et al. Pulmonary sarcoidosis: a prospective evaluation of glucocorticoid therapy. *Ann Intern Med* 1970;73:207–212.

408. Sharma OP. Pulmonary sarcoidosis and corticosteroids. *Am Rev Respir Dis* 1993;147:1598–1600.

409. Johns CJ, MacGregor MI, Zachary JB, et al. Extended experi-

ence in the long-term corticosteroid treatment of pulmonary sarcoidosis. *Ann NY Acad Sci* 1976;278:722–731.

410. DeRemee RA. The present status of treatment of pulmonary sarcoidosis: a house divided. *Chest* 1977;71:388–393.

411. Rolfe MW, Standiford TJ, Kunkel SL, et al. Interleukin-1 receptor antagonist expression in sarcoidosis. *Am Rev Respir Dis* 1993; 148:1378–1384.

412. Pinkston P, Saltini C, Muller-Quernheim J, et al. Corticosteroid therapy suppresses spontaneous interleukin-2 release and spontaneous proliferation of lung T-lymphocytes of patient with active pulmonary sarcoidosis. *J Immunol* 1987;139:755–760.

413. Israel HL, Albertine KH, Park CH, et al. Whole body gallium 67 scans-role in diagnosis of sarcoidosis. *Am Rev Respir Dis* 1991;144:1182–1186.

414. Lawrence EC, Teague RB, Gottlieb MD, et al. Serial changes in markers of disease activity with corticosteroid treatment in sarcoidosis. *Am J Med* 1983;74:747–756.

415. Ceuppens JL, Lacquet LM, Marien G, et al. Alveolar T-cells subsets in pulmonary sarcoidosis. Correlation with disease activity and effect of steroid treatment. *Am Rev Respir Dis* 1984; 129:563–568.

416. Baughman RP, Fernandez M, Boxken CH, et al. Comparison of gallium 67 scanning, bronchoalveolar lavage and serum angiotensin converting enzyme levels in pulmonary sarcoidosis. *Am Rev Respir Dis* 1984;132:65–69.

417. Hollinger WM, Statton GW, Fajman WA, et al. Prediction of therapeutic response in steroid-treated pulmonary sarcoidosis. *Am Rev Respir Dis* 1985;132:65–69.

418. Turner-Warwick M, McAllister W, Lawrence R, et al. Corticosteroid treatment in pulmonary sarcoidosis: do serial lavage lymphocyte counts, serum angiotensin converting enzyme measurements, and gallium-67 scans help management? *Thorax* 1986; 41:903–913.

419. Lawrence EG, Berger MB, Broussau KP, et al. Elevated serum levels of soluble interleukin-2 receptors in active pulmonary sarcoidosis: relative specificity and association with hypercalcemia. *Sarcoidosis* 1987;4:87–93.

420. Reynolds HY. Pulmonary sarcoidosis. Do cellular and immunochemical lung parameters exist that would separate subgroups of patients for prognosis? *Sarcoidosis* 1989;6:1–4.

421. Rankin JA, Huang SS, Sostman HD, et al. An analysis of the inter-relationships among multiple bronchoalveolar lavage and serum determinations, physiologic tests, and clinical disease activity in patients with sarcoidosis. *Sarcoidosis* 1991;8:19–28.

422. Winterbauer RH, Wu R, Springmeyer SC. Fractional analysis of the 120-ml bronchoalveolar lavage. Determination of the best specimen for diagnosis of sarcoidosis. *Chest* 1993;104:344–351.

423. Saltini C, Kirby M, Trapnell BC, et al. Biased accumulation of T lymphocytes with "Memory"-type CD45 leukocyte common antigen gene expression on the epithelial surface of the human lung. *J Exp Med* 1990;171:1123–1140.

424. Lowery WS, Whitlock WL, Dietrich RA, et al. Sarcoidosis complicated by HIV infection: three case reports and a review of the literature. *Am Rev Respir Dis* 1990;142:887–889.

425. Schatz M, Patterson R, Fink G. Immunopathogenesis of hypersensitivity pneumonitis. *J Allergy Clin Immunol* 1977;60:27–37.

426. Reynolds HY. *Clinics in chest medicine*. Philadelphia: Saunders, 1982:503–519.

427. Reynolds HY. Hypersensitivity pneumonitis: correlation of cellular and immunologic changes with clinical phases of disease. *Lung* 1991;169:S109–S128.

428. Kaltreider HB. Hypersensitivity pneumonitis. Review. *West J Med* 1993;159:570–578.

429. Malmberg P, Rask-Andersen A, Rosenhall L. Exposure to microorganisms associated with allergic alveolitis and febrile reactions to mold dust in farmers. *Chest* 1993;103:1202–1209.

430. Patterson R, Wang JLF, Fink JN, et al. IgA and IgG antibody activities of serum and bronchoalveolar fluid from symptomatic and asymptomatic pigeon breeders. *Am Rev Respir Dis* 1979; 120:1113–1118.

431. Treuhaft MW, Robert RC, Hackbarth C, et al. Characterization of precipitin response to *Micropolyspora faeni* in farmer's lung disease by quantitative immunoelectrophoresis. *Am Rev Respir Dis* 1979;119:571–578.

432. Braun SR, doPico GA, Tsiatis A, et al. Farmer's lung disease: long-term clinical and physiologic outcome. *Am Rev Respir Dis* 1979;119:185–191.

433. Sansoores R, Salas J, Chapela R, et al. Clubbing in hypersensitivity pneumonitis. *Arch Intern Med* 1990;150:1849–1851.

434. Reynolds HY. Concepts of pathogenesis and lung reactivity in hypersensitivity pneumonitis (Louis E. Siltzbach Lecture). 10th International Conference on Sarcoidosis and Other Granulomatous Disorders. *Ann NY Acad Sci* 1986;465:287–303.

435. Leatherman JW, Michael AF, Schwartz BA, et al. Lung T-cells in hypersensitivity pneumonitis. *Ann Intern Med* 1984;100: 390–392.

436. Costabel U, Bross KJ, Ruhle KH, et al. Ia-like antigens on T-cells and their subpopulations in pulmonary sarcoidosis and in hypersensitivity pneumonitis—analysis of bronchoalveolar and blood lymphocytes. *Am Rev Respir Dis* 1985;131:337–342.

437. Semanzato G, Chilosi M, Ossi E, et al. Bronchoalveolar lavage and lung histology: comparative analysis of inflammatory and immunocompetent cells in patients with sarcoidosis and hypersensitivity pneumonitis. *Am Rev Respir Dis* 1985;132:400–404.

438. Murayama J, Yoshizawa Y, Ohtsuka M, et al. Lung fibrosis in hypersensitivity pneumonitis. Association with CD4 + but not CD8 + cell dominant alveolitis and insidious onset. *Chest* 1993;104:38–43.

439. Calvanico NJ, Ambegaonkar SP, Schlueter DP, et al. Immunoglobulin levels in bronchoalveolar lavage fluid from pigeon breeders. *J Lab Clin Med* 1980;98:129–140.

440. Fournier E, Tonnel AB, Gesset P, et al. Early neutrophil alveolitis after inhalation challenge in hypersensitivity pneumonitis. *Chest* 1985;88:563–566.

441. Solal-Celigny P, Laviolette M, Hebert J, et al. Immune reactions in the lungs of asymptomatic dairy farmers. *Am Rev Respir Dis* 1982;126:964–967.

442. Cormier Y, Belanger J, Beaudoin J, et al. Abnormal bronchoalveolar lavage in asymptomatic dairy farmers—study of lymphocytes. *Am Rev Respir Dis* 1984;130:1046–1049.

443. Cormier Y, Belanger J, Laviolette M. Persistent bronchoalveolar lymphocytosis in asymptomatic farmers. *Am Rev Respir Dis* 1986;133:843–847.

444. Gariépy L, Cormier Y, Laviolette M, et al. Predictive value of bronchoalveolar lavage cells and serum precipitins in asymptomatic dairy farmers. *Am Rev Respir Dis* 1989;140:1386–1389.

445. Lalancette M, Carrier G, Laviolette M, et al. Farmer's lung. Long-term outcome and lack of predictive value of bronchoalveolar lavage fibrosing factors. *Am Rev Respir Dis* 1993;148: 216–221.

446. Cormier Y, Laviolette M, Cantin A, et al. Fibrogenic activities in bronchoalveolar lavage fluid of farmer's lung. *Chest* 1993; 104:1038–1042.

447. Tescher H, Pohl WR, Thompson AB, et al. Elevated levels of bronchoalveolar lavage vitronectin in hypersensitivity pneumonitis. *Am Rev Respir Dis* 1993;147:332–337.

448. Pérez-Arellano JL, Pedraz MJ, Fuertes A, et al. Laminin fragment P1 is increased in the lower respiratory tract of patients with diffuse interstitial lung diseases. *Chest* 1993;104: 1163–1169.

449. Koss M, Hochholzer L, Langloss J, et al. Lymphoid interstitial

pneumonia. clinicopathological and immunopathological finding in 18 cases. *Pathology* 1987;19:178–85

450. Butterworth AE, David JR. Eosinophil function. *N Engl J Med* 1981;304:154–156.
451. Crofton JW, Livingstone JL, Oswalk NC, et al. Pulmonary eosinophilia. *Thorax* 1952;7:1–35.
452. Rossing TH. Pulmonary infiltrates with eosinophilia (PIE) syndrome and asthma. *Medical Grand Rounds* 1986;4:84–93.
453. Allen J, Davis W. Eosinophilic lung diseases. *Am J Respir Crit Care Med* 1994;150:1423–1438.
454. Shannon J, Lynch J. Eosinophilic pulmonary syndromes. *Clin Pulm Med* 1995;2:19–38.
455. Allen J, Pacht E, Gadek J, et al. Acute eosinophilic pneumonia as a reversible cause of noninfectious respiratory failure. *N Engl J Med* 1989;321:569–574.
456. Badesh D, King T, Schwarz M. Acute eosinophilic pneumonia. A hypersensitivity phenomenon? *Am Rev Resp Dis* 1989;139:249–252.
457. Carrington CB, Addington WW, Goff AM, et al. Chronic eosinophilic pneumonia. *N Engl J Med* 1969;280:787–798.
458. Webb JKG, Job CK, Gault EW. Tropical eosinophilia: demonstration of microfilaria in lung, liver and lymph nodes. *Lancet* 1960;1:835.
459. Danaraj TJ, Pacheco G, Shanmugaratnum K, et al. The etiology and pathology of eosinophilic lung (tropical eosinophilia). *Am J Trop Med Hyg* 1966;15:183–189.
460. Pinkston P, Vijayan VK, Nutman TB, et al. Acute tropical pulmonary eosinophilia—characterization of the lower respiratory tract inflammation and its response to therapy. *J Clin Invest* 1987;80:216–225.
461. Nutman TB, Vijayan VK, Pinkston P, et al. Tropical pulmonary eosinophilia: analysis of antifilarial antibody localized to the lung. *J Infect Dis* 1989;160:1042–1050.
462. Rom WN, Vijayan VK, Cornelius MJ, et al. Persistent lower respiratory inflammation associated with interstitial lung disease in patients with tropical pulmonary eosinophilia following conventional treatment with diethylcarbamazine. *Am Rev Respir Dis* 1990;142:1088–1092.
463. Sederlinic PJ, Sicilian L, Gaensler EA. Chronic eosinophilic pneumonia: a report of 19 and a review of the literature. *Medicine* 1988;67:154–162.
464. Naughton M, Fahy J, Fitzgerald MX. Chronic eosinophilic pneumonia—a long term follow-up of 12 patients. *Chest* 1993;103:162–165.
465. Snider GL. In case records, Massachusetts General Hospital. *N Engl J Med* 1980;303:1218–1225.
466. McCarthy DS, Pepys J. Allergic broncho-pulmonary aspergillosis. Clinical immunology: (1) clinical features. *Clin Allergy* 1971;1:261–286.
467. Groopman JE, Golde DW. The histiocytic disorders: a pathophysiologic analysis. *Ann Intern Med* 1981;94:95–107.
468. Travis W, Borok Z, Roum J, et al. Pulmonary Langerhans cell granulomatosis (histiocytosis X). A clinicopathologic study of 48 cases. *Am J Surg Path* 17:971–986.
469. Marcy TW, Reynolds HY. Pulmonary histiocytosis. *Lung* 1985;163:129–150.
470. Strieder DJ, Mark EJ. Pulmonary eosinophilic granuloma. In case records, Massachusetts General Hospital. *N Engl J Med* 1978;298:327–332.
471. King TE, Schwarz MI, Dreisin RE, et al. Circulating immune complexes in pulmonary eosinophilic granuloma. *Ann Intern Med* 1979;98:397–399.
472. Lacronique J, Roth C, Battesti JP, et al. Chest radiologic feature of pulmonary histiocytosis X: a report based on 50 adult cases. *Thorax* 1982;37:104–109.
473. Casolaro MA, Bernaudin JF, Saltini C, et al. Accumulation of Langerhans' cells on the epithelial surface of the lower respiratory tract in normal subjects in association with cigarette smoking. *Am Rev Respir Dis* 1988;137:406–411.
474. Tazi A, Bonay M, Grandsaigne M, et al. Surface phenotype of Langerhans cells and lymphocytes in granulomatous lesions from patients with pulmonary histiocytosis X. *Am Rev Respir Dis* 1993;147:1531–1536.
475. Tazi A, Bouchonnet F, Grandsaigne M, et al. Evidence that granulocyte macrophage colony stimulating factor regulates the distribution and differentiated state of dendritic cells/Langerhans cells in human lung and lung cancers. *J Clin Invest* 1993;91:566–576.
476. Chollet S, Dournovo P, Richard MS, et al. Reactivity of histiocytosis X cells with monoclonal anti T6 antibody. *N Engl J Med* 1982;307:685–686.
477. Chollet S, Soler P, Dournovo P, et al. Diagnosis of pulmonary histiocytosis X by immunodetection of Langerhans' cells in bronchoalveolar lavage fluid. *Am J Pathol* 1984;115:225–232.
478. Hance AJ, Basset F, Saumon G, et al. Smoking and interstitial lung disease. The effect of cigarette smoking on the incidence of pulmonary histiocytosis X and sarcoidosis. In Johns C, ed. Tenth International Conference on Sarcoidosis and Other Granulomatous Disorders. *Ann NY Acad Sci* 1986;465:643–656.
479. Hance AJ, Cadranel J, Soler P, et al. Pulmonary and extrapulmonary manifestations of Langerhans' cell granulomatosis (histocytosis X). *Semin Respir Med* 1988;9:349–368.
480. Crausman R, Jennings C, Tuder R, et al. Pulmonary histiocytosis X: pulmonary function and exercise physiology. *Am Rev Respir Crit Care Med* 1996;153:426–435.
481. Taylor J, Ryu J, Colby T, et al. Lymphangioleiomyomatosis. Clinical course in 32 patients. *N Engl J Med* 1990;323:1254–1260.
482. Sullivan EJ. Lymphangioleiomyomatosis: a review. *Chest* 1998;114:1689–1703.

13

OCCUPATIONAL AND ENVIRONMENTAL LUNG DISEASE

CARRIE A. REDLICH
JOHN R. BALMES

PRINCIPLES OF OCCUPATIONAL AND ENVIRONMENTAL LUNG DISEASE
Clinical Approach to the Patient
Diagnostic Criteria

CLASSIFICATION OF OCCUPATIONAL AND ENVIRONMENTAL LUNG DISEASE MAJOR ACUTE AND SUBACUTE DISEASES
Upper Respiratory Tract Irritation
Airway Disorders
Inhalation Injury
Acute Pleural Disease

MAJOR CHRONIC DISEASES
Interstitial Fibrosing Diseases: Overview
Silicosis

Nonmalignant Asbestos-Related Pulmonary Disease
Coal Workers' Pneumoconiosis
Beryllium- and Hard Metal-Related Disease
Other Pneumoconioses
Chronic Bronchitis and Chronic Airways Disease

MALIGNANCIES OF THE RESPIRATORY TRACT AND PLEURA
Sinonasal Cancers
Laryngeal Cancer
Lung Cancer
Malignant Mesothelioma

AIR POLLUTION: NONMALIGNANT RESPIRATORY EFFECTS
Ambient Air Pollution
Indoor Air Pollution

The past decade has seen a marked increase in concern about the adverse health effects of hazardous exposures in both the workplace and elsewhere in the environment. The lung with its extensive surface area, high blood flow, and thin alveolar epithelium is an important site of contact with substances in the environment. Such agents can cause direct toxicity, can be absorbed by or deposited in the respiratory tract, or can cause an immunologic reaction. Because of the seemingly endless array of substances or lack of toxicologic, epidemiologic, or industrial hygiene expertise, many clinicians feel ill-prepared to recognize, diagnose, and treat occupational lung diseases.

This chapter discusses the major occupational respiratory tract disorders, with an emphasis on certain basic principles and the recognition and diagnosis of such disorders. The adverse health effects of environmental exposures such as passive smoking, air pollution, and domestic radon are also reviewed. Almost all respiratory diseases may be caused or exacerbated by factors in the workplace or environment. Thus, it is important to maintain a high level of suspicion when evaluating patients with any respiratory disorder. Several excellent recent occupational and environmental medi-

cine textbooks provide a more extensive review of the topic (1–5).

PRINCIPLES OF OCCUPATIONAL AND ENVIRONMENTAL LUNG DISEASE

Certain principles apply broadly to the full range of respiratory disorders caused by inhalational exposure to agents in the workplace or environment.

1. Environmental and occupational lung diseases are difficult to distinguish from those of nonenvironmental origin. Almost any defined lung disease may have an environmental cause. Conversely, few environmental lung diseases will present with obvious or pathognomonic features.
2. A given substance in the workplace or environment can cause more than one clinical or pathologic entity. For example, cobalt can cause interstitial lung disease and airways disease.
3. The etiology of many lung diseases may be multifacto-

rial, and occupational factors may interact with other factors. For example, asbestos-exposed workers who smoke have a much greater risk of developing lung cancer than those exposed to either asbestos or cigarettes alone.

4. The respiratory effects of occupational and environmental lung exposures occur following the exposure with a predictable latent interval that depends on the given exposure. For acute diseases, there is a short and usually predictable time period between exposure and resultant clinical manifestations, which should suggest an association. For chronic diseases such as cancer or most pneumoconioses, long latency between first exposure and subsequent clinical manifestations is common. Consequently, the patient's exposure to the offending agent(s) may have ceased long before the onset of the disease, making the diagnosis of such diseases much more of a challenge.

5. The dose of exposure is an important determinant of the proportion of individuals affected or the severity of disease. Higher doses usually result in more affected individuals or greater disease severity. The dose generally affects incidence in diseases with immunologic mechanisms and severity in those with nonimmunologic properties.

6. Individual differences in susceptibility to exposures exist. Adverse effects may occur in some individuals, whereas others are spared. Host factors that determine susceptibility to environmental agents are poorly understood but likely include both inherited genetic factors and acquired factors, such as diet, the presence of other lung disease, and other exposures.

There are several compelling reasons to pursue the search for an occupational or environmental cause in all cases of pulmonary disease. Knowledge of cause may affect patient management and prognosis, and may prevent further disease progression. New associations between exposure and disease may be identified, such as new agents that can cause occupational asthma. A larger population at risk that may benefit from preventive measures may be identified. Finally, establishment of cause may have significant legal and financial implications for the patient.

Clinical Approach to the Patient

There are two distinct phases in the work-up of any patient with a potential occupational or environmental lung disease. First, as with any patient presenting with a potential disorder of the respiratory tract, its nature and extent must be defined and characterized, regardless of the suspected etiology. Second, whether the disease or symptom complex is caused or exacerbated by any exposures at work or in the environment must be determined.

The initial approach to all such patients includes a de-

tailed history, physical examination, appropriate laboratory testing, chest radiograph, and pulmonary function testing. Initial exposure information can be used to direct the sequence of the work-up and to obviate unnecessary procedures when the diagnosis is fairly straightforward. If the initial evaluation does not fully explain the patient's symptomatology, other tests are available to better characterize the nature and extent of the respiratory disorder, including computed chest tomography, laryngoscopy, flow-volume loops, cardiopulmonary exercise studies, nonspecific inhalation challenge, bronchoscopy, open lung biopsy, and various immunologic studies. However, few are specific for any given occupational or environmental diagnosis.

Prior medical records can be extremely helpful in the evaluation of a patient with a potential occupational or environmental lung disease. Such records can establish the patient's earlier complaints, may provide objective data such as prior pulmonary function tests or chest radiographs for comparison, and may clarify temporal relationships between exposure and effect, an important component of biologic plausibility.

Diagnostic Criteria

After the disease process is characterized, then whether or not any occupational or environmental exposures are causative or contributory must be determined. The following criteria are used to determine whether a disease is caused or exacerbated by agents in the workplace or environment.

1. The clinical presentation and work-up are consistent with the diagnosis.
2. A causal relationship (biologic plausibility) between the exposure and the diagnosed condition has been previously established or strongly suggested in the medical or toxicologic literature. Several different types of data can be used to establish a causal relationship. Epidemiologic studies (such as cohort or case control studies) can demonstrate associations between certain exposures or jobs and adverse effects. Clinical studies or case reports of similarly exposed patients can be used to determine the adverse effects of an exposure. Such studies may also provide useful information about the magnitude of the risk, the amount of exposure necessary for disease, and the latency between exposure and disease. Data from animal toxicologic studies can also be helpful, especially when human data are not available.
3. There is sufficient exposure to cause the disease, as assessed below.
4. The details of the particular case, such as the temporal relationship between exposure and disease, are consistent with known information about the exposure–disease association.
5. There is no other more likely diagnosis.

Exposure Assessment

The occupational and environmental history is the single most helpful tool to determine whether exposure to one or more environmental agents has occurred and the magnitude and extent of the exposure. A detailed occupational history consists of a chronologic list of all jobs, including job title, a description of the job activities, potential toxins at each job, and an assessment of the extent and duration of exposure. The length of time exposed to the agent, the use of personal protective equipment such as respirators, and a description of the ventilation and overall hygiene are helpful in attempting to quantify exposure from the patient's history.

Patients should be asked whether they think their problem is related to anything in the environment. Temporal associations between the patient's symptoms and exposures and the presence of similar symptoms among coworkers should be carefully determined. Information about potential exposures outside the workplace, such as in the home or encountered with hobbies, should also be obtained.

There are a number of sources available for obtaining additional exposure information. These include Material Safety Data Sheets (MSDSs) (employers are required by federal law to provide employees with information about the potential toxicity of the materials used in the workplace); exposure records from the employer or insurance companies; information from inspections by health and regulatory agencies such as the Occupational Safety and Health Administration (OSHA), unions and community groups, and direct site visits. For recent or current exposures, a site visit is usually very helpful in providing information about the nature and extent of potential exposures and other exposed workers. Epidemiologic data on coworkers or previous workers with similar types of jobs can be used to assess the nature and extent of exposures for a given patient. Finally, further information about the patient's exposure can be obtained from certain diagnostic tests, such as a positive radioallergosorbent test (RAST) or skin test to a specific antigen or tissue mineralogic analysis. For acute diseases such as occupational asthma, reproducing the disease manifestations by re-exposure to the suspected environmental agent is additional evidence that supports the diagnosis.

Once this additional information is obtained, the clinician has to finally make a determination about whether any occupational or environmental exposures are causing or contributing to the patient's disease process. Although some diagnoses such as asbestosis are frequently very straightforward, others may be diagnostically more challenging and easily overlooked. There is always some degree of uncertainty in medical decision making. In most workers' compensation cases the standard of certainty is usually whether the patient's problem is more probably than not (a greater than 50% likelihood) related to an occupational or environmental exposure. This is a much lower standard of certainty than physicians generally use in making diagnostic decisions. Occupational or environmental diseases can be diagnosed even in the presence of a significant degree of uncertainty. Once such a diagnosis is made, the physician should consider the public health issues involved (i.e., that other individuals in that same environment may also be similarly affected), and consider appropriate action.

CLASSIFICATION OF OCCUPATIONAL AND ENVIRONMENTAL LUNG DISEASE

Environmentally induced lung diseases can be classified by several schemes. Because these diseases so closely resemble other lung diseases, it may be helpful to classify them by the clinical presentation, as shown in Table 13.1. An overview of these acute and chronic disorders, and the adverse health effects of indoor and outdoor air pollutants, can be found in this chapter, with the exception of hypersensitivity pneumonitis and infectious diseases, which are discussed in Chapters 12, Diffuse Interstitial and Alveolar Inflammatory Disease, and 15, Respiratory Tract Infections, respectively.

MAJOR ACUTE AND SUBACUTE DISEASES

Upper Respiratory Tract Irritation

Symptoms of eye, nose, and throat irritation are frequently associated with environmental exposures (6). Numerous substances can cause upper respiratory tract irritation and inflammation, including dusts such as coal or manmade vitreous fibers (MMVF); irritant gases such as ammonia, chlorine, and ozone; metal fumes; and numerous solvents. Presenting symptoms can mimic common disorders such as upper respiratory infection, rhinitis, acute bronchitis, sinusitis, or hay fever. Many of these exposures can also cause lower respiratory tract disease, including occupational asthma, toxic pneumonitis, chronic bronchitis, or interstitial lung disease, depending on the particular agent and the dose and duration of exposure.

The diagnosis usually is made on the basis of a temporal association between exposure to the irritant substance(s) and symptoms. Improvement in symptoms away from work and similar symptoms in coworkers are helpful clues. Atopic individuals appear to be at increased risk for upper respiratory tract irritation. It is important to determine whether there is any lower respiratory tract involvement, which usually can be determined by a patient's history and spirometry. RAST testing may be helpful if the history suggests IgE-mediated allergies. Successful treatment involves reducing or eliminating the offending exposures. Long-term sequelae generally do not develop.

TABLE 13.1. CLASSIFICATION OF OCCUPATIONAL LUNG DISORDERS

Disease/Problem	Example of Causative Agent
Major acute or subacute diseases	Irritant gases, solvents
Upper respiratory tract irritation	
Airway disorders	
Occupational asthma	
Sensitization	Diisocyanates, animal dander
Irritant-induced, RADS	Irritant gases
Work-aggravated asthma	Irritants
Byssinosis	Cotton dust
Grain dust effects	Grain
Inhalation injury	
Toxic pneumonitis	Irritant gases, metals
Metal fume fever	Metal oxides—zinc, copper
Polymer fume fever	Plastics
Smoke inhalation	
Hypersensitivity pneumonitis	Microbial agents
Infectious disorders	Tuberculosis
Acute pleural disease	Asbestos
Major chronic diseases	
Interstitial fibrotic diseases (pneumoconioses)	Asbestos, silica, coal
Beryllium/hard metal-related disease	Beryllium, cobalt
Chronic bronchitis/COPD	Mineral dusts, coal
Malignancies of the respiratory tract and pleura	
Sinonasal cancer	Wood dust
Laryngeal cancer	Asbestos?
Lung cancer	Asbestos, radon
Mesothelioma	Asbestos?
Air pollution	
Ambient air pollution	Sulfur oxides, particulates
Indoor air pollution	Environmental tobacco smoke

Airway Disorders

Occupational Asthma: Sensitization

Definition and Causes

Occupational asthma has been defined as variable air flow obstruction or airway hyperresponsiveness caused by a specific agent or process encountered in the workplace (7). This definition presumes nothing about pathogenic mechanism and is intended to include bronchospasm owing to nonspecific stimuli, in addition to that caused by agents to which specific "sensitization" has developed. A broader definition would include aggravation of preexisting asthma by exposures in the workplace.

Many cases of occupationally caused asthma are caused by sensitizing agents, which include both high-molecular weight (more than 1,000 daltons) and low-molecular weight compounds (Table 13.2). High-molecular weight compounds include animal, plant, and fungal proteins. Low-molecular weight compounds are usually chemicals; most common are the diisocyanates, anhydrides, and plicatic acid (the putative cause of western red cedar-induced asthma). This distinction by size is justified by the differing clinical characteristics and pathogenic features of asthma induced by agents in the respective categories. The number of agents or processes that have been shown to cause occupational

asthma is long and constantly growing (8). Environmental allergens generated by mites, cats, and cockroaches are also increasingly being recognized as important etiologic agents in asthma. The role of such environmental factors in asthma is discussed more fully in Chapter 8, Asthma.

Prevalence

The prevalence of occupational asthma is unknown, but has been estimated to be 2% to 20% of all asthma cases in developed countries (9). An occupational etiology is more likely in those asthmatics with adult onset disease. The incidence of occupational asthma in different industrial settings varies. For example, 5% to 10% of isocyanate-exposed persons, 5% to 10% of those exposed to western red cedar, and up to 26% of clam and shrimp handlers have been reported to develop occupational asthma (10).

The single most important factor determining the prevalence of occupational asthma is exposure to a sensitizing or irritant agent. Only a portion of workers exposed to a sensitizing agent ever develops asthma. However, host susceptibility factors for occupational asthma are not well understood. Atopy is often a predisposing factor for the development of asthma owing to high-molecular weight compounds such as animal- or plant-derived material (11). However, atopy does not appear to be an important risk

TABLE 13.2. OCCUPATIONAL ASTHMA[a]

Asthma-Inducing Agents	Common Occupations
High-molecular-weight compounds	
Animal-derived material (dander, excreta, secretions)	
Laboratory animals	Laboratory workers
Birds, bats	Breeders
Shellfish	Food processors
Insects	Laboratory workers
Plants and vegetable products	
Castor beans	Food processors
Coffee beans	Food processors
Grain dust	Grain handlers
Cotton dust	Textile workers
Flour	Bakers
Psyllium	Laxative manufacturers
Vegetable gums	Printers
Latex	Hospital and dental workers
Enzymes	
Alcalase	Detergent manufacturers Food processors
Papain	Pharmaceutical workers
Pancreatic extracts	
Low-molecular-weight compounds	
Wood dusts	Woodworkers, carpenters
Western red cedar	
California redwood	
Mahogany	
Oak	
Diisocyanates	(Painters, printers, foam manufacturers)
Toluene (TDI)	
Diphenylmethane (MDI)	
Hexamethylene (HDI)	
Acid anhydrides	Epoxy resin, paint, chemical workers
Trimellitic (TMA)	
Phthalic (PA)	
Maleic (MA)	
Amines	
Ethylenediamine	Plastic workers
Drugs	Pharmaceutical workers
Cimetidine	
Cephalosporins	
Psyllium	
Penicillins	
Sulfonamides	
Other chemicals	
Azo dyes	Dye workers
Formaldehyde	Nurses, laboratory workers
Glutaraldehyde	Nurses, hospital workers
Insecticides (organophosphates)	Manufacturers, farmers
Persulfates	Hairdressers
Polyvinyl chloride (decomposition)	Food wrappers
Metal fumes and salts	Metal workers, metal platers, welders
Chromium	
Cobalt	
Nickel	
Platinum salts	

[a] For a more comprehensive list see Chan-Yeung M, Malo JL. Aetiological agents in occupational asthma. *Eur Respir J* 1994;7:346–371.

factor when low-molecular weight compounds such as diisocyanates or plicatic acid are the causative agents (11). The role of cigarette smoking in the development of occupational asthma is unclear. Studies have suggested that both nonsmokers and smokers may be more susceptible (11). It remains unclear whether preexisting nonspecific airway hyperresponsiveness predisposes to occupational asthma. Most patients with occupational asthma have nonspecific airway hyperresponsiveness that probably developed after exposure to the occupational agent.

Clinical Features

The most easily recognized presentation of occupational asthma consists of wheezing and dyspnea, which occur within minutes after contact with the offending agent at the workplace and typically disappear after work, the so-called immediate reaction. Productive cough or chest tightness rather than wheezing are also common. A delayed reaction may begin up to 12 hours after exposure, so that wheeze, cough, or chest tightness at night may be the only presenting symptoms. A delayed reaction is common with low-molecular weight compounds. Patients can have both immediate and delayed symptoms (i.e., a dual reaction). Symptoms frequently worsen over the course of the work week and improve on weekends and vacation. Sensitizer-induced occupational asthma develops after a latent period that can vary from months to years following the onset of exposure.

The relationship between symptoms and exposure may be unclear. Continued exposure to the causative agent may result in persistent airway obstruction and/or hyperresponsiveness, such that symptoms may persist after cessation of exposure. Failure of symptoms to improve during periods of time off work does not exclude the diagnosis of occupational asthma. However, lack of any improvement during a vacation of several weeks is unusual. Nonspecific triggers such as upper respiratory tract infections, exercise, cold, and emotional stimuli may precipitate asthmatic attacks in patients with occupational asthma, just as in those with asthma not related to the workplace.

Diagnosis

The diagnosis of occupational asthma involves first establishing the diagnosis of asthma, and then determining whether or not it is associated with exposure to some substance or process in the workplace. There is no single simple diagnostic test for occupational asthma, and the diagnosis may be difficult to make. A high index of suspicion is key to the correct diagnosis.

A careful occupational history is the most effective, useful, and practical means of identifying workers with possible occupational asthma. The following should raise the suspicion for occupational asthma: new-onset asthma in an adult, worsening symptoms at or after work with deterioration over the course of the week, improvement away from work,

and the presence of an agent in the workplace known to cause occupational asthma. Additional helpful information is the use of any new agents or processes at the worksite, similar symptoms in other workers, and the presence of preexisting asthma or atopy.

The diagnosis of asthma is confirmed, as with any asthmatic patient, by demonstrating reversible air flow obstruction on spirometry. Tests for nonspecific airway hyperresponsiveness, such as methacholine challenge, can be used to document hyperreactive airways if spirometry is normal.

Several methods are available to document the association between air flow obstruction and exposure to the suspected agent.

1. Preshift and postshift measurement in FEV_1. Demonstration of a decrement of more than 10% in the forced expiratory volume in 1 second (FEV_1) across the workshift is a relatively specific test, but it is insufficiently sensitive because of the relatively frequent occurrence of delayed responses, and it can be logistically difficult to perform.

2. Serial measurements of peak expiratory flow rates (PEFR). Serial measurements of peak expiratory flow can be made by a worker throughout the workshift and later at home by means of a hand-held instrument, a Mini-Wright peak flowmeter. A reduction in peak flows associated with exposure to the suspected offending agent supports a diagnosis of occupational asthma. Visual interpretation is as useful as quantitative analysis. An example of a PEFR record supporting a diagnosis of occupational asthma is shown in Figure 13.1. Good-quality PEFR recordings with adequate off-work and work days may be difficult to obtain.

3. Specific inhalation challenge. Workplace challenges can be performed under actual exposure conditions, but because multiple exposures are common, they may not identify the specific agent. Specific challenge testing with the suspected agent(s) is considered the "gold standard" for diagnosing occupational asthma. A 20% fall in FEV_1 following exposure to the offending agent is diagnostic of occupational asthma. However, such testing requires a specialized chamber, carries certain risks, is time-consuming, and is not widely available, and false-negatives can occur. Specific inhalation challenge is helpful in documenting a previously unrecognized cause of occupational asthma and in establishing a specific etiologic diagnosis when the work-up has been equivocal or multiple sensitizing exposures are present. However, specific challenge is unnecessary for the diagnosis of most cases of occupational asthma.

In practice, objective evidence of variable airflow obstruction in relation to workplace exposure can be difficult to obtain for multiple reasons, especially if the patient has changed jobs. A temporal association between asthmatic symptoms and a workplace exposure may provide sufficient

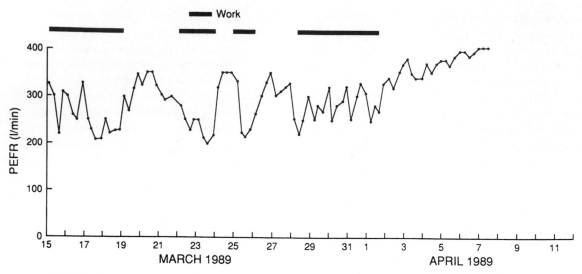

FIGURE 13.1. PEFR record of a hairdresser who developed symptoms of asthma from exposure to a bleaching reagent she used at work. PEFR showed improvement when she was away from work. (From Rosenstock L, Cullen MR. *Textbook of clinical occupational and environmental medicine.* Philadelphia: Saunders, 1994.)

evidence of work-relatedness if the suspect exposure is a documented cause of asthma (Table 13.2). One does not need to identify the specific causative agent to make a diagnosis of occupational asthma (12).

Immunologic Tests

Skin tests and detection of specific IgE antibodies to the suspected agent in the serum by immunoassays such as the RAST have varying degrees of usefulness. In the case of high-molecular weight allergens, such as flours or rodent proteins, the demonstration of a positive skin test or specific IgE antibodies is highly confirmatory of exposure. However, for low-molecular weight compounds, such as diisocyanates or plicatic acid, negative tests are common, and the application of these techniques has limited clinical utility (13).

Outcome and Management

Studies of workers with occupationally induced asthma, primarily owing to diisocyanates and western red cedar, have shown that many of these workers (up to 80%) have persistent symptoms and airway hyperresponsiveness, even after removal from further exposure (14). The factors that determine prognosis are not well defined, but persistent asthma following removal has been associated with longer duration of symptoms before diagnosis, abnormal spirometry, and more marked airway hyperresponsiveness. These patients clinically can be indistinguishable from intrinsic, nonoccupationally induced asthmatics with acute exacerbations following viral infections and nonspecific irritants. Recovery is more likely with early diagnosis and removal from further exposure.

Because many exposures that cause occupational asthma

are sensitizing agents, once symptomatic, exposure to minute quantities, even below regulatory permissible limits, can induce bronchospasm. Thus, once occupational asthma has been diagnosed, attempts should be made to remove the patient from further exposure. Respiratory protective devices are rarely effective but can be tried with close monitoring. Medications used to treat occupational asthma are the same as those used with nonoccupational asthma.

Reactive Airways Dysfunction Syndrome

The persistence of symptoms consistent with asthma and nonspecific airway hyperresponsiveness in some individuals following a single high exposure to an irritating vapor, fume, gas, or smoke has been termed reactive airways dysfunction syndrome (RADS) (15). Whether recurrent lower-level exposures to irritants can also cause asthma is somewhat controversial, but there are several reports that suggest that this can occur (15). A number of examples of irritant-induced nonallergic asthma have been reported (8). The following criteria are used to diagnose RADS.

1. Absence of preceding asthma-like respiratory disease or complaints
2. Onset of symptoms after a single or multiple high-level exposure(s) to a known irritant gas, vapor, fume, aerosol, or dust
3. Onset of symptoms shortly (within 24 hours) of the exposure and lasting for at least 3 months, usually longer
4. Symptoms and spirometric findings that simulate asthma
5. Positive methacholine challenge if spirometry is normal
6. Other asthma-like illnesses are ruled out.

The incidence of RADS is not well defined, but it is probably not uncommon. One study found that 10 of 59 workers diagnosed with occupational asthma had a history consistent with RADS (15). The evaluation of workers with RADS is similar to that for patients with sensitizer-induced occupational asthma. Exposure to respiratory irritants should be minimized. The worker may be able to return to the workplace if irritant exposures are limited. Close follow-up is necessary to monitor for persistent or progressive symptoms and air flow obstruction.

Pathogenesis of Occupational Asthma

Similar to non–work-related asthma, airway inflammation likely plays a crucial role in the pathogenesis of occupational asthma. Components of airway inflammation include alterations in airway epithelial and smooth muscle cells; airway infiltration by inflammatory cells including T lymphocytes, mast cells, eosinophils, and neutrophils; and thickening of the airway wall (16). How different exposures cause airway inflammation is not well understood but likely involves both immunologic and nonimmunologic mechanisms (13). Airways may be injured directly by intense exposure to irritant chemicals such as chlorine or sulfur dioxide, resulting in epithelial damage, airway inflammation, and hyperresponsiveness. Such a mechanism is likely involved in the pathogenesis of RADS.

In most cases of occupational asthma caused by both low-molecular weight and high-molecular weight compounds, airway inflammation likely develops through immune-mediated processes (16). The following clinical characteristics all support an immune hypersensitivity-type reaction: Asthma occurs in only a proportion of those exposed to the agent; asthma develops only after weeks to years of exposure; patients can have a dual, early, or late response; and once "sensitized," very low levels of exposure to the agent can precipitate an asthmatic response. High-molecular weight animal- and plant-derived compounds can induce specific IgE responses in a high proportion of exposed individuals. Low-molecular weight chemicals such as diisocyanates may act as haptens, which have to be conjugated to a carrier protein to form a complete antigen. However, specific IgE or IgG antibodies are detected in only a fraction of such patients. The immunologic mechanisms involved with exposure to low-molecular weight compounds are not well defined but may involve both IgE and non-IgE immune processes.

It is not uncommon for a patient with preexisting asthma to experience asthma exacerbations in response to exposure to respiratory irritants in the workplace (dusts, fumes, vapors, mists, smoke). In fact, more morbidity and lost productivity results from work-aggravated asthma than from work-induced asthma. Occupational exposure to cold and heavy exertion on the job can also cause work-aggravated asthma. Reduction of exposure to the work-related triggers of asthma usually results in improvement.

Byssinosis: Textile Dust-Related Disease

Definition

Byssinosis, an occupational lung disease of textile workers, is caused by excessive inhalation of certain vegetable fiber dusts. First described by Ramazzini almost three centuries ago, it was essentially rediscovered by Richard Schilling in England in the 1950s (17). The disease originally was recognized in cotton workers but also has been reported among other textile workers. In its early stages, byssinosis is characterized by symptoms of chest tightness, cough, wheezing, and dyspnea that are especially prominent on the first day back to work after a break in exposure. These symptoms initially tend to diminish over the first few days of the workweek, but as the disease progresses, chronic chest tightness can develop. Acute and chronic obstructive changes in pulmonary function can occur. The term byssinosis refers to both the early and late manifestations of cotton dust-induced lung disease. In addition to byssinosis, textile workers can also develop hypersensitivity pneumonitis, chronic bronchitis, and febrile syndromes such as mill fever and mattress makers' fever.

Risk Factors

The risk of developing byssinosis is related to the intensity of dust exposure, duration of exposure, job, and type of fiber. The highest incidence of disease traditionally has been found among workers involved in the dusty preparatory phases of the cotton textile manufacturing process. Workers engaged in the later phases of the process may also develop byssinosis, but the incidence is much lower. Exposure to the end product (e.g., cotton cloth) does not cause byssinosis. Several studies have found that smokers have a greater incidence of byssinosis than non-smokers do.

Clinical Features and Natural History

During the early stages of byssinosis, symptoms of chest tightness and dyspnea are often noted about 1 hour after the beginning of work. When exposure ceases, these symptoms tend to disappear. The acute symptoms of byssinosis are correlated with a reversible decline in FEV_1 across the work shift. With continued exposure, the periodic acute Monday exacerbations can progress to symptoms on every workday. After many years of textile work, respiratory symptoms can persist even in the absence of exposure, and disability may ensue (18). Several longitudinal studies have shown increased symptoms and accelerated loss of lung function in textile workers, independent of smoking history (19,20). Although byssinosis and occupational asthma share some features in common such as work-related reduction in FEV_1, byssinosis is felt by most to be a distinct entity on the basis of several features, including improvement in symptoms over the workweek.

Pathogenesis

A number of studies have investigated the possible mechanisms by which cotton and other dusts cause acute and chronic byssinosis. These studies have been complicated by the large number of potentially toxic components of cotton dust, including bacteria, fungi, inorganic material, and organic chemicals. It has been demonstrated that endotoxin is present in many cotton dusts and can cause bronchoconstriction, and that the acute symptoms and reduced lung function correlate with airborne endotoxin concentrations (21). However, there remains some uncertainty about the role of endotoxin, because inhalation of endotoxin-free cotton dust has also induced symptoms and bronchoconstriction (21).

Diagnosis

The diagnosis of byssinosis depends primarily on the occupational history of the characteristic symptom pattern in association with exposure to cotton or other natural textile dusts (18). Spirometry documenting a cross-shift decline in FEV_1 supports the diagnosis. Patients with more advanced chronic disease may have evidence of irreversible air flow obstruction.

Prevention

Attempts should be made to reduce exposures with engineering controls. In the United States, the implementation of the OSHA cotton dust standard and the closure of older mills have reduced dust levels. However, in less developed countries, very dusty conditions still exist.

Respiratory Effects of Grain Dust

Grain dust is a complex mixture consisting of various grains contaminated with fungi, mites, bacteria, insects, animal matter, endotoxins, various agricultural chemicals such as fungicides and pesticides, and inorganic matter, mainly soil. As with byssinosis acute and chronic respiratory disease in grain workers was first recognized by Ramazzini almost three centuries ago (17). Grain dust exposure can cause asthma, acute febrile syndromes, hypersensitivity pneumonitis, chronic air flow obstruction, and chronic bronchitis (22). Although it is recognized that grain workers suffer from an excess incidence of acute and chronic respiratory disease, it is not clear what percentage of this excess disease is owing to immunologically mediated "grain asthma," versus chronic irritant grain dust bronchitis. Also unclear is which constituent(s) of grain dust is responsible for these acute and chronic effects.

Risk Factors

Most grain workers who complain of respiratory symptoms do not have a history of atopy, possibly because of the healthy worker effect (23). Grain workers who are atopic are at increased risk of developing grain dust asthma (22). The combined effects of cigarette smoking and grain on lung function are probably additive (22).

Clinical Effects of Grain Dust Exposure

Grain fever presents similarly to hypersensitivity pneumonitis, but without the chest radiographic changes that are typical of that disease. Acute upper airway symptoms including conjunctivitis, rhinitis, and pharyngitis have been noted to be excessively prevalent among grain workers.

True occupational asthma can develop in grain workers, likely caused by sensitization to any of a number of different allergens present in grain dust (22). Inhalation challenge tests with grain dusts or their extracts have documented classic immediate or delayed reactions. Precipitating antibodies and positive skin tests to grain dust extracts and various fungal antigens, as well as cross-shift decrements in lung function, have been found among grain workers. However, these immunologic tests have not been found to regularly correlate with the presence or absence of acute respiratory symptoms.

A number of studies have shown that chronic grain dust exposure is associated with both chronic bronchitic symptoms and reduced lung function (22,24). Early, the initial decrements in lung function appear to be reversible, but with continued exposure, chronic irreversible changes in lung function can occur. Workers who experience acute respiratory symptoms and airway obstruction in response to grain dust may be at increased risk of developing chronic air flow obstruction (22). Evidence also exists to support a dose–response relationship for exposure to grain dust and annual decline of lung function (24). Limited postmortem pathologic examination of grain dust workers has shown both diffuse emphysematous and fibrotic changes in the lungs.

Patients with grain dust asthma should be evaluated and treated like other patients with occupational asthma. Diagnosis and management of chronic grain dust disease are similar to those for byssinosis.

Inhalation Injury

Toxic Lung Injury and Toxic Pneumonitis

Excessive inhalational exposure to a large number of different irritant gases, mists, and fumes may produce inflammation of any portion of the respiratory tract, depending on the dose and duration of exposure and the anatomic level at which the toxin is deposited or absorbed (25). The latter is determined largely by the size of the particles and the solubility of gases in water. Highly soluble gases (such as ammonia) and large particles affect the conjunctivae, pharynx, larynx, trachea, and major bronchi; small particles and insoluble gases (such as phosgene or nitrogen dioxide) affect smaller distal airways and alveoli predominantly. Common irritant gases and metals are listed in Tables 13.3 and 13.4.

Clinical Presentation and Long-Term Effects

Clinical signs appear after variable delays from the time of exposure; latency is shortest for the mucous membranes of

TABLE 13.3. COMMON IRRITANT GASES AND VAPORS

Gas	Water Solubility	Lethality
Ammonia	High	Low
Acetaldehyde	High	Low
Chlorine	Medium	Medium
Hydrogen fluoride	High	Low
Hydrogen sulfide	High	Low
Methylisocyanate	(Highly reactive)	High
Oxides of nitrogen (NO, NO_2, N_2O_4)	Low	High
Ozone	Low	Low
Phosgene	Very low	Very high
Sulfur dioxide	High	Low

the face and becomes progressively longer as one moves distally. Thus the eyes, nose, and throat are likely to become inflamed shortly after exposure, whereas evidence of pneumonitis may appear hours to days later. Because of variable latency, early results of blood gas analyses, chest radiographs, and lung function tests must be interpreted with caution.

Most patients who survive recover completely. A chronic bronchitis with fixed or reversible airway obstruction may persist after the injury, usually with gradual improvement over the course of many months. RADS can develop and persist following acute irritant exposures, as discussed. Progressive interstitial fibrosis and bronchiolitis obliterans are rare sequelae (26).

Treatment

There is no specific treatment for acute inhalational injury. Support and expectant management are the keys to treatment. Unless cardiorespiratory failure is imminent, emergency attention should proceed from the upper tract downward. Inflamed mucosal surfaces, especially the eyes, should be rinsed first. If hoarseness, stridor, or other signs are pres-

TABLE 13.4. IRRITANT METALS

Metal	Common Source of Exposure	Health Effects
Beryllium	Alloy production, metal refining	Pneumonitis, CBD
Cadmium	Smelting, brazing	Pneumonitis, COPD
Chromium	Alloy production	Pneumonitis
Mercury	Testing equipment	Pneumonitis
Manganese	Mining, welding	Metal fume fever
Nickel	Ore extraction, smelting	Asthma, pneumonitis
Osmium	Organic chemical manufacturing	Upper airway irritation
Vanadium	Chemical industry	Asthma, bronchitis
Zinc	Chemical industry	Metal fume fever

ent, the vocal cords should be visualized and endotracheal intubation considered. Bronchospasm should be treated with bronchodilators. Pneumonitis, with onset as late as 72 hours after exposure, must be anticipated, especially if bronchospasm is present. Noncardiogenic pulmonary edema due to chemical pneumonitis should be managed in the same manner as other causes of severe pneumonitis and respiratory failure.

Specific Agents

Irritant Gases

Common irritant gases are listed in Table 13.3. *Ammonia* is highly water soluble and thus extremely irritating to mucous membranes. Most cases of severe lower respiratory tract injury due to ammonia involve entrapment in confined spaces. *Sulfur dioxide* is generated during a wide range of industrial operations, including refining of petroleum products and paper manufacturing. It is relatively water soluble and causes sufficient upper respiratory tract irritation to warn anyone exposed to a high concentration. *Chlorine,* also widely used, is somewhat less soluble and is associated with a correspondingly increased risk of bronchiolitis or alveolitis. *Nitrogen dioxide,* reddish in color, is liberated whenever nitrogen-containing material is burned; it is also a byproduct of welding, store silage, and mining, as well as numerous chemical operations. It is relatively insoluble; therefore, the risk of parenchymal lung injury is high. Recurrent episodes after exposure have been reported.

Ozone is a highly toxic gas normally found in the atmosphere at very low concentrations. It can be generated by welding, and increased amounts are found at high altitude (airplanes) and in urban smog. It can cause substernal burning and transient changes in lung function (decreased FEV_1 and increased nonspecific airway responsiveness), but rarely pneumonitis or pulmonary edema. *Phosgene* is a poorly soluble gas originally developed for chemical warfare. It penetrates to the distal lung where it causes parenchymal injury.

Toxic Metal and Polymer Fumes

Table 13.4 lists irritant metals encountered in industrial environments. *Cadmium* fumes from primary smelting, electroplating, or welding can cause severe lower respiratory tract inflammation (27). Bronchitis and emphysema have been associated with chronic cadmium exposure (28). *Mercury* vapor and *beryllium* compounds can cause acute pneumonitis, and persistent symptoms can occur. Fumes and dusts of *manganese,* inhaled by welders, have been associated with acute airway and parenchymal lung inflammation.

Metal Fume Fever

Fumes of *zinc* and *copper,* generated from smelting, welding, or foundry work, contain fine particles of zinc and copper oxides. Several hours after an intense exposure, a flu-like illness with fever, myalgia, headache, and leukocytosis, called *metal fume fever,* can occur (29). Thirst and a metallic taste may also occur. In contrast to the toxic effects observed with the metals discussed, chest infiltrates are not seen, and the illness generally runs a benign 24-hour course. "Tolerance" occurs with daily or continuous exposure; workers usually get the "fever" on Mondays after a few days away from exposure. Significant chronic changes in lung function have not been detected.

Polymer Fume Fever

Closely related to metal fume fever is *polymer fume fever* from inhalation of pyrolysis products of Teflon (polytetrafluorethylene) (30). Infiltrates do occur but clear spontaneously, along with the fever and constitutional symptoms. Symptoms may persist for weeks but typically resolve completely, although long-term studies have not been performed.

Smoke Inhalation

Smoke inhalation injury is common among burn patients, including firefighters. The pulmonary effects of smoke inhalation depend on the magnitude of the exposure and the specific chemical fumes released during combustion. The major components of fire smoke are toxic irritants such as acrolein and hydrogen chloride and chemical asphyxiants such as hydrogen cyanide (Table 13.5). Less commonly, thermal injury from high temperature can also occur, especially with aerosolized liquids (i.e., steam) or particles (i.e., metallic oxides), which have a greater heat capacity than dry air and can cause thermal injury to the lower airways. Fire victims are typically exposed to a number of different toxic inhalants because of the many potentially combustible products present at the site of a fire, such as furniture, plastics, carpets, and polyurethane materials.

Evaluation and Management of Acute Smoke Inhalation

Emergency evaluation of excessive smoke inhalation should include standard emergency principles and a careful assessment of risk factors for significant exposure. Initially, all smoke-exposed individuals should receive oxygen and have samples drawn for arterial blood gas and carboxyhemoglobin determinations. Physical examination should include a careful assessment for facial or oropharyngeal burns, wheezing on chest examination, or any neurologic abnormalities. A chest radiograph, ECG, and spirometry or peak flow determination are recommended. Patients with clinically significant smoke exposures need close observation for delayed pulmonary effects, even if initially asymptomatic.

Unless anoxic damage from hypoxemia or carbon monoxide poisoning supervenes, patients who survive smoke inhalation usually recover fully. However, as with other acute irritant gas exposures, respiratory symptoms and lung function abnormalities may persist. Permanent sequelae are not common but include interstitial pulmonary fibrosis, nonspecific airway hyperresponsiveness, bronchiolitis obliterans, and chronic bronchitis. Whether firefighters are at increased risk of developing chronic air flow obstruction or other nonmalignant respiratory disease is not resolved (31). Individual firefighters can show accelerated loss of lung function, and removal from further exposure may be indicated.

Acute Pleural Disease

Asbestos exposure can result in transient pleural effusions and, less commonly, recurrent attacks of pleurisy. Asbestos-induced pleural effusions typically are exudative and may be hemorrhagic and/or eosinophilic (32,33). The diagnosis depends on the history of asbestos exposure, the presence of an effusion, no other cause for the effusion, and no development of malignancy within 3 years of diagnosis. Benign asbestos effusions are frequently asymptomatic and occur with a latency of 10 years or more. They may result in the development of diffuse pleural thickening.

MAJOR CHRONIC DISEASES

Interstitial Fibrosing Diseases: Overview

Occupational and environmental interstitial lung diseases are a group of heterogeneous lung diseases that diffusely involve the lung parenchyma with varying degrees of chronic alveolitis and fibrosis. The term pneumoconioses has traditionally been defined as the accumulation of dust in the lung and the resulting tissue reaction. Originally used to describe inorganic dust-induced diseases such as asbestosis or silicosis, the term is also used more loosely to describe diseases resulting from the inhalation of other substances that may not accumulate in the lung, such as cobalt. There are a large number of occupational and environmental

TABLE 13.5. TOXIC INHALANTS COMMONLY ENCOUNTERED IN FIRES

Chemical irritants
  Aldehydes (acrolein, formaldehyde)
  Ammonia
  Aromatic hydrocarbons (benzene)
  Hydrogen chloride
  Isocyanates
  Metals (lead, chromium, arsenic)
  Nitrogen dioxide
  Sulfur dioxide
Chemical asphyxiants
  Hydrogen cyanide
  Carbon monoxide
  Hydrogen sulfide

TABLE 13.6. MORE-COMMON CAUSES OF OCCUPATIONAL INTERSTITIAL LUNG DISEASES

Free silica
Silicates
Fibrous—asbestos
Mixed dust
Coal
Metals
Beryllium
Hard metal (cobalt)

causes of pulmonary interstitial fibrosis, which are summarized in Tables 13.6 and 13.7.

The fibrogenic potential of inorganic dusts varies considerably, with silica and asbestos having greater fibrogenic potential than coal dust or more benign agents such as iron. Most inorganic dusts, such as coal, asbestos, or silica, require prolonged exposure for at least 6 months, usually many years, at relatively high levels, for significant pulmonary disease to develop. However, disease can occur following shorter, more intense exposures (34). The response to agents such as beryllium or cobalt is much more idiosyncratic, and disease can occur after much lower exposure (35). The fibrogenic potential of a given exposure depends on various factors including the agent's ability to reach the lower respiratory tract; the dose, durability, and various physical and

TABLE 13.7. LESS COMMON CAUSES OF OCCUPATIONAL INTERSTITIAL LUNG DISEASES

Silicates
Talc
Kaolin
Diatomaceous earth
MMVF (?)
Mica
Hydrocarbon-containing sedimentary rocks
Graphite
Oil shale
Metals
Tin
Aluminum
Antimony
Barium
Iron
Titanium
Irritant gases/fumes
Sequela of toxic pneumonitis
Plastics
Polyvinyl chloride
Diisocyanates
Organic dusts
Bacteria
Fungi
Animal proteins
Paraquat
Nylon flock

chemical properties of the agent; and individual host susceptibility factors.

Airway involvement in most pneumoconioses has traditionally been felt to be nonexistent or related to smoking. However, certain exposures such as asbestos can result in peribronchial fibrosis and mild air flow obstruction, and many can cause chronic bronchitis, which may be associated with chronic airways disease.

The overall prevalence of pneumoconioses in the United States is unknown but varies significantly among different exposed populations. Historically, the most common interstitial lung diseases were owing to inhalation of mineral dusts such as silica, asbestos, and coal dust. Worldwide, silicosis remains the most common pneumoconiosis (36). With improved industrial hygiene and reduced use in the United States, heavy exposure to these dusts has declined. However, several recent reports demonstrate that high levels of exposure still exist, frequently in small uncontrolled workplaces, and can result in miniepidemics of disease (37). Even with overall improved control measures, the prevalence of these diseases remains high in many exposed populations because of the latency between exposure and disease (38).

Fibrotic lung diseases caused by agents that appear to involve immune-mediated mechanisms and which have less clear dose–response relationships, such as beryllium or hard metal, are more difficult to both diagnose and control, as disease may occur at lower exposure levels and in a more sporadic fashion.

Chest Radiography

The chest radiograph is the most important diagnostic test for occupational fibrotic disorders. It is critical that radiographs of high technical quality be obtained. The chest radiograph can be highly suggestive of a pneumoconiosis and is frequently sufficient, along with an appropriate exposure history, to establish a diagnosis. Chest radiography can be normal in approximately 10% to 20% or more of patients with interstitial lung disease (39).

An international uniform classification system, under the auspices of the International Labour Office (ILO) in Geneva, Switzerland, has evolved to evaluate chest radiographs for epidemiologic studies, clinical evaluation, and screening (40). The system classifies radiographic opacities according to shape, size, extent, and concentration. Pleural changes are also graded according to site, pleural thickening, and pleural calcification.

Computed Tomography

Much has been written about the role of computed tomography (CT) scanning in the evaluation of patients with occupational interstitial lung disease, primarily asbestosis (41). Conventional CT scanning (8- to 10-mm-thick slices) and high-resolution computed tomographic scanning (HRCT) (1- to 3-mm-thick slices) can be used to better evaluate pleural and parenchymal abnormalities. Conventional CT scanning is more sensitive than chest radiography for the diagnosis of pleural disease. It is most useful for evaluating focal pulmonary masses. In patients with suspected interstitial lung disease but a normal chest radiograph, HRCT may be helpful in identifying parenchymal abnormalities. In most cases in which the diagnosis of an occupational interstitial lung disease is clear on the basis of the chest radiograph and history, CT and HRCT scanning are not indicated.

Pulmonary Function and Cardiopulmonary Exercise Testing

Resting lung function testing is the most important tool to assess functional respiratory status. As with any interstitial fibrotic disease, physiologic testing in diffuse fibrotic occupational diseases typically shows a restrictive pattern with reduced lung volumes and decreased diffusing capacity (D_{LCO}). Air flow rates and FEV_1/FVC ratio are preserved unless there is coexisting airways disease. The findings on physiologic testing are not specific for a particular etiology, but they are important for evaluating dyspnea and assessing the degree of pulmonary impairment. In a given patient, chest radiographic findings, lung volumes, and D_{LCO} may or may not be correlated in assessing the extent of disease and functional impairment. Patients with more severe disease should be evaluated for hypoxemia at rest and with exertion.

Cardiopulmonary exercise testing is helpful in evaluating a select group of patients with dyspnea and normal pulmonary function tests or dyspnea that appears out of proportion to the changes in lung function, and can help distinguish between cardiac, pulmonary, and deconditioning causes of dyspnea. However, in most patients with occupational interstitial lung disease, exercise testing is not indicated for diagnosis or management.

Bronchoscopy

Under certain circumstances when the diagnosis is not straightforward, bronchoscopy with transbronchial biopsy and bronchoalveolar lavage (BAL) may be helpful. Transbronchial biopsies yield small tissue samples that may be adequate to diagnose the presence of interstitial fibrosis but usually can not determine specific etiology. They are most helpful in diagnosing granulomatous processes such as beryllium disease or hypersensitivity pneumonitis. Although not routinely performed in many institutions, under certain circumstances BAL can be helpful, such as in the diagnosis of beryllium disease, for which a positive lymphocyte transformation test is diagnostic. Cells obtained from BAL contain dust particles such as asbestos, which may reflect current and possibly past exposures. However, such assays primarily confirm the exposure history and have little clinical utility.

Lung Biopsy

Although frequently not needed diagnostically, open lung biopsy can be helpful when there is no clear cause of interstitial lung disease. To establish a diagnosis, histopathologic changes should be consistent with the known disease, and the suspected causative dusts or particles can, in most cases, be detectable in the lung. A number of methods to analyze dust content of tissue are available including light microscopic evaluation with polarization, bulk analytic techniques such as x-ray fluorescence, and microanalytic techniques such as scanning electron microscopy (42). If a patient with an interstitial lung disease of unclear etiology in whom an occupational or environmental cause is being considered undergoes open lung biopsy, more extensive particle analysis should be considered if light microscopic histologic examination is nondiagnostic. There are some serious limitations that should be remembered. Only particulates that are insoluble, retained in tissue, and at sufficient concentration will be detected. In addition, a positive finding indicates only some degree of exposure, not disease.

Silicosis

Silicosis is a chronic fibrosing disease of the lungs, produced by excessive inhalation of free crystalline silica dust. The ores of most minerals, from coal to gold, are generally found embedded in silica-containing rock in the earth's crust. Mining and quarrying have long been associated with a high incidence of silicosis. Hazardous exposure to silica dust also may occur in a wide variety of other industries such as foundry work, tunneling, sandblasting, pottery making, and the manufacture of glass, tiles, and bricks. Finely ground silica, used in abrasive soaps, polishes, and filters, is especially dangerous.

Silica, or silicon dioxide, can exist unbound to other minerals (free silica) and in either crystalline or amorphous states. *Silicates* are minerals containing silicon dioxide combined with other elements, such as talc, asbestos, mica, or kaolin. Inhalational exposure to most silica-containing minerals has been associated with some risk of pneumoconiosis. However, free crystalline silica dust is more likely to cause pulmonary fibrosis than either amorphous silica or nonasbestiform silicates.

Pathogenesis and Histologic Features

Respirable-sized silica particles deposited in the distal airways are readily ingested by scavenging alveolar macrophages or penetrate the interstitium. The alveolar macrophages become activated, can release a number of inflammatory mediators that initiate and perpetuate the processes of inflammation and fibrosis, and then may undergo cell death. Neutrophils, T lymphocytes, and other inflammatory cells probably contribute to the inflammatory and fibrotic processes, eventually resulting in the silicotic nodule (43,44).

Three types of silicosis have been described: (*a*) ordinary or simple chronic silicosis, in which exposure to relatively low concentrations of free silica dust has continued for 20 years or more; (*b*) accelerated silicosis, in which exposure to moderately high dust concentrations occurs, usually over a shorter period of time (4 to 8 years); and (*c*) acute silicosis, in which there is massive exposure to high concentrations of dust (44). These distinctions are important as far as clinical outcome is concerned.

Simple silicosis is characterized by the formation of silicotic nodules in the pulmonary parenchyma and the hilar lymph nodes. Particles of free silica may be demonstrated in the nodules by their birefringence under polarized light. Simple silicosis may be complicated by the development of progressive massive fibrosis (PMF). The lesions of PMF tend to be found in the upper lung zones and are composed of confluent nodules, often with obliterated blood vessels and bronchioles as well. With accelerated silicosis, the rate of progression is more rapid, and PMF occurs more frequently.

Acute silicosis is a relatively rare condition occurring only in workers exposed to very high concentrations of fine, particulate free silica dust without adequate ventilation or personal protective equipment. Unlike the situation in chronic silicosis, the lungs show consolidation without silicotic nodules, and the alveolar spaces are filled with fluid similar to that found in pulmonary alveolar proteinosis (45).

Clinical Presentation

Silicosis is most commonly a chronic disease with a long latency. The most common form of silicosis is uncomplicated simple silicosis, which is usually asymptomatic and is diagnosed on the basis of chest radiographic findings. Pulmonary function testing in patients with simple silicosis can be normal or demonstrate abnormalities consistent with mild restriction. A mild obstructive impairment is frequently found in patients with simple silicosis, presumably owing to chronic bronchitis caused by silica or other dust.

Significant dyspnea on exertion generally is seen only with patients who have complicated disease characterized by PMF. Complicated silicosis is associated with reduced lung volumes and diffusing capacity, nonreversible airflow obstruction, and arterial oxygen desaturation with exercise. Nodular lesions greater than 1 cm in diameter are seen on chest radiography and can become confluent and retract the hila upward. Constitutional symptoms such as malaise, anorexia, and weight loss can occur with complicated disease, as can respiratory failure.

The major features of accelerated silicosis are similar to

those of complicated chronic silicosis, but the course of the disease is abbreviated, and there is a greater likelihood that significant disability will develop. Patients with acute silicosis present with marked dyspnea, fever, cough, and weight loss. There usually is rapid progression to respiratory failure.

Diagnosis

The diagnosis of silicosis is based on: (*a*) a history of sufficient silica exposure; (*b*) chest radiographic abnormalities consistent with silicosis; and (*c*) absence of other illnesses that mimic silicosis. Silica exposure occurs in a number of occupational settings, and the history of exposure may not always be obvious. The presence of diffuse nodular opacities on the chest radiograph of an individual known to have sustained prolonged exposure to silica is usually sufficient (Fig. 13.2). Calcification of hilar lymph nodes and a classic "eggshell" pattern is not a consistent finding in silicosis, but when it is seen in patients with diffuse nodular lung disease, it generally excludes other diagnoses (Fig. 13.3). Histologic evaluation is usually not necessary.

Associated Illnesses

Patients with silicosis have an increased risk of mycobacterial infection (involving atypical mycobacterial organisms as well as *Mycobacterium tuberculosis*) (46). The decreased

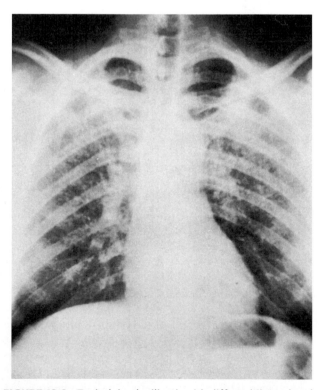

FIGURE 13.2. Typical simple silicosis with diffuse, bilateral nodular densities.

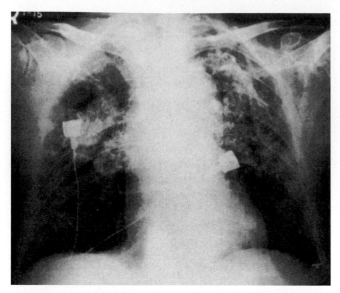

FIGURE 13.3. Eggshell calcification of hilar lymph nodes.

resistance of the silicotic lung to mycobacterial infection appears to be owing in large measure to impaired macrophage function. Tuberculosis should be suspected in any patient with silicosis whose symptoms or chest radiograph change more acutely.

Various connective tissue disorders, particularly scleroderma, have been noted to occur with greater frequency in patients with silicosis (46). Caplan's syndrome (rheumatoid arthritis and large lung nodules) occurs with silicosis as well as with coal workers' pneumoconiosis. There is an increased prevalence of circulating autoantibodies, such as antinuclear antibody and rheumatoid factor, among silicotic patients. Patients with silicosis are at increased risk of developing lung cancer (discussed in the following).

Treatment

There is no specific treatment for silicosis except removal from further exposure, which may not affect progression of the disease. Supportive therapy with the aim of preventing debilitating complications such as tuberculosis can be offered. Patients with silicosis should have annual screening for mycobacterial infection (i.e., PPD skin testing). At least 1 year of isoniazid therapy is recommended for patients with positive PPD tests without clinical evidence of active tuberculosis. Because of the decreased responsiveness of silicotuberculosis to chemotherapy, multidrug regimens including rifampin are recommended (46). Establishing the diagnosis of tuberculosis in a patient with silicosis can be challenging; a high index of suspicion remains important. Tuberculosis should be suspected if any rapid changes occur on the chest radiograph. When tuberculosis is superimposed on complicated silicosis, there may be no obvious radio-

graphic change at all. The use of induced sputum and fiberoptic bronchoscopy to obtain specimens for acid-fast staining and mycobacterial culture may increase the diagnostic yield.

The treatment of silica associated bronchitis and airflow obstruction is similar to that offered to any patient with chronic bronchitis (Chapter 9, Chronic Obstructive Pulmonary Disease, Bronchiectasis, and Cystic Fibrosis). Bronchodilator therapy can be effective for patients in whom a reversible obstructive component is present. The cessation of cigarette smoking is of obvious importance. Whole-lung lavage has been reported to be helpful in patients with acute silicosis presenting with a clinicopathologic picture consistent with pulmonary alveolar proteinosis (47).

Nonmalignant Asbestos-Related Pulmonary Disease

Asbestos is the generic name for a group of naturally occurring fibrous silicates. There are three main commercial types of asbestos, chrysotile crocidolite. Chrysotile fibers are somewhat curved or serpentine; crocidolite and amosite are needle-like or amphibole. Asbestos may cause several different types of disease involving the lungs and pleura and may also increase the risk of extrapulmonary neoplasms such as colon cancer. *Asbestosis* is a term that should be reserved for the diffuse interstitial pulmonary fibrosis caused by asbestos exposure.

Epidemiology

Although asbestos has been valued since antiquity because of its resistance to fire, only during the last century has its mining and commercial use been extensive. Not until the 1930s did the magnitude of the asbestos hazard begin to be recognized. One reason for the delayed appreciation of the fibrogenic potential of asbestos is that there is a considerable latency period between the initial exposure and the onset of clinical manifestations, often 20 to 30 years. Use of asbestos in the United States has declined since the mid-1970s, but worldwide use has not (48).

Workers with potentially significant asbestos exposure include asbestos miners and millers; many persons employed in the building trades and shipyards, such as insulation workers, pipefitters, sheet metal workers, welders, asbestos removal workers; and workers involved in the manufacture or repair of automotive friction products. Although exposure to small amounts of asbestos fiber may contribute to the risk of malignancy, it is not generally associated with clinically significant, nonmalignant, asbestos-related pulmonary disease.

Asbestos-Related Pleural Disease

Asbestos exposure can cause discrete pleural thickening (pleural plaques), diffuse pleural thickening, rounded atelectasis, and benign exudative effusions (discussed in the preceding). All types of asbestos have the potential to induce asbestos-related pleural disease.

Pleural Thickening

Circumscribed areas of pleural thickening, called pleural plaques, are the most common radiographic findings caused by chronic asbestos exposure and most commonly occur without asbestosis. Individuals with isolated pleural plaques are usually asymptomatic. Pathologically, plaques usually involve the parietal pleural surface, are composed mostly of collagen, and are accompanied by an inflammatory reaction. Pleural plaques may become calcified. They have a latency of about 15 to 20 years following first exposure. Pleural plaques most often are visible on the PA chest radiograph along the lower lateral borders of the thoracic cavity and the central portions of the hemidiaphragms. Although there are other causes of unilateral pleural thickening and calcification (empyema, hemothorax, and thoracic trauma), the presence of bilateral pleural thickening is almost always owing to asbestos exposure. Circumscribed plaques, in the absence of parenchymal asbestosis, are usually not associated with respiratory impairment. However, workers with radiographic evidence of plaques but no asbestosis can have mildly reduced lung volumes (49).

Diffuse pleural thickening, involving visceral as well as parietal pleura, is less common than circumscribed plaques but is more likely to be associated with mildly reduced lung volumes and interstitial changes on HRCT (33,50). Diffuse pleural thickening is believed to be a sequela of benign asbestos pleural effusions. Chest CT scanning provides the most sensitive and specific technique for identifying pleural plaques and diffuse pleural thickening. However, CT scanning is not required for routine clinical evaluation.

Whether asbestos-related pleural disease independent of exposure dose is a risk factor for lung cancer is an area of debate (51,52). Progression to advanced asbestosis is not common. There is no evidence that pleural plaques undergo malignant transformation to mesothelioma.

Rounded Atelectasis

Localized fibrosis of the pleura involving the visceral as well as the parietal surfaces can entrap the adjacent lung parenchyma and mimic the radiographic appearance of a solitary pulmonary nodule. This phenomenon, known as rounded atelectasis, occurs with asbestos-related pleural disease. Rounded atelectasis may be recognized radiographically by an irregular shadow that tapers toward the hilum, the so-called comet tail sign, and can usually be differentiated from a more serious mass lesion by use of CT scanning.

Asbestosis

Histologic Features and Pathogenesis

The light microscopic appearance of the pulmonary parenchyma in the early stages of asbestosis is similar to that seen with idiopathic interstitial pneumonitis. A mixed leukocyte infiltration of the interstitial spaces, accompanied by varying degrees of organizing fibrosis, is typically present. The initial areas of inflammation in asbestosis appear to center around the respiratory bronchioles. Peribronchial fibrosis may explain the observation of mild airways obstruction in nonsmoking workers exposed to asbestos dust.

Similar to silica, inhaled asbestos is phagocytosed by alveolar macrophages that become activated. Both asbestos and silica can generate reactive oxygen species such as superoxide anion, which can result in cell injury and altered function (43). Unlike silica, asbestos fibers generally are not cytotoxic to the macrophage. Activated macrophages release various cytokines and other inflammatory mediators that can directly injure the lung parenchyma or recruit additional inflammatory and mesenchymal cells, resulting in an alveolitis and fibrosis rather than normal healing. All major types of asbestos are fibrogenic, although some studies have provided support for the concept that it is the long, thin asbestos fibers that have the greatest fibrogenic potential.

Clinical Presentation, Evaluation, and Diagnosis

The clinical presentation is indistinguishable from that of other forms of interstitial pulmonary fibrosis. The most common symptom in those with asbestosis is progressive dyspnea, usually over a period of years. Cough, either nonproductive or productive, is common. The physical examination findings are nonspecific; for example, bibasilar crackles and clubbing of the fingers can occur. Signs of pulmonary hypertension and cor pulmonale may be seen in advanced cases.

The diagnosis of asbestosis is based on a history of sufficient asbestos exposure with appropriate latency, and certain clinical, radiographic, and pulmonary function findings, not all of which may be present in a particular situation. The American Thoracic Society (ATS) has attempted to develop criteria for the diagnosis of asbestosis (53). A panel of ATS experts concluded that for the diagnosis of asbestosis to be made in the absence of pathologic examination of lung tissue (i.e., the usual situation), it is necessary that there be: (*a*) a reliable history of exposure; and (*b*) an appropriate time interval between exposure and detection (typically more than 15 years). The panel also regarded the following clinical criteria to be of recognized value: (*a*) chest radiographic evidence of small, irregular opacities; (*b*) a restrictive pattern of lung impairment; (*c*) a diffusing capacity below the lower limit of normal; and (*d*) bilateral late or paninspiratory crackles at the posterior lung bases not cleared with cough. Of these clinical criteria, the chest radiographic evidence is the most important. There is some controversy regarding the level of abnormality of the radiographic images needed for the diagnosis of asbestosis. Some require an ILO grade of 1/1 or 1/0 on chest radiograph, whereas others consider HRCT evidence of interstitial fibrosis sufficient radiographic evidence. The certainty of the diagnosis of asbestosis increases as more of the criteria are met.

The occupational history of asbestos exposure is critical to the diagnosis of asbestosis. The onset, duration, and intensity of exposure are important to determine. There is a characteristic latency of 15 or more years between first exposure and disease manifestation. Exposure durations of less than 6 months rarely can result in asbestosis. The intensity of asbestos exposure can be determined by information on the job, industry, and use of personal protective equipment. Overall, exposures since the mid-1970s have been much reduced, although there are exceptions.

Radiography

Chest radiograph and determination of lung volumes and diffusing capacity are usually sufficient to make a diagnosis of asbestosis once a history of occupational exposure is obtained. The characteristic chest radiograph shows irregular or linear opacities distributed throughout the lung fields but more prominent in the lower zones (Fig. 13.4). There can be loss of definition, or "shagginess," of the heart border. The most useful finding in the differential diagnosis of asbestosis is the presence of pleural thickening (Fig. 13.4). Diaphragmatic or pericardial calcification is almost a pathognomonic sign of asbestos exposure. However, asbestosis can occur without any visible pleural changes on chest radiography.

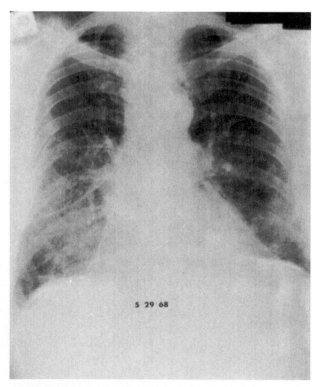

FIGURE 13.4. Typical asbestosis with "shaggy heart" and pleural plaques with diaphragm calcification.

Histologic fibrosis can occur with a normal appearing chest radiograph. HRCT is more sensitive than either plain chest radiographs or conventional CT for the detection of parenchymal abnormalities (41). However, when the diagnosis is clear on the basis of the chest radiograph and history, HRCT usually is not necessary for either the diagnosis or the management of such patients.

Pulmonary Function

Pulmonary function abnormalities usually indicate the presence of a restrictive defect with decreased lung volumes, decreased lung compliance, and decreased exercise tolerance. More recent studies suggest that asbestos, in the absence of cigarette smoking, can result in a mild degree of air flow obstruction (54). Although in population studies there is a correlation between pulmonary function and radiographic severity of asbestosis, in individual cases such correlation may not be present. The presence of a marked obstructive ventilatory defect usually indicates the influence of other factors, notably cigarette smoking. Because asbestosis and chronic air flow obstruction exert opposite effects on total lung capacity, the total lung capacity is an insensitive measure of impairment in patients with both asbestosis and obstructive airways disease (55).

Other Tests

Patients with asbestosis may have abnormal gallium uptake. However, such findings are not particularly sensitive or specific, and gallium scanning is not recommended in the evaluation of patients with asbestosis. Bronchoscopy and lung biopsy are rarely necessary to make the diagnosis of asbestosis, but may be indicated in atypical presentations. BAL and transbronchial biopsy can rule out other causes of abnormality such as infection, sarcoidosis, or hypersensitivity pneumonitis, and can document the presence of an alveolitis. Histopathologic material from lung biopsy can be used to identify and grade the presence of fibrosis and identify and quantify asbestos bodies or fibers. The presence of numerous asbestos bodies in a biopsy specimen confirms the exposure history and suggests that the pulmonary fibrosis seen is related to asbestos exposure (Fig. 13.5). However, asbestos bodies may also be found in lung tissue from individuals without significant histories of exposure (42).

Prognosis and Treatment

The natural history of patients with asbestosis is variable. Marked accelerated loss of pulmonary function can occur, but more stable disease with minimal or mild progression is more common (56,57). The risks that parenchymal scarring will develop and progress appears to increase with cumulative asbestos exposure and ILO score (57). Progression of disease can occur following removal from exposure. A major concern is the increased risk of lung cancer, which is discussed below. In addition to its synergistic effects on lung cancer, it is possible cigarette smoking may also act to

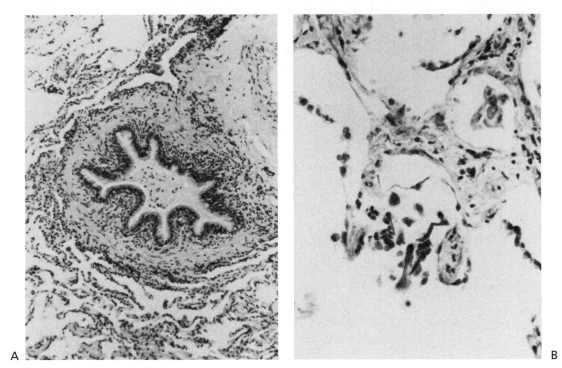

FIGURE 13.5. A: Lung biopsy from a patient with asbestos showing peribronchiolar fibrosis. **B:** Intraalveolar asbestos bodies.

increase the fibrotic response to inhaled asbestos. Smoking cessation for active smokers is crucial.

Further asbestos exposure should be minimized. Steroids and immunosuppressor therapy probably have little beneficial effect on the course of the disease, although no controlled trials have been reported in the literature. Appropriate therapy of superimposed respiratory tract infections is important, although it is not clear that patients with asbestosis are more susceptible to such infection. Bronchodilator therapy is indicated if there is evidence of a reversible obstructive component. Although there is no evidence that ongoing medical surveillance with annual chest radiography and spirometry is beneficial, such surveillance is commonly recommended.

Coal Workers' Pneumoconiosis

Two different respiratory diseases can develop from the chronic excessive inhalation of coal dust: coal workers' pneumoconiosis (CWP) and chronic bronchitis. Chronic bronchitis and reduced lung function secondary to coal dust is treated in a separate section of this chapter, but it should be mentioned that this problem is more common among coal workers than CWP (58).

CWP occurs in either simple or complicated forms. Only a small percentage of miners with simple CWP ever develop complicated disease (59). The chest radiographic pattern of simple CWP is typically one of small nodular opacities. The opacities visible on chest radiographs of simple CWP are owing to the presence of coal macules in the lungs. The diagnosis of complicated CWP is made when larger opacities (1 cm or larger in diameter) are seen on chest radiograph (Fig. 13.6). These large opacities represent masses of confluent fibrous tissue and may undergo cavitation secondary to either ischemic necrosis or superimposed tuberculous infection.

History and Epidemiology

Pneumoconiosis was associated with coal mining in Great Britain early in the nineteenth century. The problem of respiratory disease in coal miners was given scant attention in the United States until the 1960s. Since 1969, there have been extensive efforts by the National Institute for Occupational Safety and Health (NIOSH) at surveillance of respiratory disease among coal miners. A heavy dust load usually is required to cause CWP. It is unusual to see significant pneumoconiosis in miners who have spent less than 20 years underground. Bronchitic symptoms from inhalation of coal dust are common among miners.

Pathology and Pathogenesis

The initial response to the inhalation of coal dust into the terminal respiratory units involves phagocytosis of the deposited dust by alveolar macrophages. Coal appears to be

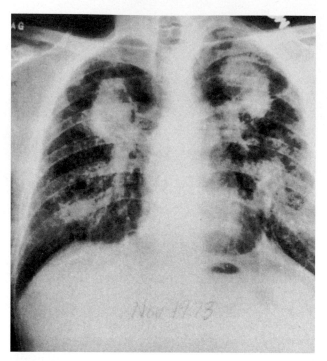

FIGURE 13.6. Coal workers' pneumoconiosis with progressive massive fibrosis.

less fibrogenic than asbestos or silica, but similar to these exposures, coal dust can result in increased reactive oxygen species, and macrophage activation with production of various cytokines and growth factors (60). The factors that determine whether simple CWP progresses to complicated CWP are not well understood. The presence of silica in the retained dust and superimposed tuberculous infection can stimulate fibrosis. However, cases of complicated CWP can occur in the absence of either of these factors.

Clinical Evaluation and Diagnosis

Simple CWP is usually a relatively benign process unless superimposed pulmonary infections or other concomitant disease is present. Respiratory symptoms of cough and dyspnea are common among coal miners in general and may be present in a given individual miner regardless of whether the chest radiograph shows pneumoconiosis. Complicated disease is now uncommon. Once the process of complicated disease begins, however, it generally results in PMF, even if there is no further exposure to coal dust. Miners with PMF are usually dyspneic to the point of being disabled. Pulmonary hypertension and cor pulmonale may be late sequelae.

The results of pulmonary function testing vary with the stage of CWP. With simple CWP, there are usually no gross abnormalities. However, statistically significant reductions in lung function in coal miners (compared with control

populations) have been documented in a number of large epidemiologic studies (58,61). Decline in FEV_1 and the presence of irregular opacities have been correlated with cumulative dust exposure. Miners with complicated CWP can have obstructive, restrictive, or mixed ventilatory defects. There is an increased prevalence of autoantibodies in the serum of miners with CWP, usually without clinical manifestation of collagen-vascular disease. Caplan's syndrome was first described in conjunction with CWP.

A diagnosis of CWP can usually be made on the basis of the exposure history and characteristic chest radiograph findings. A lung biopsy is rarely needed. Bronchitis and COPD can occur from exposure to coal mine dust in the absence of complicated pneumoconiosis or smoking (59). Miners with CWP or bronchitis should try to minimize further mining exposures but do not necessarily have to leave mining, depending on the extent of their disease. Bronchospasm should be treated with standard bronchodilator therapy. For miners who smoke, smoking cessation should be strongly recommended.

Beryllium and Hard Metal-Related Disease

Beryllium and cobalt are both metals that may cause interstitial lung disease, probably through immunologically mediated mechanisms. Although more is known about the pathogenesis of chronic beryllium disease than about hard metal (cobalt)-related lung disease, these diseases share several features in common: Only a fraction of exposed workers appear to be susceptible; disease can occur at relatively low exposure levels, compared with those necessary to cause traditional pneumoconioses such as asbestosis; and the exposure history is frequently less obvious than with exposures such as asbestos or coal dust. Thus, both the diagnosis and prevention of beryllium- and hard metal-related disease can be more challenging than with the traditional pneumoconioses.

Chronic Beryllium Disease

Chronic beryllium disease (CBD) is a chronic pulmonary and systemic granulomatous disease that is similar to sarcoidosis but is caused by chronic beryllium exposure. Acute high beryllium exposures can cause an acute pneumonitis, which is not commonly seen.

Epidemiology

Chronic granulomatous lung disease and systemic illness was first recognized in the United States among employees frosting fluorescent light bulbs with beryllium oxide (BeO) during World War II (62). As beryllium use has increased in aerospace, electronics, and other high technology industries, cases have become more widely dispersed. The reported prevalence of CBD in exposed workers is low, around 5% in most settings, but can be higher (63,64). As exposure is decreased, the incidence, but not necessarily the severity, appears to decrease. Cases of CBD from a metal refinery where exposures may have been below OSHA standards have been reported (35). Beryllium is usually present as an alloy with other metals such as copper, aluminum, and nickel, and workers may not be aware of beryllium exposure.

Pathogenesis and Pathology

Noncaseating granulomas identical to those seen in sarcoidosis are the pathologic hallmark of CBD (Fig. 13.7). Although predominantly seen in the lung, these granulomas can be found in numerous peripheral sites such as the liver and skin. CBD is believed to be a disorder involving cell-mediated immunity, a beryllium-specific cell mediated immune response. This is supported by a number of findings, including lung and lymph node histology similar to that of other cell-mediated disorders, the presence of delayed hypersensitivity to beryllium salts, and animal models characterized by antigen-specific T-lymphocyte sensitization to beryllium (65,66). Beryllium can be phagocytosed by macrophages that present beryllium antigen to lymphocytes, resulting in sensitization and proliferation of beryllium-specific CD4+ T cells. Beryllium-activated T cells may release various cytokines and other inflammatory mediators, resulting in granuloma formation.

Why only a small percentage of an exposed population becomes sensitized to beryllium is not well understood. Recent studies have found genetic markers for CBD involving polymorphisms in MHC genes (67,68).

Clinical Evaluation and Diagnosis

The most common symptom with CBD is progressive exertional dyspnea. The latency between exposure and manifestations of disease is more variable than with traditional

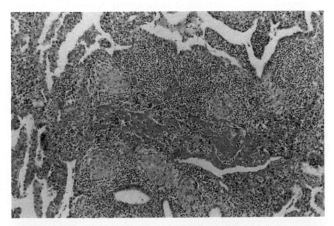

FIGURE 13.7. Lung biopsy from a patient with chronic beryllium disease showing lymphocytic alveolitis and noncaseating granulomas (H&E).

pneumoconioses and can range from months to over 20 years. Nonproductive cough and systemic complaints such as fatigue or weight loss are common.

Chest radiographs typically show diffuse interstitial infiltrates, and bilateral hilar adenopathy in less than half the cases. Obstructive, restrictive, or mixed restrictive-obstructive patterns are seen on pulmonary function testing.

Newman and coworkers have proposed the following diagnostic criteria for CBD: (*a*) history of beryllium exposure; (*b*) beryllium-specific cell mediated immune response; (*c*) consistent lung histopathology; and (*d*) clinical presentation including either respiratory symptoms, compatible abnormalities on chest radiograph or chest CT scan, or altered pulmonary physiology (restrictive or obstructive defects or reduced diffusing capacity on pulmonary function testing or ventilatory impairment on exercise testing) (66,69).

The history of beryllium exposure can be difficult to obtain, because beryllium is frequently present as an alloy with other metals. Furthermore, because of the latency between exposure and clinical presentation, the relevant exposure history may have occurred many years in the past. A history of CBD in coworkers is very helpful in documenting exposure. Beryllium exposure can also be documented by measuring beryllium in tissues (especially in lung and lymph nodes) or in urine. Elevated tissue levels reflect body burden rather than recent exposure, and they document exposure, not disease. Adequate amounts of lung tissue for beryllium analysis can usually only be obtained from open lung biopsy, not from transbronchial biopsy. Urinary excretion of beryllium can be determined but usually indicates ongoing, rather than past, exposure.

A beryllium-specific cell mediated immune response can be documented by demonstrating the proliferation of either peripheral blood lymphocytes or lymphocytes obtained from BAL in response to beryllium salts *in vitro* (i.e., a positive lymphocyte proliferation test). The test is more sensitive when performed on BAL lymphocytes (close to 100% sensitivity) than on peripheral blood lymphocytes (60% to 95%) (70,71). The peripheral blood lymphocyte proliferation test has been used to detect preclinical disease and to screen exposed workers for beryllium sensitization and early disease (66,69). The beryllium patch test is not recommended because it can cause hypersensitivity and exacerbate existing disease.

Clinically CBD can be difficult to distinguish from sarcoidosis. The presence of uveitis, erythema nodosum, and asymptomatic hilar adenopathy favor a diagnosis of sarcoidosis; a history of beryllium exposure and evidence of beryllium hypersensitivity strongly support the diagnosis of CBD.

Prognosis and Treatment

The natural history and prognosis with CBD can be quite variable and difficult to predict. CBD can progress to advanced, irreversible disease, even in the absence of ongoing exposure (69). Spontaneous improvement after removal from further exposure can also occur, and patients may respond to corticosteroids (66,69). Earlier milder disease may be more reversible. Patients with symptomatic CBD should be removed from further exposure, which may lead to improvement. Therapy follows the principles for sarcoidosis, including a trial of systemic steroids for symptomatic disease.

Hard Metal Disease

Exposure to hard metal, a cemented alloy of tungsten carbide with cobalt, can result in interstitial pulmonary fibrosis or asthma (72). Cobalt is probably the etiologic agent for both processes, but may require the concomitant inhalation of other compounds such as metallic carbides or diamond dust (73). Cobalt dust has been shown experimentally to cause acute alveolitis, fibrosis, and bronchitis, whereas tungsten carbide without cobalt appears to be nontoxic (72). Diamond workers exposed to cobalt without any tungsten carbide have developed an interstitial disease histologically identical to hard metal disease, as well as specific airway sensitization to cobalt (74,75).

Epidemiology and Pathogenesis

Exposure to cobalt is not uncommon and can occur during production or use of hard metal tools, and in industries such as diamond polishing. However, the reported prevalence of interstitial disease in exposed workers is relatively low, ranging from less than 1% (most studies) to 12.8% (72). Cobalt-induced asthma is probably more common, around 5% to 10%. Although usually occurring separately, cobalt-induced interstitial lung disease and asthma can occur in the same patient. A strong association of hard metal disease with an HLA polymorphism has been reported (76).

The histologic finding is a fibrosing alveolitis, with characteristic multinucleated giant cells consisting of macrophages and alveolar epithelial cells. Multinucleated macrophages can be seen on BAL but can be a nonspecific finding.

Clinical Presentation, Diagnosis, and Management

Cobalt-exposed workers can present with symptoms of occupational asthma, slowly progressive interstitial lung disease, or rapidly progressive interstitial pneumonitis. Severe respiratory insufficiency can occur. The latency from exposure to onset of hard metal disease is variable, from a few to over 20 years. Chest radiographs in patients with hard metal disease typically demonstrate a diffuse reticulonodular pattern that tends to be more prominent in the mid- and lower lung fields. Most commonly restrictive, but also obstructive or mixed, defects can be seen on pulmonary function testing.

A high level of suspicion and a careful occupational history are key to the diagnosis of hard metal disease. An open lung biopsy may be required. The characteristic lung pathol-

ogy showing multinucleated giant cells is helpful. The detection of tungsten on lung biopsy confirms exposure. Cobalt, because it is more soluble than tungsten, is usually not detected. Cobalt in the blood and urine indicates current or recent exposure.

Hard metal disease can progress after removal from exposure. Removal from further exposure, steroids, and bronchodilator therapy if air flow obstruction is present are the mainstay of therapy.

Other Pneumoconioses

A number of other silicates, dusts, and metals that are less common causes of pneumoconioses are listed in Table 13.7. Several of these are discussed in the following.

Talcosis

Talc is a hydrated magnesium silicate that is chemically related to asbestos. Because asbestos and silica are found in conjunction with talc, there is some uncertainty about the magnitude of the fibrogenic potential of pure talc (77).

Pulmonary fibrosis can occur after many years of exposure to high concentrations of talc dust, usually in the course of mining soapstone. Significant talc exposure also can occur during the manufacture of ceramics, roofing materials, and rubber goods. Cases of talcosis have been reported to result from heavy exposure to commercial talcum powder (78). Pulmonary fibrosis also may result from a microembolization process secondary to the intravenous injection of talc-containing pills by drug abusers. Pathologically, lesions similar to those of silicosis and asbestosis as well as foreign-body granulomas containing talc particles may be seen.

The clinical presentation is one of progressive dyspnea and productive cough. The initial chest radiographic appearance of talcosis is similar to that of asbestosis: The upper lung zones tend to be relatively spared, and mild pleural thickening and calcification may occur. However, talcosis may progress in a manner similar to that of silicosis with regard to the coalescence of lesions and the ultimate development of PMF. Studies of pulmonary function in patients with talcosis have demonstrated decreases in both lung volumes and diffusing capacity.

Kaolin Pneumoconiosis

Kaolin, also called China clay, is a hydrated aluminum silicate used in the manufacture of ceramics, paint, paper, and cement. Epidemiologic studies are somewhat conflicting, but it appears that radiographic changes owing to excessive kaolin dust exposure (diffuse nodular opacities) are more prominent than clinical manifestations of disease. However, cases of kaolin-associated PMF have been reported (79).

Other Silicates

Fuller's earth (attapulgite) is an absorbent aluminum silicate clay now used primarily in oil refining and in the building of foundry molds. Although massive fibrosis can occur, the pneumoconiosis associated with Fuller's earth generally runs a relatively benign course (80).

Micas are a group of complex aluminum silicates that have been associated with the development of interstitial pulmonary fibrosis in heavily exposed workers (81). Mica also has been associated with pleural thickening. It is unclear whether these findings may be caused by contamination with silica or asbestos (81).

Mixed-dust pneumoconiosis refers to lung disease seen in workers exposed to crystalline silica and other dusts, such as coal or iron oxides. The disease is similar to silicosis, the amount of fibrosis depending on the amount of free silica exposure.

Manmade Vitreous Fibers

A variety of synthetic silicate mineral fibers (manmade vitreous fibers, MMVFs) have increasingly been used in substitution for asbestos. There are several types of MMVFs: mineral (slag or rock) wools, glass fibers, and ceramic fibers. Most common are mineral wools and glass fiber, which can cause skin and respiratory tract irritation and bronchitis but have not been shown to cause a pneumoconiosis (82,83). There is concern that the less common refractory ceramic fibers may be more fibrogenic and carcinogenic, based on animal data and fiber shape (82). A possible relationship between refractory ceramic fiber exposure and both pleural plaques and a small reduction in FVC has been reported (84,85). In view of the massive substitution of fiberglass for asbestos in insulation materials, it is understandable that there is concern about the long-term health risks of exposure to MMVF. Thus far, epidemiologic studies in populations exposed to MMVF have not revealed evidence that symptomatic pneumoconiosis is a consequence of such exposure, although there may not yet be adequate follow-up time to entirely exclude the possibility. The carcinogenic potential are discussed below.

Graphite Pneumoconiosis

Graphite is pure crystallized carbon that can be either natural or synthetic. Most natural deposits are contaminated with some free silica, whereas synthetic graphite is relatively pure. Graphite is used in the manufacture of steel, pencils, electrical equipment, and in the printing industry. Excessive graphite dust exposure may lead to chest radiographic changes identical to those of simple CWP, and concomitant silica exposure has been implicated as the cause for the more severe pulmonary fibrosis occasionally seen in graphite-exposed workers (86). An uncommon pneumoconiosis has also been associated with inhalation of pure synthetic graphite dust (87).

Aluminum Pneumoconiosis

Aluminum is produced from bauxite, a naturally occurring hydrous aluminum oxide ore. Pulmonary fibrosis has been reported in workers exposed to aluminum oxide dust and fumes. This condition, known as Shaver's disease, typically presents as progressive dyspnea, and has been attributed to free silica contamination (88). However, exposure to aluminum powder that does not contain silica can result in pulmonary fibrosis and is associated with an increased incidence of spontaneous pneumothorax (88). The pathologic features of this uncommon pneumoconiosis are interstitial fibrosis, initially in the upper lobes, and emphysematous bleb formation on pleural surfaces. The aluminum content in the lung is greatly increased. Pulmonary function testing reveals a restrictive disorder.

Work in aluminum potrooms has been associated with obstructive lung disease, termed potroom asthma, although the exact causative agent is not clear (89).

Flock Worker's Lung

Recently a new and unique form of work-related interstitial lung disease has been reported in workers in nylon flock plants (90). Nylon flock is finely cut nylon filaments used to make velvet-like fabrics, such as upholstery covering. Exposed workers have developed interstitial lung disease with typical symptoms, reduced lung volumes and DLCO, and increased interstitial markings on chest radiographs. Histopathologic findings have revealed a characteristic lesion, a lymphocytic bronchiolitis and peribronchiolitis with lymphoid hyperplasia (90,91). Most have improved away from work although recovery has not always been complete. Recent clinical, epidemiologic and toxicologic studies suggest that the causative agent is respirable fragments of nylon.

Miscellaneous Dusts

Exposure to the dusts of such metals as *iron, barium, tin, antimony,* and *titanium* may lead to radiographically visible deposits in the lungs without corresponding parenchymal fibrosis and pulmonary function impairment. Pneumoconiosis can also occur as a result of chronic exposure to dusts of synthetic materials such as *Bakelite* and polyvinyl chloride, but there is some controversy about the degree of functional impairment that may result (92,93).

Chronic Bronchitis and Chronic Airways Disease

Occupational or industrial bronchitis is defined as bronchitis that is caused or aggravated by exposures at work. The

TABLE 13.8. PARTIAL LIST OF AGENTS THAT CAUSE CHRONIC BRONCHITIS

Minerals
  Coal
  Oil mist
  Silica
  Silicates
  MMVF
Metals
  Welding fumes
Organic substances
  Cotton
  Grain
  Wood
Irritant gases
  Sulfur dioxide
  Chlorine
  Nitrogen dioxide
Smoke
Diesel exhaust

pathophysiology and interrelationships between chronic bronchitis, emphysema, and asthma, all of which are associated with air flow obstruction, are discussed in Chapters 8, Asthma, and 9, Chronic Obstructive Pulmonary Disease, Bronchiectasis, and Cystic Fibrosis. A wide range of different occupational exposures can cause bronchitic symptoms, including gases, mineral dusts, metals, fumes, and organic substances (Table 13.8). Irritant exposures can cause airway inflammation and mucus hypersecretion, both of which can be associated with air flow obstruction.

Whether occupational exposure to chronic irritant exposures can cause air flow obstruction or accelerated loss of ventilatory function and not just bronchitic symptoms is an important question that has been a source of debate (94). This has been difficult to determine because of the high prevalence of smoking, the limited size of some cohort studies, and the potential bias of the healthy worker effect in cross-sectional studies. A number of both community- and workforce-based epidemiologic studies have shown an association between chronic irritant exposures and air flow obstruction or accelerated loss of lung function in populations occupationally exposed to dusts and fumes, such as miners or cotton workers (94,95). However, this occupational effect is usually of lesser magnitude than the detrimental effect of cigarette smoke on lung function. Cigarette smoke is the major cause of bronchitic symptoms and chronic obstructive airways disease. Epidemiologic studies suggest that the interaction between smoking and occupational exposures in causing bronchitic symptoms and reduced lung function may be additive or multiplicative (94,95). Certain host susceptibility factors such as preexisting nonspecific airway hyperresponsiveness may predispose certain workers to chronic airways obstruction. The presence of airway hyper-

responsiveness is associated with a more rapid than expected annual rate of decline in lung function in certain exposed populations (96). However, it has been more difficult to determine whether the presence of industrial bronchitis itself causes air flow obstruction or is a marker for some other risk factor.

Pathologic data support the notion that occupational exposure to certain dusts is capable of causing chronic air flow obstruction. Coal miners, for example, had more centrilobular emphysema than controls in an autopsy study, and severity of emphysema was related to lung burden of coal dust (97).

Common exposures that can cause chronic bronchitis and which have also been clearly documented to cause accelerated loss of lung function include asbestos, silica, coal, grain, wood, and cotton dusts. Chronic exposures that can cause chronic bronchitic symptoms and that are suspected of causing respiratory impairment include *MMVFs, welding fumes, firefighting exposures, irritant gases,* and *diesel exhaust.*

Clinical Evaluation

The clinical evaluation of a patient with suspected occupational bronchitis is similar to that of any patient with chronic bronchitic symptoms. It is important to assess whether bronchitic symptoms alone are present or whether asthma, emphysema, or some other pulmonary process is involved. Any environmental or occupational exposures that may be causing or exacerbating the pulmonary condition should be identified. No specific diagnostic tests are available for occupational bronchitis, and a causal role for occupational exposures can be difficult to establish, especially in a smoker. The presence of eye and upper respiratory tract irritation and inflammation, a temporal association between symptoms and workplace exposures (especially early in the course), and coworkers with similar symptoms suggest work-relatedness. Chronic bronchitic symptoms can persist after removal from exposure.

Pulmonary function testing, including D$_{LCO}$, is useful both diagnostically and to assess level of impairment. Methacholine challenge testing may be indicated if the history suggests asthma and spirometry is normal. Chest radiography should also be performed.

When a patient's bronchitis is suspected to be work-related, interventions to reduce or eliminate exposure to the putative agent(s) or process are justified. Engineering controls are preferable to the use of respirators. If the patient improves with such intervention, then the diagnosis of work-relatedness is supported. However, symptoms may persist after cessation of exposure. Commonly, bronchitis is of multifactorial etiology with smoking playing a role. Smoking cessation is key. Medical surveillance to detect accelerated loss of ventilatory function or airway hyperresponsiveness is recommended. The medical management of work-related chronic bronchitis is similar to that caused by smoking alone.

Data available concerning prognosis in patients with irritant-induced chronic bronchitis are limited. However, as discussed, exposure to inhaled irritants may be associated with both symptoms of chronic bronchitis and small decrements in lung function.

MALIGNANCIES OF THE RESPIRATORY TRACT AND PLEURA

This section addresses the occupational and environmental causes of lung carcinoma and other cancers of the respiratory tract and pleura. (See Chapter 14, Lung Neoplasms, for a more extensive discussion of the pathogenesis, evaluation, and treatment of lung cancer.)

Sinonasal Cancers

Squamous carcinoma and adenocarcinoma of the sinuses are rare in the general population but have been associated with several different exposures. Occupational exposures to nickel and wood dust are considered to be established risk factors for sinonasal cancers (98,99). Increased risk of sinonasal cancers has been reported with exposure to chromium, and formaldehyde (100,101). Cigarette smoking and alcohol use are not major causes of sinonasal cancers.

Laryngeal Cancer

Squamous carcinoma of the larynx usually is attributed to tobacco smoke and alcohol exposure. Data from several large cohorts, including insulators and friction product manufacturing workers, have provided evidence supporting a contributory role for asbestos fibers, possibly a twofold relative risk (102). Because synergism between asbestos exposure and cigarette smoking has been documented for lung cancer, it is possible that such synergism might apply to this related epithelial cancer. Several recent studies have found an increased risk of laryngeal cancer with exposure to metal working fluids (103).

Lung Cancer

Lung cancer, once a rare tumor, is now the leading cause of cancer death in both men and women in the United States. The dramatic increase in the incidence of lung cancers in the past 50 years has encouraged study of the modern environment for possible causal factors. Starting with the demonstration by Doll in the 1950s of a causal role for cigarette smoke, epidemiologic techniques have identified a number of respiratory tract carcinogens (104,105). Although cigarette smoking is the single greatest risk factor for lung cancer, occupational and environmental exposures

TABLE 13.9. KNOWN OCCUPATIONAL LUNG CARCINOGENS

Substance	Examples of Exposure Settings
Asbestos	Insulation workers, shipyard workers
Arsenic	Smelting of copper, zinc, lead; pesticide production
Beryllium	Beryllium production, processing
Chloromethyl ether	Production workers
Chromium	Chromate production, pigment manufacture, electroplating
Mustard gas	Production workers, soldiers
Nickel	Nickel refining, plating
Polycyclic aromatic hydrocarbons	Coke oven workers, rubber workers, aluminum reduction workers, roofers
Radon	Uranium mining, hard rock mining
Silica	Mining, foundries

are important preventable causes. Estimates of the percentage of lung cancers attributable to occupational and environmental factors have varied widely, ranging from 5% to over 30% of all cases (104–106). A number of agents are considered to be either known or suspected human lung carcinogens (Tables 13.9 and 13.10). Additionally, studies have shown an excess risk of lung cancer among members of several trades and industries, although identification of specific carcinogenic agents has not been possible.

There is considerable evidence that diet is also an important factor in the etiology and prevention of lung cancer. Most consistently, a diet high in fruit and vegetables has been shown to be associated with a reduced risk of lung cancer (107). What component(s) of such a diet, beta-carotene, retinoids, or other nutrient, produce(s) the protective effect remains unclear. Clinical chemoprevention trials of vitamin A and beta-carotene in preventing lung cancer among high-risk smokers and asbestos-exposed workers have found either no effect or increased risk of lung cancer in those taking the vitamin supplementation (108,109).

From a public health standpoint, recognition of causal connections provides the first step in cancer control, reducing ongoing exposure to human carcinogens. For those already exposed, recognition of the degree of risk allows the

TABLE 13.10. SUSPECTED OCCUPATIONAL LUNG CARCINOGENS

Substance	Examples of Exposure Settings
Acrylonitrile	Plastics, petrochemicals
Cadmium	Smelting, battery production
Formaldehyde	Production formaldehyde resins
Synthetic fibers (MMVF)	Production, insulating
Vinyl chloride monomer	Polyvinyl chloride, plastic production

intelligent application of smoking cessation and other interventions to reduce risk of lung cancer or screening strategies to identify early curable tumors.

Clinical Evaluation and Management

The evaluation of any patient with lung cancer should include a careful occupational and environmental exposure history. To determine whether a given exposure caused the patient's cancer, the following guidelines are recommended. The clinician must determine what potential lung carcinogens the patient was exposed to and assess dose of exposure and latency as best as possible. A thorough smoking history is essential. When more than one carcinogen is present, it can be difficult to specify etiology, and one usually concludes that both exposures contributed to the patient's cancer. The management of a patient with occupationally induced lung cancer is similar to that of any patient with lung cancer.

Known Lung Carcinogens

Arsenic

Arsenic has been shown to increase lung cancer risk in workers engaged in smelting, pesticide manufacturing, and other industries with arsenic exposure (110). A clear dose–response relationship has been shown. The latency from onset of exposure to lung cancer is about 25 years on average. Arsenic is believed to be a late-stage promoter of lung cancer rather than an initiator.

Asbestos

Asbestos was established as a cause of lung cancer in the 1950s (111). Lung cancer is a far more important cause of death than mesothelioma in asbestos-exposed workers, affecting up to 40% of those with asbestosis (112). Although numerous studies have confirmed a causal relationship between asbestos and lung cancer, several areas of controversy remain, including the carcinogenic potential of different types of asbestos fibers, the magnitude of the synergistic effect between asbestos and cigarette smoke, whether asbestosis or asbestos exposure is the risk factor, whether a safe threshold exists, and the risks of low-level exposures.

There are no distinctive features of asbestos-related lung cancer to distinguish it from lung cancer owing to smoking alone or other causes. Latency between exposure and disease peaks at 20 to 30 years. Although at one time it appeared that adenocarcinoma was the predominant histologic type, current data indicate a distribution of cell types comparable to that among the general population (113). Although the location of tumors is more frequently in the lower lobes, this feature is insufficiently specific to determine etiology in an individual patient. Persons with asbestosis are clearly at highest risk (114). However, some studies have shown that individuals with occupational asbestos exposure without parenchymal changes also have an increased risk of lung cancer (115).

Although the exact quantitative interaction may be debatable, cigarette smoke clearly potentiates the carcinogenic effects of asbestos. It is generally stated that asbestos and cigarette smoke act synergistically to increase risk for lung cancer. Some studies have shown more of an additive rather than a synergistic effect of asbestos and cigarettes. Among nonsmoking workers exposed to asbestos, the relative risk is increased by a factor of approximately five; among smokers who have not been exposed to asbestos, the risk is increased by a factor of approximately ten. However, among smoking asbestos workers, the relative risk is increased by a factor of at least 15 (additive) to greater than 50 (synergistic) (116). Cessation of smoking, therefore, is the most important step in cancer prevention for previously exposed individuals, although control of asbestos exposure is also imperative.

The data from epidemiologic studies of heavily exposed cohorts demonstrate a nearly linear relationship between estimates of exposure and mortality from lung cancer at high levels of asbestos exposure (117). However, the dose–response relationship at low levels of exposure is less clear. In some cohort studies the dose–response relationship does not include zero risk, suggesting that there is no threshold or "safe" level of exposure. There are also arguments that favor the existence of a safe threshold, including cohort mortality studies showing no increased risk at low exposure, low-dose animal studies, negative studies among residents with low-level asbestos exposure, and data suggesting that asbestos-related lung cancers only occur in those with asbestosis. If there is an increased risk of lung cancer at low doses, the risk is small.

The mechanism of asbestos-related carcinogenesis is not clear but is probably linked to the processes of lung inflammation and fibrosis. Asbestos is a lung carcinogen that probably acts primarily as a promoting, rather than an initiating, agent. There is mounting evidence that both the physical dimensions and surface chemical characteristics of the fibers are important. All major forms of asbestos appear to be associated with an increased risk of lung cancer, although chrysotile may be less hazardous than the amphiboles (amosite, crocidolite, and tremolite).

Beryllium

The epidemiological data linking beryllium to lung cancer have been controversial, primarily because of questions concerning small relative risks, exposure misclassification, lack of adequate smoking data, and other confounders. However, the relative risks that have been identified have been generally consistent from study to study, and the association between beryllium and lung cancer has been supported by numerous animal studies. Following a 1993 review of this data, the International Agency for Research on Cancer classified beryllium as "definitely carcinogenic to humans" (118).

Chloromethyl Ethers and Mustard Gas

Alkylating agents used in the chemical and pharmaceutical industries, including bischloromethyl ether (BCME) and mustard gas (bis[2-chloroethyl] sulfide), are highly carcinogenic (119). A number of studies have documented that BCME exposure is strongly associated with an increased risk of lung cancer, especially small-cell carcinomas at a young age. Smoking does not appear to further increase the risk of cancer among BCME-exposed workers.

Chromium

Hexavalent chromium, used in chromate production, electroplating, pigment manufacture, and the ferrochromium industry, has been associated with an increased relative risk of lung cancer (120).

Nickel

Nickel exposure (among nickel mining and refinery workers) has been associated with excess lung cancer rates, with a mean latency of about 20 years (106). Metallic nickel has not been associated with an increased risk of lung cancer.

Polyaromatic Hydrocarbons

Polyaromatic hydrocarbons (PAHs) are a complex mix of a number of widespread substances generated during the incomplete combustion of carbonaceous products such as coal, oil, pitch, and tar. PAHs are also present in cigarette smoke and diesel exhaust. Workers exposed to PAHs—including coke oven workers, printers, roofers, aluminum production workers, railroad workers and truck drivers—have been found to have significant excess lung cancer rates (121–123).

Radon

Radon is an inert gas that is a decay product of uranium-238. Radon decays with alpha particle emission to various short-lived radon daughters. Underground uranium miners exposed to radon and its decay products have a marked increased risk of developing lung cancer, with a preponderance of small cell carcinoma, although other cell types are also increased (124). Cigarette smoke and radon most likely interact more than additively in increasing the risk for lung cancer (124). Excess lung cancer rates have been found in other types of miners including tin, iron, and lead miners (125). The potential risk of domestic radon is discussed in the following.

Silica

Traditionally, silica has not been viewed as a human carcinogen. However, there has been increasing evidence of an excess of lung cancer associated with silica exposure. In 1996 the International Agency for Research on Cancer (IARC)

reclassified silica as a definite human carcinogen (126). Several recent studies have reported an increased risk of lung cancer among miners, foundry workers, and other silica-exposed workers (46,127). The risk of lung cancer is highest in those with chronic silicosis compared to those with only silica exposure.

Suspected Lung Carcinogens

Vinyl chloride monomer and *acrylonitrile*, both animal carcinogens, are suspected human respiratory tract carcinogens. Excess mortality because of lung cancer in human populations exposed to acrylonitrile has been shown, but the magnitude of the effect is relatively small and variable (106). There is also evidence that *cadmium* exposure as well as occupational exposure to diesel exhaust is associated with increased risk of lung cancer (106).

Manmade vitreous fibers (MMVFs) include rock and slag wool, glass fibers, and ceramic fibers. Some excess lung cancer risk has been reported in MMVF-exposed cohorts, but without a strong dose–response relationship (82,127). Ceramic fibers, when instilled in the pleural space, can cause malignant mesothelioma in rodents, but there are insufficient human data.

A recent study of a large cohort of industrial workers exposed to *formaldehyde* showed a small increase risk of lung cancer (128).

Workers in several industries including foundries, rubber industry, welding, and printing have been shown to be at increased risk of lung cancer in some studies (129). However, the etiologic agents are unclear, and confounding by smoking and other exposures can limit the findings.

Risk Factors for Lung Cancer in the Environment

There has been increasing interest in the role of environmental exposures such as environmental tobacco smoke, air pollution, and domestic radon in the causation of lung cancer. The nonmalignant respiratory effects of these and other exposures present in indoor and ambient air are discussed in the final section of this chapter.

Domestic Radon

The potential risk of lung cancer from exposure to radon in homes, derived primarily from rock, soil, and drinking water, is receiving increasing attention. Average domestic radon exposures in the United States range from 0.8 to 1.5 picocuries per liter (pCi/L), well below the levels experienced by miners. However, cumulative lifetime exposures comparable to those of miners are likely to exist in a small percentage of American homes. It is believed that radon may act more than additively as a risk factor for lung cancer in smokers, possibly because radon decay particles can attach to respirable particles such as cigarette smoke (124).

Most estimates of the risk of domestic radon are based

on extrapolations from studies of miners to lower indoor levels (124). These risk assessments estimate that about 5,000 to 20,000 deaths annually in the United States (approximately 3% to 15% of all lung cancer deaths) are attributable to radon (130). Case-control studies have found an increased relative risk of lung cancer associated with increased domestic radon levels (131). However, other case-control studies have found no increased relative risk of lung cancer in relation to domestic radon exposure (132). In smokers, the best way to reduce the risk of lung cancer is to stop smoking, regardless of domestic radon levels. If very high domestic radon measurements are found (e.g., above 5 to 10 pCi/L in a living area), it would be reasonable to consider home mitigation techniques such as improved ventilation.

Environmental Tobacco Smoke

Environmental tobacco smoke (ETS) contains sidestream smoke (SS) released from the burning cigarette and mainstream smoke (MS) exhaled by the smoker. Passive smokers are exposed to the same carcinogenic constituents of tobacco smoke as smokers, although generally at lower doses and in different relative concentrations. A number of epidemiologic studies have consistently shown a statistically significant increase risk of lung cancer in nonsmokers from exposure to ETS ranging from 20% to 100% (133,134). Because of the large number of people exposed to ETS and the relatively high incidence of lung cancer, a small increase in lung cancer risk owing to ETS risk is of great public health importance.

Air Pollution

Outdoor air pollution is a complex and variable mixture of natural and manmade pollutants including sulfur oxides, particulates, carbon monoxide, and photochemical pollution. Specific compounds found in air pollution are potentially carcinogenic, and there may be a small increased risk of lung cancer associated with air pollution (135). In particular, recent meta-analyses of occupational studies have suggested that ambient exposure to diesel exhaust may pose a potential problem (121,122). However, it has been difficult to confirm an air pollution-associated risk for lung cancer using epidemiologic data. There are numerous methodologic difficulties in attempting to determine whether air pollution is associated with an increased risk of lung cancer, including quantifying exposures and controlling for confounders such as cigarette smoking and occupational exposures.

Another concern is whether *indoor air pollution* such as household coal smoke or other heating or cooking smoke increases the risk of lung cancer. Studies from China suggest that household coal smoke may increase this risk (136).

Asbestos in Buildings

Low-level asbestos exposure is ubiquitous. Exposures in buildings, especially schools and public buildings, which frequently contain friable and decaying asbestos, have created great anxiety. The primary concern about low-level exposure is the risk of mesothelioma and lung cancer. As discussed, the magnitude of this risk, if any, is an area of controversy. Although the risk of cancer from such exposures is undoubtedly quite low, it is unlikely to be zero. In considering public policy and personal decisions, the risks of low-level asbestos exposure should be considered in the context of other risks in life, and the costs of remediation likewise need to be weighed against other costs and financial decisions.

Malignant Mesothelioma

Malignant mesotheliomas are rare tumors of the pleura or peritoneum that in at least 80% of cases are associated with a history of asbestos exposure. Although there is some dose–response relationship between asbestos exposure and risk of mesothelioma, mesotheliomas may occur with relatively short-term and low-level exposures. Mesotheliomas have been reported to occur in family members of asbestos workers and persons living near shipyards. Many patients will be free of obvious radiographic evidence of asbestos exposure, unlike the situation with asbestos-related lung cancer (137). The latency period is in the range of 30 to 40 years. Pleural cases are more common than peritoneal.

The relative carcinogenicity of the different asbestos fiber types is an area of debate. Although all types probably can cause mesothelioma, chrysotile, the most common fiber type in the United States, is the least likely to cause mesothelioma, whereas the amphiboles crocidolite and amosite appear to have the highest potential for inducing mesotheliomas (127). In contrast to what has been observed with bronchogenic carcinoma, cigarette smoking does not increase the risk of mesothelioma.

The most common presenting symptom in patients with pleural mesothelioma is chest pain. Dyspnea, weight loss, and cough may also be present. A pleural effusion is frequently seen on the chest radiograph. CT scanning is frequently performed to confirm the presence of a pleural-based mass(es). The pleural fluid is exudative, and cytologic examination frequently is insufficiently sensitive or specific to confirm the diagnosis. Histologic differentiation from poorly differentiated adenocarcinoma metastatic to the pleura or reactive mesothelial cells is frequently difficult. Open pleural biopsy with adequate tissue specimens and an experienced pathologist capable of performing electron microscopic and histochemical studies are often required to make the diagnosis. Mesotheliomas extend locally and can also metastasize. New therapeutic options are under investigation, but the prognosis remains poor (138).

AIR POLLUTION: NONMALIGNANT RESPIRATORY EFFECTS

There has been increasing concern about the adverse health effects of both outdoor ambient and indoor air pollution. Patients and the public frequently turn to physicians with questions concerning the risks of radon, environmental tobacco smoke, ozone, other air pollutants, and for advice on what to do about such exposures. This section reviews the known nonmalignant pulmonary health effects of ambient (outdoor) and indoor air pollution and which populations may be more susceptible to these effects. The role of these exposures in contributing to lung cancer is addressed in the preceding section.

Ambient Air Pollution

Numerous natural and manmade sources contribute to outdoor air pollution. There are four broad groups of exposures that may have adverse health effects: (*a*) combustion of sulfur-containing fossil fuels (sulfur oxides, particulates, acidic aerosols); (*b*) photochemical pollution (ozone and oxides of nitrogen); (*c*) carbon monoxide; and (*d*) toxic air pollutants (fossil fuel combustion and industrial products). The EPA has categorized pollutants as "criteria" pollutants and "hazardous" pollutants (primarily carcinogens such as asbestos, benzene, or polyaromatic hydrocarbons), the levels of which are regulated by the Clean Air Act (Table 13.11). Investigators have tried to determine the adverse effects of air pollution with both large-scale epidemiologic studies and experimental exposure chambers. It should be remembered that these exposures almost always occur as part of a complex mix of pollutants, not individually, and that interactions between different exposures probably exist but are difficult to determine.

TABLE 13.11. UNITED STATES AMBIENT AIR QUALITY CRITERIA POLLUTANTS AND PRINCIPAL HEALTH EFFECTS AT AMBIENT LEVELS

Pollutant	Health Effects
Ozone	Acute respiratory symptoms, decrements in lung function, respiratory tract inflammation, and asthma exacerbation
Particulate matter ($PM_{2.5}$, PM_{10})	Asthma, COPD exacerbation, increased cardiopulmonary mortality
Sulfur oxides	Asthma exacerbation
Nitrogen dioxide	? Asthma/COPD exacerbation; ? Increased susceptibility to respiratory tract infections
Carbon monoxide	Ischemic heart disease exacerbation
Lead	Decreased cognitive function in children

Epidemiologic studies have shown that air pollution can be associated with increased respiratory symptoms and exacerbations of asthma and bronchitis, although which particular component, such as fine particulates or ozone, is responsible can be difficult to determine from epidemiologic studies (139,140). Multiple studies have shown an association between air pollution (primarily fine particulates) and daily mortality, largely from cardiopulmonary causes (141). Longitudinal cohort studies have also shown an association between particulate pollution and mortality, thereby strengthening the likelihood that the association is real (142,143).

The effects of specific pollutants at ambient levels of exposure are summarized (144).

Sulfur oxides and *particulate matter* are produced by sulfur-containing fuels such as coal and petroleum and can exacerbate the status of patients with asthma and COPD and increase respiratory symptoms in children. Children and asthmatics also appear susceptible to *acid aerosols* (such as sulfuric acid and nitric acid).

Acute exposure to ambient levels of *ozone* has been shown to result in lung inflammation and transient reductions in lung function. However, the chronic effects of such exposures remain unclear. Persons with asthma appear to have enhanced airway inflammatory responses to ozone and multiple epidemiologic studies have demonstrated increased risk of asthma exacerbations after exposure to high levels of ambient ozone (145,146).

Carbon monoxide (CO) can bind to hemoglobin and carboxyhemoglobin, reducing oxygen delivery to tissues. In patients with coronary artery disease, CO may exacerbate myocardial ischemia and arrhythmias (147,148).

In summary, current data suggest that ambient levels of certain pollutants may increase respiratory symptoms and exacerbate underlying respiratory or cardiac diseases, primarily in children, asthmatics, and persons with COPD, ischemic heart disease, or congestive heart failure. Cigarette smoking may have additive or synergistic effects with air pollutants, and exercise may also increase the likelihood of adverse effects.

Indoor Air Pollution

Increasing concern is being raised about the adverse health effects of indoor air, and various symptoms have been attributed to exposures in the indoor environment. Illnesses that have been related to building exposures include allergic respiratory diseases such as sinusitis, rhinitis, asthma, and hypersensitivity pneumonitis due to exposures to molds, spores, chemicals, or other substances (149). Building-related infectious diseases such as Legionnaires' disease are well recognized. It is important to obtain a careful occupational and environmental exposure history in any patient presenting with such an illness. Nonindustrial environments should not be assumed to be clean and free of significant exposures.

Sick Building Syndrome (SBS)

Since the 1970s, nonspecific symptoms among employees in indoor, non-industrial environments have increasingly come to medical attention. Because many SBS complaints are related to the respiratory tract, pulmonary physicians should be aware of this syndrome. The term SBS refers to nonspecific complaints that usually involve mucous membrane and upper respiratory irritative symptoms, headaches, fatigue, difficulty concentrating, and odor complaints, and that are associated with a particular building(s) (149,150). Symptoms generally improve away from that indoor environment. Similar symptoms in coworkers are common. Other causes for the patient's complaints should be evaluated and ruled out. The cause of SBS is likely multifactorial. Inadequate ventilation systems are an important contributing factor in most cases. However, other factors such as indoor air pollutants (i.e., ETS, particulates, and cleaning agents), job satisfaction, and work stress are frequently involved. Physician recommendations concerning the workplace environment may facilitate ventilation improvements or other beneficial interventions in the work environment.

Environmental Tobacco Smoke

As mentioned earlier, ETS contains most of the ingredients inhaled by the active smoker, but at lower concentrations. A number of studies have demonstrated that children of parents who smoke are at increased risk of respiratory infections, respiratory symptoms, asthma exacerbations, and reduced lung function, compared with children of nonsmoking parents (151,152). More recently ETS exposure has been associated with respiratory tract disease in adults, including exacerbation of asthma, sensory irritation symptoms, lower respiratory tract symptoms, and lung function impairment (153,154).

Biomass and Fossil Fuels

Indoor use of wood, coal, kerosene, or gas for heating and cooking release various combustion products. Epidemiologic studies have shown an association between these exposures and childhood respiratory symptoms and also possibly an increased risk of childhood infections, asthma, and reduced lung function (136,155,156).

Carbon Dioxide

Carbon dioxide, which is produced primarily by human respiration, is frequently measured as an indicator of adequate indoor ventilation CO_2 results are not uncommonly presented to physicians caring for patients with complaints of SBS. Normal CO_2 levels are frequently measured despite inadequate ventilation, and such measurements are frequency not helpful in managing complaints of inadequate indoor air quality or SBS (150).

REFERENCES

1. Rosenstock L, Cullen MR, eds. *Textbook of clinical occupational and environmental medicine.* Philadelphia: Saunders, 1994.
2. Rom WN, ed. *Environmental and occupational medicine,* 3rd ed. Boston: Little, Brown & Co, 1998.
3. Parker JR, Banks DE, eds. *Occupational lung disease: an international perspective.* Philadelphia, Lippincott Williams & Wilkins, 1999.
4. Parkes WR. *Occupational lung disorders.* Oxford: Butterworth-Heinemann, 1994.
5. Harper P, Schenker M, Balmes J, eds. *Occupational and environmental respiratory disease.* St. Louis: Mosby-Year Book, 1996.
6. Cullen MR, Cherniack MG, Rosenstock L. Medical progress: occupational medicine. *N Engl J Med* 1990;322:594–601, 675–683.
7. Bernstein IL, Bernstein DI, Chan-Yeung M, et al. Definition and classification of asthma. In Bernstein IL, Chan-Yeung M, Malo J-L, et al., eds. *Asthma in the workplace.* New York: Marcel Dekker, 1999:1–4.
8. Chan-Yeung M, Malo JL. Aetiological agents in occupational asthma. *Eur Respir J* 1994;7:346–371.
9. Blanc PD, Cisternas, Smith S, et al. Occupational asthma in a community-based survey of adult asthma. *Chest* 1996;109:56–57s.
10. Becklake MR, Malo J-L, Chan-Yeung M. Epidemiological approaches in occupational asthma. In Bernstein IL, Chan-Yeung M, Malo J-L, et al. eds. *Asthma in the workplace.* New York: Marcel Dekker, 1999:27–65.
11. Venables KM, Chan-Yeung M. Occupational asthma. *Lancet* 1997;349:1465–1469.
12. Cullen MR. Clinical surveillance and management of occupational asthma. *Chest* 1990;98:196S–201S.
13. Raulf-Heimsoth M, Baur X. Pathomechanisms and pathophysiology of isocyanate-induced diseases: summary of present knowledge. *Am J Ind Med* 1998;34:137–143.
14. Perfetti L, Cartier A, Ghezzo H, et al. Follow-up of occupational asthma after removal from or diminution of exposure to the responsible agent: relevance of the length of the interval from cessation of exposure. *Chest* 1998;114:398–403.
15. Alberts WM. Reactive airways dysfunction syndrome. *Chest* 1996;109:1618–1626.
16. Fabbri LM, Boschetto P, Caramori G, et al. Pathophysiology. In Bernstein IL, Chan-Yeung M, Malo J-L, et al., eds. *Asthma in the workplace.* New York: Marcel Dekker, 1999:27–65.
17. Ramazzini B. *De morbis artificum diatriba* (1713). Wright WC (trans). New York: Hafner, 1964.
18. Schachter EN. Byssinosis and other textile dust-related lung diseases. In Rosenstock L, Cullen MR, eds. *Textbook of clinical occupational and environmental medicine.* Philadelphia: Saunders, 1994.
19. Glindmeyer HW, Lefante JJ, Jones RN, et al. Exposure-related declines in the lung function of cotton workers: relationship to current workplace standards. *Am Rev Respir Dis* 1991;144:675–683.
20. Christiani DC, Wegman DH, Eisen EA, et al. Pulmonary function among cotton textile workers. *Chest* 1994;105:1713–1721.
21. Castellan RM. Cotton dust. In Harber P, Schenker MB, Balmes

JR, eds. *Occupational and environmental respiratory disease.* St. Louis: Mosby, 1996:401–419.

22. Chan-Yeung M, Enarson DA, Kennedy SM. State of the art: the impact of grain dust on respiratory health. *Am Rev Respir Dis* 1992;145:476–487.

23. Grzybowski S, Chan-Yeung M, Ashley JA. Atopy and grain dust exposure. In Dosman JA, Cotton DA, eds. *Occupational pulmonary disease: focus on grain dust and health.* New York: Academic Press, 1980.

24. Huy T, Schipper KD, Chan-Yeung M, et al. Grain dust and lung function: dose-response relationships. *Am Rev Respir Dis* 1991;144:1314–1321.

25. Schwartz DA. Acute inhalational injury. *Occup Med* 1987;2(2): 297–318.

26. Epler GR, Colby TV, McLoud TC, et al. Bronchiolitis obliterans organizing pneumonia. *N Engl J Med* 1985;312:152–158.

27. Barnhart S, Rosenstock L. Cadmium chemical pneumonitis. *Chest* 1985;86:789–791.

28. Davison AG, Newman Taylor AJ, Darbyshire J, et al. Cadmium fume inhalation and emphysema. *Lancet* 1988;1:663–667.

29. Sperkazza SJ, Beckett WS. The respiratory health of welders: state of the art. *Am Rev Respir Dis* 1991;143:1134–1148.

30. Williams N, Smith FK. Polymer fume fever: an elusive diagnosis. *JAMA* 1972;219:1587–1589.

31. Rosenstock L, Demers P, Heyer NJ, et al. Respiratory mortality among firefighters. *Br J Ind Med* 1990;47(7):462–465.

32. Epler GR, McCloud TG, Gaensler EA. Prevalence and incidence of benign asbestos pleural effusion in a working population. *JAMA* 1982;247:617–622.

33. Rudd RM. Occupational lung disease: 2—New developments in asbestos-related pleural disease. *Thorax* 1996;51(2):210–216.

34. Talcott JA, Thurber WA, Kantor AF, et al. Asbestos-associated diseases in a cohort of cigarette-filter workers. *N Engl J Med* 1989;321:1220–1223.

35. Kreiss K, Mroz MM, Zhen B, et al. Risks of beryllium disease related to work processes at a metal, alloy, and oxide production plant. *Occup Environ Med* 1997;54:605–612.

36. van Sprundel MP. Pneumoconioses: the situation in developing countries (review). *Exp Lung Res* 1990;16:5–13.

37. Nugent K, Perrotta D, Dodson RF, et al. A cluster of silicosis in sandblasters [Letter]. *Am Rev Respir Dis* 1990;142:1466.

38. Rosenman KD, Reilly MJ, Kalinowski DJ, et al. Silicosis in the 1990s. *Chest* 1997;111(3):779–786.

39. Epler GR. Normal chest roentgenograms in chronic diffuse infiltrative lung disease. *N Engl J Med* 1978;27:934–939.

40. International Labour Office. Guidelines for the use of ILO International Classification of Radiographs of Pneumoconioses. *Occup Safety Health Series* No 22 (revised) Geneva, 1980.

41. Begin R. Computed tomography in the early detection asbestosis. *Br J Ind Med* 1993;50:689–698.

42. Churg A, Green FHY, eds. *Pathology of occupational lung disease,* 2nd ed. New York: Igaku-Shoin, 1998.

43. Mossman BT, Churg A. Mechanisms in the pathogenesis of asbestosis and silicosis. *Am J Respir Crit Care Med* 1998;157: 1666–1680.

44. Weber SL, Banks DE. Silicosis. In Rosenstock L, Cullen MR, eds. *Clinical occupational and environmental medicine.* Philadelphia: Saunders, 1994:264–274.

45. Xipell JM, Ham KN, Price CG, et al. Acute silicolipoproteinosis. *Thorax* 1977;32:104–111; American Thoracic Society. Adverse effects of crystalline silica exposure. *Am J Respir Crit Care Med* 1997;155:761–765.

46. Beckett W, Abraham J, Becklake M, et al. Adverse effects of crystalline silica exposure. *Am J Respir Crit Care Med* 1997;155: 761–765.

47. Costello JF, Moriarty DC, Branthwaite MA, et al. Diagnosis

and management of alveolar proteinosis: the role of electron microscopy. *Thorax* 1975;30:121–132.

48. Wagner GR. Asbestosis and silicosis. *Lancet* 1997;349(9061): 1311–1315.

49. Schwartz DA, Fuortes LJ, Galvin JR, et al. Asbestos-induced pleural fibrosis and impaired lung function. *Am Rev Respir Dis* 1990;141:321–326.

50. Schwartz DA, Galvin JR, Yagla SJ, et al. Restrictive lung function and asbestos-induced pleural fibrosis. A quantitative approach. *J Clin Invest* 1993;91:2685–2692.

51. Weiss W. Asbestos-related pleural plaques and lung cancer. *Chest* 1993;103:1854–1859.

52. Nurminen M, Tossavainen A. Is there an association between pleural plaques and lung cancer without asbestosis? *Scand J Work Environ Health* 1994;20:62–64.

53. Murphy RL, Becklake MR, Brooks SM, et al. The diagnosis of nonmalignant diseases related to asbestos: official statement of the American Thoracic Society. *Am Rev Respir Dis* 1986;134: 363–368.

54. Griffith DE, Garcia JG, Dodson RF, et al. Airflow obstruction in non-smoking, asbestos- and mixed dust-exposed workers. *Lung* 1993;141:213–224.

55. Barnhart S, Hudson LD, Mason SE, et al. Total lung capacity: an insensitive measure of impairment in patients with asbestosis and chronic obstructive pulmonary disease? *Chest* 1988;93: 299–302.

56. Beckett WS. Diagnosis of asbestosis. *Chest* 1997;111: 1427–1428.

57. Markowitz SB, Morabia A, Lilis R, et al. Clinical predictors of mortality from asbestosis in the North American Insulator Cohort, 1981–1991. *Am J Crit Care Med* 1997;156(1): 101–108.

58. Lapp NL, Parker JE. Coal workers' pneumoconiosis. In Epler GR, ed. *Clinics in chest medicine: occupational lung diseases.* Philadelphia: Saunders, 1992:243–252.

59. Coggon D, Newman TA. Coal mining and chronic obstructive pulmonary disease: a review of the evidence. *Thorax* 1998;53(5): 398–407.

60. Schins RP, Borm PJ. Mechanisms and mediators in coal dust induced toxicity: a review. *Ann Occup Hygiene* 1999;43(1): 7–33.

61. Attfield MD, Hodous TK. Pulmonary function of U.S. coal miners related to dust exposure estimates. *Am Rev Respir Dis* 1992;145:605–609.

62. Hardy HL, Tabershaw IR. Delayed chemical pneumonitis occurring in workers exposed to beryllium compounds. *J Ind Hyg Toxicol* 1946;28:197–211.

63. Kreiss K, Mroz Mm, Zhen B, et al. Epidemiology of beryllium sensitization and disease in nuclear workers. *Am Rev Respir Dis* 1993;148:985–991.

64. Kreiss K, Wasserman S, Mroz MM, et al. Beryllium disease screening in the ceramics industry. Blood lymphocyte test performance and exposure-disease relations. *J Occup Med* 1993;35: 267–274.

65. Newman LS. Beryllium lung disease: the role of cell-mediated immunity in pathogenesis. In Dean JH, Luster MI, Munson AE, et al. eds. *Immunotoxicology and immunopharmacology.* New York: Raven, 1994.

66. Newman LS, Kreiss K, King TE, et al. Pathologic and immunologic alterations in early stages of beryllium disease: re-examination of disease definition and natural history. *Am Rev Respir Dis* 1989;139:1479–1486.

67. Richeldi L, Sorrentino R, Saltini C. HLA-DPB1 glutamate 69: a genetic marker of beryllium disease. *Science* 1993;262:242–243.

68. Newman LS. To Be2 + or not to be2 +: immunogenetics and occupational exposure (comment). *Science* 1993;262:197–198.

69. Maier LA, Newman LS. Beryllium disease. In Rom WN, ed. *Environmental and Occupational Medicine,* 3rd ed. Philadelphia: Lippincott-Raven, 1998:1021–1035.

70. Mroz Mm, Kreiss K, Lezotte DC, et al. Reexamination of the blood lymphocyte transformation test in the diagnosis of chronic beryllium disease. *J Allergy Clin Immunol* 1991;88: 54–60.

71. Rossman MD, Kern JA, Elias JA, et al. Proliferative response of bronchoalveolar lymphocytes to beryllium: a test for chronic beryllium disease. *Ann Intern Med* 1988;108:687–693.

72. Cugell DW. The hard metal diseases. In Epler GB, ed. *Clinics in chest medicine: occupational lung diseases.* Philadelphia: Saunders, 1992:269–279.

73. Lison D, Lauwerys R, Demedts M, et al. Experimental research into the pathogenesis of cobalt/hard metal lung disease. *Euro Respir J* 1996;9(5):1024–1028.

74. Demedts M, Gheysens B, Nagels J, et al. Cobalt lung in diamond polishers. *Am Rev Respir Dis* 1984;130:130–135.

75. Gheysens B, Auwerx J, Van den Eeckhout A, et al. Cobalt-induced bronchial asthma in diamond polishers. *Chest* 1985; 88:740–744.

76. Potolicchio I, Mosconi G, Forni A, et al. Susceptibility to hard metal lung disease is strongly associated with the presence of glutamate 69 in HLA-DP beta chain. *Eur J Immunol* 1997; 27(10):2741–2743.

77. Gibbs AE, Pooley FD, Griffiths DM, et al. Talc pneumoconiosis: a pathologic and mineralogic study. *Hum Pathol* 1992; 23(12):1344–1354.

78. Nam K, Gracey DR. Pulmonary talcosis from cosmetic talcum powder. *JAMA* 1972;221:492–493.

79. Kennedy T, Rawlings W Jr, Baser M, et al. Pneumoconiosis in Georgia kaolin workers. *Am Rev Respir Dis* 1983;127:215–220.

80. Sakula A. Pneumoconiosis due to fuller's earth. *Thorax* 1961; 16:176–180.

81. Skulberg KR, Gylseth B, Skaug V, et al. Mica pneumoconiosis—a literature review. *Scand J Work, Environ Health* 1985; 11(2):65–74.

82. De Vuyst P, Dumortier P, Swaen GM, et al. Respiratory health effects of man-made vitreous (mineral) fibers. *Eur Respir J* 1995; 8(12):2149–2173.

83. Lockey JE, Wiese NJ. Health effects of synthetic vitreous fibers. *Clin Chest Med* 1992;13:329–339.

84. Lockey JE, Levin LS, Lemaster GK, et al. Longitudinal estimates of pulmonary function in refractory ceramic fiber manufacturing workers. *Am J Respir Crit Care Med* 1998;157(4 Pt 1): 1226–1233.

85. Lockey J, Lemasters G, Rice C, et al. Refractory ceramic fiber exposure and pleural plaques. *Am J Respir Crit Care Med* 1996; 154:1405–1410.

86. Hanoa R. Graphite pneumoconiosis. A review of etiologic and epidemiology aspects. *Scand J Work, Environ Health* 1983;9(4): 303–314.

87. Lister WB, Wimborne D. Carbon pneumoconiosis in a synthetic graphite worker. *Brit J Ind Med* 1972;29(1):108–110.

88. Mitchell J, Manning GB, Molyneux M, et al. Pulmonary fibrosis in workers exposed to finely powered aluminum. *Br J Ind Med* 1961;18:10–20.

89. Kongerud J, Boe J, Soyseth V, et al. Aluminum potroom asthma: the Norwegian experience. *Eur Resp J* 1994;7:165–172.

90. Kern DG, Crausman RS, Durand KT, et al. Flock worker's lung: chronic interstitial lung disease in the nylon flocking industry. *Ann Int Med* 1998;129:261–272.

91. Eschenbacher WL, Kreiss K, Lougheed MD, et al. Nylon flock-associated interstitial lung disease. *Am J Respir Crit Care Med* 1999;159:2003–2008.

92. Pimental JC. A granulomatous lung disease produced by Bakelite. *Am Rev Respir Dis* 1973;108:1303–1310.

93. Soutar CA, Copland LH, Thornly PE, et al. Epidemiological study of respiratory disease in workers exposed to polyvinyl chloride dust. *Thorax* 1980;35:644–652.

94. Oxman AD, Muir DCF, Shannon HS, et al. Occupational dust exposure and chronic obstructive pulmonary disease: a systemic overview of the evidence. *Am Rev Respir Dis* 1993;148:38–48.

95. Becklake MR. Chronic airflow limitation: its relationship to work in dusty occupations. *Chest* 1985;88:608–617.

96. Pham QT, Mur JM, Chan N, et al. Prognostic value of acetylcholine challenge test: a prospective study. *Br J Ind Med* 1984; 41:267–271.

97. Cockcroft A, Seal RME, Wagner JC, et al. Postmortem studies of emphysema in coalworkers and noncoalworkers. *Lancet* 1980; 2:600–603.

98. Colin D, Matos E, et al. Pooled reanalysis of cancer mortality among five cohorts of workers in wood-related industries. *Scand J Work, Environ Health* 1995;21(3):179–190.

99. Doll R, Mathews JD, Morgan LG. Cancers of the lung and nasal sinuses in nickel workers: a reassessment of the period of risk. *Br J Ind Med* 1977;34:102–105.

100. Satoh N, Fukuda S, Takizawa M, et al. Chromium-induced carcinoma in the nasal region. *Rhinology* 1994;32(1):47–50.

101. Luce D, Gerin M, Leclerc A, et al. Sinonasal cancer and occupational exposure to formaldehyde and other substances. *Int J Cancer* 1993;53(2):224–231.

102. Smith AH, Handley MA, Wood R. Epidemiological evidence indicates asbestos causes laryngeal cancer. *J Occup Med* 1990; 32:499–507.

103. Calvert GM, Ward E, Schnorr TM, et al. Cancer risks among workers exposed to metalworking fluids: a systematic review. *Am J Ind Med* 1998;33(3):282–292.

104. Doll R, Peto R. The causes of cancer: quantitative estimates of avoidable risks of cancer in the United States today. *JNCI* 1981; 66:1192–1308.

105. Vallyathan V, Green F, Ducatman B, et al. Roles of epidemiology, pathology, molecular biology, and biomarkers in the investigation of occupational lung cancer. *J Toxicol Environ Health* 1998;Part B 1:91–116.

106. Steenland K, Loomis D, Shy C, et al. Review of occupational lung carcinogens. *Am J Ind Med* 1996;29(5):474–490.

107. Willett WC. Micronutrients and cancer risk. *Am J Clin Nutr* 1994;59:1162S–1165S.

108. Omenn GS, Goodman GE, Thornquist MD, et al. Effects of a combination of beta carotene and vitamin A on lung cancer and cardiovascular disease. *N Engl J Med* 1996;24(18): 1150–1155.

109. The Alpha-Tocopherol, Beta-Carotene Cancer Prevention Study Group. The effect of vitamin E and beta carotene on the incidence of lung cancer and other cancers in male smokers. *N Engl J Med* 1994;330:1029–1035.

110. Blot WJ, Fraumeni JF. Arsenic and lung cancer. In Samet JM, ed. *Epidemiology of lung cancer.* New York: Marcel Dekker, 1994:207–218.

111. Doll R. Mortality from lung cancer in asbestos workers. *Br J Ind Med* 1955;12:81–86.

112. Berry G. Mortality of workers certified by pneumoconiosis medical panels as having asbestosis. *Br J Ind Med* 1981;38:130–137.

113. Brodkin CA, McCullough J, Stover B, et al. Lobe of origin and histologic type of lung cancer associated with asbestos exposure in the Carotene and Retinol Efficacy Trial (CARET). *Am J Ind Med* 1997;32(6):582–591.

114. Weiss W. Asbestosis: a marker for the increased risk of lung cancer among workers exposed to asbestos. *Chest* 1999;115: 536–549.

115. Hillerdal G, Henderson DW. Asbestos, asbestosis, pleural plaques and lung cancer. *Scand J Work Environ Health* 1997; 23:93–103.

116. Hammond EC, Selikoff IJ, Seidman H. Asbestos exposure, cigarette smoking, and death rates. *Ann NY Acad Sci* 1979;33: 473–490.

117. Hughes JM, Weill H. Asbestos and man-made fibers. In Samet JM, ed. *Epidemiology of lung cancer.* New York: Marcel Dekker, 1994:185–205.

118. Meeting of the IARC working group on beryllium, cadmium, mercury, and exposures in the glass manufacturing industry. *Scand J Work Environ Health* 1993;19:360–363.

119. McCallum RI, Wooley V, Petrie A. Lung cancer associated with chloromethyl methyl ether manufacture: an investigation at two factories in the United Kingdom. *Br J Ind Med* 1983;40: 384–389.

120. Hayes RB. The carcinogenicity of metals in humans. *Cancer Causes Control* 1997;8(3):371–385.

121. Bhatia R, Lopipero P, Smith A. Diesel exhaust exposure and lung cancer. *Epidemiology* 1997;9:84–91.

122. Lipsett M, Campleman S. Occupational exposure to diesel exhaust and lung cancer: a meta-analysis. *Am J Public Health* 1999; 89(7):1009–1017.

123. Mastrangelo G, Fadda E, Marzia V. Polycyclic aromatic hydrocarbons and cancer in man. *Environ Health Perspect* 1996; 104(11):1166–1170.

124. Darby SC, Samet JM. Radon. In Samet JM, ed. *Epidemiology of lung cancer.* New York: Marcel Dekker, 1994:219–243.

125. Reger RB, Morgan WK. Respiratory cancers in mining. *Occup Med* 1993;8:185–204.

126. IARC Reevaluates Silica and Related Substances. Meeting Report. *Environ Health Perspec* 1997;105(7):756–759.

127. Steenland K, Stayner L. Silica, asbestos, man-made mineral fibers, and cancer. *Cancer Causes Control* 1997;8:491–503.

128. Partanen T. Formaldehyde exposure and respiratory cancer—a meta-analysis of the epidemiologic evidence. *Scand J Work, Environ Health* 1993;19:8–15.

129. Coultas DB, Samet JM. Occupational lung cancer. In Epler GR, ed. *Clinics in chest medicine: occupational lung diseases.* Philadelphia: Saunders, 1992:341–354.

130. Samet JM. Indoor radon and lung cancer—estimating the risks. *West J Med* 1992;156:25–29.

131. Pershagen G, Akerblom G, Axelson O, et al. Residential radon exposure and lung cancer in Sweden. *N Engl J Med* 1994;330: 159–164.

132. Létoumeau EA, Krewski D, Choi NW, et al. Case control study of radon and lung cancer in Winnipeg, Manitoba, Canada. *Am J Epidemiol* 1994;140:310–322.

133. Hackshaw AK. Lung cancer and passive smoking. *Stat Meth Med Res* 1998;7(2):119–136.

134. Pershagen G. Passive smoking and lung cancer. In Samet JM, ed. *Epidemiology of lung cancer.* New York: Marcel Dekker, 1994:109–130.

135. Speizer FE, Samet JM. Air pollution and lung cancer. In Samet JM, ed. *Epidemiology of lung cancer.* New York: Marcel Dekker, 1994:131–150.

136. Smith KR, Youcheng L. Indoor air pollution in developing countries. In Samet JM, ed. *Epidemiology of lung cancer.* New York: Marcel Dekker, 1994:151–184.

137. Antman DH. Natural history and epidemiology of malignant mesothelioma. *Chest* 1993;103:373s–376s.

138. Sterman DH, Kaiser LR, Albelda SM. Advances in the treatment of malignant mesothelioma. *Chest* 1999;116:504–520.

139. Schwartz J. Air pollution and the duration of acute respiratory symptoms. *Arch Environ Health* 1992;47:116–122.

140. Pope CA. Respiratory disease associated with community air pollution and a steel mill, Utah valley. *Am J Public Health* 1989; 79:623–628.

141. Pope CA, Dockery DW. Epidemiology of particle effects. In Holgate St, Samet JM, Koren HS, et al, eds. *Air pollution and health.* New York: Academic Press, 1999:673–705.

142. Dockery DW, Pope CA, Xu X, et al. An association between air pollution and mortality in six U.S. cities (see comments). *N Engl J Med* 1993;329:1753–1759.

143. Pope CA, Thun MJ, Namboodiri MM, et al. Particle air pollution as a predictor of mortality in a prospective study of U.S. adults. *Am J Respir Crit Care Med* 1995;151:669–674.

144. American Thoracic Society. State of the art: health effects of outdoor air pollution. *Am J Respir Crit Care Med* 1996;153: 3–50, 477–498.

145. Scannell C, Chen L, Aris RM, et al. Greater ozone-induced inflammatory responses in subjects with asthma. *Am J Respir Crit Care Med* 1996;154:24–29.

146. Delfino RJ, Murphy-Moulton AM, Burnett RT, et al. Effects of air pollution on emergency room visits for respiratory illnesses in Montreal, Quebec. *Am J Respir Crit Care Med* 1997;155: 568–576.

147. Allred EN, Bleecker ER, Chaitman BR, et al. Short-term effects of carbon monoxide exposure on the exercise performance of subjects with coronary artery disease. *N Engl J Med* 1989;321: 1426–1432.

148. Sheps DS, Herbst MC, Hinderliter AL, et al. Production of arrythmias by elevated carboxyhemoglobin in patients with coronary artery disease. *Ann Intern Med* 1990;113:343–351.

149. Menzies D, Bourbeau J. Building-related illnesses. *N Engl J Med* 1997;337(21):1524–1531.

150. Redlich CA, Sparer J, Cullen MR. Sick-building syndrome. *Lancet* 1997;349:1013–1016.

151. Cook DG, Strachan DP. Health effects of passive smoking. 3. Parental smoking and prevalence of respiratory symptoms and asthma in school age children. *Thorax* 1997;52(12): 1081–1094.

152. Cook DG, Strachan DP. Health effects of passive smoking-10: summary of effects of parental smoking on the respiratory health of children and implications for research. *Thorax* 1999;54(4): 357–366.

153. Coultas DB. Health effects of passive smoking. 8. Passive smoking and risk of adult asthma and COPD: an update. *Thorax* 1998;53(5):381–387.

154. Eisner MD, Yelin EH, Henke J, et al. Environmental tobacco smoke and adult asthma. The impact of changing exposure status on health outcomes. *Am J Respir Crit Care Med* 1998; 158(1):170–175.

155. Lambert WE, Samet JM. Indoor air pollution. In Harber P, Schenker MB, Balmes JR, eds. *Occupational and environmental respiratory disease.* St. Louis: Mosby, 1996:784–807.

156. Brauer M, Kennedy SM. Gas stoves and respiratory health [comment]. *Lancet* 1996;347(8999):412.

14

LUNG NEOPLASMS

RICHARD A. MATTHAY
LYNN T. TANOUE
DARRYL C. CARTER

EPIDEMIOLOGY

ETIOLOGY
Tobacco Smoking
Gender
Atmospheric Pollution
Occupational Factors

PATHOLOGY
Bronchogenic Carcinoma
Other Pulmonary Neoplasms

CLINICAL MANIFESTATIONS
Symptoms and Signs
Metabolic Manifestations
Neuromuscular Manifestations
Skeletal Manifestations
Dermatologic Manifestations
Vascular Manifestations

DIAGNOSIS
Screening Techniques for Early Diagnosis of Lung Cancer

Chest Imaging
Sputum Cytology
Bronchoscopy
Needle Aspiration Biopsy
Pleural Biopsy

STAGING CLASSIFICATION

STAGING PROCEDURES
Thoracic Imaging Techniques
Invasive Staging Techniques
Evaluation for Extrapulmonary Metastasis

APPROPRIATE INVESTIGATION OF A SOLITARY PERIPHERAL PARENCHYMAL MASS

TREATMENT
Surgery
Radiation Therapy
Chemotherapy
Laser Therapy, Brachytherapy, and Endobronchial
    Prostheses

EPIDEMIOLOGY

Lung cancer is the most common malignant neoplasm in men throughout the world (1–4). Lung cancer constitutes 16% of all malignant tumors and accounts for 28% of all cancer deaths (35% in men and 19% in women) and about 6% of all deaths (1,2,4,5). In the year 2,000, the World Health Organization (WHO) has projected that there will be 2 million cases of lung cancer annually worldwide, resulting in enormous health costs (6–9).

In the United States, lung cancer is the leading cause of cancer mortality in men and women, accounting for 31% of all cancer deaths in men and 25% in women in the year 2000 (1). The relative significance of lung cancer as a cause of mortality in the United States can be appreciated when the annual death rates are compared with those for the second ranking sites in men and women, respectively, namely, prostate 13%

and breast 16% (1). An estimated 164,100 Americans will die of lung cancer in 2000—789,500 men and 74,600 women (1). The average patient with carcinoma of the lung is a heavy cigarette smoker in the sixth or seventh decade of life. Other age groups are affected, but less than 5% of patients are under 40 years of age. In the past, lung cancer was a problem primarily confined to men. There has been a decrease in lung cancer incidence and death rates among men in the United States since the early 1990s, whereas the incidence and mortality from this disease has increased steadily in women for the past several decades (Figs. 14.1 and 14.2) (1). The declining male to female ratio appears to parallel the well-documented increase in the number of women smokers (8).

The economic costs of lung cancer are enormous (9). In the United States, lung cancer-associated medical costs are estimated to exceed $10 billion and represent 1.5% of the total national cost of illness. Twenty percent of the cost is for

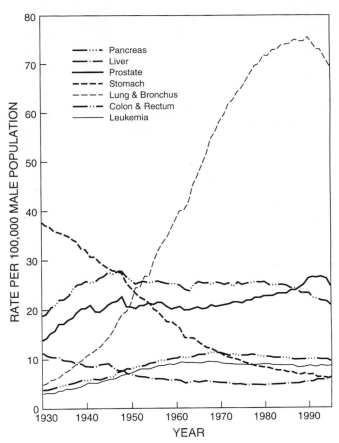

FIGURE 14.1. Age-adjusted cancer death rates for selected sites, males, United States, 1930–1990. Age-adjusted to the 1970 U.S. standard population. (Adapted with permission from Boring CC, Squire TS, Tong T, Montgomery S. Cancer statistics, 1994. *CA* 44:7–26, 1994.)

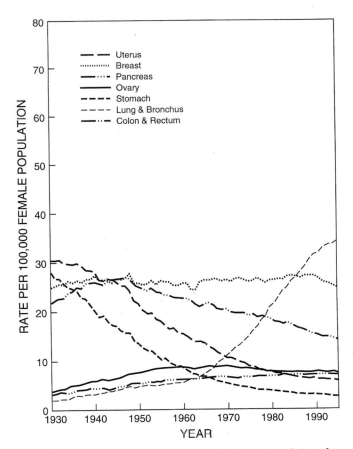

FIGURE 14.2. Age-adjusted cancer deaths for selected sites, females, United States, 1930–1990. Age-adjusted to the 1970 U.S. standard population. (Adapted with permission from Boring CC, Squire TS, Tong T, Montgomery S. Cancer statistics, 1994. *CA* 44:7–26, 1994.)

direct health care, whereas lost wages and productivity account for 80%. The potentially greater costs of other cigarette-related illnesses, such as heart disease and chronic obstructive lung disease, are not even taken into account in this figure.

ETIOLOGY

Tobacco Smoking

A vast amount of statistical evidence has incriminated smoking of tobacco, especially cigarettes, as the main cause of the progressive rise in mortality from bronchial carcinoma (4,5,7,10). Retrospective and a steadily increasing body of prospective data indicate that a dose–response relationship exists between cigarette smoking and lung cancer; the demographic distribution of this cancer correlates with long-term smoking habits; reduced lung cancer rates are found among exsmokers; and lung cancer has been induced by the administration of tar or inhaled cigarette smoke in experimental animals (4,8,11).

For both men and women, the risk of developing lung cancer is related directly to total exposure to cigarette smoke as measured by the number of cigarettes smoked, the duration of smoking in years, the age of initiation of smoking, the depth of inhalation, and the tar and nicotine levels in the cigarettes smoked (9). Worldwide prospective epidemiologic studies confirm these associations and indicate that in comparison with nonsmokers, average cigarette smokers have approximately a 9- to 10-fold increased risk of developing lung cancer, and heavy smokers at least a 10- to 25-fold increased risk (4,8,11,12). In a review of 3,070 new patients with lung cancer, the Edinburgh Lung Cancer Group found only 74 lifelong nonsmokers (2.4%), of whom 19 were men (0.6%) and 55 were women (1.8%) (13). Among smokers, the presence of airway obstruction is an additional risk factor for lung cancer, after adjustment for pack-years smoked (14,15).

In one of the more persuasive studies, all male doctors over 35 years of age in Britain were asked to state their smoking habits, and the proportion of these dying from carcinoma of the bronchus was determined during the later years (16). The risk of dying from carcinoma of the bronchus increased with the amount smoked and was highest for those who smoked cigarettes only. The risk for pipe smokers was considerably higher than for nonsmokers but was less than for cigarette smokers. An encouraging finding was that the risk decreased rapidly in those who stopped smoking, and it was halved in those who had stopped for 1 to 5 years. Moreover, data compiled in the United States indicate that the risk of lung cancer among exsmokers declines progressively from 2 to 15 years following discontinuation of smoking, after which it approaches the risk of lifelong nonsmokers (16).

The number of smokers in the United States is estimated to be more than 50 million (9). However, the percentage of white men still smoking has been decreasing steadily since 1964 when the Surgeon General of the United States issued the first major report linking smoking to lung cancer, and in 1982–1983, for the first time in over 50 years, new cases of lung cancer in adult white men dropped by 4%. In contrast, new lung cancer cases in US women did not plateau until 1995, because the smoking rate in women did not begin to decline until 1976 (1,9). Brown and Kessler have projected reductions in lung cancer mortality in the twentieth century that depend primarily on the effectiveness of current efforts to reduce smoking prevalence (17). Figure 14.3 shows their projections of the US age-adjusted lung cancer death rate with *(solid lines)* and without *(dashed lines)*

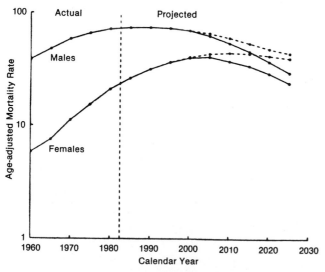

FIGURE 14.3. Actual (up to 1982) and projected age-adjusted lung cancer mortality rates for U.S. white men and women, 1960–2025. *Solid line* indicates projections based on current trends in smoking prevalence, per capita consumption, initiation, age, and cigarette tar content. *Dotted lines* represent projections assuming achievement of a reduction in overall smoking prevalence to 15% of U.S. adults in 1990, according to the National Cancer Institute Year 2000 Project. (This national goal in smoking cessation was not reached in 1990). (From Brown CC, Kessler LG. Projections of lung cancer mortality in the United States: 1986–2025. *JNCI* 80:43–51, 1988.)

additional successful interventions targeted at smoking prevention. In men, the higher current rate of lung cancer deaths plateaued and began to decline in the 1990s, whereas in women, the rate will not peak and start to decline until after the year 2010 (1,17).

An extremely controversial area is that of "passive smoking," or environmental tobacco smoke (ETS). Studies have shown that sidestream smoke actually has higher concentrations of carcinogens than mainstream smoke, and nonsmokers exposed to ETS may have measurable levels of carbon monoxide or urinary continence, an indication of significant smoke inhalation (18). Several studies have examined the risk of lung cancer developing in passive smokers, and the weight of evidence now shows that there is an increased, albeit small, risk of lung cancer in passive smokers (4,19,20). An average lifetime passive smoke exposure to a smoking spouse increases a nonsmoker's low risk by about 35% compared with the risk of 1000% (tenfold) for a lifetime of active smoking (4,5).

Lung cancer does, of course, exist in nonsmokers, but two features make it distinct: the considerably lower incidence of the disease in nonsmokers and a different histologic distribution among them (21). Thus, smoking is associated chiefly with squamous cell carcinoma and, to a lesser degree, with the small cell type (7,21). In nonsmokers, the predominant cell type is adenocarcinoma, although this tumor is more prevalent in smokers (20).

Gender

Since 1950, a greater than 500% increase in lung cancer mortality has been noted in women (4). Although most of this increase has been attributed to the dramatic increase in the prevalence of cigarette smoking among women since the 1940s, several additional disturbing facts have emerged. The first is that dose for dose women appear to have an increased susceptibility to carcinogens when compared with men. This in turn may translate into an increased risk for lung cancer. A number of studies suggest that women may be more vulnerable to tobacco carcinogens than men (22–26). In a case control study by Risch and colleagues, male–female differences in lung cancer covering the period 1981 to 1985 in Ontario, Canada were assessed (25). Among individuals with 40-pack-years of cigarette smoking relative to lifelong nonsmoking, the odds ratio for women developing lung cancer was 27.9, versus 9.6 in men. In another large case control study, Zang and Wydner showed that the dose–response odds for development of lung cancer in women were 1.2- to 1.7-fold higher in women than men (26). In both studies, the increase in lung cancer risk was present in all major histologic types. This gender difference in susceptibility may be related to a number of factors, including hormonal effects, sex-related differences in nicotine metabolism, or metabolic activation or detoxification of lung carcinogens (26).

Although women have enhanced susceptibility to the carcinogenic effects of tobacco, lung cancer also appears to occur more commonly in nonsmoking women than in nonsmoking men (4,10,26). In their recent case control study, Zang and Wynder evaluated 1889 lung cancer subjects and 2,070 control subjects, and the proportion of never-smoking lung cancer patients was more than twice as high in women than men (26). Although the reasons for this are not clear, women may have a greater susceptibility to nontobacco environmental carcinogens, have increased exposure to environmental tobacco smoke, or have sex-linked differences in metabolism of nontobacco environmental carcinogens (26). Whether hormone supplements in postmenopausal women enhance susceptibility to lung cancer requires study.

Atmospheric Pollution

Both in the United States and the United Kingdom, mortality is higher in urban areas than in rural regions and increases with the degree of urbanization, even if allowance is made for differences in smoking habits (27). This fact suggests an etiologic role for atmospheric pollution in the development of lung carcinoma, yet such a role is difficult to elucidate. Various carcinogenic agents, such as 3,4-benzpyrene, 1:12-benzperylene, arsenious oxide, radioactive substances, nickel and chromium compounds, and non-combustible aliphatic hydrocarbons, are present in the atmosphere (28). There may be synergism between air pollutants such as these and tobacco smoke, because when extracts of filtered air pollutants and tobacco smoking condensate are applied to mouse skin, their carcinogenicity is at least additive (21).

Occupational Factors (Also see Chapter 13)

Specific agents found in industrial exposure have been related to the development of bronchial carcinoma and are listed in Table 14.1 (5). The most notorious ones are radioactive material, asbestos, chromates, nickel, mustard gas, isopropyl oil, hydrocarbons, arsenic, hematite, vinyl chloride, and bis(chloromethyl) ether (4,5,11,26–32).

Radioactive Materials

All types of radiation may be carcinogenic. The lung cancer risk is increased from three to 30 times, depending on the degree of exposure (27). The latent period (interval between beginning of exposure and onset of lung cancer) is more than 10 years, the mean value being 16 to 17 years. There is a strong association between exposure to uranium and development of bronchogenic carcinoma, particularly small cell carcinoma (29–32). It is well documented that the combination of smoking and uranium exposure markedly increases the risk of developing lung cancer (Fig. 14.4) (4,29–32).

TABLE 14.1. SUBSTANCES ENCOUNTERED IN WORKPLACE EXPOSURES CATEGORIZED AS CAUSATIVE FOR BRONCHOGENIC CARCINOMA

Arsenic
Asbestos
Bis(chloromethyl) ether and chloromethyl methyl ether
Chromium and certain chromium compounds (hexavalent chromium)
Ionizing radiation, gamma radiation x-rays
Manmade mineral fibers (certain kinds only)
Mustard gas
Nickel in nickel refining
Radon progeny (decay products)
Soots, tars, mineral oils (polycyclic aromatic hydrocarbons)
Vinyl chloride

Source: Beckett WS. Epidemiology and etiology of lung cancer. *Clin Chest Med* 1993;14:1–15, with permission.

Asbestos

Asbestos is now a universally recognized carcinogen and appears to be the most frequent occupational cause of human lung cancer (4,5,28,33,34). Among asbestos workers, one death in five is owing to lung cancer, one of 10 to pleural or peritoneal mesotheliomas, and one of 10 to gastrointestinal carcinomas (28). The latent period is usually 20 years or more (28,33).

There are differences in carcinogenic potential of the various types of asbestos. Men exposed to chrysotile asbestos have a respiratory tract cancer mortality two to four times higher than controls, whereas those exposed to a combina-

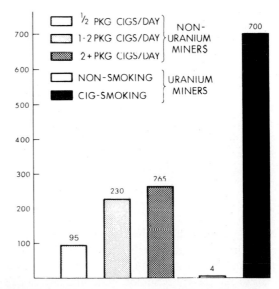

FIGURE 14.4. Lung cancer due to smoking and uranium exposure. (Adapted from Wright ES, Hammond EC. Radiation-induced carcinoma of the lung—the St. Lawrence tragedy. *J Thorac Cardiovasc Surg* 74:496, 1977.)

tion of chrysotile and crocidolite asbestos have a mortality rate 5.3 times higher than controls. For amosite asbestos, the death rate owing to respiratory cancer is more than 10 times higher than in controls.

Tobacco is a critical cofactor (4,5,7,28,34). Most cases of lung cancer in occupationally exposed workers occur in smokers with asbestosis, and the distribution of cell types is about the same as that of smokers (7). Lung cancer in asbestos-exposed nonsmokers is uncommon (7).

Asbestos exposure is more than an occupational hazard confined to such industries as shipbuilding and the manufacture and installation of brake lining and insulation (28,33). Asbestos fibers (ferruginous bodies) have been found in the lungs of 100% of city dwellers in France, and the atmosphere in New York City contains 10×10^{-9} g of asbestos per cubic meter of air, which corresponds to millions of submicroscopic fibrils (28). The significance of prolonged exposure to such concentrations of asbestos remains uncertain.

Other Occupational Factors

Workers engaged in the handling of chromates from chromium-containing iron ore have approximately a four to 15 times greater incidence of lung cancer than the general population (28). There is usually a long latent period, similar to the 20 years that commonly elapses between asbestos exposure and tumor occurrence (28). Nickel refinery workers were once noted to have a three- to five-fold increased lung cancer mortality and a 150-fold increased risk of nasal cancer. Nickel dust was the likely responsible carcinogen, although generally adopted changes in the refinery process made before World War II not only drastically reduced nickel dust levels but also reduced worker exposure to arsenic. Arsenic is a known carcinogen that has been implicated in the development of lung cancer in individuals given arsenic-containing drugs or engaged in the manufacture and use of pesticides.

The mining of hematite (an iron ore containing ferric oxide and silica) is associated with an increased risk of lung cancer (28). In addition, a number of other industrial operations in which exposure to iron and silica is common may be responsible for a poorly quantified but increased risk of lung cancer. These include metal grinding, sandblasting, and iron and steel foundry work.

Diet

Several epidemiologic studies have shown a relation between greater dietary intake of vegetables and modestly lower risk for lung and other cancers (4,5,35,36). Beta-carotene (a precursor to the class of retinoids, including retinol or vitamin A, which are found in many green, yellow, and orange fruits and vegetables) may be the substance associated with lower lung cancer risk (4,5,35). The protective effect is par-

ticularly evident in current or past cigarette smokers (5). A variety of studies in several countries have shown: (a) low dietary intake of these fruits and vegetables is associated with an increased lung cancer risk; and (b) a low serum level of beta-carotene is associated with risk for later development of lung cancer (Fig. 14.5) (5,35–37).

Three important prospective, randomized, controlled large-scale epidemiologic studies were performed recently to address whether supplemental beta-carotene and vitamin A might be useful as cancer chemopreventive agents (36,38,39). Unfortunately, none of these trials established that administration of either beta-carotene or vitamin A decreased mortality owing to lung cancer. In fact, in the study from Finland there was an unsuspected higher than expected mortality owing primarily to lung cancer and heart disease in a group receiving beta-carotene (38). Similarly, in the study by Omenn and colleagues, patients receiving both vitamin A and beta-carotene experienced a 17% increase in mortality and a 28% increase in the number of lung cancers compared with the placebo group (39). The study by Hennekins and colleagues evaluating the effects of beta-carotene revealed neither benefit nor harm in terms of malignancy or cardiovascular disease (36). Based on the findings of these three trials, the use of supplemental beta-carotene and vitamin A should be discouraged. Instead, a balanced dietary intake of fruits and vegetables, including those containing beta-carotene, should be encouraged.

Genetic Factors

A minority of heavy cigarette smokers (approximately one in eight) develops lung cancer, suggesting that other factors are important in determining risk (5). Family studies have shown repeatedly a slightly greater lung cancer risk, two- to threefold, in nonsmokers who are relatives of lung cancer patients, compared with nonsmokers who have no family history of lung cancer (40–43). Environmental factors are probably superimposed on genetic patterns that predispose to lung cancer (5). In fact, genetic factors may exert an influence on the development of lung cancer equal to that of cigarette smoking (26,44–47).

The genetically determined ability to metabolize carcinogens may have a direct role in lung cancer risk (5). One such inherited variant in xenobiotic metabolism is the aryl-hydrocarbon hydroxylase system (5). The inducible enzyme aryl hydrocarbon hydroxylase (AHH) converts the polycyclic hydrocarbons of cigarette smoke into epoxides, compounds that are highly carcinogenic (5,29,44,45). The inducibility of AHH by polycyclic hydrocarbons appears to be controlled by a single gene. The degree of inducibility of this enzyme in lymphocytes from patients with and without lung cancer not only has been correlated with the presence or absence of lung cancer, but also with cigarette smoking, independent of the presence of lung cancer (48).

Moreover, several genetic changes have been associated

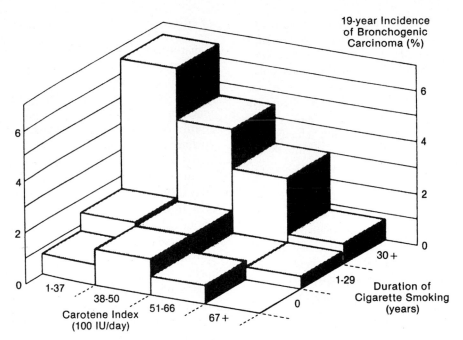

FIGURE 14.5. Association of an index of dietary beta-carotene and the duration of cigarette smoking with the 19-year index of cigarette smoking in the Western Electric study. Dietary index was based on questionnaires about food intake during the previous 28 days given to 2100 men aged 40 to 55 years at examinations separated by 1 year. Intake of preformed retinol (vitamin A) and other nutrients was not significantly associated with lung cancer risk. (From Shekelle RB, Liu S, Raynor WJ, et al. Dietary vitamin A and risk of cancer in the Western Electric Study. *Lancet* 2:1185–1190, 1981; with permission.)

with small cell and non-small cell carcinomas of the lung (5,7,46,47). These include loss of DNA sequences on the short arm of chromosome 3 (3p) or 11 (11p) and amplification of a number of oncogenes (tumor-promoting genes), including the *myc* family (C-*myc*, N-*myc*, L-*myc*) and the *ras* family (K-*ras*, H-*ras*, N-*ras*). Such genetic markers, it should be emphasized, are not necessarily heritable and may represent markers for the effects of carcinogens such as those in tobacco (5).

It is likely, therefore, that the etiology of lung cancer is multifactorial, involving far more than a simple association with smoking. Undoubtedly, other environmental carcinogens have additive, even synergistic, effects, and certain genetic characteristics probably increase susceptibility to these environmental carcinogens (21,43,46,47,49).

PATHOLOGY

Bronchogenic Carcinoma

Classification

A committee of pathologists convened by the World Health Organization (WHO) established the standard classification system for lung cancer (50,51). As new data become available on the natural history of treated and untreated lung cancer, this comprehensive system continues to be updated (7,50–65). According to this classification, the four major cell types of lung cancer and their approximate relative incidence include adenocarcinoma (31% to 34%), squamous cell carcinoma (30%), small cell carcinoma (20% to 25%), and large cell carcinoma (10% to 16%). Bronchioloalveolar carcinomas (so-called alveolar cell carcinomas) are considered adenocarcinomas; as a group, they comprise approximately 3% to 4% of all lung carcinomas (53,54).

Pathogenesis

Squamous cell bronchogenic carcinomas arise most commonly in segmental and subsegmental bronchi in response to repetitive carcinogenic stimuli, inflammation, or irritation (57). The mucosal lining is most susceptible to injury, particularly at the bifurcation of bronchial structures. Ciliary mechanisms and superficial columnar lining cells tend to shed or become denuded, a process abetted by the physiologically altered air flow and reduced mucus flow rates at these sites. Carcinogenic agents are more likely to be deposited, absorbed, and retained in these zones. Basal (reserve) cells are stimulated to proliferate.

Hyperplasia of mucin-secreting columnar epithelial cells is followed, in some cases, by replacement of the bronchial lining by an orderly arrangement of metaplastic, stratified squamous epithelium. Metaplasia is a response to injury by either carcinogenic or noncarcinogenic agents. In the course of carcinogenesis, the basal half of the metaplastic epithelium may become disorganized. Cells lose their usual polarity and individual cells develop atypical, irregular, hyperchromatic nuclei. Abnormal mitoses may be identified, whereas the superficial layers of the mucosa retain a stratified, flattened, but unified pattern. These changes are termed atypical metaplasia or dysplasia (60). Eventually, the entire thickness of the mucosa may be replaced by proliferating neoplastic cells (carcinoma *in situ*).

Infiltrating neoplasms may develop at some unpredictable future time when the integrity of the basal membrane has been lost. This mechanism pertains particularly to bronchial squamous cell malignancies in experimental animals as well as humans. Factors associated with these changes include smoking and occupational exposure to arsenic, uranium, chromium, asbestos, or other minerals (5,11). The pathogenesis of small cell carcinoma is not as well understood, but this tumor may also originate in the basal cells of the bronchial epithelium.

Multiple exogenous and endogenous factors are associated with adenocarcinomas, which probably arise from the mucin-secreting cells in the more peripheral bronchi. Among the exogenous factors are tobacco smoke, asbestos, cadmium, chromium, beryllium, and pneumoconiotic dusts. Endogenous conditions include chronic interstitial pneumonitis and fibrosis and progressive systemic sclerosis (scleroderma).

Histology

Squamous Cell Carcinoma

Squamous cell carcinoma is the second most common bronchogenic carcinoma (Figs. 5.23, 14.6, and 14.7) (7,50,51, 57,60). These tumors are composed predominantly of flattened or polygonal neoplastic epithelial cells that tend to stratify, form intercellular bridges, and elaborate keratin on an individual cell basis or in the complex of an epithelial pearl. Based on the degree of differentiation, these tumors are divided into three subtypes: well-differentiated, moderately differentiated, and poorly differentiated. They usually arise from the mucosa of large bronchi and are frequently associated with adjoining foci of intraepithelial malignancy or dysplasia. In about two-thirds of cases, they present as a proximal or hilar lesion, and it is uncommon for them to metastasize early (7). The tumors tend to be bulky, to encroach on bronchial lumen, with the production of obstructing intraluminal granular or polypoid masses, and to invade cartilage and adjoining lymph nodes. One-half of differentiated squamous cell lung carcinomas are confined to the thorax at autopsy (62). Gail et al. found squamous cell carcinomas to have the most favorable prognosis of the non-small cell carcinomas (58).

Small Cell Carcinoma

Small cell carcinomas have been divided by WHO into two groups: pure small cell and combined (Fig. 14.8) (51,63). Histologic variants include oat cell (lymphocyte-like) carci-

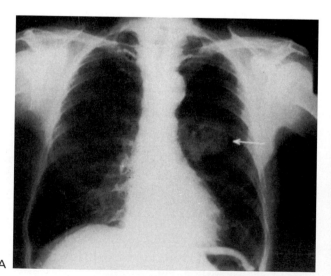
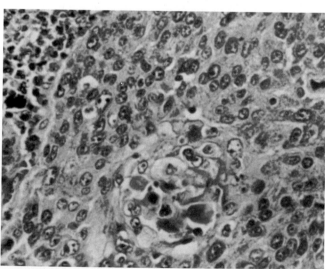

FIGURE 14.6. **A,** Squamous cell carcinoma. A posterior-anterior (PA) chest radiograph shows a 3-cm mass adjacent to the left hilum *(arrow).* **B,** Squamous cell carcinoma histology. Squamous cell carcinomas are characterized by the presence of keratin in the cytoplasm of the malignant cell. The malignant cells are frequently connected by an extensive series of intercellular bridges and may form small "pearls" in which the squamous cells are arranged in small groups. In this figure, the cells at the periphery do not show differentiation, but the central portion contains some cells with markedly hyperchromatic nuclei and keratinized cytoplasm characteristic of squamous cell carcinoma.

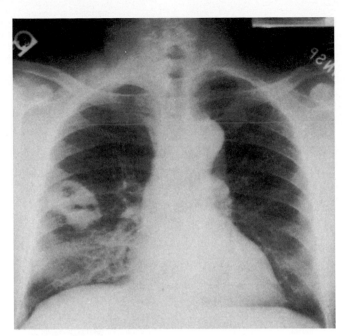

FIGURE 14.7. Squamous cell carcinoma. PA chest radiograph shows a large cavitating peripheral squamous cell carcinoma in the right hemithorax.

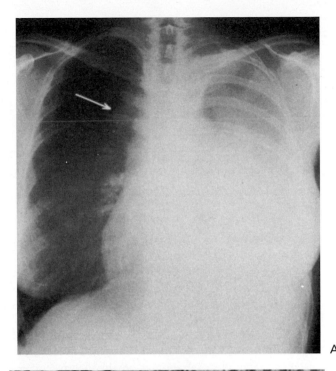

A

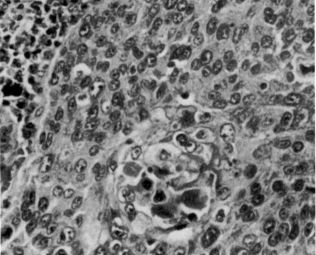

B

noma, which is composed of cells with round-to-oval nuclei. The nucleoli are always indistinct, and the cytoplasm is scanty. The intermediate (polygonal) variant is the most common and is characterized by cells with somewhat larger, fusiform or spindled nuclei. Nuclear chromatin has a dense but even distribution, and nucleoli are usually absent and always indistinct. Cytoplasm is minimal. In the combined type, small cell carcinoma is combined with a non-small cell type—large cell, squamous cell or adenocarcinoma. The most important combined variant is the small cell plus large cell variant (64,65).

Although 75% to 80% of the small cell carcinomas present as proximal lesions, they may arise in any part of the tracheobronchial tree; they tend to lift the mucosa slightly to form a velvety, thickened lining, rapidly invade vascular channels, mediastinal lymph nodes, and soft tissue, and disseminate widely, often before pulmonary symptoms are recognized or provoked. In contrast to squamous cell carcinoma, the lumen is usually not filled with tumor but is compressed externally through the submucosa and by hilar lymph node spread.

Small cell carcinoma is extrathoracic when discovered in 70% of cases, with little chance of 5-year survival (7). When limited to the thoracic cavity, small cell carcinoma has a complete response to chemotherapy and radiation therapy in more than half the cases with approximately 30% of these remissions sustained beyond 2 years. The most common sites of metastatic involvement at initial presentation are listed in Table 14.2 (66).

FIGURE 14.8. **A,** Small cell carcinoma. PA chest radiograph showing a large left pleural effusion opacifying the left hemithorax. Note the mediastinal adenopathy manifested on the chest radiograph by a density in the right paratracheal area *(arrow).* Pleural fluid analysis revealed malignant cells, and bronchoscopy revealed a large endobronchial mass identified as small cell carcinoma on biopsy. **B,** Histology of small cell carcinoma. The nucleus of small cell carcinoma is different from that of other types of lung cancer. It is characterized by the relatively even distribution of chromatin throughout the nucleus. There is no clearing of the chromatin, and nucleoli are never prominent. The cytoplasm of the cell varies from the small rim of cytoplasm seen in the oat cell variant (shown in this photomicrograph) to a moderate amount of eosinophilic cytoplasm seen in the polygonal variant. The subtyping of various types of small cell carcinoma has been shown to have a profound effect on prognosis or response to therapy.

TABLE 14.2. SITES OF METASTASES IN PATIENTS PRESENTING WITH SMALL CELL LUNG CANCER

Site	Percentage
Bone	35
Liver	25
Bone marrow	20
Brain	10
Extrathoracic lymph nodes	5
Subcutaneous masses	5

Source: Johnson BE. Management of small cell lung cancer. *Clin Chest Med* 1993;14:173–187, with permission.

Adenocarcinoma

Adenocarcinoma, the most prevalent carcinoma of the lung in both sexes, forms acinar or glandular structures (Fig. 14.9) (7,51,55–57,60). Histologically, this tumor is divided broadly into well-differentiated, moderately well-differentiated, poorly differentiated, and bronchioloalveolar types.

Fifty-five to sixty percent of adenocarcinomas are limited to the periphery of lung, not obviously related to any bronchus. Peripheral adenocarcinomas are frequently circumscribed and subpleural with central pigmented fibrotic cores. Classic bronchioloalveolar carcinomas, whether single, multicentric, or lobar in type, tend to use existing alveolar septa as a framework for their growth and are not scar-associated.

The liver, adrenals, bone, and central nervous system (CNS) are frequent sites of metastases (7). In over half the cases studied at autopsy the brain is involved, and in 12% the brain is the sole site of metastasis (67).

Large Cell Carcinoma

Large cell carcinoma, also called undifferentiated carcinoma, includes all tumors that show no evidence of differentiation to small cell, squamous cell, or adenocarcinoma (Fig. 14.10) (7,57,60). In general, these tumors are composed of pleomorphic cells with variably enlarged nuclei and prominent nucleoli with abundant cytoplasm. The tumors tend to form large, bulky, somewhat circumscribed and necrotic masses, are frequently subpleural in origin, invade locally, and disseminate widely. About 60% are limited to the periphery of the lung. The metastatic pattern of large cell carcinoma is similar to that of the adenocarcinomas, with cerebral metastases in over half the cases (7).

The giant cell variant of large cell carcinoma is composed of huge, multinucleated, bizarre cells that are frequently associated with an extensive inflammatory cell infiltrate (7). These tumors are usually large and peripheral, aggressive, and most often found at a late stage, but are amenable to surgical cure when resected in stage I or II (68). They show an ability to metastasize widely, curiously with a predilection for the small intestine (7,69).

Other Pulmonary Neoplasms

Carcinoid Tumor (Bronchial Adenoma)

Bronchopulmonary carcinoid tumors constitute 1% to 4% of all primary lung neoplasms (70). These highly vascularized lesions arise in submucosal glands in the bronchial wall, grow slowly, invade locally, and occasionally metastasize to the lymph nodes, mediastinum, vertebra, and liver (7,71). The red or pink carcinoid appears as a polypoid or

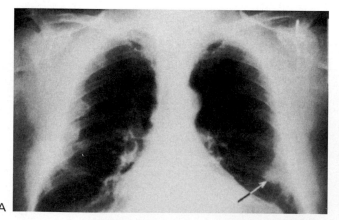

A

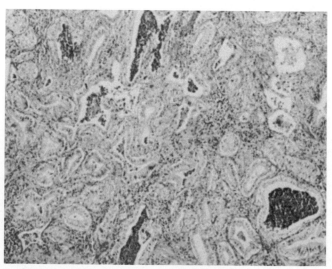

B

FIGURE 14.9. A, Adenocarcinoma. PA chest radiograph shows a 1.5-cm solitary lesion in the lingula *(arrow)*. Note also rib fractures in the right hemithorax, a finding due to previous trauma. **B,** Histology of adenocarcinoma. Adenocarcinomas of the lung are characterized by gland formation in a fibrous background. Numerous glands are formed in this well-differentiated adenocarcinoma.

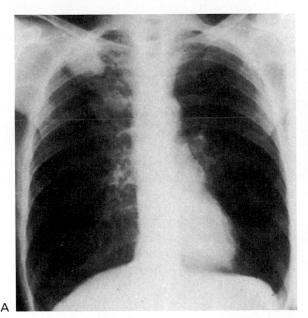
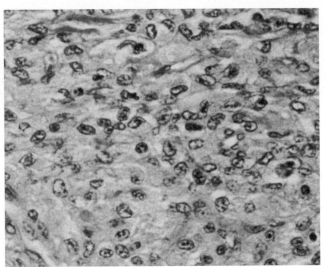

A

B

FIGURE 14.10. A, Large cell carcinoma. PA chest radiograph shows a right apical density adjacent to the pleura and chest wall and a proximal density adjacent to the right tracheal wall. **B,** Histology of large cell carcinoma. The cells of a large cell undifferentiated carcinoma are characterized by a moderate amount of cytoplasm, nuclei that are usually oval or round with some chromatin clearing, and the presence of one or several nucleoli, which may be markedly irregular in shape. These cells contain neither keratin nor mucin.

sessile mass protruding from the bronchial wall and is covered by intact bronchial mucosa. Of these lesions, 90% of typical carcinoids are located in a major or segmental bronchus, and about 10% present as peripheral lesions. Carcinoids are composed of small uniform cuboidal cells with fine granular homogeneous cytoplasm. The nuclei are round or oval and deeply staining and are usually in the center of the cell. Little pleomorphism is seen, and mitoses and necrosis are absent. Neuroendocrine markers—chromogranin, syntoptophysin, or hormones are demonstrable by immunohistochemistry and dense core granules are evident ultrastructurally.

Carcinoids occur slightly more frequently in women (71). Most patients are in their thirties and have had symptoms for over 5 years prior to diagnosis. Signs and symptoms are secondary to bronchial obstruction or the extreme vascularity of the tumor. Hemoptysis occurs in one-third of patients, but signs and symptoms of pulmonary infection behind the obstructed bronchus are more frequently noted (72). Occasionally, a patient is asymptomatic and the tumor is discovered after routine radiography of the chest.

Three types of chest radiographic abnormalities are seen in patients with carcinoid tumor (71). Most frequently there is a pneumonia or the sequela of such an infection, with poor bronchial drainage. A smooth, rounded hilar mass may be present, or rarely, a peripheral nodule is seen.

The diagnosis is usually made on the basis of the history of frequent hemoptysis or repeated bouts of pneumonia and observation of the characteristic tumor by bronchoscopy. Biopsy is usually inadvisable because of the possibility of severe hemorrhage. Also, it may be difficult to make a definite histologic diagnosis from the small pieces of tissue obtained by bronchial biopsy. Cytologic study of sputum or bronchial washings is usually not diagnostic, because the mucous membrane over the tumor is usually intact. Operative removal is indicated, because this is the only means of preventing the severe hemoptysis and infection that can accompany these tumors. Moreover, early removal may prevent the late metastatic spread that occurs in a few instances (71). The 5-year survival rate after resection is over 90% (7).

Atypical Carcinoid Tumors

In 1972, Arrigoni and coworkers described an atypical carcinoid tumor that accounted for most but not all of the mortality of pulmonary carcinoids (73). Half of these lesions were large and peripherally located. Histologically, they are carcinoids with necrosis, numerous mitotic figures, and more anaplastic nuclei of the large cell type (73–75). A 41% survival rate has been reported (7). Travis et al. have divided the atypical carcinoids into low grade, which they call atypical carcinoid, and high-grade, which they refer to as large cell neuroendocrine carcinoma (LCNEC) (76). The 5-year survival of LCNEC is poor.

Bronchial Tumors of the Salivary Gland Type

Neoplasms that are similar to those of the major and minor salivary glands infrequently arise in bronchial submucosal glands. These include mucoepidermoid carcinoma, adenoid cystic carcinoma, and pleomorphic adenomas (77–79). All present as endobronchial or endotracheal masses. The mucoepidermoid carcinomas are divided into high- and low-grade, according to both size and histology. High-grade mucoepidermoid carcinomas are larger and more invasive with both epidermoid glandular and intermediate cell elements that have more anaplastic nuclei, numerous mitotic figures, and foci of necrosis. Treatment is resection; survival is good for low-grade but not as good for high-grade lesions (80). Adenoid cystic carcinomas are composed of cells that form a characteristic cylindromatous pattern of regular glands (77). Resection is the preferred treatment, if possible, and 5-year survival is good (85%), lower at 10 years (55%), and poor at 20 years (20%) (70,77,81).

Papillomas of the Bronchus

Papillomas are exceedingly rare lung tumors that are often associated with generalized papillomatosis of the upper respiratory tract (71). They are usually wart-like growths and have a well-developed connective tissue stroma (82). Bronchial papillomas in adults are often solitary growths but may be associated with papillomas elsewhere in the bronchial tree (83,84). Approximately 50% of the solitary adult tumors become malignant (84). They are associated with human papilloma virus immunohistochemically demonstrated in these tumors (82,85).

Sclerosing Hemangioma

In 1956, Liebow and Hubbell described a lesion of the periphery of the lung, often found in women and at a younger age than is usual for adenocarcinoma (86). Because of the strikingly vascular pattern associated with the lesion, it was named a sclerosing hemangioma. Grossly, the lesions are usually sharply circumscribed and present a hemorrhagic appearance.

Microscopically, there are three distinct patterns, which include the vascular pattern with numerous small and large spaces filled with red blood cells, a papillary pattern, and a solid pattern. The cells making up the lesion are large, with centrally placed nuclei which often contain small nucleoli. Although the lesion is quite cellular, mitotic figures are rarely, if ever, seen. The mingling of patterns, cellularity, and vascularity may suggest a diagnosis of malignancy, especially adenocarcinoma. The histogenesis of the lesion was debated primarily because of the original designation as a hemangioma. Electron microscopic studies showed the cells lining the blood filled space to be type II pneumocytes (87). Subsequently, immunohistochemical studies have con-

firmed their epithelial nature (88,89). Although it is unusual, it is important to recognize this lesion because it has a benign course, distinctly different from the much more common adenocarcinoma, which it mimics.

Alveolar Adenoma

In 1986, Yousem and Hochholzer described six cases of an alveolar adenoma (90). These presented as solitary nodules in basically asymptomatic patients, were resected by wedge biopsy or lobectomy, and all of the patients did well. Grossly, the lesions were strikingly well circumscribed. Histologically, they were composed of proliferating alveolar pneumocytes, far less cellular than those seen in the sclerosing hemangioma, and were accompanied by an interstitial spindle cell component of benign appearing stromal cells.

Intravascular Bronchioloalveolar Tumor

In 1983, Dail and Liebow described a lesion with the name intravascular bronchioloalveolar tumor (91). This lesion occurs predominantly in women, with an age range of 12 to 60. Most patients present with cough, dyspnea, and chest pain. On chest radiograph, multiple peripheral, usually bilateral pulmonary nodules, measuring up to 3 cm in diameter are seen. Grossly, the lesions are circumscribed and often multiple, even in a small wedge biopsy. Microscopically, the polygonal tumor cells are characterized by nuclei with an evenly dispersed chromatin pattern and rare mitotic figures. They are often found in a slightly basophilic matrix, apparently filling the alveolar spaces in a polypoid fashion. Despite the epithelial appearance of the cells, it has been shown both ultrastructurally and immunohistochemically that the lesion is endothelial in character. Corrin et al. described the presence of Weibel-Palade Bodies characteristic of endothelial cells and several studies have immunohistochemically demonstrated the presence of factor VIII-related antigen (92). Its appearance is similar to that of the histiocytoid hemangioma, or epithelioid hemangioendothelioma, another vascular lesion that may be mistaken for carcinoma. The clinical course is one of slow progression with a 40% mortality rate overall.

Mesodermal Tumors of the Bronchi and Lung

Mesodermal tumors of the lung as a group are rare and account for a small percentage of all pulmonary neoplasms (71). The following is a classification of these neoplasms (93).

1. *Benign parenchyma tumors:* hamartomas
2. *Benign intrabronchial tumors:* chondroma, osteochondroma, lipoma, leiomyoma
3. *Malignant intrabronchial tumors:* fibrosarcoma, leiomyosarcoma
4. *Malignant parenchyma tumors:* sarcomas, lymphomas

Hamartoma

Hamartomas are the most common benign tumors of the lung (70). They are composed of disorganized elements of tissue normally present in the lung (71,84,94). The term hamartoma is applied inappropriately to an interstitial mesenchymal tumor composed primarily of cartilage with focal ossification in some cases. Septae of connective tissue extend from the periphery to the central portion of the nodule, near the edge of which bronchial or alveolar epithelium is entrapped. No capsule is present, and the tumor does not invade the surrounding tissue. The cartilage found within the tumor is not related to the cartilage found normally in bronchi, but 8% to 10% of the lesions arise within a major or segmental bronchus; the remainder are found in the periphery of the lung.

Most hamartomas are discovered on routine chest radiography (71). Characteristically, the lesion is round, has sharply defined margins, and varies in size from a few millimeters to 4 to 5 cm in diameter. As it grows, it may become lobulated. On chest radiograph, it is most likely to be confused with a tuberculoma or metastatic lesion from elsewhere in the body. Calcification is evident on chest radiograph in 10% and appears as small flecks throughout the lesion rather than in a ring form (70).

Definite diagnosis can be made only by histologic examination of the lesion (94–96). Adequate tissue can be obtained through the bronchoscope or by transthoracic needle biopsy; however, often thoracotomy is required. The lesion does not start to grow and become large enough to be seen on radiographs until later in life.

Histologic confirmation is necessary to eliminate the possibility of a malignant lesion. Simple excision of the lesion is adequate, but follow-up has been undertaken in small, slowly growing, well-documented hamartomas.

Chondroma and Osteochondroma

Chondromas and osteochondromas are very rare neoplasms that arise in the trachea or a major bronchus in association with normal cartilaginous rings (71,97,98). They are usually slow growing but may reach great size and cause obstruction and destruction of the pulmonary parenchyma. Histologically, they differ from hamartoma in containing only cartilage. If extensive lung destruction distal to the tumor has occurred, pulmonary resection is indicated.

Lipoma

Lipomas originate from fatty tissue normally present in fibrous tissue external to cartilaginous plates and to a lesser extent in connective tissue and muscular layers of the bronchi (71,99,100). They occur more frequently in men than women, usually in the fifth or sixth decade of life and are more common in the left bronchial tree (99,100). They present as soft, smooth, often lobulated masses. Removal of the tumor can usually be accomplished through the straight-tube bronchoscope with satisfactory results, unless bronchial obstruction has produced destruction of lung tissue.

Leiomyoma

Nearly all of the smooth muscle tumors in the lung are well-differentiated metastases from leiomyosarcomas of the uterus. Primary leiomyoma is extremely rare (101–103). In one series of 14 cases, 12 were in women. This tumor probably arises from the smooth muscle of the interstitium and is composed of bands of amitotic smooth muscle cells. Surgical removal is the treatment of choice.

Sarcomas

Sarcomas in the lung show the spectrum of histologies seen in malignant tumors of soft tissue from which they are more often metastatic than primary in the lung. Two sarcomas, malignant fibrous histiocytoma and leiomyosarcoma, are mentioned briefly here. As in soft tissue, the most common sarcoma is malignant fibrous histiocytoma. On histologic examination, this tumor is composed of elongated spindle-shaped malignant cells, many of which are arranged in bands (104–106). A variable component of histiocytes is present. The tumor is relatively slow growing and metastasizes late. If complete removal of the primary tumor can be accomplished surgically, the prognosis is good (105–107).

In a study of 20 patients with pulmonary leiomyosarcoma, the age at presentation varied from 4 to 83 years, with 11 patients over 40 (108). Signs and symptoms of bronchial obstruction had been present from 1 month to 3½ years. Most of the tumors were encapsulated and on cut surface had a gray or white surface. Histologically, leiomyosarcomas are composed of spingle-shaped cells with elongated nuclei and abundant cytoplasm with myofibrils. Mitotic figures are frequent. Five of the patients had metastases at the time the cases were reported. Of the 11 patients in whom the tumor was resected, nine were alive and well 6 years after operation. Radiation therapy in two patients had no effect on their disease (103).

Lymphoma

Most lymphomas occur in several sites and secondary pulmonary involvement is a frequent finding (71). Lymphomas primary in the lung include the so-called lymphomatoid granulomatosis (LYG) and low-grade lymphomas of bronchial mucosa associated lymphoid tissue (Baltomas) of B cell type (109,110). LYG occurs over a broad age range, presents with cough, fever, and shortness of breath, and may also involve skin, CNS sinuses, and peripheral nerves. Lymph node involvement is unusual. Radiographically, it presents with multiple often cavitary nodules. Histologically, it is characterized by necrosis secondary to vascular invasion and destruction by abnormal lymphocytes. LYG has been separated into three grades according to increasing numbers of malignant lymphocytes which mark as both clonal B cells with evidence of Epstein-Barr virus and a larger number of non-clonal T-lymphocytes, although some histologically and clinically similar cases mark as clonal T cells. Outcome is generally poor (111).

Baltomas are often found radiographically in asymptomatic patients, although symptomatic patients may present with cough, fever, and shortness of breath. Most cases (70%) present as solitary masses and are localized to the lung without nodal involvement, but multiple pulmonary nodules may be present. Histologically, there are sheets of small round lymphocytes that may be admixed with plasma cells and germinal centers with features of the previously diagnosed pseudolymphoma. The B cells are monoclonal and lack CD-5 and CD-10 staining, and do not show BCL-1 gene rearrangement. The 5-year survival is excellent, with or without chemotherapy, but progression to higher-grade lymphoma has been observed.

Large cell lymphomas also occur primarily in the lung but are more often secondary to lymph node-based lymphomas. Lymphomas in the setting of transplant patients are often associated with Epstein-Barr virus residues.

CLINICAL MANIFESTATIONS

Symptoms and Signs

Approximately 5% of patients with lung cancer are asymptomatic, and the tumor is discovered on routine radiographic examination of the chest (112). Other patients have one or more symptoms and signs related to the presence of the tumor, although the symptomatology may not be specific to lung cancer. Shields and Ritts have divided these symptoms and signs into the following categories: bronchopulmonary, extrapulmonary intrathoracic, extrathoracic metastatic, and extrathoracic nonmetastatic (112). Presence of symptoms is a less favorable prognostic sign. Shimizu and colleagues reported a 5-year survival of only 25% among patients with lung cancer who presented with symptoms, contrasted with 56% for asymptomatic patients detected by screening (113).

Bronchopulmonary Symptoms

Cough is the most common symptom in patients with lung cancer, present in between 45% and 75% of patients (114). Irritation of the bronchus induces the cough, which may be productive or nonproductive and is frequently described by the patient as being a "cigarette cough." Ulceration of the tumor results in hemoptysis, which most often presents as episodic blood streaking of the sputum. Hemoptysis occurs in approximately 60% of patients; massive hemoptysis is rare (112,114). Airway obstruction, complete or partial, may lead to wheezing, dyspnea, and occasionally, stridor. The obstruction may lead to atelectasis with infection of the distal pulmonary parenchyma. The inflammatory process, obstructive pneumonitis, or abscess formation leads to febrile respiratory symptoms, which may be present in as many as one-third of patients (112). Unfortunately, the febrile episode may be misinterpreted by the physician, because it may be ameliorated by antibiotic therapy and thus lead to delay in diagnosis.

Vague chest pains, often described as a dull ache, occur in up to 50% of patients (112,114). This chest pain may be caused by inflammatory involvement of the parietal pleura and chest wall.

Extrapulmonary Intrathoracic Symptoms and Signs

Approximately 15% of patients complain of symptoms caused by growth of the tumor outside the lung into the pleura, chest wall, mediastinal structures, and contiguous nerves (112). Hoarseness, owing to involvement of the left or rarely the right recurrent laryngeal nerve, and the superior vena caval syndrome both occur in approximately 5% of patients with carcinoma of the lung (112). The latter syndrome is owing to compression or invasion of the superior vena cava by neoplastic tissue from related lymph nodes or is sometimes owing to direct invasion by a primary growth in the right upper lobe. A sensation of fullness in the head and dyspnea are the most frequent presenting features. Cough, pain, and dysphagia occur less often (115). Physical signs include dilated neck veins, a prominent venous pattern on the anterior chest wall, upper-extremity and facial edema, and a plethoric appearance (114).

Pleural effusion of varying amounts occurs in 7% to 10% of patients, and most commonly indicates obstruction to pulmonary lymph flow or metastatic involvement of the pleura (112,114,116).

Partial obstruction of the esophagus by tumor in paraesophageal lymph nodes causes dysphagia in approximately 1% of patients with lung cancer, as does massive pleural effusion from metastatic involvement of the pleura (112). Malignant pleural effusions may be serous, serosanguineous, or grossly bloody in appearance and are more common in patients with adenocarcinoma (114,117). Involvement of the branches of the brachial plexus from tumors located in the superior sulcus can cause pain and weakness of the arm and shoulder. Horner's syndrome also may be present in the latter situation (112).

Extrathoracic Metastatic Symptoms and Signs

Symptoms caused by metastatic spread of the tumor outside the thorax account for a small percentage of the presenting complaints of lung carcinoma patients (112). By histologic type, small cell lung carcinoma has the highest propensity for involvement of the central nervous system and squamous cell carcinoma has the least (118). Neurologic abnormalities caused by intracranial metastases are present in 3% to 6%. These include hemiplegia, epilepsy, personality changes, confusion, speech defects, or only headache. Bone pain and pathologic fracture from metastatic involvement are noted on presentation in 1% to 2% (112). Rarely, jaundice, ascites, or an abdominal mass is a major complaint. Neck, muscle, or subcutaneous tissue masses are present infrequently.

Extrathoracic Nonmetastatic Manifestations (Paraneoplastic Syndromes)

Approximately 2% of patients with bronchial carcinoma seek medical advice for systemic symptoms and signs not related to metastatic spread of the tumor, the so-called paraneoplastic syndromes (Table 14.3) (7,112,114,119,120). These manifestations are not specific, and they may occur in association with malignant lesions other than bronchogenic carcinoma. In the following section, we emphasize several of the most common syndromes.

Metabolic Manifestations

The majority of metabolic manifestations are the result of secretion of endocrine or endocrine-like substances by the tumor. At times, these syndromes may be produced by tumors that are still resectable, and treatment of the primary tumor may result in complete or partial remission of the paraneoplastic syndrome. Most of the syndromes are found in association with small cell carcinoma (66,112,114,121).

Cushing's Syndrome

Approximately 50% of patients with paraneoplastic Cushing's syndrome have bronchogenic carcinoma, with small cell lung cancer and bronchial carcinoid being the most commonly associated tumor types (122). In patients with lung carcinoma, this syndrome differs from the classic syndrome (112,121). In small cell carcinoma patients, for instance, it is characterized by reversal of the sex ratio, an older age incidence, the prominence of hypokalemic alkalosis, fewer physical stigmata of typical Cushing's syndrome, and a more rapid, fulminating course. This syndrome is clinically apparent in approximately 2% to 5% of patients with small cell carcinoma (66,114). Adrenocorticotropic hormone (ACTH) has been demonstrated in the tumor tissue and blood of many of these patients. This ectopic ACTH is indistinguishable from the normal hormone, although the tumors have physiologic autonomy, since dexamethasone fails to suppress the levels of ACTH end products in the urine. Excessive quantities of hydroxycorticosteroids (17-OHCS) are demonstrable in the urine. Treating the carcinoma is the most important therapy for patients with ectopic ACTH production.

TABLE 14.3. CLASSIFICATION OF EXTRAPULMONARY MANIFESTATIONS OF CARCINOMA OF THE LUNG

Endocrine and metabolic
  Carcinoid syndrome
  Cachexia
  Antidiuretic hormone secretion
  Hypercalcemia
  Ectopic adrenocorticotropic hormone secretion
  Ectopic gonadotropic stimulating hormone secretion
  Gynecomastia
  Insulinlike activity
Neuromuscular
  Hoarseness
  Horner's syndrome
  Seizures
  Cranial nerve abnormalities
  Carcinomatous myopathy
  Peripheral neuropathies
  Eaton-Lambert syndrome
  Cortical-cerebellar degeneration
  Encephalomyelopathy
  Autonomic overactivity
  Dementia, psychosis
Skeletal
  Clubbing
  Pulmonary hypertrophic osteoarthropathy
  Monarticular arthritis
Dermatologic
  Acanthosis nigricans
  Scleroderma
  Dermatomyositis, polymyositis
Cardiovascular
  Migratory thrombophlebitis
  Nonbacterial verrucous endocarditis
  Arterial thrombosis
Hematologic
  Anemia
  Thrombocytosis
  Red cell aplasia
  Fibrinolytic purpura
  Nonspecific leukocytosis
  Polycythemia
  Gastrointestinal
  Jaundice
  Abnormal liver function tests
Renal
  Proteinuria
  Nephrotic syndrome

Antidiuretic Hormone

The syndrome of inappropriate antidiuretic hormone secretion (SIADH) with excessive antidiuretic hormone secretion is associated with symptoms of water intoxication—anorexia, nausea, and vomiting accompanied by increasingly severe neurologic complications (121–125). SIADH is characterized by hyponatremia (serum sodium concentration less than 135 mmol/L), hyposmolality (plasma osmolality less than 275 mOsm/kg), and impaired water excretion in the absence of hypovolemia, hypotension, ineffective intravascular volume, or abnormalities of cardiac, renal, thyroid, and adrenal function (114,123). Small cell lung cancer is estimated to account for more than 75% of all tumors associated with SIADH (124,125). Treating the carcinoma is the most important therapy for patients with paraneoplastic SIADH (125). Fluid restriction (less than 800 mL/day) to produce a negative water balance usually causes a modest rise in serum sodium (114,125,126). If hyponatremia persists, chronic daily furosemide with sodium chloride tablets, urea, mannitol, or glycerol has been used in outpatients with variable success.

Carcinoid Syndrome

Carcinoid syndrome is a well-defined clinical entity characterized by cutaneous, cardiovascular, gastrointestinal, and respiratory manifestations (7,112). Neurosecretory granules have been described in small cell tumors that are similar to those seen in carcinoid tumors and thought to be the source of this and other materials (127). Classically, the syndrome includes episodic signs and symptoms related to the release of various vasoactive amines. Flushing or edema, or both, of the face and upper body, hyperperistalsis and diarrhea, tachycardia, wheezing, pruritus, paresthesia, and vasomotor collapse may occur in varying combinations. Many vasoactive substances in addition to serotonin (5-hydroxytryptamine), which was originally thought to be the cause of the clinical features, have been shown to be produced by these tumors. These include 5-hydroxytryptophan, bradykinin and its precursor enzyme kallikrein, and various catecholamines (112).

Treatment of the manifestations of the carcinoid syndrome, which is usually identified with small cell carcinoma, is only palliative. In addition to irradiation and cytotoxic chemotherapy, corticosteroids, phenothiazines, antihistamines, and kallikrein inhibitors have been used in the management of flushing, with varying degrees of success (112).

Hypercalcemia

Hypercalcemia may be caused by bony metastases (20% of cases) or excessive secretion by the tumor of parathyroid hormone-related protein (PTHRP), so-called humoral hypercalcemia of malignancy (80% of cases) (128,129). An accompanying hypophosphatemia is found frequently. Most of the lung tumors associated with hypercalcemia have been squamous cell in type (7,112,128–131). Clinically, the hypercalcemic patient may have somnolence and mental changes as well as anorexia, nausea, vomiting, and weight loss. In resectable cases, removal of the tumor has resulted in calcium blood levels returning to normal. Among treatments used to control hypercalcemia in patients with lung cancer are saline diuresis, calcitonin, plicamycin, etidronate, pamidronate, and gallium nitrate (128,129).

Ectopic Gonadotropin

Ectopic gonadotropin production has been found rarely in association with carcinoma of the lung. Most of these tumors have been large cell carcinomas. Usually, the patient is a man with tender gynecomastia, often with hypertrophic osteoarthropathy, in whom production of gonadotropin has been documented (112,121).

Hypoglycemia

Hypoglycemia, the result of increased insulin or insulin-like activity, has been described in association with squamous cell carcinoma and may be relieved after resection of the tumor (132).

Neuromuscular Manifestations

Carcinomatous neuromyopathies are the most frequent extrathoracic, nonmetastatic manifestations of carcinoma of the lung, occurring in approximately 15% of these patients (112,129). In one combined series of patients with such manifestations, 56% had small cell carcinoma, 22% squamous cell carcinoma, 16% large cell tumors, and 5% adenocarcinoma (133). Half of the patients had no other symptoms of the lung tumor, and in one-third, the neuromyopathy preceded by 1 year or more the symptoms or the diagnosis of the carcinoma (112). Thus, neuromyopathic complications are not related to metastases, and their pathogenesis is uncertain. The following main varieties occur (114,129).

1. *Mental abnormalities.* Progressive dementia, sometimes with depression, is the most common manifestation. Confusion, stupor, or emotional instability may occur.
2. *Cerebellar degeneration.* This is manifested by ataxia, vertigo, and dysarthria.
3. *Sensory neuropathy.* This often starts with numbness and sometimes pain in the face and limbs, gradually progressing to loss of all forms of sensibility throughout the body, loss of reflexes, and occasionally deafness.
4. *Motor neuropathy.* This is manifested by progressive wasting, weakness, and fasciculation.
5. *Polyneuritis.* This is associated with mixed motor and sensory changes.
6. *Myopathy.* This is manifested by atrophic pareses, especially of the muscles of the limb girdles and the proximal limbs, often accompanied by a smooth, red tongue.
7. *Polymyositis.* This is characterized by weakness and marked fatigability of the proximal muscles of the extremities, particularly those of the pelvic girdle and thighs. Muscular wasting is prominent, and there is a primary degeneration of muscle fibers.
8. *Autonomic system abnormalities.* Those described include postural hypotension.

Skeletal Manifestations

The most frequent peripheral sign of bronchial carcinoma is clubbing of the fingers, which at times is associated with generalized hypertrophic pulmonary osteoarthropathy (112,114). This clinical syndrome consists of swelling of the soft tissues of the terminal phalanges, with curvature of the nails, pain and swelling of the joints, and periostitis, with elevation of the periosteum and new bone formation. The mechanism of development of the tissue changes is not well known, although an increase in blood flow in the affected portions of the limbs has been reported. A prompt fall in the blood flow to normal levels occurs following successful treatment of the underlying condition. The cause of increased flow is unknown.

Both humoral and neurogenic factors have been implicated as the cause of the osteoarthropathy. Elevated levels of estrogen have been described, but the significance of this finding has been questioned. An efferent and afferent neurologic reflex has been postulated, with the afferent fibers running in the vagus or the intercostal nerves. This theory is supported by the observation that the osteoarthropathy may be reversed by cutting either the vagi or intercostal nerves without removal of the underlying disease (134,135).

The incidence of hypertrophic pulmonary osteoarthropathy in patients with carcinoma of the lung has been reported to be from 2% to 12% (112,136). It occurs only rarely, if ever, in small cell tumors. Its occurrence is distributed equally among the other three major cell types (squamous, adenocarcinoma, and large cell).

The removal of the pulmonary lesion may give dramatic remission of the arthralgia and peripheral edema; however, osseous radiographic changes regress much more slowly. Recurrence of the pulmonary neoplasm does not necessarily indicate return of the symptoms of osteoarthropathy.

Dermatologic Manifestations

The development of acanthosis nigricans may be associated with bronchial adenocarcinoma (112). Scleroderma, erythema gyratum, acquired ichthyosis, and nonspecific dermatoses also may occur in patients with bronchial carcinoma (112).

Vascular Manifestations

Thrombophlebitis, recurrent or migratory, may be the first indication of the presence of bronchial tumor (7,112). It occurs in approximately 0.3% of all patients with lung cancer (119). The incidence of operability is low in these individuals, and after resection the incidence of death from pulmonary embolism is high (112,114).

Nonbacterial, verrucous, marantic endocarditis, characterized by deposition of sterile fibrin plaques on the heart valves, and resultant arterial embolization, may occur (112).

The mechanism by which these complications take place is unknown.

DIAGNOSIS

Screening Techniques for Early Diagnosis of Lung Cancer

Recently, emphasis has been placed on the role of screening high-risk patients (male smokers over the age of 45) for the early diagnosis of lung cancer, because the best chance for therapeutic cure is surgical removal of the small, localized tumor. Techniques include serial chest radiographs and sputum cytology. The National Cancer Institute Cooperative Early Lung Cancer Detection Program at the Mayo Clinic, Memorial Sloan-Kettering Cancer Center, and Johns Hopkins University conducted a multiyear trial assessing the benefit of the chest radiograph and sputum cytology to detect lung cancer early (137). Five-year follow-up results from this large screening trial indicate that: *(a)* the prevalence rate of lung carcinoma increases in individuals over the age of 55; *(b)* there is an additive value of sputum cytology and chest radiographs in detecting central squamous cell carcinomas and peripheral adenocarcinomas; and *(c)* screening patients with stage I tumors augments survival (137–142). However, survival was poor for patients with stage II and stage III tumors, and overall survival was not significantly improved by these screening modalities. The failure of this trial to demonstrate a survival benefit for early lung cancer detection is likely attributable to the limitations of conventional sputum cytology and especially chest radiography to detect lung cancer while it is localized. Whether or not mass screening programs will ultimately have a beneficial impact on augmenting survival for lung cancer is not clear. At this time, there are no official recommendations that advocate screening high-risk patients for lung carcinoma. In 1999 the Early Lung Cancer Action Project (ELCAP) reported promising preliminary data on screening low dose chest computed tomography (CT) for detecting early lung cancers (143). In 1,000 volunteers, aged 60 years or older, with at least 10 pack years of cigarette smoking, noncalcified nodules were detected in 233 (23%) participants by low-dose CT at baseline, compared with 68 (7%) by chest radiography. Malignant disease was detected in 27 (2.7%) by CT and seven (0.7%) by chest radiography. Twenty-three of the 27 CT-detected cancers and four of the seven chest radiography detected lesions were stage I. These data suggest low-dose CT can greatly improve the detection of lung cancer at an earlier and potentially curable stage. Further trials assessing this approach are underway.

Chest Imaging

Most lung cancers are detected by the standard chest radiograph. Although a small percentage of patients have a stage

0 lesion (endobronchial tumor and negative chest film), most will have a detectable lesion on chest radiograph. It is possible to visualize lesions as small as 3 mm, but generally lesions less than 5 to 6 mm in diameter are unlikely to be detected (138,139). It is usually difficult to differentiate between benign and malignant lesions on a chest radiograph, yet certain radiographic signs may suggest malignancy (144,145). Spiculation or poorly defined smooth margins of lesions are more indicative of a malignancy; however, a sharply defined smooth margin does not rule out malignancy (146–148). The presence of calcification within a lesion suggests a benign diagnosis when it is central, homogeneous, ring-like, or popcorn-like in distribution (149). Eccentric calcification may occur in bronchogenic carcinoma.

Certain radiographic patterns characterize the different cell types (84,146,147). Squamous cell carcinoma is centrally located two-thirds of the time but may arise in the lung periphery, often as a cavitating lesion (Fig. 14.7). In fact, it is the lung cancer cell type that cavitates most frequently. Small cell carcinoma is also a central lesion in most cases, often with central adenopathy at presentation (Fig. 14.8). It is peripheral in less than 20% of cases and does not cavitate. As stated, in 55% to 60% of cases adenocarcinoma is a peripheral lesion (Fig. 14.9). Frequently, there is associated pleural involvement, and in 50% of patients, hilar or mediastinal adenopathy is identified at initial presentation. Bronchioloalveolar carcinoma, a subtype of adenocarcinoma, may have a variety of radiographic manifestations. Most commonly, it appears as a solitary peripheral nodule on the chest radiograph, but it may present as numerous small nodules resembling metastatic disease or as a consolidation with air bronchograms. Large cell carcinomas are more likely to be peripheral than central and are sharply defined, lobulated masses that occasionally cavitate (Fig. 14.10).

Sputum Cytology

Sputum cytology may be particularly helpful in diagnosing central squamous cell and small cell carcinomas (150,151). However, there are several potential problems in accurately interpreting sputum cytology specimens. Among these are an inexperienced cytologist, inadequate sample number (less than 3 or 4), inadequate specimen sample (without alveolar macrophages), purulent sputum causing degeneration of malignant cells prior to examination, and poor sample preparation. Accordingly, a negative sputum cytologic examination in a suspicious setting should never terminate further evaluation. Sputum immunostaining with monoclonal antibodies offers considerable promise in detecting early, localized cancers.

Bronchoscopy

Flexible fiberoptic bronchoscopy is used widely for diagnosing both central airway and peripheral parenchymal lesions (152–159). For endobronchial lesions that are endoscopically visible, bronchial washings have a diagnostic yield of 79%, bronchial brushing 92%, and forceps biopsy 93% (154). Occasionally, in the setting of deeper submucosal lesions (e.g., small cell carcinoma), false-negative results occur because of an inability to grasp and bite tissue with biopsy forceps. Transbronchial needle aspiration in association with transbronchial biopsy may improve the diagnostic yield in these lesions (155,159). Bronchoscopy is less helpful in peripheral lesions, particularly lesions less than 2 cm in diameter (153,156,157). For lesions less than 2 cm, the diagnostic yield is in the range of 20% or less; however, lesions larger than 4 cm may be diagnosed in 50% to 80% of cases (153,156–158).

Complications of fiberoptic bronchoscopy have been minimal. In one report, among 24,521 bronchoscopies performed by 192 bronchoscopists, mortality was only 0.1% and there were no deaths in a series of 600 procedures performed by Zavala (160,161). Other potential complications include laryngospasm (0.13%), pneumothorax (0.1%), hypoxemia (0.3%), and significant hemorrhage (0.2%) (159–161).

Needle Aspiration Biopsy

Transbronchial needle aspiration for both central and peripheral lesions was introduced for use with the fiberoptic bronchoscope by Wang and Terry (162). When used in conjunction with transbronchial biopsy, the diagnostic yield may be as high as 95% for central lesions and somewhat lower for peripheral lesions. Complications of this procedure are few and include minor bleeding or pneumothorax.

Percutaneous transthoracic thin-needle aspiration biopsy has proven to be a safe and reliable method for diagnosing nonendobronchial lung carcinomas (153,163,164). A 95% or greater accuracy for diagnosing malignant lesions has been reported (164,165). CT or fluoroscopy is used to guide most biopsies. A positive cytologic examination appears to be diagnostic for lung malignancy, because there have been only a few reported cases of false-positive results.

However, because false-negative results may occur, a negative cytologic examination cannot be called a "benign lesion" unless the pathologist can provide a specific benign diagnosis such as "hamartoma." Twenty-nine percent of lesions initially diagnosed as negative on percutaneous needle aspiration were subsequently found to be malignant in one recent study (166). In most of these cases, the initial needle aspiration biopsy reading was nonspecifically benign (i.e., no specific benign diagnosis, such as hamartoma or granuloma, could be made). Also in this study, a specific benign diagnosis or granulomatous inflammation was associated with malignancy. Thus, serial follow-up chest radiographs must be obtained in patients with a specific benign diagnosis by transthoracic needle biopsy. When a high-risk patient has a nonspecific diagnosis by percutaneous needle biopsy, a further invasive diagnostic work-up is necessary until either malignancy or a specific benign process has been diagnosed.

Pneumothorax, the major complication of transthoracic needle aspiration, develops in 25% to 30% of patients and usually resolves spontaneously (153,164,167). The most important contributing factor for the development of a pneumothorax is the presence of chronic obstructive pulmonary disease (COPD) (164). In one study, there was a 46% incidence of pneumothorax in patients with COPD, compared with a 7% incidence in patients without COPD (168). The placement of a chest tube or small catheter connected to a Heimlich (one-way) valve may be required (164). Other infrequent complications include hemoptysis and transient parenchyma hemorrhage (164). Cardiac tamponade and fatal air embolism are rare complications. There have been only two reports of implantation of the needle tract with malignant cells (169,170).

Pleural Biopsy

Combined thoracentesis and pleural biopsy will provide up to a 90% yield in patients with carcinoma of the lung and malignant pleural involvement (171). Thoracoscopy, which involves introduction of either a flexible or a rigid bronchoscope into the pleural space with biopsy taken under direct vision, may augment the diagnostic yield in patients with pleural effusions (172).

STAGING CLASSIFICATION

After the tissue diagnosis of lung carcinoma is made, the disease is staged to assess extent, to select correct therapy, and to determine prognosis (173–176). The most widely accepted staging system for non-small cell carcinoma is the tumor-node-metastasis (TNM) classification originally proposed in 1946 by Denoix (175). In 1986 and 1997, the TNM classification was revised and updated (174,176). The details of each subset under the new system are given in Table 14.4 and stage groupings for TNM subsets and outcome by clinical and surgical-pathologic stage are given in Table 14.5 (176). The TNM system can be employed at any time from the initial clinical diagnosis to the time of autopsy (173–176). The critical distinction is between clinical staging (TNM) made prior to the institution of any therapy and surgical-pathologic staging determined from histologic examination of resected specimens (173–176). The recent changes in TNM classification were designed to include within stage groupings and subgroupings tumor with somewhat similar outcomes (176). It has long been recognized that patients with T1NM0 (stage IA) lesions have significantly better survival than patients with T2N0M0 (stage IB) lesions. Clinical estimates of extent of disease reveal that 61% of patients with clinical stage IA and

TABLE 14.4. DEFINITIONS IN THE REVISED INTERNATIONAL STAGING SYSTEM FOR LUNG CANCER

Primary tumor (T)

TX	Primary tumor cannot be assessed, or tumor proven by the presence of malignant cells in sputum or bronchial washings but not visualized by imaging or bronchoscopy
T0	No evidence of primary tumor
Tis	Carcinoma *in situ*
T1	Tumor ≤3 cm in greatest dimension, surrounded by lung or visceral pleura, without bronchoscopic evidence of invasion more proximal than the lobar bronchus[a] (i.e., not in the main bronchus)
T2	Tumor with any of the following features of size or extent: >3 cm in greatest dimension; Involves main bronchus, ≥2 cm distal to the carina; Invades the visceral pleura; Associated with atelectasis or obstructive pneumonitis that extends to the hilar region but does not involve the entire lung.
T3	Tumor of any size that directly invades any of the following: chest wall (including superior sulcus tumors), diaphragm, mediastinal pleura, parietal pericardium; or tumor in the main bronchus <2 cm distal to the carina, but without involvement of the carina; or associated atelectasis or obstructive pneumonitis of the entire lung
T4	Tumor of any size that invades any of the following: mediastinum, heart, great vessels, trachea, esophagus, vertebral body, carina; or tumor with a malignant pleural or pericardial effusion,[b] or with satellite tumor nodule(s) within the ipsilateral primary-tumor lobe of the lung

Regional lymph nodes (N)

NX	Regional lymph nodes cannot be assessed
N0	No regional lymph node metastasis
N1	Metastasis to ipsilateral peribronchial and/or ipsilateral hilar lymph nodes, and intrapulmonary nodes involved by direct extension of the primary tumor
N2	Metastasis to ipsilateral mediastinal and/or subcarinal lymph node(s)
N3	Metastasis to contralateral mediastinal, contralateral hilar, ipsilateral or contralateral scalene, or supraclavicular lymph node(s)

Distant metastasis (M)

MX	Presence of distant metastasis cannot be assessed
M0	No distant metastasis
M1	Distant metastasis present[c]

[a] The uncommon superficial tumor of any size with its invasive component limited to the bronchial wall, which may extend proximal to the main bronchus, is also classified T1.
[b] Most pleural effusions associated with lung cancer are owing to tumor. However, there are a few patients in whom multiple cytopathologic examinations of pleural fluid show no tumor. In these cases, the fluid is nonbloody and is not an exudate. When these elements and clinical judgment dictate that the effusion is not related to the tumor, the effusion should be excluded as a staging element and the patient's disease should be staged T1, T2, or T3. Pericardial effusion is classified according to the same rules.
[c] Separate metastatic tumor nodule(s) in the ipsilateral nonprimary-tumor lobe(s) of the lung also are classified M1.
Source: Mountain CF. Revisions in the International system for staging lung cancer. *Chest* 1997;111:1710–1717, with permission.

TABLE 14.5. STAGE GROUPING OF TNM SUBSETS AND OUTCOME BY CLINICAL AND PATHOLOGIC STAGE

Stage	TNM Subset	5 Years After Treatment (cumulative % surviving)	
		Clinical Stage[a]	Surgical Pathology Stage[b]
IA	T1N0M0	61	67
IB	T2N0M0	38	57
IIA	T1N1M0	34	55
IIB	T2N1M0	24	39
	T3N0M0	22	38
IIIA	T3N1M0	9	25
	T1N2M0		
	T2N2M0	13	23
	T3N2M0		
IIIB	T4N0M0		
	T4N1M0	7	ND
	T4N2M0		
	T1N3M0		
	T2N3M0	3	ND
	T3N3M0		
IV	ANY T ANY N M1	1	ND

ND, No Data.
[a] Percentage distribution of cell types: adenocarcinoma, 47.2% (2,466/5.230); squamous cell carcinoma, 33.9% (1,773/5.230); large cell carcinoma, 3.1% (163/5.230); small cell carcinoma, 11.9% (624/5.230); NOS (carcinoma not specified), 3.9% (204/5.230).
[b] Percentage distribution of cell types: adenocarcinoma, 53.0% (1,012/1,910); squamous cell carcinoma, 41.6% (794/1,910); large cell carcinoma, 3.6% (68/1,910); NOS (carcinoma not specified), 1.9% (36/910).
Source: Moutain CF. Revisions in the Internationl system for staging lung cancer. *Chest* 1997;111:1710–1717, with permission.

38% of patients with clinical stage IB tumors are expected to survive 5 years or more after treatment (Table 14.5) (176). Similarly, within stage II, patients with T1N1M0 (stage IIA) lesions have a significantly better survival than patients with T2N1M0 or T3N0M0 (stage IIB) lesions. Thirty-four percent of patients with clinical T1N0M0 tumors (stage IIA) and 24% of those who have clinical T2N1M0 (stage IIB) disease are expected to survive 5 or more years after treatment (Table 14.5) (176). The substantial difference in survival between clinical and surgical stage represents the under appreciation of extent of disease with our current clinical staging techniques. Surgical staging reveals occult disease not appreciated in clinical staging methods. By either clinical or surgical stage, patients with stage IA (T1N0M0) lesions have the best overall survival and stage IV patients with distant metastasis (M1) have the worst survival (Table 14.5) (176). Most pleural effusions associated with lung cancer are caused by tumor. There are, however, a few patients in whom multiple cytopathologic examinations (on more than one specimen) are negative for tumor; the fluid is nonbloody and is not an exudate. In such cases where these elements and clinical judgment dictate that the effusion is not related to the tumor, the patient should be staged

T1, T2, or T3, excluding effusion as a staging element (176). Pericardial effusion is classified according to the same rules.

The TNM classification has been less useful in staging small cell carcinoma because of the rapid extrathoracic spread of tumor (66,177,178). At the time of diagnosis, more than 85% of patients are stage III or stage IV, and even for those considered to be stage I or stage II, the prognosis is poor because of the frequent presence of undetected metastatic disease (177). The staging system most commonly used for small cell carcinoma is that of the Veterans Administration Lung Cancer Study. Group, in which disease is simply classified as either limited or extensive (66,177,178). Limited disease refers to tumor confined to the ipsilateral hemithorax with or without superior vena caval obstruction or involvement of supraclavicular nodes. Extensive disease is defined as spread beyond the ipsilateral hemithorax and adjacent lymph nodes, recurrent disease after radiation to the primary tumor, or cytologically positive pleural effusion. With limited stage disease, complete response to therapy and prolonged survival are more likely, although fewer than one-third of patients fall into this category at the time of diagnosis.

STAGING PROCEDURES

The staging process commences with a complete history and physical examination; attention is given to signs and symptoms related to CNS, bone, liver, chest wall, or mediastinal involvement (153,179). A full laboratory examination should include a complete blood count, liver function tests, and determination of calcium level. Hematologic abnormalities such as anemia, thrombocytopenia, or leukoerythroblastic peripheral blood may result from direct bone marrow involvement by the tumor. Hypercalcemia may be owing to metastatic spread of tumor to bone or, more commonly, parathyroid-like hormone released by the malignancy (128–131). Abnormal liver function may reflect intrahepatic spread or extrahepatic obstruction.

Thoracic Imaging Techniques (Also see Chapter 5)

The crucial element in staging is determining whether mediastinal involvement has occurred (153). Except in special cases, the presence or absence of mediastinal metastases will determine whether surgery is performed. The conventional chest radiograph is only about 40% sensitive for detecting mediastinal lymph node involvement (180). Tomography may increase the yield, but the most sensitive, widely utilized technique is the chest CT scan, which is up to 60% to 75% sensitive for detecting malignant mediastinal disease (153,179,181). Many thoracic surgeons take patients directly to thoracotomy for tumor resection when the mediastinum appears to be without disease on chest CT. However, patients with enlarged mediastinal lymph nodes detected by CT scan require histologic examination of the nodes, because enlarged lymph nodes may be the result of an inflammatory, nonneoplastic process (182). Prior to thoracotomy, these patients should undergo further invasive staging procedures such as mediastinoscopy, percutaneous needle aspiration biopsy, or transbronchial needle aspiration (153,164,182).

Magnetic resonance imaging (MRI) has also been evaluated for imaging the mediastinum (148,153,183). However, because the sensitivity of MRI appears to be similar to that of CT, CT remains the initial procedure of choice for evaluating the mediastinum, and MRI is reserved for patients in whom CT results are equivocal. MRI is the procedure of choice for evaluating superior sulcus tumors and for assessing chest wall extension of lung cancer (Fig. 5.23). Moreover, tumor invasion of the pericardium or heart (the latter indicating tumor unresectability) is best demonstrated with MRI (148). Multiplanar imaging capability provides accurate evaluation of involvement of the brachial plexus, spinal canal, chest wall, and subclavian artery by such tumors (153).

Recently, positron emission tomography (PET) has been introduced as a useful noninvasive method for diagnosing and staging lung cancer (184,185). Malignant tissue demonstrates increased glucose metabolism that can be observed by using PET and [18F]fluoro-deoxy-2 D-glucose (FDG). Images are based on measurements of uptake of positron emitting radiotracers such as (^{18}F) FDG, a glucose analog that is utilized to track glucose uptake and phosphorylation. When it is transported into the cells and phosphorylated by hexokinase, FDG does not undergo further significant metabolism or diffusion out of the cell. Therefore, PET imaging is a functional test that can identify malignancy by demonstrating increased FDG uptake in metabolically malignant cells (184). PET has been shown to be more accurate than CT and MRI in diagnosing lung cancers. The diagnostic sensitivity has ranged from 95% to 100% and the specificity has ranged from 78% to 100% (184).

Occasional false-negative PET findings have been reported in patients with a solitary, slow growing bronchioloalveolar lung carcinoma (186,187). Increased FDG uptake has been described in patients with pneumonia, tuberculosis, aspergillus lung disease, and acute necrotizing inflammatory granulomas (188).

PET combined with CT is superior to CT alone for intrathoracic lymph node staging in nonsmall cell lung cancer (184,185). A study by Vansteen-kiste et al. (185) showed that utilizing PET plus CT scanning for staging the mediastinum improved the sensitivity of CT scanning alone from 75% to 93%. Moreover, the specificity was improved from 63% for CT alone to 95% for PET plus CT. Since PET is a whole body test, it is effective for extrathoracic staging of lung cancer. PET can detect metastases in brain, bones, and adrenal glands. Two important limitations of PET scanning include the lack of wide availability of PET scanners and the high current cost of the test.

Invasive Staging Techniques

Bronchoscopy and Needle Aspiration Biopsy

Several procedures are available to stage the extent of disease after a primary tumor diagnosis has been established. Tumor proximity to carina is assessed, and tumors involving the carina or located within 1 to 2 cm of the carina are often considered to be nonoperable because of the technical difficulty of the surgical resection and a poorer prognosis with lesions in this location.

Transbronchoscopic needle aspiration biopsy has been used as a mediastinal staging technique (153,158,159,162). The sensitivity of this procedure varies, but a positive result indicates malignant involvement of peritracheal or subcarinal lymph nodes. Percutaneous needle aspiration biopsy has been used to diagnose enlarged mediastinal and hilar nodes as well as peripheral lesions (164).

Lymph Node Biopsy

Biopsy of lymph nodes in the supraclavicular fossa or in the mediastinal is necessary in some cases to obtain a tissue diagnosis and in others to assess the resectability of the tumor (112). Excision of lymph nodes in the scalene triangle should only be performed in patients with carcinoma of the lung when these lymph nodes are palpable. The biopsy of nonpalpable lymph nodes is not indicated because the yield is 10% or less (189).

Mediastinoscopy and Mediastinotomy

Mediastinoscopy and mediastinotomy are two techniques used for direct exploration or sampling of tissues from the mediastinum (153,179,190–192). In general, only the superior aspects of the mediastinum can be fully evaluated by cervical mediastinoscopy because of the presence of large vessels, airways, and nerves. Lesions that involve the subcarinal and left anterior (periaortic) regions may be palpable, but biopsy specimens may be difficult to obtain. Anterior mediastinoscopy or mediastinotomy (Chamberlain procedure) is helpful for the latter situation (182,190,192). The procedure of choice depends largely on the site of the primary lesion, and selection may be guided by CT scan results.

The indication for mediastinoscopy in patients with carcinoma of the lung is to determine the presence or absence of metastatic tumor in the mediastinal nodes (Fig. 14.11). Such information may be of considerable prognostic significance and also may be helpful in planning the appropriate therapeutic approach. Contralateral positive lymph nodes (N3) are regarded as an absolute contraindication to thora-

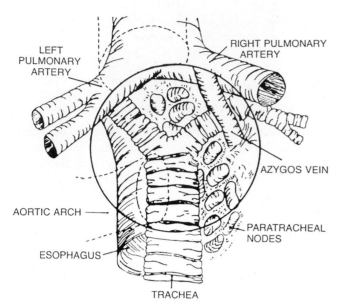

FIGURE 14.11. Representation of the view through a mediastinoscope at the level of the tracheal bifurcation with subcarinal lymph nodes and right pulmonary artery and azygous vein. (From Straus MJ. *Lung Cancer: Clinical Diagnosis and Treatment.* New York, Grune & Stratton, 1977, p 123.)

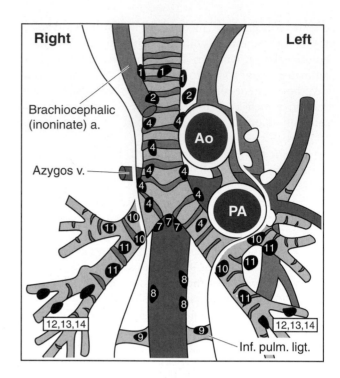

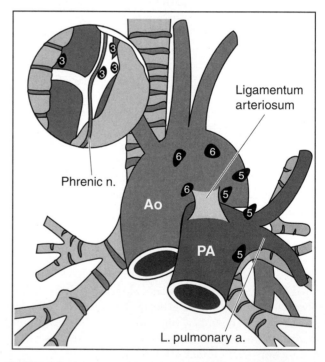

FIGURE 14.12. Regional lymph node stations for lung cancer staging. *Source:* Mountain CF, Dresler CM. Regional lymph node classification for lung cancer staging. *Chest* 1997;111:1718–1723, with permission.

cotomy. Contralateral spread is more likely to occur in patients with left lower lobe lesions (120). When ipsilateral mediastinal lymph nodes are involved (stage N2), opinion remains divided as to whether or not pulmonary resection with radical node dissection is recommended. In such patients, preoperative chemotherapy, with or without radiation therapy, in such patients is often administered.

Opinion is also divided as to whether or not mediastinoscopy should be performed in all patients with clinically resectable disease. Most surgeons believe it should be performed when a hilar mass or mediastinal lymph node enlargement is apparent either on the standard chest radiograph, on laminograms of the chest, on chest CT, or on PET. Also, mediastinoscopy should be performed when a thoracotomy is not indicated because of the general condition of the patient and when all other simpler diagnostic methods have failed to give a positive histologic diagnosis of the tumor. Recently, a specific schema has been established for mediastinal lymph nodes (Fig. 14.12) (193).

Generally, mediastinoscopy is contraindicated in patients who have received mediastinal irradiation or who have had a tracheotomy. The highest positive yield is in patients with small cell tumors, the next highest with large cell carcinoma, and the least with squamous cell tumors (194). False-negative results are reported in only 4% to 6% of patients (194). Most often this is owing to involvement of lymph nodes present in nonaccessible areas of the mediastinum.

Anterior mediastinotomy, a limited parasternal thoracot-

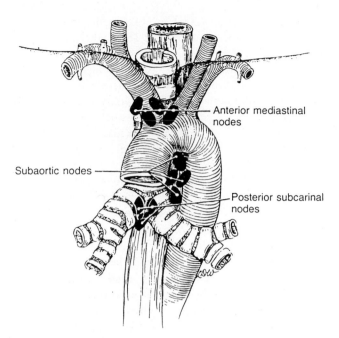

FIGURE 14.13. Diagrammatic representation of thoracic lymph nodes inaccessible to mediastinoscopy. The anterior mediastinal lymph nodes and subaortic lymph nodes may be reached by anterior mediastinotomy (Chamberlain procedure). (From Shields TW, Ritts RE. *Bronchial Carcinoma.* Springfield, IL, Charles C Thomas, 1974.)

Labels on figure: Anterior mediastinal nodes; Subaortic nodes; Posterior subcarinal nodes

omy, provides a more direct approach to the mediastinal lymph nodes than mediastinoscopy. This approach is most popular for left-lung tumors when the major lymph node groups to be evaluated are in the subaortic anterior mediastinal areas. Neoplasms of the left upper lobe in particular may spread directly to the anterior mediastinal group or lymph nodes without involving the inferior tracheal bronchial, superior tracheal bronchial, or paratracheal nodal chain. Routine surgical mediastinoscopy does not sample the anterior mediastinal group (Fig. 14.13) (192,195).

Thoracotomy for Diagnosis and Staging

Historically, 5% to 20% of patients with bronchial carcinoma underwent surgery without a positive histologic or cytologic diagnosis. Today, because of widespread use of bronchoscopy and needle biopsy techniques, at least 95% of patients with lung cancer who undergo thoracotomy should have a histologic or cytologic diagnosis established prior to surgery. Thoracotomy should not be used for establishing the diagnosis when there appears to be no hope that the lesion is resectable; this is especially true in the elderly patient or one with limited functional pulmonary reserve (112).

A formal thoracotomy for diagnosis alone is usually not justified in patients with a superior sulcus tumor or superior

vena caval syndrome. In the former situation, a tissue diagnosis may be obtained prior to institution of a therapeutic regimen by a bronchoscopy with fluoroscopic guidance, percutaneous needle aspiration biopsy, or one of three open surgical procedures: a posterior, axillary, or cervical approach. In patients with superior vena caval obstruction, tissue diagnosis may usually be obtained by bronchoscopy or mediastinotomy; however, mediastinoscopy could be hazardous, owing to increased pressure in large veins (112).

Evaluation for Extrapulmonary Metastasis

Prior to instituting therapy, particularly surgical resection for non-small cell lung cancer, it is important to assess whether disease has spread to extrathoracic organs (153,182). Metastases can be detected by CT scan, PET scan, or radionuclide scan of specific organs. A CT scan of the head or PET scan is useful for detecting CNS spread and may reveal asymptomatic metastasis. CT scanning of the liver and adrenal glands or a PET scan may also detect metastatic lesions (182,184,196). Bone scans and radionuclide liver-spleen scans are sensitive indicators of tumor spread; however, in asymptomatic patients with non-small cell carcinoma and normal laboratory tests, the routine use of these scans is unnecessary, and results may be potentially misleading (197,198). Positive liver or bone scan findings may represent nonmalignant disease (e.g., old fracture, inflammation) and unnecessarily delay surgery while necessitating an invasive, costly further evaluation. The best screen for extrathoracic spread continues to be a thorough history and physical examination along with laboratory data, including calcium and alkaline phosphatase levels and liver function tests. Any abnormality should be followed by the appropriate radionuclide or CT scans (182). If available, the PET scan provides an excellent technique for combined diagnosis, intrathoracic staging and extrathoracic staging of lung cancer (184,185,188).

As with non-small cell lung cancer, the radiographic staging of small cell tumors focuses on the presence or absence of extrathoracic disease. The approach remains the same as that for non-small cell tumors, but some clinicians recommend routine multiorgan (i.e., head, bone, liver, adrenal) scanning because of the frequent spread of disease. In addition, many investigators recommend routine bone marrow investigation with bone marrow aspiration and biopsy, because bone marrow involvement occurs in up to 50% of cases, even in the absence of peripheral blood abnormalities or a bone scan with positive findings. Certainly, patients who are considered for locoregional therapy (chest radiotherapy and/or surgical resection) or participation in clinical trials should undergo these additional staging studies to identify asymptomatic metastatic sites (66).

APPROPRIATE INVESTIGATION OF A SOLITARY PERIPHERAL PARENCHYMAL MASS

A circumscribed, solitary, peripheral lung mass (the pulmonary coin lesion) in the asymptomatic patient frequently represents a relatively early primary carcinoma of the lung. However, it may be an inflammatory mass, a vascular lesion, a benign tumor, or even a solitary metastasis to the lung. On chest radiograph, the actual margins of the lesion may vary from ill-defined to sharply demarcated, and the size may vary, although in general no lesion greater than 3 cm in diameter should be included in this category (153,199,200). Table 14.6 shows some of the benign causes of the solitary pulmonary nodule.

The percentage of benign and malignant lesions in any given series of coin lesions varies with patient selection and the definition of such a lesion. In the general population, 5% of such masses discovered by a routine radiographic survey are carcinomas. However, in series in which resections have been performed, 50% of such masses in patients over 50 years of age are carcinomas (112). Further, this percentage increases with advancing age of the patient group.

Of the malignant lesions, approximately 8% to 10% are metastatic (112). Less than 0.5% of all patients with coin lesions have metastatic disease in the lungs from an unknown, asymptomatic tumor elsewhere in the body (201). Consequently, in a patient with a coin lesion, any extensive radiographic examination for a possible primary tumor hidden in another organ system has little potential reward. As stated, investigation of a specific organ system is indicated only when the patient has a history of a previous malignant tumor or symptoms related to that system or when the routine laboratory studies reveal an abnormality that suggests the presence of a silent tumor (112,182). Since the sensitivity of PET ranges from 95% to 100%, the failure to demonstrate increased FDG uptake in a solitary lung lesion (greater than or equal to 1 cm in widest diameter), in most cases warrants watchful waiting. If the solitary lesion contains an air bronchogram, suggesting a bronchioloalveolar cell carcinoma, the PET scan may be false negative, and further investigations (e.g., transthoracic needle aspiration biopsy or surgical removal) may be warranted (186,187).

In the evaluation of a coin lesion, following a standard history, physical examination, and routine laboratory and radiographic studies of the chest, skin tests should be performed for *Mycobacterium tuberculosis* and other suspected infectious agents. Sputum smears for detection of acid-fast organisms and cytologic studies should be carried out. Chest CT should be performed to confirm that the lesion is solitary and to assess for presence of calcification, and any available previous radiographs of the chest should be reviewed. When the lesion is found to have been present and unchanged for a period of 24 months or more or when any one of four specific types of calcification (central, ring-like, homogeneous, or popcorn-like) is seen, the lesion may be judged to be benign and may be observed radiographically at periodic intervals (144,153,182). When acid-fast organisms are demonstrated in the sputum, the patient should receive appropriate antituberculous chemotherapy, and the lesion should be reevaluated within 2 to 3 months. When none of these features is present, particularly when the patient is over 40 years of age, the lesion should be removed to permit diagnosis and treatment (112,200).

TABLE 14.6. COMMON NONMALIGNANT LESIONS PRESENTING AS SOLITARY PULMONARY NODULES

Very common
    Granulomas
        Histoplasmoma, tuberculoma, coccidioidoma
        Cryptococcosis, blastomycosis, actinomycosis
        Unidentified granulomas
Common
    Lung abscess before evacuation into a bronchus
    Slowly resolving circumscribed pneumonia
    Lipoid pneumonia
    Hamartoma
Less common
    Bronchogenic cyst
    Pulmonary infarct
    Bronchial adenoma
    Arteriovenous fistula
    Enlarged pulmonary artery
    Infected, fluid-filled bulla
    Rheumatoid nodule

TREATMENT

Lung cancer therapy varies depending on the cell type, the stage of the cancer, and multiple host factors such as age, general condition, and the presence of concomitant diseases, particularly chronic obstructive lung disease and coronary heart disease (182). Current modalities, used in various combinations, are surgical resection, radiation therapy, chemotherapy, immunotherapy, and laser therapy. Despite the aggressive application of these modalities, the 5-year survival of large groups of patients with lung cancer remains only 11% to 14%. Obviously, improvement is needed in the management of this disease.

Surgery

Indications for Resection

Surgical resection of the tumor is the primary modality of therapy for non-small cell lung cancer (182,202–206). This remains true for all age groups, although surgical morbidity and mortality may be higher in older populations (204).

The best long-term results have been obtained in patients who have true (i.e., pathologic staging) stage I disease and small primary tumors (T1N0M0) (176,182,202–206). Mountain (Table 14.5) and Naruke et al. have reported 67.5% and 75.5% 5-year survivals, respectively, in this subgroup (176,203). Patients with tumors larger than 3 cm (stage IB, T2N0M0) have a lower 5-year survival than patients with tumors equal to or less than 3 cm (stage IA, T2N0M0) (Table 14.5) (176). Following complete resection of stage I non-small cell lung cancer in 598 patients, Martini reported the overall 5- and 10-survival rates were 75% and 67%. Survival rates in patients with T1 tumors were 82% at 5 years and 74% at 10 years, contrasted with 68% at 5 years and 60% at 10 years for patients with T2 tumors. Hence, the smaller the tumor, the better the survival. The prognostic significance of the specific cell type (i.e., adenocarcinoma, squamous cell, or large cell) is debated. Some data suggest that with or without lymph node involvement, patients with adenocarcinoma do less well than those with squamous cell carcinoma (58,182).

The usual surgical procedure is lobectomy, although patients with central lesions may require pneumonectomy. Procedures that spare pulmonary parenchyma (segmentectomy, wedge resection, or bronchial sleeve resection) have been used more frequently because of the common coexistence of chronic obstructive lung disease with lung cancer (182,205). Patients with stage II non-small cell tumors also are considered eligible for complete resection, although they may require a more extensive surgical procedure, such as pneumonectomy, and have a poorer prognosis (Table 14.5) (176).

According to the new revised staging classification for lung cancer, nonsmall cell lung cancer with a direct extension into the chest wall, but negative lymph nodes (T3N0M0) is considered stage IIB with an approximate 39% 5-year survival (Tables 14.4 and 14.5) (176). However, when N1 and N2 disease is present in addition to chest wall involvement (T3N1M0, T3N2M0), the 5-year survival rate drops precipitously (176,182).

The role of surgery in more extensive, stage IIIA non-small cell carcinoma is controversial (182,207). Some groups have claimed that patients with certain types of patterns may benefit from resectional surgery (206). Among stage IIIA (N2) patients there is an important distinction between occult N2 disease discovered at thoracotomy and evidence preoperatively of bulky N2 disease by chest radiograph or chest CT scan. The former group has a 5-year survival following complete surgical resection of 20% to 30%, whereas the latter group of patients has a poor survival, less than 10% (182). Accordingly, investigators have been assessing neoadjuvant chemotherapy with or without radiation therapy, followed by surgery in patients with clinically evident N2 disease (206,208–211). Two promising randomized controlled trials suggest this approach may enhance survivorship in patients with stage IIIA (N2) lung cancer (208,209).

The role of surgery in small cell carcinoma has been undergoing reevaluation (182,212). In general, surgery has not been shown to improve outcome because of the frequent presence of microextrathoracic or macroextrathoracic metastasis at the time of tumor diagnosis. However, there is renewed enthusiasm for operating on patients with limited-stage disease because removal of the primary tumor combined with chemotherapy may limit local chest relapse. Several prospective trials of primary surgery and surgery as an adjuvant to chemotherapy for small cell lung cancer are underway. As yet, surgical removal of small cell lung tumors has not been conclusively shown to favorably alter outcome (182).

Medical Contraindications to Resection

Almost all medical contraindications to resection of malignant lesions are related to either the lungs or the heart. Rarely does advanced age alone or the presence of other systemic disease preclude surgical resection. At times, the determination of what constitutes insufficient pulmonary reserve for tolerance of the required pulmonary resection is, at best, difficult to make. However, data suggest that in patients with borderline pulmonary reserve (preoperative forced expiratory volume in 1 second less than 2,000 mL), the preoperative combination of simple spirometric analysis and quantitative perfusion lung scanning can permit an accurate assessment of postoperative lung function in most cases (179,182,213).

Cardiac contraindications include recent myocardial infarction, a changing pattern of angina pectoris, and uncontrolled or uncontrollable heart failure (182).

General Summary of Surgical Therapy

Most authorities agree that surgical resection is the proper treatment of lung cancer whenever there is a reasonable chance of removing all the cancer with an acceptable risk of morbidity and mortality. Thus, stages I and II non-small cell lung cancers are usually resected. Small cell lung cancer requires chemotherapy, with or without radiation therapy, and perhaps removal of solitary peripheral lesions (182). Some stage IIIA non-small cell lung cancers are resected if there is a reasonable probability that all the cancer can be removed (e.g., peripheral carcinomas with direct invasion of the chest wall without metastases to lymph nodes or T1 or T2 lesions with metastases to distal ipsilateral paratracheal lymph nodes) (182,206). Patients with clinical stage IIIA lesions are currently considered candidates for preoperative chemotherapy, with or without radiation therapy, followed by surgical resection and additional radiation therapy. Further randomized control trials are awaited to determine the best therapy for stage IIIA disease.

Radiation Therapy

Curative

Radical radiation therapy (local dosage of 50 to 65 Gy) is capable of sterilizing carcinoma of the lung (214–216). Thus, potential local control of a bronchial carcinoma may be accomplished. The various cell types respond differently to irradiation. Small cell carcinomas are moderately radio-sensitive and may be eradicated by a dose of 35 to 40 Gy. Squamous cell tumors require a higher dose (50 to 55 Gy). Adenocarcinoma responds to similar dosage levels, but the response is sometimes said to be less favorable than that of squamous cell tumors. Large cell undifferentiated tumors respond least favorably of all. Response, of course, also depends on the size of the lesion as well as the presence of extraparenchymal intrathoracic spread of the tumor. The selection of radiation therapy as the curative modality is indicated in an occasional patient with stage I or stage II disease. This is either the patient in whom resection is contraindicated because of inadequate pulmonary or cardiac reserve or the patient who refuses the operation (216–219). Patients who seem to benefit most from this approach are those with small peripheral lesions (T1N0M0), the same group with the best survival outcome from surgical resection (219). Approximately 15% of these patients will be long-term survivors, 25% will die of intercurrent disease, 30% will die of distant metastatic disease, and 30% will die after local failure only (219).

One special circumstance in which radiation may play a curative role is that of the superior sulcus tumor. Up to a 50% 5-year survival may be achieved in patients treated with a combination of preoperative radiation and en bloc resection of the chest wall, including the involved lung, ribs, thoracic vertebrae, and brachial plexus (220).

Small cell carcinoma of the lung is extremely sensitive to radiation, but chemotherapy remains the treatment of choice because of the frequency of extrathoracic metastases at the time of therapy (166,221,222). However, local radiation has been combined with chemotherapy because of the high incidence of local chest relapse in patients receiving chemotherapy alone (223). The current treatment of choice for patients with limited-stage small cell carcinoma is combined chemotherapy and radiation therapy (66,221, 222,224). Patients with extensive disease may derive local benefit from chest irradiation, but survival does not appear to improve because of the involvement of extrathoracic organ by tumor (66).

The second role for radiation in small cell carcinoma is in treating cranial involvement (66). CNS spread occurs in more than 50% of patients at some time during the course of their disease and may provide a sanctuary from chemotherapeutic agents because of the blood–brain barrier. Cranial irradiation reduces the development of CNS metastases but has little effect on survival because of concomitant spread of disease to other sites (225,226). Thus, prophylactic cranial irradiation is reserved for patients who are judged to have a complete response to chemotherapy. Treatment is usually given 2 to 4 months after the beginning of chemotherapy.

Palliative Radiation Therapy

Most, if not all, patients with tumor spread beyond the confines of the ipsilateral hemithorax are candidates for radiotherapy, if only for the relief of distressing symptoms (66,227,228). When the tumor is obviously incurable, no attempt at long-term control is indicated, and the routine use of radiation therapy other than for control of symptoms cannot be defended from the present data in the literature. Longevity appears not to be increased, and unless irradiation is given with care, appreciable morbidity as well as shortened life span may occur (229).

In most cases, complications such as hemoptysis, superior vena caval obstruction, bone invasion, chest pain, and dyspnea can be controlled (66,227,228). Ventilation–perfusion relationships of the lung may improve rapidly after a course of radiation therapy (230).

Complications of Radiation Therapy

The primary complication of radiation therapy is an acute pneumonitis, usually occurring 1 to 3 months after radiation (231,232). Patients usually present with complaints of a nonproductive cough and dyspnea and on physical examination have evidence of either pulmonary consolidation or pleural inflammation. Typically, the chest radiograph shows a sharply demarcated alveolar or interstitial parenchymal infiltrate limited to the radiation port (Fig. 14.14). Significant pleural effusions are uncommon. These patients gradually improve over several weeks, with a minority progressing to severe respiratory insufficiency. It is unclear whether corticosteroids are beneficial in these cases.

Other less common complications include esophagitis, pericarditis, and myelitis.

Chemotherapy

Non-Small Cell Carcinoma

In the past, there was considerable pessimism regarding chemotherapy for patients with non-small cell lung cancer. However, randomized trials from the 1980s showed that Cisplatin based chemotherapy improved patient survival, improved quality of life assessed by the patient and relieved symptoms in the majority of symptomatic patients (233,234).

Drugs that appear to have the best activity against non-small cell lung cancer include cisplatin, VP-16, taxines, paclitaxel, and doctaxel (233,234). Most current regimens

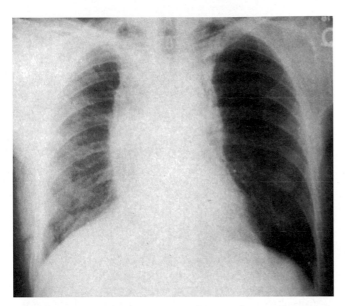

FIGURE 14.14. Radiation pneumonitis. PA chest radiograph illustrates profound radiation pneumonitis noted 3 months after irradiation (3500 rads) was completed to the central thorax for a squamous cell carcinoma invading the main carina. Note the well-demarcated, paramediastinal density and decreased lung volume in the right hemithorax.

include cisplatin and one or more additional agents, such as vindesin or VP-16 (etoposide) (233,234). Complete and partial response rates are at best in the range of 30% to 50% (233,234). Toxicity may be significant and in patients with advanced nonsmall cell lung cancer, those with the best performance status appear most appropriate for this therapy. Factors that appear to correlate best with response to chemotherapy are extent of disease and performance status. Whether a particular histologic subtype of tumor may respond better to chemotherapy has not been demonstrated consistently. Currently, the most realistic recommendation is to use chemotherapy as part of a protocol in patients with a reasonably modest tumor burden and good performance (232–235). As stated, the role of chemotherapy as a neoadjuvant treatment in patients with stage IIIA disease prior to surgical resection appears promising in early studies (206,208,209).

Small Cell Carcinoma

Chemotherapy is the treatment of choice for small cell lung cancer (66,221,222). Survival has been increased from between 2 and 3 months in untreated patients to between 8 and 14 months and sometimes longer in patients treated with combination chemotherapy. A variety of drug regimens are effective, but the most effective include cisplatin plus etoposide alone in alternation with cyclophosphamide, doxorubicin, and vincristine (221). Several studies have documented overall response rates in the range of 80% to 95% (221,222,236,237). However, only 10% of patients with small cell lung cancer will have a significant long-term survival (221).

Patients with extensive disease at initial treatment have a poorer initial response and long-term survival than those with limited disease (66,221,222). In 25% of patients, complete response rates are achieved, and median survival ranges from 8 to 9 months. Long-term disease-free survival is achieved in only a minority of patients (1% to 3%).

As stated, combined-modality therapy using chemotherapy with radiation for the primary chest tumor is advocated (66,221–223). This appears to improve the percentage of complete responses in patients with limited disease, diminish local tumor relapse, and increase overall survival. Among the newer approaches being tested are the use of non–cross-resistant chemotherapeutic agents to overcome tumor resistance, more aggressive "leukemia-style" induction and consolidation chemotherapy, autologous bone marrow transplantation with high-dose chemotherapy infusion, new drug development, and better *in vitro* cell cloning assays for prediction of chemotherapeutic efficiency (66,235–237). As yet, there is no defined role for dose increased treatment of small cell lung cancer (221).

Laser Therapy, Brachytherapy, and Endobronchial Prostheses

Local approaches to the treatment of malignant endobronchial lesions have included laser therapy with or without hematoporphyrin derivative and brachytherapy with endobronchial radioisotopic implantation (238–240). These treatments have been used for *in situ* premalignant lesions as well as palliative therapy for advanced endobronchial disease. Although laser therapy may be curative for patients with *in situ* lesions, laser therapy and brachytherapy generally are palliative therapies and do not affect overall survival.

Many patients present with malignant large airway obstruction owing to extrinsic compression from either tumor or enlarged lymph nodes. When surgical resection is not an option and radiotherapy has not adequately improved airway caliber, several endobronchial prosthetic devices (expandable metal wire, molded silicone, or combination of both) are now available as an alternative to disabling dyspnea (240,241).

REFERENCES

1. Greenlee RT, Murray T, Bolden S, et al. Cancer statistics, 2000. *CA Cancer J Clin* 2000;50:7–33.
2. Haskell CM, Holmes EC. Non-small cell lung cancer. *DM* 1988;34:53–108.
3. Smoking and Health. *A Report of the Surgeon General.* Washington, DC, US Department of Health and Human Services, 1980.
4. Tanoue LT, Matthay RA. Lung cancer: epidemiology and carcinogenesis. In Shields TW. *General thoracic surgery,* 5th ed. Philadelphia: Lippincott Williams & Wilkins, 2000:1215–1228.

5. Beckett WS. Epidemiology and etiology of lung cancer. *Clin Chest Med* 1993;14:1–15.

6. Stjernsward J, Stanley K. A world-wide health problem. *Lung Cancer* 1988;4(Suppl):11–24.

7. Yesner R. Pathogenesis and pathology (of lung cancer). *Clin Chest Med* 1993;14:17–30.

8. Stolley PD. Lung cancer: unwanted equality for women (Editorial). *N Engl J Med* 1977;297:886–887.

9. Loeb LA, Ernster VL, Warner KE, et al. Smoking and lung cancer: an overview. *Cancer Res* 1984;44:5940–5948.

10. Wyndner EL, Graham EA. Tobacco smoking as a possible etiologic factor in bronchogenic carcinoma. A study of 684 proved cases. *JAMA* 1950;143:329–338.

11. Morgan WKC, Andrews CE. Bronchogenic carcinoma. In Morgan WNC, ed. *Textbook of pulmonary diseases,* 2nd ed. Boston: Little, Brown & Co, 1974:755.

12. Gazdar AF, Carney DN, Minna JD. The biology of non-small cell lung cancer. *Semin Oncol* 1983;10:3–19.

13. Capewell S, Sankaran R, Lam D, et al. Lung cancer in lifelong nonsmokers. Edinburgh Lung Cancer Group. *Thorax* 1991;46:565–568.

14. Skillrud D, Offord K, Miller R. Higher risk of lung cancer in chronic obstructive pulmonary disease. A prospective matched, controlled study. *Ann Intern Med* 1986;105:503–507.

15. Tockman M, Anthonisen N, Wright E, et al. Airways obstruction and the risk of lung cancer. *Ann Intern Med* 1987;106:512–518.

16. Doll R, Hill AB. Mortality in relation to smoking: 10 years' observation of British doctors. *Br Med J* 1964;1:1399–1410.

17. Brown CC, Kessler LG. Projections of lung cancer mortality in the United States. 1985–2025. *J Natl Cancer Inst* 1988;80:43–51.

18. Sandler DP, Everson RB, Wilcox AJ. Passive smoking in adulthood and cancer risk. *Am J Epidemiol* 1985;121:37–48.

19. Matsukura S, Taminato T, Kitano N, et al. Effects of environmental tobacco smoke on urinary cotinine excretion in nonsmokers. Evidence for passive smoking. *N Engl J Med* 1984;311:828–832.

20. Hirayama T. Non-smoking wives of heavy smokers have a higher risk of lung cancer: a study from Japan. *Br Med J* 1981;282:183–185.

21. Holmes EC. Lung cancer. In Simmons DH, ed. *Current pulmonology.* Boston: Houghton Mifflin, 1979:239–250.

22. Brownson R, Chang J, David J. Gender and histologic type variations in smoking-related risk of lung cancer. *Epidemiology* 1992;3:61–64.

23. Lubin J, Qiao Y, Taylor P, Yao S, et al. Quantitative evaluate of the radon and lung cancer association in a case control study of Chinese miners. *Cancer Res* 1990;50:174–180.

24. McDuffie H, Klaasen D, Dosman J. Female-male differences in patients with primary lung cancer. *Cancer* 1987;59:1825–1830.

25. Risch H, Howe G, Jain M, et al. Are female smokers at higher risk for lung cancer than male smokers? A case-control analysis by histologic type. *Am J Epidemiol* 1993;138:281–293.

26. Zang E, Wynder E. Differences in lung cancer risk between men and women: examination of the evidence. *J Natl Cancer Inst* 1996;88:183–192.

27. Brown LM, Pottern LM, Blot WJ. Lung cancer in relation to environmental pollutants emitted from industrial sources. *Environ Res* 1984;34:250–261.

28. Chahinian AP, Chretien J. Present incidence of lung cancer: epidemiologic data and etiologic factors. In Israel L, ed. *Lung cancer—Natural history, prognosis, and therapy.* New York: Academic Press, 1976:1–22.

29. Frank AL. The epidemiology and etiology of lung cancer. *Clin Chest Med* 1982;3:219–228.

30. Samet JM, Kutvirt DM, Waxweiler RJ, et al. Uranium mining and lung cancer in Navajo men. *N Engl J Med* 1984;310:1481–1484.

31. Radford EP, Renard KGSC. Lung cancer in Swedish iron miners exposed to low doses of radon daughters. *N Engl J Med* 1984;310:1485–1494.

32. Wright ES, Couves CM. Radiation-induced carcinoma of the lung—the St. Lawrence tragedy. *J Thorac Cardiovasc Surg* 1977;74:495–498.

33. Selikoff IJ, Hammond EC. Asbestos-associated disease in United States shipyards. *Cancer J Clin* 1978;28:87–89.

34. Craighead JE, Mossman BT. The pathogenesis of asbestos-related diseases. *N Engl J Med* 1982;306:1446–1455.

35. Shekelle RB, Liu S, Raynor WJ, et al. Dietary vitamin A and risk of cancer in the Western Electric study. *Lancet* 1981;2:1185–1190.

36. Hennekens C, Buring J, Manson J, et al. Lack of effect of long-term supplementations with beta carotene on the incidence of malignant neoplasms and cardiovascular disease. *N Engl J Med* 1996;334:1145–1149.

37. Samet JM, Skipper BJ, Humble CG, et al. Lung cancer risk and vitamin A consumption in New Mexico. *Am Rev Respir Dis* 1985;131:198–202.

38. Alpha-tocopherol beta carotene cancer prevention study group. The effect of vitamin E and beta carotene on the incidence of lung cancer and other cancers in male smokers. *N Engl J Med* 1994;330:1029–1035.

39. Omenn G, Goodman G, Thornquist M, et al. Effects of a combination of beta carotene and vitamin A of lung cancer and cardiovascular disease. *N Engl J Med* 1996;334:1150–1155.

40. Sellers TA, Bailey-Wilson JE, Elston RC, et al. Evidence for mendelian inheritance in the pathogenesis of lung cancer. *J Natl Cancer Inst* 1990;82:1272–1279.

41. Tokuhata GK, Lilienfeld AM. Familial aggregation of lung cancer in humans. *J Natl Cancer Inst* 1963;30:289–312.

42. Kern JA, Filderman AE. Oncogenes and growth factors in human lung cancer. *Clin Chest Med* 1993;14:31–41.

43. Schottenfeld D. Epidemiology of lung cancer. In Pass HI, Mitchell JB, Johnson DH et al. *Lung cancer principles and practice.* Philadelphia: Lippincott-Raven, 1996:305–321.

44. Kazazian JH. A geneticist's view of lung disease. *Am Rev Respir Dis* 1976;113:261–266.

45. Kellerman G, Shaw CR, Layten-Kellerman M. Aryl-hydrocarbon-hydroxylase inducibility in bronchogenic carcinoma. *N Engl J Med* 1973;289:934–937.

46. Brauch H, Johnson B, Hovis J, et al. Molecular analysis of the short arm of chromosome 3 in small-cell and non-small cell carcinoma of the lung. *N Engl J Med* 1987;317:1109–1113.

47. Rodenhuis S, Van de Wetering ML, Mooi WJ, et al. Mutational activation of the K-*ras* oncogene. A possible pathogenic factor in adenocarcinoma of the lung. *N Engl J Med* 1987;317:929–935.

48. Karki NT, Pokela R, Nuutineu L, et al. Aryl hydrocarbon hydroxylase in lymphocytes and lung tissue from lung cancer patients and controls. *Int J Cancer* 1987;39:565–570.

49. Cohen MH. Natural history of lung cancer. *Clin Chest Med* 1982;3:229–241.

50. World Health Organization. The WHO histological typing of lung tumors. Second edition. *Am J Clin Pathol* 1982;77:123–126.

51. Shimosato Y. Pulmonary neoplasms. In Steinberg SS. *Diagnostic surgical pathology.* Philadelphia: Lippincott Williams & Wilkins, 1999:1114–1115.

52. Yesner R. Classification of lung cancer histology. *N Engl J Med* 1985;312:652–653.

53. Travis WD, Linder J, Mackay B. Classification, histology, cytology, and electron microscopy. In Pass HI, Mitchell JB, Johnson

DH, et al. *Lung cancer principles and practice.* Philadelphia: Lippincott-Raven, 1996:359–395.

54. Matthews MJ, Mackay B, Lukeman J. The pathology of non-small cell carcinoma of the lung. *Semin Oncol* 1983;10:34–55.

55. Kodama T, Biyajima S, Watanabe S, et al. Morphometric study of adenocarcinomas and hyperplastic epithelial lesions in the peripheral lung. *Am J of Clin Pathol* 1986;85:146–151.

56. Kurokawa T, Matsuno Y, Noguchi M, et al. Surgically curable "early" adenocarcinoma in periphery of the lung. *Am J of Surg Pathol* 1994;18:431–438.

57. Matthews MJ. Problems in morphology and behavior of bronchopulmonary malignant disease. In Israel L, ed. *Lung cancer—Natural history, prognosis, and therapy.* New York: Academic Press, 1976.

58. Gail MH, Eagan RT, Feld R, et al. Prognostic factors in patients with resected Stage I non-small cell lung cancer: a report from the Lung Cancer Study Group. *Cancer* 1984;54:1802–1813.

59. Woolner LB, Fontana RS, Cortese DA, et al. Roentgenographically occult lung cancer: pathologic findings and frequency of multicentricity during a 10-year period. *Mayo Clin Proc* 1984; 59:453–466.

60. Matthews MJ. Morphologic classification of bronchogenic carcinoma. *Cancer Chemother Rep* 1973;4(Suppl):229–230.

61. Hirsch FR, Matthews MJ, Aisner S, et al. Histopathologic classification of small cell lung cancer: changing concepts and terminology. *Cancer* 1988;62:973–977.

62. Yesner R, Carter D. Pathology of carcinoma of the lung: Changing Patterns. *Clin Chest Med* 1982;3:257–289.

63. World Health Organization. In Shimosato Y, Subin L, Spencer H, et al, eds. *Histological typing of lung tumours,* 2nd ed. Geneva: World Health Organization, 1981.

64. Radice PA, Matthew MJ, Ihde DK, et al. The clinical behavior of "mixed" small cell/large cell bronchogenic carcinoma compared to "pure" small cell subtypes. *Cancer* 1982;50: 2894–2902.

65. Aisner SC, Finkelstein DN, Ettinger DS, et al. The clinical significance of variant morphology small cell carcinoma of the lung. *J Clin Oncol* 1990;8:402–408.

66. Johnson BE. Management of small cell lung cancer. *Clin Chest Med* 1993;14:173–187.

67. Cox JD, Yesner RA. Adenocarcinoma of the lung: recent results from the Veterans Administration Lung Group. *Am Rev Respir Dis* 1979;120:1025–1029.

68. Ginsberg SS, Buzaid AC, Stern H, et al. Giant cell carcinoma of the lung. *Cancer* 1992;70:606–610.

69. Razzak MA, Urschel HC Jr, Albers JE, et al. Pulmonary giant cell carcinoma. *Ann Thorac Surg* 1976;21:540–545.

70. Arroliga AC, Carter D, Matthay RA. Other primary neoplasms of the lung. In Bone RC, Dantzker DR, George RB, et al, eds. *Pulmonary and critical care medicine.* St. Louis: Mosby-Year Book, 1993:H2–H6.

71. Andrews CE, Morgan WKC. Tumors of the lung other than bronchogenic carcinoma. In Morgan WKC, ed. *Textbook of pulmonary diseases,* 2nd ed. Boston: Little, Brown & Co, 1974: 789.

72. Kee JL Jr. Bronchial adenoma. In Shaw RR, Paulson DL, Kee JS Jr, eds. *Treatment of bronchial neoplasms.* Springfield, IL: Charles C Thomas, 1955:103–121.

73. Arrigoni MG, Woolner LB, Bernatz PE. Atypical carcinoid tumors of the lung. *J Thorac Cardiovasc Surg* 1972;64:413–421.

74. Carter D, Yesner R. Carcinomas of the lung with neuroendocrine differentiation. *Semin Diagn Pathol* 1985;2:235–255.

75. Mills SE, Cooper PH, Walker AN, et al. Atypical carcinoid of the lung: a clinicopathologic study of 17 cases. *Am J Surg Pathol* 1982;6:643–654.

76. Travis WD, Linnoila I, Tsokos MG, et al. Neuroendocrine tumors of the lung with proposed criteria for large cell neuroendocrine carcinoma: an ultrastructural, immunohistochemical, and flow cytometric study of 35 cases. *Am J Surg Pathol* 1991; 15:529–555.

77. Reid JD. Adenoid cystic carcinoma of the trachea (cylindroma) of the bronchial tree. *Cancer* 1952;5:685–694.

78. Turnball AD, Hu AG, Goodner JT, et al. Mucoepidermoid tumors of bronchial glands. *Cancer* 1971;28:539–544.

79. Ashmore PG. Papilloma of the bronchus. *J Thorac Surg* 1954; 27:293–294.

80. Yousem SA, Hochholzer L. Mucopidermoid tumors of the lung. *Cancer* 1987;60:1346–1352.

81. Moran CA, Suster S. Primary adenoid cystic carcinoma of the lung: a clinicopathologic and immunohistochemical study of 16 cases. *Cancer* 1994;73:1390–1397.

82. Helmuth RA, Strate RW. Squamous carcinoma of the lung in a nonirradiated, nonsmoking patient with juvenile laryngotracheal papillomatosis. *Am J Surg Pathol* 1987;11:643–650.

83. Miura H, Tsuchida T, Kawate N, et al. Asymptomatic solitary papilloma of the bronchus: review of occurrence in Japan. *Eur Respir J* 1993;6:1070–1073.

84. Spencer H. *Pathology of the lung.* Philadelphia: Saunders, 1977: 773–859.

85. Bejui-Thivolet F, Liagre N, Chignol MC, et al. Detection of human papilloma virus. *Human Pathol* 1990;21:111–116.

86. Liebow AA, Hubbell DS. Sclerosing hemangioma of the lung. *Cancer* 1956;9:53–75.

87. Hill GS, Eggleston JC. Electron microscopic study of so-called "pulmonary sclerosing hemangioma." Report of a case suggesting epithelial origin. *Cancer* 1972;30:1092–1106.

88. Nagata N, Dairku M, Sueishi K, et al. Sclerosing hemangioma of the lung: an epithelial tumor composed of immunohistochemically heterogeneous cells. *Am J Clin Pathol* 1987;88: 552–559.

89. Sugio K, Kaneko S, Ishida T, et al. Sclerosing hemangioma of the lung: radiographic and pathological study. *Ann Thorac Surg* 1992;53:295–300.

90. Yousem SA, Hocholzer L. Alveolar adenoma. *Human Pathol* 1986;17:1066–1071.

91. Dail DH, Liebow AA, Gmelich JJ, et al. Intravascular, bronchiolar, and alveolar tumor of the lung (IVBAT): an analysis of twenty cases of a peculiar sclerosing endothelial tumor. *Cancer* 1983;51:452–464.

92. Corrin B, Manners B, Millard M, et al. Histogenesis of the so called "intravascular bronchioloalveolar tumor." *J Pathol* 1979; 128:163–167.

93. Liebow AA. Tumors of the lower respiratory tract. In Liebow AA, ed. *Atlas of tumor pathology.* Washington, DC: Armed Forces Institute of Pathology, 1952.

94. Bateson EM. So-called hamartoma of the lung—a true neoplasm of fibrous connective tissue of the bronchi. *Cancer* 1973; 31:1458–1467.

95. Hochberg LA, Schacter B. Benign tumors of the bronchus and lung. *Am J Surg* 1955;89:415–438.

96. Pastlethwait RW, Hagerty RF, Trent JC. Endobronchial polypoid hamartochondroma. *Surgery* 1948;24:732–738.

97. Sun CJ, Kroll M, Miller JE. Primary chondrosarcoma of the lung. *Cancer* 1982;50:1864–1866.

98. Chan K, Ma Fine G, Lewis J, et al. Benign mixed tumor of the trachea. *Cancer* 1979;44:2260–2266.

99. Watts CF, Clagett OT, McDonald JR. Lipoma of the bronchus: discussion of benign neoplasms and a report of endobronchial lipoma. *J Thorac Surg* 1946;15:131–144.

100. McCall RE, Harrison W. Intrabronchial lipoma: a case report. *J Thorac Surg* 1955;29:317–322.

101. Agnos JW, Starkey GWB. Primary leiomyosarcoma and leiomy-

oma of the lung: review of the literature and report of two cases of leiomyosarcoma. *N Engl J Med* 1958;158:12–17.

102. Guccion JG, Rosen SH. Bronchopulmonary leiomyosarcoma and fibrosarcoma. *Cancer* 1972;30:836–847.

103. Gal AA, Brooks JSJ, Petra GG. Leimoyomatous neoplasms of the lungs: a clinical, histologic and immunohistochemical study. *Modern Pathol* 1989;2:209–216.

104. Misra DP, Sunderrajan EV, Rosenholt MJ, et al. Malignant fibrous histiocytoma in the lung masquerading as recurrent pulmonary thromboembolism. *Cancer* 1983;51:53–541.

105. Lee JT, Shelburne JD, Linder J. Primary malignant fibrous histiocytoma of the lung: a clinicopathologic and ultrastructural study of five cases. *Cancer* 1984;53:1124–1130.

106. Stuart AP. Fibrosarcoma: malignant tumor of fibroblasts. *Cancer* 1948;1:30–63

107. McDonnell T, Kyriakos M, Robert C, et al. Malignant fibrous histiocytoma of the lung. *Cancer* 1988;61:137–145.

108. Noehren TH, McKee FW. Sarcoma of the lung. *Dis Chest* 1954; 25:663–678.

109. Koss MN, Hochholzer L, Nichols PW, et al. Primary non-Hodgkin's lymphoma and pseudolymphoma of the lung: a study of 161 patients. *Human Pathol* 1982;14:1024–1038.

110. L'Hoste RJ JR, Filippa DA, Lieberman PH, et al. Primary pulmonary lymphoma. A clincopathologic analysis of 36 cases. *Cancer* 1984;54:1397–1406.

111. Donner LR, Dobin S, Harrington D, et al. Angiocentric immunoproliferative lesion (lymphomatoid/granulomatosis): a cytogenetic, immunophenotypic and genotypic study. *Cancer* 1990; 65:249–254.

112. Shields TW, Ritts RE. *Bronchial carcinoma.* Springfield, IL: Charles C Thomas, 1974.

113. Shimizu N, Ando A, Teramoto S, et al. Outcome of patients with lung cancer detected via mass screening as compared to those presenting with symptoms. *J Surg Oncol* 1992;50:7–11.

114. Midthun DE, Jett JR. Clinical presentation of lung cancer. In Pass HI, Mitchell JB, Johnson DH, et al. *Lung cancer principles and practice.* Philadelphia: Lippincott-Raven, 1996:421–435.

115. Parish JM, Marschke RF, Dines DE, et al. Etiologic considerations in superior vena cava syndrome. *Mayo Clin Proc* 1981; 56:407–413.

116. Chernow B, Sahn SA. Carcinomatous involvement of the pleura: an analysis of 96 patients. *Am J Med* 1977;63:695–702.

117. Johnston WW. The malignant pleural effusions. A review of cystopathologic diagnoses of 584 specimens from 472 consecutive patients. *Cancer* 1985;56:905–909.

118. Newman SJ, Hansen HH. Proceedings: frequency, diagnosis and treatment of brain metastasis in 247 consecutive patients with bronchogenic carcinoma. *Cancer* 1974;33:492–496.

119. LeRoux BT. Bronchial carcinoma. *Thorax* 1968;23:136–143.

120. Shields TW. Carcinoma of the lung. In Shields TW, ed. *General thoracic surgery.* Philadelphia: Lea & Febiger, 1972:797–845.

121. Merrill WW, Bondy PK. Production of biochemical marker substances by bronchogenic carcinomas. *Clin Chest Med* 1982; 3:307–320.

122. Patel AM, Bavila OG, Peters SG. Paraneoplastic syndromes associated with lung cancer. *Mayo Clin Proc* 1993;68:278–287.

123. Kovacs L, Robertson GL. Syndromes of inappropriate antidiuresis. *Endocrinol Metab Clin NA* 1992;21:859–875.

124. DeTroyer A, Demanet JC. Clinical biological and pathogenic features of the syndrome of inappropriate secretion of antidiuretic hormone. *Q J Med* 1976;45:521–531.

125. List AF, Hainsworth JD, Davis BW, et al. The syndrome of inappropriate secretion of antidiuretic hormone in small cell lung cancer. *J Clin Oncol* 1986;4:1191–1198.

126. Berl T. Treating hyponatremia: damned if we do and damned if we don't. *Kidney Int* 1990;37:1006–1018.

127. Bensch KG, Corrin B, Pariente R, et al. Oat-cell carcinoma of the lung. *Cancer* 1968;22:1163–1172.

128. Gaich G, Burtis WJ. The diagnosis and treatment of malignancy associated hypercalcemia. *Endocrinologist* 1991;1:371–378.

129. Arroliga AC, Matthay RA. Paraneoplastic syndromes in bronchogenic carcinoma. *Clin Pulm Med* 1994;1:322–332.

130. Bender RA, Hausen H. Hypercalcemia in bronchogenic carcinoma: a prospective study of 200 patients. *Ann Intern Med* 1974;80:205–208.

131. Mundy GR, Ibbotson KJ, D'Soufa SM, et al. The hypercalcemia of cancer. Clinical implications and pathogenic mechanisms. *N Engl J Med* 1984;310:1718–1727.

132. Daughtry DC, Chesney JG, Spear HC, et al. Unexplained systemic manifestations of malignant lung tumors. *Dis Chest* 1967; 52:632–639.

133. Morton DL, Itabashi HH, Grimes OF. Non-metastatic neurological complications of bronchogenic carcinoma. *J Thorac Cardiovasc Surg* 1966;51:14–29.

134. Hollings HE, Brody RS, Boland HC. Pulmonary hypertrophic osteoarthropathy. *Lancet* 1961;2:1269–1273.

135. Holman CW. Osteoarthropathy in lung cancer: disappearance after section of intercostal nerves. *J Thorac Cardiovasc Surg* 1963;45:679–681.

136. Stenseth JH, Clagett OT, Woolner LB. Hypertrophic pulmonary osteoarthropathy. *Dis Chest* 1967;52:62–68.

137. Early Lung Cancer Cooperative Study Group. Early lung cancer detection summary and conclusions. *Am Rev Respir Dis* 1984; 130:565–570.

138. Frost SK, Ball WC, Levin ML, et al. Early lung cancer detection: results of the initial (prevalence) radiologic and cytologic screening in the Johns Hopkins Study. *Am Rev Respir Dis* 1984;150: 549–554.

139. Flehringer BJ, Melamed MR, Zaman MB, et al. Early cancer detection: results of the initial (prevalence) radiologic and cytologic screening in the Memorial Sloan Kettering Study. *Am Rev Respir Dis* 1984;130:555–560.

140. Fontana RS, Sanderson DR, Taylor WF, et al. Early lung cancer detection: results of the initial (prevalence) radiologic and cytologic screening in the Mayo Clinic Study. *Am Rev Respir Dis* 1984;130:561–565.

141. Melamed MR, Flehinger BJ, Zaman MB, et al. Detection of true stage 1 lung cancer in a screening program and its effect on survival. *Cancer* 1981;47:1182–1187.

142. Melamed MR, Flehinger BJ. Should asymptomatic smokers have annual chest x-rays after age 55 years? *Debates Med Yearbook* 1990;3:123–124.

143. Henschke CI, McCauley DI, Yankelevitz DF, et al. Early Lung Cancer Project: overall design and findings from baseline screening. *Lancet* 1999;354:99–105.

144. Heitzman ER. *The lung: radiologic-pathologic correlations.* St. Louis: Mosby, 1984.

145. Heitzman ER. Bronchogenic carcinoma: radiologic-pathologic correlations. *Semin Roentgenol* 1977;12:165–174.

146. Filderman AE, Shaw C, Matthay RA. Lung cancer: part I. Etiology, pathology, natural history, manifestations, and diagnosis. *Invest Radiol* 1986;21:80–90.

147. Theros EG. 1976 Caldwell Lecture. Varying manifestations of peripheral pulmonary neoplasms: a radiologic-pathologic correlative study. *AJR* 1977;128:893–914.

148. White CS, Templeton PA. Radiologic manifestations of bronchogenic cancer. *Clin Chest Med* 1993;14:55–67.

149. O'Keefe ME Jr, Good CA, McDonald JR. Calcification in solitary nodules of the lung. *AJR* 1957;77:1023–1033.

150. Savage P, Donovan WN, Dellinger RP. Sputum cytology in the management of patients with lung cancer. *South Med J* 1984; 777:840–842.

151. Mehta AC, Marty JJ, Lee FYW. Sputum cytology. *Clin Chest Med* 1993;14:68–85.
152. Shaw GL, Mulshine JL. General strategies for early detection: new ideas and future directions. In Pass HI, Mitchell JB, Johnson DH, et al. *Lung cancer principles and practice.* Philadelphia: Lippincott-Raven, 1996:329–340.
153. American Thoracic Society/European Respiratory Society Official Statement. Pretreatment evaluation of non-small-cell lung cancer. *Am J Respir Crit Care Med* 1997;156:320–332.
154. Martini N, McCormick PM. Assessment of endoscopically visible bronchial carcinomas. *Chest* 1978;73:718–720.
155. Shure D, Fedullo PF. Transbronchial needle aspiration in the diagnosis of submucosal and peribronchial bronchogenic carcinoma. *Chest* 1985;88:49–51.
156. Stringfield JT, Markowitz DJ, Bentz RR, et al. The effect of tumor size and location on diagnosis by fiberoptic bronchoscopy. *Chest* 1977;72:474–476.
157. Wallace JM, Deutsch AL. Flexible fiberoptic bronchoscopy and percutaneous needle aspiration for evaluating the solitary nodule. *Chest* 1982;81:655–671.
158. Arroliga AC, Matthay RA. The role of bronchoscopy in lung cancer. *Clin Chest Med* 1993;14:87–98.
159. Shure D. Tissue procurement: bronchoscopic techniques for lung cancer. In Pass HI, Mitchell JB, Johnson DH, et al. *Lung cancer principles and practice.* Philadelphia: Lippincott-Raven, 1996:471–479.
160. Credle WF, Smiddy JF, Eliott RC. Complications of fiberoptic bronchoscopy. *Am Rev Respir Dis* 1974;109:67–72.
161. Zavala DC. Diagnostic fiberoptic bronchoscopy: techniques and results of biopsy in 600 patients. *Chest* 1975;68:12–19.
162. Wang KP, Terry PB. Transbronchial needle aspiration in the diagnosis and staging of bronchogenic carcinoma. *Am Rev Respir Dis* 1983;127:344–347.
163. Westcott JL. Direct percutaneous needle aspiration of localized pulmonary lesions: results in 422 patients. *Radiology* 1980;137: 31–35.
164. Salazar AM, Westcott JL. The role of transthoracic needle biopsy for the diagnosis and staging of lung cancer. *Clin Chest Med* 1993;14:99–110.
165. Khouri NF, Stitik FP, Erozan YS, et al. Transthoracic needle aspiration biopsy of benign and malignant lung lesions. *AJR* 1985;144:281–288.
166. Calhoun P, Feldman PS, Armstrong P, et al. The clinical outcome of needle aspirations of the lung when cancer is not diagnosed. *Ann Thorac Surg* 1986;41:592–596.
167. Poe RH, Kallay MC, Wicks CM, et al. Predicting risk of pneumothorax in needle biopsy of the lung. *Chest* 1984;85:232–235.
168. Fish GD, Stanley JH, Miller KS, et al. Post-biopsy pneumothorax: estimating the risk by chest radiography and pulmonary function tests. *Am J Roentgenol* 1988;150:71–74.
169. Sinner WN, Zajicek J. Implantation metastasis after percutaneous transthoracic needle aspiration biopsy. *Acta Radiol (Diagn) (Stockh)* 1976;17:473–480.
170. Muller NL, Bergin CJ, Miller RR, et al. Seeding of malignant cells into the needle tract after lung and pleural biopsy. *J Can Assoc Radiol* 1986;37:192–194.
171. Salyer WR, Eggleston JC, Erozan YS. Efficacy of pleural needle biopsy and pleural fluid cytopathology in the diagnosis of malignant neoplasm involving the pleura. *Chest* 1975;67:536–539.
172. Boutin C, Cargnino P, Viallet JR. Thoracoscopy in the early diagnosis of malignant pleural effusions. *Endoscopy* 1980;12: 155–160.
173. Mountain CF. Lung cancer staging classification. *Clin Chest Med* 1993;14:43–51.
174. Mountain CF. A new international staging system for lung cancer. *Chest* 1986;89:225S–233S.
175. Denoix PF. Enquete permanente dans les centres anticancereux. *Bull Inst Natl Hyg* 1946;1:70–75.
176. Mountain CF. Revisions in the international system for staging lung cancer. *Chest* 1997;111:1710–1717.
177. Hande KR, Des Prez RM. Current perspectives in small cell lung cancer. *Chest* 1984;85:669–677.
178. Hansen HH, Dombernowsky P, Hirsch FR. Staging procedures and prognostic features in small cell anaplastic bronchogenic carcinoma. *Semin Oncol* 1978;5:280–287.
179. Filderman AE, Shaw C, Matthay RA. Lung cancer: Part II. Staging and therapy. *Invest Radiol* 1986;21:173–185.
180. Swett HA, Nagel JS, Sostman HD. Imaging methods in primary lung carcinoma. *Clin Chest Med* 1982;3:331–351.
181. Inouye SK, Sox HC Jr. Standard and computed tomography in the evaluation of neoplasms of the chest. *Ann Intern Med* 1986;105:906–924.
182. Shields TW. Surgical therapy for carcinoma of the lung. *Clin Chest Med* 1993;14:121–147.
183. Webb WR, Jensen BG, Sollitto R. Bronchogenic carcinoma. Staging with MR compared with staging with CT and surgery. *Radiology* 1985;156:117–124.
184. Scott WJ, Dewan NA. Use of positron emission tomography to diagnose and stage lung cancer. *Clin Pulm Med* 1999;6: 198–204.
185. Vansteenkiste JF, Stroobants SG, DeLeyn PR, et al. Lymph node staging in non-small cell lung cancer with FDG-PET scan: a prospective study on 690 lymph node stations from 68 patients. *J Clin Oncol* 1998;16:2142–2149.
186. Higashi K, Ueda Y, Seki H, et al. Fluorine-18-FDG PET imaging is negative in bronchioloalveolar lung carcinoma. *J Nucl Med* 1998;39:1016–1020.
187. Kim BT, Kim Y, Lee KS, et al. Localized form of bronchioloalveolar carcinoma; FDG-PET findings. *AJR* 1998;170: 935–939.
188. Strauss LG, Conti PS. The application of PET in clinical oncology. *J Nucl Med* 1991;22:623–628.
189. Brantigan JW, Brantigan CO, Brantigan OC. Biopsy of nonpalpable scalene lymph nodes in carcinoma of the lung. *Am Rev Respir Dis* 1973;107:962–974.
190. Hashim SW, Baue AE, Geha AS. The role of mediastinoscopy and mediastinotomy in lung cancer. *Clin Chest Med* 1982;3: 353–359.
191. Nohl-Oser HC. Lymphatics of the lung. In Shields TW, ed. *General thoracic surgery.* Philadelphia: Lea & Febiger, 1972: 74–85.
192. Straus MJ. *Lung cancer: clinical diagnosis and treatment.* New York: Grune & Stratton, 1977:123.
193. Mountain CF, Dresler CM. Regional lymph node classification for lung staging. *Chest* 1997;111:1718–1723.
194. Sarin CG, Nohl-Oser HG. Mediastinoscopy. *Thorax* 1969;24: 585–588.
195. Bowen TE, Zajtchuk R, Green DC, et al. Value of anterior mediastinotomy in bronchogenic carcinoma of the left upper lobe. *J Thorac Cardiovasc Surg* 1978;76:269–271.
196. Sandler MA, Pearlberg JL, Madrazo BL, et al. Computed tomographic evaluation of the adrenal gland in the preoperative assessment of bronchogenic carcinoma. *Radiology* 1982;145: 733–736.
197. Hooper G, Beechler CR, Johnson MC. Radioisotope scanning in the initial staging of bronchogenic carcinoma. *Am Rev Respir Dis* 1978;118:279–286.
198. Ramsdell JW, Peters RM, Taylor AT, et al. Multiorgan scans for staging lung cancer. Correlation with clinical evaluation. *J Thorac Cardiovasc Surg* 1977;73:653–659.
199. Stoller JK, Ahmad M, Rice TW. Solitary pulmonary nodule. *Cleve Clin J Med* 1988;55:68–74.

200. Lillington GA, Caskey CI. Evaluation and management of solitary and multiple pulmonary nodules. *Clin Chest Med* 1993; 14:111–119.

201. Steel JD. Solitary pulmonary nodule. *J Thorac Cardiovasc Surg* 1963;46:21–39.

202. Martini N, Beattie EJ Jr. Results of surgical treatment in stage I lung cancer. *J Thorac Cardiovasc Surg* 1977;74:499–505.

203. Naruke T, Goya T, Tsuchiya T, et al. Prognosis and survival in resected lung carcinoma based on the new international staging system. *J Thorac Cardiovasc Surg* 1988;96:440–447.

204. Yellin A, Benfield JR. Surgery for bronchogenic carcinoma in the elderly. *Am Rev Respir Dis* 1985;131:197–198.

205. Luketich JD, Ginsberg RJ. Limited resection versus lobectomy for Stage I non-small cell lung cancer. In Pass HI, Mitchell JB, Johnson DH, et al. *Lung cancer principles and practice.* Philadelphia: Lippincott-Raven, 1996:561–566.

206. Martini N, Kris MG, Ginsberg RJ, et al. The role of multimodality therapy in local regional non-small cell lung cancer. *Surg Oncol Clin N Am* 1997;6:769–791.

207. Martini N, Flehinger BJ, Zaman MB, et al. Prospective study of 445 lung carcinomas with mediastinal lymph node metastases. *J Thorac Cardiovasc Surg* 1980;80:390–399.

208. Rosell P, Gomez-Codina J, Camps C, et al. A randomized trial comparing preoperative chemotherapy plus surgery with surgery alone in patients with non-small-cell lung cancer. *N Engl J Med* 1994;330:153–158.

209. Roth JA, Fossella F, Komaki R, et al. A randomized trial comparing peri-operative chemotherapy and surgery with surgery alone in resectable stage IIIA non-small-cell lung cancer. *J Natl Cancer Inst* 1994;86:673–680.

210. Lung Cancer Study Group. Effects of postoperative mediastinal radiation on completely resected stage II and stage III epidermoid cancer of the lung. *N Engl J Med* 1986;315:1377–1381.

211. Lung Cancer Study Group. Surgical adjuvant therapy for stage II and III adenocarcinoma and large-cell undifferentiated carcinoma. *J Clin Oncol* 1986;4:710–715.

212. Friess GG, McCracken JD, Troxell ML, et al. Effect of initial resection of small-cell carcinoma of the lung: a review of Southwestern Oncology Group Study 7628. *J Clin Oncol* 1985;3: 964–968.

213. Olsen GN, Block AJ, Tobias JA. Prediction of postpneumonectomy pulmonary function using quantitative macroaggregate lung scanning. *Chest* 1984;66:13–16.

214. Sause WT, Turrisi AT. Principles and applications of preoperative and standard radiotherapy for regionally advanced nonsmall cell lung cancer. In Pass HI, Mitchell JB, Johnson DH et al. *Lung cancer principles and practice.* Philadelphia: Lippincott-Raven, 1996:697–710.

215. Bloedern FG, Cowley RW, Cuccia CA, et al. Combined therapy: irradiation and surgery in the treatment of bronchogenic carcinoma. *Am J Roentgenol* 1961;85:875–885.

216. Coy P, Kennelly GM. The role of curative radiotherapy in the treatment of lung cancer. *Cancer* 1980;45:698–702.

217. Smart J, Hilton G. Radiotherapy of cancer of the lung: results in a selected group of cases. *Lancet* 1956;270:880–881.

218. Cooper JD, Pearson G, Todd TRJ, et al. Radiotherapy alone for patients with operable carcinoma of the lung. *Chest* 1985; 87:289–292.

219. Silbey GS. Radiotherapy for patients with medically inoperable Stage I nonsmall cell lung cancer—a review. *Cancer* 1998;82: 432–438.

220. Hilaris BS, Luomanen RK, Beattie EJ. Integrated irradiation and surgery in the treatment of apical lung cancer. *Cancer* 1971; 27:1369–1373.

221. Sandler AB. Current management of small cell lung cancer. *Semin Oncol* 1997;24:463–476.

222. Bunn PA JR, Carney DN. Overview of chemotherapy for small cell lung cancer. *Semin Oncol* 1997;24(2 suppl 7):S7-69–S7-74.

223. Hansen HH, Elliott JA. Patterns of failure in small cell lung cancer: implications for therapy. Recent results. *Cancer Res* 1984;92:43–57.

224. Perry MC, Eaton WL, Propert KJ, et al. Chemotherapy with or without radiation therapy in limited small-cell carcinoma of the lung. *N Engl J Med* 1987;316:912–918.

225. Rosen ST, Makuch RW, Lichter AS, et al. Role of prophylactic cranial irradiation in prevention of central nervous system metastases in small cell lung cancer. Potential benefit restricted to patients with complete response. *Am J Med* 1983;74:615–624.

226. Ball DL, Matthews JP. Prophylactic cranial irradiation in small cell lung cancer. In Pass HI, Mitchell JB, Johnson DH, et al. *Lung cancer principles and practice.* Philadelphia: Lippincott-Raven, 1996:761–773.

227. Murren JR, Buzaid AC. Chemotherapy and radiation for the treatment of non-small cell lung cancer: a critical review. *Clin Chest Med* 1993;14:161–171.

228. Sullivan FJ. Palliative radiotherapy for lung cancer. In Pass HI, Mitchell JB, Johnson DH, et al. *Lung cancer principles and practice.* Philadelphia: Lippincott-Raven, 1996:775–789.

229. Roswit B, Patno ME, Rapp R, et al. The survival of patients with inoperable lung cancer: a large scale randomized study of radiation therapy versus placebo. *Radiology* 1968;90:688–697.

230. Cox JD. Radiotherapeutic management of complications of carcinoma of the lung. *Clin Chest Med* 1982;3:415–421.

231. Gross NJ. Pulmonary effects of radiation therapy. *Ann Intern Med* 1977;86:81–92.

232. Travis EL, Komaki R. Treatment related to lung damage. In Pass HI, Mitchell JB, Johnson DH, et al. *Lung cancer principles and practice.* Philadelphia: Lippincott-Raven, 1996:285–301.

233. Bunn PA JR, Kelly K. New chemotherapeutic agents prolong survival and improve quality of life in non-small cell lung cancer: a review of the literature and future directions. *Clin Cancer Res* 1998;5:1087–1110.

234. Sweeney CJ, Sandler AB. Treatment of advanced (stage III and IV) non-small-cell lung cancer. *Current Problems in Lung Cancer* 1998;222:85–132.

235. Souhami R. Chemotherapy in non-small cell bronchial carcinoma. *Thorax* 1985;40:641–645.

236. Aisner J, Alberto P, Bitran J, et al. Role of chemotherapy in small cell lung cancer: a consensus report of the International Association for the Study of Lung Cancer Workshop. *Cancer Treat Rep* 1983;67:37–43.

237. Ihde DC. Current status of therapy for small cell carcinoma of the lung. *Cancer* 1984;54:2722–2728.

238. Hetzel MR, Nixon C, Edmonstone WM, et al. Laser therapy in 100 tracheobronchial tumors. *Thorax* 1985;40:341–345.

239. Cortese DA, Edell ES. Role of phototherapy, laser therapy and prosthetic stents in the management of lung cancer. *Clin Chest Med* 1993;14:149–159.

240. Mostovych M, Mathisen DJ. Management of malignant airway obstruction. In Pass HI, Mitchell JB, Johnson DH, et al. *Lung cancer principles and practice.* Philadelphia: Lippincott-Raven, 1996:663–669.

241. Dasgupta A, Dolmatch BL, Abi-Saleh WJ, et al. Self-expandable metallic airway stent insertion employing flexible bronchoscopy. *Chest* 1998;114:106–109.

15

RESPIRATORY TRACT INFECTIONS

MICHAEL S. NIEDERMAN
GEORGE A. SAROSI

EPIDEMIOLOGY OF RESPIRATORY INFECTIONS

DEFINITIONS

BACTERIOLOGY OF THE RESPIRATORY TRACT
The Normal Respiratory Tract

SPECIFIC INFECTIOUS SYNDROMES—CLINICAL FEATURES AND THERAPY
The Upper Respiratory Tract
Airway Infections
Parenchymal Lung Infections
Fungal Lung Disease: Normal Host
Opportunistic Fungal Infections

In spite of the sophistication and advances in modern medicine, respiratory tract infections remain a major source of morbidity, mortality, and economic cost in our society. The availability of new and potent antibiotics, the development of rapid and elegant diagnostic methods, the emergence of effective vaccines for certain infections, and the appreciation of the role of newly recognized organisms in causing disease have not reduced the scope of the problem presented by respiratory tract infections. In fact, the current ability of modern medicine to extend life and the application of novel life-sustaining therapies have created patient populations with specific impairments in their ability to resist infection and have thereby added to the problem of one specific infection: pneumonia. The patient at risk for pneumonia is always changing, and we now have individuals with novel forms of immunosuppressive illness as the result of organ transplantation or infection with the HIV virus. Although our therapeutic armamentarium is ever expanding, the organisms responsible for respiratory infections continue to adapt to the selective pressure of antibiotics. In the new millennium, we have multiple-drug-resistant tuberculosis, penicillin-resistant pneumococci, β-lactamase-producing *Haemophilus influenzae,* and highly resistant Gram-negative enteric bacteria. The changing epidemiology and ecology of respiratory infections make these illnesses an ongoing challenge.

EPIDEMIOLOGY OF RESPIRATORY INFECTIONS

The common cold is a viral infection of the upper respiratory tract that accounts for 20% of all acute disabling conditions annually in the United States and for 40% of all acute respiratory conditions. Adults have more than 100 million disabling colds annually, leading to 250 million days of restricted activity and 30 million lost days of work, amounting to a staggering economic impact (1). Furthermore, more than 1 billion dollars are spent annually on over-the-counter cold remedies. In spite of these data, a preventative vaccine for the common cold is unlikely because more than 200 different viruses lead to this type of infection. Similarly, the common cold is an unavoidable annual event for most adults because, even with four colds per year, it would take at least 50 years to contract an infection with every available cold virus and to develop immunity to each one.

Pneumonia, or infection of the lung parenchyma, is also common and occurs in as many as 6 million Americans annually. Pneumonia can occur in the community or in the hospital, and different types of individuals have varying susceptibilities to this infection. It has been estimated that there are 1.1 million cases of community-acquired pneumonia requiring hospitalization each year, at an estimated cost of $8.0 billion (2). Community-acquired infections may be viral, bacterial, or, rarely, fungal and parasitic. Nosocomial or hospital-acquired pneumonia occurs yearly in at least 275,000 individuals and is the most important hospital-acquired infection because it is associated with the highest mortality rate of nosocomial infections that contribute causally to death (3). Most nosocomial pneumonias are bacterial in origin, although hospital-acquired viral infections can also occur, particularly if personnel come to work carrying such an illness. In addition to direct patient care costs, pneumonia is responsible for over 50 million days of restricted activity from work and (in concert with influenza) is the sixth leading cause of death in this country, with a mortality rate of 13.4 per 100,000 (4,5). In 1991 there were an estimated 129.6 million episodes of influenza which accounted for over 450 million restricted-activity days (5).

Certain patient populations have an enhanced risk for pneumonia that reflects their disease-associated impairments in respiratory tract host defenses. Among the elderly, pneumonia is the fourth leading cause of death, with a mortality rate of 169.7 per 100,000 (6). Similarly, 80% of the excess deaths from influenza are in individuals above the age of 65 (5). This enhanced rate of dying from respiratory infection with advancing age has been recognized for a long time, and Sir William Osler called pneumonia the "friend of the aged" that allowed the elderly an escape from "those 'cold gradations of decay' that make the last state of all so distressing" (7).

Among the elderly, the risk of pneumonia varies with an individual's general health and is often reflected by his or her place of residence. Thus pneumonia occurs in 25 to 44 per 1,000 noninstitutionalized elderly individuals and in 68 to 114 per 1,000 residents of chronic care institutions. At any one time, as many as 3.2% of all nursing home residents will have pneumonia (8). In the hospital, the elderly have a threefold greater incidence of pneumonia than younger patients, with 1.6% of all hospital admissions in the elderly being complicated by lung infection (8). In one study, patients over the age of 60 represented only 23% of all hospitalized patients, yet they accounted for 64% of all nosocomial infections (9). In the National Nosocomial Infection Surveillance (NNIS) study, 54% of more than 100,000 nosocomial infections were seen in patients over the age of 55. Pneumonia was more common in the elderly than in younger patients and accounted for 48% of all infection-related mortality in the elderly (10).

Among critically ill patients treated with mechanical ventilation, nosocomial pneumonia develops in 20% to 55% of all patients, depending on the type of illness that led to the need for mechanical ventilation. Patients who have had general surgery and require mechanical ventilation in an intensive care unit (ICU) have at least a 10% incidence of pneumonia; a general medical ICU population has a 20% incidence; and patients with the acute respiratory distress syndrome (ARDS) have a 55% incidence of secondary pneumonia (11). Particularly with ARDS, the mortality implications of this infection can be striking. In one study, if ARDS was complicated by pneumonia, only 12% of patients survived, while if the ARDS patient remained free of infection, survival rate was 67% (12). In contrast, in one recent study, the mortality rate of patients with ARDS and pneumonia was high, but it was no higher than for ARDS patients without pneumonia (11). These data raise the question of "attributable mortality," namely whether some patients are so ill that pneumonia does not add further to their risk of dying. Although not all populations, particularly surgical trauma patients, have an attributable mortality from nosocomial pneumonia, recent data have shown that many patients do not die merely with nosocomial pneumonia but in fact they actually die because of nosocomial pneumonia,

with up to half of all deaths being the direct effect of infection and not comorbid illness (13,14).

Other groups at increased risk for pneumonia include patients with cardiac disease, alcoholism, chronic obstructive lung disease, malnutrition, head injury, cystic fibrosis or bronchiectasis, splenic dysfunction, malignancy, cirrhosis, diabetes, renal failure, sickle cell disease, and any immunosuppressive therapy or disease state. Recognition of the increased risk of infection in all of these patient groups should prompt the use of available vaccines to prevent respiratory infection.

Bronchitis—infection of the large bronchi—can be caused by either viruses or bacteria. In children, more than 40% of episodes of acute bronchitis are viral and the remainder are bacterial. Viral bronchitis in children may lead to transient or even persistent airway hyperreactivity and thereby may be a risk factor for subsequent adult asthma. Chronic bronchitis is an adult disease characterized by a persistent inflammatory state of the large airways, generally caused by cigarette smoking, and found in 12.5 million Americans (5,15–17). Patients with this condition frequently have acute infectious bronchitis (viral or bacterial) superimposed on their chronic condition, with such exacerbations happening on average three times per year (18). Bronchiolitis is an acute infection, usually viral, of the small airways that occurs in children usually between the ages of one month and one year, with an attack rate in this age group of six to seven cases per 100 children per year (19).

In recent years, particularly with the application of immunosuppressive therapy for a variety of illnesses, with the emergence of the acquired immune deficiency syndrome (AIDS), and with an increasing number of institutionalized elderly individuals, tuberculosis and fungal and parasitic lung infections have emerged once again as important and common infections. Mycobacterial illnesses frequently complicate AIDS or occur in nursing homes, and fungal infections may emerge from a dormant state in patients living in endemic areas when a disease such as AIDS develops. From 1985 to 1992, the incidence of tuberculosis increased, but this trend has recently reversed, with the case rate falling below 10 per 100,000. Certain populations are at increased risk for tuberculosis, particularly blacks, Hispanics, and immigrant populations. Minority groups now account for as many as 70% of all tuberculosis cases in the United States, even though they represent only one-quarter of the population (5,20). An additional concern today is the emergence of multiple-drug-resistant disease, a phenomenon that is particularly common in certain areas of the country such as large cities in the Northeast.

DEFINITIONS

The respiratory tract can be anatomically divided into an upper and lower system, with the vocal cords serving as the dividing line between them. Infections of the upper respiratory tract include the common cold, sinusitis, pharyngitis, tonsillitis, and epiglottitis. Influenza is a viral infection that can involve the epithelial cells of both the upper and lower respiratory tract, and some patients have predominantly upper-respiratory infectious symptoms while others have more marked lower-airway signs and symptoms.

Infections of the lower respiratory tract can involve the airways, lung parenchyma, or pleural space. When infection involves the large airways, it is termed bronchitis, and symptoms are a reflection of this localization, with patients complaining of cough, sputum production, and often wheezing. If the infection involves smaller, more peripheral airways, it is termed bronchiolitis; this infection primarily involves children, but recently an adult version, possibly initiated by an infectious agent, has been recognized and is termed "bronchiolitis obliterans with organizing pneumonia." One chronic airways disease, bronchiectasis, is often a consequence of preceding respiratory infection and is frequently characterized by multiple episodes of infection in the areas of diseased airways. Bronchiectasis is characterized pathologically by abnormal and permanent dilation of subsegmental airways, which are inflamed and usually filled with secretions (20). It is these areas of stagnant secretions that frequently become infected. Similarly, chronic bronchitis, a disease usually caused by cigarette smoking, is often complicated by bouts of acute infectious bronchitis.

Pneumonia is an infection of the lung parenchyma itself, involving the alveolar space with microbial invasion. In the immunocompetent individual, this type of infection is accompanied by a brisk filling of the alveolar space with inflammatory cells and fluid. When this alveolar infection involves an entire anatomic lobe of the lung, it is termed "lobar pneumonia," and more than one lobe can be involved in some instances. When the alveolar process occurs in a distribution that is patchy and is adjacent to bronchi without filling an entire lobe, it is termed a "bronchopneumonia." From a clinical perspective, pneumonias have been classified as being "typical" or "atypical," depending on their mode of clinical presentation. Although the "typical" pneumonia syndrome is characterized by sudden onset of fever, chills, pleuritic chest pain, and productive cough, this type of presentation can be expected only if the patient has an intact immune response system and if the infection is due to a bacterial pathogen such as *Streptococcus pneumoniae, H. influenzae, Klebsiella pneumoniae, Staphylococcus aureus,* aerobic Gram-negative bacilli, or anaerobes. If a patient is infected by one of these organisms but has an impaired immune response, the classic pneumonia symptoms may be absent, as can be the case with the elderly and debilitated patient. The atypical pneumonia syndrome, characterized by preceding upper respiratory symptoms, fever without chills, nonproductive cough, headache, myalgias, and mild leukocytosis, is often the result of infection with viruses, *Mycoplasma pneumoniae, Legionella* organisms and other un-usual infectious agents (as in psittacosis and Q fever). In clinical practice it is often very difficult to use this type of classification to predict the microbial etiology of pneumonia. In fact, clinical features may be at best only 40% accurate in distinguishing *M. pneumoniae,* pneumococcus, and other pathogens (22). Another classification system that is often applied to pneumonias is their place of origin, and thus the infection can be community-acquired or hospital-acquired (nosocomial). Patients who develop pneumonia while receiving immunosuppressive therapy or having abnormal immune systems are referred to as compromised hosts, and the infectious possibilities will vary with the localization of the immune defect.

When a parenchymal lung infection leads to necrosis and breakdown of lung tissue and a cavity is evident within the pneumonic area, the infection is termed a lung abscess. These infections are usually caused by anaerobes, but other etiologic agents include *S. aureus, K. pneumoniae, Escherichia coli,* and *Pseudomonas aeruginosa.* Empyema is an infection of the pleural space characterized by grossly purulent material and usually caused by anaerobes, Gram-negative bacilli, or *S. aureus.*

BACTERIOLOGY OF THE RESPIRATORY TRACT

The Normal Respiratory Tract

Certain sites in the respiratory tract are sterile under normal conditions, and the isolation of a microorganism from these sites generally connotes infection; other sites may contain organisms because they are colonized but not infected. When organisms persist at a particular body site without evidence of a host response or without adverse effects to the host, it is termed colonization. When organisms lead to a host response or adverse tissue effects, then an infection is present. Respiratory tract sites that are sterile in normal individuals include the paranasal sinuses and the lower respiratory tract. Although bacteria can colonize the proximal tracheobronchial tree of smokers and others with impaired host defenses, the more distal areas of the lung are normally sterile unless infection is present. On the other hand, the nasopharynx and oropharynx are normally colonized and have an endogenous microflora; it is the identity of these colonizing organisms that changes when disease is present.

The Upper Airway

The oropharynx is normally colonized by a mixture of aerobic and microaerophilic bacteria as well as by anaerobic organisms. The "normal" oral flora can include *S. mitis, Streptococcus salivarius, Staphylococcus epidermidis, Neisseria* species, pneumococcus, *Candida* species and lactobacilli. Colonizing anaerobes include *Veillonella* species, *Fusobacte-*

TABLE 15.1. COMMON PATHOGENS FOR UPPER RESPIRATORY TRACT INFECTIONS

Pharyngitis
  Group A streptococci
  Viruses
    Adenovirus
    Enteroviruses
    Influenza
    Epstein-Barr virus
    Herpesvirus hominis
Laryngitis
  Viruses
Common cold
  Viruses
    Rhinovirus
    Adenovirus
    Coronavirus
    Influenza
Sinusitis
  Haemophilus influenzae
  Pneumococcus
  Anaerobes
  Rhinovirus
Epiglottitis
  H. influenzae
  Haemophilus parainfluenzae
  Staphylococcus aureus
  Group A streptococcus
Croup
  Viruses
    Parainfluenza virus
    Respiratory syncytial virus
    Adenovirus
Mycoplasma pneumoniae

rium species, anaerobic streptococci and micrococci, and certain *Bacteroides* species (19,23). Conspicuously absent from this group of bacteria are the enteric Gram-negative bacilli. Multiple investigators have shown that normal individuals are not colonized by these Gram-negative bacteria, but patients with serious illness of any type may harbor these organisms in the oropharynx. The likelihood that a given individual will have upper-airway colonization by these bacteria is directly related to the severity and duration of illness. Patients with "moderate" illness will harbor Gram-negative organisms in the oropharynx 35% of the time, while 73% of "moribund" individuals will be colonized (24). Most patients develop colonization of the oropharynx when they enter a hospital, usually by the third hospital day. Risk factors for upper-airway colonization include alcoholism, endotracheal intubation, neutropenia, prior antibiotic use, azotemia, coma, hypotension, smoking, surgery, prior viral illness, and malnutrition (23–25).

The microbial ecology of the upper airway changes with infection, and the bacteriology of infection is different, depending on the site (Table 15.1). This tendency of specific organisms to cause infection at one airway site but not an-

other can be described as a "tissue tropism," or preference, of certain organisms for certain epithelial locations. The reason for tissue tropisms is not fully known, but their existence would suggest that colonization and infection proceed in unique ways for each mucosal site, making some sites more susceptible to the effects of a particular organism than are others.

The Tracheobronchial Tree

The lower respiratory tract is sterile in healthy individuals but may become colonized when illness is present (26). Smokers commonly will have *H. influenzae* recovered from tracheobronchial secretions, even when there is no evidence of an acute bronchitis. In patients with chronic bronchitis, tracheobronchial colonization is common and can include *H. influenzae,* pneumococci, *Moraxella catarrhalis,* and occasionally enteric Gram-negative bacteria (23). Gram-negative colonization becomes a particularly common event if

TABLE 15.2. COMMON PATHOGENS FOR LOWER RESPIRATORY TRACT INFECTIONS

Bronchitis
  Haemophilus influenzae
  Pneumococcus
  Moraxella catarrhalis
  Mycoplasma pneumoniae
  Viruses
    Adenovirus
    Influenza
    Rhinovirus
    Respiratory syncytial virus
Bronchiolitis
  Viruses
    Respiratory syncytial virus
    Parainfluenza virus
    Adenovirus
    Rhinovirus
Pneumonia
  Pneumococcus
  Legionella pneumophilia
  M. pneumoniae
  C. pneumoniae
  H. influenzae
  Anaerobes
  Staphylococcus aureus
  Enteric Gram-negatives
  Viruses
    Influenza
    Respiratory syncytial virus
    Adenovirus
  Chlamydia psittaci
  Pneumocystis carinii
Bronchiectasis
  Pseudomonas aeruginosa
  S. aureus
  Mucoid *Escherichia coli*
  H. influenzae

the patient has one of a variety of acute or chronic illnesses, including ciliary dysfunction (cystic fibrosis and bronchiectasis), corticosteroid therapy, immunodeficiency, tracheostomy, prior antibiotic therapy, viral infection, malnutrition, and endotracheal intubation (23,25). Most bacteria enter the lower airway via aspiration from a previously colonized oropharynx, and thus there is frequently congruence of organism identity at the two respiratory tract sites. Occasionally, organisms reach the lung hematogenously from nonrespiratory sites of infection. Inhalation is not a major route of bacterial entry to the lung, with the exception of certain organisms such as *Legionella pneumophila viruses* and *Mycobacterium tuberculosis*. More recently, the intestinal tract has been identified as another potential source of organism entry to the lung. Either by reflux or by passage along a nasogastric tube, gastric bacteria can enter the oropharynx and then be aspirated into the lung. Although many studies have documented the presence of this route of infection, controversy exists as to how commonly this route of entry actually operates in the ICU patient (27). Also, in critically ill patients treated with an endotracheal tube or tracheostomy, certain organisms, such as *P. aeruginosa,* can enter the lower airway directly from environmental sources, and colonization can follow (28).

With infectious illness, as with the upper respiratory tract, the lower airway and lung parenchyma can also become infected with different organisms at different sites. These "tropisms" of specific organisms causing specific illnesses are summarized in Table 15.2.

SPECIFIC INFECTIOUS SYNDROMES—CLINICAL FEATURES AND THERAPY

The Upper Respiratory Tract

The Common Cold

The common cold is a symptom complex caused by one of more than 200 viral agents. The most common viral etiologic agent is a rhinovirus, of which there are at least 100 types (29). Other common agents causing this infection are adenovirus, coronavirus, parainfluenza virus, respiratory syncytial virus, and influenza A, B, and C viruses. Less common viral pathogens include enterovirus, Epstein-Barr, and herpes simplex viruses. Typical symptoms include nasal congestion and discharge, sneezing, sore throat, and cough. In contrast to some other viral illnesses, upper-respiratory tract symptoms predominate, while systemic symptoms are mild or absent, and fever is not usually high. The incubation period of the illness varies for each virus, but is generally 48 to 72 hours (30). The illness may last up to one week, but up to one-quarter of patients will be ill for up to two weeks. When symptoms persist, consideration must be given to the occurrence of a secondary bacterial infection

such as sinusitis (in 0.5% of cases) or pharyngitis. Other complications can include bacterial otitis media (in 2% of cases) and persistent bronchospastic cough. Physical findings are generally confined to the upper respiratory tract and include nasal mucosal swelling and exudation and pharyngeal erythema. Only a few viral "colds" will be accompanied by an exudative pharyngitis, most notably those caused by adenovirus.

Most adults develop two to four colds per year, while children may have six to eight such infections. Smokers have more frequent and more severe viral respiratory illnesses (31). Illness is more common in the fall and winter, helping to distinguish a cold from seasonal allergies, which are more common in the spring and early fall. The major route of viral transmission is person to person via the hand-nose-hand inoculation route, but there is some evidence that cold viruses can also be spread via droplet nuclei generated by sneezing (32).

Therapy is entirely symptomatic and supportive unless a secondary bacterial infection supervenes. Nasal decongestants, warm saline gargles, cough suppressants, and antipyretics are generally effective, along with bed rest. Aspirin should be used cautiously in children and adolescents because of its association with Reye's syndrome, especially after influenza and varicella infection. Antibiotics should not be routinely administered unless bacterial infection is present. Therapy with vitamin C is unproven. Echinacea has also been studied, and compared to placebo was not able to decrease the incidence, duration or severity of colds and respiratory infections (33). Some data have shown that zinc lozenges can reduce the duration of symptoms in adults, but this therapy has not proven of benefit to children and adolescents (34). Prevention of cold transmission can be achieved by careful hand-washing after contact with an infected individual. Experimental prophylactic approaches have included the use of virucidal-impregnated tissues to wipe the nose of infected individuals and the application of intranasal interferon alpha-2 (35).

Sinusitis

Infection of one or more of the paranasal sinuses can be a cryptogenic event (5% of cases) or can be associated with other conditions such as viral upper-respiratory infection, allergic rhinitis, or mechanical obstruction of the sinuses. There are four different paranasal sinuses; they are ordinarily sterile but they can fill with serous fluid when the ostia are obstructed as the result of inflammation or infection. The fluid-filled sinus can in turn become infected by viruses (especially rhinovirus), pneumococcus, *H. influenzae, M. catarrhalis,* or anaerobes. Most cases result from the common cold or from allergic rhinitis leading to ostial obstruction, but 10% to 15% of cases can arise from a dental abscess. The maxillary sinus is most frequently infected in both adults and children; the frontal sinus is the second most commonly infected site in adults (29).

If the maxillary or frontal sinuses are affected, the patient may note facial pain and tenderness to percussion over these areas. Purulent nasal discharge and low-grade fever are common symptoms. Infection of the ethmoid sinus can result in retro-orbital pain, tearing, and headache that worsens in the supine position. Sphenoidal sinusitis may lead to a vertex headache that is most severe at night.

A clinical diagnosis of sinusitis can be made with typical headache pain and other associated findings, particularly if they arise after a viral upper-respiratory tract infection. Transillumination of the sinuses can also lead to a diagnosis. To perform this maneuver for the maxillary sinus, a light is placed over the orbital rim, and transmission to the hard palate is observed. Opacity by this maneuver is highly related to bacterial infection, while bright transillumination makes sinus infection unlikely (36). Sinus radiographs may also confirm the diagnosis. In fact a four-view radiographic series is 72% to 96% as accurate for demonstrating maxillary sinusitis as is sinus aspiration and culture (37). When sinus radiographs are used to define the illness, certain clinical findings can be elicited that correlate highly with the presence of radiographic abnormalities. In a logistic regression model (37), patients were likely to have sinusitis if they had at least four of the following signs or symptoms: maxillary toothache, poor response of symptoms to nasal decongestants, a history of colored nasal discharge, purulent nasal secretions, and an abnormal transillumination of the sinuses. Sinus tenderness is only present in about half of all patients with sinusitis. In addition to acute sinusitis, some patients can have resolution and then recurrent acute sinusitis, while others can have chronic sinusitis. The latter is defined as purulent or mucopurulent sinus discharge for at least three months, usually due to chronic inflammatory changes initiated by a preceding acute infection.

Bacteriologic studies have shown that sinusitis is caused by *H. influenzae,* pneumococcus, and anaerobes, with viruses (rhinovirus, influenza virus, parainfluenza virus) being found occasionally. Less common are *S. aureus,* Gram-negative bacteria, and fungi (36). Patients with chronic sinusitis can have any of these organisms, with many having staphylococci, although the bacteria may be commensals and not true pathogens. Based on this spectrum, therapy of acute sinusitis is usually with an oral antimicrobial agent for 10 to 14 days. Some clinical improvement should be seen within 48 hours of therapy, but if the findings are not completely resolved by two weeks, then an additional week of therapy may be used. Appropriate therapy can be achieved with ampicillin, 2 g daily, or trimethoprim-sulfamethoxazole. Use of β-lactamase-resistant agents may also be appropriate if resistance to ampicillin is encountered, an increasingly likely possibility with many of the etiologic organisms producing β-lactamase enzymes. The fluoroquinolones may also be effective therapy, and these agents generally cover the spectrum of likely pathogens. Adjunctive therapy can include analgesics and decongestants. When antibiotic therapy does not work, complications such as osteomyelitis, facial cellulitis, intracranial abscess, cavernous sinus thrombosis, and even meningitis must be considered.

Epiglottitis

Acute swelling and inflammation of the epiglottis and aryepiglottic folds caused by an infectious agent can be a life-threatening illness, particularly in children. This infection does not descend into the lower airway and is usually bacterial, with *H. influenzae* type B being the most common etiologic pathogen (38–41). The seriousness of this infection is related to its potential to cause sudden upper-airway obstruction and asphyxiation. The disease is more common in children than adults, with the incidence greatest between the ages of two and four and with a peak around the age of three and a half. There is no seasonal predisposition. Adults can develop this illness, with an incidence as high as 9.7 cases per million (38).

Patients with epiglottitis fall into one of three age ranges: below the age of two, above the age of two, and adults. Children above the age of two present with "classic" epiglottitis (40), with symptoms of sore throat or mild upper-respiratory symptoms that can rapidly progress to high fever, drooling, dysphagia, and lethargy (42). The symptoms can be described as the "four Ds" of dysphagia, dysphonia, dyspnea, and drooling (40). Generally, all patients have respiratory distress, and breathing can be noisy with signs of inspiratory stridor. Unlike the case with croup, there is not a prominent cough, stridor is lower-pitched, and patients are generally older (the peak age for croup is two years).

When adults develop this disease, sore throat is the most common symptom, with less than one-half of the patients having respiratory distress and approximately one-quarter having drooling. Both infants (below the age of 2) and adults have a similar form of illness that is more a supraglottitis than an epiglottitis. In infants the illness is similar to croup but with a more severe clinical course. In adults, the infection is also primarily a supraglottitis, and the disease can be either gradual or accelerated (43). Factors associated with a more accelerated illness and the need for intubation are bacteremia and tachycardia (41). The most common pathogens in adults are type B *H. influenzae, S. aureus,* and *Klebsiella* species (40). In adults, abscess formation can be a complication, and the bacteriology of these lesions includes *S. aureus* and a variety of streptococci.

The diagnosis is usually made by recognition of typical signs and symptoms. An attempt at direct or indirect visualization of the epiglottis may reveal the presence of a swollen, cherry-red epiglottis projecting over the back of the tongue. The patient should never be examined with a tongue blade, as this may precipitate total airway obstruction. A lateral neck radiograph can confirm the diagnosis when the "thumb sign" of an enlarged epiglottis is seen, but this technique may be negative even with life-threatening disease. In adults, the findings may be more subtle, with only mild erythema or even pale edema of the epiglottis. In one series, lateral neck radiographs were abnormal in 79% of affected adults (38). Recently, other radiographic signs of epiglottitis have been described. In one series, epiglottic width in relation to epiglottic height or in relation to the width of the third cervical vertebra has been described as a sensitive and specific diagnostic finding (44). In adults, laryngoscopy (direct, indirect, or flexible) can establish the diagnosis and generally can be preformed safely and without complications (41). Other diseases to be considered in the differential diagnosis are angioedema, bacterial tracheitis, croup, foreign body aspiration, and peritonsillar abscess.

Management is directed at maintenance of a patent airway to minimize mortality. With the use of a prophylactic artificial airway, mortality in children has fallen below 1%. In adults, mortality was 7% in one series in which routine establishment of an artificial airway was not used. In that series, 15 of 56 patients had airway compromise and differed from less ill patients with a higher incidence of respiratory difficulty and positive blood cultures. All deaths were within 6 hours of hospital admission, indicating how rapidly progressive this illness may be. It is currently recommended that all affected children have an artificial airway established via orotracheal or nasotracheal intubation, usually under general anesthesia, and only if this cannot be done is a tracheostomy needed. Routine intubation in adults is controversial, and management must be individualized, with careful observation being essential in the early hours of illness. In one series of 30 adults seen over a 10-year period, no patient required intubation or tracheostomy (43).

Other adjunctive measures include humidified oxygen and antibiotics. The pediatric illness is almost always caused by *H. influenzae,* and in adults *H. influenzae* is still the predominant organism, being recovered in 56% of patients in one series (38). Blood cultures are positive, usually for *H. influenzae,* in up to 75% of children and 23% of adults. As mentioned, other possible infecting agents include pneumococcus, *S. aureus, H. parainfluenzae, Fusobacterium* spp., and group A streptococcus. With this bacteriologic spectrum in mind, therapy is usually with ampicillin (200 mg per kg per day in six divided doses), ampicillin/sulbactam (if β-lactamase-resistant strains are suspected), or alternatively, a second- or third-generation cephalosporin. The use of corticosteroids in conjunction with an antibiotic is of unproven benefit but may be helpful just prior to removal of an endotracheal tube to prevent laryngeal edema after extubation.

Other Upper Respiratory Tract Infections

Pharyngitis

Pharyngitis may occur with or without symptoms of the common cold. Etiologic agents may be viral or bacterial, with pharyngitis due to group A beta-hemolytic streptococci (GABHS) being potentially the most important to recognize and treat. In the first two years of life infection by group A streptococci is uncommon, but the incidence rises between the ages of five and 10. In children GABHS accounts for one-third of all cases of pharyngitis. In college-age students, one-quarter of cases are streptococcal, but viral pharyngitis is seen in 38% (45). In those over the age of 35, streptococcal infection is present in only 5% of those with pharyngitis (29). In children and adults, other common infecting agents besides streptococci include adenovirus, respiratory syncytial virus, rhinovirus, coronavirus, influenza and parainfluenza viruses, Epstein-Barr virus, herpesvirus hominis, and *M. pneumoniae.* Less common agents include *Neisseria gonorrhoeae* and *Neisseria meningitides, H. influenzae, Corynebacterium diphtheriae,* and anaerobes in a mixed pattern.

It may be difficult to distinguish the responsible pathogen from clinical features, but streptococcal pharyngitis onset may be sudden, with high fever, pharyngeal and uvular edema, yellowish pharyngeal exudate, along with red follicular lesions with yellow centers being found on the uvula. However, infections with the Epstein-Barr virus, herpesviruses, adenoviruses, and enteroviruses may also present with similar findings.

Streptococcal pharyngitis should be treated with penicillin VK, 500 mg every six hours for 10 days, or another antibiotic such as erythromycin if the patient is allergic. Therapy provides four benefits: reduction in illness duration, avoidance of spread to others, prevention of suppurative complications (such as peritonsillar and retropharyngeal abscess), and prevention of rheumatic fever (but probably not glomerulonephritis) (46).

Croup

Croup, or acute laryngotracheobronchitis, is a disease of young children usually between the ages of three months and three years, with a peak incidence in the second year of life. The etiology is usually viral, and this complication may occur in certain individuals while others infected with the same virus develop only a mild upper-respiratory illness. Some children develop recurrent episodes whenever they acquire a viral upper-respiratory infection, and in these instances the disease is termed "spasmodic croup." Parainfluenza virus type 1 is the most common cause, but the disease may also result from influenza viruses, respiratory syncytial virus, adenovirus, mycoplasma, or rhinoviruses (45). Patients with croup present with acute dyspnea following an upper-respiratory illness. A barking cough is seen, followed by symptoms of hoarseness and stridor. The stridor may be accompanied by severe dyspnea, and the course may be fluctuating, with improvement in the daytime. Airway edema is less severe than with epiglottitis, and thus acute upper-airway obstruction is less likely. Treatment is supportive, with inhalation of moist cold air, racemic epinephrine, and possibly steroids, the latter being controversial. Antibiotics are not needed unless the patient has secondary bacterial infection.

Airway Infections

Bronchitis

In the Previously Healthy Adult

Bronchitis is acute infection and inflammation of the large conducting airways and may be viral or bacterial in origin. When this infection occurs in a previously normal host, the resulting acute bronchitis will present in a manner very similar to a mild form of pneumonia, and the responsible pathogens will be similar for both illnesses. In the presence of chronic respiratory disease or chronic inflammatory bronchitis, the manifestations and etiologic agents will differ from those seen with acute bronchitis in the normal host.

Acute bronchitis in the normal host may be due to viruses in at least 40% of cases and these include adenovirus, influenza A and B virus, coronavirus, rhinovirus, herpes simplex, respiratory syncytial virus, and parainfluenza virus. The role of bacteria in acute bronchitis is difficult to establish, particularly in those with chronic bronchitis, because it may be difficult to distinguish colonization from infection. Bacterial agents implicated include *H. influenzae,* both typable and nontypable strains, and pneumococcus. *M. pneumoniae* may account for 10% of infections. Newer agents identified as causing bronchitis are *M. catarrhalis* and *Chlamydia pneumoniae* (also called the TWAR agent) (47).

Patients with bronchitis have symptoms of cough, purulent sputum, low-grade fever, chest burning, and substernal discomfort. These lower-respiratory symptoms usually follow a preceding upper respiratory infection. Hemoptysis can also occur, and acute bronchitis is the most common cause of this symptom. Dyspnea is generally mild, and the physical examination may demonstrate diffuse adventitious sounds such as crackles, rhonchi, and wheezes. Diagnosis is made by discovering appropriate clinical features in the absence of a lung infiltrate on chest film. Sputum Gram stain will show numerous polymorphonuclear cells and possibly bacterial pathogens. Therapy is supportive, with cough suppressants, liquids, and antipyretics. There is no clear role for antibiotics in this illness, and use in this setting can be reduced with patient education, an intervention that may help prevent antibiotic resistance and which is not associated with any adverse patient outcomes (48). Many patients with acute bronchitis will develop the frustrating complication of postinfectious bronchospasm. This is characterized by persistent dry cough and wheezing lasting four to six weeks after the acute infection subsides. Symptoms are treated with bronchodilators and sometimes corticosteroids, and only rarely will the airway reactivity persist and lead to chronic asthma. Some data indicate that children who have multiple episodes of acute viral bronchitis are at risk for developing adult chronic airways disease and asthma (49).

In the Patient with Chronic Lung Disease

Patients with chronic bronchitis and chronic lung disease frequently have episodes of acute bronchitis, but the clinical picture and bacteriology differ from those seen in the normal host. These episodes of acute airway infection occur every 20 to 78 weeks, with most studies reporting an exacerbation of chronic bronchitis on average three times per year (18). With infection, patients may note increasing dyspnea, purulent sputum, wheezing, fever, and general malaise. The three cardinal symptoms of an exacerbation—dyspnea, increased sputum purulence, and increased sputum volume—can be counted and used to grade the severity of an exacerbation. Patients with all three symptoms have the most severe exacerbation, a type 1 exacerbation (50). It has been estimated that 80% of all exacerbations are accompanied by two or three of these cardinal symptoms (50).

Examination may reveal diffuse crackles, rhonchi, or wheezes, and the chest radiograph shows no acute infiltrate. Exacerbations in this setting may be viral or bacterial, with some investigators believing that viral causes are most common. It is very difficult to reach such a conclusion with any certainty, since patients with chronic bronchitis have bacterial colonization of the tracheobronchial tree in the absence of acute infection, and thus the recovery of bacterial pathogens from their sputum may represent either colonization or infection. However, in one study that used quantitative bacteriologic methods in patients with severe exacerbation, nearly half of all patients had bacteria present in concentrations equal to that seen in the presence of pneumonia (51). Even with less severe exacerbations, bronchoscopic studies have reported that half of all episodes are bacterial in origin. The clinical features of exacerbation (fever, hypoxemia, leukocytosis) are similar for bacterial and nonbacterial episodes, making it difficult to identify the responsible pathogen on clinical grounds. Common viral pathogens are adenovirus, influenza, rhinovirus, coronavirus, herpes simplex, and respiratory syncytial virus. The most common bacterial pathogens are *H. influenzae,* pneumococcus, and *M. catarrhalis.* Other recently recognized pathogens include *Chlamydia pneumoniae* and *M. pneumoniae* (47). *Moraxella* spp. are neisseria-like organisms that have only recently been recognized as pathogens after being appreciated as simply part of the "normal" flora in the past (47,52). More than 90% of *Moraxella* spp. produce β-lactamase enzymes and are resistant to β-lactam antibiotics such as amoxicillin. Similarly, up to 40% of *H. influenzae* produce β-lactamase enzymes or are resistant to ampicillin via other mechanisms. Most patients with *Moraxella* infections have abnormal host defenses, with up to 77% being smokers and 84% having preexisting cardiopulmonary disease (52).

The role of antibiotics in treating acute bronchitic exacerbations of chronic bronchitis is controversial (16,53). The benefits of such therapy are uncertain in many studies, possibly because many episodes are viral. However, a recent meta-analysis has examined nine placebo-controlled studies and has concluded that antibiotics do speed the resolution of symptoms and the return of peak flow rates, especially if the patient has at least two of the cardinal symptoms of exacerbation (increased dyspnea, increased sputum volume, increased sputum purulence) (54). In addition, antibiotics can eradicate organisms and thus reduce the host inflammatory response to the presence of bacteria, thereby preventing inflammatory injury to the airway (16). In doing so, antibiotics may disrupt the "vicious cycle" of infection, inflammation, and further infection (53). In the past, amoxicillin, 500 mg three times a day for 10 days, or ampicillin were appropriate antibiotic choices, but now with the emergence of *M. catarrhalis* and β-lactamase-producing *H. influenzae* as pathogens, amoxicillin combined with a β-lactamase inhibitor (amoxicillin/clavulanate 500 mg every eight hours), a new cephalosporin, one of the new macrolides (azithromycin or clarithromycin), tetracycline, or a fluoroquinolone is an appropriate choice. Trimethoprim-sulfamethoxizole is no longer reliable against pneumococcus and erythromycin does not cover *H. influenzae,* and thus these agents should not be used. Because the bacteriology of exacerabation becomes more complex with the presence of comorbid illness, severe airway obstruction, and frequent exacerbations, these patients may need broader spectrum therapy than less complicated patients with acute exacerbations. For these more complex patients, therapy should focus on the quinolones and other β-lactamase resistant agents.

In patients treated with chronic tracheostomy or mechanical ventilation, an illness termed febrile tracheobronchitis may develop (55). Clinically the disease is similar to nosocomial pneumonia with fever, leukocytosis, and purulent respiratory secretions. In some individuals bacteremia may occur. Unlike with pneumonia, the patient has no new parenchymal lung infiltrate. The disease is diagnosed if the patient has a compatible clinical picture and no new parenchymal lung infiltrate. The etiology is usually enteric Gram-negative bacteria, particularly *P. aeruginosa* in the most seriously ill patients, and occasionally nontypable *H. influenzae.* Therapy is usually with systemic antibiotics directed against the responsible pathogen, but aerosolized antibiotics may be effective in patients without systemic toxicity.

Bronchiolitis

Bronchiolitis, an infection of the small airways, is primarily a viral infection of children, seen in the first year of life. Respiratory syncytial virus, parainfluenza virus type 3, influenza virus, adenovirus, and rhinovirus are the most common causes (19). Other infectious agents leading to bronchiolitis include *M. pneumoniae, L. pneumophila, Nocardia asteroides,* and *Pneumocystis carinii* (56). Children present with fever, tachypnea, wheezing, cough, and malaise. Therapy is supportive, with hydration, oxygen, and possibly bronchodilators. Recently, aerosolized ribavirin has been advocated to treat respiratory syncytial virus, a common cause of bronchiolitis in the midwinter and spring.

An adult form of this infection has been recognized and termed "bronchiolitis obliterans with organizing pneumonia" (BOOP). Although bronchiolitis obliterans can result from any viral bronchiolitis, the adult disease may present in an indolent fashion, with cough and dyspnea and no evident acute infection. Because of distal atelectasis beyond the inflamed airways, segmental infiltrates may be seen, in what has been termed the "proliferative" form of bronchiolitis (56). BOOP may be of viral origin or may be the result of inhalational injury, drug effects, or inflammation from a noninfectious systemic illness such as rheumatoid arthritis (56,57). Therapy is generally with corticosteroids.

Influenza

This acute respiratory infection results from an RNA virus of either type A or B, with the disease from type A being generally more severe (58). Influenza A virus is the most important respiratory virus on a global scale, with the highest overall morbidity and mortality. The virus has two major surface glycoprotein antigens, the hemagglutinin (H) and neuraminidase (N), which can change yearly, and thus the disease appears in epidemics annually. Both antigenic drift and waning immunity make this infection a yearly threat, particularly to those who have underlying cardiac or respiratory illnesses, the elderly, and pregnant women. The virus has an incubation period of two to four days and is spread via aerosol or mucosal contact with infected secretions. Epidemics occur yearly in the late fall and extend into the early spring. Influenza A can coexist with other viral infections including respiratory syncytial virus and parainfluenza virus, particularly in the elderly (59,60).

The virus has its main site of infection in the respiratory mucosa, leading to desquamation of the respiratory mucosa with cellular degeneration, edema, and airway inflammation with mononuclear cells (61). Although up to half of the infections are subclinical, the typical illness lasts three days and is characterized by sudden onset of fever, chills, severe myalgia, malaise, and headache. As the major symptoms recede, respiratory symptoms dominate, with dry cough and substernal burning which may persist for several weeks. Laboratory data and physical examination are not specific, and diagnosis is made by noting the presence of typical symptoms during the time of a known epidemic. Serologic evaluation, using hemagglutinating-inhibiting antibody or ELISA testing, and viral cultures can confirm the diagnosis. The illness can be more severe in smokers, the elderly, those under the age of one, pregnant women, and patients with chronic cardiorespiratory disease.

Influenza viruses can interfere with many aspects of respiratory host defenses and thus may be complicated by secondary bacterial pneumonia. The virus can interfere with mucociliary clearance, can promote tracheal bacterial colonization, and can interfere with the function of polymorphonuclear cells and macrophages. Respiratory complications include obliterative bronchiolitis, airway hyperreactivity, exacerbation of chronic bronchitis, primary viral pneumonia, and secondary bacterial pneumonia. When viral pneumonia develops, the disease follows the classic three-day illness without a hiatus and is characterized by cough (dry or productive) and severe dyspnea. Chest radiograph reveals bilateral infiltrates, and mortality is high. Bacterial pneumonic superinfection follows the primary influenza illness with a hiatus of patient improvement for three to four days before the pneumonia begins. In this setting, pneumonia is usually lobar, and the most common pathogens are pneumococcus, *H. influenzae,* enteric Gram-negative organisms, and *S. aureus.* Other serious complications include myocarditis and pericarditis, seizures, neuritis, coma, transverse myelitis, toxic shock, and renal failure (58).

Therapy of influenza is mainly symptomatic, with antipyretics, bed rest, and fluids. Amantadine can ameliorate the illness caused by influenza A if given within the first 24 to 48 hours. This medication may also be used prophylactically during an epidemic in high-risk individuals in doses of 100 mg twice a day until the epidemic passes or for two weeks until vaccination can be given and become effective. Dosage must be reduced with renal insufficiency, and confusion may occur in 3% to 7% of treated individuals. Rimantadine, a derivative of amantadine, is also effective for the therapy and prevention of influenza A infection (62). Rimantidine can be given once daily because of its long half-life, and it has fewer central nervous system and other side effects than amantadine. A new class of influenza agents, the neuraminidase inhibitors, is effective against both influenza A and B, and these agents appear to be effective for either therapy or prophylaxis. The recently-approved neuraminidase inhibitors Zanamivir and Oseltamivir can be used during acute infection and will reduce the duration of symptoms if given within 36–48 hours. Immunization should be given to all high-risk patients yearly with a vaccine prepared against the strains most likely to be epidemic. If an epidemic of influenza A develops in a closed environment (e.g., a nursing home) among nonimmunized patients, antiviral therapy should be given along with vaccination, and antiviral therapy is continued for two weeks until the vaccine takes effect.

Bronchiectasis

Bronchiectasis is another chronic airway disease that can be complicated by intermittent bouts of airway infection. In addition, the disease itself and its progression may be the result of airway infection. The disease is characterized pathologically by an abnormal and permanent dilation of subsegmental airways (21). In this condition, the airways are dilated and inflamed, and they become obstructed by thick secretions that may intermittently become infected. The actual shape of the abnormal airways has led to a classification system that characterizes the involvement as being either cylindrical, varicose, or saccular.

The causes of bronchiectasis are multiple, and in years past it was most often the result of a preceding respiratory infection such as tuberculosis or a virulent bacterial, fungal, or viral illness. A localized process can lead to focal bronchiectasis, while a more extensive process or a systemic illness can lead to diffuse bronchiectasis. Some of the diseases that may be complicated by bronchiectasis include cystic fibrosis, rheumatoid arthritis, influenza, lung abscess, foreign body aspiration, hypoglobulinemia, immotile cilia syndrome, and allergic bronchopulmonary aspergillosis.

The major symptom of bronchiectasis is cough, which is generally productive but may be dry. In severe disease, patients may expectorate more than 150 mL of sputum daily. Dyspnea and hemoptysis are also common, with massive hemoptysis at times of acute infection in some patients. The disease is accompanied by chronic bacterial colonization of the lower respiratory tract. When the quantity of sputum increases and the sputum becomes purulent, usually in association with fever and dyspnea, infection is present and requires antibiotics. In some settings, patients are given monthly antibiotics to prevent recurrent bouts of airway infection. The usual pathogens are bacterial and include pneumococcus and *H. influenzae.* Patients with cystic fibrosis may have *S. aureus.* In more advanced forms of bronchiectasis and cystic fibrosis, airway infection is with mucoid variants of *E. coli* or *P. aeruginosa.* Recovery of these mucoid variants should immediately prompt consideration of the diagnosis of bronchiectasis if it has not been previously recognized, because these organisms are not ordinarily found in the absence of chronic airway infection.

Some investigators (63) have found evidence for progression of the airway damage as a result of recurrent infection episodes. When airway infection occurs, it is accompanied by a brisk inflammatory response, with the release of neutrophilic proteases that can damage the airways and lead to more bronchiectasis. Observations such as these have prompted the suggestion that airway infection be treated promptly and possibly in a prophylactic fashion to limit disease progression. Episodes of airway infection are treated with antibiotics similar to those used in exacerbations of chronic bronchitis; it may not be necessary to treat every pathogen recovered from the sputum because some organisms may be colonizers and not infecting agents. One effective regimen is amoxicillin 500 to 1,000 mg three times a day for 14 days, but when *P. aeruginosa* is present, ciprofloxacin should be used. In cystic fibrosis and bronchiectasis, the use of aerosolized aminoglycosides in a prophylactic fashion may be effective in preventing acute episodes of airway infection, and these agents may also be used for the therapy of airway infection. In cystic fibrosis patients, DNAse has

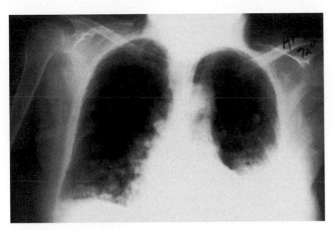

FIGURE 15.1. This patient had long-standing bronchiectasis with chronic increased markings in both lower-lung zones. The typical increased markings of this disease are seen in the right lower lobe, while the left lower lobe had evidence of pneumonia due to *Pseudomonas aeruginosa*.

been used via aerosol to help in sputum clearance and to prevent exacerbations. Other adjunctive therapies include chest physical therapy with percussion and postural drainage, bronchodilators, oxygen, pneumococcal vaccine, and yearly influenza vaccine. In cases of severe hemoptysis or localized recurrent infections due to bronchiectasis, surgical resection of the involved lung may be considered.

When bronchiectasis is suspected by history, it should be confirmed by high-resolution computed tomography of the chest. Routine chest radiographs (Fig. 15.1) may show areas of increased airway markings, atelectasis, dilated bronchi, "tramlines," or cavities. Physical examination may show clubbing, nasal polyposis, and adventitious breath sounds (rhonchi, rales, and wheezes). If the history is appropriate, a workup for hypogammaglobulinemia (immunoglobulin quantitation), immotile cilia syndrome (electron microscopy of nasal cilia), or cystic fibrosis (sweat chloride) may be indicated. Although cystic fibrosis is an inherited disease that usually appears in childhood, recognition in adolescence and longevity into adulthood are increasingly common.

Parenchymal Lung Infections

Pathogenesis of Pneumonia

Bacteria commonly enter the lower airway and do not lead to pneumonia because of the presence of an intact, elaborate, host defense system. When pneumonia does occur, it is the result of an exceedingly virulent organism, a large inoculum, and/or an impaired host defense system. In the nonhospitalized person, bacteria reach the lung by one of four routes: inhalation from ambient air, hematogenous spread, direct inoculation from contiguous infected sites, or aspiration from a previously colonized upper airway. Criti-

cally ill patients in the hospital may acquire organisms from a colonized gastrointestinal tract (particularly if a nasogastric tube is present to direct bacteria from the stomach to the oropharynx), or bacteria may reach the lung directly down the endotracheal tube from a contaminated hospital environment (27,28). Aspiration is the major route of acquisition for most forms of pneumonia, but in fact, very few individuals who do aspirate contaminated oropharyngeal secretions actually develop pneumonia. As many as 45% of normals and 70% of obtunded patients aspirate oral secretions, and the effectiveness of the normal respiratory tract defenses prevents most from becoming ill (64).

The upper airway is normally colonized, as mentioned above, and with increasing degrees of systemic illness, the flora become dominated by enteric Gram-negative bacteria. In healthy individuals, these organisms are unable to colonize the oropharynx because they are repelled by salivary proteases, lysozyme, and IgA (23). In addition, the "normal" flora of the oropharynx inhibit the growth of pathogens through a process termed "bacterial interference," whereby unfavorable growth conditions for pathogens are created. The absence of Gram-negative organisms in the oral flora of normals may also reflect the fact that these organisms have a poor ability to adhere, or bind, to the surface of normal upper-airway epithelial cells. This process—bacterial adherence—is a bacterial-mucosal interaction in which organisms bind irreversibly to cell surfaces and form a nidus from which overt colonization may follow (23,65) (Fig. 15.2). In many mucosal sites throughout the

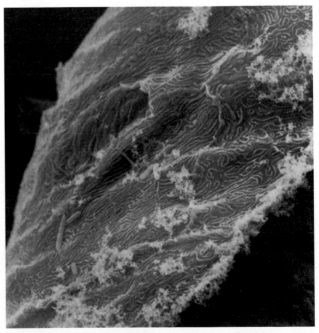

FIGURE 15.2. This scanning electron micrograph shows the bacterial adherence interaction between *Pseudomonas aeruginosa* and the surface of tracheal cells.

body, adherence is the first step leading to colonization. With systemic illnesses such as starvation, uremia, and surgical stress, salivary proteases are released into the oral cavity, and they act upon the mucosa to remove from it a glycoprotein—fibronectin—and thereby expose previously covered epithelial cell receptors for Gram-negative bacteria. An increase in oral mucosal cell receptivity for bacteria has been observed in individuals with acute illness and has been correlated with the clinical finding of Gram-negative colonization of the oropharynx in such settings (23).

Once bacteria reach the lower airway, they encounter a variety of specific (organism-directed) and nonspecific defense mechanisms. The nonspecific physical barriers include cough, reflex bronchoconstriction, angulation of the airways (favoring impaction and subsequent transport upward), and the mucociliary escalator. Immune defenses in the lower airway include bronchus-associated lymphoid tissue, phagocytosis (by polymorphonuclear cells and macrophages), immunoglobulins A and G, complement, cytokines, surfactant, and cell-mediated immunity by T lymphocytes. Bacterial adherence also plays a role in colonization of the lower airway, and normal tracheal cells have the capacity to bind to Gram-negative bacteria such as *P. aeruginosa*. It is likely that when bacteria have prolonged contact with the tracheobronchial mucosa, as is the case when mucociliary clearance is reduced (bronchiectasis, cystic fibrosis, endotracheal intubation), then the potential interaction of organisms with the tracheobronchial mucosa will occur. In the lower airway, adherence would be a particularly useful way for bacteria to "stick" to the mucosa and resist the constant flow of air and secretions. In tracheostomized patients, colonization by Gram-negative organisms has been correlated with an increase in tracheal cell capacity to bind bacteria (66). In intubated patients, an increase in tracheal cell bacterial adherence has been correlated with the occurrence of ventilator-associated pneumonia (67).

Colonization of both the oropharynx and the tracheobronchial tree with Gram-negative bacteria is an important harbinger of pneumonia, particularly when it arises in an ill, hospitalized individual. In one study, 23% of ICU patients with Gram-negative bacteria in the oropharynx developed pneumonia, in contrast to only 3.3% of patients without this finding (68). Similarly, lower airway colonization by these organisms is a risk factor for pneumonia because bacteria have gained a foothold in the tracheobronchial tree from which they can propagate downward toward the alveoli. Many clinical features have been correlated with colonization, but a general principle is that colonization is a "marker" of a patient with systemic illness who has impairments in the host defense system at multiple sites throughout the respiratory tract. As mentioned, bacterial adherence is a cellular interaction that has been correlated with colonization, and it may represent one mechanism whereby systemic illness alters a specific cellular behavior, making the patient more receptive to invasion by bacteria. Thus when

TABLE 15.3. RISK FACTORS FOR AIRWAY COLONIZATION BY ENTERIC GRAM-NEGATIVE BACILLI

Oropharyngeal colonization
Underlying serious illness
Prior antibiotic therapy
Coma
Diabetes
Renal failure
Malnutrition
Hypotension
Advanced age
Recent surgery
Underlying lung disease
Cigarette smoking
Tracheobronchial colonization
Advanced age
Tracheostomy
Malnutrition
Endotracheal intubation
Prior antibiotics
Neurologic disease
Bronchiectasis, cystic fibrosis
Acute lung injury (ARDS)
Chronic bronchitis
Corticosteroid therapy
Prolonged hospitalization
Recent surgery

a malnourished patient develops airway colonization by Gram-negative bacteria, one reason may be that an impaired nutritional status has made the patient's epithelial cells more receptive to binding by these organisms. Other clinical risk factors for colonization of either the oropharynx or tracheobronchial tree include antibiotic therapy, azotemia, diabetes, coma, hypotension, endotracheal intubation, corticosteroid therapy, smoking, chronic bronchitis, cystic fibrosis, and viral infection (Table 15.3).

When an organism of low virulence or a small inoculum enters the lung, containment is by phagocytosis and killing by the alveolar macrophage, and lung inflammation does not result. With more virulent insults, a complex inflammatory response is required for containment (69). This mechanism requires a variety of chemotactic factors (complement, alveolar macrophage cytokine products such as IL-8 and others) to attract polymorphonuclear cells to the alveolus and generate an inflammatory response to prevent the growth of any invading pathogens. Phagocytosis of bacteria by polymorphonuclear cells and macrophages can then occur, but this step requires opsonization by immunoglobulins, complement, or surfactant. In addition, effective phagocytosis by macrophages may require activation of these cells by T helper lymphocytes. Thus all the components of lower respiratory tract defenses can be integrated to deal with large inocula of bacteria or organisms of intrinsic virulence that reach them. When this inflammatory response has been studied in patients with unilateral pneumonia, the response has generally been contained at the site of infection and has not "spilled over" to the uninvolved lung or to the serum. This type of contained response explains why most patients with pneumonia have a focal process and only rarely develop bilateral inflammation in the form of ARDS.

An understanding of the normal host defense system will allow the clinician to understand why pneumonia results in specific patient settings. In addition, with an understanding of any specific patient's immune function, a likely guess about the responsible pathogen is possible. Thus, if a previously healthy patient develops pneumonia, it will usually be with a pathogen of intrinsic virulence such as pneumococcus, *Legionella* species, or *M. pneumoniae.* Patients with certain specific host impairments may become infected by *H. influenzae, S. aureus,* tuberculosis, or Gram-negative bacteria.

Certain organisms are known to predominate in specific clinical settings, and these associations should always be considered when such a patient is encountered (Table 15.4). For example, alcoholics may develop pneumonia with *K. pneumoniae;* those with chronic bronchitis can be infected with *H. influenzae* or *M. catarrhalis;* cystic fibrosis patients may be infected by *S. aureus* or *P. aeruginosa;* cardiac patients may develop pneumococcal infection; splenectomized patients become infected by encapsulated bacteria; the elderly have enteric Gram-negative bacteria causing pneumonia in 20% to 40% of all cases, and infection with *H. influenzae* and anaerobes is also common (70); postinfluenza patients may develop infection with *S. aureus, H. influenzae,* or pneumococcus; leukemics have Gram-negative and fungal pneumonias; and mechanically ventilated and tracheostomized patients often have Gram-negative pneumonias, particularly with *P. aeruginosa,* and if a Gram-positive organism is present, it is usually methicillin-resistant *S. aureus* (MRSA). Similarly, if helper T lymphocyte function is impaired, as is the case with AIDS, then macrophage activation will be abnormal, and organisms usually contained by cell-mediated immunity will predominate.

When a patient is evaluated for the risk of developing pneumonia, several factors should be considered. First, the patient's primary medical status should be evaluated so that diseases associated with an increased risk of infection can be identified. These might include cardiac disease, advanced age, ARDS, or diabetes. Other associated illnesses, in addition to the primary disease, should also be recognized. For example, hypotension, cancer, stroke, head injury, sepsis, hypophosphatemia, hypoxia, and ethanol intake all have associated specific impairments in lower-airway defenses. Another factor that may increase the risk of lung infection—and one that is frequently overlooked—is the therapeutic interventions that patients undergo while receiving medical care. Many medications can interfere with the lung's handling of bacteria, including oxygen, aspirin, digoxin, calcium channel blockers, morphine, cimetidine, antacids, corticosteroids, antibiotics, and β-blockers. The last factor to be considered is the patient's nutritional status, since malnutrition can interfere with cell-mediated and humoral immunity in the lung, in addition to increasing epithelial cell receptivity for bacteria. Table 15.5 shows how many of these factors can interact with the respiratory host defenses in one population of patients—the elderly—thereby partially explaining the increased incidence of pneumonia in these individuals.

Community-Acquired Pneumonia: General Clinical Features

The distinction between "typical" and "atypical" presentations of pneumonia has been referred to above. Although some clinicians have used this distinction in patterns of clinical presentation to predict the etiology of community-acquired pneumonia (CAP), in recent studies this approach does not work very well (22,71). There are two reasons why clinical features correlate poorly with the etiology of pneumonia. First, certain pathogens, such as *Legionella* and *C. psittaci,* can have a clinical picture that overlaps both syndromes, with high fever, chills, prodromal symptoms, dry cough, leukocytosis, and relative bradycardia (71,72). Secondly, if the host is not normal because of comorbid illness or advanced age, then the clinical features may be altered, even in the presence of a bacterial pathogen that should lead to the "typical" pneumonia syndrome. Thus in one study, clinical features were only 40% accurate in telling the difference between pneumococcal, mycoplasma, and other pneumonic infections (22). Similarly, in a study of

TABLE 15.4. PATHOGENS CAUSING PNEUMONIA IN SPECIFIC SETTINGS

Setting	Pathogens
Elderly	Enteric Gram-negative bacilli, *Haemophilus influenzae,* pneumococcus
Cardiac disease	Pneumococcus, Gram-negative bacilli
Alcoholism	*Klebsiella pneumoniae, H. influenzae, M. tuberculosis,* pneumococcus
Cystic fibrosis	*Pseudomonas aeruginosa, Staphylococcus aureus*
Postinfluenza	Pneumococcus, *H. influenzae, S. aureus*
Mechanical ventilation, ARDS	*P. aeruginosa,* other enteric Gram-negative bacilli
Chronic bronchitis	*H. influenzae,* pneumococcus, *Moraxella catarrhalis*
Splenectomy	Pneumococcus, *H. influenzae,* staphylococcus
Neutropenia	*P. aeruginosa, Aspergillus,* Gram-negative bacilli
AIDS	*Pneumocystis carinii, Mycobacterium avium,* cytomegalovirus, *Salmonella, Cryptococcus*

TABLE 15.5. HOST DEFENSES AND AGING FEATURES

Defense Mechanism	Impairments Related to Age, Comorbid Illness or Drug Therapy
Upper airway	
Nasal filtration	Bypassed by endotracheal tube, tracheostomy
Oropharyngeal bacterial adherence	Severe coexisting illness, increased oral proteases, xerostomia with a fall in intraoral pH, malnutrition, viral illness, smoking, ? aging
Bacterial interference	Prior antibiotic therapy, altered colonization patterns resulting from aging
Epiglottis	Sedating medications, stroke, feeding tube, endotracheal tube, carcinoma of the upper airway
Lower airway	
Cough	Sedating medications, stroke, neuromuscular illness, malnutrition, chronic bronchitis
Mucociliary transport	Aging, cigarette smoking, chronic bronchitis, bronchiectasis, dehydration, vitamin A deficiency, decreased airway pH, airway inflammatory proteases, morphine, atropine, hyperoxia
Immunoglobulins: IgG, IgA, IgM	Malnutrition, aging, vitamin deficiency (B_6, folate), zinc deficiency, malignancy
Complement	Normal with aging
Polymorphonuclear cells	Aging, hypothermia, cytotoxic therapy, diabetes, corticosteroids, ethanol, salicylates, malnutrition, hypophosphatemia
T cells	Aging, zinc deficiency
Tracheal cell adherence	Malnutrition, inflammatory proteases, viral illness, endotracheal intubation, ? zinc excess
Alveolar macrophages	Viral illness, malnutrition, ? aging, corticosteroids, cytotoxic therapy, salicylates

From Niederman MS, Fein AM. Pneumonia in the elderly. *Clin Geriatr Med* 1986;2:247, with permission.

196 patients with CAP, multilobar disease, pleural effusion, lung collapse, and cavitation were sufficiently common in patients with pneumococcal pneumonia, Legionnaires' disease, mycoplasma, and psittacosis that the radiograph could not be used to determine etiology (73). Because it is usually impossible to recognize a specific pathogen by its clinical presentation or radiographic picture, a judicious use of epidemiology, laboratory data, and clinical findings is needed in approaching therapy, and often more than one potential pathogen is targeted for therapy. The American Thoracic Society has presented an approach to initial empiric therapy of CAP that is based on an assessment of disease severity, place of therapy, and advanced age (over 60 years) and comorbid illness (71). In developing this approach, the use of

clinical features to predict microbial pathogens was rejected as being unhelpful.

As mentioned, many patient populations present with bacterial pneumonia with unusual patterns and clinical features. When the elderly develop bacterial pneumonia, fever, rigors, and pleuritic chest pain are less common than in younger patients. In the elderly, pneumonia may present with such nonspecific findings as confusion, lethargy, worsening of an underlying chronic medical condition, or raised respiratory rate. Certain medications such as aspirin and corticosteroids can mask the expected features of pneumonia. Coexisting illness such as chronic obstructive pulmonary disease can interfere with expected physical findings, while congestive cardiac failure may be associated with lung infiltrates that mimic or hide pneumonia (70).

Pneumonia can be caused by a wide variety of pathogens, but the responsible agent will vary depending on the status of the patient's underlying host defenses, which is often reflected in the place of residence. Community-acquired infection has a specific etiologic agent identified in approximately 50% of cases. The exact incidence of viral pneumonia in the community setting is unclear, but these agents may account for up to one-third of all such pneumonias. The most common bacterial pathogen for community-acquired infection is pneumococcus for all types of patients. The bacteriology varies for different populations, and one approach is to define likely pathogens on the basis of the severity of initial presentation, the need for hospitalization, the presence of advanced age or comorbidity, and the presence of risk factors for drug-resistant organisms (pneumococcus and Gram-negatives) (71) (Fig. 15.3). Risk factors for penicillin-resistant *S. pneumoniae* (PRSP) include: age over 65 years, beta-lactam therapy within three months, alcoholism, or immune suppression. In patients with mild

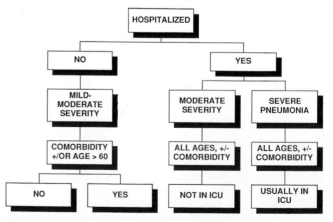

FIGURE 15.3. Shown here is an approach to stratifying patients with community-acquired pneumonia. Patients fall into one of four groups, each with its own likely pathogens and suggested therapy. The groups are defined by the need for hospitalization, severity of illness on initial presentation, and the presence of advanced age (over 60 years) and/or comorbid illness.

to moderate pneumonia treated out of the hospital, pathogens vary depending on the presence of advanced age or comorbidity. For those without advanced age or comorbidity, after pneumococcus the most common pathogens are *M. pneumoniae,* respiratory viruses, *Chlamydia pneumoniae, H. influenzae,* and miscellaneous pathogens such as enteric Gram-negative bacteria, *Legionella* spp., anaerobes, and *S. aureus.* Unusual pathogens in this setting should be suspected if the patient has an unusual travel or exposure history. In these circumstances, pneumonia may be a presentation of tularemia (in hunters), plague (from exposure to small animals), anthrax (in wool sorters and tanners), cryptococcosis (from pigeon droppings), histoplasmosis (from river valleys or bat droppings), coccidioidomycosis (from travel to the southwestern United States), psittacosis (from infected birds), or parasitic infestation (from foreign travel to the tropics). If the patient has mild to moderate pneumonia but either advanced age, comorbidity, a smoking history, or risk factors for Gram-negatives (such as coming from a nursing home or chronic corticosteroid therapy), then the most common pathogens are pneumococcus, respiratory viruses, *H. influenzae,* aerobic Gram-negative bacilli, *S. aureus,* and other miscellaneous organisms.

When the patient is hospitalized, a distinction is made between pneumonia treated out of the ICU and severe pneumonia requiring admission to the ICU. As mentioned below, the bacteriology of severe CAP is predictable but subtly different from that for CAP in general. Criteria for severe pneumonia include the presence of two of the following three: hypoxemia defined as a PaO_2/FiO_2 ratio less than 250 mm Hg, bilateral or multilobar infiltrates, or systolic blood pressure under 90 mm Hg; or one of the following two: need for mechanical ventilation, or septic shock (74). The mortality rate for severe CAP varies from 25% to 50% or higher, with the greatest death rates being found in populations that have the most patients treated with mechanical ventilation (71,75). Other prognostic factors indicating a poor outcome for hospitalized patients with CAP include advanced age, the presence of comorbidity, hospitalization within the last year, altered mental status on presentation, fever above 101°F, BUN above 19.6 mg per dL, and extrapulmonary seeding of infection (71,76).

If the patient is hospitalized but not in the ICU, then the likely pathogens are pneumococcus, *H. influenzae,* polymicrobial infection (including anaerobes), *Legionella* spp., *S. aureus, C. pneumoniae,* viruses, and other miscellaneous pathogens. In patients with severe CAP requiring admission to the ICU, the most likely pathogens are pneumococcus, *Legionella* spp., and enteric Gram-negative bacteria (including *P. aeruginosa*). It is important to consider *Legionella* as a likely pathogen in patients with severe CAP, because many studies of this illness document the importance of this pathogen (75,77). Other pathogens that can cause severe CAP include *M. pneumoniae,* respiratory viruses, and *H. influenzae.*

In the past several years, the role of atypical pathogens in CAP has been redefined. Many studies have shown that these organisms are common, being present in up to 40% of all CAP patients, often as copathogens along with bacterial organisms (78). When mixed infection is present, it can be found in patients of all ages and may lead to a more complex course than if monomicrobial infection is present. If coinfection is indeed common, routine therapy of atypical pathogens may be necessary in most patients.

Community-Acquired Pneumonia: Specific Illnesses

Streptococcus Pneumoniae

This Gram-positive, lancet-shaped diplococcus is the most common cause of CAP and can be found in all age groups and all clinical settings. There are 84 different serotypes, each with a distinct antigenic polysaccharide capsule, but 85% of all infections are caused by one of 23 serotypes, which are now included in a vaccine. Type 3 pneumococcus is a particularly virulent serotype and is also one of the most commonly encountered (79). Infection is most common in the winter and early spring, which may relate to the finding that up to 70% of patients have a preceding viral illness (80). Spread is from person to person, but the organism commonly colonizes the oropharynx of patients before it leads to pneumonia. Carriage rates vary from 5% in childless adults to 60% in infants, and rates also vary throughout the year. Pneumonia develops when colonizing organisms are aspirated into a lung that is unable to contain the aspirated inoculum. Infection is more common in the elderly; those with asplenia, multiple myeloma, congestive heart failure, alcoholism; after influenza; and in patients with chronic lung disease. In patients with AIDS, pneumococcal pneumonia with bacteremia is more common than in healthy populations of the same age.

Clinically, patients with an intact immune response present with the "typical" pneumonia syndrome of abrupt onset of illness accompanied by a toxic appearance, pleuritic chest pain, and rusty-colored sputum. In the past, a lobar pattern was most common, and patients with this finding will have consolidation by physical examination with bronchial breath sounds, egophony, dullness to percussion, and increased tactile fremitus (Fig. 15.4). More recently, it has been recognized that pneumococcus can cause bronchopneumonia, and in some series, this is the most common pattern (81). Bacteremia can occur in 15% to 25% of all patients and will increase the mortality rate of the illness (70,79). In patients with AIDS, the incidence of bacteremia may exceed 50% but is not associated with an enhanced mortality rate. Laboratory data are not specific but will usually show leukocytosis and slight liver function abnormalities. With overwhelming infection, neutropenia may occur. In the absence of a positive blood culture, diagnosis is often empiric and epidemiologic, based on finding appropriate

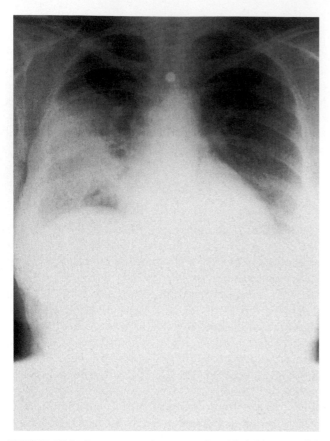

FIGURE 15.4. Pneumococcal pneumonia with lobar consolidation in the right lower lobe and a patchy bronchopneumonia in the left lower lobe.

clinical features in a compatible setting. Sputum Gram stain may show pneumococci, but this finding can be absent in half of infected patients, while it may be present when there is oropharyngeal colonization without infection. Counter-immunoelectrophoresis can be applied to urine, serum, and sputum to detect pneumococcal antigen and may thus help establish the diagnosis.

Recently, penicillin and multi-drug-resistant pneumococci have been identified with an ever increasing frequency. Currently, at least 40% of all pneumococci may be penicillin-resistant, but most of this is "intermediate" and not high-level resistance. The clinical impact of resistance is uncertain, since the outcome of patients with resistant organisms is the same as the outcome of patients who have sensitive organisms (82). Penicillin resistance may coexist with resistance to other agents including the macrolides, trimethoprim-sulfamethoxizole, and possibly even the quinolones. With current definitions of resistance, patients with PRSP can be successfully treated with high doses of penicillins, carbapenems, or with selected cephalosporins such as cefotaxime or ceftriaxone. The new antipneumococcal quinolones (levofloxacin, gatifloxacin, moxifloxacin) are also highly active against these resistant organisms. If meningeal

involvement with PRSP is suspected or proven, then vancomycin should be used. Although the incidence of resistance is rising, empiric therapy should be focused on these organisms mainly in patients with clinical risk factors for resistance which include age over 65 years or under five years, beta-lactam therapy within the past three months, alcoholism, immune suppression, or multiple medical comorbidities (83).

With effective therapy, clinical improvement follows in 24 to 48 hours, but fever may persist for five to seven days. Most patients are treated for five to seven days, but patients with AIDS should be treated longer. Radiographic improvement may lag behind clinical response, and only about 70% of patients have a normal radiograph after two months (84). Mortality is age-related, with 4% below the age of 40 dying, and 26% dying if they are between ages 40 and 69 (70). More recent data have questioned these age-related mortality statistics and suggested that mortality could well be a function of coexisting diseases seen in the aged rather than the aging process itself. Diseases that can increase the mortality of pneumococcal infection are cardiac illness, pulmonary disease, cirrhosis, malignancy, and asplenia. Mortality is also greater with bacteremia, multilobar involvement, and extrapulmonary spread of infection. In patients with advanced illness, antibiotic therapy may be of no benefit because mortality in the first 36 hours of illness is unchanged by therapy (85). Extrapulmonary involvement may be seen with meningitis, arthritis, endocarditis, brain abscess, and pericarditis and should be suspected if the patient fails to improve in the expected time period. Although pleural effusion is common and may be seen in 25% of patients, empyema is less common.

Patients at risk for pneumococcal infection should be considered for prophylaxis with the currently available pneumococcal vaccine (85–87). This injection is active against 23 serotypes of pneumococcus that account for 85% of all cases. At the present time, the vaccine is not being utilized in many of the at-risk population for a variety of unsound reasons. There are no major side effects of immunization, and although the efficacy of vaccination has been questioned, the current consensus is that the vaccine is effective, particularly if the patient is immunocompetent and if the vaccine is given before the patient is ill enough to be unable to have an adequate immune response (87). In patients with an abnormal immune response (the immunecompromised patient), one revaccination after five years, is recommended.

Legionella pneumophila

This small, weakly staining, Gram-negative bacillus was first characterized after it led to an epidemic of pneumonia in Philadelphia in 1976 that was known as Legionnaires' disease. Since this initial recognition, it has become clear that *L. pneumophila* is not a new bacterium but one that has only recently been recognized. It is one species of legionellae, of which more than 30 species have been identified. Legionellae have been isolated since as early as 1943, and retrospective serum analysis has shown that *L. pneumophila* has caused human disease since at least 1965 (88). At present, 12 different serogroups of the species *L. pneumophila* have been described, and these account for 90% of all cases of Legionnaires' disease, with serogroup 1 causing the most cases. The other species that commonly causes human illness is *Legionella micdadei.*

Infection by *Legionella* spp. can be in an epidemic fashion, and in the Philadelphia experience more than 200 individuals were infected, with a mortality of at least 16%. The organism is water borne and can emanate from air conditioning equipment, drinking water, lakes and riverbanks, water faucets, and showerheads. When a water system becomes infected in an institution, endemic outbreaks may occur, as has been the case in some hospitals. In addition to these patterns, *Legionella* infection can be in the form of sporadic cases and may account for 7% to 15% of all cases of CAP (89,90). In some studies, *Legionella* is the most common cause of CAP, a possible artifact of careful testing for this organism. *Legionella* has consistently emerged as a common pathogen in severe CAP. In a number of series (71,75), *Legionella* has been the second most commonly identified pathogen for severe CAP, leading some to advocate empiric *Legionella* therapy for any patient with severe CAP (71).

Infection is caused by inhalation of an infected aerosol generated by a contaminated water source. Person-to-person spread has not been documented, nor has infection via aspiration from a colonized oropharynx. It is also possible that infection can develop after subclinical aspiration of contaminated water. Incubation period is two to 10 days, and disease may occur in normal hosts, as some organisms have significant virulence. Other strains are less virulent and infect impaired hosts with risk factors for infection, including renal transplantation, dialysis, malignancy, smoking, chronic lung disease, diabetes, age greater than 50, male sex, and alcoholism. In hospitalized patients, the most important risk factor for nosocomial *Legionella* pneumonia is the use of corticosteroids, but an environmental source is needed for this type of nosocomial infection to occur (91). Once the organism is inhaled, it localizes intracellularly to the alveolar macrophage and multiplies, generating an inflammatory response that involves neutrophils, lymphocytes, and antibody. Since cell-mediated immunity is needed to contain infection, the disease can occur in compromised hosts and may relapse if not treated long enough.

Patients with *Legionella* pneumonia commonly have high fever, chills, headache, myalgias, and leukocytosis. Features that can suggest the diagnosis specifically are the presence of a pneumonia with preceding diarrhea, along with mental confusion, hyponatremia, relative bradycardia, and liver function abnormalities, but this syndrome is usually not present. Symptoms are rapidly progressive, and the patient may appear to be quite toxic. As mentioned, the presence of severe forms of CAP should automatically prompt consideration of *Legionella* spp. The patient may have purulent sputum, pleuritic chest pain, and dyspnea. The chest radiograph is not specific and may show bronchopneumonia, unilateral or bilateral disease, lobar consolidation, or rounded densities with cavitation. Up to 15% will have pleural effusion, but empyema is uncommon. Proteinuria is common, and some patients have developed glomerulonephritis and acute tubular necrosis. Myocarditis and cerebellar dysfunction have been reported as rare complications of *Legionella* pneumonia.

Diagnosis can be made serologically by detecting a serial rise in antibody titer to the organism. Using indirect immunofluorescence, a fourfold rise in titer, with samples collected six to eight weeks apart during and after the illness, to 1:128 or greater is diagnostic, as is a single titer greater than 1:512. This method may not be useful clinically, since it may take up to nine weeks to make a diagnosis. When patients with proven infection are studied at the time of initial presentation, a single acute serum titer is usually not diagnostic, but testing for urinary antigen is the most sensitive test, being positive in over half of all patients in this setting. The urinary antigen test can detect only *L. pneumophila* serotype 1 but has a high sensitivity and specificity for this organism, which causes more than 80% of clinically evident *Legionella* infections. The organism can also be identified in culture using special medium such as buffered charcoal-yeast extract. Direct fluorescent antibody staining of sputum or bronchoscopy specimens may lead to the diagnosis by detecting *Legionella* antigen. In most clinical settings, the direct fluorescent antibody technique is available, and all appropriate clinical specimens should be tested with it, although it will not be positive in all cases. A DNA probe for the *Legionella* genome has also become available for use.

Once the diagnosis is suspected, therapy should be with erythromycin in doses of 500 to 1000 mg every six hours intravenously until fever is gone for two days. Then a daily dose of 2 g orally is continued for a total of two weeks in immunocompetent patients and for three weeks in immunocompromised patients. With severe infection, rifampin should be added in doses of 600 mg every 12 hours. Alternatives to erythromycin are tetracycline and azithromycin. Clarithromycin has been reported to be effective when other agents have failed (92). Quinolone antibiotics, such as ciprofloxacin or the newer agents, may also be effective (92,93). With therapy, decline in fever may be slow, and high spikes in temperature may continue for one week after starting appropriate therapy. Mortality is less than 5% in normal hosts but may be as high as 25% in compromised hosts (89).

Aspiration Pneumonia

Pulmonary aspiration occurs in specific patient populations who are at risk of having material enter the lung because of impaired consciousness or altered respiratory tract anatomy. Aspiration can be in one of three forms: gastric acid or other toxic fluids may enter the lung and cause a chemical pneumonitis; inert substances such as water or solid particles can reach the lung and lead to drowning or airway obstruction, respectively; or pathogenic bacteria from the stomach or oropharynx can enter the lung and cause pneumonitis or lung abscess (94,95). Risk factors for aspiration include uncontrolled seizures, stroke, drug intoxication, shock, acute neurologic illness, tracheoesophageal fistula, esophageal diverticulum or dysmotility, tracheostomy, intestinal obstruction, and nasogastric tube use. When aspiration occurs, it is generally in a dependent lung segment, and in a supine prone patient this will be the superior segment of the lower lobe or the posterior segment of the upper lobe, with the right side being affected more often than the left because of the relatively straighter takeoff of the right mainstem bronchus.

If gastric contents are aspirated and solid material obstructs the airway, patients may develop cough and atelectasis and later on may have secondary bacterial infection distal to the obstruction in the form of lung abscess, bronchiectasis, or even empyema. If gastric acid or other toxic material is aspirated, then a chemical pneumonitis results, which may be complicated by secondary infection. Acutely, patients who inhale gastric acid with a pH below 2.4 may have dyspnea, bronchospasm, hypotension, hypoxemia, frothy sputum, and pulmonary edema. When aspiration involves primarily bacteria, acute infectious pneumonitis may follow. This process may be indolent and is characterized by fever and purulent sputum, followed by necrosis and possibly lung abscess one to two weeks later. When aspiration occurs out of the hospital, infection is usually with anaerobes that have colonized the mouth, including *Prevotella* (formerly *Bacteroides*) *melaninogenicus* and *Bacteroides fragilis, Fusobacterium* spp., peptococci, and peptostreptococci. Pneumococci and staphylococci may also be aspirated in this setting. In the hospital, aspiration is usually with both anaerobes and aerobes, usually *S. aureus* and enteric Gram-negative bacilli (96).

When aspiration is witnessed, the major therapy is to suction the airway, provide oxygen, and support the patient. The use of corticosteroids and prophylactic antibiotics is of no proven value. If an infiltrate is present, it should develop within 24 hours of the aspiration event, and then antibiotics are indicated. In cases of aspiration out of the hospital, penicillin G (up to 12 million units per day) or clindamycin (600 mg every six hours) can be used. Nosocomial aspiration is best treated with a second- or third-generation cephalosporin or another aagent active against enteric Gram-negatives, combined with clindamycin. Alternatively, a beta-lactam/beta-lactamase inhibitor combination can be

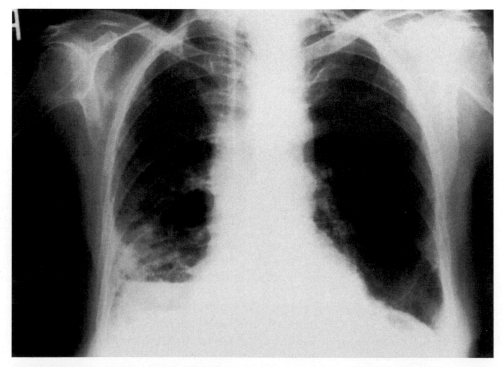

FIGURE 15.5. Aspiration pneumonia in the right lower lobe of an alcoholic with a seizure disorder. A patchy pneumonitis is evident in the right lower lobe, along with two lung abscesses and a pleural effusion due to empyema. A thick-walled cavity is present in the right perihilar area, while an air-fluid level—due to an abscess that has ruptured into the pleural space and caused an empyema—is present in the lower-lung zone.

used alone. Failure to respond to therapy should prompt a search for continued aspiration conditions, airway obstruction by a foreign body, or lung abscess.

Lung Abscess

This is a necrotizing parenchymal lung infection generally caused by aspiration of anaerobic bacteria. When a lung abscess arises in this manner, it is termed a primary or simple abscess, and it follows the anatomic distribution of aspiration discussed above. By definition, the radiograph will show a cavity of at least 2 cm. The cavity may contain an air-fluid level and may be associated with or preceded by a pneumonitis (Fig. 15.5). The cavities may be multiple, and generally average 4 to 5 cm (97). Empyema is often associated with lung abscess. The risk factors and microbiology of lung abscess are similar to those of out-of-hospital aspiration, and lung abscess is itself a complication of aspiration. Patients present with low-grade fever, weight loss, and cough with foul-smelling sputum. When lung abscess arises in the absence of a predisposing condition or in a patient without teeth (which can harbor the growth of anaerobes in the periodontal area), then lung cancer or another bronchial obstruction should be suspected. Even without these findings, many patients present with such an indolent course and with weight loss so that malignancy is part of the differential diagnosis. Therapy is with penicillin G or clindamycin, in the doses stated above, with some data to suggest that the latter is more effective (98). With therapy, the patient may improve within a week, with a decline in fever. However, it may take one month for the cavity to close and up to two months for the radiograph to clear, and therapy should be continued until the infection has cleared on chest film. Generally, therapy is intravenous until the patient is improving and then is continued orally for four to eight weeks. Complications of lung abscess include empyema, bronchopleural fistula, and brain abscess.

If lung abscess arises unrelated to aspiration, other pathogens besides anaerobes should be considered. Cavitary pneumonias can result from infection with tuberculosis, fungi, *S. aureus, K. pneumoniae, P. aeruginosa,* and group A streptococci. Another clinical situation that may be confused with lung abscess is periemphysematous infection of lung bullae. In this setting, pneumonia develops in a diseased lung with preexisting bullae due to emphysema. As these air sacs become infected, they fill with fluid and simulate a lung abscess. This type of infection can be distinguished from lung abscess if prior radiographs show bullae. In addition, the bullae are thin-walled, in contrast to the thick and irregular walls of a true lung abscess (Fig. 15.6).

Haemophilus influenzae

This Gram-negative coccobacillary rod can occur in either a typable, encapsulated form or a nontypable, unencapsulated form; either can cause pneumonia. The nontypable organisms are also a common cause of bronchitis and a frequent

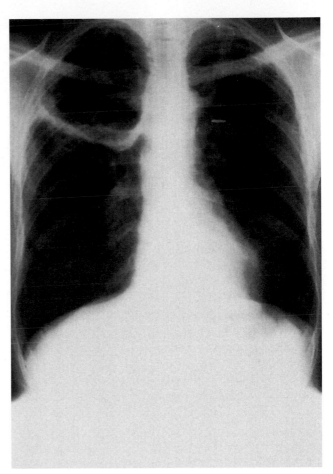

FIGURE 15.6. Periemphysematous bullous infection in a preexisting upper-lobe bulla. Unlike a lung abscess, the location is the entire upper lobe, there is no air-fluid level, and the wall of the bulla are thin, unlike the thick and irregular walls of an abscess.

colonizer in patients with COPD. The encapsulated organism can be one of seven types, but type B accounts for 95% of all invasive infections. Opsonizing IgG antibody is required to phagocytose the encapsulated organisms; this may not be the case for the unencapsulated bacteria. It has been suggested that since encapsulated organisms require a more elaborate host response, they are more virulent than unencapsulated organisms. However several studies have shown that in adults, particularly those with COPD, infection with unencapsulated bacteria is more common than infection with encapsulated organisms, and that opsonizing antibody is needed to control unencapsulated bacteria as well (99). It is probably safe to assume that pneumonia from these bacteria results if there is some impairment in host defense, which may include both humoral immunity and local phagocytic dysfunction.

When pneumonia is present, the organism may be bacteremic in some patients, particularly in those with segmental pneumonias as opposed to those with bronchopneumonia. It has been estimated (100) that 15% of cases are segmental, but that up to 70% of these patients have bacteremia, while only 25% of bronchopneumonia cases are bacteremic. The encapsulated type B organism is more common in patients with segmental pneumonia than in those with bronchopneumonia. Because pneumonia with *H. influenzae* represents a host defense failure, most patients have some underlying illness and half may be alcoholics. In patients with COPD, bronchopneumonia is more common than segmental pneumonia.

Patients with segmental pneumonia present with a sudden onset of fever and pleuritic chest pain along with a sore throat. Those with bronchopneumonia will have a slightly lower fever, tachypnea, and constitutional symptoms. Multilobar, patchy bronchopneumonia is the most common radiographic pattern, and pleural reaction is also common, being seen in more than half with segmental pneumonia and in approximately 20% with bronchopneumonia (Fig. 15.7). Overall, the adult mortality is 30%, a reflection of the type of impaired host who develops the illness. Complications include empyema, lung abscess, meningitis, arthritis, pericarditis, epiglottitis, and otitis media, particularly in children.

Therapy is usually with ampicillin, but recently resistance to this antibiotic has been reported in up to 40% of nontypable *H. influenzae* isolates and in up to 50% of type B

organisms as a result of bacterial production of β-lactamase enzymes. Other effective antibiotics are the third-generation cephalosporins, the beta-lactam/beta-lactamase inhibitor combinations, the newer macrolides (azithromycin more active than clarithromycin), and the fluoroquinolones. A vaccine against type B organisms is available but its use is limited, and it is best used in young children over the age of two to prevent invasive infection such as meningitis (86). Adults who are chronically colonized by *H. influenzae* achieve this condition in spite of the presence of antibodies to this organism and they are often infected with an unencapsulated organism, and thus it is unlikely that the vaccine will have utility in this type of adult population.

Mycoplasma pneumoniae

Although this organism closely resembles a bacterium, it lacks a cell wall and is surrounded by a three-layer membrane. Most of the respiratory infections caused by *M. pneumoniae* are minor and in the form of upper respiratory tract illness or bronchitis. Although pneumonia occurs in only 3% to 10% of all mycoplasma infections, this organism is still a common cause of pneumonia. In the general population, it may account for 20% of all pneumonia cases and up to 50% in certain closed populations, such as college students (101). The disease is seen year-round, with a slight

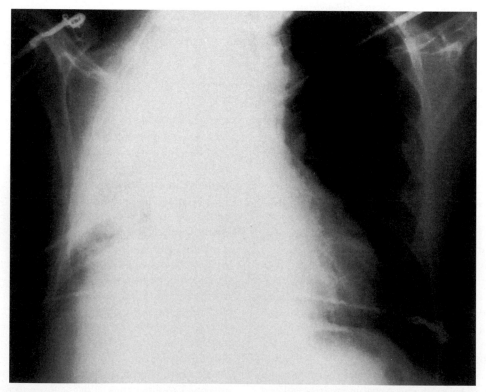

FIGURE 15.7. This patient with advanced chronic bronchitis had bacteremic *Haemophilus influenzae* from this extensive segmental pneumonia. A dense pleural reaction accompanied the pneumonia.

increase in the fall and winter. All age groups are affected, and although it is common in those less than 20 years of age, it is also a common cause of CAP, even in older adults.

Respiratory infection occurs after the organism is inhaled and then binds via neuraminic acid receptors to the airway epithelium. An inflammatory response with neutrophils, lymphocytes, and macrophages then follows, accompanied by the formation of IgM and then IgG antibody. Some of the observed pneumonitis may be mediated by the host response to the organism rather than by direct tissue injury by the mycoplasma. Up to 40% of infected individuals will have circulating immune complexes (102).

When pneumonia is present, it is usually in the form of an "atypical" pneumonia. Patients commonly have a dry cough, fever, chills, headache, and malaise after a two- to three-week incubation period. Up to half will have upper respiratory tract symptoms, including sore throat and earache. Some of the patients with earache will have hemorrhagic or bullous myringitis. Pleural effusion is quite common, being seen in at least 20% of patients with pneumonia, although it may be small. Chest radiograph will show interstitial infiltrates, which are usually unilateral and in the lower lobe but can be bilateral and multilobar, although the patient usually does not appear as ill as suggested by the radiographic picture. Rarely, patients will have a severe illness with respiratory failure or a necrotizing pneumonia, but most cases resolve in seven to 10 days in an uncomplicated fashion (75).

Infection with *M. pneumoniae* is often characterized by its extrapulmonary manifestations. These include neurologic illness such as meningoencephalitis, meningitis, transverse myelitis, and cranial nerve palsies, which can be seen in 7% of hospitalized patients (101). The most common extrapulmonary finding is an IgM autoantibody that is directed against the I antigen on the red blood cell and causes cold agglutination of the erythrocyte. Although up to 75% of patients may have this antibody and a positive Coombs' test, clinically significant autoimmune hemolytic anemia is uncommon. Other systemic complications include myocarditis, pericarditis, hepatitis, gastroenteritis, erythema multiforme, arthralgias, pancreatitis, generalized lymphadenopathy, and glomerulonephritis. The extrapulmonary manifestations may follow the respiratory symptoms by as long as three weeks.

Diagnosis is made by finding a compatible clinical picture and radiograph in a host with pneumonia and possibly some extrapulmonary findings. Confirmation can be made by isolating the organism in culture from respiratory tract secretions. Serologic diagnosis is made by finding a fourfold rise in specific antibody to *M. pneumoniae* by complement fixation test, although a single titer of 1:64 is suggestive of infection. If this finding is present with a cold agglutinin titer of 1:64, then the diagnosis is made. Recently testing for IgM antibody has also been used to define infection. Using these methods, some investigators have found that

M. pneumoniae can be a copathogen along with bacterial agents in patients with CAP. Once the diagnosis is made, therapy is given with erythromycin (2 g per day), a newer macrolide (azithromycin or clarithromycin), a quinolone, or tetracycline, which can reduce the duration and severity of the illness. Therapy is usually given for 10 to 14 days.

Chlamydia Species

Psittacosis is a pneumonia due to *C. psittaci,* an agent transmitted by inhaling infected excrement from avian species; the infectious bird does not need to be ill to transmit disease. Patients commonly have headache, high fever, splenomegaly and dry cough, all of insidious onset after a one- to two-week incubation period (103). A macular rash similar to that of typhoid fever may also be seen, along with relative bradycardia. Other extrapulmonary involvement may occur, including hepatitis, encephalitis, hemolytic anemia, and renal failure. Diagnosis is on the basis of a compatible contact history and can be confirmed serologically. Treatment is with tetracycline (2 to 3 g per day) or chloramphenicol for 10 to 14 days.

Recently another *Chlamydia* species, *C. pneumoniae,* has been found to cause respiratory infection. In some series this organism is a common cause of CAP in patients of all ages, and can also be present as a coinfecting pathogen, potentiating the severity of pneumococcal pneumonia. This organism is not transmitted by birds and has been designated as the TWAR agent. Antibody to TWAR has been found in 25% to 45% of adults, and the organism can cause up to 12% of pneumonias in a student population and 6% of pneumonias in an elderly population (104,105). In one report, the organism led to an epidemic of respiratory infection, including pnemonia in patients residing in nursing homes (105). The disease has no specific features but is commonly seen with laryngitis and pharyngitis. Patients have fever, chills, pleuritic chest pain, headache, and cough, and can occasionally have respiratory failure. Therapy is with tetracycline (2 g per day), but erythromycin, as well as the newer macrolides and fluoroquinolones, may also be effective; therapy should continue for 14 to 21 days.

Although all the agents of atypical pneumonia have not been thoroughly discussed, the clinical features of the most important infections are summarized in Table 15.6.

Klebsiella pneumoniae

This enteric Gram-negative rod can cause both CAP and nosocomial pneumonia. When it arises out of the hospital, it can be an explosive illness with up to a 50% mortality, and it generally affects debilitated individuals (106). Known as Friedlander's pneumonia, after the physician who first observed this illness, patients are predominantly male and usually middle-aged or older, with alcoholism being the most common coexisting condition. Other patients at risk are diabetics, the elderly in nursing homes, those with malignancy, and patients with chronic cardiopulmonary or renal

TABLE 15.6. DIAGNOSTIC FEATURES OF THE ATYPICAL PNEUMONIAS

Key Characteristics	*Mycoplasma* Pneumonia	Legionnaires' Disease/LLO	Psittacosis	Q Fever	Tularemia	TWAR Agent *Chlamydia*
Symptoms						
Mental confusion	±	+	−	−	−	−
Prominent headache	−	−	+	+	−	−
Meningismus	−	−	+	−	−	−
Myalgias	+	+	+	+	−	±
Ear pain	±	−	−	−	−	−
Pleuritic pain	±	+	−	−	−	−
Abdominal pain	−	+	−	−	−	−
Diarrhea	±	+	−	−	−	−
Signs						
Rash	± (E. multiforme)	± (Pretibial rash)	± (Horder's spots)	−	−	−
Raynaud's phenomenon	±	−	−	−	−	−
Nonexudative pharyngitis	+	−	+	−	±	+[a]
Hemoptysis	−	+	+	−	−	−
Lobar consolidation	±	±	±	±	±	−
Cardiac involvement	± (Myocarditis/ heart block/ pericarditis)	−	± (Myocarditis)	± (Endocarditis)	−	−
Splenomegaly	−	−	+	−	−	−
Relative bradycardia	−	+	+	−	−	−
Chest film						
Infiltrate	Patchy	Patchy/ consolidation[b]	Patchy/ consolidation	Perihilar pattern	"Ovoid bodies"	Single "circumscribed" lesions
Bilateral hilar adenopathy	−	−	−	−	+	−
Pleural effusion	± (Small)	±	−	−	+ (Bloody)	±
Laboratory abnormalities						
WBC count	↑/N	↑	↓	↑/N	↑/N	N[a]
Hyponatremia/ hypophosphatemia	−	+	−	−	−	−
Increase in SGOT/SGPT	−	+	+	+	−	−
Cold agglutinins	+	−	−	−	−	−
Microscopic hematuria	−	+	−	−	−	−
Diagnostic tests						
Direct isolation (culture)	±	±	±	−	−	+
Serology (specific)	CF	IFA	CF	CF	TA	CF
Psittacosis CF titers	−	↑	↑	−	−	↑
Legionella IFA titers	−	↑	−	−	↑	−

[a] Often associated with laryngitis.
[b] Asymmetric, rapidly progressive infiltrates are characteristic. *L. micdadei* pneumonia is suggested by a nodular infiltrate.
From Cotton EM, Strampfer MJ, Cunha BA. *Legionella* and mycoplasma pneumonia—a community hospital experience with atypical pneumonias. *Clin Chest Med* 1987;8:443, with permission.

disease. The onset is sudden with productive cough, pleuritic chest pain, rigors, and prostration. Sputum may be thick and purulent with blood as well, or it may be thin with a "currant jelly" appearance. Patients appear toxic, with high fever and tachycardia, and examination reveals signs of lobar consolidation. The radiographic finding that is most distinct is consolidation in the upper lobe with a fissure bulging downward because of the dense infiltrate. Lung abscess and bronchopneumonia may also occur. Other complications include pericarditis, meningitis, and empyema. Diagnosis is suspected by finding Gram-negative rods in the sputum in a patient with a compatible illness and risk factors. Therapy should be for two weeks, and usually two drugs that are active against the bacteria are used to avoid emerging resistance and to provide antibacterial synergy. There is some debate about the need for combination therapy, but if third-generation cephalosporins are used alone, resistance may emerge during therapy (107). Effective agents in addition to third-generation cephalosporins include an aminoglycoside, an antipseudomonal penicillin, aztreonam, imipenem, or a fluoroquinolone.

Staphylococcus aureus

S. aureus may account for up to 5% of CAPs but may also arise in the hospital. In the community setting, it is most common in the elderly and in residents of nursing homes. Pneumonia is also seen after influenza or in patients with chronic lung disease. Hematogenous pneumonia with this organism can be seen in drug addicts with right-sided endocarditis. Clinical features include sudden onset of fever, tachypnea, and cough with purulent sputum. The radiograph may show pleural effusion, cavitary bilateral infiltrates, lung abscess, or pneumatoceles (Fig. 15.8). Empyema is common, being found in eight of 31 patients in one

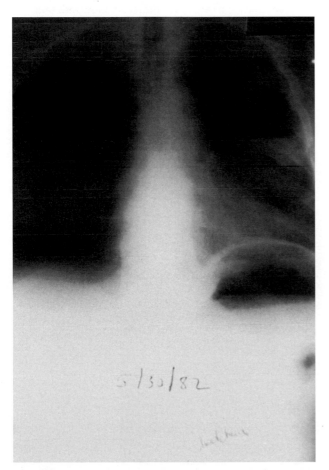

FIGURE 15.8. Multiple necrotizing lung cavities due to *Staphylococcus aureus.*

series (108). In that series, which included both CAP and nosocomial pneumonia, infiltrates were typically multilobar and bilateral, and involved the lower lobes. Pleural effusion was common (48%), but abscess was infrequent (16%). Therapy is with an antistaphylococcal penicillin, a first-generation cephalosporin, or vancomycin; it should be continued for four to six weeks in complicated infections. Reinfection can occur, and a mortality rate of 32% was reported for all infected patients in one study (108). Strains resistant to methicillin have become increasingly common and require therapy with vancomycin. These organisms are especially common in patients with ventilator-associated pneumonia, and emerge in the setting of late-onset infection (after day five of mechanical ventilation) and in patients with chronic lung disease, those on corticosteroids, and after prior antibiotic therapy. Extrapulmonary complications include endocarditis and meningitis.

Viruses

The exact incidence of viral pneumonia is difficult to estimate because careful serologic testing for viruses is not done in most cases of lung infection. However, viral pneumonia probably accounts for 20% or more of all cases of CAP. The common agents causing lower respiratory infection may be spread by aerosol or via person-to-person contact through infected secretions (Table 15.7) and include adenovirus, influenza virus, herpes group viruses (which include cytomegalovirus), parainfluenza virus, and respiratory syncytial virus.

Viral lower-respiratory infections are usually in the tracheobronchial tree or small airways, but primary pneumonia may also occur. The virus first localizes to the respiratory epithelial cell and causes destruction of the cilia and mucosal surface. The resulting loss of mucociliary function may then predispose the patient to a secondary bacterial pneumonia (109). If the infection reaches the alveoli, there may be hemorrhage, edema, and hyaline membrane formation, and the physiology of ARDS may follow. The initial host response to viral invasion is via the alveolar macrophage, which can have a variety of actions: it can phagocytose the virus; it can produce antiviral cytokines such as interferon gamma; and it can present the viral antigen to lymphocytes in the bronchus-associated lymphoid tissue. Lymphocytes can in turn lead to viral-specific antibody of the IgM, G, and A classes, activated T cells, and natural killer cells (109).

Viral lower-respiratory-tract involvement can be in the form of an airway infection with a normal chest radiograph, a primary viral pneumonia, a bacterial superinfection, or a combined viral and bacterial pneumonia. As was discussed with influenza, primary viral pneumonia may be a severe illness, with diffuse infiltrates and extensive parenchymal injury along with severe hypoxemia (Fig. 15.9). This pattern is often seen in those with underlying cardiopulmonary disease, immunosuppression, or pregnancy. However, many patients with primary viral pneumonia get only a mild

TABLE 15.7. CHARACTERISTICS OF COMMON RESPIRATORY VIRUSES CAUSING LOWER RESPIRATORY TRACT INFECTION

Agent	Genetic Structure	Mode of Transmission	Epidemiology	Clinical Syndromes
Adenovirus group (41 serotypes)	Linear double-stranded DNA	Aerosol, direct person-to-person contact	Ubiquitous agent, no seasonal prevalence	Epidemic pneumonia in closed populations (e.g., military recruits), disseminated disease in immunosuppressed hosts
Coronavirus	Single-strand RNA	Presumed person-to-person contact	Commoner in winter and spring, clusters within families	Occasional pneumonia, exacerbation of asthma, bronchitis
Herpes group (CMV, HSV, VZV)	Double-stranded DNA	Venereal route, blood products, transplanted organs, aerosol (VZV)	Immunosuppressed host	Tracheobronchitis (HSV), interstitial pneumonitis
Influenza virus (types A, B)	Seven single RNA strands	Small particle aerosol	Peak prevalence in winter and early spring, highest attack rates at extreme ages of life	Tracheobronchitis, pneumonia with or without bacterial superinfection
Parainfluenza	Single-strand RNA	Direct person-to-person spread	Late fall to early winter peaks, severe infection commonest between 6 months and 6 years	Croup (serotypes 1–3), pneumonia and bronchitis (type 1–2)
Respiratory syncytial virus	Single-strand RNA	Self-inoculation with fomites	Outbreaks in winter and spring, most serious infection in 1st 2 years of life	Pneumonia and bronchitis (infants), bronchitis and pneumonia (adults)

From Rose RM, Pinkston P, O'Donnell C, et al. Viral infections of the lower respiratory tract. *Clin Chest Med* 1987;8:406, with permission.

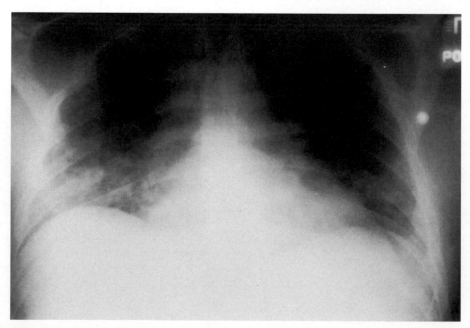

FIGURE 15.9. Primary viral pneumonia due to varicella-zoster in a 35-year-old male with an extensive vesicular rash and a clinical syndrome of chickenpox.

"atypical" pneumonia with dry cough, fever, and a radiograph that is more severely affected than the patient. When bacterial superinfection is present, the illness is biphasic, with initial improvement from the primary viral infection followed by sudden increase in fever along with purulent sputum and lobar consolidation. Another common complication of viral lower-airway infection is bronchial hyperreactivity, and asthma and chronic airflow obstruction may occur.

The major clinical distinctions between the many viral agents that can cause pneumonia are in the type of host who becomes infected and in the type of extrapulmonary manifestations that accompany the pneumonia. Immunocompromised hosts with AIDS, malignancy, and major organ transplantation are often infected by cytomegalovirus, varicella-zoster, and herpes simplex virus. Children are most affected by respiratory syncytial virus and parainfluenza virus, which can cause both airway and parenchymal lung infections. Children and military recruits develop pneumonia with adenovirus, while influenza pneumonia can develop in adults, particularly the debilitated elderly. Extrapulmonary signs may suggest a specific viral agent. Rash may be seen with varicella-zoster, cytomegalovirus, measles, and enterovirus infections (Fig. 15.9). Pharyngitis may accompany infection by adenovirus, influenza, and enterovirus. Hepatitis may be seen with cytomegalovirus and infectious mononucleosis (Epstein-Barr virus).

The diagnosis of viral illness can be clinical or it can be confirmed by specific laboratory methods. Viruses can be isolated with special culture techniques if specimens are properly collected and prepared. Upper-airway swabs, sputum, bronchial washes, rectal swabs, and tissue samples should be placed in viral transport media as early in the patient's illness as possible, while viral shedding is still prominent. These samples are then cultured on certain laboratory cell lines, and viral growth may be detected in five to seven days. More recently, the shell vial culture method has allowed for identification of viruses within one to two days. In this method, a clinical specimen is centrifuged onto a tissue culture monolayer and then stained with virus-specific antibodies (110). Viral illness can also be rapidly diagnosed by using immunofluorescence or ELISA assays to test patient samples for viral antigens. Immunofluorescent tests are available for influenza, parainfluenza, respiratory syncytial virus, adenovirus, measles, rubella, coronavirus, and herpesvirus. ELISA assays are also available for most of these agents (110). Serology can be used retrospectively to diagnose a suspected viral infection, but this technique may be a "shot in the dark" if specific viruses are not suspected and sought directly. A new technique that shows promise is the use of genetic probes to detect specific viral DNA or RNA. Such methodology is now available for cytomegalovirus, varicella-zoster virus, herpes simplex, and adenovirus.

With the current interest and understanding of viral infections, some specific therapy with antiviral agents has become available. Pneumonia from herpes simplex and varicella-zoster can be treated with acyclovir. Influenza A can be treated or prevented by the use of amantadine 200 mg orally per day or the new neuraminidase inhibitors (also active ageainst Influenza B). Ribavirin aerosol has been used to treat respiratory syncytial virus and influenza B. Patients with cytomegalovirus infection have been successfully treated by the acyclovir analog, DHPG (ganciclovir).

Hospital-Acquired Pneumonia

The epidemiology and pathogenesis of nosocomial pneumonia have been discussed above. When pneumonia arises in the hospitalized or institutionalized patient, the bacteriology shifts, and Gram-negative organisms are responsible for most cases. In addition to the enteric Gram-negative bacilli, other common causes of nosocomial pneumonia are *S. aureus* (including methicillin-resistant organisms), *H. influenzae,* pneumococcus, aspiration with anaerobes, *Legionella* spp. in certain places, and viruses in certain hosts or in settings of an epidemic among the staff (69). It should be emphasized that nosocomial pneumonia is an opportunistic occurrence that preys upon the sickest patients in a hospital. In one study, nosocomial infections in general were seen in 2% of all hospitalized patients but in nearly one-quarter of those with an underlying fatal illness (111). In patients with ARDS, as many as 55% have secondary pneumonia, and this complication may adversely affect survival (11,12,112) (Fig. 15.10). The responsible pathogen is usually an enteric Gram-negative bacillus, particularly *P. aeruginosa* in the most ill individuals; it is the impairment of the host response

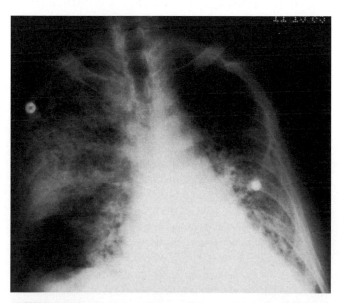

FIGURE 15.10. Acute respiratory distress syndrome with bilateral diffuse infiltrates and a complicating nosocomial pneumonia in the right upper lobe. Distinguishing pneumonia from the primary lung process is very difficult, although asymmetry can be a clue, as it was in this case.

to bacterial challenge and not usually the intrinsic virulence of the organism that leads to this infection. Much of the current research in this field is focused on prevention, and this approach arises out of a thorough understanding of pathogenesis.

There is still considerable difficulty in determining whether nosocomial pneumonia is present, because many noninfectious illnesses may present a similar clinical picture, particularly in the critically ill patient. An accepted definition of this infection is onset after 48–72 hours of hospitalization, with development of a new or progressive lung infiltrate on radiograph plus two of the following: fever, leukocytosis, and purulent tracheobronchial secretions (113,114). This diagnosis may be particularly difficult to make in the mechanically ventilated patient with coexisting ARDS or congestive heart failure because either illness is associated with lung infiltrates and the other clinical features of infection may be the result of tracheobronchitis and not pneumonia. Conversely, the elderly and the immunocompromised patient may have pneumonia in the absence of clear-cut signs and symptoms of infection because of the absence of adequate inflammation. In these patients, fever and purulent sputum may not be present.

Risk factors for nosocomial pneumonia can be categorized as being one of four types: acute illness (such as ARDS, sepsis, hemorrhagic shock) with its attendant alterations in a variety of lower-airway defense mechanisms; coexisting illnesses such as diabetes, smoking, chronic cardiac or pulmonary disease, recent intraabdominal surgery, advanced age, shock, intraabdominal infection, uremia, and other systemic illnesses; therapeutic interventions; and impaired nutritional status (112). The area of therapeutic interventions that predispose to pneumonia is particularly interesting, because an appreciation of these factors will prompt the physician to minimize therapies that increase the chance of developing infection. Such therapies include antacids, possibly H_2-blocking drugs, high oxygen concentrations, sedating drugs, corticosteroids, nasogastric tube use, broad-spectrum antibiotics, and endotracheal intubation (112).

The diagnosis of nosocomial pneumonia is hampered by the problems cited above. It is common practice to both underdiagnose and overdiagnose this illness in certain populations. For example, in patients with ARDS, one-third of all autopsy-proven cases of pneumonia had been unrecognized, while one-fifth of uninfected patients were treated for pneumonia (115). It is likely that this degree of misdiagnosis is common in other settings because of the imprecision of the clinical diagnosis of this illness. Some studies have reported that only one of three mechanically ventilated patients with a clinical diagnosis of pneumonia had microbiologic confirmation of the diagnosis (116). Although this estimate may be overly pessimistic, it is likely that pneumonia is overdiagnosed in mechanically ventilated patients. Many hospitalized patients are colonized by potential pathogens, and thus their recovery from the lower airway

does not always represent invasive infection. However, it is unlikely that if pneumonia is present, the organism responsible would not be found in the culture of a tracheal aspirate. Thus in the ventilated patient, a sputum (tracheal aspirate) culture is sensitive, but not specific for the etiologic organisms of pneumonia.

In an effort to improve the accuracy of diagnosing nosocomial pneumonia, several invasive techniques have been developed (116). With these methods, lower-respiratory secretions are sampled, either bronchoscopically or via endotracheal suction, and the recovered material is cultured quantitatively. The bacteriologic results are then used to determine whether pneumonia is present on the basis of how many organisms are recovered. Invasive methods have involved the use of special "protected" brushes or bronchoalveolar lavage for the recovery of secretions for culture. Debate continues about the accuracy and clinical utility of invasive methods (116). Concern about invasive methods centers around the potential arbitrariness of thresholds selected to separate pneumonia from nonpneumonia. In addition, there are concerns about the reproducibility of the methods, the potential for these techniques to overlook early infection, and the limited value of the methods if the patient is on antibiotics at the time of testing. Studies of ventilator-associated pneumonia have shown that the major determinant of outcome is the timeliness and accuracy of initial therapy, and that unless invasive methods add to the accuracy of initial empiric therapy, it is unlikely that they can affect outcome (117).

Therapy is with antimicrobial agents directed at the likely pathogens, which fall into a "core" group of bacteria including *Klebsiella* spp., *Enterobacter* spp., *E. coli, Proteus* spp., *Serratia marcescens, S. pneumoniae, H. influenzae,* and *S. aureus* (113,114). Some patients with nosocomial pneumonia have infection with a polymicrobial flora, and up to 40% of nosocomial pneumonia in mechanically ventilated patients is polymicrobial (114). Patients with certain comorbidities or therapies can be at risk for other organisms in addition to the core bacteria. *S. aureus* (including its methicillin-resistant form) is more likely in patients who are in coma, as well as in those with head injury, renal failure, and recent influenza. MRSA is a particular concern in patients with pneumonia of late onset (after day 5 of mechanical ventilation), and in those on corticosteroid therapy or after a recent course of antibiotics. *Legionella* spp. are more likely in patients receiving corticosteroids or cytotoxic chemotherapy, and *Aspergillus* spp. are more likely if patients have received antibiotics or corticosteroids (118). Patients with recent thoracoabdominal surgery or witnessed aspiration are at risk for anaerobic organisms. *P. aeruginosa* is a concern in patients who have severe nosocomial pneumonia and in those who develop pneumonia in the setting of prolonged mechanical ventilation, prior broad-spectrum antibiotics, corticosteroid use, malnutrition, or chronic structural lung disease (such as bronchiectasis).

Therapy should be directed at the core bacteria for all patients, with modifications if specific other organisms are suspected or documented. The core organisms can be treated with a second-generation cephalosporin, a nonpseudomonal third-generation cephalosporin, a β-lactam/β-lactamase inhibitor combination, or a fluoroquinolone. If anaerobic organisms are likely, clindamycin should be added to one of these agents, or a β-lactam/β-lactamase inhibitor combination can be used alone. If methicillin-resistant *S. aureus* is suspected, and the Gram stain of a tracheal aspirate shows Gram-positive organisms, vancomycin should be added. If *P. aeruginosa* is suspected, dual antipseudomonal therapy should be initiated, since monotherapy of infection by this organism is often complicated by the emergence of resistance during therapy. The antipseudomonal antibiotics include the antipseudomonal penicillins (piperacillin, azlocillin, mezlocillin), certain third-generation cephalosporins (ceftazidime), the fourth-generation cephalosporin cefepime, aztreonam, imipenem/cilastatin, meropenem, piperacillin/tazobactam ticarcillin/clavulanic acid, ciprofloxacin, and the aminoglycosides.

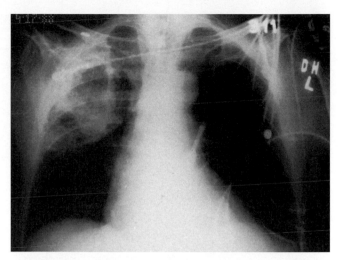

FIGURE 15.11. Nosocomial pneumonia due to *Pseudomonas aeruginosa* in a patient treated chronically with corticosteroids. Necrotization is evident, with a cavity in the right upper lobe.

Pseudomonas aeruginosa

This aerobic Gram-negative bacillus is the most common cause of nosocomial pneumonia, accounting for up to 15% of all cases, and colonizes the airway of up to 40% of all mechanically ventilated patients (28). The bacteria reach the lung by aspiration, direct entry via the endotracheal tube, or hematogenously. Patients most at risk for infection are those with cystic fibrosis, bronchiectasis, burns, corticosteroid therapy, neutropenia, tracheostomy, and mechanical ventilation. A necrotizing pneumonia is common, with alveolar septal necrosis, microabscesses, and vascular thrombosis. In postoperative patients, the mortality from pseudomonal pneumonia is over 70% (119). The virulence of the organism can be enhanced by production of a slime layer in its surface capsule, endotoxin lipopolysaccharide, pili, exotoxins, and proteases. Exotoxin A, phospholipase, fibrinolysin, and elastase help to mediate the lung injury that accompanies infection. Patients with this infection may be quite toxic and have confusion, fever, chills, and productive cough, along with relative bradycardia, leukocytosis, and hemorrhagic pleural effusion. Bilateral bronchopneumonia, particularly in the lower lobes, nodular infiltrates, and cavitation may be seen (Fig. 15.11). With bacteremia in the neutropenic patient, a characteristic skin lesion—ecthyma gangrenosum—may be seen. With bacteremic infection, combination therapy is associated with improved survival compared to monotherapy.

Pneumonia in Special Settings

The Immunocompromised Host

Patients with specific immune impairments related to an underlying primary illness (often malignancy or HIV infection) or arising as a consequence of medical therapy (most typically chemotherapy or transplant-related immunosuppression) may develop respiratory infections; these individuals are referred to as immunocompromised hosts (ICHs) (110,120). More recently, AIDS has led to a large and important population of ICH patients who may develop pneumonia. In any ICH, a new infiltrative pulmonary process may be infectious or noninfectious (such as an adverse drug reaction). Pneumonia may be a life-threatening infection in patients with malignancy or immunosuppressive therapy, and efforts at making a specific etiologic diagnosis are often necessary. As shown in Table 15.8, the spectrum of possible infections is broad and will vary with the nature of the immune deficit.

Often it is possible to narrow down the infectious possibilities with an understanding of the basic immune impairment (Table 15.8). Thus patients who have had a splenectomy (including those with sickle cell anemia and autosplenectomy) are usually infected by encapsulated bacteria such as pneumococcus, staphylococci, *H. influenzae,* and *N. meningitides.* Patients with chemotherapy-induced neutropenia may be infected with *P. aeruginosa,* other Gram-negative bacteria, and *Aspergillus* species. Patients with abnormal T-lymphocyte function, such as those with certain lymphomas or AIDS, may be infected by bacteria such as *Listeria monocytogenes, Salmonella* species, *Legionella* spp., *Mycobacterium avium,* or *M. tuberculosis;* fungi such as *Cryptococcus neoformans, Histoplasma capsulatum,* or *Coccidioides immitis;* viruses such as cytomegalovirus and herpes simplex; or parasites such as *P. carinii, Toxoplasma gondii,* or *Cryptosporidium* spp. (121,122). In the HIV-infected patient, the type of infection that develops is directly related to the degree of immune dysfunction, as reflected by the patient's CD4 lymphocyte count. Those with little immune

TABLE 15.8 TYPE OF IMMUNOLOGIC DEFECT AND ASSOCIATED MICROORGANISMS

Defect or Factor	Microorganism			
	Bacteria	Fungi	Viruses	Parasites
Abnormal T lymphocyte function lymphoma, AIDS	Listeria monocytogenes Nocardia Salmonella (species other than S. typhi) Mycobacteria Legionella	Cryptococcus neoformans Histoplasma capsulatum Coccidioides immitis Candida Trichosporon	Cytomegalovirus Varicella-zoster Herpes simplex	Pneumocystis carinii Toxoplasma gondii Strongyloides stercoralis
Abnormal B lymphocyte function myeloma, primary and acquired deficiency	Streptococcus pneumoniae Haemophilus influenzae			
Neutropenia (<500 neutrophils/mm³): Myeloproliferative disease, lymphoma cytotoxic therapy, alcoholism, sickle cell disease	Pseudomonas aeruginosa Escherichia coli Klebsiella Serratia Aeromonas Other Gram-negative bacilli	Aspergillus Zygomycetes		
Splenectomy	S. pneumoniae H. influenzae E. coli Staphylococcus aureus Neisseria meningitis			
Decreased serum complement	S. pneumoniae			
Primary, collagen vascular disease	H. influenzae Neisseria spp.			
Use of corticosteroid therapy equivalent to >20 mg of prednisone daily or cytotoxic therapy (or both)	S. aureus L. monocytogenes Mycobacteria P. aeruginosa Nocardia Other Gram-negative bacilli	Aspergillus Zygomycetes H. capsulatum C. neoformans C. immitis	Cytomegalovirus Varicella-zoster Herpes simplex	P. carinii T. gondii Strongyloides stercoralis

From Rosenow EC, Wilson WR, Cockerill FR. Pulmonary disease in the immunocompromised host. *Mayo Clin Proc* 1985; 60:612, with permission.

dysfunction and a CD4 count above 500 per mm^3 usually do not develop opportunistic infection, and their predominant pneumonia is bacterial, especially pneumococcal. As the CD4 count falls, the risk of opportunistic infection rises, and patients with a count above 200 per mm^3 are at particular risk for such infections as *P. carinii* (122).

Immunocompromised patients should have a careful clinical examination with attention to the skin, gastrointestinal tract, central nervous system, optic fundi, liver, and lungs. Respiratory symptoms may be minimal, with fever as the only finding, or the patient may have cough and dyspnea. Certain extrapulmonary findings in conjunction with a specific immune defect can suggest an etiologic agent. Skin lesions are common with infections caused by *P. aeruginosa*, *M. tuberculosis*, nocardia, varicella-zoster, herpes simplex, *Cryptococcus*, and *Blastomyces*. The central nervous system may be affected by *Nocardia*, pneumococcus, *H. influenzae*, *P. aeruginosa*, *M. tuberculosis*, *Legionella*, *Aspergillus*, *Cryptococcus*, *Toxoplasma*, varicella-zoster, and cytomegalovirus. Liver function abnormalities can be seen with cytomegalovirus, *Legionella*, and *Nocardia* infection, tuberculosis, histoplasmosis, toxoplasmosis, and *S. aureus* and *P. aeruginosa* infection. Diarrhea can occur with *Legionella*, *Cryptosporidium*, cytomegalovirus, or herpes simplex (120).

Patients who have received organ transplants represent an expanding population of ICH individuals. Infections in this population can be related to hospitalization, the presence of serious illness, and transplant immunosuppression. Within the first month of transplant, patients get the usual bacterial nosocomial pneumonias. In the period from one to six months after transplant, infection is related to immunosuppression and can be with cytomegalovirus, *P. carinii*, fungal agents, *L. monocytogenes*, and *Legionella* spp. After six months, these same pathogens may still lead to infection in patients who are heavily immunosuppressed, while chronic viral infection can develop in those less heavily immunosuppressed (123).

Chest radiography is often the way that the diagnosis of pneumonia is made, since many patients will have only fever and no respiratory complaints or findings. Focal lung lesions can be seen with bacterial, fungal, and mycobacterial illness. Diffuse infiltrates are seen with *P. carinii*, cytomegalovirus, *Legionella* infection, miliary tuberculosis, viral pneumonia, *Aspergillus*, and *Candida*. After a careful clinical examination, samples of sputum and blood should be collected and cultured for bacteria, fungi, *M. tuberculosis*, and viruses. Special stains for *M. tuberculosis*, *Legionella*, and *P. carinii* can be applied to respiratory tract secretions. Based on all available data, the patient is usually given empiric antibiotic therapy directed at the most likely pathogens. If improvement occurs, therapy is continued for two to three weeks. If there is no improvement, an invasive procedure is performed. If the patient has an adequate platelet count, the procedure is either a transbronchial or an open-lung biopsy. With inadequate platelets, bronchoalveolar lavage without biopsy can be performed or transfusion and biopsy can be undertaken. The decision between bronchoscopic and surgical lung biopsy is made on the basis of how rapidly the patient is deteriorating and on the expected yield and risks of bronchoscopy. In all patients who are immunocompromised, consideration must be given to drug-induced lung disease, malignant involvement of the lung, heart failure, and pulmonary hemorrhage, in addition to the possibility of opportunistic infection (120).

Lung Infection in the Patient with AIDS

Patients with AIDS have impairment of T-cell function but also have humoral immune dysfunction. Thus infections with bacteria, fungi, viruses, and parasites have all been seen in this population. The T-cell deficiency can lead to pneumonia caused by *P. carinii,* cytomegalovirus, and *Mycobacterium, Legionella,* and *Nocardia* spp. (122). The humoral immune dysfunction has been responsible for infections by pneumococcus and *H. influenzae.* As mentioned, the degree of T-lymphocyte depletion will determine which infections the patient is most likely to develop.

The most common pneumonias in immunosuppressed patients with HIV infection are caused by *P. carinii* (PCP) and pneumococcus. PCP is probably a fungus that can exist in cyst form containing sporozoites or in free form as a trophozoite. The organism can be recognized by methenamine silver stain or by Giemsa stain, usually of lung tissue or bronchoalveolar lavage fluid. Infection may represent endogenous reactivation of latent infection present in early childhood. Most patients probably acquired *Pneumocystis* from natural sources prior to the onset of AIDS and contained it within the lung. Once AIDS develops, these latent stores of organism may become reactivated, but new primary infection or reinfection are also possible. Most patients present with a subacute course of fever, cough, dyspnea, and weight loss. Chest pain, malaise, fatigue, and night sweats may also occur, and some patients are even asymptomatic. Chest radiograph usually shows bilateral diffuse interstitial or alveolar infiltrates (Fig. 15.12). Asymmetric or focal infiltrates may occasionally be seen, as can predominantly upper-lobe disease and solitary pulmonary nodules (124). Less common findings include pneumothorax and pleural effusion. Upper-lobe disease and pneumothorax have been reported to be more likely in patients who have received aerosolized pentamidine for prophylaxis of *P. carinii* infection.

The diagnosis of *Pneumocystis* may be elusive, since it may be the first presentation of AIDS for many individuals.

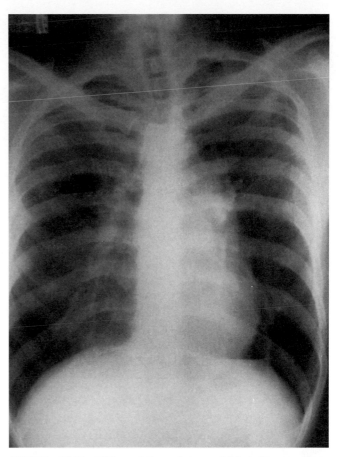

FIGURE 15.12. Diffuse bilateral interstitial infiltrates in a "ground glass" pattern in a 33-year-old intravenous drug abuser. This pattern is typical for *Pneumocystis carinii.*

Therefore all patients with pneumonia, particularly one that is subacute, should be questioned for AIDS risk factors, and if these are present, *Pneumocystis* should be considered in the differential diagnosis. Findings that suggest the diagnosis are a compatible radiograph, leukopenia and lymphopenia, elevated serum LDH, oral candidiasis, and a widened alveolar-arterial oxygen tension gradient. When this infection arises in an AIDS patient, it is usually associated with a more prolonged course, lower fever, less tachypnea, and less hypoxemia than when it occurs in other immunocompromised patients, such as those with lymphoma. In AIDS patients, *Pneumocystis* may coexist with cytomegalovirus, toxoplasmosis, or mycobacterial illness. Diagnosis is usually made by bronchoalveolar lavage or transbronchial biopsy, and in some centers, the induction of sputum for expectoration has led to the diagnosis in up to half of all patients.

With therapy, improvement is slower in the AIDS patient than in other ICHs with *Pneumocystis* infection. Fever may persist for seven to 10 days, and overall survival from the infection is as high as 90%. Survival is more likely if the clinical manifestations are mild, the organism burden is not large, and if the infection is the first episode of *P.*

carinii. Therapy is begun with intravenous trimethoprim-sulfamethoxazole (15 to 20 mg per kg per day of trimethoprim and 75 to 100 mg per kg per day of sulfamethoxazole), but as many as half of all AIDS patients will not be able to tolerate therapy because of adverse reactions. These patients, as well as those who do not respond to trimethoprim-sulfamethoxazole, are then treated with pentamidine (4 mg per kg per day). Other effective agents are trimethoprim/dapsone, or for mild-to-moderate infections, atovaquone (750 mg orally three times daily). Trimetrexate and aerosolized pentamidine have been tried but are generally less effective than standard therapy (125,126). Therapy with most regimens is continued for 21 days. If the illness leads to hypoxemia, with a room-air arterial PO_2 below 70 mm Hg, then corticosteroids should be added to ameliorate the host inflammatory response to the killing of organisms that accompanies therapy. Corticosteroids are given in a dose of prednisone 40 mg twice daily for five days, followed by 20 mg twice daily for five days, and then 20 mg once daily for 11 days (122). After recovery from pneumonia, patients should receive chemoprophylaxis against recurrent infection, which can be done with oral trimethoprim/sulfamethoxazole or aerosolized pentamidine.

Approach to the Patient with Pneumonia

History and Physical Examination

Although it may be impossible to identify a specific etiologic agent on clinical grounds alone, a careful evaluation can help guide initial therapy. As shown in Figure 15.3, patients with CAP should have initial empiric therapy selected by assessing three factors: the need for hospitalization; advanced age (over 60 years) or comorbid illness (especially chronic cardiac or pulmonary disease); and the severity of the patient's illness (71). In addition, therapeutic selection should be made with a consideration of the presence of smoking history, and risk factors for PRSP and Gram-negatives. Based on these assessments, a likely set of pathogens can be identified, and from this list therapeutic choices follow. In the statement by the American Thoracic Society, an empiric approach utilizing these three determinations was endorsed; other approaches were discussed and found to have only limited value. For example, the use of clinical features to predict microbial etiology, the use of sputum Gram stain to guide initial therapy, and the routine use of extensive diagnostic testing were all regarded as not useful (71).

The initial history and physical examination can be used to define how ill the patient is and whether hospitalization will be needed (71). Indicators of more severe pneumonia include a respiratory rate above 30 per minute, diastolic hypotension (under 60 mm Hg), systolic hypotension, oliguria, need for vasopressors, or the presence of respiratory failure. Examination can also reveal other findings indicating a poor prognosis, including altered mental status, high fever, or evidence of extrapulmonary spread of infection. Other historical information may help in determining the probable etiologic pathogen. Thus patients should be specifically questioned about rash, diarrhea, headache, myalgias, change in mentation, and nausea. Travel history, pets, unusual occupations, and unusual hobbies can also help raise suspicion about certain of the less common infectious agents. If aspiration pneumonia is suspected, the patient should be asked about neurologic disease, esophageal disease, and alcohol use. In addition, an allergic history should be obtained before antimicrobial therapy is prescribed.

Physical examination can also help identify certain etiologic pathogens and disease complications. Respiratory examination can reveal consolidation, pleural effusion, and bronchopneumonia. Examination of the skin, fundi, liver, heart, and neurologic system can help point to specific etiologic diagnoses. In some patients, the examination may be the first clue to the presence of pneumonia. In the elderly, the most reliable physical finding for pneumonia, because of the abnormal inflammatory response in this population, is elevation of the respiratory rate above 25 per minute (127). Patients should also be evaluated for their ability to cough and expectorate sputum, so that individuals with impaired cough can receive physical therapy to aid in tracheobronchial toilet.

When a patient has nosocomial pneumonia, the same assessments of comorbidity and severity of illness should be made, and these factors can be used to guide initial therapy (113,114). However, since many patients develop nosocomial pneumonia because of impaired host defenses, nosocomial pneumonia is commonly present in the absence of fever or other classic respiratory features of pneumonia.

Chest Radiograph

In many patients, the history and examination may suggest pneumonia, but the diagnosis is firmly established by finding a new parenchymal lung infiltrate. The infiltrate should be lobar, interstitial, nodular, cavitary, or bronchopneumonic. Bilaterality, pleural effusion, and multiple lobe involvement should also be noted. Multilobar infiltrates, cavitation, and rapidly expanding infiltrates (over 50% increase in 48 hours) all predict an increased mortality from CAP (71,75). The location of the infiltrate can also be helpful: apical disease can suggest tuberculosis, disease in dependent segments is compatible with aspiration, and consolidation of the upper lobe suggests infection with *K. pneumoniae* or pneumococcus. In some patients, early in the course of infection, focal physical findings of pneumonia may be present but the chest radiograph can be normal.

The chest film can also be used to follow the patient during therapy of pneumonia to detect any complications. Cavitation and empyema should be suspected and sought if the patient develops a new or persistent fever during treatment. Serial radiographs can also be used to determine the duration of a pneumonia and whether it is resolving appropriately. When radiographs fail to show improvement, this may suggest an unusual or unsuspected organism *(M. tuberculosis* or fungus), an antibiotic-resistant organism, a noninfectious inflammatory disease (such as Wegener's granulomatosis), an impaired host (with a normally slow response to therapy), or an unsuspected malignancy (128). Before a pneumonia is termed unresolving, the natural course of radiographic improvement for each infection should be appreciated. Both pneumococcal and *Legionella* infections may have radiographic deterioration in up to half of all patients during the initial week of a successful course of therapy. In each of these infections, radiographic clearing will begin in the first two weeks of treatment, but the chest film may not be entirely normal for three to six months.

Diagnostic Methods

Many techniques are available to identify the etiologic agent in lower respiratory tract infection, including sputum Gram stain and culture, blood culture, transtracheal aspirate culture, bronchoscopic specimen culture (protected brush samples, bronchoalveolar lavage, transbronchial biopsy, bronchial wash), open-lung biopsy, and immunologic methods (129). For most patients, collection of sputum is the primary diagnostic test, along with blood cultures (which are positive in no more than 15% of all cases of pneumonia) and a careful clinical evaluation. In spite of these assessments, many patients require empiric therapy, with modifications being made after the results of diagnostic testing become available. If there is no response or if a specific diagnosis is required (as in certain ICHs), then more invasive tests are done.

Sputum samples are not always the source of reliable data. Culture of expectorated sputum may be of no help because the sample can be contaminated by oral flora as it passes through the oropharynx; the sample may not contain the responsible pathogen; or the sample may contain pathogens that are colonizing the patient but not causing the invasive infection. A sputum sample should be assessed for quality by microscopic examination. If there are fewer than 10 squamous epithelial cells and more than 25 neutrophils per low-power field, the sample is probably a good representation of the lower airway's secretions. Samples with more than 25 squamous epithelial cells are too contaminated by oral secretions to be useful. The value of sputum Gram stain is widely debated (71). Although Gram staining can show a dominant organism, the sensitivity and specificity vary widely depending on the criteria used to define a sample as "positive." Often the test is performed by individuals who cannot correlate the findings with the clinical picture, or else it is performed by clinicians with limited technical expertise. All of these practical considerations limit the utility of a sputum Gram stain. The difficulty with sputum Gram stain data is highlighted by finding false-positive rates of up to 88% and false-negative rates of 50% (129). With pneumococcal pneumonia, up to half of the sputum Gram

stains will be negative. Given all of these considerations, it is possible to use a Gram stain to broaden empiric therapy to include organisms seen on the stain which were not initially included in therapy, but it is probably not possible to narrow therapy based on the findings.

A high false-positive rate of both Gram stain and sputum culture may result from the fact that many patients who have pneumonia also have airway colonization by enteric Gram-negative organisms. The exact role of these cultured organisms in causing any pneumonia in such a colonized patient is unclear. For example, up to 40% of the elderly are colonized by Gram-negative organisms, and up to 75% of hospitalized patients can harbor these organisms in their airway even without pneumonia. Certain organisms can be recovered on stain or culture of sputum whose presence alone is diagnostic, since these organisms never colonize without causing infection; they include *M. tuberculosis, P. carinii,* certain fungi, and *L. pneumophila.* A sputum culture should be obtained from any CAP patient who is suspected of having one of these unusual organisms or a drug-resistant organism.

Of the noninvasive techniques, immunologic methods can be applied to many patients with varying degrees of sensitivity and rapidity of receiving diagnostic information. Serologic titers for viral, fungal, *Legionella,* and certain atypical agents can be diagnostic, but there is often a delay in receiving results and often convalescent titers must be collected. Thus this method is of little use in the acute management of patients and is more helpful for epidemiologic studies. Immunologic staining of respiratory secretions for bacterial or viral antigens can occasionally be useful. Counterimmunoelectrophoresis can detect small amounts of pneumococcal antigen in the sputum, serum, or urine of up to half of the patients with pneumococcal pneumonia. Direct fluorescent antibody staining of sputum for *L. pneumophila* can be positive in 70% of cases, and testing for urinary antigen is positive in over half of all patients at the time of initial evaluation (129). Genetic probes for the nucleic acids of *Legionella* and certain viruses are increasingly available.

Of the invasive techniques, open-lung biopsy is generally reserved for the immunocompromised patient or for the patient with an unresolving pneumonia. The most commonly used invasive procedure is bronchoscopy, and it should be used only if its risks are less than the risks of empiric therapy or if empiric therapy is not successful. Transbronchial biopsy allows histologic examination and culture for mycobacteria, *Pneumocystis,* fungi, and viral agents. Bronchoscopy has its greatest utility in the ICH and (as mentioned) is controversial and of uncertain value in patients with suspected nosocomial pneumonia (130,131). In patients with CAP, it should be reserved for the nonresponding patient. Bronchoalveolar lavage has been used in the ICH and has had a diagnostic yield of over 60% (130). By wedging the bronchoscope and instilling 210 mL of saline in 30 mL aliquots, the lavage fluid can be returned and collected for culture and staining. This method has detected ICHs with infections caused by *Pneumocystis*, viruses, fungi, and mycobacteria.

Therapy of Pneumonia

Antibiotics represent the mainstay of pneumonia therapy and may be viewed as specific in contrast to many of the other therapies, which are primarily supportive. Antibiotic therapy is organism-directed, but if a specific pathogen is not identified, empiric therapy directed at the most likely pathogens is commonly used and will be selected after a careful epidemiologic assessment of the patient. The supportive measures that are not specific to any organism are adjunctive therapy and include supplemental oxygen, intravenous hydration, and measures to promote tracheobronchial toilet such as mucolytic and mucokinetic agents, bronchodilators, and bronchoscopy.

Indications for Hospitalization of CAP Patients

Individuals who have moderate to severe illness generally require intravenous antibiotics, hydration, and supplemental oxygen (arterial oxygen tension less than 60 mm Hg on room air), and these therapies require admission to the hospital. In addition, those with serious coexisting illness or multiple risk factors for a poor outcome should also be treated in an inpatient setting. Risk factors for a complicated course of illness include the presence of coexisting diseases such as congestive heart failure, obstructive lung disease, diabetes, renal failure, hospitalization within the last year, and neurologic illness; age above 65 years; certain physical findings such as tachypnea, hypotension, or high fever; hypoxemia or hypercarbia (PaO_2 less than 60 mm Hg or $PaCO_2$ above 50 mm Hg) on room air; and evidence of sepsis or end-organ dysfunction (71). Recently, scoring systems have been developed to predict mortality from CAP, and these can be used to guide the admission decision. However, the use of such systems in place of clinical judgment has not yet been proven to be safe or cost-effective (132).

In addition to offering specific therapy that is unavailable to outpatients, hospitalization allows observation of the patient's course during therapy. Individuals with serious comorbidity may have deterioration of their underlying illness in response to infection, their pneumonia may progress rapidly, and on initial evaluation they may appear less ill than they actually are because of an impaired host inflammatory response. Hospitalization is also able to provide specific therapy for patients who are in respiratory failure (severe hypoxemia or hypercarbia), as well as for those with an impaired cough reflex and copious sputum (so that they may receive adequate tracheobronchial toilet), those with atelectasis, and those with systemic sepsis.

Antibiotic Therapy

If a specific pathogen is identified, therapy should be as narrowly directed as possible, with the agents mentioned above for each organism. If no etiology can be established, empiric therapy is required, with full appreciation of the pitfalls of this approach. With empiric regimens, multiple antibiotics are often required, not all likely pathogens can be covered, and some combination therapies are nephrotoxic.

Therapy for community-acquired infection is directed toward pneumococcus, *M. pneumoniae,* and *C. pneumoniae* if the patient has no host impairment (71). If the patient is elderly, has aspirated, is an alcoholic, or has serious coexisting illness, then in addition to these organisms the empiric regimen must also cover enteric Gram-negative organisms, *H. influenzae, S. aureus,* and anaerobes. Hospitalized patients should be treated for pneumococcus, enteric Gram-negative organisms, *H. influenzae, S. aureus,* anaerobes, and possibly *Legionella*. Those with severe CAP should be treated for pneumococcus, *Legionella,* enteric Gram-negative organisms (including *P. aeruginosa),* and possibly *M. pneumoniae* and *H. influenzae*. PRSP should be covered in patients with risk factors such as age over 65 years, β-lactam therapy within the last three months, immunosuppressive illness, alcoholism, and multiple medical comorbidities.

When antibiotics are used, precautions are necessary in certain settings. With renal or hepatic failure, certain drugs will have their elimination interfered with, and dosage must be adjusted. Renally cleared drugs include the aminoglycosides, certain cephalosporins, quinolones, penicillins, and other β-lactams. Liver-excreted drugs include erythromycin, chloramphenicol, and nafcillin. In patients with a reduction in lean body mass and an increase in body fat, such as the elderly, there may be a rise in drug levels if they are given on a per-kilogram basis. With a reduction in serum albumin, the free concentration of certain drugs that are ordinarily highly protein-bound may rise. Some drugs, particularly the penicillins, have a high sodium content, which should be considered if the patient has coexisting heart failure.

Some antibiotics penetrate poorly into bronchial secretions, and topical antibiotics may be indicated to increase antibiotic levels in the lung. This approach is not a standard one, but it has been used successfully to treat *P. aeruginosa* airway infections in patients with cystic fibrosis. It may also be indicated to treat patients with severe Gram-negative infections that have not responded to parenteral antibiotics. When topical therapy is given, it may be via direct intratracheal injection or aerosolization and should be preceded by bronchodilator treatment to avoid reflex bronchospasm. The drugs most commonly used in this manner are polymyxin and the aminoglycosides. Some evidence suggests that topical antibiotics can be used prophylactically in critically ill patients to prevent nosocomial pneumonia.

Once the patient has responded to initial therapy, a rapid switch to oral therapy followed by prompt hospital discharge is recommended. Criteria for switch to oral therapy include subjective improvement in cough, sputum and dyspnea; resolution of fever (afebrile, two occasions, eight hours apart); improvement in leukocytosis; and ability to take oral medications. In many patients, this switch can be safely achieved by the third or fourth hospital day.

Oxygenation and Mechanical Ventilation

Endotracheal intubation and mechanical ventilation are required in patients with refractory hypoxemia (arterial oxygen tension less than 60 mm Hg on maximal mask oxygen) or hypercarbic respiratory failure with acute respiratory acidosis, and in patients who cannot adequately clear secretions (to allow deep airway suctioning). When patients have severe hypoxemia and a unilateral pneumonia, their oxygenation can be improved by positioning them with the unaffected lung in a gravity-dependent position. This maneuver increases perfusion to the normal lung relative to the diseased lung, and thereby minimizes ventilation-perfusion mismatches.

Tracheobronchial Toilet

Chest physiotherapy can be used to promote clearance of respiratory secretions. This therapy, which employs components of postural drainage, chest percussion, vibration, coughing, and forced expiratory breathing, is best used for patients with copious secretions (more than 30 mL per day) who have a reduced ability to cough. These physical methods may be no more effective than a good cough, but many patients are unable to provide this, and assistance may be required (133).

Agents that reduce the viscosity and consistency of sputum are termed mucolytic; those that increase mucociliary clearance are termed mucokinetic (134). Mucolytic therapy can be achieved with hydration, aerosolized saline, and inhaled *N*-acetylcysteine. The use of mucolytic agents is best reserved for patients with retained secretions who have developed atelectasis. Mucokinetic drugs are rarely used, but some agents that may be used for other purposes have mucokinetic effects. These include β-agonist bronchodilators and theophylline. Another technique that may be helpful for some patients with mucus plugging and retained secretions is bronchoscopy. If atelectasis is present without an air bronchogram, there may be a large central airway plug, and bronchoscopy can be used for suction removal under direct vision. Bronchoscopy can also be used in patients with unresolving pneumonia to evaluate for the presence of a tumor or aspirated foreign body. For patients with nosocomial pneumonia, secretions may also be mobilized by endotracheal suctioning. Another approach is to place the patient on an oscillating bed that rotates from side to side. Although it is unclear whether this approach can help pneumonia resolve more rapidly, there are data suggesting that this type of intervention can prevent pneumonia in high-risk patients, possibly by mobilizing secretions (135).

Tuberculosis

Epidemiology and Pathogenesis

Tuberculosis (TB) may be a pulmonary disease, an extrapulmonary disease, or both, and is caused by Koch's bacillus, *M. tuberculosis.* The organism is a nonmotile, acid-fast staining, Gram-positive rod with a high lipid content. It is an obligate aerobe which is not pigmented (in contrast to some of the other mycobacterial species) and is normally contained by cell-mediated immunity. Patients with impaired cellular immune responses, such as the elderly, diabetics, patients treated with immunosuppressives, patients with renal failure, those with hematologic malignancy, and individuals with AIDS, are thus at increased risk of illness from this organism. Disease is spread from person to person via inhalation of droplet nuclei produced by infected persons when they talk, cough, or sneeze. Casual contacts of infected persons are not usually infected, but those with prolonged and close contact, particularly in areas of poor ventilation, are most at risk. This mode of spread, which favors disease in crowded, small spaces, may contribute to the predominance of this illness among those of lower socioeconomic status and in persons living in underdeveloped nations.

In the United States, there were about 15 new cases per 100,000 population during the 1970s, and the incidence declined at a rate of 6.7% annually until 1985. Beginning in 1986 and continuing until 1992, the incidence of new cases began to rise, which has been attributed to the frequent infection of AIDS patients with the tubercle bacillus (20,136). With aggressive measures of disease control and directly observed therapy, this rise was reversed in 1993. In 1990, it was estimated that 4.3% of HIV-infected persons had TB infection (20). In addition, tuberculosis remains an important infection in many immigrants to this country, among the homeless, and in the elderly who are confined to nursing homes. Currently, more than two-thirds of TB cases occur in nonwhite racial and ethnic groups. One-quarter of all cases in the United States occur in the foreign-born, but still one-third of cases occur in middle- and upper-income groups (20). Among patients aged 25 to 44 years, most are nonwhites and Hispanics, while whites predominate in the elderly population of TB patients. One other recent change in TB epidemiology has been the emergence of organisms that are multiply resistant to traditional TB medications. Multidrug-resistant tuberculosis (MDR-TB) is a particular problem among HIV-infected individuals and those with a history of prior TB therapy. In New York City, as many as 23% of all previously untreated TB patients had primary drug resistance to at least one drug in the early 1990's (137).

Most individuals who encounter the tubercle bacillus become infected with it, contain the organism within the lung by developing an adequate immune response, and thus do not develop clinical illness. Those with the clinical disease "tuberculosis" are either individuals who cannot contain the primary infection or persons who have reactivated a previously contained and dormant infection. Thus much of the literature makes a distinction between "infection" and "disease" due to *M. tuberculosis.* Many people have had the infection, but fewer than 10% of infected individuals will develop the disease.

The initial infection with the organism, the primary infection, is usually in the middle or lower zones of the lung. Since these areas receive the most ventilation with each breath, it is not surprising that an airborne organism would localize in this fashion. Over the next few weeks, the organisms multiply and spread via lymphatics to the regional lymph nodes, particularly in the hilum. The combination of a primary peripheral lung lesion with an enlarged hilar lymph node is termed a Ghon complex. During this time, some organisms may disseminate via the bloodstream to extrapulmonary sites, where they are usually contained but may reactivate at a later date. The favored sites for secondary seeding and growth of these aerobic bacteria are ones with high tissue oxygen content such as the apex of the lung, the renal parenchyma, and the growing ends of long bones.

Within three to six weeks of primary infection, sensitized T lymphocytes release lymphokines that can attract monocytes and macrophages to the infected area in the lung to phagocytose the bacteria. Lymphocytes are also attracted, and during this time, the host develops immunity to reinfection, which becomes detectable by conversion of the tuberculin skin test to positive. Once the skin test becomes positive, the host can usually kill any other organisms that are inhaled, but it may not always be able to eliminate the organisms already within the lung and lung macrophages. Thus most cases of active tuberculosis are in patients with positive skin tests and are due to progressive primary disease or reactivation disease; they are less commonly due to reinfection after exposure to another infected patient with active disease. However, in the HIV-infected patient, superinfection with a resistant TB strain during TB therapy for infection with another strain has been reported (138).

The initial tissue response to infection involves mononuclear cells which may crowd together with their lipid-rich cytoplasm and form a tubercle made up of cells that are described as epithelioid. The tubercle may contain multinucleated giant cells, called Langhans cells, and it is surrounded by fibroblasts, lymphocytes, and more monocytes to form a granuloma, which is characteristic of tuberculosis. This granulomatous reaction must be distinguished from other granulomatous tissue reactions such as those seen with sarcoidosis and fungal disease. When a host cannot contain the organism by this inflammatory response, the organism continues to multiply, and the center of the granuloma undergoes a process of liquefaction necrosis, termed caseation. The progression to this necrotizing process does not occur in most infected patients, but only in those who cannot contain the organism. The caseous material is full of living organisms that can spread within the lung. The necrotic, caseating granuloma then becomes a tuberculous cavity, which may contain up to 10^9 organisms (139). Without caseation, a granuloma has many fewer organisms. When large quantities of caseous material are spread along the bronchi from a cavity to another part of the lung, a tuberculous pneumonia may develop. When granulomas finally do heal, they often develop calcification, particularly if caseation has occurred.

About 5% of patients with primary infection will not be able to contain the organism and will develop progressive primary disease within two years of infection. Rates of progressive primary disease may be higher with HIV infection, reaching as high as 38% in the first year, and averaging 8% per year afterwards (140), as the onset of illness is accelerated by the HIV coinfection. As primary infection usually involves the lower-lung zones, the patient with progressive primary disease may manifest with lower-lobe tuberculosis (Fig. 15.13). The failure to contain the organism may be related to the size of inoculum and the status of the host defense system. Patients at risk for progressive primary infection are the very young, the elderly, the malnourished, blacks, diabetics, alcoholics, and those with immunosuppressive medications or illnesses (including HIV infection). An additional 5% will develop disease more than two years after infection, which will be due to reactivation of live bacilli that had been contained and dormant within healed granulomas. This reactivation illness usually develops in sites where the organism was hematogenously disseminated during the primary infection. The lung apex is a common site for reactivation disease, particularly in the apical posterior segment (Fig. 15.14). Thus, based on this pathogenetic schema, lower-lobe tuberculosis is usually a progressive primary disease, while upper-lobe disease may represent reactivation. In either situation, the patient with tuberculous disease has been unable to contain the organism, whereas most people who are infected do not develop disease because they can contain the organism. For this reason, a deficit in host defense should be sought in all patients with active tuberculosis, and HIV testing should be considered in all patients with active tuberculosis. Extrapulmonary disease may occur as a result of progressive primary infection or with reactivation.

Clinical Features

With primary infection, most patients are asymptomatic or may have mild, nonspecific symptoms of a transient lower-respiratory-tract infection. When disease is present, symptoms are usually chronic and may cause respiratory symptoms as well as systemic manifestations. Many patients note simply malaise, headache, fever, night sweats, and weight loss. Some patients may have abdominal pain and anorexia. Pulmonary symptoms are common but not specific. Persistent cough may be present, with or without mucoid sputum, and occasionally hemoptysis is present. Hemoptysis can be the result of tuberculous pneumonia but is more commonly due to cavitary disease or rupture of an artery in an old

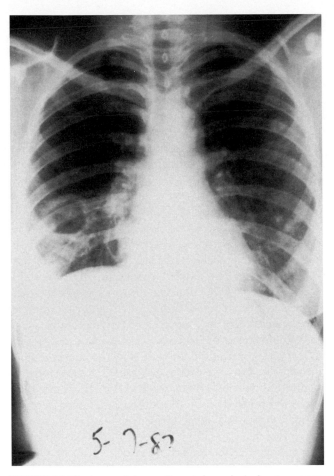

FIGURE 15.13. Lower-lobe cavitary tuberculosis due to progressive primary disease in a 46-year-old black diabetic man.

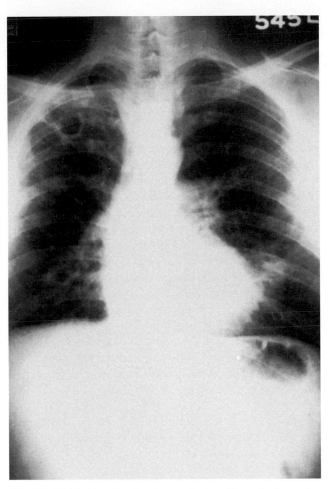

FIGURE 15.14. Reactivation tuberculosis with cavity formation and infiltrate in the upper lobe and endobronchial spread from an upper-lobe cavity to the lower lobes.

tuberculous cavity (Rasmussen's aneurysm). Several late posttuberculous complications can cause hemoptysis, including bronchiectasis, broncholithiasis, or the presence of an aspergilloma in a prior tuberculous cavity. Another pulmonary symptom can be chest pain, particularly pleurisy-type pain, when a pleural effusion is present. Tuberculous effusions usually result when a small number of organisms from a subpleural granuloma, early in the course of the illness, rupture into the pleural cavity and the patient has a hypersensitivity response to this material. Because most of the pleural fluid is inflammatory, not many organisms are present, and culture of the pleural fluid yields the tubercle bacillus in no more than 20% to 40% of cases. Because the pleural response is a hypersensitivity one, it usually correlates with a positive tuberculin test. Much less commonly, a large inoculum of organisms can reach the pleural space and cause a tuberculous empyema. Dyspnea may occur as a result of extensive parenchymal disease, pneumothorax, or a large pleural effusion. Both the systemic and pulmonary symptoms are usually chronic, having been present for weeks to months prior to diagnosis, but occasionally an acute pneumonia presentation is seen, and acute respiratory

failure may result (141). The elderly generally have less dramatic symptoms than do younger patients (142).

Extrapulmonary disease is seen in up to 16% of tuberculosis cases in the United States. However, in patients with AIDS, this pattern is much more common and may occur in 60% to 70% of all tuberculosis cases in this population (143,144). When extrapulmonary involvement is present, the patient may present with a skin lesion that is slow to heal or a chronic draining cervical lymph node (scrofula, or cervical lymph node tuberculosis). When genital tuberculosis is present, men may have epididymal involvement with a slightly painful scrotal mass, while women may have pelvic pain or infertility. Renal tuberculosis is usually without symptoms, but patients will have "sterile" pyuria or hematuria on urinalysis. Tuberculous meningitis may cause dementia, coma, cranial nerve abnormalities (because the base of the brain is involved), focal neurologic deficits, or headache. Abdominal pain, fever, ascites, and anorexia can be manifestations of tuberculous peritonitis. Chest pain, fever, and dyspnea may result from pericardial involvement. Tuberculous involvement of the skeleton may cause bone pain or spine collapse with spinal cord compression. When the disease is fulminant and hematogenously disseminated, it is termed "miliary" because of the millet seed appearance of the multiple pulmonary lesions that are seen on chest radiograph. Miliary disease may occur with progressive primary infection or reactivation but is the result of bloodstream invasion and dissemination of large numbers of bacteria that overcome host defenses at multiple sites. Miliary tuberculosis may cause fever, malaise, cough, dyspnea, weight loss, anorexia, and headache. The lungs, liver, adrenals, kidneys, and spleen are often involved, and diagnosis may require lung or bone marrow biopsy, although organisms may be recovered from bronchoalveolar lavage or urine.

Physical findings are not specific, and patients may show signs of pneumonitis (rales), pleural effusion (dullness to percussion and reduced breath sounds), or specific extrapulmonary involvement. Laboratory data may reveal anemia, leukopenia, or severe leukocytosis. Hyponatremia and hypercalcemia are also common findings. Liver function tests may be abnormal with disseminated infection. Pleural fluid is usually an exudate with lymphocytosis, low glucose, and low pH. Spinal fluid may show low glucose, high protein, and lymphocytes if meningitis is present.

Diagnosis

The chest radiograph is an important clue to the presence of tuberculosis. Lower-lobe involvement with infiltrates or cavitation may occur in progressive primary disease, but most patients have evidence of apical involvement, particularly in the posterior segments. Apical scarring may indicate prior infection, and a change in a previously stable upperlobe pattern may indicate reactivation. Cavitation is common with reactivation and may accompany a parenchymal, reticular upper-lobe infiltrate (Fig. 15.14). Some patients will have extensive nodular lung involvement in conjunction with one or multiple cavities, and this pattern of extensive parenchymal infection is the result of endobronchial dissemination of bacteria from a caseating cavitary lesion. Nodal enlargement in the hilum and mediastinum as well as nodal calcification can result from tuberculosis. Solitary nodules may occasionally represent a tuberculoma, and sometimes these lesions can cavitate. Other radiographic findings can include a miliary pattern with bilateral, diffuse, small densities or pleural effusion with or without an evident parenchymal lesion. In one series (145), patients with primary tuberculosis had pulmonary consolidation in the lower-lung zones or anteriorly in the upper lobe (50%), cavitation (29%), miliary disease (6%), or a normal radiograph (15%). Those with reactivation disease had a different pattern, with 91% having apical and posterior fibrous infiltrates, 45% having cavities, and 21% having bronchogenic spread of disease.

Clinical and radiographic features may be different when HIV infection is present. As mentioned, fewer HIV-infected patients than other infected individuals have only pulmonary disease. With lung involvement, HIV-infected patients with TB have lower-lobe infiltrates and adenopathy and infrequently have cavitation. Even with bacteriologically confirmed pulmonary TB, HIV-infected persons can have a normal chest radiograph (136). In general, the more classic, typical, radiographic patterns are seen in HIV-infected persons who are early in their disease and are relatively intact immunologically. The severely immune-suppressed HIV patient tends to have more unusual TB manifestations, and infection with *M. avium intracellulare* is also frequently present.

A definitive diagnosis of tuberculosis disease is made by isolating the organism from a clinical specimen such as sputum, urine, a biopsy of involved tissue, pleural fluid, bone marrow aspirate, spinal fluid, ascites fluid, or bronchoscopic lavage. Sputum is best sampled by collecting the first sample produced in the early morning. In some patients, gastric aspirates can be collected and cultured, and these samples may contain organisms that have been expectorated and swallowed. Clinical specimens can be stained for organisms by the acid-fast method or with the rhodamine fluorochrome stain. Gastric aspirates may give a false-positive stain as some gastric saprophytes are acid-fast. If a patient has pulmonary involvement and sputum samples are negative, bronchoscopy should be performed with lavage, as the diagnostic yield may exceed 90%. Newer diagnostic modalities are becoming available, and they have the advantage of identifying a mycobacterial organism more rapidly than more traditional methods. With radiometric culture techniques and nucleic acid probes, organisms can be identified in a week or less, and fewer bacteria are needed than with traditional diagnostic methods (136).

Tuberculous infection (but not disease) is diagnosed by finding a positive skin test response to tuberculin antigen. The standard Mantoux test uses purified protein derivative (PPD) of tuberculin, and a dose of 5 tuberculin units in 0.1 mL is administered intradermally. The degree of induration at 48 to 72 hours is measured, and a positive test is defined in relation to the individual's relative risk of being infected with the tuberculosis bacterium (20,146). A reaction of 5 mm or more is defined as positive for patients who are HIV-positive or have HIV risk factors and are of unknown HIV status, those who are close contacts of an active case, and those who have a chest radiograph consistent with old, healed tuberculosis. A reaction of 10 mm or more is defined as positive in patients who do not fall in any of the above categories but who are foreign-born from highprevalence countries, intravenous drug users, in minority or medically underserved groups, residents of a chronic care facility or correctional institution, and patients with medical conditions that increase the risk of tuberculosis. Such medical conditions include silicosis, gastrectomy, ileal bypass, chronic renal failure, diabetes mellitus, high-dose corticosteroids or immunosuppressive therapy or illness, and malnutrition. All other persons who do not fit into any of these groups are defined as positive only if the skin test reaction is 15 mm or more (143,144,146).

Over 90% of patients with tuberculous disease will have a positive skin test, and those that do not are either anergic due to overwhelming illness or are too early in the course of disease to have converted the skin test to positive. If a skin test reaction increases in size by 10 mm or more in a previously negative person under the age of 35, a "conversion" is said to have occurred, and this indicates infection during the time between the two skin tests. For persons over the age of 35, an increase of 15 mm or more is needed to define a conversion if the patient was previously negative (146). In some populations, particularly the elderly, a false-negative skin test can occur because of a "loss of immunologic memory." In such patients, a second skin test will be positive because the antigenic exposure of the first skin test "boosted" the immune response that had been present but suppressed. When comparing the first and second skin test, one should not conclude that these patients have converted from a negative test to a positive one, but rather that they have had their false-negative result unmasked by the so-called "booster effect." It is important in mass screening programs to account for this phenomenon by giving a second skin test to all negative reactors one to two weeks after the first test so that a boosted response will be recognized and not confused with a new conversion.

Treatment

Antituberculous therapy can be given to individuals with infection who are at high risk of developing active disease; this practice, which can prevent illness, is called prophylactic therapy. In addition, patients with active tuberculosis are treated with medications that are generally able to cure the disease effectively.

Prophylactic therapy is given with isoniazid 10 mg per kg per day (up to a maximum of 300 mg) for six to nine months (143,144). Those with AIDS may require prophylaxis for 12 months (143,144). Since any person with a positive PPD skin-test has been infected with the tubercle bacillus and can develop disease, prophylactic therapy should be considered for all skin-test reactors. However, isoniazid can cause hepatotoxicity, and the incidence of this complication rises with age, particularly above the age of 35. Thus prophylactic therapy is recommended only for those whose risk of developing disease exceeds their risk of liver toxicity. A positive tuberculin test (as defined above) indicates the need for prophylaxis regardless of age if the patient falls into one of the following groups: (a) known or suspected HIV infection; (b) close contact with an active case; (c) recent convertor (defined above); (d) radiographic evidence of prior tuberculosis; (e) presence of a medical condition that increases the risk of TB (listed above). Prophylaxis is offered to other people only if they are under the age of 35 and fall into the following categories: (a) for-

eign-born from a high-risk area; (b) medically underserved, low-income populations; (c) residents of long-term care facilities or correctional institutions; (d) patients with no risk factors but a skin test of more than 15 mm.

Active tuberculosis, both pulmonary and extrapulmonary, should be treated with isoniazid 300 mg daily along with rifampin 600 mg daily for six months, combined with pyrazinamide (25 mg per kg) for the first two months if the organism is not drug-resistant (147). This regimen combines the most active antituberculous medications and is the most widely used today. An alternative is to use isoniazid and rifampin together for nine months for drug-sensitive organisms. Both isoniazid and rifampin are bactericidal for the tubercle bacillus, and when used together they can eliminate the organism rapidly and usually prevent relapse due to resistant bacteria. Rifampin is rapidly bactericidal to tubercle bacilli that exist in any of the three populations present in the body: actively growing extracellular organisms, slowly growing intracellular (in macrophages) organisms at acid pH, and slowly growing extracellular organisms. Isoniazid is bactericidal against the first two of these populations; streptomycin kills only actively growing extracellular bacteria; and pyrazinamide kills slowly growing intracellular bacteria. Two active drugs are needed for therapy because naturally occurring drug-resistant mutants are present in most patients. It has been estimated that one in 10^5 organisms is resistant to isoniazid and one in 10^9 is resistant to rifampin. Since an active tuberculous cavity has no more than 10^8 to 10^9 organisms, the combination therapy will effectively kill any naturally occurring drug-resistant mutants. If drug combinations other than isoniazid, rifampin, and pyrrazinamide are used, therapy must be extended to 18 to 24 months, because other drugs are not as active. These regimens are used if the patient develops toxicity to one of the standard drugs or if drug-resistant disease is documented or suspected (as is common in certain immigrant populations). Ethambutol and streptomycin are commonly used in these extended regimens; second-line drugs include capreomycin, ethionamide, cycloserine, and PAS. Compliance can be improved with intermittent regimens given under direct supervision three to five times per week. In some communities, directly observed therapy has become the standard of care and can reduce the incidence of tuberculosis, especially drug-resistant disease.

The current concerns about MDR-TB have changed the initial approach to therapy in many parts of the country. When the possibility of resistance is entertained, patients are started on a four-drug regimen of isoniazid, rifampin, pyrazinamide, and ethambutol (148). If susceptibility patterns reveal that the organism is not drug-resistant, ethambutol is stopped, pyrazinamide is continued for a total of two months, and isoniazid is continued along with rifampin for a total of six months. In this way, short-course therapy can be achieved while still protecting against the possibility of resistant disease. If MDR-TB is identified, therapy is continued with at least two active first-line drugs. These include INH, pyrazinamide, ethambutol, and rifampin. If the organism is not sensitive to at least two of these agents, second-line drugs should be used, but at least three will be required (137). Some patients with MDR-TB require multiple drugs for prolonged periods of time, and occasionally drug therapy must be supplemented with resectional surgery. To improve the outcome of therapy of MDR-TB in certain populations, directly observed therapy has been recommended (148).

Mycobacteria Other Than Tuberculosis

Mycobacteria other than tuberculosis (MOTT) are generally slow-growing mycobacteria that, unlike *M. tuberculosis,* are niacin-negative (i.e., they metabolize and do not accumulate niacin) in the laboratory. Although some of the MOTT are niacin-positive and some are rapid growers, most human disease is caused by species that do not fit this pattern. MOTT differ from the tubercle bacillus in several other important ways. They are not spread from person to person, and they are not always pathogens when isolated from human samples. In fact, most normal individuals can effectively resist infection by these organisms without tissue invasion occurring, while others may become colonized but not infected. MOTT can cause illnesses very similar to tuberculosis, but usually only in abnormal hosts. Because of the similarities and differences that these organisms and their manifestations have to the tubercle bacillus, they are sometimes called "atypical mycobacteria." In recent years, the incidence of infection by these organisms has risen, particularly in the AIDS population, where disseminated infection with *M. avium* complex (MAC) has occurred. There are multiple species of MOTT, many of which rarely cause human disease. The species that are potentially pathogenic in humans include MAC, *M. kansasii, M. fortuitumchelonei, M. scrofulaceum, M. xenopi, M. szulgai, M. simiae, M. marinum, M. ulcerans,* and *M. haemophilum* (149).

The diseases caused by MOTT may cause findings in the lungs, the cervical lymph nodes (lymphadenitis), the skin (abscess or nonhealing ulcer), or occasionally systemically. The pulmonary disease may appear radiographically (Fig. 15.15) like tuberculosis but may differ in that cavities can be thin-walled with little surrounding infiltrate. In addition, bronchogenic spread is unusual, pleural disease is uncommon, and preexisting chronic pulmonary disease is often present (150). Symptoms are more slowly progressive than in tuberculosis but may include cough, dyspnea, weight loss, and occasionally hemoptysis and fever. The pulmonary disease is usually indolent, and when it occurs, it commonly affects older patients with chronic obstructive pulmonary disease. This pattern can occur with MAC, *M. kansasii,* or others of the MOTT group. Recently a much more virulent and disseminated form of disease, caused by MAC, has been found in AIDS patients (144). Up to one-

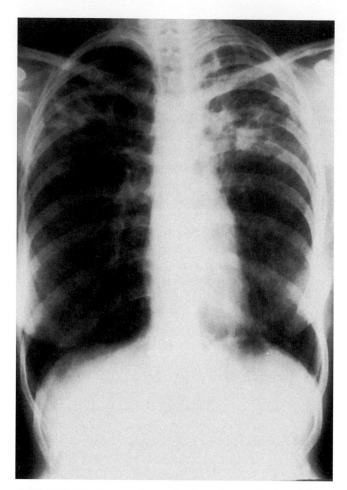

FIGURE 15.15. Chest radiograph of a patient with chronic bronchitis and slowly progressive cavitary disease in both upper lobes due to *M. avium* complex.

quarter of AIDS patients may have disseminated MAC disease diagnosed antemortem, while half will have it at autopsy. Mortality from this infection is high, and symptoms are not specific and commonly include fever, weight loss, abdominal pain, malabsorption, and diarrhea. Pulmonary symptoms may also be present but not in every case. Patients may have generalized lymphadenopathy and hepatosplenomegaly. Diagnosis of disseminated MAC infection in the AIDS patient can be made by finding the organism in bone marrow, liver, urine, lymph nodes, or blood cultures.

In general, the diagnosis of MOTT infections is difficult, because simple isolation of the organisms from sputum is not sufficient to establish infection since these bacteria may colonize diseased lungs yet not cause invasive infection. A diagnosis of pulmonary disease by MOTT is made by having a compatible clinical picture and radiograph in a patient with repeated isolation of organisms from sputum or with evidence of tissue invasion by organisms on biopsy. If cavitary disease is present, the diagnosis can be made by finding the organisms on two or more sputum samples, provided that other diagnoses have been excluded. If cavitary disease is absent, the diagnosis requires the above findings plus a failure to convert sputum samples to negative with either bronchial hygiene or two weeks of specific drug therapy (151). If the sputum is nondiagnostic, the diagnosis can also be established by finding the organisms in a biopsy specimen. Skin testing is not widely available or clinically useful in diseases caused by these bacteria. In the AIDS patient, the recovery of MAC organisms from blood or stool in a patient with a compatible illness will establish the diagnosis of disseminated infection. Once the diagnosis of MOTT infection is made, therapy is started with multiple antituberculous drugs, but the success rate, particularly in the AIDS patient, may be quite low because the organisms are usually resistant to most available medications. Some newer agents that may be active against some of the MOTT organisms are clarithromycin, azithromycin, ciprofloxacin, ofloxacin, and rifabutin.

Fungal Lung Disease: Normal Host

The dimorphic fungi *Histoplasma capsulatum, Blastomyces dermatitides, Coccidioides immitis, Paracoccidioides brasiliensis,* and *Sporothrix schenckii* are all soil-growing organisms. With the exception of *Sporothrix,* they are sharply defined in their endemic areas. Again with the exception of *S. schenckii,* their primary mechanisms of infection are via the lungs; *S. schenckii* may also invade the host via the lungs but the usual manifestation of the illness is lymphocutaneous. Moreover, most infections are asymptomatic, and only a certain percentage of infected individuals go on to develop clinically recognizable illness. Occasionally, following the acute illness, chronic or disseminated disease may develop.

After the infecting spores are inhaled, these organisms convert at body temperature to their pathogenic forms, which in all but *C. immitis* is a yeast. *C. immitis* at body temperature converts to giant spherules. While the yeast multiply by binary fission, giant spherules multiply by endosporulation.

The underlying state of immunity of the host will determine the extent and nature of human illness. Normal hosts are usually able to localize the illness to the lungs, and spontaneous recovery is the rule. However, when the disease occurs in patients who are immunocompromised, either by another underlying illness or because of the administration of cytotoxic agents or glucocorticoids, dissemination to multiple organs is the rule.

Histoplasmosis

The endemic area for *H. capsulatum* includes most of the Midwestern and South-Central United States, extending down to the Gulf Coast in Texas and to the St. Lawrence Valley in Canada (152). The organism occurs in microfoci in nature, and grows in soil enhanced by organic nitrogen,

usually by droppings of birds or bats. In nature the organism grows as a mold, and when the sites are disturbed, an infecting aerosol is produced, leading to inhalation of the spores.

Following inhalation, the spores produce an area of pneumonitis in the lung after conversion to the yeast form. After spread to the hilar nodes, the organism gains access to the bloodstream and disseminates throughout the body. Cells of the reticuloendothelial (RE) system remove the organism from circulation, and once specific delayed hypersensitivity develops, the "armed" macrophages will destroy the organisms, leading to granuloma formation. Frequently, healing causes necrosis, which over the years may undergo calcification.

In abnormal hosts such as infants, the very elderly, or patients who are immunosuppressed by underlying disease or by administration of various agents, progressive disseminated disease frequently occurs (153). In these individuals adequate cell-mediated immunity fails to develop and the organism begins to replicate within cells of the RE system.

The vast majority of primary infections with *H. capsulatum* are either asymptomatic or minimally symptomatic. Only a small fraction of patients will ever visit a physician because of the onset of acute histoplasmosis. Those who are symptomatic usually have a "flulike" illness, with arthralgias and myalgias as well as a nonproductive cough. Fever is usually low-grade. Chest roentgenograms may be normal or show extensive bilateral nodular disease with hilar adenopathy. In addition, erythema nodosum may accompany the onset of clinical illness (154).

The primary infection in patients with altered lung anatomy, such as seen with centrilobular emphysema of smokers, looks different from that seen in normal hosts. In these patients the acute infection may surround these abnormal air spaces, giving the roentgenographic appearance of cavity formation. It is important to remember that the vast majority of these patients probably also recover spontaneously, and only in rare instances will the upper-lobe disease become progressive and require treatment (155).

Symptoms of progressive upper-zone histoplasmosis are chronic illness with low-grade fever, weight loss, anorexia, and a cough productive of mucopurulent sputum. Because of the great similarity of the symptoms and the chest roentgenogram to tuberculosis, many of these patients are initially thought to have tuberculosis (Fig. 15.16) (156). Among the other residuals following primary infection, the most common is the "coin lesion" caused by rounding off and hardening of the area of previous pneumonitis. The main significance of these lesions is that they frequently occur in patients otherwise at high risk for bronchogenic neoplasms.

An unusual complication of acute histoplasmosis is the development of mediastinal fibrosis, which is probably an abnormal host response rather than an unusual effect of the parasite (Fig. 15.17) (157).

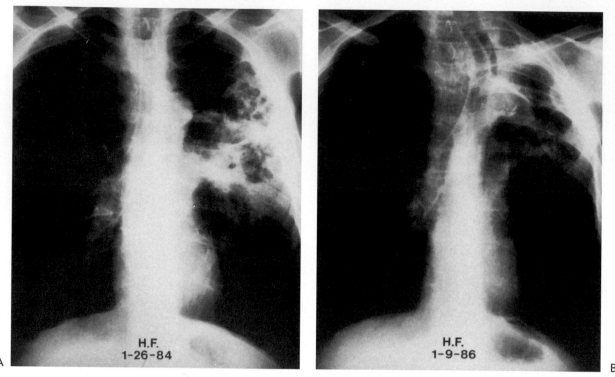

FIGURE 15.16. **(A)** Chronic pulmonary histoplasmosis. Note the extensive left upper-lobe infiltrate with apparent cavitation. This patient received 400 mg ketoconazole daily for nine months. **(B)** Follow-up chest roentgenogram shows clearing 15 months after completion of successful drug therapy. Note extensive retraction of the lobe with marked tracheal shift.

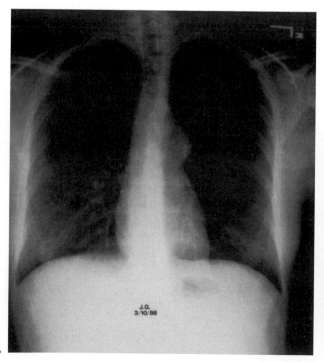

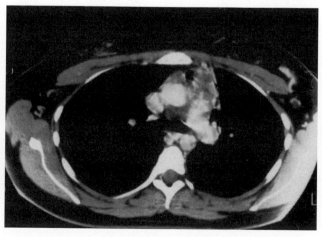

FIGURE 15.17. **(A)** Chest roentgenogram of a 33-year-old woman with minimal respiratory symptoms. There is a large left-sided anterior mediastinal mass. **(B)** Computed tomographic scan showing the full extent of the mass. Open biopsy showed healing granulomatous lesions. Histopathologic examination confirmed histoplasmosis.

In patients in whom the original dissemination of *Histoplasma* becomes progressive, a life-threatening illness occurs. As a rule, cell-mediated immunity is either weak or does not develop at all (153). In patients with the most severe form of immunodeficiency, such as those with AIDS or with Hodgkin's disease, progressive disseminated histoplasmosis (PDH) follows a fulminant course. Manifestations include fever, weight loss, and hepatosplenomegaly as well as the appearance of severe bone marrow involvement with anemia, leukopenia, and thrombocytopenia. Histopathologic examination of affected tissues reveals complete absence of granulomata, and all one sees are macrophages containing multiple organisms (153,158).

In patients in whom partial cell-mediated immunity still remains, PDH follows a much more subacute or chronic course. Histopathologically, the disease is characterized by the appearance of granulomata with a relative scarcity of organisms. Clinical symptoms in these patients are primarily those of a chronic illness; special areas of *Histoplasma* involvement include oropharyngeal, rectal, and genital ulcers as well as hepatosplenomegaly (153). Adrenal gland involvement may occur, and occasionally this adrenal gland involvement may lead to frank Addison's disease (159).

With the emergence of the AIDS epidemic, PDH became recognized as a frequent opportunistic infection in individuals infected by the human immunodeficiency virus (HIV). The nearly total deficiency of T-lymphocyte-mediated immune function, which is the hallmark of AIDS, renders every HIV-positive individual uniquely susceptible to developing PDH. Two potential pathogenic mechanisms exist. First is the progression from primary infection. When immunocompromised individuals become infected with *H. capsulatum,* progressive dissemination will develop in most of them (160). Thus it is to be anticipated that when patients with AIDS become exposed to the fungus, the outcome will be the development of PDH.

The second mechanism is reactivation of previously dormant foci of infection. Following recovery from the primary infection, after development of specific cell-mediated immunity has successfully localized the fungus, healing with granuloma formation takes place. Resected specimens of such granulomas frequently show persisting organisms. Such dormant foci may reactivate when immunosuppressive treatment is given (161). During progression of HIV infection, most T-cell-mediated immunity wanes, and when an individual harboring dormant foci of histoplasmosis reaches the critical level of waning immunity, the fungus begins to multiply and PDH will develop. Most likely both mechanisms are operative in HIV-infected patients.

The second mechanism is probably the more important consideration for physicians who reside outside the usual endemic area for histoplasmosis. The first mechanism (as well as reactivation disease) is more likely to occur in the endemic area. As Wheat and coworkers have pointed out, the diagnosis of PDH should prompt one to evaluate the patient's HIV status (160).

In Houston, which is on the fringe of the endemic area, fully 5% of patients with AIDS have developed PDH (162). However, in more endemic areas, the risk is far greater. In Indianapolis almost 27% of HIV-infected patients developed PDH (163). Experience during the early years of the HIV panendemic from both the East Coast and the West Coast have documented a rapidly increasing incidence of PDH among HIV-infected individuals, most of whom resided in endemic areas for histoplasmosis prior to moving to either New York (164) or California. Remember that in addition to Central United States, both Central America and the Caribbean are endemic areas. Since the advent of protease inhibitors, the incidence of PDH among HIV-infected patients has decreased rapidly.

The clinical manifestation of PDH in AIDS is a severe febrile illness. Over half of the patients will not have had the diagnosis of AIDS established prior to the onset of PDH. Symptoms are those of a febrile illness with anorexia and weight loss. Physical examination is often normal, but hepatosplenomegaly may be present in up to one-third of patients. The chest roentgenogram may show diffuse interstitial changes with multiple small nodules, but is often negative (Fig. 15.18) (162). Pancytopenia is frequently present but it is a nonspecific finding, since HIV-infected patients receiving zidovudine or other similar agents may have bone marrow suppression.

Rapid diagnosis is facilitated by remembering that any febrile individual at high risk for HIV infection may have PDH. Blood cultures and bone marrow examination and culture are the best tests (Fig. 15.19), and the fungus may be seen on examination of the buffy coat, where circulating phagocytes may be parasitized (165).

Isolation of the fungus from biologic material or visualization of the organism in histopathologic sections remains the gold standard. Proper handling of biologic specimens will yield a high frequency of positive cultures. Depending on inoculum size, a tentative diagnosis may be offered as early as five days, but usually this takes much longer—up to four to six weeks. When PDH is suspected, the best organ to sample is the bone marrow. Multiple blood cultures are frequently useful, especially when they are processed with the lysis-centrifugation system.

Skin testing for the diagnosis of histoplasmosis no longer has any role. While the skin test is still an outstanding epidemiologic tool, it simply cannot be used for the diagnosis of acute histoplasmosis.

In acute illness, serodiagnosis is the mainstay of diagnosis. Of the currently available serologic tests, complement fixation (CF) remains the best. Unfortunately, it suffers from the fact that it is seldom timely enough, since it frequently takes two weeks or more before a fourfold rise can be demonstrated. The immunodiffusion (ID) test, although highly specific, is relatively insensitive. In a recent outbreak,

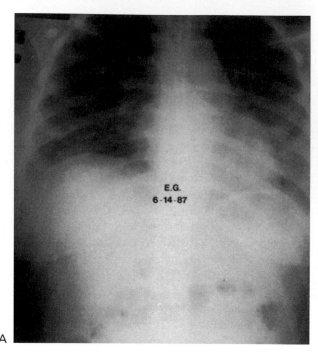

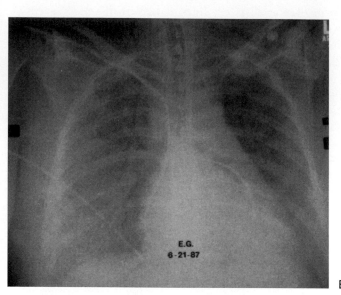

FIGURE 15.18. **(A)** Admission chest radiograph of a 26-year-old, HIV-positive pregnant woman showing interstitial infiltrates bilaterally. The main complaint was shortness of breath and fever. Bronchial washings showed small, 2-to-4 μm round organisms thought to be *P. carinii.* **(B)** One week later, in spite of aggressive therapy, infiltrates have progressed. Blood cultures obtained on the day of admission yielded *H. capsulatum.*

it was positive in only 50% of the proven cases (166). The best available test is the measurement of the *Histoplasma* polysaccharide antigen (167). The test is also helpful in following the course of treatment and detecting relapses (168).

Acute histoplasmosis, unless it results in significant interference with gas exchange, does not require treatment. Pa-

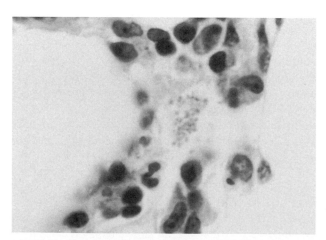

FIGURE 15.19. Bone marrow biopsy of an AIDS patient with progressive disseminated histoplasmosis. Note the large number of organisms inside a macrophage (hematoxylin and eosin stain × 1,000).

tients with severe, life-threatening, acute histoplasmosis will respond readily to intravenous administration of amphotericin B (AMB) (152).

Upper-lobe cavitary disease, when progressive, will respond to 400 mg ketoconazole daily. The recently introduced oral triazole, itraconazole, is also highly effective and is much better tolerated than ketoconazole (169). The much lower price of ketoconazole, however, makes it the agent of choice. Treatment failures may occur with both oral agents, and in these patients, AMB in a total dose of 35 mg per kg is effective (170). PDH is best treated with full courses of AMB until the patient's clinical condition has stabilized. This stabilization occurs somewhere between 500 and 1000 mg of AMB. Following stabilization, our practice has been to switch to itraconazole. This form of combination therapy was worked out carefully in HIV-infected patients with PDH and is extremely effective. Itraconazole should be continued for life in HIV-infected patients. Although its use makes excellent sense, this form of combination therapy has not been tested in HIV-negative patients with PDH. Our practice has been to treat with AMB until stable, then follow up with at least one year of 400 mg per day itraconazole therapy. Itraconazole may be used as primary therapy for patients with PDH if the tempo of the illness is slow and the patient is clinically stable. Following successful primary therapy with itraconazole, lifelong suppression with smaller doses of itraconazole (200 mg per day) is indicated.

Resected solitary pulmonary nodules containing *Histoplasma* need no treatment.

Blastomycosis

The endemic area of blastomycosis overlaps that of histoplasmosis but extends farther north. Besides humans, dogs are frequently victims of the disease, and veterinary practitioners are usually quite knowledgeable about blastomycosis (171). Much less is known about the epidemiology of blastomycosis than about that of histoplasmosis. It appears that the organism exists in microfoci in nature, usually in areas well watered by streams (172). Disturbance of the mycelial growth results in the formation of the infecting aerosol, following which the infecting particles are inhaled into the lung. Once in the lung, conversion to the yeast phase takes place, and propagation begins by binary fission.

The portal of entry is the lung. In the original area of pneumonitis, the initial cellular exudate is primarily polymorphonuclear (PMN). Once delayed hypersensitivity develops, macrophages move in, but the PMN component of the infiltrate never disappears completely. The organism is frequently restricted to the lungs by the establishment of cell-mediated immunity, but in some instances blood-borne dissemination may occur. The organs most commonly involved are the skin, bone, prostate, and meninges (171).

Acute pulmonary blastomycosis may be a severe, febrile illness, with cough productive of mucopurulent sputum. Frequently it is accompanied by arthralgia and myalgia. Chest roentgenogram usually reveals single or multiple areas of pneumonitis. Pleural involvement is more common than in histoplasmosis. Acute blastomycosis is frequently self-limited (173) (Fig. 15.20). Progressive pulmonary disease may occur, as well as dissemination outside the confines of the lung (Fig. 15.21). Frequently, the original pulmonary infiltrate may resolve spontaneously while the extrapulmonary components of the disseminated disease progress at the same time. Recently a number of HIV-infected patients with blastomycosis have been described. The illness is usually rapidly progressive and is frequently widely disseminated, including frequent involvement of the meninges (174).

Visualization of the organism, either on histopathologic sections or in sputum, as well as culture of the organism, is the only means of diagnosing blastomycosis reliably. The simplest and most effective diagnostic test is the examination of sputum (or aspirated pus) after digestion with 10% potassium hydroxide (KOH) (175). Under reduced light the characteristic large, double-refractile, thick-walled yeasts are readily identifiable. The daughter cell is attached by a broad neck. On histopathologic sections the organism is readily seen either by the periodic acid-Schiff (PAS) stain or by one of the silver stains. Culture identification is not difficult but may take time. A small inoculum usually takes up to 30 days before positive identification is possible. There is no commercially available skin test.

The serodiagnosis of blastomycosis is not well developed. Of the currently available serologic tests, complement fixation (CF) and immunodiffusion (ID) are more specific but far less sensitive; the recently introduced enzyme immunoassay (EIA) is far more sensitive but much less specific (176). At the present time a positive serodiagnostic test for blastomycosis does not establish the diagnosis of the disease. Nevertheless, a positive serologic test should serve as a strong indicator that the disease may be present (177)

In most instances, acute pulmonary blastomycosis re-

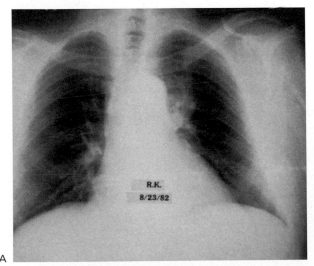 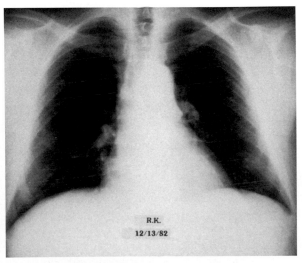

FIGURE 15.20. **(A)** Active self-limited blastomycosis with left upper lobe infiltrate. Sputum digestion with 10% potassium hydroxide was positive for *B. dermatitidis.* **(B)** Four months later, the infiltrate had diminished in size. Sputum examination no longer showed the fungus.

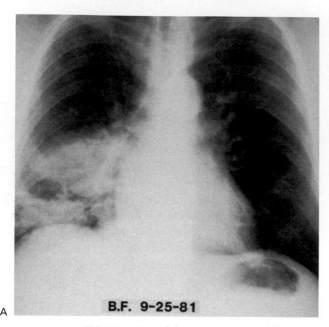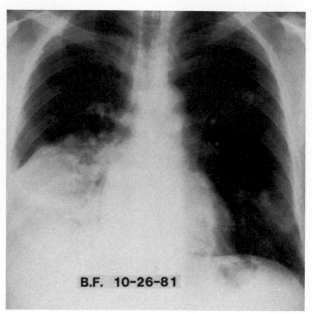

FIGURE 15.21. **(A)** Extensive right lower-lobe pneumonia due to *B. dermatitidis.* **(B)** One month later, cultures are reported growing the fungus. Note worsening right lower-lobe consolidation and spread of the infection to the left.

solves spontaneously (178). In rapidly progressive disease or in patients coinfected with HIV, especially when air exchange problems develop, AMB to a total of 2 g is the agent of choice (171). Similarly, meningeal involvement requires prompt intravenous AMB treatment. In more chronic or subacute forms of the illness, both pulmonary and disseminated, ketoconazole in a dose of 400 mg daily has proved to be an excellent drug (179,180). Itraconazole is highly effective and is far less difficult to administer than ketoconazole (169).

Coccidioidomycosis

The endemic area in the United States for coccidioidomycosis includes the Southwestern states of Texas, New Mexico, Arizona, Nevada, and California. In addition, the disease is also found in Central and South America. The organism usually resides several inches below the surface, and following the brief rainy season, rapid growth occurs. Disruption of these microfoci results in the production of the infecting aerosol (181). Since much of the endemic area is dry, dusty desert, wind-borne outbreaks of coccidioidomycosis have been noted (182,183).

Although primary cutaneous inoculations may occur, the usual portal of entry for most patients is the lung. Following inhalation of the arthrospores, germination occurs in the alveoli, leading to the production of giant spherules. Following maturity of the giant spherule, it bursts and releases a large number of endospores that in turn lead to the formation of new giant spherules. Histopathologically, the inflam-

matory exudate involves PMNs as well as macrophages, and the PMN component seldom disappears completely even after the development of cell-mediated immunity (181).

Following the successful development of cell-mediated immunity, the infection is contained. In certain high-risk groups this localization is not successful, leading to either progressive pulmonary or extrapulmonary disease. Diabetics, immunosuppressed individuals, members of the dark-skinned races—blacks especially—and men in general localize the disease poorly, and these "high-risk" groups provide most patients in whom progressive extrapulmonary spread occurs.

The primary infection is very similar to that seen in other soil-dwelling fungal infections. It is usually an influenzalike illness with a dry cough. Pleuritic chest pain is often severe. Arthralgias and myalgias are common. Erythema nodosum is a frequent accompaniment to these symptoms, leading to the characteristic "Valley fever" or "desert rheumatism." Chest roentgenogram may show single or multiple densities with involvement of the hilar nodes.

Resolution of the primary symptoms with clearing of the chest roentgenogram is the most common fate of acute infection. Occasionally, especially in members of the high-risk groups, resolution is slow or incomplete, and progressive pulmonary or extrapulmonary illness may develop. Extrapulmonary spread involves the skin, bones, and visceral organs. In about one-third of these patients, the meninges are also involved. Dissemination, when it occurs, is usually a relatively early event. It is uncommon to see stable disease that leads to dissemination after one year. Coccidioidomy-

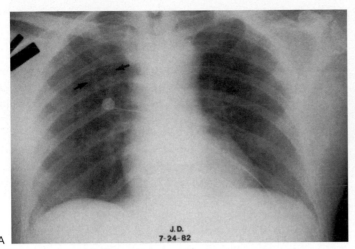 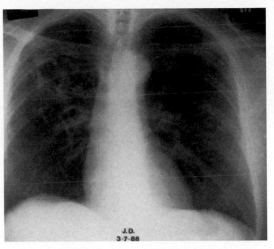

FIGURE 15.22. (A) Residual thin-walled cavity in right upper lobe *(arrows)*. Sputum is positive for *C. immitis*. **(B)** After almost six years and several courses of therapy with both amphotericin B and ketoconazole, the cavity still persists, and sputum is still intermittently positive for the organism. This patient declined surgery.

cosis occurring in HIV-positive individuals produces a severe, relentlessly progressive disease with widespread dissemination (184,185).

In an occasional patient, the pulmonary lesions may persist. The characteristic lesion is a thin-walled cavity (Fig. 15.22). Under observation, the vast majority of these cavities will close. Occasionally, however, the cavities grow and may reach the pleural surface, where they may rupture, leading to a bronchopleural fistula (186). Rarely, progressive pulmonary coccidioidomycosis involves the upper zones, mimicking tuberculosis (187).

Although cultural identification is not difficult, extreme care must be taken when working with biologic material suspected of harboring *C. immitis*. In most laboratories, cultural identification no longer takes place, but cultures are processed for the presence of the characteristic exoantigen. In any event, clinicians suspecting coccidioidomycosis should alert the laboratory, to prevent laboratory-borne infections.

Although excellent skin test antigens exist, skin tests are seldom used to establish the diagnosis of coccidioidomycosis. In disseminated disease the skin test is frequently negative, while in endemic areas a positive skin test could easily have been acquired prior to the onset of the clinical illness in question.

Unlike the other fungal illnesses, serodiagnostic tests are not only diagnostic but frequently produce excellent prognostic information (188). Early on, determination of IgM antibodies, either by the tube precipitation or by the latex agglutination method, is extremely helpful. CF antibodies are readily measured, and a rising titer frequently signifies impending dissemination. The CF test is extremely useful in suspected meningitis, and any CF activity in cerebrospinal fluid (CSF) should be considered proof of disease (186).

Most recently, the more easily performed immunodiffusion test has replaced the time-honored but cumbersome tests for IgM and IgG antibody. Our practice is to screen patients with the immunodiffusion test and then follow up the positive test by CF testing performed at a reference laboratory for prognostic purposes.

Regrettably, coccidioidal infections are much more difficult to deal with than either histoplasmosis or blastomycosis. Some authorities recommend treating stable pulmonary disease in members of the high-risk group. It is thought that a brief course of 0.5 to 1.5 g of AMB might prevent subsequent dissemination. Even though this is common clinical practice, proof of efficacy is lacking. Disseminated disease not involving the meninges can usually be treated with large doses of AMB intravenously (186). Treatment courses of up to 3.5 g are not uncommon. Since AMB is far less effective in the treatment of coccidioidomycosis than it is in either histoplasmosis or blastomycosis, alternative treatments are needed. Ketoconazole, although originally thought to be effective, produces lasting benefit in less than a third of the patients (189). The recently introduced oral triazoles fluconazole and itraconazole appears to be a significant improvement over ketoconazole, both in reported lower toxicity and increased efficacy (190). In a recently completed study, fluconazole and itraconazole were compared in patients with stable, nonmeningeal coccidioidomycosis. Both drugs performed well, with itraconazole showing a slight edge over fluconazole in some subgroups of patients.

The treatment of coccidioidomycosis in HIV-infected patients has been difficult and generally not successful. Most patients are treated initially with AMB until stabilization occurs. Fluconazole has been used successfully in several patients, especially those who are not critically ill initially, and it is especially helpful in meningeal coccidioidomycosis (191).

Coccidioidal meningitis requires both intravenous and intrathecal administration of AMB. Most authorities recommend long-term intrathecal therapy, even after all apparent disease activity has ceased in the central nervous system. Fluconazole is highly effective in the treatment of meningeal coccidioidomycosis and is now the treatment of choice for stable patients (191). It is important to remember that fluconazole should not be discontinued after apparently successful resolution of coccidioidomycotic meningitis. The risk of relapse, even in not obviously immunocompromised patients, is very high, necessitating lifelong suppressive therapy with fluconazole (192). In the event that surgery is attempted for an enlarging coccidioidal granuloma, some surgeons prefer to perform the surgery with pre- and postoperative administration of AMB. Although this is common practice, proof of efficacy is lacking.

Paracoccidioidomycosis

Paracoccidioides brasiliensis is the most common dimorphic fungus in Latin America. The endemic area stretches from Mexico to Argentina. Occupational exposure to the soil is common, and males are most commonly affected. Interestingly, point-source epidemics have not been reported, perhaps because of the rudimentary health care system in the endemic area.

As with all the other dimorphic fungi, the lung is probably the portal of entry. Inhalation of the infecting particles leads to the production of an area of pneumonitis, with granuloma formation occurring later. The organism may remain localized to the lung or may disseminate to the skin, mucous membranes, or organs with RE cells (193). Commonly, disseminated paracoccidioidomycosis occurs in younger patients in whom the major manifestations of the disease involve the RE system, leading to hepatosplenomegaly and hilar adenopathy. This form of the disease is referred to as the juvenile type. The adult form may present many years after the primary infection. Chronic pulmonary manifestations may still be present, and symptoms are those of low-grade chronic illness. Characteristic lesions involve the oropharynx, lips, and gums, and frequently involve the skin, leading to ulcerations. Draining lymph nodes are frequent, and adrenal involvement may occur in up to half of the patients.

Recovery of the organism from culture or visualization in KOH-digested specimens is relatively easy. The characteristic "pilot wheel" appearance of the yeast is diagnostic in sputum or pus.

Ketoconazole in 200 mg doses is currently one of the drugs of choice (194). In cases that are difficult to treat, AMB or sulfadiazine may be used. Itraconazole is also highly effective at doses of 100 mg daily for six months (195).

Sporotrichosis

By far the most common form of sporotrichosis is lymphocutaneous disease. Pulmonary involvement is rare, with perhaps less than 50 cases reported in the literature. The disease appears as a chronic pulmonary infection, indistinguishable by symptoms or by roentgen appearance from tuberculosis.

Diagnosis is usually by recovery of the fungus from sputum, although a serologic test is also available.

Although many authors recommend AMB as the initial treatment, it is far from certain that it is as effective as in the other fungal illnesses (196,197). The other treatment modality is oral administration of saturated solution of potassium iodide. There have been numerous patients reported in whom drug therapy failed but resection of the involved tissues proved to be curative. The recently introduced oral agent itraconazole has shown considerable success in treating this infection (198).

Cryptococcosis

The encapsulated yeast *Cryptococcus neoformans* is the one truly cosmopolitan fungus. The disease has been reported from all continents, and the fungus is easily recovered from pigeon droppings. Disturbance of the dried pigeon guano produces the infecting aerosol (199).

The portal of entry is the lung. Following inhalation the yeasts begin to germinate and form large capsules. This polysaccharide capsule is antiphagocytic. Histopathologic examination of tissue confirms the antiphagocytic nature of encapsulated cryptococci: large clumps of the yeast are surrounded by essentially no inflammatory exudate. In addition to the ability of the organism to resist phagocytosis and killing by PMNs, cell-mediated immunity also figures prominently into the normal host defenses for dealing with cryptococcal infection. Long before cytotoxic chemotherapy or glucocorticoid administration produced large numbers of immunocompromised hosts, the literature was replete with instances of cryptococcal disease complicating such naturally occurring immunocompromised states as Hodgkin's disease. To emphasize further the role of T-cell-mediated protection against the cryptococcus, AIDS patients have an unusually high incidence of cryptococcal disease (200,201).

Cryptococcal pulmonary disease in normal hosts is rapidly dealt with by the development of granulomatous inflammatory response and clearing of the infiltrate. It appears that the natural history of cryptococcal pulmonary disease in normal hosts is usually complete resolution.

Occasionally, however, even in immunologically competent hosts, the organism gains access to the bloodstream and establishes itself in extrapulmonary tissues, most commonly in the meninges. There is as yet no clear understanding of the remarkable tropism of cryptococci for the central nervous system.

Cryptococcal pulmonary infection in immunocompromised patients, on the other hand, is a severe, potentially life-threatening, and almost always disseminated illness. The general rule of thumb should be that anyone who is immunocompromised will develop disseminated disease following pulmonary infection by the fungus (202).

The acute pulmonary infection is relatively uncommon. Symptoms include acute onset of fever followed by chest pain and cough. Frequently, however, patients present with cryptococcal meningitis. In these instances, the inference is that an asymptomatic pulmonary infection preceded the obvious meningeal disease. Chest radiographic findings are variable but usually consist of patchy areas of consolidation involving the lower lung fields, often bilateral. Some lesions appear as nodules with associated areas of infiltration. Pleural effusions are uncommon.

The cornerstone of diagnosis in pulmonary cryptococcosis is the recovery of the fungus from respiratory secretions. A confounding variable is the frequent presence of cryptococci in patients with other, unrelated pulmonary diseases in whom *Cryptococcus* in respiratory secretions frequently represents colonization only.

Immunodiagnosis of cryptococcal disease is highly refined. Determination of cryptococcal antigen by the latex agglutination method is highly reproducible, and when the results are corrected for the possible presence of rheumatoid factor, false positives are remarkably infrequent.

The diagnosis of cryptococcal meningitis may be established by visualization of the large encapsulated yeasts on India ink preparation. Moreover, determination of the cryptococcal antigen on all cerebrospinal fluid samples will further hasten diagnosis. Cultural recovery of the organism is also relatively simple, and the organism grows in three to five days.

It is uncertain whether occasional isolates of *Cryptococcus* from sputum in patients with chronic pulmonary disease merit treatment. It was previously thought that acute cryptococcal disease in immunocompetent hosts can be observed with relative safety once the absence of central nervous system involvement has been documented by a negative lumbar puncture. The reason for this belief was that at the time Kerkering's original manuscript was published (202), the only available treatment for cryptococcal disease was AMB. Given this option, it seemed reasonable to observe patients, since a large majority of immunocompetent patients would likely recover without antifungal treatment. Today, with the availability of both fluconazole and itraconazole, it makes more sense to treat such patients to prevent the occasional deterioration or dissemination (203). In the unlikely event that treatment is deemed necessary, AMB 0.7 mg per kg per day should be administered along with 5-fluorocytosine (5-FC), 100 mg per kg per day in four divided doses, for a total of four weeks. Meningeal disease should also be treated with a combination of AMB and 5-FC in the same doses for a minimum of four weeks in nonimmunocompro-

mised patients, and six weeks or longer in non-HIV-infected immunocompromised individuals (204).

Since the advent of the HIV endemic, cryptococcal meningitis has increased in frequency 20-fold to become the most common fungal complication of HIV infection. It usually occurs late during the course of the HIV infection. With the availability of fluconazole, with its excellent penetration into the CSF, AIDS-related cryptococcal meningitis has frequently been treated with this agent. In a carefully randomized, controlled study, fluconazole performed about as well (but both with a high failure rate) as AMB, making fluconazole appear attractive due to the presence of fewer side affects. Subsequent review of this study, however, identified the fact that one of the reasons for the unacceptably high failure rate was that the dose of AMB used was smaller than it should have been (205). In a second, smaller study from a single institution, larger doses of AMB clearly outperformed fluconazole (206). The observations led to the last multicenter study, which established the new standard for the treatment of cryptococcal meningitis (207). On the basis of these studies the recent recommendations are to use 0.7 mg per Kg per day of AMB with 5-FC at 100 mg per Kg per day until the cerebrospinal fluid is sterile, followed by 400 mg of fluconazole. In the above-mentioned study, fluconazole was compared with itraconazole after CSF sterilization, showing fluconazole to be more effective, but also showing that itraconazole may be used in **the case of intolerance to fluconazole.**

Opportunistic Fungal Infections

The preceding subsections describe the normally pathogenic fungi which, although frequently infecting immunocompromised individuals, are also capable of infecting immunologically normal hosts. The following subsections deal with infections due to opportunistic fungi: *Aspergillus* species, *Mucorales,* and *Pseudallescheria boydii.*

Aspergillosis

Members of the genus *Aspergillus* are widespread in nature. They are readily recoverable from decomposing organic matter, and the fungi are capable of withstanding extreme environmental conditions. Although well over 100 species of this genus have been identified in human illness, the vast majority of human illness is caused by *Aspergillus fumigatus.* Other *Aspergillus* species that occasionally cause human disease are *Aspergillus niger, Aspergillus terreus, Aspergillus flavus,* and *Aspergillus nidulans.* It is thought that initiation of the illness follows inhalation of spores from the fruiting head into the lungs.

Aspergillus causes a vast array of human illness, and thus a unitary hypothesis for its pathogenesis is difficult, if not impossible. A form of aspergillosis usually seen in asthmatics, allergic bronchopulmonary aspergillosis, is discussed in Chapter 8, Asthma.

Aspergillomas, or fungus balls, occur in air spaces in the lungs. These air spaces may be the residua of healed tuberculosis, other fungal diseases, sarcoidosis, or tumor. The fungi grow within these epithelialized cavities as a mycelial mat, deriving their nourishment from the wall of the cavity. The most frequent symptom is hemoptysis, with occasional life-threatening result (208).

The other major form of aspergillosis involves granulocytopenic hosts. This illness is most frequently seen in patients with hematologic malignancies and leukemias who are undergoing intense cytotoxic chemotherapy. Aspergillosis has also emerged as the most feared complication of organ transplantation, especially bone marrow transplantation.

It appears that in these individuals the organism gains access to the lungs where, following multiplication in the alveolar spaces, the fungus invades blood vessels. The hallmark of this disease is the appearance of rapidly progressive, large pulmonary infiltrates accompanied by high fever and pleuritic chest pain. Frequently, a great deal of confusion exists because of the appearance of these infiltrates, which closely mimic pulmonary emboli with infarction. Indeed, histopathologically these lesions are pulmonary infarctions secondary to the growth of the organism within vascular channels. In the vast majority of patients, invasive aspergillosis restricted to the lungs alone is capable of killing the host. Occasionally, however, apparent blood-borne dissemination takes place with dissemination of the organism. The most common sites of dissemination include the brain, the myocardium, and the thyroid gland (209).

Recent reports have described an admixture of the fungus ball and invasive aspergillosis. Most affected patients, in addition to underlying chronic lung disease, had mild immunosuppression, resulting from either diabetes or the administration of chronic glucocorticoid therapy. The disease appears as a chronic, low-grade infection in which most of the symptoms are those of the underlying lung disease. Radiographically there is an aspergilloma with a slowly progressive infiltrate surrounding it. Treatment with AMB appears to slow down the progression of the illness, but it is not yet certain whether the process can be arrested or cured (210). Itraconazole also appears to be effective (211).

Diagnosis of aspergillomas is relatively easy. The chest roentgenogram is characteristic, showing a round, freely movable density within a previously existing cavity. Sputum culture is frequently positive for the fungus, and serologic diagnosis is very helpful since the vast majority of patients with aspergillomas have positive serum precipitins against *Aspergillus*. One must remember, however, that precipitins are species-specific, which accounts for the occasionally negative precipitin tests observed in patients with an obvious aspergilloma.

Disseminated aspergillosis or acute invasive aspergillosis is usually a difficult diagnosis. Although the disease is fre-

quently suspected on clinical grounds alone, attempts to recover the organism from respiratory secretions or bronchoscopic material frequently fail. Occasionally, however, positive cultures can be obtained from respiratory secretions. Although these positive cultures do not definitely establish the etiology of the infection, they frequently serve to point one in the right direction.

Although aspergillosis was originally listed among the agents causing opportunistic infections complicating HIV infection, this fungus was removed from the list soon after because of the paucity of reported patients. Recently, however, an increasing number of patients have been reported with various forms of aspergillosis complicating the late course of HIV infection. While most reported patients had the usual predisposing conditions to aspergillosis, such as drug-induced neutropenia or glucocorticoid administration, a sizable number of patients did not (212,213). All previously reported forms of aspergillosis have been seen in HIV-infected individuals, and two new forms have been added. These new forms are obstructing endobronchial aspergillosis and pseudomembranous aspergillosis.

Most authorities consider the diagnosis of aspergillosis definite only when the organism is seen invading host tissues. This usually requires either bronchoscopic biopsy or open-lung biopsy. Blood cultures are usually sterile.

Clinical and roentgenographic features of the infection are relatively nondiagnostic. The roentgenogram may show single or multiple areas of rapidly advancing pulmonary infiltrates, which do not cavitate until the granulocyte count begins to return toward normal.

Drug therapy is not indicated for the treatment of aspergillomas, since it universally fails. In patients with life-threatening hemoptysis, surgery is the only reasonable choice of therapy. Unfortunately, the majority of such patients have severely compromised pulmonary function, rendering surgery difficult if not impossible (208).

Treatment of acute invasive aspergillosis is frequently futile. AMB is the drug of choice, and the recommendation is that early and large doses of the agent be used. Our practice has been to aim at a minimum of 1 mg per kg per day for the acute phase of the illness and, after stabilization, to reduce the dose or switch to an alternate-day dosage regimen. Recently, especially in institutions dealing with large numbers of patients with hematologic malignancies, the custom has been to begin AMB treatment after three to seven days of a febrile course not responding to routine antibiotic treatment (214). Although definite proof of the success of this regimen is still lacking, it appears to have significantly reduced the incidence of invasive aspergillosis at postmortem examination.

The recently introduced triazole, itraconazole, has been used in some patients with different forms of aspergillosis with good results. While it is uncertain whether rapidly progressive invasive disease is likely to improve, it appears that the more chronic indulin forms of aspergillosis infections can be treated with itraconazole and can be expected to respond (211).

Mucormycosis

Members of the genus *Mucorales,* like *Aspergillus,* are widespread in nature. Although much less is known and understood about mucormycosis than of aspergillosis, it appears to be quite similar to aspergillosis. The organism has a high affinity for invasion of blood vessels and will frequently produce extensive tissue necrosis because of occlusion of blood vessels.

Clinical manifestations are very similar to those of aspergillosis, as is the chest roentgenogram, which usually shows multiple, large pulmonary infiltrates extending to the pleura, mimicking pulmonary embolization with infarction. The diagnosis requires identifying the invading broad, nonseptate fungus either in histopathologic material or by culture. There are no immunologic tests available. Blood culture and sputum culture are seldom, if ever, positive.

Treatment of mucormycosis is similar to that of aspergillosis and requires large doses of AMB. Early starting of the treatment is essential, and the best results have been in patients in whom treatment was started very early in the course of the illness.

Pseudallescheriasis

The organism *Pseudallescheria boydii* is an occasionally identified saprophyte. Clinically and histopathologically the illness is indistinguishable from invasive aspergillosis. Cultural identification is extremely important because it appears that miconazole, rather than AMB, is the drug of choice in this illness.

REFERENCES

1. Couch RB. The common cold: control? *J Infect Dis* 1984;150: 167–173.
2. Niederman MS, McCombs J, Unger A, et al. The cost of treating community-acquired pneumonia. *Clin Ther* 1998;20: 820–837.
3. Vincent JL, Behari DJ, Sueter PM, et al. The prevalence of nosocomial infection in intensive care units in Europe. *JAMA* 1995;274:634–644.
4. Garibaldi RA. Epidemiology of community-acquired respiratory tract infections in adults: incidence, etiology, and impact. *Am J Med* 1985;78[Suppl 6B]:32–37.
5. *Lung disease data 1994.* New York: American Lung Association, 1994:37–42.
6. Schneider EL. Infectious diseases in the elderly. *Ann Intern Med* 1983;98:395–400.
7. Gleckman RA, Roth RM. Community-acquired bacterial pneumonia in the elderly. *Pharmacotherapy* 1984;4:81–88.
8. Niederman MS. Nosocomial pneumonia in the elderly patient: chronic care facility and hospital considerations. *Clin Chest Med* 1993;14:479–490.
9. Gross PA, Van Antwerpen C. Nosocomial infections and hospital deaths: a case-control study. *Am J Med* 1983;75:658–662.
10. Emori TG, Banerjee SN, Culver DH, et al. Nosocomial infections in elderly patients in the United States, 1986–1990. *Am J Med* 1991;91(3):289S–293S.
11. Chastre J, Trouillet JL, Vuagnat A, et al. Nosocomial pneumonia in patients with acute respiratory distress syndrome. *Am J Respir Crit Care Med* 1998;157:1165–1172.
12. Seidenfeld JJ, Pohl DF, Bell RD, et al. Incidence, site, and outcome of infections in patients with the adult respiratory distress syndrome. *Am Rev Respir Dis* 1986;134:12–16.
13. Fagon JY, Chastre J, Hance A, et al. Nosocomial pneumonia in ventilated patients: a cohort study evaluating attributable mortality and hospital stay. *Am J Med* 1993;94:281–288.
14. Fagon JY, Chastre J, Vaugnat A, et al. Nosocomial pneumonia and mortality among patients in intensive care units. *JAMA* 1996;275:866–869.
15. Kronenberg RS. Chronic bronchitis: significant infection or social annoyance? *Semin Respir Infect* 1988;3:1–4.
16. Niederman MS. Evaluating the difficult management issues in chronic bronchitis. *Contemp Intern Med* 1993;5(11):8–16.
17. Niederman MS. Chronic obstructive pulmonary disease (COPD): The role of infection. *Chest* 1997;112(6):301S–302S.
18. Ball P, Harris JM, Lowson D, et al. Acute infective exacerbations of chronic bronchitis. *Q J Med* 1995;88:61–68.
19. Penn RL, George RB. Respiratory infections. In: Matthay RA, Light RM, George RB, eds. *Chest medicine,* 1st ed. New York: Churchill Livingstone, 1983:403–479.
20. American Thoracic Society. Control of tuberculosis in the United States. *Am Rev Respir Dis* 1992;146:1623–1633.
21. Barker AF, Bardana EJ. Bronchiectasis: update of an orphan disease. *Am Rev Respir Dis* 1988;137:969–978.
22. Farr BM, Kaiser DL, Harrison BDW, et al. Prediction of microbial aetiology at admission to hospital for pneumonia from presenting clinical features. *Thorax* 1989;44:1031–1035.
23. Niederman MS. Gram-negative colonization of the respiratory tract: pathogenesis and clinical consequences. *Semin Respir Infect* 1990;5:173–184.
24. Johanson WG, Pierce AK, Sanford JP. Changing pharyngeal flora of hospitalized patients: emergence of Gram-negative bacilli. *N Engl J Med* 1969;281:1137–1140.
25. Palmer LB. Bacterial colonization: pathogenesis and clinical significance. *Clin Chest Med* 1987;8:455–466.
26. Laurenzi GA, Potter RT, Kass EH. Bacteriologic flora of the lower respiratory tract. *N Engl J Med* 1961;265:1273–1278.
27. Niederman MS, Craven D. Devising strategies for nosocomial pneumonia prevention: should we ignore the stomach? *Clin Infect Dis* 1997;24:320–323.
28. Niederman MS, Mantovani R, Schoch P, et al. Patterns and routes of tracheobronchial colonization in mechanically ventilated patients: the role of nutritional status in colonization of the lower airway by *Pseudomonas* species. *Chest* 1989;95:155–161.
29. Rabinowitz HK. Upper respiratory tract infections. *Prim Care* 1990;17:793–809.
30. Gwaltney JM. The common cold: epidemiology and strategies for prevention. In: Sande MA, Hudson LD, Root RK, eds. *Respiratory infections.* New York: Churchill Livingstone, 1986: 139–147.
31. Blake GH, Abell TD, Stanley WG. Cigarette smoking and upper respiratory infection among recruits in basic combat training. *Ann Intern Med* 1988;109:198–202.
32. Dick EC, Jennings LC, Mink KA. Aerosol transmission of colds. *J Infect Dis* 1987;156:442–448.
33. Grimm W, Muller HH. A randomized controlled trial of the effect of fluid extract of Echinacea purpurea on the incidence

and severity of colds and respiratory infections. *Am J Med* 1999; 106:138–143.

34. Macknin ML, Piedmonte M, Claendine C, et al. Zinc gluconate lozenges for treating the common cold in children: a randomized controlled trial. *JAMA* 1998;279:1962–1967.

35. Douglas RM, Moore BW, Miles HB, et al. Prophylactic efficacy of intranasal alpha 2-interferon against rhinovirus infections in the family setting. *N Engl J Med* 1986;314:65–70.

36. Evans FO, Syndor JB, Moore WEC, et al. Sinusitis of the maxillary antrum. *N Engl J Med* 1975;293:735–739.

37. Williams JW, Simel DL. Does this patient have sinusitis? Diagnosing acute sinusitis by history and physical examination. *JAMA* 1993;270:1242–1246.

38. MayoSmith MF, Hirsch PJ, Wodzinski SF, et al. Acute epiglottitis in adults: an eight-year experience in the state of Rhode Island. *N Engl J Med* 1986;314:1133–1139.

39. Baker AS, Eavey RD. Adult supraglottitis (epiglottitis). *N Engl J Med* 1986;314:1185–1186.

40. Loos GD. Pharyngitis, croup and epiglottitis. *Prim Care* 1990; 17:335–345.

41. Solomon P, Weisbrod M, Irish JC, et al. Adult epiglottitis: the Toronto Hospital experience. *J Otolaryngol* 1998;27:332–336.

42. Ashcraft CK, Steele RW. Epiglottitis: a pediatric emergency. *J Respir Dis* 1988;9(7):48–60.

43. Wolf M, Strauss B, Kronenberg J, et al. Conservative management of adult epiglottitis. *Laryngoscope* 1990;100:183–185.

44. Rothrock SG, Pignatiello GA, Howard RA. Radiologic diagnosis of epiglottitis: objective criteria for all ages. *Ann Emerg Med* 1990;19:978–982.

45. Hall CB, McBride JT. Upper respiratory tract infections: the common cold, pharyngitis, croup, bacterial tracheitis and epiglottitis. In: Pennington JE, ed. *Respiratory infections: diagnosis and management.* New York: Raven Press, 1988:97–118.

46. Centor RM, Meier FA. Throat cultures and rapid tests for diagnosis of group A streptococcal pharyngitis. *Ann Intern Med* 1986;105:892–899.

47. Wallace RJ Jr. Newer oral antimicrobials and newer etiologic agents of acute bronchitis and acute exacerbations of chronic bronchitis. *Semin Respir Infect* 1988;3:49–54.

48. Gonzales R, Steiner JF, Lum A, et al. Decreasing antibiotic use in ambulatory practice: impact of a multidimensional intervention on the treatment of uncomplicated bronchitis in adults. *JAMA* 1999;281:1512–1519.

49. Schroeckenstein DC, Busse WW. Viral bronchitis in childhood: relationship to asthma and obstructive lung disease. *Semin Respir Infect* 1988;3:40–48.

50. Anthonisen NR, Manfreda J, Warren CPW, et al. Antibiotic therapy in exacerbations of chronic obstructive pulmonary disease. *Ann Intern Med* 1987;106:196–204.

51. Fagon JY, Chastre J, Trouillet JL, et al. Characterization of distal bronchial microflora during acute exacerbation of chronic bronchitis: use of the protected specimen brush technique in 54 mechanically ventilated patients. *Am Rev Respir Dis* 1990; 142:1004–1008.

52. Karnad A, Alvarez S, Berk SL. *Branhamella catarrhalis* pneumonia in patients with immunoglobulin abnormalities. *South Med J* 1986;79:1360–1362.

53. Murphy TF, Sethi S. Bacterial infection in chronic obstructive pulmonary disease. *Am Rev Respir Dis* 1992;146:1067–1083.

54. Saint S, Bent S, Vittinghoff E, et al. Antibiotics in chronic obstructive pulmonary disease exacerbations: a meta-analysis. *JAMA* 1995;273:957–960.

55. Niederman MS, Ferranti RD, Ziegler A, et al. Respiratory infection complicating long-term tracheostomy: the implication of persistent Gram-negative tracheobronchial colonization. *Chest* 1984;85:39–44.

56. King TE Jr. Overview of bronchiolitis. *Clin Chest Med* 1993; 14:607–610.

57. Epler GR, Colby TV, McLoud TC, et al. Bronchiolitis obliterans organizing pneumonia. *N Engl J Med* 1985;312:152–158.

58. Cox NJ, Fukuda K. Influenza. *Infect Dis Clin North Am* 1998; 12:27–38.

59. Mathur U, Bentley DW, Hall CB. Concurrent respiratory syncytial virus and influenza A infections in the institutionalized elderly and chronically ill. *Ann Intern Med* 1980;93:49–52.

60. Gross PA, Rodstein M, LaMontagne JR, et al. Epidemiology of acute respiratory illness during an influenza outbreak in a nursing home: a prospective study. *Arch Intern Med* 1988;148: 559–561.

61. Hayden FG, Gwaltney JM. Viral infections. In: Murray JF, Nadel JA, eds. *Textbook of respiratory medicine.* Philadelphia: WB Saunders, 1988:769–778.

62. Van Voris LP, Newell PM. Antivirals for the chemoprophylaxis and treatment of influenza. *Semin Respir Infect* 1992;7:61–70.

63. Stockley RA. Bronchiectasis—new therapeutic approaches based on pathogenesis. *Clin Chest Med* 1987;8:481–494.

64. Huxley EJ, Viroslav J, Gray WR, et al. Pharyngeal aspiration in normal subjects and patients with depressed consciousness. *Am J Med* 1978;64:565–568.

65. Beachey EH. Bacterial adherence: adhesin-receptor interactions mediating the attachment of bacteria to mucosal surfaces. *J Infect Dis* 1981;143:325–345.

66. Niederman MS, Merrill WW, Ferranti RD, et al. Nutritional status and bacterial binding in the lower respiratory tract in patients with chronic tracheostomy. *Ann Intern Med* 1984;100: 795–800.

67. Todd TRJ, Franklin A, Mankinen-Irvin P, et al. Augmented bacterial adherence to tracheal epithelial cells is associated with Gram-negative pneumonia in an intensive care unit population. *Am Rev Respir Dis* 1989;140:1585–1589.

68. Johanson WG Jr, Pierce AK, Sanford JP, et al. Nosocomial respiratory infections with Gram-negative bacilli: the significance of colonization of the respiratory tract. *Ann Intern Med* 1972;77:701–706.

69. Toews GB. Nosocomial pneumonia. *Clin Chest Med* 1987;8: 467–479.

70. Fein AM, Feinsilver SH, Niederman MS. Atypical manifestations of pneumonia in the elderly. *Clin Chest Med* 1991;12: 319–336.

71. Niederman MS, Bass JB, Campbell GD, et al. Guidelines for the initial management of adults with community-acquired pneumonia: diagnosis, assessment of severity, and initial antimicrobial therapy. *Am Rev Respir Dis* 1993;148:1418–1426.

72. Wollschlager CM, Khan FA, Khan A. Utility of radiography and clinical features in the diagnosis of community-acquired pneumonia. *Clin Chest Med* 1987;8:393–404.

73. MacFarlane JT, Miller AC, Smith WH, et al. Comparative radiographic features of community-acquired Legionnaires' disease, pneumococcal pneumonia, mycoplasma pneumonia, and psittacosis. *Thorax* 1984;39:28–33.

74. Ewig S, Ruiz M, Mensa J, et al. Severe community-acquired pneumonia: Assessment of severity criteria. *Am J Respir Crit Care Med* 1998;158:1102–1108.

75. Torres A, Serra-Batlles J, Ferrer A, et al. Severe community-acquired pneumonia. Epidemiology and prognostic factors. *Am Rev Respir Dis* 1991;144:312–318.

76. Farr BM, Sloman AJ, Fisch MJ. Predicting death in patients hospitalized for community-acquired pneumonia. *Ann Intern Med* 1991;115:428–436.

77. Pachon J, Prados MD, Capote F, et al. Severe community-acquired pneumonia. Etiology, prognosis, and treatment. *Am Rev Respir Dis* 1990;142:369–373.

78. Porath A, Schlaeffer F, Lieberman D. The epidemiology of community-acquired pneumonia among hospitalized adults. *J Infect* 1997;34:41–48.

79. Mufson MA. Pneumococcal infections. *JAMA* 1981;246:1942–1948.

80. Johnson CC, Finegold SM. Pyogenic bacterial pneumonia, lung abscess, and empyema. In: Murray JF, Nadel JA, eds. *Textbook of respiratory medicine.* Philadelphia: WB Saunders, 1988:803–841.

81. Ort S, Ryan JL, Barden G, et al. Pneumococcal pneumonia in hospitalized patients: clinical and radiological presentations. *JAMA* 1983;249:214–218.

82. Plouffe JF, Breiman RF, Facklam RR. Bacteremia with Streptococcus pneumoniae. Implications for therapy and prevention. Franklin County Pneumonia Study Group. *JAMA* 1996;275:194–198.

83. Clavo-Sánchez AJ, Girón-González JA, López-Prieto D, et al. Multivariate analysis of risk factors for infection due to penicillin-resistant and multidrug-resistant Streptococcus pneumoniae: a multicenter study. *Clin Infect Dis* 1997;24:1052–1059.

84. Jay SJ, Johanson WG, Pierce AK. The radiographic resolution of *Streptococcus pneumoniae* pneumonia. *N Engl J Med* 1975;293:798–801.

85. Austrian R. A reassessment of pneumococcal vaccine. *N Engl J Med* 1984;310:651–653.

86. Arunabh, Niederman, MS. Strategies for prevention of community-acquired pneumonia. *Sem Respir Infect* 1998;13:68–78.

87. Centers for Disease Control and Prevention. Prevention of pneumococcal disease: recommendations of the Advisory Committee on Immunization Practice. *MMWR* 1997;46(RR-8):1–24.

88. Brenner DJ. Classification of the legionellae. *Semin Respir Infect* 1987;4:190–205.

89. Davis GS, Winn WC. Legionnaires' disease: respiratory infections caused by *Legionella* bacteria. *Clin Chest Med* 1987;8:419–439.

90. Yu VL, Kroboth FJ, Shonnard J. Legionnaires' disease: new clinical perspective from a prospective pneumonia study. *Am J Med* 1982;73:357–361.

91. Carratala J, Gudiol F, Pallares R, et al. Risk factors for nosocomial *Legionella pneumophila* pneumonia. *Am J Respir Crit Care Med* 1994;149:625–629.

92. Muder RR, Yu VL. Legionella. In: Niederman MS, Sarosi GA, Glassroth J, eds. *Respiratory infections: a scientific basis for management,* 1st ed. Philadelphia: WB Saunders, 1994:319–330.

93. Edelstein PH. Antimicrobial chemotherapy for Legionnaires disease: time for a change. *Ann Intern Med* 1998;129:328–330.

94. Bartlett JG, Gorbach SL. The triple threat of aspiration pneumonia. *Chest* 1975;68:560–566.

95. Wynne JW, Modell JH. Respiratory aspiration of stomach contents. *Ann Intern Med* 1977;87:466–474.

96. Mier L, Dreyfuss D, Darchy B, et al. Is penicillin G an adequate initial treatment for aspiration pneumonia? A prospective evaluation using a protected specimen brush and quantitative cultures. *Intensive Care Med* 1993;19:279–284.

97. Bartlett JG, Finegold SM. Anaerobic infections of the lung and pleural space. *Am Rev Respir Dis* 1974;110:56–77.

98. Levison ME, Mangura CT, Lorber B, et al. Clindamycin compared with penicillin for the treatment of anaerobic lung abscess. *Ann Intern Med* 1983;98:466–471.

99. Musher DM, Kubitschek KR, Crennan J, et al. Pneumonia and acute febrile tracheobronchitis due to *Haemophilus influenzae. Ann Intern Med* 1983;99:444–450.

100. Smith AL. *Haemophilus influenzae* pneumonia. In: Pennington JE, ed. *Respiratory infections: diagnosis and management.* New York: Raven Press, 1988:364–380.

101. Cassell GH, Cole BC. Mycoplasmas as agents of human disease. *N Engl J Med* 1981;304:80–89.

102. Tuazon CU, Murray HW. Atypical pneumonias. In: Pennington JE, ed. *Respiratory infections: diagnosis and management.* New York: Raven Press, 1988:341–363.

103. Cotton EM, Strampfer MJ, Cunha BA. *Legionella* and mycoplasma pneumonia—a community hospital experience with atypical pneumonias. *Clin Chest Med* 1987;8:441–453.

104. Grayston JT, Kuo CC, Wang SP, et al. A new *Chlamydia psittaci* strain, TWAR, isolated in acute respiratory tract infections. *N Engl J Med* 1986;315:161–168.

105. Troy CJ, Peeling RW, Ellis AG, et al. Chlamydia pneumoniae as a new source of infectious outbreaks in nursing homes. *JAMA* 1997;277:1214–1218.

106. Pierce AK, Sanford JP. Aerobic Gram-negative bacillary pneumonias. *Am Rev Respir Dis* 1974;110:647–658.

107. Meyer KS, Urban C, Eagan JA, et al. Nosocomial outbreak of *Klebsiella* infection resistant to late-generation cephalosporins. *Ann Intern Med* 1993;119:353–358.

108. Kaye MG, Fox MJ, Bartlett JG, et al. The clinical spectrum of *Staphylococcus aureus* pulmonary infection. *Chest* 1990;97:788–792.

109. Rose RM, Pinkston P, O'Donnell C, et al. Viral infections of the lower respiratory tract. *Clin Chest Med* 1987;8:405–418.

110. Shellhammer J, Gill VJ, Quinn TC, et al. The laboratory evaluation of opportunistic pulmonary infections. *Ann Intern Med* 1996;124:585–599.

111. Britt MR, Schleupner CJ, Matsumiya S. Severity of underlying disease as a predictor of nosocomial infection. *JAMA* 1978;239:1047–1051.

112. Niederman MS, Fein AM. Sepsis syndrome, the adult respiratory distress syndrome, and nosocomial pneumonia: a common clinical sequence. *Clin Chest Med* 1990;11:633–656.

113. Mandell LA, Marrie TJ, Niederman MS. Initial antimicrobial treatment of hospital acquired pneumonia in adults. a conference report. *Can J Infect Dis* 1993;4:317–321.

114. Campbell GD, Niederman MS, Broughton WA, et al. Hospital-acquired pneumonia in adults: diagnosis, assessment of severity, initial antimicrobial therapy, and preventative strategies: A consensus statement. *Am J Respir Crit Care Med* 1996;153:1711–1725.

115. Andrews CP, Coalson JJ, Johanson WG Jr. Diagnosis of nosocomial bacterial pneumonia in acute diffuse lung injury. *Chest* 1981;80:254–258.

116. Niederman MS, Torres A, Summer W. Invasive diagnostic testing is not needed routinely to manage suspected VAP. *Am J Respir Crit Care Med* 1994;150:565–569.

117. Luna CM, Vujacich P, Niederman M, et al. Impact of bronchoalveolar lavage data on the therapy and outcome of ventilator-associated pneumonia. *Chest* 1997;1997;111:676–685.

118. Rodrigues J, Niederman MS, Fein AM, et al. Nonresolving pneumonia in steroid-treated patients with obstructive lung disease. *Am J Med* 1992;93:29–34.

119. Stevens RM, Teres D, Skillman JJ, et al. Pneumonia in an intensive care unit: a 30-month experience. *Arch Intern Med* 1974;134:106–111.

120. Rosenow EC, Wilson WR, Cockerill FR. Pulmonary disease in the immunocompromised host. *Mayo Clin Proc* 1985;60:473–487.

121. Rankin JA, Collman R, Daniele RP. Acquired immune deficiency syndrome and the lung. *Chest* 1988;94:155–164.

122. Gallant JE, Chaisson RE. Respiratory infections in persons infected with human immunodeficiency virus. In: Niederman MS, Sarosi GA, Glassroth J, eds. *Respiratory infections: a scientific basis for management,* 1st ed. Philadelphia: WB Saunders, 1994:199–215.

123. Hibberd PL, Rubin RH. Renal transplantation and related infections. *Semin Respir Infect* 1993;8:216–224.

124. Levine SJ, White DA. *Pneumocystis carinii*. *Clin Chest Med* 1988;9:395–423.

125. Conte JE, Hollander H, Golden JA. Inhaled or reduced-dose intravenous pentamidine for *Pneumocystis carinii* pneumonia: a pilot study. *Ann Intern Med* 1987;107:495–498.

126. Allegra CJ, Chabner BA, Tuazon CU, et al. Trimetrexate for the treatment of *Pneumocystis carinii* pneumonia in patients with the acquired immunodeficiency syndrome. *N Engl J Med* 1987;317:978–985.

127. McFadden JP, Price RC, Eastwood HD, et al. Raised respiratory rate in elderly patients: a valuable physical sign. *Br Med J* 1982;1:626–627.

128. Fein AM, Feinsilver SH, Niederman MS, et al. When pneumonia doesn't get better. *Clin Chest Med* 1987;8:529–541.

129. Tobin MJ. Diagnosis of pneumonia: techniques and problems. *Clin Chest Med* 1987;8:513–527.

130. Stover DE, Zaman MB, Hajdu SI, et al. Bronchoalveolar lavage in the diagnosis of diffuse pulmonary infiltrates in the immunosuppressed host. *Ann Intern Med* 1984;101:1–7.

131. Chastre J, Fagon JY, Bornet M, et al. Diagnosis of nosocomial bacterial pneumonia in intubated patients undergoing ventilation: comparison of the usefulness of bronchoalveolar lavage and the protected specimen brush. *Am J Med* 1988;85:499–506.

132. Atlas SJ, Benzer TI, Borowsky LH, et al. Safely increasing the proportion of patients with community-acquired pneumonia treated as outpatients: an interventional trial. *Arch Intern Med* 1998;158:1350–1356.

133. Graham WGB, Bradley DA. Efficacy of chest physiotherapy and intermittent positive-pressure breathing in the resolution of pneumonia. *N Engl J Med* 1978;299:624–627.

134. Wanner A, Rao A. Clinical indications for and effects of bland, mucolytic and antimicrobial aerosols. *Am Rev Respir Dis* 1980;122:79–87.

135. de Boisblanc BP, Castro M, Everret B, et al. Effect of air-supported, continuous, postural oscillation on the risk of early ICU pneumonia in nontraumatic critical illness. *Chest* 1993;103:1543–1547.

136. Glassroth J. Tuberculosis. In: Niederman MS, Sarosi GA, Glassroth J, eds. *Respiratory infections: a scientific basis for management,* 1st ed. Philadelphia: WB Saunders, 1994:449–458.

137. Hirschtick RE, Glassroth J. Multidrug-resistant tuberculosis: epidemiology, treatment, and prevention. *Clin Pulm Med* 1994;1:78–83.

138. Small PM, Shafer RW, Hopewell PC, et al. Exogenous reinfection with multidrug-resistant *Mycobacterium tuberculosis* in patients with advanced HIV infection. *N Engl J Med* 1993;328:1137–1144.

139. Bates JH. Transmission and pathogenesis of tuberculosis. *Clin Chest Med* 1980;1:167–174.

140. Daley CL, Small PM, Schecter GM, et al. An outbreak of tuberculosis with accelerated progression among persons infected with human immunodeficiency virus: an analysis using restriction-fragment-length polymorphisms. *N Engl J Med* 1992;326:231–235.

141. Levy H, Kallenbach JM, Feldman C, et al. Acute respiratory failure in active tuberculosis. *Crit Care Med* 1987;15:221–225.

142. Alvarez S, Shell C, Berk SL. Pulmonary tuberculosis in elderly men. *Am J Med* 1987;82:602–606.

143. Bass JB Jr, Farer LS, Hopewell PC, et al. Treatment of tuberculosis and tuberculosis infection in adults and children. *Am J Respir Crit Care Med* 1994;149:1359–1374.

144. American Thoracic Society. Mycobacteriosis and the acquired immunodeficiency syndrome. *Am Rev Respir Dis* 1987;136:492–496.

145. Woodring JH, Vandiviere HM, Fried AM, et al. Update: the radiographic features of pulmonary tuberculosis. *AJR* 1986;497–506.

146. American Thoracic Society. Diagnostic standards and classification of tuberculosis. *Am Rev Respir Dis* 1990;142:725–735.

147. Grosset J. Bacteriologic basis of short-course chemotherapy for tuberculosis. *Clin Chest Med* 1980;1:231–241.

148. Nardell EA. Beyond four drugs: public health policy and the treatment of the individual patient with tuberculosis. *Am Rev Respir Dis* 1993;148:2–5.

149. Woods GL, Washington JA. Mycobacteria other than *Mycobacterium tuberculosis:* review of microbiologic and clinical aspects. *Rev Infect Dis* 1987;9:275–294.

150. Tellis CJ, Bombenger. Pulmonary disease caused by nontuberculous mycobacteria. In: Pennington JE, ed. *Respiratory infections: diagnosis and management.* New York: Raven Press, 1988:544–569.

151. American Thoracic Society. Diagnosis and treatment of disease caused by nontuberculous mycobacteria. *Am J Respir Crit Care Med* 1997;156:S1–S25.

152. Goodwin RA, DesPrez RM. Histoplasmosis: state of the art. *Am Rev Respir Dis* 1978;117:929–956.

153. Goodwin RA, Shapiro JL, Thurman GH, et al. Disseminated histoplasmosis: clinical and pathologic correlations. *Medicine* 1980;59:1–33.

154. Goodwin RA, Loyd JE, DesPrez RM. Histoplasmosis in normal hosts. *Medicine* 1981;60:231–266.

155. Davies SF, Sarosi GA. Acute cavitary histoplasmosis. *Chest* 1978;73:103–105.

156. Goodwin RA, Owens FT, Snell JD, et al. Chronic pulmonary histoplasmosis. *Medicine* 1976;55:413–452.

157. Loyd JE, Tillman BF, Atkinson JB, et al. Mediastinal fibrosis complicating histoplasmosis. *Medicine* 1988;67:295–310.

158. Davies SF, McKenna RW, Sarosi GA. Trephine biopsy of the bone marrow in disseminated histoplasmosis. *Am J Med* 1979;67:617–622.

159. Sarosi GA, Voth DW, Dahl BA, et al. Disseminated histoplasmosis: results of long term follow-up. A Center for Disease Control Cooperative Mycose Study. *Ann Intern Med* 1971;75:511–516.

160. Wheat LJ, Slama TG, Norton JA, et al. Risk factors for disseminated or fatal histoplasmosis. *Ann Intern Med* 1982;96:159–163.

161. Davies SF, Khan M, Sarosi GA. Disseminated histoplasmosis in immunologically suppressed patients. *Am J Med* 1978;64:94–100.

162. Johnson PC, Khardori N, Najjar AF, et al. Progressive disseminated histoplasmosis in patients with acquired immunodeficiency syndrome. *Am J Med* 1988;85:152–158.

163. Wheat LJ, Connolly-Stringfield PA, Baker RL, et al. Disseminated histoplasmosis in the acquired immune deficiency syndrome: clinical findings, diagnosis and review of the literature. *Medicine (Baltimore)* 1990;69:361–374.

164. Mandell W, Goldberg DM, Neu HC. Histoplasmosis in patients with the acquired immune deficiency syndrome. *Am J Med* 1986;81:974–978.

165. Sarosi GA, Johnson PC. Disseminated histoplasmosis in patients infected with human immunodeficiency virus. *Clin Infect Dis* 1992;14[Suppl]1:60–67.

166. Davies SF. Serodiagnosis of histoplasmosis. *Semin Respir Infect* 1986;1:9–15.

167. Wheat LJ, Kohler RB, Tewari RP. Diagnosis of disseminated histoplasmosis by detection of *Histoplasma capsulatum* antigen in serum and urine specimens. *N Engl J Med* 1986;314:83–88.

168. Wheat LJ, Connolly-Stringfield P, Kohler RB, et al. *Histoplasma capsulatum* polysaccharide antigen detection in diagnosis and

management of disseminated histoplasmosis in patients with acquired immunodeficiency syndrome. *Am J Med* 1989;87: 396–400.

169. Dismukes WE, Bradsher RW Jr, Cloud GC, et al. Itraconazole therapy for blastomycosis and histoplasmosis: NIAID Mycosis Study Group. *Am J Med* 1992;93:489–497.

170. Parker JD, Sarosi GA, Doto IL, et al. Treatment of chronic pulmonary histoplasmosis. A National Communicable Disease Center Cooperative Mycoses Study. *N Engl J Med* 1970;283: 225–229.

171. Sarosi GA, Davies SF. Blastomycosis: state of the art. *Am Rev Respir Dis* 1979;120:911–938.

172. Klein BS, Vergeront JM, Weeks RJ, et al. Isolation of *Blastomyces dermatitidis* in soil associated with a large outbreak of blastomycosis in Wisconsin. *N Engl J Med* 1986;314:529–534.

173. Sarosi GA, Hammerman KJ, Tosh FE, et al. Clinical features of acute pulmonary blastomycosis. *N Engl J Med* 1974;290: 540–543.

174. Pappas PG, Pottage JC, Powderly WG, et al. Blastomycosis in patients with the acquired immunodeficiency syndrome. *Ann Intern Med* 1992;116:847–853.

175. Sanders JS, Sarosi GA, Nollet DJ, et al. Exfoliative cytology in the rapid diagnosis of pulmonary blastomycosis. *Chest* 1977; 72:193–196.

176. Klein BS, Vergeront JM, Kaufman L, et al. Serological tests for blastomycosis: assessments during a large point source outbreak in Wisconsin. *J Infect Dis* 1987;155:262–268.

177. Bradsher RW, Pappas PG. Detection of specific antibodies in human blastomycosis by enzyme immunoassay. *South Med J* 1995;88(12):1256–1259.

178. Sarosi GA, Davies SF, Phillips JR. Self-limited blastomycosis: a report of 39 cases. *Semin Respir Infect* 1986;1:40–44.

179. National Institute of Allergy and Infectious Diseases Mycoses Study Group. Treatment of blastomycosis and histoplasmosis with ketoconazole. *Ann Intern Med* 1985;103:861–872.

180. Bradsher RW, Rice DC, Abernathy RS. Ketoconazole therapy for endemic blastomycosis. *Ann Intern Med* 1985;103: 872–879.

181. Drutz DJ, Catanzaro A. Coccidioidomycosis: state of the art. Part I. *Am Rev Respir Dis* 1978;117:559–585.

182. Galgiani JN. Coccidioidomycosis. *West J Med* 1993;159: 153–171.

183. Stevens DA. Coccidioidomycosis. *N Engl J Med* 1995;332: 1077–1082.

184. Fish DG, Ampel NM, Galgiani JN, et al. Coccidioidomycosis during human immunodeficiency virus infection. A review of 77 patients. *Medicine* 1990;69:384–391.

185. Singh VR, Smith DK, Lawrence J, et al. Coccidioidomycosis in patients infected with human immunodeficiency virus: review of 91 cases from a single institution. *Clin Infect Dis* 1996;23: 563–568.

186. Drutz DJ, Catanzaro A. Coccidioidomycosis: state of the art. Part II. *Am Rev Respir Dis* 1978;117:727–771.

187. Sarosi GA, Parker JD, Doto IL, et al. Chronic pulmonary coccidioidomycosis. *N Engl J Med* 1970;283:325–329.

188. Smith CD, Saito MT, Beard RR, et al. Serologic tests in the diagnosis and prognosis of coccidioidomycosis. *Am J Hyg* 1950; 52:1–21.

189. Galgiani JN, Stevens DA, Graybill JR, et al. Ketoconazole therapy of progressive coccidioidomycosis. *Am J Med* 1988;84: 603–610.

190. Graybill JR, Stevens DA, Galgiani JN, et al. Itraconazole treatment of coccidioidomycosis. *Am J Med* 1990;89:282–290.

191. Galgiani JN, Catanzaro A, Cloud GA, et al. Fluconazole therapy for coccidioidal meningitis. *Ann Intern Med* 1993;119:28–35.

192. Dewsnup DH, Galgiani JN, Greybill JR. Is it ever safe to stop azole therapy for coccidioides immitis meningitis? *Ann Intern Med* 1996;124:305–310.

193. Restrepo A, Robledo M, Giraldo R, et al. The gamut of paracoccidioidomycosis. *Am J Med* 1976;61:33–42.

194. Cuce LC, Wroclawski EL, Sampaio SAP. Treatment of paracoccidioidomycosis with ketoconazole. *Rev Inst Med Trop Sao Paulo* 1981;23(2):82–85.

195. Restrepo A, Gomez I, Robledo J, et al. Itraconazole in the treatment of paracoccidioidomycosis: a preliminary report. *Rev Infect Dis* 1987;9[Suppl 1]:551–553.

196. Gerding DN. Treatment of pulmonary sporotrichosis. *Semin Respir Infect* 1986;1:61–65.

197. Pluss JL, Opal SM. Pulmonary sporotrichosis: review of treatment and outcome. *Medicine* 1986;65:143–153.

198. Sharkey-Mathis PK, Kauffman CA, Graybill JR, et al. Treatment of sporotrichosis with itraconazole: NIAID Mycoses Study Group. *Am J Med* 1993;95:279–285.

199. Powell KE, Dahl BA, Weeks RJ, et al. Airborne *Cryptococcus neoformans*: particles from pigeon excreta compatible with alveolar deposition. *J Infect Dis* 1972;125:412–415.

200. Kovacs JA, Kovacs AA, Polis M, et al. *Cryptococcus* in the acquired immunodeficiency syndrome. *Ann Intern Med* 1985; 103:533–538.

201. Zuger A, Louie E, Holzman RS, et al. Cryptococcal disease in patients with the acquired immunodeficiency syndrome. *Ann Intern Med* 1986;104:234–240.

202. Kerkering TM, Duma RD, Shadmy S. The evolution of pulmonary cryptococcosis. *Ann Intern Med* 1981;794:611–616.

203. Sarosi GA. Cryptococcal lung disease in patients without HIV infection. *Chest* 199;115(3):610–611.

204. Dismukes WE, Cloud G, Gallis HA, et al. Treatment of cryptococcal meningitis with combination amphotericin B and flucytosine for four as compared with six weeks. *N Engl J Med* 1987;317:334–341.

205. Saag MS, Powderly WG, Cloud GA, et al. Comparison of amphotericin B with fluconazole in the treatment of acute AIDS-associated cryptococcal meningitis. *N Engl J Med* 1992;326: 83–9.

206. Larsen RA, Leal MAE, Chan LS. Fluconazole compared with amphotericin B plus Flucytosine for cryptococcal meningitis in AIDS. A randomized trial. *Ann Intern Med* 1990;113:183–87.

207. Van der Horst CM, Saag MS, Cloud GA, et al. Treatment of cryptococcal meningitis associated with acquired immunodeficiency syndrome. *N Engl J Med* 1997;337:15–21.

208. Varkey B, Rose HD. Pulmonary aspergilloma—a rational approach to treatment. *Am J Med* 1976;61:626–631.

209. Young RC, Bennett JE, Vogal CL, et al. Aspergillosis: the spectrum of the disease in 98 patients. *Medicine* 1970;49:147–173.

210. Binder RE, Faling LJ, Pugatch RD, et al. Chronic necrotizing pulmonary aspergillosis: a discrete clinical entity. *Medicine* 1982;60:109–124.

211. Denning DW, Tucker RM, Hanson LH, et al. Treatment of invasive aspergillosis with itraconazole. *Am J Med* 1989;86: 791–800.

212. Denning DW, Follansbee SE, Scolaro M, et al. Pulmonary aspergillosis in the acquired immunodeficiency syndrome. *N Engl J Med* 1991;324:654–662.

213. Minamoto GY, Barlam TF, Vander Els NJ. Invasive aspergillosis in patients with AIDS. *Clin Infect Dis* 1992;14:66–74.

214. Pizzo PA, Robichaud KJ, Gill FA, et al. Empiric antibiotic and antifungal therapy for cancer patients with prolonged fever and granulocytopenia. *Am J Med* 1982;72:101–111.

16

PULMONARY COMPLICATIONS IN THE IMMUNOSUPPRESSED PATIENT

WENDY J. MANGIALARDI
ROBERT J. MANGIALARDI

INTRODUCTION

CHEMOTHERAPY/BONE MARROW TRANSPLANT
Evaluation
Bacterial Infections
Fungal Infections
Viral Infections
Other Pulmonary Infections
Diseases Specific to Bone Marrow Transplant Recipients
Prevention

PATIENTS INFECTED WITH HUMAN IMMUNODEFICIENCY VIRUS
Evaluation
Pneumocystis carinii Pneumonia
Bacterial Infections
Tuberculosis
Other Mycobacteria
Fungal Infections
Prevention

INTRODUCTION

Physicians encounter the immunocompromised host with increasing frequency because of three phenomena: the acquired immunodeficiency syndrome (AIDS) epidemic, advances in cancer chemotherapy, and expanding organ transplantation. Such individuals have impairment in host defenses such that they are at risk of developing infections with both true pathogens and opportunistic pathogens (those that do not cause disease in normal hosts). Defects in host defense mechanisms include failure of the primary defenses (skin and mucosa) and secondary defenses (humoral and cellular immune mechanisms). The defects in the secondary defenses may relate to either the underlying disease or the therapy used to treat it (Tables 16.1 and 16.2).

TABLE 16.1. INFECTIONS ASSOCIATED WITH IMMUNE DEFECTS

Immune Defect	Causes
Granulocytopenia	Acute and chronic myelocytic leukemia
T-cell defects	AIDS, Hodgkin's and non-Hodgkin's lymphoma
B-cell defects	Multiple myeloma, acute and chronic lymphocytic leukemia, non-Hodgkin's lymphoma

TABLE 16.2. IMMUNE DYSFUNCTION ASSOCIATED WITH MEDICATIONS

Immune Defect	Agents
Neutrophil dysfunction	Steroids, radiation
Defective antibody production	Methotrexate, cyclophosphamide, L-asparaginase, 6-mercaptopurine
Macrophage dysfunction	Steroids, cyclophosphamide, dactinomycin
Lymphocyte dysfunction	Steroids, cyclophosphamide, methotrexate, 5-fluorouracil, fludarabine, cytarabine, L-asparaginase, dactinomycin, hydroxyurea

This chapter will review the evaluation and management of pulmonary complications in these patient populations.

CHEMOTHERAPY/BONE MARROW TRANSPLANT

The lung is the most frequent site of serious infections in immunocompromised patients. In one series of patients with acute myelogenous leukemia, 73% of fatal infections originated in the lung (1). The job of diagnosis is made

TABLE 16.3. NONINFECTIOUS CAUSES OF PULMONARY DISEASE

Drug-induced pneumonitis
Alveolar hemorrhage
Recurrent tumor
Radiation lung injury
Leukoagglutinin transfusion reaction
Alveolar proteinosis
Pulmonary emboli
Pulmonary edema
Graft-versus-host disease (bone marrow transplant patients)

arduous not only by the broadened differential diagnosis but also by the altered presentations of routine conditions due to impairment of the normal inflammatory response. There are also numerous noninfectious conditions that cause pulmonary infiltrates (Table 16.3) and many of these processes often cause deadly secondary infections (2). Other infections, such as cytomegalovirus, compound the problem by further suppressing the immune system. Finally, it is not uncommon for these patients to have two pulmonary processes occurring simultaneously.

Evaluation

History And Physical

The first step in the evaluation of the immunocompromised patient with pulmonary infiltrates is to determine the timing and the extent of the immune defect. A pulmonary problem early in the course of chemotherapy (i.e., early neutropenia) most often represents a bacterial infection or possibly cancer metastases rather than infection with an opportunistic pathogen. Later, after prolonged neutropenia—and often after broad-spectrum antibacterials—fungal infections become common. Infection with opportunistic organisms such as cytomegalovirus (CMV) occurs late and typically in the bone marrow transplant recipient who has two to three months of profound immune function impairment.

Similarly, the illness's mode of onset and rate of progression are clues to the diagnosis. Rapid onset and progression suggest bacterial infection, pulmonary edema, pulmonary embolus, or pulmonary hemorrhage. Progression over several weeks suggests fungal, mycobacterial, radiation, or drug-induced damage.

The clinician should obtain an exposure history of both those outside and inside the hospital, as this history often provides diagnostic clues. Community exposures of importance include geographic exposures. Systemic mycosis with the so-called "geographic fungi" (histoplasmosis, blastomycosis, and coccidiomycosis) and cryptococcosis as well as tuberculosis can present as progressive primary infection, reactivation with secondary dissemination, or reinfection with dissemination. Even remote residence in endemic areas including the Southeastern United States puts a patient at risk for disease from the parasite *Strongyloides stercoralis* when cell-mediated immune function is depressed. Possible zoonotic infections include toxoplasmosis from cats and psittacosis from birds. Finally, adenovirus, influenza, and respiratory syncytial virus acquired from close community contacts can cause significant illness and subsequently lead to superinfection with bacterial pathogens.

Nosocomial pathogens are also a common cause of pneumonia in immunocompromised hosts. *Pseudomonas aeruginosa, Klebsiella pneumoniae,* other Enterobacteriaceae, and *Legionella* are the more common causative agents. Although less frequent, *Nocardia asteroides* and the *Aspergillus* species should be considered due to the high morbidity and mortality rate associated with their infection. Many outbreaks of aspergillosis have been associated with construction in or near hospitals caring for immunocompromised (3,4). The fungal spores have the ability to travel by air currents to distant sites, only to be concentrated by air-handling systems that lack adequate filtration.

Although the lung exam itself is often unhelpful, associated physical findings may give clues to a specific agent. Fungi such as *Aspergillus* may produce skin lesions in association with pulmonary disease. Some Gram-negative organisms, especially *P. aeruginosa,* may be associated with skin lesions, including ecthyma gangrenosum. *Nocardia,* as well as fungi, may disseminate to the central nervous system and lead to meningoencephalitis or brain abscesses producing neurologic findings. Finally, the presence of abdominal signs and diarrhea may be associated with infection from *Legionella* and cytomegalovirus.

Serologic testing to diagnose active infection has been shown to have limited benefit (5). However, these tests are useful to determine a patient's past exposures. A negative antibody test for varicella-zoster identifies the patient as being at high risk for varicella pneumonia. Similarly, an organ transplant recipient who is CMV-negative and who receives a transplant from a CMV-positive donor can be expected to develop CMV disease. The lack of previous exposure to the Epstein-Barr virus, although very rare among adults, places a bone marrow transplant (BMT) patient at very high risk of developing lymphoproliferative disease.

Diagnostic Testing

A chest radiograph should be the initial test obtained, and its appearance can help the clinician form a differential diagnosis (Table 16.4). In addition to the radiographic appearance at presentation, the radiographic progression may be characteristic for certain infections. Cavitation suggests a necrotizing process such as that caused by *Staphylococcus aureus, Klebsiella,* and *Pseudomonas,* as well as *Nocardia* and various fungi (2). Cancers may also cavitate, but they tend to do so at a slower rate. It is important to remember that

TABLE 16.4. RADIOGRAPHIC APPEARANCE OF LUNG DISEASE IN THE IMMUNOCOMPROMISED PATIENT

Alveolar	Interstitial	Nodular
Bacterial	Viral	Fungal
Hemorrhage	*Pneumocystis*	*Nocardia*
	Pulmonary Edema	Mycobacteria
	Radiation	Tumor

patients with severe neutropenia may have a significantly diminished inflammatory response and thus may exhibit minimal radiographic changes even in the face of severe infection. Paradoxically, as the neutrophil count returns, there may be significant radiographic worsening despite appropriate antimicrobial therapy (6).

Computerized tomography (CT) of the chest has been shown to detect pulmonary infections in immunocompromised patients with normal-appearing chest radiographs (7). In addition, CT scans can aid in the localization of the pulmonary process so the appropriate invasive diagnostic procedure can be performed. For peripheral nodules, the procedure of choice is often a CT-guided needle biopsy or a thoracoscopic lung biopsy. Most centrally situated lesions are amenable to bronchoscopy, and CT determination of the involved lung segment can improve the diagnostic yield by 50% (8).

Attempts should be made to obtain good-quality expectorated or induced sputum (under 25 epithelial cells and, if not neutropenic, over 25 white blood cells per field at 100 times magnification), as a diagnosis obtained by this method may obviate the need for more invasive diagnostic testing. It is important to remember that neutropenic patients frequently do not produce sputum and if they do, it may be contaminated with upper respiratory flora altered by previous or ongoing antibiotic therapy. A few organisms, however, never colonize the airways, and their identification on either stain or culture can be assumed to be the cause of disease: *Pneumocystis, Cryptococcus,* the geographic fungi, *Mycobacterium tuberculosis, Nocardia,* and *Legionella.* Also, in the immunocompromised patient with pulmonary infiltrates, the isolation of *Aspergillus* should not be ignored.

Although immunocompromised patients will often not develop a fever with their pulmonary infection, blood cultures should still be obtained as part of the initial work-up. The blood should be cultured for aerobic and anaerobic bacteria, fungi, and mycobacteria. For the latter two groups of organisms, the lysis centrifuged specimen technique will result in a higher yield. Exudative material from skin lesions should also be stained and cultured, as this easy procedure may provide the diagnosis. Patients who are found to have cryptococcal lung disease require a cerebrospinal fluid examination, as central nervous infection expands the treatment.

If an etiologic agent has not been identified by these methods, more invasive testing must be undertaken. Fiberoptic bronchoscopy with bronchoalveolar lavage (BAL), bronchial brushings, and possibly transbronchial biopsy is the procedure of choice. The diagnostic yield is greatest when diffuse pulmonary infiltrates are present. BAL, which provides evaluation of the alveolar space, can diagnose opportunistic infections in up to 83% of cases, though the yield for malignancies and drug toxicity is not as high (9). Cytological examination of BAL fluid is especially useful to visualize the pneumocystis organisms as well as the inclusion bodies of CMV. Transbronchial biopsy allows for the evaluation of tissue samples. The likelihood of obtaining a specific etiologic diagnosis ranges from 35% to 65%. As the samples are small, processes such as drug toxicities and metastatic malignancies are often difficult to diagnose. Bleeding and pneumothorax are the major complications and occur in less than 3% and 5%, respectively.

If the lung disease is peripherally located or at the pleural surface, transthoracic needle biopsy may be useful, especially when infection is the primary concern. An aspiration needle biopsy usually obtains adequate diagnostic material for stain and culture, and the diagnostic yield is greater if the lesion has cavitated.

An alternative to fine needle aspiration is the thoracoscopic or open lung or pleural biopsy. This procedure has been shown to be well tolerated in the immunocompromised patient and generally yields a greater quantity of material than either bronchoscopy or needle aspiration (10). Specific diagnoses are made in 70% to 80% of cases and the information is consistent with postmortem diagnoses (11). The complication rate (hemorrhage and pneumothorax) with the open-lung biopsy is 5% to 10%. Making the diagnosis of a treatable pneumonia by this method, however, does not necessarily improve the overall outcome. In one series, survival to hospital discharge was 53% in those patients with treatable infection and 50% in those with an untreatable or no diagnosis (12).

Bacterial Infections

Common bacterial infections in the neutropenic host originate from colonization with pyogenic Gram-positive *(S. pneumonia* and *S. aureus)* and Gram-negative *(P. aeruginosa,* the Enterobacteriaceae, and *S. maltophilia)* organisms. Therapy in most patients, however, must be initiated prior to identification of the offending organism(s). Choices should be based on the resistance pattern in the institution (i.e., vancomycin if methacillin-resistant *S. aureas* incidence is high). Although some studies have shown success with monotherapy using broad-spectrum agents such as ceftazidime or imipenem, most practitioners still use combination therapies to provide broader coverage and to limit the emergence of antibiotic resistance. Most importantly, the therapy should continue for at least two to three weeks after the patient has shown a response.

In the bone marrow transplant population, early bacterial pneumonias are uncommon, most likely due to the extensive use of empiric antibacterial drugs for early febrile episodes. In one series, only six of 55 cases of nosocomial pneumonia were bacterial in origin (13). Four or more months after the transplant, the incidence of bacterial pneumonia increases, with encapsulated organisms being the most common. This phenomenon is likely due to a persistent deficiency in antibacterial antibodies.

Fungal Infections

Aspergillus is the most common serious fungal infection in the granulocytopenic patient. The only chance for a favorable outcome is the combination of prompt diagnosis, aggressive antifungal treatment, and recovery of the granulocyte count (14). Although this organism is ubiquitous in the environment and may colonize the respiratory tract, its presence in the granulocytopenic patient should never be ignored. The species most commonly recovered are *A. fumigatus* and *A. flavus,* the latter commonly in infections that originate from the nose or paranasal sinuses.

Invasive *Aspergillus* is suggested by fever followed by the development of one or more areas of focal, dense, radiological lung infiltrates. As the patient's neutrophil count improves, these areas often cavitate. Hemoptysis and pneumothorax are possible complications. During prolonged granulocytopenia, the organism may disseminate to the brain, liver, skin, and other organs. A definitive diagnosis comes from growth in culture or demonstration of the organism in tissue specimen. Unfortunately, the fungus is essentially never isolated from blood, nor are serologic tests useful.

Amphotericin B, at doses of at least 1 mg per kg daily, remains the drug of choice for invasive pulmonary aspergillosis. Surgical resection of solitary pulmonary lesions has been advocated by some (15), but is not currently widely performed. Several studies have evaluated itraconazole, but its utility in immunocompromised patients has not been determined (16).

Viral Infections

Without prophylaxis, CMV disease occurs in up to 50% of allogeneic BMT recipients. The usual timing of the infection is eight to 10 weeks after the transplant; and it occurs more often in older patients, those who received total body irradiation (TBI), and those with graft-versus-host disease (17).

Early detection is the key to both preventing the development of CMV pneumonia and successfully treating the infection. Blood antigen testing has replaced culture and shell vial in most institutions as the initial test of choice. In BMT patients, treatment of low-grade viremia (more than one positive cell per slide for allograft or more than four positive cells per slide for autografts) can prevent the development of CMV disease. First-line therapy remains intravenous ganciclovir, usually combined with CMV-specific immune globulin.

During the winter months, respiratory syncytial virus (RSV) and influenza should be considered in the differential diagnosis of pneumonia. Patients with these illnesses often present with fever, cough, and rhinorrhea with rales or rhonchi on examination. Chest radiograph findings may include diffuse interstitial or lobar infiltrates. Treatment with ribavirin for RSV or amantadine for influenza should be considered, though there are no large clinical trials proving efficacy. These patients are also at risk for developing secondary bacterial infections.

Other Pulmonary Infections

Fortunately, *Pneumocystis carinii* pneumonia (PCP) has been virtually eliminated from the bone marrow transplant population due to the use of trimethoprim/sulfamethoxazole or pentamidine prophylaxis. Use of the former also makes infection with *Toxoplasmosis gondii* and *Nocardia* significantly less likely. Even with a remote exposure, disease from the parasite *Strongyloides stercoralis* may occur. Pulmonary illness comes from either the parasite delivering bacteria to the lung or by direct tissue injury from larvae that have metamorphosed to adults in the lung. In severe cases hemorrhagic pulmonary infiltrates and the adult respiratory distress syndrome may result (18).

Diseases Specific To Bone Marrow Transplant Recipients

A disease unique to the bone marrow transplant recipient is graft-versus-host disease (GVHD). It is a process whereby the donor lymphocytes attack antigenically distinct host cells primarily in the skin, liver, and gastrointestinal tract. The acute form of GVHD occurs in up to 60% of recipients usually within the first three months after transplantation; the chronic form appears after posttransplant day 100 and may additionally involve the ophthalmic and sinopulmonary systems. Not only does the development of this condition delay recovery of the immune system itself, but its cytotoxic therapy intensifies the patient's immunosuppression. Patients with both forms are at increased risk of infectious pneumonitis. Patients with chronic GVHD are at increased risk for obstructive airway disease. Interestingly, the lung pathology in these patients is similar to bronchiolitis obliterans, which may suggest direct immune-mediated damage by the donor lymphocytes (19).

Interstitial pneumonitis occurs in the early posttransplant period in up to 50% of allogeneic transplant recipients and is the cause of death in 40% (20). It presents within the first 90 days after transplantation, and manifestations include fever, dyspnea, dry cough, and hypoxia. In some cases, an infectious agent such as CMV and less frequently herpes simplex virus (HSV) or varicella-zoster virus (VZV) is identified, but the rest remain labeled "idiopathic." Several studies have evaluated risk factors for the development of this disease, and it is felt the lung injury represents the cumulative effect of chemotherapy and radiation on the lung.

Prevention

The most important and yet the most ignored strategy for the prevention of infections with resistant organisms is strict adherence to hand-washing precautions (21). Other more aggressive measures, such as reverse isolation, have been attempted but have not been found to be any more effective (22). The use of high-efficiency particulate air (HEPA) filters, in addition to other control measures during periods of construction near patient care areas, may decrease the incidence of invasive aspergillosis. Water purification systems may be useful if *Legionella* colonization is suspected.

Prophylactic antimicrobials have been the subject of many clinical trials. The use of quinolones has been shown to delay the time to fever and the need for empiric antibiotic therapy. As would be anticipated, though, their use does allow for the emergence of resistant organisms, thus limiting the drugs' usefulness at the time of a documented infection (23). Similarly, the use of prophylactic antifungals such as fluconazole has been shown to decrease the rate of serious candidal infections, though possibly at the cost of overgrowth of more resistant species such as *Aspergillus* (24). Acyclovir is very effective in preventing both mucocutaneous and visceral infection with HSV. Ganciclovir appears to prevent CMV infection when used prophylactically (25).

The hematopoietic growth factors granulocyte colony-stimulating factor (G-CSF) and granulocyte-macrophage colony-stimulating factor (GM-CSF) have not only been shown to decrease the length of neutropenia, but have also been associated with fewer infections (26). Additionally, these drugs may also increase neutrophil bactericidal and fungicidal activity.

Most patients who are transiently neutropenic from cancer chemotherapy should receive routine immunizations as scheduled once their cell lines have recovered. In the bone marrow transplant recipients, most centers reimmunize all patients once they are free from GVHD for one year. The vaccines that are included are as follows: tetanus toxoid, diphtheria toxoid, inactivated polio vaccine, pneumococcal polysaccharide, *H. influenzae* type B polysaccharide, and influenza.

PATIENTS INFECTED WITH HUMAN IMMUNODEFICIENCY VIRUS

Highly active antiretroviral therapy (HAART) has dramatically changed the lives and the care of patients with HIV

TABLE 16.5. NONINFECTIOUS PULMONARY COMPLICATIONS IN HIV

Lymphocytic alveolitis
Primary pulmonary hypertension
Nonspecific interstitial pneumonitis
Lymphoid interstitial pneumonitis
Lymphoma
Lung cancer
Pulmonary edema due to HIV cardiomyopathy

and AIDS. For the first time in the epidemic, morbidity and mortality have fallen (27). Whether this is a temporary change or a trend that will continue remains to be seen. Unfortunately, the rate of new infections has remained steady, and thus there will continue to be a large number of immunocompromised patients in need of care. Also, the long-term side effects of these powerful medications remain to be seen. It should be emphasized that there are many noninfectious pulmonary complications in HIV patients (Table 16.5).

Evaluation

As with other immunocompromised patients, the initial step in evaluating a patient infected with HIV presenting with a pulmonary process is to determine their current immune status. HAART has been shown to suppress HIV viral load, which results in immune recovery. This recovery does not, however, appear to be immediate. For the first several months after HAART initiation, the increased number of CD4+ cells is due to expansion of preexisting memory T cells. After that, there is a more gradual rise in the CD4+ cells due mostly to new naïve cells, indicating a true recovery of the immune system (28). So, while the patient's current CD4 count should be determined, it is important to also know his or her CD4 nadir.

Previous exposures should also be elicited. All patients infected with HIV should have a tuberculin skin test with controls placed on their initial evaluation. A test resulting in 5 mm of induration or more is considered positive and indicative of tuberculous infection in individuals coinfected with HIV. A negative tuberculin skin test, however, does not rule out the infection. The responsiveness to delayed-type hypersensitivity skin test antigens declines as the HIV infection progresses and the number of CD4 cells decreases. In one study of patients with known tuberculosis, tuberculin skin tests were found to be positive in 64% of HIV-infected patients with more than 100 CD4 cells per mm^3 but in none of 13 patients with less than 100 CD4 cells per mm^3 (29). Delayed-type hypersensitivity skin testing with *Candida*, mumps, or tetanus toxoid antigens as controls has been advocated at the time of PPD testing. A negative tuberculin skin test with a positive control makes tuberculous infection unlikely. A negative PPD with negative controls (anergy) does not exclude tuberculosis, and further diagnostic evaluation should be undertaken.

Chest radiography may be helpful in forming a differential diagnosis. Hilar adenopathy, pleural effusions, and cavitation suggest a diagnosis of tuberculosis, as they are rare findings in PCP or cytomegalovirus pneumonitis. Kaposi's sarcoma and lymphoma can present with hilar adenopathy and pleural effusion; however, extrapulmonary evidence of these diseases is usually present. Fungal infections such as coccidioidomycosis, histoplasmosis, and cryptococcosis can present with chest roentgenogram findings similar to those of tuberculosis, but diffuse infiltrates are more typical, extrapulmonary manifestations are common, and serologic tests help in the differential diagnosis. A miliary pattern on chest roentgenogram suggests tuberculosis, but other interstitial processes such as PCP, cytomegalovirus pneumonitis, fungal infections, and noninfectious pneumonitis should be considered. Upper lobe infiltrates, although frequent in tuberculosis, can also be found in patients developing PCP while receiving prophylaxis with aerosolized pentamidine. If chest radiographs are negative, but lung disease is still suspected, gallium scanning may be useful, as the test has a low false-negative rate.

Sputum examination should always be attempted for organism isolation prior to more invasive testing. Sputum induction (ultrasonic nebulizer delivery of 3% to 5% saline into the airway) may be used if the patient is unable to produce an adequate sample. Although some centers report yields as high as 75% for the identification of PCP, in practice the overall sensitivity is around 20%. The yield for tuberculosis appears to be somewhat higher, around 55%, even in a patient with normal chest radiographs (30).

If induced sputum fails to produce a diagnosis, further invasive testing needs to be considered. There has been much discussion about empiric treatment versus bronchoscopy in the patient suspected of having PCP. Although some studies have shown no difference in mortality between these two groups, the number of clinically significant alternative diagnoses that are identified makes the procedure justified (31). The diagnosis of bacterial infections by bronchoscopy remains problematic, with both high false-positive as well as false-negative rates. The isolation of CMV from BAL fluid is also not synonymous with infection. Interestingly, there is greater three-to-six month mortality in those patients in whom the virus is isolated even without the diagnosis of viral pneumonia (32).

Pneumocystis Carinii Pneumonia

Despite the widespread use of prophylaxis, PCP remains one of the most common pulmonary infections in patients infected with HIV. There are two theories relating to the transmission of PCP. First, it has been hypothesized that the *Pneumocystis carinii* infection results from reactivation of a previously dormant infection acquired during childhood. Evidence for this theory is based upon the fact that most healthy children by the age of four have antibodies to *Pneu-*

mocystis carinii (33). The second theory is that the organism is transmitted among susceptible individuals by the airborne route. There are two lines of evidence to support airborne transmission: (a) in animal studies, susceptible animals that share the same airspace can become infected (34); and (b) clustering of PCP cases occurs in persons with close contact (35).

The usual clinical presentation is one of gradually increasing fatigue, fevers, chills, sweats, dyspnea, nonproductive cough, and chest tightness. The mean duration of symptoms prior to diagnosis is usually weeks. On physical examination, the patient appears ill with tachypnea and tachycardia, though the lung exam itself is most often normal. Patients receiving prophylaxis often present with milder signs and symptoms.

Most patients have CD4 counts in the range of 50 to 75 cells per mm^3 at the time of diagnosis of their first episode of PCP, and more than 90% of PCP episodes occur when the CD4 count is below 200 cells per mm^3 (36). Routine laboratory testing is usually remarkable only for the findings of an acute pneumonia. PCP rarely occurs without an elevation of the LDH. Arterial blood gas analysis usually reveals a respiratory alkalosis with a widened alveolar-to-arterial oxygen pressure difference (37).

Typical chest radiographic findings are those of diffuse bilateral interstitial infiltrates without a pleural effusion. As the disease progresses, alveolar infiltrates may also develop. Although abnormal chest radiographs have been reported in up to 90% of patients, normal chest radiographs may occur (38). Many other less common chest radiographic findings have been reported, including focal infiltrates, nodules, cystic lesions, and pneumothoraces. Atypical radiographic findings are more commonly found in patients who have other underlying lung disease, have had previous episodes of PCP, or are receiving pentamidine prophylaxis (39).

Empiric treatment for suspected PCP should be initiated as soon as the diagnosis is expected. Large numbers of *Pneumocystis carinii* cysts and trophozoites remain in lung tissues and pulmonary secretions for weeks to months after the initiation of therapy (40). Sputum should be collected, as this method is successful in up to 60%, thus sparing more invasive testing. If the sputum is unrevealing, bronchoscopically guided BAL is the principal method of diagnosis. Transbronchial biopsy performed during bronchoscopy has a sensitivity and specificity similar to those of BAL alone (9) but should be considered in patients receiving prophylaxis or in those who have unusual chest radiographic findings, as the organism burden may be lower in these patients.

In patients clinically suspected of having PCP, the first-line antibiotic regimen is trimethoprim/sulfamethoxazole (TMP/SMX). The usual dose of TMP/SMX is 15 to 20 mg per kg per day orally or parenterally at six- or eight-hour intervals daily for 21 days. TMP/SMX has the added benefit of antibacterial properties that are beneficial in patients with concurrent or misdiagnosed bacterial pneumonia. It is common for patients who ultimately recover from PCP to deteriorate during the initial two to three days of treatment; thus it has been recommended that alternate medications should not be started until the patient has received at least five to seven days of therapy (41). Second-line agents include intravenous pentamidine, clindamycin/primaquine, TMP/dapsone, reduced-dose TMP/SMX, and atovaquone.

Several studies have shown that corticosteroids are beneficial as adjunctive therapy in the treatment of moderate to severe PCP (42). If the PaO$_2$ is less than 60 mm Hg, prednisone at a dose of 40 mg a day should be initiated. No benefit from the addition of corticosteroids was found when they were added more than 72 hours after the start of antipneumocystis therapy.

Pneumothorax with bronchopleural fistula is a life-threatening condition in patients infected with HIV. The pneumothorax may be due to an acute episode of PCP, may be associated with aerosolized pentamidine prophylaxis, or may be related to a chronic form of PCP in which lung cavitation and honeycombing can occur (43). The persistent air leak will rarely heal on its own and may require surgical or thoracoscopically guided closure, which may or may not be successful. HIV-infected patients who present with pneumothoraces should be suspected of having PCP.

Bacterial Infections

It is important to remember that patients infected with HIV have defects in their humoral as well as their cellular immunity; thus routine bacterial infections also occur at an elevated rate. The most common pathogens are the encapsulated organisms *Streptococcus pneumoniae* and *Haemophilus influenzae.* Other reported bacterial organisms include group B streptococci, *Staphylococcus aureus, Moraxella catarrhalis, Mycoplasma pneumoniae,* and *Rhodococcus equi.*

The clinical presentation of acute bacterial pneumonia in HIV-infected patients is similar to that in the seronegative population. Patients present with productive cough, fever, and pleuritic chest pain (44). Bacteremia is frequently present. Chest radiographs commonly reveal diffuse infiltrates with *H. influenzae* infection and lobar infiltrates with *S. pneumoniae* infection. Signs and symptoms in patients with bacterial pneumonia are usually more acute than those in patients with PCP alone.

Tuberculosis

The resurgence of tuberculosis has been at least in part due to the HIV epidemic. The diseases are linked not only biologically but also socioeconomically. There are currently an estimated 6,000 to 9,000 new cases annually in the United States (45). In immunocompetent individuals newly infected with *M. tuberculosis,* only 10% will develop clinical

disease at the time of infection with another 5% developing clinically apparent tuberculosis within two years. After close contact with a tuberculous patient, 37% of HIV-infected persons develop disease within five months (46). The risk of reactivation of tuberculosis in HIV-infected patients is 8% to 10% per year.

In the United States, a rise in resistant tuberculosis has paralleled the overall increase in tuberculosis since the mid-1980s (47). Historically, most patients with resistant tuberculosis acquired resistant *M. tuberculosis* organisms through ineffective courses of treatment (often because of erratic compliance with therapy). Since 1990, several outbreaks of multidrug-resistant tuberculosis have occurred in institutions. *M. tuberculosis* organisms resistant to isoniazid, rifampin, and up to seven antimycobacterial agents were transmitted to contacts in New York and Florida hospitals as well as in New York state prisons (48). The fact that many HIV-infected individuals develop active tuberculosis soon after being infected with *M. tuberculosis* contributed to the rapid nosocomial spread of multidrug-resistant tuberculosis among HIV-infected persons.

The clinical and radiographic manifestations of tuberculosis vary with the severity of HIV-induced immunodeficiency. In patients with less advanced HIV infection, extrapulmonary tuberculosis is uncommon, tuberculin skin tests are usually positive, and the chest roentgenogram findings are often suggestive of reactivation tuberculosis with upper-lobe infiltrates and cavitations. In contrast, patients with advanced HIV infection frequently have extrapulmonary disease, negative tuberculin skin tests, and chest roentgenogram changes typical of primary tuberculosis, with hilar adenopathy and interstitial or miliary infiltrates (49). Recently, it has been reported that patients with tuberculosis who are treated with HAART have paradoxical worsening of their tuberculosis. They may develop increasing pleural effusions, adenopathy, and fevers (50).

The diagnosis of tuberculosis relies upon the isolation of *M. tuberculosis* on culture. Acid-fast smears of sputum are positive in 31% to 82% of HIV-infected persons with tuberculosis; sputum cultures are positive in 88% to 100% of cases (50). New tests that can identify *M. tuberculosis* RNA or DNA have been approved for testing on specimens that are positive for mycobacterium by acid-fast testing. Their utility on stain-negative specimens is still to be determined (51). Aspiration biopsy of tuberculous lymphadenopathy reveals acid-fast organisms in 67% to 90% of HIV-infected patients. Blood cultures prepared by the lysis-centrifugation system are positive in up to 40% of patients (52).

In response to the increase in drug-resistant tuberculosis in the United States, the Centers for Disease Control has recommended a four-drug regimen including isoniazid (INH), rifampin (RIF), pyrazinamide (PZA), and ethambutol (EMB) as the initial empiric treatment of tuberculosis in all patients, including those infected with HIV (47). This four-drug regimen should be continued for two months, at which time the treatment can be altered according to drug-susceptibility results. Those patients who have susceptible *M. tuberculosis* organisms should receive INH and RIF for an additional seven months (a total of nine months) or for six months after cultures have converted to negative, whichever is longer. A prolonged treatment of tuberculosis is advocated in patients infected with HIV because the efficacy of a six-month regimen remains unproven in this population.

Multidrug-resistant tuberculosis in patients with HIV infection should be treated empirically with six drugs until the drug susceptibility results are available. If the resistance pattern of a source case is known or once the drug susceptibilities of the patient's isolate are available, four effective agents should be used for at least 24 months. Antituberculous medications that can be used in the treatment of multidrug-resistant tuberculosis include amikacin, kanamycin, streptomycin, and capreomycin as injectable agents and ethionamide, cycloserine, aminosalicylic acid, and ofloxacin or ciprofloxacin as oral agents.

Other *Mycobacteria*

The *M. avium* complex (MAC) includes two species of mycobacteria classified within Runyon's group III: *M. avium* and *M. intracellulare*. MAC organisms are ubiquitous in the environment and are commonly isolated from water and soil, thus colonization of the respiratory or GI tracts with MAC organisms is not uncommon in patients with AIDS and is a risk factor for disseminated MAC (53). Typically, in patients with AIDS, MAC infection disseminates widely and causes a wasting syndrome with fever, night sweats, anorexia, hepatosplenomegaly, and bone marrow suppression. There may be pulmonary complaints, but they are minimal in comparison to the other symptoms.

Disseminated infections with mycobacteria other than *M. tuberculosis* or MAC occasionally occur in HIV-infected patients. *M. kansasii* infection usually presents as a pulmonary disease with or without concomitant extrapulmonary involvement. Chest radiographs show diffuse interstitial involvement, focal upper-lobe disease and/or thin-walled cavities (54).

Fungal Infections

The yeastlike fungus *Cryptococcus neoformans* is distributed worldwide in the environment and can be isolated from soil, fruits, and other sources in nature. Human infection probably results from the inhalation of the aerosolized yeast. *C. neoformans* is a pathogen of relatively low virulence, and severe immunosuppression is required for cryptococcal disease to occur. Most HIV-infected patients with cryptococcosis have CD4 cell counts below 100 per mm^3.

Cryptococcosis in patients with HIV infection presents as a meningitis in 85% of cases, though concomitant or isolated pneumonia occurs in up to 50% of patients (55). Symptoms of pulmonary cryptococcal disease include fever, shortness of breath, pleuritic chest pain, and productive cough. Chest roentgenographic findings most often consist of diffuse or focal interstitial infiltrates. Nodular infiltrates, intrathoracic adenopathy, focal alveolar consolidation, cavitation, and isolated pleural effusion are less common findings (56).

The definitive diagnosis of cryptococcosis relies upon the isolation of *C. neoformans* from body fluids or tissue. A positive sputum culture indicates disease even in the absence of radiographic changes (41). The serum cryptococcal antigen is a very sensitive test that is positive in 75% to 99% of patients with AIDS-related cryptococcosis (55).

Treatment usually consists of an initial induction course of amphotericin B alone (0.7 to 0.8 mg per kg per day) or amphotericin B (0.3 to 0.5 mg per kg per day) combined with 5-flucytosine (100 mg per kg per day in four divided doses) for a period of two weeks or until the patient's condition stabilizes. Treatment can then be continued with oral fluconazole 400 mg daily for eight to 10 weeks. Daily maintenance therapy with fluconazole 200 mg per day is very effective in preventing relapse of cryptococcal disease in HIV-infected patients (57).

Histoplasmosis

H. capsulatum is endemic in the Central and South-Central states of the United States, southern Mexico, Central America, South America, and the Caribbean. It clinically presents as a disseminated disease in HIV-infected patients. Evidence suggests that both newly acquired infection with *H. capsulatum* as well as reactivation of latent foci of infection lead to dissemination in patients with HIV infection (58).

Symptoms of disseminated histoplasmosis in HIV-infected patients include fevers, chills, and weight loss, often lasting for weeks. Cough and dyspnea are present in 50% of patients (58). Diffuse interstitial infiltrates are the most common chest radiographic abnormalities. Occasional patients will present with a fulminant illness manifested by hypotension, acute renal failure, adult respiratory distress syndrome, and disseminated intravascular coagulation (59).

The recovery of *H. capsulatum* on culture or the visualization of the organism in histopathologic material is necessary for the diagnosis of histoplasmosis. Blood cultures using the lysis-centrifugation method are positive in 90% of cases. A rapid diagnosis is possible in more than a third of patients when *H. capsulatum* organisms are identified in a smear of peripheral blood or bone marrow. The *H. capsulatum* polysaccharide antigen (HPA) appears to be an excellent marker for early diagnosis and is now available (58).

Amphotericin B is very effective in the treatment of histoplasmosis in HIV-infected patients and is the drug of choice in patients with severe disease. Itraconazole at a dose of 200 mg orally, three times a day for three days, then twice a day for 12 weeks is very effective as primary therapy in patients with mild-to-moderate disease (58). Maintenance therapy with itraconazole 200 mg orally twice a day prevented relapse of histoplasmosis in 95% of patients over a median follow-up period of 109 weeks (60).

Coccidioidomycosis

The fungus *Coccidioides immitis* is a soil organism endemic to the semiarid regions of the Southwestern United States, northern Mexico, and some areas of Central and South America. In HIV-infected patients, coccidioidomycosis can present either as a primary progressive infection or as reactivated disease. A diagnosis of AIDS, a CD4 cell count below 250 cells per mm^3, or residing in an endemic area are risk factors for developing coccidioidomycosis.

Most HIV-infected patients with coccidioidomycosis present with fever and pulmonary symptoms such as cough and dyspnea. Both focal and diffuse pulmonary disease can occur. Other sites of involvement include the meninges, the skin, the lymph nodes, and the liver. Chest radiographic findings consist of focal alveolar infiltrates, diffuse interstitial infiltrates, and, less commonly, nodules, hilar lymphadenopathy, or pleural effusions (61).

Demonstrating the organisms on stain or culture from an infected site makes the diagnosis of coccidioidomycosis. Bronchoscopy with BAL and transbronchial biopsy is usually helpful in making a diagnosis. The tube precipitin immunodiffusion or the complement fixation serologic tests are helpful as they are positive in 90% of patients with active disease. The coccidioidin or spherulin skin tests are not helpful because they are positive in less than 20% of patients with active disease (61).

Amphotericin B is the treatment of choice in HIV-infected patients with life-threatening coccidioidomycosis. Less severe forms of the disease may be treated with fluconazole at 400 to 1200 mg per day or itraconazole at 400 mg per day. Both of these agents have also been used for maintenance therapy.

Prevention

Without prophylaxis, patients with CD4 counts below 200 cells per mm^3 have a risk of developing PCP that is 8.4% at six months, 18.4% at 12 months, and 33% at 36 months (36). The medications best tested for prophylaxis are TMP/SMX (TMP 160 mg and SMX 800 mg) once daily or aerosolized pentamidine 300 mg every four weeks. TMP/SMX is recommended as the first-line medication for prophylaxis, although up to 30% of patients develop side effects that require substitution of another medication. Other medications used prophylactically are dapsone, intermittent parenteral pentamidine, oral dapsone/pyrimethamine, oral clindamycin/primaquine, and oral atovaquone. Whether or not prophylaxis can be discontinued when the patient's CD4 count increases is still being evaluated.

Prophylaxis with INH, 300 mg per day for 12 months, is recommended for all HIV-infected patients with a positive tuberculin skin test, regardless of age, unless specifically contraindicated. Anergic HIV-infected patients who have (a) close contacts with contagious tuberculous patients, (b) a previously untreated positive tuberculin skin test, (c) chest roentgenographic changes suggesting previous untreated tuberculosis, or (d) a history of inadequately treated tuberculosis should receive INH prophylaxis as well. Other anergic patients infected with HIV who should be considered for prophylaxis include intravenous drug users, the homeless, and foreign-born persons from countries with a high endemicity of tuberculosis (47). Patients exposed to drug-resistant tuberculosis should receive prophylaxis according to the drug susceptibility pattern of the source case.

The pneumococcal vaccine is recommended by the Centers for Disease Control for primary prevention of pneumococcal pneumonia in HIV-infected patients, although its efficacy in this population has not been proven (62). Similarly, most providers administer the influenza vaccine yearly despite no evidence of effectiveness.

REFERENCES

1. Estey EH, Keating MJ, McCredie KB, et al. Causes of initial remission induction failure in acute myelogenous leukemia. *Blood* 1982;60(2):309–315.
2. Ramsey PG, Rubin RH, Tolkoff-Rubin NE, et al. The renal transplant patient with fever and pulmonary infiltrates: etiology, clinical manifestations, and management. *Medicine (Baltimore)* 1980;59(3):206–222.
3. Lentino JR, Rosenkranz MA, Michaels JA, et al. Nosocomial aspergillosis: a retrospective review of airborne disease secondary to road construction and contaminated air conditioners. *Am J Epidemiol* 1982;116(3):430–437.
4. Opal SM, Asp AA, Cannady PB Jr, et al. Efficacy of infection control measures during a nosocomial outbreak of disseminated aspergillosis associated with hospital construction. *J Infect Dis* 1986;153(3):634–637.
5. Filice G, Yu B, Armstrong D. Immunodiffusion and agglutination tests for Candida in patients with neoplastic disease: inconsistent correlation of results with invasive infections. *J Infect Dis* 1977;135(3):349–357.
6. Sickles EA, Greene WH, Wiernik PH. Clinical presentation of infection in granulocytopenic patients. *Arch Intern Med* 1975; 135(5):715–719.
7. Graham NJ, Muller NL, Miller RR, et al. Intrathoracic complications following allogeneic bone marrow transplantation: CT findings. *Radiology* 1991;181(1):153–156.
8. Naidich DP, Sussman R, Kutcher WL, et al. Solitary pulmonary nodules. CT-bronchoscopic correlation. *Chest* 1988;93(3): 595–598.
9. Stover DE, Zaman MB, Hajdu SI, et al. Bronchoalveolar lavage in the diagnosis of diffuse pulmonary infiltrates in the immunosuppressed host. *Ann Intern Med* 1984;101(1):1–7.
10. Dijkman JH, van der Meer JW, Bakker W, et al. Transpleural lung biopsy by the thoracoscopic route in patients with diffuse interstitial pulmonary disease. *Chest* 1982;82(1):76–83.
11. McKenna RJ Jr, Mountain CF, McMurtrey MJ. Open lung biopsy in immunocompromised patients. *Chest* 1984;86(5): 671–674.

12. Haverkos HW, Dowling JN, Pasculle AW, et al. Diagnosis of pneumonitis in immunocompromised patients by open lung biopsy. *Cancer* 1983;52(6):1093–1097.

13. Pannuti CS, Gingrich RD, Pfaller MA, et al. Nosocomial pneumonia in adult patients undergoing bone marrow transplantation: a 9-year study. *J Clin Oncol* 1991;9(1):77–84.

14. Burch PA, Karp JE, Merz WG, et al. Favorable outcome of invasive aspergillosis in patients with acute leukemia. *J Clin Oncol* 1987;5(12):1985–1993.

15. Moreau P, Zahar JR, Milpied N, et al. Localized invasive pulmonary aspergillosis in patients with neutropenia. Effectiveness of surgical resection. *Cancer* 1993;72(11):3223–3226.

16. Denning DW, Tucker RM, Hanson LH, et al. Treatment of invasive aspergillosis with itraconazole. *Am J Med* 1989;86(6 Pt 2):791–800.

17. Meyers JD, Flournoy N, Thomas ED. Risk factors for cytomegalovirus infection after human marrow transplantation. *J Infect Dis* 1986;153(3):478–488.

18. Scowden EB, Schaffner W, Stone WJ. Overwhelming strongyloidiasis: an unappreciated opportunistic infection. *Medicine (Baltimore)* 1978;57(6):527–544.

19. Clark JG, Schwartz DA, Flournoy N, et al. Risk factors for airflow obstruction in recipients of bone marrow transplants. *Ann Intern Med* 1987;107(5):648–656.

20. Weiner RS, Bortin MM, Gale RP, et al. Interstitial pneumonitis after bone marrow transplantation. Assessment of risk factors. *Ann Intern Med* 1986;104(2):168–175.

21. Albert RK, Condie F. Hand-washing patterns in medical intensive-care units. *N Engl J Med* 1981;304(24):1465–1466.

22. Nauseef WM, Maki DG. A study of the value of simple protective isolation in patients with granulocytopenia. *N Engl J Med* 1981;304(8):448–453.

23. Kotilainen P, Nikoskelainen J, Huovinen P. Emergence of ciprofloxacin-resistant coagulase-negative staphylococcal skin flora in immunocompromised patients receiving ciprofloxacin. *J Infect Dis* 1990;161(1):41–44.

24. Goodman JL, Winston DJ, Greenfield RA, et al. A controlled trial of fluconazole to prevent fungal infections in patients undergoing bone marrow transplantation [See comments]. *N Engl J Med* 1992;326(13):845–851.

25. Schmidt GM, Horak DA, Niland JC, et al. A randomized, controlled trial of prophylactic ganciclovir for cytomegalovirus pulmonary infection in recipients of allogeneic bone marrow transplants; The City of Hope-Stanford-Syntex CMV Study Group [See comments]. *N Engl J Med* 1991;324(15):1005–1011.

26. Lieschke GJ, Burgess AW. Granulocyte colony-stimulating factor and granulocyte-macrophage colony-stimulating factor (1). *N Engl J Med* 1992;327(1):28–35.

27. Palella FJ Jr, Delaney KM, Moorman AC, et al. Declining morbidity and mortality among patients with advanced human immunodeficiency virus infection. HIV Outpatient Study Investigators [See comments]. *N Engl J Med* 1998;338(13):853–860.

28. Kaufmann D, Pantaleo G, Sudre P, et al. CD4-cell count in HIV-1-infected individuals remaining viraemic with highly active antiretroviral therapy (HAART). Swiss HIV Cohort Study [Letter]. *Lancet* 1998;351(9104):723–724.

29. Jones BE, Young SM, Antoniskis D, et al. Relationship of the manifestations of tuberculosis to CD4 cell counts in patients with human immunodeficiency virus infection [See comments]. *Am Rev Respir Dis* 1993;148(5):1292–1297.

30. Greenberg SD, Frager D, Suster B, et al. Active pulmonary tuberculosis in patients with AIDS: spectrum of radiographic findings (including a normal appearance). *Radiology* 1994;193(1):115–119.

31. Huang L, Hecht FM, Stansell JD, et al. Suspected Pneumocystis carinii pneumonia with a negative induced sputum examination. Is early bronchoscopy useful? *Am J Respir Crit Care Med* 1995;151(6):1866–1871.

32. Hayner CE, Baughman RP, Linnemann CC Jr, et al. The relationship between cytomegalovirus retrieved by bronchoalveolar lavage and mortality in patients with HIV [See comments]. *Chest* 1995;107(3):735–740.

33. Pifer LL, Hughes WT, Stagno S, et al. Pneumocystis carinii infection: evidence for high prevalence in normal and immunosuppressed children. *Pediatrics* 1978;61(1):35–41.

34. Hughes WT, Bartley DL, Smith BM. A natural source of infection due to pneumocystis carinii. *J Infect Dis* 1983;147(3):595.

35. Goesch TR, Gotz G, Stellbrinck KH, et al. Possible transfer of Pneumocystis carinii between immunodeficient patients [Letter] [See comments]. *Lancet* 1990;336(8715):627.

36. Phair J, Munoz A, Detels R, et al. The risk of Pneumocystis carinii pneumonia among men infected with human immunodeficiency virus type 1. Multicenter AIDS Cohort Study Group [See comments]. *N Engl J Med* 1990;322(3):161–165.

37. Kovacs JA, Hiemenz JW, Macher AM, et al. Pneumocystis carinii pneumonia: a comparison between patients with the acquired immunodeficiency syndrome and patients with other immunodeficiencies. *Ann Intern Med* 1984;100(5):663–671.

38. DeLorenzo LJ, Huang CT, Maguire GP, et al. Roentgenographic patterns of Pneumocystis carinii pneumonia in 104 patients with AIDS. *Chest* 1987;91(3):323–327.

39. Jules-Elysee KM, Stover DE, Zaman MB, et al. Aerosolized pentamidine: effect on diagnosis and presentation of Pneumocystis carinii pneumonia. *Ann Intern Med* 1990;112(10):750–757.

40. Shelhamer JH, Toews GB, Masur H, et al. NIH conference. Respiratory disease in the immunosuppressed patient. *Ann Intern Med* 1992;117(5):415–431.

41. Murray JF, Mills J. Pulmonary infectious complications of human immunodeficiency virus infection. Part I. *Am Rev Respir Dis* 1990;141(5 Pt 1):1356–1372.

42. Bozzette SA, Sattler FR, Chiu J, et al. A controlled trial of early adjunctive treatment with corticosteroids for Pneumocystis carinii pneumonia in the acquired immunodeficiency syndrome. California Collaborative Treatment Group [See comments]. *N Engl J Med* 1990;323(21):1451–1457.

43. Wassermann K, Pothoff G, Kirn E, et al. Chronic Pneumocystis carinii pneumonia in AIDS. *Chest* 1993;104(3):667–672.

44. Witt DJ, Craven DE, McCabe WR. Bacterial infections in adult patients with the acquired immune deficiency syndrome (AIDS) and AIDS-related complex. *Am J Med* 1987;82(5):900–906.

45. Markowitz N, Hansen NI, Hopewell PC, et al. Incidence of tuberculosis in the United States among HIV-infected persons. The Pulmonary Complications of HIV Infection Study Group. *Ann Intern Med* 1997;126(2):123–132.

46. Daley CL, Small PM, Schecter GF, et al. An outbreak of tuberculosis with accelerated progression among persons infected with the human immunodeficiency virus. An analysis using restriction-fragment-length polymorphisms. *N Engl J Med* 1992;326(4):231–235.

47. Centers for Disease Control and Prevention. Initial therapy for tuberculosis in the era of multidrug resistance: recommendations of the Advisory Council for the Elimination of Tuberculosis. *JAMA* 1993;270(6):694–698.

48. Centers for Disease Control. Nosocomial transmission of multidrug-resistant tuberculosis among HIV-infected persons—Florida and New York, 1988–1991. *JAMA* 1991;266(11):1483–1485.

49. Perlman DC, el-Sadr WM, Nelson ET, et al. Variation of chest radiographic patterns in pulmonary tuberculosis by degree of human immunodeficiency virus-related immunosuppression. The Terry Beirn Community Programs for Clinical Research on AIDS (CPCRA). The AIDS Clinical Trials Group (ACTG). *Clin Infect Dis* 1997;25(2):242–246.

50. Havlir DV, Barnes PF. Tuberculosis in patients with human immunodeficiency virus infection. *N Engl J Med* 1999;340(5): 367–373.

51. Barnes PF. Rapid diagnostic tests for tuberculosis: progress but no gold standard [Editorial; Comment] [published erratum appears in *Am J Respir Crit Care Med* 1997;156(3 Pt 1):1022]. *Am J Respir Crit Care Med* 1997;155(5):1497–1498.

52. Kramer F, Modilevsky T, Waliany AR, et al.Delayed diagnosis of tuberculosis in patients with human immunodeficiency virus infection [See comments]. *Am J Med* 1990;89(4):451–456.

53. Horsburgh CR Jr, Metchock BG, McGowan JE Jr, et al. Clinical implications of recovery of Mycobacterium avium complex from the stool or respiratory tract of HIV-infected individuals [Letter]. *AIDS* 1992;6(5):512–514.

54. Levine B, Chaisson RE. Mycobacterium kansasii: a cause of treatable pulmonary disease associated with advanced human immunodeficiency virus (HIV) infection [See comments]. *Ann Intern Med* 1991;114(10):861–868.

55. Chuck SL, Sande MA. Infections with Cryptococcus neoformans in the acquired immunodeficiency syndrome [See comments]. *N Engl J Med* 1989;321(12):794–799.

56. Wasser L, Talavera W. Pulmonary cryptococcosis in AIDS. *Chest* 1987;92(4):692–695.

57. Bozzette SA, Larsen RA, Chiu J, et al. A placebo-controlled trial of maintenance therapy with fluconazole after treatment of cryptococcal meningitis in the acquired immunodeficiency syndrome. California Collaborative Treatment Group. *N Engl J Med* 1991; 324(9):580–584.

58. McKinsey DS, Spiegel RA, Hutwagner L, et al. Prospective study of histoplasmosis in patients infected with human immunodeficiency virus: incidence, risk factors, and pathophysiology. *Clin Infect Dis* 1997;24(6):1195–1203.

59. Wheat LJ, Connolly-Stringfield PA, Baker RL, et al. Disseminated histoplasmosis in the acquired immune deficiency syndrome: clinical findings, diagnosis and treatment, and review of the literature. *Medicine (Baltimore)* 1990;69(6):361–374.

60. Wheat J, Hafner R, Wulfsohn M, et al. Prevention of relapse of histoplasmosis with itraconazole in patients with the acquired immunodeficiency syndrome. The National Institute of Allergy and Infectious Diseases Clinical Trials and Mycoses Study Group Collaborators. *Ann Intern Med* 1993;118(8):610–616.

61. Fish DG, Ampel NM, Galgiani JN, et al. Coccidioidomycosis during human immunodeficiency virus infection. A review of 77 patients. *Medicine (Baltimore)* 1990;69(6):384–391.

62. Simberkoff MS, El Sadr W, Schiffman G, et al. Streptococcus pneumoniae infections and bacteremia in patients with acquired immune deficiency syndrome, with report of a pneumococcal vaccine failure. *Am Rev Respir Dis* 1984;130(6):1174–1176.

DISEASES OF THE PLEURA, MEDIASTINUM, CHEST WALL, AND DIAPHRAGM

RICHARD W. LIGHT

DISEASES OF THE PLEURA
Anatomy of the Pleural Space
Physiology of the Pleural Space
Pleural Effusions
Transudative Pleural Effusions
Exudative Pleural Effusions
Chylothorax and Pseudochylothorax
Hemothorax
Pleural Diseases Not Associated with Effusion
Pneumothorax

DISEASES OF THE MEDIASTINUM
Mediastinal Masses
Mediastinitis
Mediastinal Emphysema

DISEASES OF THE CHEST WALL
Kyphoscoliosis
Ankylosing Spondylitis
Pectus Excavatum (Funnel Chest) and Pectus Carinatum
   (Pigeon Breast)
Fractures of Single Ribs
Fractures of Multiple Ribs

DISEASES OF THE DIAPHRAGM
Unilateral Paralysis of the Diaphragm
Bilateral Paralysis or Paresis of the Diaphragm
Eventration
Hiccup

DISEASES OF THE PLEURA

The pleural space is not really a space but rather a potential space between the lung and chest wall. It is a crucial feature of the breathing apparatus, since it serves as a coupling system between the lung and chest wall. There is normally a very thin layer of fluid (from 2 to 10 μm thick) between the two pleural surfaces. The pleural space and the fluid within it are not under static conditions. During each respiratory cycle the pleural pressures and the geometry of the pleural space fluctuate widely. Fluid constantly enters and leaves the pleural space. In this section are discussed the anatomy and physiology of the pleural space, as well as the etiology, diagnosis, and treatment of various diseases that affect it.

Anatomy of the Pleural Space

The serous membrane covering the lung parenchyma is called the *visceral pleura*. The remainder of the lining of the pleural cavity is designated the *parietal pleura*. The parietal pleura includes the diaphragmatic pleura, the mediastinal pleura, and the costal pleura, which cover the diaphragm, mediastinum, and thoracic skeleton, respectively. The vis-

ceral pleura and the parietal pleura meet at the lung root at the hilum.

The parietal pleura receives its blood supply from the systemic capillaries. The visceral pleura is supplied predominantly by branches of the bronchial artery in humans and in large animals with thick visceral pleura such as sheep or horses (1). The lymphatic vessels in the parietal pleura are in direct communication with the pleural space by means of stomata (2). These stomata are the only route through which cells and large particles can leave the pleural space and are the primary route through which liquid exits the pleural space. Although there are abundant lymphatics in the visceral pleura, these lymphatics do not appear to participate in the removal of particulate matter from the pleural space.

Physiology of the Pleural Space

Fluid can enter the pleural space from the capillaries in the parietal or visceral pleura or from the interstitial spaces or lymphatics in either pleural surface. The passage of protein-free liquid across the pleural membranes is dependent on

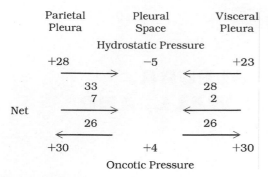

FIGURE 17.1. Diagrammatic representation of the pressures involved in the formation and absorption of pleural fluid.

the hydrostatic and oncotic pressures across them (Fig. 17.1). When the capillaries in the parietal pleura are considered, the net hydrostatic pressure favoring the movement of fluid from these capillaries to the pleural space is the systemic capillary pressure (28 cm H_2O) minus the negative pleural pressure (5 cm H_2O), or 33 cm H_2O. Opposing this is the oncotic pressure in the blood (30 cm H_2O) minus the oncotic pressure in the pleural fluid (4 cm H_2O), or 26 cm H_2O. The resulting net pressure difference of 7 cm H_2O (33 − 26) favors movement of fluid from the parietal pleura into the pleural space.

The only difference between the visceral and the parietal pleura in the scheme outlined in Figure 17.1 is that the capillaries of the visceral pleura have a slightly lower hydrostatic pressure because they drain into the low-pressure pulmonary veins. The net force across the visceral pleura is 2 cm H_2O, again favoring the formation of pleural fluid.

In recent years it has become apparent that the origin of much pleural fluid is the interstitial spaces of the lung. The pleural membranes are leaky to both liquid and protein (3). The pleural pressure is lower than the interstitial pressure, and this pressure difference produces a gradient for fluid to move from the interstitium to the pleural space (4). When the acute respiratory distress syndrome is induced in sheep with the intravenous injection of oleic acid, 20% of the edema fluid exits the lung via the pleural space (5). When high-pressure pulmonary edema is induced in sheep with fluid overload, again about 20% of the edema fluid is cleared via the pleural space (6). Patients with heart failure are much more likely to have pleural effusions if there is radiologic evidence of pulmonary edema (7).

The rate of pleural fluid formation in each pleural space in normal animals with a thick visceral pleura is approximately 0.01 mL per kg per hour or 15 mL per 24 hours for a 60 kg individual. There is a small amount of protein in this fluid. Normally, the pleural space is maintained nearly fluid-free because the filtered fluid is removed from the pleural space by the pleural lymphatics, which can remove over 0.20 mL per kg per hour from each pleural space (8). Pleural fluid will accumulate, producing a pleural effu-

sion when the rate of pleural fluid formation exceeds the capacity of the lymphatics in the parietal pleura to remove the fluid. Pleural effusions can also develop when chyle escapes from the thoracic duct (chylothorax), when blood vessels are disrupted (hemothorax), or when there is free fluid in the peritoneal cavity if there are holes in the diaphragm.

Pleural Effusions

Pathophysiology

Pleural fluid will accumulate when the rate of pleural fluid formation is greater than the rate of pleural fluid removal by the lymphatics. Pleural fluid will continue to accumulate until another equilibrium is reached. Pleural effusions have classically been divided into transudative and exudative pleural effusions. A transudative pleural effusion occurs when alterations in the systemic factors that influence pleural fluid movement result in a pleural effusion. Examples are increased pulmonary interstitial fluid and elevated visceral pleural capillary pressure with left heart failure, elevated parietal pleural capillary pressure with right heart failure, and decreased serum oncotic pressure with the nephrotic syndrome. In contrast, exudative pleural effusions occur when local factors are altered in such a way that pleural fluid accumulates. Inflammation of the lung or the pleura leading to increased flux of fluid from the capillaries of the lung or the pleura into the pleural space is the most common cause of exudative pleural effusions. However, exudative effusions can also occur with decreased lymphatic flow or with a more negative pleural pressure, as with atelectasis.

Clinical Manifestations

The symptoms of a patient with a pleural effusion are to a large extent dictated by the underlying process causing the effusion. Many patients have no symptoms referable to the effusion. When symptoms are related to the effusion, they arise either from inflammation of the pleura or from compromise of pulmonary mechanics. Pleuritic chest pain is the usual symptom of pleural inflammation. Since there are pain fibers only in the parietal pleura, pleuritic chest pain indicates inflammation of the parietal pleura. Some patients with pleural effusion experience dull, aching chest pain. This symptom is particularly common if the underlying process directly involves the parietal pleura, as with metastatic tumor or lung abscess. Irritation of the pleural surfaces may also result in a dry, nonproductive cough.

Physical examination of a patient with pleural effusion reveals decreased expansion, decreased or absent tactile fremitus, dullness to percussion, and diminished breath sounds over the site of the effusion. Bronchial breath sounds and egophony are frequently present immediately above the effusion.

A pleural effusion acts as a space-occupying process in the thoracic cavity and therefore reduces all subdivisions of lung volumes. However, the increase in lung volumes after a therapeutic thoracentesis is much less than the volume of fluid removed (9). With larger effusions, dyspnea results from lung compression. Even though an entire lung may be compressed when the pleural effusion occupies a complete hemithorax, blood gases usually remain nearly normal owing to a reflex reduction in perfusion to the unventilated lung.

Radiographic Appearance

Since pleural fluid is more dense than the lung, the fluid tends to go to the lowermost parts of the thoracic cavity as the lung floats in the fluid. In contrast, with pneumothorax the air is lighter than the lung, so it tends to rise to the uppermost part of the thoracic cavity. The other factor governing the radiologic appearance of a pleural effusion is the inherent tendency of the lung to maintain its usual shape at all stages of collapse.

The first fluid accumulates in the lowest portion of the thoracic cavity, which is the posterior costophrenic angle. Therefore, the earliest radiologic sign of a pleural effusion is blunting of the posterior costophrenic angle on the lateral chest radiograph. After several hundred milliliters of fluid accumulate, the fluid spills out into the costophrenic sinuses laterally and anteriorly. At this time the lateral costophrenic angle on the posteroanterior radiograph is obliterated. Blunting of the posterior and lateral costophrenic angles also occurs as a result of previous inflammation or chronic obstructive pulmonary disease (COPD). Pleural fluid can be differentiated from these entities by obtaining lateral decubitus radiographs. If a posteroanterior radiograph is obtained with the patient lying on the affected side, free pleural fluid will gravitate inferiorly and a pleural fluid line (see Fig. 7.2 in Chapter 7, Invasive Diagnostic Procedures) will be visible. If the film is obtained with the patient lying on the contralateral side, the angle will clear if the blunting is caused by fluid. Alternatively, if the blunting is not due to fluid, neither a pleural fluid line nor clearing of the blunted angle will be observed.

Pleural fluid is said to be *loculated* when it does not shift freely in the pleural space as the patient's position is changed. Loculated pleural effusions occur when there are adhesions between the visceral and parietal pleurae. Such adhesions result from marked inflammation of the pleura. It follows that loculated pleural effusions are more common with empyema or hemothorax. At times the differentiation of loculated pleural fluid from pleural thickening or parenchymal disease is quite difficult. Both ultrasound and computed tomography have proved useful in making this differentiation (10).

Approach to the Patient with Pleural Effusion

There are many different diseases that can be associated with pleural effusion (Table 17.1). When a pleural effusion is discovered, two questions need to be answered: (a) Is the effusion a transudate (i.e., is it due to systemic factors) or

TABLE 17.1. DIFFERENTIAL DIAGNOSIS OF PLEURAL EFFUSION

Transudative pleural effusions
  Congestive heart failure
  Cirrhosis
  Pulmonary embolism
  Pericardial disease
  Nephrotic syndrome
  Myxedema
  Peritoneal dialysis
Exudative pleural effusions
Infectious diseases
  Bacterial infections
  Tuberculosis
  Fungal infections
  Viral infections
  Parasitic infections
Neoplastic diseases
  Metastatic disease
  Mesotheliomas
Collagen vascular diseases
  Systemic lupus erythematosus
  Rheumatoid pleuritis
Pulmonary embolism
Gastrointestinal diseases
  Acute pancreatitis
  Pancreatic pseudocyst
  Esophageal perforations
  Intraabdominal abscess
Iatrogenic pleural effusion
  Post–coronary artery bypass surgery
  Post–abdominal surgery
  Post–lung transplant
  Post–liver transplant
  Post–endoscopic esophageal sclerotherapy
Drug hypersensitivity
  Nitrofurantoin
  Methysergide
  Dantrolene
  Bromocriptine
  Procarbacine
  Amiodarone
Miscellaneous diseases
  Pulmonary embolism
  Asbestos exposure
  Meigs' syndrome
  Uremia
  Post–cardiac injury syndrome
  Trapped lung
  Yellow nail syndrome
  Sarcoidosis
  Urinary tract obstruction
Hemothorax
Chylothorax
  Traumatic
  Nontraumatic
  Pulmonary and lymph node myomatosis

is it an exudate (i.e., is it due to disease of the pleura itself)? (b) If the effusion is an exudate, what is the disease responsible for its production? Answers to these two questions can be obtained only by examining the pleural fluid.

Nearly every patient with a pleural effusion should have a diagnostic thoracentesis. No difficulty should be encountered in obtaining fluid if the pleural fluid is more than 10 mm in thickness on the lateral decubitus roentgenogram. The performance of the diagnostic thoracentesis, the separation of transudates from exudates, and the utility of various diagnostic tests on the pleural fluid are discussed in Chapter 7, Invasive Diagnostic Procedures.

Transudative Pleural Effusions

Congestive Heart Failure

Congestive heart failure is probably responsible for more pleural effusions than any other disease entity. The accumulation of pleural fluid can be secondary to increases in the hydrostatic pressures in either the systemic or the pulmonary circulation. Clinically, however, pleural effusion due to congestive heart failure usually occurs only when the pulmonary wedge pressure is elevated (7). It is thought that the origin of the increased pleural fluid is the interstitial spaces of the lung. The pleural effusion is usually bilateral, but if it is unilateral it is more commonly on the right (11). A large unilateral effusion is uncommon in uncomplicated congestive heart failure and suggests malignancy, pulmonary emboli, or other complicating disease.

The diagnosis is usually suggested by the clinical picture of congestive heart failure. With appropriate treatment of the heart failure, the effusion will resolve rapidly in most cases. When the patient is first evaluated, a thoracentesis is indicated if the effusions are not bilateral and comparable in size, if the patient has pleuritic chest pain, or if the patient is febrile. If the pleural effusion persists after treatment, a diagnostic thoracentesis should be performed. In congestive heart failure, the pleural fluid is a transudate, and its characteristics change very little with diuresis (12).

Cirrhosis

The incidence of pleural effusion with cirrhosis varies from 0.5% to 10%. The predominant mechanism leading to a pleural effusion in a patient with cirrhosis and ascites appears to be the movement of the ascitic fluid from the peritoneal cavity through a diaphragmatic defect into the pleural space (13). The decreased plasma oncotic pressure is only a secondary factor.

The clinical picture is of cirrhosis and ascites, although at times the ascites may be minimal. The effusions are most common on the right side but may be bilateral or left-sided. At times the effusions may be very large, occupying almost an entire hemithorax. These large effusions may induce re-

spiratory symptoms. Therapeutic thoracentesis is of virtually no use, since the fluid reaccumulates very rapidly and the thoracentesis further depletes the patient's protein stores.

The initial management of the pleural effusion associated with cirrhosis and ascites should be directed toward treatment of the ascites with a low-salt diet and diuretics. If the ascites cannot be controlled with conservative measures, more aggressive measures are indicated. The optimal treatment is liver transplantation, but the implantation of a transjugular intrahepatic portal systemic shunt (TIPS) usually controls the ascites and the effusion (14). If neither TIPS nor liver transplantation is feasible, the best alternative is probably videothoracoscopy with closure of the diaphragmatic defects and pleurodesis (15).

Other Causes of Transudative Pleural Effusions

Pericardial Disease

The incidence of pleural effusion in patients with pericardial disease is about 30% (16). Most of the effusions are left-sided or bilateral and are small to moderate in size. The pleural effusion is usually transudative and results from either elevated capillary pressures or pericardial inflammation.

Nephrotic Syndrome

Patients with the nephrotic syndrome commonly have an associated pleural effusion. The mechanism responsible for the effusion is probably decreased plasma oncotic pressure secondary to the hypoproteinemia in combination with the increased hydrostatic pressure due to salt retention producing hypervolemia (17). The fluid is a typical transudate. Treatment is aimed at the nephrotic syndrome in an attempt to increase the serum proteins.

Myxedema

A pleural effusion sometimes occurs as a complication of myxedema. Most patients with myxedema and pleural effusion have a concomitant pericardial effusion, in which case the pleural effusion is a transudate. The rare isolated pleural effusion seen in conjunction with myxedema can be either a transudate or an exudate (18).

Peritoneal Dialysis

Approximately 1% to 2% of patients on continuous ambulatory peritoneal dialysis will develop a pleural effusion. The mechanism is probably the same as that with cirrhosis and ascites. The peritoneal dialysis increases the intraabdominal pressure, and the dialysate flows from the peritoneal cavity into the pleural cavity through pores in the diaphragm. The pleural fluid in such instances is similar to the dialysate. The treatment of choice is thoracoscopy with closure of the diaphragmatic defects, followed by pleurodesis (19).

Exudative Pleural Effusions

Parapneumonic Effusion

Any pleural effusion associated with bacterial pneumonia, lung abscess, or bronchiectasis is a parapneumonic effusion. Parapneumonic effusions are common, since more than one million cases of pneumonia occur annually in the United States and 40% of these have an associated parapneumonic effusion (20). The amount of fluid varies from a few milliliters, in which case the fluid is usually not detected, to several liters. The character of the fluid varies from a clear, straw-colored fluid with a few hundred white blood cells per cubic millimeter to frank pus. Parapneumonic effusions that require tube thoracostomy or which are culture-positive are designated *complicated parapneumonic effusions.*

Natural History of Parapneumonic Effusions

The evolution of a parapneumonic effusion can be divided into three stages (18). The first stage is the *exudative* stage, in which a focus of parenchymal infection leads to increased pulmonary interstitial fluid which traverses the visceral pleura and results in the accumulation of pleural fluid. In this stage the pleural fluid is characterized by a relatively low lactate dehydrogenase (LDH) level and a normal glucose and pH.

The second stage is the *fibropurulent* stage, which is characterized by the invasion of the pleural fluid by bacteria. As this stage progresses, the pleural fluid becomes increasingly cloudy and viscous since it contains large amounts of fibrin, cellular debris, and white blood cells. In this stage, there is a progressive tendency toward loculation of the fluid and the formation of limiting membranes. Although the loculation prevents extension of the pleural infection, it makes drainage of the pleural space difficult.

The third stage is the *organization* stage, in which fibroblasts grow into the exudate from both the visceral and parietal pleural surfaces to produce an inelastic membrane called the *pleural peel.* This peel encases the lung and renders it virtually functionless. At this stage the exudate is very thick, and if the patient has remained untreated the fluid may drain spontaneously through the chest wall *(empyema necessitatis)* or into the lung, in which case a bronchopleural fistula will be produced.

Initial Management of Patients with Parapneumonic Effusion

When a patient with acute bacterial pneumonia is initially evaluated, the physician should determine whether or not a parapneumonic effusion is present. If the posterior costophrenic angles are not blunted on the lateral chest radiograph, one can assume that there is not a clinically significant pleural effusion unless the chest radiograph reveals loculated fluid elsewhere in the chest. If the posterior costophrenic angles are blunted or if the diaphragm is obscured by the infiltrate, then a lateral decubitus chest roentgeno-gram should be obtained with the suspicious side down. The amount of pleural fluid can be semiquantitated on the decubitus film by measuring the distance between the inside of the chest wall and the bottom of the lung. If this measurement is less than 10 mm, it can be assumed that the effusion is not clinically significant and thoracentesis is not indicated (20).

If the thickness of the fluid is greater than 10 mm on the decubitus x-ray film, a therapeutic thoracentesis should be performed with removal of all the pleural fluid. If the fluid is removed completely with the therapeutic thoracentesis and does not reaccumulate, no additional therapy need be directed toward the effusion. At the time of the initial therapeutic thoracentesis, the pleural fluid should be Gram-stained and cultured and analyzed for leukocyte count, LDH, glucose, and pH levels. Indicators of a poor prognosis in order of increasing seriousness are the presence of pus, a glucose level less than 40 mg per dL, a pH less than 7.00, and an LDH level more than three times the upper limit of normal (21).

If the therapeutic thoracentesis removes all the pleural fluid and the fluid recurs, the next step is guided by the initial pleural fluid findings. If none of the poor prognostic indicators listed above are present, no invasive procedures are indicated if the patient is doing well clinically. If any of the poor prognostic indicators were present at the initial thoracentesis, a second therapeutic thoracentesis should be performed and the pleural fluid reanalyzed. If the pleural fluid accumulates a third time, a small (8 to 13 French) chest tube should be inserted into the pleural space unless none of the poor prognostic factors were present at the time of the second thoracentesis (21).

The presence of a pleural effusion does not affect the choice or the dosage of antibiotics since the antibiotic levels in the pleural fluid are comparable with those in the serum (22).

Loculated Pleural Fluid

If the pleural fluid cannot be removed completely with a therapeutic thoracentesis or with a small chest tube, it is probably loculated. The loculation indicates a high level of inflammation in the pleural space. The majority of loculated pleural effusions require drainage. If the pleural fluid is loculated and if any of the poor prognostic factors listed above are present, efforts should be made to break down the loculations in order to obtain complete drainage of the pleural space.

The two primary means by which the loculations can be broken down are with thrombolytics or with thoracoscopy. There have been two recent randomized controlled studies which showed that thrombolytics were superior to tube thoracostomy alone in breaking down adhesions (23,24). One study (23) used streptokinase 250,000 U, while the other study (24) used 100,000 U urokinase. Since the availability of urokinase is limited at the present time, streptokinase is presently the preferred thrombolytic.

The alternative approach to the patient with loculated pleural effusions is thoracoscopy with the breakdown of adhesions. One study (25) concluded that proceeding directly to thoracoscopy was more cost effective than using an intermediate step with thrombolytics. One advantage of thoracoscopy is that the chest tube can be positioned in the most dependent part of the empyema cavity. Before thoracoscopy is performed, a CT scan should be obtained. This examination will provide information about the size and extent of the empyema cavity that will guide the planned procedure. A thickened visceral pleural peel without septations suggests that the empyema may be chronic and probably will not be amenable to thoracoscopic debridement alone (26).

When faced with a patient with a loculated parapneumonic effusion, should thrombolytics be administered intrapleurally or should thoracoscopy be performed? It is recommended that patients with loculated parapneumonic effusions and poor prognostic indicators in the pleural fluid be treated initially with thoracoscopy if the expertise for this procedure is available locally. If the expertise is not available locally, then a trial of thrombolytics is warranted. If there is not substantial improvement with the thrombolytics within a few days, one should proceed to more invasive procedures.

Thoracotomy with Decortication

This is the most invasive procedure for the treatment of parapneumonic effusions and empyema. With decortication, all the fibrous tissue is removed from the visceral pleura and all pus is evacuated from the pleural space. The primary indication for decortication is a trapped lung; loculations are better treated with thoracoscopy. This procedure allows the underlying lung to reexpand and obliterate the pleural space. Some thoracic surgeons recommend decortication in all cases in which a thick pleural peel remains after either closed or open drainage of a pleural infection. However, since the pleural peel frequently improves substantially in the months after the drainage, it is recommended that decortication be delayed for at least six months if the infection has been controlled and the lung reexpanded. After this time, decortication should be performed only if the patient has limited exercise capacity and if close evaluation of the patient's pulmonary status suggests that the procedure will improve pulmonary function.

Tuberculous Pleural Effusions

In many parts of the world, the most common cause of an exudative pleural effusion is tuberculosis. However, in the United States the annual incidence of tuberculous pleural effusion is only about 1,000 cases. Of all the patients with tuberculosis, approximately one in every 30 cases is a case

of tuberculous pleuritis (27). In some countries, however, the percentage of patients with tuberculosis who have a pleural effusion exceeds 30% (28).

Pathogenesis

The exudative pleural effusion associated with pleural tuberculosis appears to be predominantly a manifestation of delayed hypersensitivity to tuberculous protein. Frequently it is difficult to demonstrate the tubercle bacillus in either the pleural fluid or the pleural tissue. It is probable that granulomatous pleuritis results any time a patient with a positive tuberculin purified protein derivative (PPD) skin test gets tubercle bacillus protein into their pleural space. It should be emphasized that many patients with tuberculous pleuritis have a negative PPD test when first seen. The possible explanations for the negative PPD test in these individuals are that there are circulating adherent cells that suppress the delayed hypersensitivity reaction to the PPD in the skin or that the specifically sensitized lymphocytes are sequestered in the pleural space (29).

Clinical Manifestations

A pleural effusion as a manifestation of tuberculosis has been likened to a primary chancre as a manifestation of syphilis. Both are self-limited and of little immediate concern, but both may lead to serious disease at a later date. Most cases of isolated tuberculous effusion will resolve spontaneously without treatment, but active tuberculosis will subsequently develop in a large percentage of patients. Patiala (30) followed 2,816 members of the Finnish armed forces who developed pleural effusion during World War II before antituberculous drugs were available. Over 40% of these individuals developed active tuberculosis during the seven-year follow-up period. Accordingly, when managing a patient with a pleural effusion, it is the physician's obligation either to treat the patient for tuberculous pleuritis or to exclude this diagnosis.

At the onset of tuberculous pleuritis, most patients have symptoms of an upper respiratory tract infection, and many also have pleuritic chest pain. Most but not all patients also have a temperature elevation not uncommonly in the 103° to 105°F range. Subsequently the patient develops a chronic illness characterized by anorexia, weight loss, and a low-grade fever. Without treatment most patients will recover completely, only to develop active tuberculosis at another site later. Most patients with tuberculous pleuritis do not have radiologically evident parenchymal infiltrates. In those without parenchymal infiltrates, the effusion is almost always unilateral.

Diagnosis

The diagnosis of tuberculous pleuritis should be considered in every patient with an exudative pleural effusion. The diagnosis of tuberculous pleuritis depends on the demonstration of a positive marker for tuberculosis in the pleural fluid, tubercle bacilli in the sputum, pleural fluid, or pleura, or of granulomas in the pleura. As mentioned earlier, a negative PPD test when the patient is first seen certainly does not rule out the diagnosis. Although the sputum is usually negative for tubercle bacilli unless there are parenchymal infiltrates, it should be analyzed for the tubercle bacillus.

Pleural fluid analysis in tuberculous pleuritis is useful. The fluid is invariably an exudate. Frequently the pleural fluid protein is over 5.0 g per 100 mL, and this finding is very suggestive of tuberculous pleuritis. In most cases, the differential white cell count reveals more than 80% lymphocytes, but if symptoms have been present less than one week, neutrophils at times predominate. A pleural effusion that contains more than 10% eosinophils at the time of the initial thoracentesis is seldom, if ever, tuberculous. The pleural fluid glucose level may be reduced with tuberculous pleuritis, but the majority of patients have a pleural fluid glucose level above 60 mg per dL (18). Cultures of the pleural fluid for tubercle bacilli are positive in less than 20% of cases (31).

As discussed in detail in Chapter 7, Invasive Diagnostic Procedures, in the last few years three tests on pleural fluid have been developed which can establish the diagnosis of tuberculous pleuritis, namely, adenosine deaminase (ADA), gamma interferon, and polymerase chain reaction (PCR) for tuberculous DNA. A pleural fluid ADA level which exceeds 47U per L is seen in virtually all patients with tuberculous pleuritis unless they are immunologically compromised (32). The other two diseases which are associated with an elevated pleural fluid ADA are rheumatoid pleuritis and empyema, and these should be easy to differentiate from tuberculous pleuritis clinically (31). The primary problem with using the level of ADA in the pleural fluid to establish the diagnosis of tuberculous pleuritis is that presently there is no commercial laboratory in the United States which measures the ADA levels reliably (31). The level of gamma interferon is higher in patients with tuberculous pleuritis than it is in pleural fluids due to other etiologies. In one recent study, a pleural fluid gamma interferon level of 3.7 U per mL had a sensitivity of 0.99 and a specificity of 0.98 in a series of 388 pleural effusions (33). Accurate gamma interferon levels are available in the United States. Pleural fluid PCR analysis holds promise for the diagnosis of tuberculous pleuritis, but gamma interferon is just as good and is less expensive and less difficult technically (34). In patients with lymphocytic pleural effusions, an elevated level of one of the pleural fluid TB markers is sufficient for the diagnosis of tuberculous pleuritis.

For the past 50 years, pleural biopsy has been the most common way to establish the diagnosis of tuberculous pleuritis. However, the pleural fluid tests for tuberculosis markers, as discussed above, are at least as sensitive as the needle biopsy of the pleura. Hence, needle biopsy of the pleura is being used less and less frequently to establish the diagnosis of tuberculous pleuritis (31).

Treatment

Patients with tuberculous pleuritis should be treated with the same antituberculous treatment regimens as are patients with pulmonary tuberculosis, as discussed in Chapter 15, Respiratory Tract Infections. With treatment, patients generally become afebrile within about two weeks, and the pleural effusion resolves within six weeks. Repeated pleural fluid aspiration has not been shown to be beneficial in preventing chronic pleural thickening. The administration of corticosteroids will rapidly relieve the patient's symptoms of pleuritic chest pain, malaise, and fever and does not lead to dissemination of the tuberculosis. Markedly symptomatic patients should be started on prednisone 40 mg per day and then gradually tapered over several weeks.

Actinomycosis

Over 50% of patients with thoracic actinomycosis have pleural involvement. The characteristic chest radiographic finding is a localized lung lesion extending to the chest wall, with pleural thickening or effusion. The presence of chest wall abscesses or draining sinus tracts suggests the diagnosis, as do bone changes consisting of periosteal proliferation or bone destruction. The definitive diagnosis is established with the demonstration of *Actinomyces israelii* by anaerobic cultures. The appropriate treatment is high doses of penicillin or another suitable antimicrobial agent for prolonged periods.

Nocardiosis

Pleural effusions develop in nearly 50% of patients with pulmonary nocardiosis. When pleural involvement does occur, grossly purulent pleural fluid and draining sinuses are common. The diagnosis is established by demonstrating the organism on aerobic culture. Since the organism is slow-growing, cultures should be maintained for four weeks to exclude the diagnosis. Frequently with pleural nocardiosis, tuberculosis is wrongly diagnosed because the organisms are acid-fast. The drug treatment of choice is the combination of trimethoprim and sulfamethoxazole (Bactrim), two tablets twice a day for at least two months.

Fungal Diseases of the Pleura

Aspergillosis

Pleural aspergillosis usually occurs in one of two settings. Pleural aspergillosis may complicate lobectomy or pneumonectomy, in which situation a bronchopleural fistula is almost always present. Once the diagnosis is established, a chest tube should be inserted, and the pleural space should be irrigated daily with amphotericin B 25 mg or nystatin

75,000 units. The diagnosis of pleural aspergillosis should also be suspected in any patient with a history of artificial pneumothorax therapy for tuberculosis who has signs and symptoms of a chronic infection. The diagnosis is established by demonstrating the organisms on stains or cultures of the pleural fluid. The optimal treatment for pleural aspergillosis in this situation is surgical removal of the involved pleura and resection of the involved lobe or the entire ipsilateral lung if necessary (35).

Blastomycosis

Approximately 10% of patients with blastomycosis will have a pleural effusion. The clinical picture with pleural blastomycosis is identical to that with pleural tuberculosis. The diagnosis is established by demonstrating the organism in the pleural fluid or histologic sections. The treatment of choice is an azole, such as iatraconazole, or amphotericin B if the patient is immunosuppressed or has CNS blastomycosis.

Coccidioidomycosis

Pleural effusions of two types occur in association with coccidioidomycosis. The incidence of pleural effusion with symptomatic primary coccidioidomycosis is about 7%, and 50% of the patients with pleural effusion will also have a coexisting parenchymal infiltrate. Most patients are febrile and have pleuritic chest pain, and nearly 50% have either erythema nodosum or erythema multiforme. The pleural effusion is a lymphocyte-predominant exudate. Pleural fluid cultures are positive in about 20%, while cultures of pleural biopsy specimens are almost always positive. Most patients with primary coccidioidal pleural effusion require no systemic antifungal therapy. Only patients who are immunosuppressed or who have a negative skin test or other evidence of dissemination need be treated with antifungal therapy (36).

Hydropneumothoraces develop in 1% to 5% of patients with chronic cavitary coccidioidomycosis. These patients should undergo tube thoracostomy immediately to drain the air and fluid from the pleural space. Most patients will require a thoracotomy with a partial or total lobectomy, and most will require some degree of decortication. The administration of antifungal drugs does not appear to be required (37).

Cryptococcosis

Pleural involvement with cryptococcosis appears to result from extension of a primary subpleural cryptococcal nodule into the pleural space. The majority of patients who have a cryptococcal pleural effusion are immunosuppressed and many have AIDS (38). The pleural fluid is usually a lymphocyte-predominant exudate. Immunosuppressed patients should be treated with a combination of amphotericin B (0.4 mg per kg) and 5-flucytosine (100 mg per kg) daily for six weeks, as should patients with cryptococcal antigen

in either their blood or their cerebrospinal fluid. If none of these criteria are met, then the patient probably does not need to be treated. However, if the effusion increases in size, if the LDH levels in the effusion tend to increase, or if antigens appear in the blood or cerebrospinal fluid, treatment should be initiated (18).

Histoplasmosis

On rare occasions patients with histoplasmosis will have a lymphocyte-predominant exudative pleural effusion. The pleural biopsy will reveal noncaseating granulomas. No systemic treatment is necessary unless the patient is immunosuppressed or the effusion persists for more than four weeks.

Viral Diseases of the Pleura

Viral infections are probably responsible for a sizable percentage of undiagnosed exudative pleural effusions. However, the diagnosis is rarely established because it depends on isolation of the virus or the demonstration of a significant increase in the antibodies to the virus. The incidence of pleural effusion with primary atypical pneumonia is as high as 20% (39).

Parasitic Diseases of the Pleura

Amebiasis

Pleural involvement with the parasite *Entamoeba histolytica* is almost invariably secondary to a liver abscess. Most patients present with fever and right upper-quadrant tenderness. Right-sided pleuritic chest pain is common and it is frequently referred to the right shoulder as a manifestation of diaphragmatic irritation. Thoracentesis can yield either "chocolate-sauce" fluid or a serous exudate that develops in response to the diaphragmatic irritation. The expectoration of "chocolate-sauce" sputum is nearly pathognomonic and indicates that a bronchohepatic fistula has developed. The discovery of "chocolate sauce" in either the sputum or the pleural space serves as an indication for therapy with metronidazole, 750 mg three times a day for five to 10 days (40). Tube thoracostomy should be performed if "chocolate sauce" is found on thoracentesis.

Paragonimiasis

This diagnosis should be suspected in patients with undiagnosed pleural effusion who have recently been in the Orient, since the oriental lung fluke, *Paragonimus westermani*, at times produces pleural disease. Patients with pleural paragonimiasis present with a chronic illness. The pleural fluid in patients with pleural paragonimiasis is quite characteristic in that it is an exudate with a glucose level less than 10 mg per dL, an LDH level above 1,000 IU per L, a pH below 7.10, and a differential revealing a high percentage of eosinophils (41). The pleural fluid findings are virtually pathognomonic, but the diagnosis is established by demonstrating the typical operculated eggs in the sputum, pleural fluid, or stool. The treatment of choice is praziquantel, 25 mg per kg body weight three times a day for three days (40). At times thoracotomy with decortication is necessary for resolution of the process.

Echinococcosis

Pleural disease from *Echinococcus granulosus* usually results from rupture of either a pulmonary or a hepatic hydatid cyst into the pleural space. When the cyst ruptures the patient experiences the abrupt onset of chest pain, fever, and systemic toxicity. Diagnosis is dependent on the demonstration of hooklets from scolices in the sputum or pleural fluid. The treatment of choice is surgical excision of the cyst combined with tube drainage of the pleural space. After surgery, patients should be treated with albendazole 400 mg twice a day for several weeks (42).

Pleural Effusions Secondary to Neoplasms

Pathogenesis

Neoplasms are responsible for a high percentage of pleural effusions. Along with congestive heart failure, they account for the majority of pleural effusions in patients over the age of 50 years. Pleural effusions associated with neoplasms arise through at least five different mechanisms:

1. The pleural surfaces may be involved by the tumor, which leads to increased permeability of the pleural membranes, possibly due to vascular endothelial growth factor (VEGF) (43).
2. The neoplasm may obstruct the lymphatics or veins draining the pleural space, leading to the accumulation of pleural fluid.
3. An endobronchial tumor may completely obstruct a bronchus, leading to atelectasis and decreasing the pleural pressure.
4. A pneumonitis distal to a partially obstructed bronchus may lead to a parapneumonic effusion.
5. The neoplasm may disrupt the thoracic duct, leading to a chylothorax.

Pleural effusions in patients with known malignancy may not be related to the malignancy itself; these patients may also develop heart failure, pulmonary emboli, pneumonia, hypoproteinemia, pericardial disease, or tuberculosis, any of which may be responsible for the effusion. It should be noted that not all patients with metastases to the pleura develop pleural effusions. Meyer (44) reviewed 52 cases of metastatic carcinoma to the pleura and found that only 14 of these patients had had recognized pleural effusions during their lifetime. He found that the development of an effusion is closely related to neoplastic infiltration of the mediastinal lymph nodes and that in all types of tumors the visceral pleura is involved much sooner and more extensively than is the parietal pleura. Pleural involvement with most bronchogenic tumors arises from pulmonary arterial emboli, while pleural involvement with nonbronchogenic tumors usually represents tertiary spread from established hepatic metastases.

Bronchogenic carcinomas in men and breast carcinomas in women are the leading types of tumors causing neoplastic effusions. The lymphomas and leukemias are the third leading type of malignancy with secondary effusions. However, many other tumors, predominantly carcinomas, are associated with metastases to the pleura and pleural effusions.

Diagnosis

The diagnosis of a malignant effusion should be considered in all patients with exudative pleural effusions. The diagnosis is established by demonstrating malignant cells by cytopathologic studies or by pleural biopsy. Although there is nothing absolutely characteristic about the pleural fluid secondary to malignancy, several generalizations can be made.

The pleural fluid is almost always an exudate. A grossly bloody pleural fluid is suggestive of malignancy, but nearly 50% of malignant effusions have pleural fluid RBC counts of less than 10,000. The pleural fluid WBC count is usually between 500 and 25,000 and the differential can be characterized by a predominance of polymorphonuclear leukocytes, small lymphocytes, or other mononuclear cells. The pleural fluid glucose level is usually similar to the corresponding serum level, but is occasionally less than 50 mg per dL. The pleural fluid amylase level is elevated in approximately 10% of malignant pleural effusions. In such cases the primary tumor is usually not in the pancreas and the amylase has a salivary rather than a pancreatic isoenzyme pattern. The pleural fluid pH may be normal or reduced. A low pleural fluid pH usually occurs in conjunction with a low pleural fluid glucose, and this combination indicates a poor prognosis because it is due to a large tumor burden in the pleural space. Pleural fluid carcinoembryonic antigen (CEA) levels are above 10 ng per mL in about one-third of patients with malignant pleural effusions, but since these are usually the effusions with the positive cytology, the routine use of this test or other tumor markers is not recommended (45).

The diagnosis of a malignant pleural effusion is most commonly established by cytologic examination of the pleural fluid. When specimens from three separate thoracenteses are submitted for cytologic examination, the diagnosis can be established in approximately 80% of individuals who have pleural metastases (46). Almost all adenocarcinomas will be diagnosed with cytology, but the yield is less with mesothelioma, squamous cell carcinoma, Hodgkin's disease, and sarcomas.

At times no diagnosis will be obtained despite at least two cytologies on the pleural fluid. How aggressive should one be in attempting to establish the diagnosis of malignancy in these patients? Only about 20% of such patients have pleural malignancy, and almost all who do have a pleural malignancy will have a clinical picture suggestive of malignancy (47). Accordingly, if the patient is symptomatic from the effusion and the symptoms are tending to increase, thoracoscopy or thoracotomy with pleural biopsy should be performed. If thoracoscopy is performed, a procedure such as pleural abrasion should be performed to effect a pleurodesis at the time of thoracoscopy (48).

In a patient with a known neoplasm and pleural effusion, the key questions are whether the pleural effusion is secondary to the malignancy and, if so, by what mechanism. Again, cytopathologic study and pleural biopsy can demonstrate direct involvement of the pleura. The chest x-ray is useful in delineating the responsible mechanisms. If the mediastinum is shifted toward the contralateral side, the pleural surfaces are probably involved. If the mediastinum is shifted toward the ipsilateral side and the bronchi are not outlined by air on the routine chest radiograph, total bronchial obstruction with resulting atelectasis and effusion is the probable explanation. A parapneumonic effusion is suggested by a high white cell count, predominantly neutrophils, in the pleural fluid. A mediastinal mass on the chest x-ray film suggests lymphatic obstruction or dysruption. Protein analysis of peripheral blood demonstrates hypoproteinemia. A globular cardiac shadow suggests pericardial involvement and pericardial effusion. Not uncommonly, more than one of these mechanisms are involved.

Treatment

The initial step in the management of a patient with a malignant pleural effusion is to attempt to identify the site of the primary tumor in order to decide whether to administer systemic chemotherapy. Patients who have primary tumors that are responsive to systemic chemotherapy, such as small-cell carcinoma of the lung, breast carcinoma, and lymphoma, should be given chemotherapy to treat the primary disease. Prior to chemotherapy it is best to drain the pleural effusion.

The proper therapy for a pleural effusion associated with malignancy depends on the mechanism responsible for it. If an endobronchial tumor is responsible for complete bronchial obstruction, the obstruction should be treated with a stent or laser therapy. If pneumonitis behind a partial obstruction is present, the patient should be treated with appropriate antibiotics and postural drainage in combination with therapy for the obstruction. If the pleural effusion is due to lymphatic blockage in the mediastinum, radiotherapy to the mediastinum may be effective in controlling the effusion, particularly with lymphomas.

When the effusion is due to pleural metastases, consideration should be given to obliterating the pleural space with a pleurodesis. Patients who are subjected to this procedure should meet the following two criteria. First, the patient should have the quality of his or her life diminished by dyspnea. Second, a therapeutic thoracentesis should cause

improvement in the patient's dyspnea. Many patients with malignant pleural effusions do not meet the above two criteria and therefore should not be subjected to pleurodesis.

If the above two conditions are met, a pleurodesis should be attempted. With chemical pleurodesis an irritant (e.g., doxycycline) is injected into the pleural space, which creates intense pleural inflammation and leads to fusion of the visceral and parietal pleura. Many different agents have been used as pleural sclerosants, but doxycycline 500 mg is the agent recommended by me at the present time. The only two agents approved for pleurodesis by the FDA are talc and bleomycin. Talc is not recommended because it causes a fatal acute respiratory distress syndrome (ARDS) in about 1% of patients and nonfatal ARDS in another 5% (49,50). Bleomycin is not recommended because it is less effective than doxycycline (51), is more expensive, and does not effect a pleurodesis in animals (52).

The following procedure is recommended for pleurodesis. A chest tube is inserted into the pleural space to drain the fluid. Before the sclerosant is injected, the patient should be given systemic medications such as lorazepam or midazolam to produce conscious sedation because the procedure can be very painful (53). As soon as the underlying lung has reexpanded, doxycycline 500 mg in 50 mL saline is injected through the chest tube into the pleural space. After the injection the chest tube is clamped for the next 60 to 90 minutes. There appears to be no need to place the patient into various positions after the injection (54). The chest tube is then unclamped and negative pressure is applied through the chest tube for 48 to 72 hours or until the drainage becomes less than 15 mL per hour. At this time the chest tube is removed. The intense inflammation induced by the sclerosant results in fusion of the visceral and parietal pleural surfaces when they are brought into close approximation by the negative pressure of the chest tubes. Pleurodesis performed in this manner is effective in obliterating the pleural space and controlling the pleural effusion about 75% of the time (51).

At the present time pleurodesis is usually attempted on inpatients. It would be preferable, however, to perform pleurodesis as an outpatient since the life expectancy of a patient with a malignant pleural effusion is only about 90 days and a mean hospitalization of five days is required for pleurodesis (55). The feasibility of outpatient therapy has been demonstrated by Patz and coworkers (56), who drained the effusions via gravity drainage into a collection bottle, and by Putnam and coworkers (55), who drained the effusions by connecting the indwelling catheter to suction bottles on a PRN basis. If outpatient therapy is selected, the sclerosant can be injected through the indwelling catheter after the volume of the drainage is less than 100 mL per day. If no sclerosant is injected, with the vacuum bottle system a spontaneous pleurodesis will occur in approximately 50% of patients at a median time of 25 days after the indwelling catheter is inserted (57).

An alternative to pleurodesis is the implantation of a pleuroperitoneal shunt (58). The shunt, which can be placed with local anesthesia, consists of two catheters connected by a pump chamber containing two one-way valves. Fluid flows from the pleural space to the pump chamber and then from the pump chamber to the peritoneal cavity. The patient pumps on the reservoir daily to move fluid from the pleural space to the peritoneal space.

Mesothelioma

Malignant mesothelioma is an uncommon disease that is highly malignant and has been shown to be associated with exposure to asbestos. It is thought that asbestos exposure is responsible for most mesotheliomas, but no history of significant asbestos exposure can be obtained in approximately one-third of patients with mesothelioma (59). Mesotheliomas are thought to arise from the cells that line the pleural cavity.

Once the tumor is present, it spreads rapidly along the pleural surfaces. Eventually, the entire visceral and parietal pleural surfaces become infiltrated by a continuous layer of tumor encasing the entire lung. Metastases to regional lymph nodes are common, but distant metastases are rare. Histologically, diffuse mesotheliomas frequently contain large amounts of fibrous tissue. The predominant cellular type may be either mesenchymal or epithelial, and the majority of these tumors have both cell types.

Most patients with malignant mesothelioma present with either chest pain or dyspnea. The chest pain is nonpleuritic, aching, and frequently referred to the upper abdomen or shoulder. When the patient initially presents, the chest film almost invariably reveals a unilateral pleural effusion. The prognosis of patients with mesothelioma is poor, with a median survival time of slightly more than 12 months after diagnosis (60), but it should be noted that this is significantly better than the survival with other malignant pleural effusions.

It is difficult definitely to establish the diagnosis of malignant mesothelioma. Although cytologic smears, needle biopsies, and sections from cell blocks of pleural fluid can establish the diagnosis of malignancy, they usually cannot distinguish between a metastatic adenocarcinoma and a mesothelioma. Thoracoscopy is probably the best procedure with which to establish the diagnosis of mesothelioma (61). At thoracostomy, a small portion of the specimen should be placed in glutaraldehyde for electron microscopy in any patient suspected of having mesothelioma (62). In addition, attempts should be made to create a pleurodesis using pleural abrasion or some other procedure at the time of thoracoscopy.

Three techniques are available that help establish the diagnosis of mesothelioma with greater certainty. Most adenocarcinomas are positive with the periodic acid-Schiff (PAS) stain after diastase digestion, while all mesotheliomas are negative. Electron microscopy is also useful in differentiating mesothelioma from metastatic adenocarcinoma in that mesotheliomas are characterized by long, lush microvilli. Lastly, when immunohistochemical studies are performed using CEA, B72.3 and Leu-M, the diagnosis of adenocarcinoma is established if two or more of the stains are positive while the diagnosis of mesothelioma is established if all three stains are negative (63).

There is no satisfactory treatment for malignant mesothelioma, and it is unclear whether any of the available treatments prolong life (64). If the patient appears to have resectable disease, surgery should probably be performed. Chemical pleurodesis should be attempted if the patient is dyspneic from a large pleural effusion, and sufficient analgesics, including opiates when necessary, should be given to alleviate the pain.

Localized Benign Pleural Mesothelioma

Benign fibrous mesotheliomas are localized pleural tumors with an excellent prognosis. Their occurrence does not appear to be related to previous asbestos exposure. These tumors appear radiologically as solitary, sharply defined, discrete masses located at the periphery of the lung or related to a fissure. The most frequent symptoms are cough, chest pain, and dyspnea, but approximately 50% of patients are asymptomatic. Hypertrophic pulmonary osteoarthropathy occurs in approximately 20% of patients with benign mesotheliomas, and in such instances the tumor is usually greater than 7 cm in diameter. The association of hypertrophic osteoarthropathy and a large pleural-based intrathoracic mass should strongly suggest the possibility of a localized pleural mesothelioma. Symptomatic hypoglycemia occurs in about 4% of patients with benign mesothelioma. The treatment is surgical excision and the prognosis is excellent (65).

Primary Effusion Lymphoma

Primary effusion lymphomas grow in body cavities and present as malignant lymphomatous effusions without an identifiable continuous tumor mass (66). These tumors usually occur in homosexual patients with AIDS and contain the Kaposi's sarcoma–associated herpes virus (KSHV or HHV8); the majority are also characterized by the presence of the Epstein-Barr virus. The primary effusion lymphoma has a distinctive morphology bridging large-cell immunoblastic lymphoma and anaplastic large-cell lymphoma. The pleural fluid is a lymphocytic exudate characterized by a very high LDH level. No effective treatment is known.

Pyothorax-Associated Lymphoma

Pyothorax-associated lymphoma occurs almost exclusively in patients who several decades previously received artificial pneumothorax for the treatment of pleural tuberculosis (67). Accordingly, these lymphomas should actually be named pneumothorax-associated lymphoma. These lymphomas are of B-cell lineage, and the Epstein-Barr virus genome has been detected in all of the tumors tested. CT scans reveal pleural masses without effusions in the majority of patients.

Pleural Effusions Secondary to Collagen Vascular Disease

Systemic Lupus Erythematosus

The pleura is frequently involved in systemic lupus erythematosus (SLE). Pleurisy without effusion is more common than pleurisy with effusion. In one series of patients observed for prolonged periods, 72% had pleuritic chest pain and 40% had pleural effusions some time during their course (67). The effusions are frequently bilateral but may be unilateral and change from one side to the other. Pericardial effusions are frequently present concomitantly with the pleural effusions.

The diagnosis of systemic lupus erythematosus should be considered in all patients with undiagnosed pleurisy or pleural effusion. The pleural fluid is typically a serous exudate, and the differential may reveal predominantly lymphocytes, neutrophils, or mesothelial cells. The pleural fluid in the majority of cases is characterized by a normal pH and glucose level and an LDH is below 500 IU per L (68). Measurement of the pleural fluid antinuclear antibody does not appear to be useful in diagnosing lupus pleuritis (69). The diagnosis of lupus pleuritis is established by using the diagnostic criteria published by the American Rheumatism Association for SLE.

Patients with lupus pleuritis should be treated with oral prednisone, 80 mg every other day, with rapid tapering once the symptoms are controlled.

Rheumatoid Pleuritis

Approximately 20% of patients with rheumatoid arthritis will at some time have pleuritic chest pain and about 4% will have a pleural effusion. The pleuritic chest pain may occur before, be coincident with, or occur after the onset of arthritis. The pleural effusion usually occurs after the onset of the arthritis, frequently in conjunction with an arthritic flare-up. Most rheumatoid pleural effusions occur in men, and the majority of patients with rheumatoid effusions also have subcutaneous rheumatoid nodules. The effusion may be on either side and is sometimes bilateral. It is usually small to moderate in size and only occasionally does it produce symptoms, including fever and pleuritic chest pain (68).

The diagnosis is suggested by the clinical picture of rheumatoid arthritis and the presence of a pleural effusion. The pleural fluid with rheumatoid pleuritis is very distinctive in that it is characterized by a glucose level less than 30 mg

per dL, an LDH level above 700 IU per L, a pH less than 7.20, low levels of complement, and the presence of immune complexes (68). The other condition that is likely to yield similar pleural fluid findings is a complicated parapneumonic effusion. Since patients with rheumatoid disease tend to have a high incidence of complicated parapneumonic effusion, the differentiation of the two entities is important and is dependent on the Gram stain and culture of the pleural fluid.

The optimal therapy for rheumatoid pleural effusions remains unclear. Although the majority of such effusions resolve spontaneously over several months, in some the effusion persists, leading to the development of a thick peel covering the visceral pleura and producing a severe restrictive ventilatory defect. No studies have demonstrated that systemic antiinflammatory therapy has any influence on the course of rheumatoid pleuritis, and the results after intrapleural corticosteroids have not been conclusive (70).

Other Collagen Vascular Diseases

An eosinophilic pleural effusion with a very high LDH level, a low glucose level, and a low pH may occur with the Churg-Strauss syndrome, which is characterized by hypereosinophilia and systemic vasculitis in the patient with asthma. Patients with Wegener's granulomatosis, familial Mediterranean fever, and immunoblastic lymphadenopathy also at times get pleural effusions. The effusions in these situations rarely dominate the clinical picture (18).

Pleural Effusions Secondary to Pulmonary Embolism

The diagnosis of pulmonary embolism should be considered in every patient with an undiagnosed pleural effusion. Nearly 50% of patients with pulmonary emboli have a pleural effusion (71). There are two separate mechanisms by which pulmonary emboli can produce pleural effusion. First, the vascular obstruction associated with the emboli can lead to elevated intravascular pressures in the lung or pleura, which can produce a transudative pleural effusion. Second, the ischemia and release of the vasoactive amines secondary to the embolus can increase the permeability of the capillaries in the lung, leading to an increased amount of interstitial fluid and an exudative pleural effusion.

Most pleural effusions associated with pulmonary emboli are small; in one recent study, 48 of 56 patients (86%) had only blunting of the costophrenic angle, and no patient had an effusion that occupied more than one-third of a hemithorax (71). The effusions are usually unilateral, but a recent study with chest CT scan demonstrated bilateral pleural fluid in six of 13 patients with pulmonary emboli (72). The pleural fluid may be either a transudate or an exudate, depending on which of the two mechanisms is responsible for its formation, and the fluid is frequently not bloody. Patients with undiagnosed pleural effusions should have the possibility of pulmonary embolism investigated with a spiral CT scan (73). The spiral CT will not only identify vascular filling defects which are highly suggestive of pulmonary embolism, but it will also demonstrate concomitant parenchymal abnormalities and mediastinal lymphadenopathy.

The treatment of choice for the patient with pleural effusions secondary to pulmonary embolism is adequate anticoagulation (see Chapter 11, Pulmonary Thromboembolism and Other Pulmonary Vascular Diseases). The presence of blood in the pleural fluid does not serve as a contraindication for anticoagulation. Tube thoracostomy for a bloody pleural effusion secondary to pulmonary emboli should be performed only if the hematocrit of the pleural fluid is above 20%.

Pleural Effusions Secondary to Gastrointestinal Conditions

Acute Pancreatitis

The prevalence of pleural effusion was 66% in a recent study of acute pancreatitis (74). In this study, the effusion was bilateral in 51 (77%), unilateral left-sided in 10 (15%) and unilateral right-sided in five (8%). The mechanism responsible for the pleural effusion associated with pancreatitis appears to be inflammation of the diaphragmatic pleura secondary to the transdiaphragmatic transfer of pancreatic enzymes. The clinical picture is usually dominated by abdominal symptoms; however, at times respiratory symptoms consisting of pleuritic chest pain and dyspnea may predominate. In addition to the small- to-moderate-sized pleural effusion, the chest radiograph may reveal an elevated diaphragm and basilar infiltrates. The diagnosis is confirmed with demonstration of an elevated pleural fluid amylase level. Patients with pancreatitis and a pleural effusion should be treated for their pancreatitis in the usual manner, but it should be noted that patients with acute pancreatitis and a pleural effusion tend to have more severe disease and are more likely to subsequently develop a pseudocyst (74).

Chronic Pancreatic Pleural Effusion

Patients with a pancreatic pseudocyst at times develop a large chronic pleural effusion. The pathogenesis of the large pleural effusion is a sinus tract that runs from the pancreas retroperitoneally into the mediastinum and then into the pleural space. The clinical picture is usually dominated by chest symptoms, and most patients do not have abdominal symptoms because the pancreaticopleural fistula decompresses the pseudocyst. The pleural effusion is usually massive and recurs rapidly after thoracentesis. It most commonly is left-sided but it may be right-sided or bilateral. The diagnosis is supported by a markedly elevated pleural fluid amylase level. This is an important diagnosis to consider, because most patients with this entity look as though they have malignancy. Accordingly, the pleural fluid amy-

lase level should be measured in all patients with large, unexplained, chronic pleural effusions. The diagnosis is established with CT scan of the abdomen. Treatment consists of total parenteral nutrition plus drainage of the pleural space. Some patients also require surgical drainage of the pancreas or decortication (75).

Esophageal Perforations

Most esophageal perforations are associated with either a pleural effusion or a hydropneumothorax. Since the mortality associated with this condition approaches 100% if it remains undiagnosed for several days, it should be considered in every patient with a pleural effusion who appears acutely ill. Esophageal perforations occur in three different settings: (a) as a complication of endoscopy, esophageal dilation, thoracic surgery, or the insertion of a Blakemore-Sengstaken tube; (b) spontaneously (Boerhaave's syndrome) when there is a sudden explosive rise in intraabdominal pressure, usually in association with vomiting; and (c) as a complication of esophageal carcinoma.

The clinical picture associated with esophageal rupture is impressive and is highly suggestive of the diagnosis. Pain is the most striking symptom and is characteristically excruciating, unremitting, and unrelieved by opiates. Thirst is a prominent symptom, and most patients show at least some degree of circulatory collapse. A pathognomonic triad of physical signs consists of rapid respiration, abdominal rigidity, and subcutaneous emphysema in the suprasternal notch. The chest radiograph usually reveals a pleural effusion or hydropneumothorax.

The diagnosis is not difficult if it is considered. The pleural fluid amylase level is usually very high (greater than 2,500 units). The amylase in this condition has a salivary origin, and the high pleural fluid amylase level is due to the saliva leaking from the esophagus into the pleural space (76). The pleural fluid pH is usually low (below 7.00) owing to the mediastinal and pleural infection. Both Gram stain and culture of the pleural fluid usually reveal organisms. If there is any doubt as to the diagnosis, it can be substantiated by having the patient swallow methylene blue, in which case the pleural fluid will turn blue if there is an esophageal perforation. Immediate thoracotomy with drainage of the mediastinum and pleural space is indicated once the diagnosis is made. A delay of only several hours is associated with a much higher mortality than if treatment is initiated promptly. The tear in the esophagus should be repaired and high doses of systemic broad-spectrum antibiotics should be administered (77).

Intraabdominal Abscess

Pleural effusions frequently occur with intraabdominal abscesses. The incidence of pleural effusion is approximately 80% with subphrenic, 40% with pancreatic, 33% with splenic, and 20% with intrahepatic abscess. The possibility of intraabdominal abscess should be considered in any patient with an undiagnosed exudative pleural effusion containing predominantly polymorphonuclear leukocytes, particularly when there are no pulmonary parenchymal infiltrates. The diagnosis of intraabdominal abscess is best established with abdominal CT scanning or ultrasound. The appropriate treatment is drainage of the abscess combined with parenteral antibiotics (78).

Postsurgical Procedures

Post–Coronary Artery Bypass Surgery
In the few days immediately following coronary artery bypass graft surgery (CABG), the prevalence of pleural effusion exceeds 50% (79). Most of these effusions are small, left-sided and resolve without intervention. However, about 8% of patients who undergo CABG develop effusions that occupy more than 25% of their hemithorax (80). The great majority of these effusions are left-sided and occur in patients who have received internal mammary artery grafts (80–82). These large symptomatic pleural effusions can be separated into two categories—those that occur within 30 days of surgery and those that occur more than 30 days after surgery (81). In general the primary symptom produced by these effusions is dyspnea; fever and pleuritic chest pain are uncommon. The early effusions are usually bloody (mean hematocrit 20%) with marked eosinophilia (mean over 40%). They are probably due to postoperative bleeding into the pleural space, and resolve with one or two therapeutic thoracenteses. The late effusions tend to be clear exudates with relatively low LDH levels and predominantly lymphocytes on the differential. Their etiology is unknown but they quite possibly represent a limited form of the postcardiac injury syndrome (82). Their treatment is more difficult than the early occurring effusions and may include tube thoracostomy with pleurodesis or thoracoscopy with removal of a thin fibrous coating from the visceral pleura.

Post–Abdominal Surgery
Nearly 50% of patients who have undergone abdominal surgery will develop a pleural effusion postoperatively (83). The incidence of pleural effusion is higher after upper abdominal surgery, in patients with postoperative atelectasis, and in patients with free abdominal fluid at surgery. Most of the effusions are exudates and are thought to be due to diaphragmatic irritation or atelectasis. Nevertheless, a diagnostic thoracentesis should be performed if the effusion is more than minimal in size to rule out a complicated parapneumonic effusion. Pleural effusions developing several days after abdominal surgery suggest either pulmonary embolism or subphrenic abscess.

Post–Lung Transplantation
The amount of pleural fluid which is formed in the immediate postoperative period in patients who receive lung transplantation is markedly increased because the lymphatics which normally drain the lung are severed during the transplantation. Accordingly, all the fluid that enters the interstitial spaces of the lung must exit the lung via the pleural space. The amount of pleural fluid does slow dramatically during the first week postoperatively. Nevertheless, patients who develop complications post–lung transplantation frequently have a pleural effusion. Pleural effusions occurred in 14 of 19 (74%) episodes of acute rejection, seven of eight (88%) instances of chronic rejection, six of 11 (55%) episodes of infection, and three of four (75%) instances of lymphoproliferative disease in one study (84).

Post–Liver Transplantation
The prevalence of pleural effusion in patients who undergo orthotopic liver transplantation approaches 100% (85). The effusions are bilateral in about 30%, but the effusion on the right side is almost always larger. The effusions are large enough to require therapeutic thoracentesis or tube thoracostomy in a sizeable percentage of patients. These effusions tend to increase in size over the first few postoperative days and then gradually resolve over several weeks to months. These effusions are probably due to injury or irritation of the right hemidiaphragm caused by the extensive right upper-quadrant dissection. If a fibrin sealant is sprayed on the undersurface of the diaphragm around the insertion of the liver ligaments at the time of the transplantation, the development of the effusions can largely be prevented (86).

Post–Endoscopic Variceal Sclerotherapy
Small pleural effusions complicate this procedure approximately 50% of the time. The effusion is thought to result from extravasation of the sclerosant into the esophageal mucosa, which results in an intense inflammatory reaction in the mediastinum and pleura. If the effusion persists for more than 24 to 48 hours and is accompanied by fever, or if the effusion occupies more than 25% of the hemithorax, a thoracentesis should be done to rule out an infection or an esophagopleural fistula (87).

Pleural Effusions Due to Drug Reactions

Pleural effusions have been reported definitely to occur as a complication of the administration of six different drugs, namely nitrofurantoin, methysergide, dantrolene, bromocriptine, procarbazine, and amiodarone (18). Other drugs have been reported to cause pleural effusion, but the association is less definite (88). In addition, many other drugs may cause drug-induced lupus erythematosus, which frequently has an associated pleural effusion.

Nitrofurantoin
The administration of nitrofurantoin is occasionally associated with the development of a syndrome characterized by chills, fever, and cough, soon followed by dyspnea, malaise, and pleuritic chest pain. The chest x-ray is characterized by

bilateral interstitial infiltrates, and a pleural effusion is present in about 25% of the cases. This diagnosis should be suspected in any patient taking nitrofurantoin who has a pleural effusion associated with bilateral pulmonary infiltrates. If the drug is discontinued, the symptoms and radiologic abnormalities resolve within a few days.

Methysergide
The administration of methysergide for migraine headaches can be complicated by the development of pleuritis with effusion without parenchymal infiltrates. The pleural effusions are bilateral in nearly 50% of the patients. They develop within three weeks to three years after starting the drug. Discontinuation of the drug early in the course results in complete resolution. However, if the pleuritis has been present for several months, pleural thickening may remain after the drug is discontinued.

Dantrolene
Dantrolene sodium is a long-acting skeletal muscle relaxant used in treating patients with spastic neurologic disorders. It is structurally similar to nitrofurantoin. Its administration is at times associated with the development of sterile exudative pleural effusions without parenchymal infiltrates. Patients with this syndrome have both peripheral and pleural eosinophilia. The syndrome develops only after at least two months of therapy with dantrolene and may be complicated by the presence of pericardial effusion. The pleural effusion and eosinophilia typically take several months to resolve after the drug is discontinued.

Bromocriptine
The long-term administration of bromocriptine mesylate, a dopamine receptor agonist, which is sometimes used in the long-term treatment of Parkinson's disease, can lead to pleuropulmonary changes. Patients who have taken the drug for more than six months many develop pleural thickening and/or a pleural effusion. The natural history of pleuropulmonary disease during bromocriptine therapy is unclear, as the disease progresses only in some of the patients who continue taking the drug (18).

Procarbazine
There have been two detailed case reports in which pleuropulmonary reactions consisting of chills, cough, dyspnea, and bilateral pulmonary infiltrates with pleural effusion occurred after treatment with procarbazine. In both cases symptoms redeveloped within hours of rechallenge (18).

Amiodarone
Amiodarone is an antiarrhythmic that may produce severe pulmonary toxicity. Pleural effusions occur as a complication of amiodarone administration, but pulmonary infiltrates are much more common. Most cases with pleural effusion have concomitant parenchymal involvement (18).

Exudative Pleural Effusions Due to Other Diseases

Asbestos Pleural Effusion
Asbestos exposure that may have been brief, intermittent, and in the immediate or distant past may lead to a pleural effusion. Epler and coworkers (89) reviewed the medical histories of 1,135 asbestos workers whom they had observed for several years and found that 35 of the workers (3%) had pleural effusions for which there was no other explanation. The heavier the asbestos exposure, the more likely the patient is to develop a pleural effusion. The pleural effusion sometimes develops within five years of the initial exposure but sometimes may not develop until more than 30 years after the initial exposure (90). Most patients with benign asbestos pleural effusions are asymptomatic. The pleural fluid is an exudate and frequently has more than 10% eosinophils (18).

The diagnosis of benign asbestos pleural effusion is one of exclusion and requires the following: (a) a history of exposure to asbestos; (b) exclusion of other causes, notably infection, pulmonary embolism, and malignancy; and (c) a follow-up of at least three years to verify that the effusion is benign. There is no known treatment for benign asbestos pleural effusion but it does resolve spontaneously with time.

Meigs' Syndrome
By definition, Meigs' syndrome is the presence of a pleural effusion and ascites in association with an ovarian tumor that is solid, benign, and characteristically a fibroma. Resection of the tumor must effect resolution of the ascites and pleural effusion with no recurrence. The basic abnormality with Meigs' syndrome appears to be fluid loss from the benign tumor into the peritoneum (91). At laparotomy, these tumors are frequently noted to be oozing serous fluid. The effusion is usually on the right side but may be bilateral or left-sided. The size of the pleural effusion is largely independent of the amount of ascites. The pleural fluid may be either a transudate or an exudate. The diagnosis is made at laparotomy with the demonstration of the benign tumor and is confirmed when the ascites and pleural fluid disappear postoperatively. Although Meigs' syndrome is uncommon, it is important to remember it so that patients with a pelvic mass, pleural effusion, and ascites are not labeled as having disseminated ovarian malignancy without histologic proof.

Pulmonary Lymphangiomyomatosis
This rare condition (92) is characterized by the widespread proliferation of smooth muscle in the lymph nodes and lungs, resulting in a honeycomb lung and frequently a chylothorax. All the cases have been in females, and most of the patients present with dyspnea, which is usually due to chylothorax. The chylothorax results from obstruction of the lymphatics by the smooth muscle proliferation. Pneu-

mothorax is also very common with this condition. The chest radiograph reveals bilateral pulmonary infiltrates with hyperinflation. The diagnosis is strongly suggested by the high-resolution CT scan, which reveals numerous air-filled cysts surrounded by normal lung parenchyma. Diagnosis is made by lung biopsy. Treatment in general is unsatisfactory; most patients die within 10 years of onset. There is some evidence that the smooth muscle proliferation is hormonally dependent. It is therefore recommended patients be treated with medroxyprogesterone intramuscularly at a dose of 400 to 800 mg per month for at least one year. Other therapies that can be tried if the medroxyprogesterone fails are oophorectomy or tamoxifen (92). In general, these therapies are at best marginally effective, and accordingly many patients have been subject to lung transplant. However, the disease has recurred in the transplanted lung in some of the recipients (93).

Uremia

A fibrinous pleurisy occasionally occurs in the course of uremia (94). The pathogenesis of the pleuritis is probably similar to that of the pericarditis seen with uremia. More than half of the patients with uremic pleuritis also have uremic pericarditis. The blood urea nitrogen concentration has borne little relationship to the occurrence of the pleuritis. The prevalence of pleural abnormalities in patients undergoing hemodialysis is high. In a recent study of 117 patients who had been receiving hemodialysis for a mean of 48 months and had a CT scan for pulmonary symptoms, the prevalence of pleural effusion was 51% (more than half bilateral) and the prevalence of pleural thickening was 22% (95). The pleural fluid with uremic pleuritis is an exudate, which is frequently bloody with many eosinophils. The diagnosis is made by excluding other causes of exudative pleural effusions in patients with uremia.

Trapped Lung

As a result of inflammation, a fibrous peel may form over the visceral pleura. The peel can prevent the underlying lung from expanding and can lead to a chronic decrease in the pleural pressure. From Figure 17.1 it is easily seen how a more negative pleural pressure could lead to pleural fluid accumulation. The effusion usually becomes evident several months after the initial insult, which can be pneumonitis, thoracic surgery, pneumothorax, trauma, or any other condition producing intense inflammation of the pleura. The pleural fluid with trapped lung usually meets the criteria for an exudate. The diagnosis of trapped lung is best made by measuring the pleural pressures as fluid is withdrawn during a therapeutic thoracentesis (96). If the pleural pressure drops more than 2 cm H_2O for each 100 mL of pleural fluid withdrawn, the patient in all probability has a trapped lung. If the patient is asymptomatic, no therapy is necessary. If the patient is symptomatic from the effusion, a decortication should be considered.

Post–Cardiac Injury Syndrome

The post–cardiac injury (Dressler's) syndrome is characterized by pericarditis with effusion, pleuritis, and pneumonitis following myocardial infarction, cardiac surgery, or cardiac trauma (97). This syndrome occurs between one and 12 weeks following the initiating event and complicates about 1% of myocardial infarctions. The pleural effusions that occur after CABG possibly represent a variant of this syndrome. The pleural effusions may be either unilateral or bilateral and are usually small to moderate in size. The pleural fluid is an exudate that is often bloody. The diagnosis is established by excluding other causes of pleural effusion in the patient with a recent history of myocardial insult. The treatment of choice is NSAIDS if the patient is not excessively symptomatic, since the syndrome is self-limiting. If the patient is distressed, corticosteroids are rapidly effective in relieving symptoms.

Yellow Nail Syndrome

Pleural effusions are frequently associated with congenital abnormalities of the lymphatics. The most common syndrome is characterized by yellow nails, lymphedema, and chronic pleural effusion (98). Often the pleural effusion does not appear until the patient reaches middle age. Examination of the pleural fluid reveals an exudate that is not chylous. The diagnosis can be made by examining the fingernails. When the patient is symptomatic from a large effusion, pleurodesis with a sclerosing agent such as doxycycline should be considered.

Sarcoidosis

The incidence of pleural effusion with sarcoidosis is probably between 1% and 2%. The pleural effusions are usually small, and the pleural fluid is an exudate with predominantly small lymphocytes. The pleural biopsy with sarcoid pleural effusion may reveal noncaseating granulomas. The pleural effusion secondary to sarcoidosis may resolve spontaneously, or corticosteroid therapy may be required for its resolution. It is important to rule out the diagnosis of tuberculous pleuritis in patients with known sarcoid and an exudative pleural effusion, especially if they have been on immunosuppressive therapy (99).

Urinary Tract Obstruction

Obstruction of the urinary tract, with its associated retroperitoneal urine collection, can lead to a pleural effusion. It is believed that the urine moves directly retroperitoneally into the pleural space. The diagnosis is established by the demonstration that the pleural fluid creatinine level is higher than the serum creatinine level. The pleural effusion will rapidly disappear when the urinary tract obstruction is relieved (100).

Chylothorax and Pseudochylothorax

Pleural fluid is occasionally found to be milky or at least turbid. When this cloudiness persists after centrifugation, it is almost always due to a high lipid content in the pleural fluid. Two different situations bring about the accumulation of high levels of lipid in the pleural fluid. In the first, chyle enters the pleural space as a result of disruption of the thoracic duct, producing a *chylothorax* or a *chylous* effusion. In the second, large amounts of cholesterol or lecithin-globulin complexes accumulate in a long-standing pleural effusion to produce a *pseudochylothorax* or a *chyliform* pleural effusion.

Chylothoraces can be traumatic or nontraumatic in origin. The most common traumatic cause is a cardiovascular surgical procedure, but penetrating injuries or nonpenetrating injuries in which the spine is hyperextended can lead to chylothorax. Tumors, most commonly lymphomas, are the most common cause of nontraumatic chylothorax. Other diseases associated with chylothorax include pulmonary lymphangiomyomatosis (discussed earlier in this chapter), abnormalities of the lymphatic vessels such as intestinal lymphangiectasis, filariasis, lymph node enlargement, lymphangitis of the thoracic duct, and tuberous sclerosis (18). If no etiology can be found for the chylothorax, it is labeled as idiopathic. Before attaching this label, however, lymphoma should be excluded.

Patients with chylothorax present with large pleural effusions. Pleuritic chest pain is very rare because chyle is not irritating to the pleura. The pleural fluid with chylothorax is distinctive in that it looks like milk and has no odor. At times the pleural fluid may be blood-tinged or frankly bloody. Patients who have a chylothorax have a pleural fluid triglyceride level above 110 mg per dL (1.24 mmol per L), a ratio of the pleural fluid to the serum triglyceride of greater than 1.0, and a ratio of the pleural fluid to the serum cholesterol of less than 1.0 (101). If doubt remains as to whether a patient has a chylothorax, lipoprotein analysis of the pleural fluid should be obtained. The demonstration of chylomicrons in the pleural fluid by lipoprotein analysis establishes the diagnosis of chylothorax.

The primary danger to the patient with chylothorax is malnutrition and a compromised immunologic status caused by the removal of large amounts of chyle, with its high levels of protein, fat, electrolytes, and lymphocytes, with repeated thoracenteses or chest tube drainage. Therefore it is important to undertake definitive treatment for the chylothorax before the patient becomes too cachectic to tolerate the treatment. Most patients with traumatic or idiopathic chylothorax should originally be treated with a pleuroperitoneal shunt (102). The shunt takes the chyle with its nutrients and leukocytes from the pleural space to the peritoneal cavity, where it is absorbed. This treatment keeps the patient from becoming malnourished and allows the thoracic duct time to heal, which it will do spontaneously in the majority of patients. If the chylothorax persists for more than four weeks, consideration should be given to surgical exploration with ligation of the thoracic duct (18). Patients with nontraumatic chylothorax can also

be treated with the pleuroperitoneal shunt, and this is probably the treatment of choice if the patient's life expectancy is limited. If the patient has mediastinal lymphoma, the chylothorax will usually resolve after radiotherapy or effective chemotherapy. If the patient has benign disease, consideration should be given to chemical pleurodesis or surgical exploration with ligation of the thoracic duct.

The diagnosis of pseudochylothorax is usually easy. The patient has usually had a pleural effusion for five years or longer, and the pleura is thickened or calcified. Most patients with pseudochylothorax either have rheumatoid pleuritis or have been treated by artificial pneumothorax therapy for tuberculosis. Chemical analysis of the pleural fluid usually reveals cholesterol crystals or pleural fluid cholesterol levels above 250 mg per dL. If the patient's exercise capacity is limited by shortness of breath, a therapeutic thoracentesis should be performed because some patients will improve markedly. If the patient is symptomatic and the underlying lung is believed to be functional, a decortication should be considered (103).

Hemothorax

A hemothorax is said to be present when the hematocrit of the pleural fluid is greater than 50% of the peripheral hematocrit. Most hemothoraces are due to trauma. A spontaneous hemothorax occasionally occurs with malignancy. Other causes of hemothorax include a leaking aortic aneurysm or pulmonary arteriovenous malformations, a complication of overzealous anticoagulation for pulmonary emboli, or as a complication of splenoportography. There are several other rare causes of hemothorax, and at times the etiology of the hemothorax remains unknown despite exploratory thoracotomy.

One would think that the diagnosis of a hemothorax is simple. However, frequently pleural fluid will appear to be pure blood when in fact the hematocrit of the fluid is less than 5%. Accordingly, when bloody pleural fluid is obtained on thoracentesis, a hematocrit should be obtained. The diagnosis of hemothorax should be made only when the pleural fluid hematocrit is more than 50% that of the peripheral blood. At times it may be difficult to determine whether the bloody fluid obtained is venous or arterial blood or pleural fluid. However, blood that has been present in the pleural space for more than a few minutes will not clot, while both venous and arterial blood will clot.

Patients with traumatic hemothoraces should be initially managed by inserting a chest tube (104). Not only can the blood be removed by the chest tube, diminishing the likelihood of a subsequent fibrothorax, but the drainage from the chest tube will allow an assessment of persistent bleeding and will serve as a guide as to whether a thoracotomy is necessary for control of the bleeding. If persistent bleeding is not observed but more than one-third of the hemithorax is occupied by a blood clot, thoracoscopy should probably be performed to remove the retained blood (105).

Pleural Diseases Not Associated with Effusion

Fibrothorax

A dense layer of fibrous tissue may be deposited over the pleural surface when there is intense inflammation in the pleural space, most commonly following empyema or hemothorax. The fibrous tissue creates a cast for the lung and renders it immobile and essentially unavailable for air exchange. On physical examination, the affected side is fixed and does not move with respiration. Breath sounds are absent and the percussion note is dull. The treatment of fibrothorax is to remove the fibrous peel from the visceral pleura in an operation called a decortication. If the underlying lung is intact, decortication may result in spectacular improvement in the subjective feeling and in the pulmonary functions of the patient. This improvement can occur even if the fibrothorax has been present 10 or more years.

Pleural Thickening Associated with Asbestos Exposure

The pleura of patients exposed to asbestos may develop plaques or diffuse thickening. The pleural disease is thought to be the result of short, submicroscopic asbestos fibers entering the pleural space. The small asbestos fibers lodge in the pleural lymphatics and, in conjunction with appropriate inflammatory cells, create inflammation that eventually leads to plaque formation or diffuse fibrosis (103). Pleural calcification usually occurs only 20 or more years after the initial exposure to asbestos. Patients with pleural thickening or calcification are usually asymptomatic. The pleural involvement with asbestos exposure is usually bilateral, but if it is unilateral, the left hemithorax is more frequently involved. The detection of pleural thickening or calcification is significant only as an indication of previous exposure to asbestos. However, since it is known that heavy asbestos exposure is associated with a markedly higher incidence of bronchogenic carcinomas and mesotheliomas, the presence of these abnormalities should alert the clinician to these possibilities.

Pneumothorax

Pneumothorax is the presence of gas in the pleural space. A *spontaneous* pneumothorax is one that occurs without antecedent trauma to the thorax. These pneumothoraces can be subdivided into *primary* spontaneous pneumothorax, for which there is no underlying predisposing disease, and *secondary* spontaneous pneumothorax, for which there is an underlying disease such as chronic obstructive pulmonary disease or cystic fibrosis. A *traumatic* pneumothorax occurs as a result of penetrating or nonpenetrating chest injuries. An iatrogenic pneumothorax occurs as a consequence of a diagnostic or therapeutic maneuver. A *tension* pneumothorax is a pneumothorax in which the pressure in the pleural space is positive throughout the respiratory cycle.

Pathogenesis

The pressure in the pleural space is negative with respect to the atmospheric pressure and the alveolar pressure. Therefore, if there is a communication either between the alveoli and the pleural space or between the outside of the thoracic cavity and the pleural space, air will continue to enter the pleural space until the pleural pressure becomes atmospheric or the communication is closed. The increase in the pleural pressure will result in both a hyperexpanded hemithorax and a collapsed lung. Occasionally, when the communication is between the alveoli and the pleural space, a "ball-valve" effect is present, resulting in a one-way flow of air into the pleural space. Since the alveolar pressure becomes very positive with respect to atmospheric pressure during expiration, especially when there is coughing, the pleural pressure may become quite positive, producing a tension pneumothorax.

Primary Spontaneous Pneumothorax

Approximately 8,600 individuals in the United States develop a primary spontaneous pneumothorax each year (18). Tall, thin individuals appear to be more susceptible to this entity, and almost all affected individuals are smokers. Primary spontaneous pneumothoraces are usually due to the rupture of apical pleural blebs. These are small cystic spaces, seldom exceeding 1 to 2 cm in diameter, which lie within or immediately under the visceral pleura. The main symptoms associated with a spontaneous pneumothorax are chest pain and dyspnea. The symptoms start abruptly in about two-thirds of the cases and insidiously in the remainder. In the majority of cases the symptoms start while the patient is sedentary. The diagnosis is established with the demonstration of a visceral pleural line on the chest radiograph.

The recommended initial treatment for primary spontaneous pneumothorax is simple aspiration (106). A 16-gauge needle with an overlying polyethylene catheter is inserted into the second anterior intercostal space at the midclavicular line after local anesthesia. After the needle is inserted, it is extracted from the cannula. Then a three-way stopcock and a 60-mL syringe are attached to the catheter and air is manually withdrawn until no more can be aspirated. If the total volume of air aspirated exceeds 4 L and no resistance has been felt, it can be assumed that no expansion has occurred and a chest tube should be inserted or an immediate thoracoscopy should be performed (106).

The recurrence rate for primary spontaneous pneumothorax after the initial occurrence is between 30% and 50% over five years if no attempts are made to produce a pleurodesis (106). Once a patient has one recurrence, subsequent recurrences are even more common. Patients who have a recurrent primary spontaneous pneumothorax and those in whom the initial aspiration is unsuccessful are best managed with thoracoscopy with stapling of blebs and pleural abrasion (107). If thoracoscopy is not available, one can attempt to induce a pleurodesis by the intrapleural injection of doxycycline (5 to 10 mg per kg) (106). The intrapleural injection of a tetracycline derivative will decrease the subsequent risk of a pneumothorax by about 50% (53). Talc slurry is not recommended because of its propensity to induce ARDS (50), and bleomycin is not recommended because it does induce a pleurodesis when the pleural space is normal (52). Another alternative is open thoracotomy with stapling of blebs and abrasion of the parietal pleura, but this is a bigger surgical procedure.

Secondary Spontaneous Pneumothorax

COPD is responsible for more secondary spontaneous pneumothoraces than is any other disease. The occurrence of a pneumothorax in these patients is more life-threatening than it is in a normal individual on account of their limited pulmonary reserve. Owing to the diminished breath sounds and lung hyperinflation of these patients, the diagnosis, both by physical examination and radiographically, is much more difficult than it is in the normal individual. The possibility of a pneumothorax should be considered in all patients with an exacerbation of their COPD, and the chest radiograph should be closely examined for a pleural line. Since small pneumothoraces can lead to marked respiratory embarrassment, all patients should be treated with tube thoracostomy. We routinely recommend thoracoscopy with the stapling of blebs and pleural abrasion or instill doxycycline into the pleural space of such patients in an attempt to prevent a recurrence. If after four days of tube thoracostomy the lung remains collapsed or a bronchopleural fistula persists, thoracoscopy should be considered (106).

Secondary spontaneous pneumothoraces complicate about 1% of parenchymal tuberculosis cases. Such cases should be treated with tube thoracostomy. Frequently, multiple tubes are necessary for long periods to effect resolution of the process. Bacterial pneumonia, particularly that due to *Staphylococcus aureus*, may be complicated by pneumothorax. In this situation there is usually a complicating empyema. Such cases should have two chest tubes inserted: one high to drain the air and the other one low to drain the pus. Secondary spontaneous pneumothoraces have also been reported in association with AIDS and *Pneumocystis carinii* pneumonia, asthma, cystic fibrosis, lymphangioleiomyomatosis, scleroderma, histiocytosis X, tuberous sclerosis, interstitial pneumonitis, sarcoidosis, pulmonary embolism, rheumatoid disease, hydatid disease, silicosis, metastatic malignancy, and primary carcinoma of the lung.

Tension Pneumothorax

A tension pneumothorax is present when the intrapleural pressure exceeds the atmospheric pressure throughout expiration and often during inspiration as well. The positive pleural pressure is life-threatening, not only because ventilation is severely compromised, but also because the positive pressure is transmitted to the mediastinum, resulting in decreased venous return to the heart and reduced cardiac output. In addition, patients with tension pneumothorax are usually markedly hypoxemic. Tension pneumothorax most commonly occurs in patients who are receiving positive pressure to their airways (mechanical ventilation or resuscitation). In patients not receiving positive airway pressure, the positive pressure in the pleural space is sustained by a "ball-valve" mechanism. Strong inspiratory efforts promote the entry of air into the pleural space, but the check valve prevents its egress, so the pressure continues to increase in the pleural space.

Patients with tension pneumothorax are acutely ill with dyspnea, tachycardia, and tachypnea. The neck veins are distended and the decreased venous return results in a thready pulse and hypotension. The trachea is deviated toward the side contralateral to the pneumothorax. The side with the tension pneumothorax is hyperexpanded and moves poorly with respiration. Tactile fremitus and breath sounds are absent, and the percussion note is hyperresonant on the side with the pneumothorax.

The treatment of a tension pneumothorax is a medical emergency. If the tension in the pleural space is not relieved, the patient is likely to die from inadequate cardiac output or marked hypoxemia. The diagnosis is made with the physical examination. Valuable time should not be wasted in the acutely ill patient in obtaining radiologic confirmation. If the diagnosis is suspected, a large-bore needle should be inserted immediately into the pleural space through the second anterior intercostal space. If large amounts of gas come forth through the needle after its insertion, the diagnosis is confirmed. Observation of this phenomenon is facilitated by attaching the needle to a syringe containing sterile saline. With the plunger removed from the syringe, bubbling of air through the saline will establish the diagnosis. If a tension pneumothorax is present, the needle should be left in place until a thoracostomy tube can be inserted. In contrast, if air passes from the atmosphere into the pleural space, a tension pneumothorax is not present and the needle should be immediately withdrawn.

DISEASES OF THE MEDIASTINUM

The mediastinum is the region between the pleural sacs. It is bounded laterally by the mediastinal pleura and extends

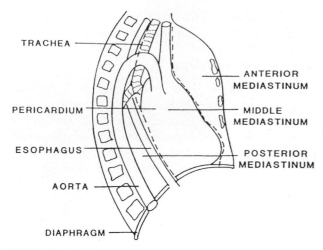

FIGURE 17.2. Subdivisions of the mediastinum. The dashed lines separate the middle mediastinum from the anterior and the posterior mediastinum.

from the thoracic inlet superiorly to the diaphragm inferiorly and from the sternum anteriorly to the spine posteriorly. The mediastinum contains the heart; the thoracic aorta and its proximal branches; the venae cavae; the azygos and proximal innominate veins; the thoracic duct; the lymph nodes and lymphatics; the esophagus; the trachea; the thymus; and the vagus, phrenic, posterior intercostal, and sympathetic nerves. Anatomically the mediastinum is divided into three compartments (Fig. 17.2). The anatomical boundaries, the normal contents, and the lesions that occur in the three compartments are shown in Table 17.2.

Mediastinal Masses

Mediastinal masses may be discovered as a result of routine chest radiographs or in the evaluation of symptoms suggestive of mediastinal disease. Regardless, the differential diagnosis involves an abnormal shadow in the mediastinum on a radiograph. Since a given mediastinal lesion tends to be located in one mediastinal compartment, the first step in evaluating a mediastinal lesion is to place it in one of three mediastinal compartments. The lesions that tend to appear in the various compartments are given in Table 17.2, and the following discussion of mediastinal masses is organized according to the three compartments. It should be emphasized that the locations listed in Table 17.2 are those in which the various masses are most likely to occur. For example, lymph node involvement in lymphoma occurs almost as frequently in the anterior as in the middle compartment. Aortic aneurysms may be situated in any of the three compartments.

It is evident from Table 17.2 that there are many different abnormalities that can produce abnormal mediastinal shadows. The relative incidence of the more common primary mediastinal tumors and cysts is outlined in Table 17.3. This table was compiled by combining nine series of adult patients and five series of pediatric patients (108). The incidence is heavily dependent on the patient's age. Thymomas are the most common abnormality in adults but are rare in children. Neurogenic tumors occur very frequently in children, while mesothelial cysts and endocrine (thyroid, parathyroid) tumors are very uncommon in children.

It should be emphasized that the majority of abnormal mediastinal shadows do not represent primary mediastinal

TABLE 17.2 THE ANATOMICAL BOUNDARIES, THE NORMAL CONTENTS, AND THE LESIONS THAT OCCUR PREDOMINANTLY IN THE THREE DIFFERENT MEDIASTINAL COMPARTMENTS

	Anterior Compartment	Middle Compartment	Posterior Compartment
Anatomical boundaries	Manubrium and sternum anteriorly; pericardium, aorta, and brachiocephalic vessels posteriorly	Anterior mediastinum anteriorly; posterior mediastinum posteriorly	Pericardium and trachea anteriorly; vertebral column posteriorly
Contents	Thymus gland, anterior mediastinal lymph nodes, internal mammary arteries and veins	Pericardium, heart, ascending and transverse arch of aorta, superior and inferior venae cavae, brachiocephalic arteries and veins, phrenic nerves, trachea and main bronchi and their contiguous lymph nodes, pulmonary arteries and veins	Descending thoracic aorta, esophagus, thoracic duct, azygous and hemiazygos veins, sympathetic chains, and the posterior group of mediastinal lymph nodes
Common abnormalities	Thymoma, lymphomas, teratomatous neoplasms, thyroid masses, parathyroid masses, mesenchymal tumors, giant lymph node hyperplasia, hernia through foramen of Morgagni	Metastatic lymph node enlargement, granulomatous lymph node enlargement, pleuropericardial cysts, bronchogenic cysts, masses of vascular origin	Neurogenic tumors, meningocele, meningomyelocele, gastroenteric cysts, esophageal diverticula, hernia through foramen of Bochdalek, extramedullary hematopoiesis

TABLE 17.3 RELATIVE FREQUENCY OF VARIOUS PRIMARY MEDIASTINAL TUMORS AND CYSTS IN ADULTS AND CHILDREN

Tumor or Cyst	Adults		Children	
	Number	%	Number	%
Neurogenic tumor	384	21	135	39
Thymoma	387	21	0	0
Lymphoma	242	13	68	19
Teratomatous neoplasm	201	11	42	12
Primary carcinoma	65	4	16	5
Mesenchymal tumor	134	7	35	10
Endocrine tumor	115	6	0	0
Pleuropericardial cysts	126	7	0	0
Bronchogenic cysts	126	7	28	8
Enteric cysts	57	3	24	7
	1832	100	349	100

From Jones KW, Pietra GG, Sabiston DC Jr. Primary neoplasms and cysts of the mediastinum. In: Fishman AP, ed. *Pulmonary diseases and disorders.* New York: McGraw-Hill, 1980, with permission of McGraw-Hill Book Co.

cysts or tumors. In a review of 782 cases of mediastinal masses, Lyons and coworkers (109) found that neoplasms accounted for the most mediastinal masses (41.6%), followed closely by inflammatory diseases (35.7%) such as sarcoidosis, histoplasmosis, and tuberculosis, and then by vascular abnormalities (10.6%), hernias, diverticula, and achalasia (5.4%), cysts (2.8%), and miscellaneous disorders (3.9%).

The diagnostic approach to disorders of the mediastinum may be divided into imaging techniques (computed tomography, magnetic resonance imaging, radionuclide studies, and barium studies) and procedures for obtaining tissue samples (needle aspiration and biopsy, thoracoscopy and mediastinoscopy). Computed tomographic (CT) imaging of the mediastinum is the most valuable imaging technique. The accurate cross-sectional information provided by CT can be very useful when a mediastinal mass cannot be accurately delineated by conventional radiographic methods, as illustrated in Figure 17.3. With thoracic CT, normal variations and benign neoplasms such as fat and fluid-filled cysts can be distinguished from other processes, and the site of origin of masses can be better identified. Magnetic resonance imaging (MRI) is usually reserved for clarifying problems encountered on CT or to examine patients who cannot tolerate IV administration of contrast material (110). At times, barium studies of the gastrointestinal tract are indicated, since hernias, diverticula, and achalasia are readily diagnosed in this manner.

In many patients with mediastinal masses, a definitive diagnosis can be obtained with radiologically guided percutaneous needle biopsy of the mass. In a recent series of 95 patients, the diagnosis of malignancy was established with greater than 90% sensitivity and 100% specificity (111).

Fine needle aspiration techniques usually suffice for carcinomatous lesions, but a cutting-needle biopsy should be performed whenever possible when lymphoma, thymoma, or neural masses are suspected, to obtain larger specimens for more accurate histologic diagnosis. At times mediastinoscopy (112), endoscopic ultrasound-guided fine needle aspiration, thoracoscopy, or anterior mediastinotomy (113) is necessary to establish the diagnosis.

Mediastinal Masses Located Primarily in the Anterior Compartment

Thymoma

Thymic tumors are the most common tumors in the anterior mediastinum and account for about 20% of all primary mediastinal tumors. About 25% are malignant and are invasive by direct extension rather than by distant metastasis. The differentiation between benign and malignant tumors must be made at surgery, since they cannot be distinguished histologically. However, a higher grade of malignancy is suggested if infiltration of local tissues is demonstrated with a CT scan (114).

The peak incidence of thymomas is between the ages of 40 and 60; they are rare in children. Benign tumors are usually discovered on routine chest radiography, since they are asymptomatic. Malignant thymomas produce symptoms by invading contiguous structures. Substernal chest pain and dyspnea are the most frequent symptoms.

There are several paraneoplastic syndromes that occur in patients with thymomas (114). The most common is myasthenia gravis. Approximately 40% of patients with thymic tumors have myasthenia gravis, while 15% of patients with myasthenia have thymomas. Since thymectomy will lead to improvement of the myasthenia gravis in approximately two-thirds of patients with myasthenia and thymoma, mediastinal CT is indicated in all patients with myasthenia gravis. Patients with thymoma should have a serum antiacetylcholine receptor antibody level test preoperatively to exclude myasthenia gravis even if they are asymptomatic (114). Thymomas have also been linked to the occurrence of hypogammaglobulinemia, red cell aplasia, and various other autoimmune disorders and tumors.

Radiologically, thymomas present as well-defined, rounded, or lobulated anterior-superior mediastinal masses on one or both sides of the superior mediastinal shadow (Fig. 17.4). At times they are visible only in the lateral views, where they appear as a rounded or elongated shadow in the anterior part of the upper mediastinum. The upper pole of a thymoma can usually be seen clearly in the posterior-anterior (PA) film, and this differentiates it from retrosternal goiter.

All thymomas should be treated surgically, but surgery is not always curative. In one series of 70 patients who had their thymomas surgically removed, 25 patients subse-

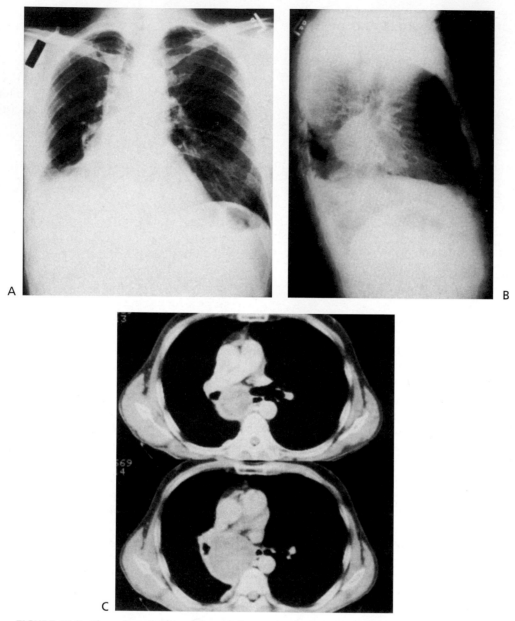

FIGURE 17.3. The value of CT scanning of the mediastinum in delineating mediastinal masses. Posteroanterior **(A)** and lateral **(B)** radiographs of a patient, demonstrating a mediastinal mass or a right lower-lobe mass. Mediastinal CT scan **(C)** reveals that the mass is in the middle and posterior mediastinum and is separate from the right lower lobe. The patient had a bronchogenic cyst.

quently died from progression of their thymoma and four other patients had evidence of recurrence (115). Radiotherapy is usually recommended for invasive or incompletely excised tumors. Postoperative chemotherapy should also be administered to patients in whom the tumor cannot be resected completely (114).

Lymphomatous Tumors
Lymphomas as a group are the second most common kind of tumor in the anterior mediastinum and are the third

most frequently encountered kind of primary neoplasm of the entire mediastinum after neurogenic tumors and thymomas (116). Lymph node enlargement with lymphomas is most common in the anterior mediastinum but occurs frequently in the middle mediastinum and sometimes in the posterior mediastinum (Fig. 17.5). Any of the several types of lymphatic tumors may arise in the mediastinal nodes, but Hodgkin's disease and non-Hodgkin's lymphoma are seen most frequently. Of patients with peripheral lymphoma and mediastinal involvement, 50% to 70%

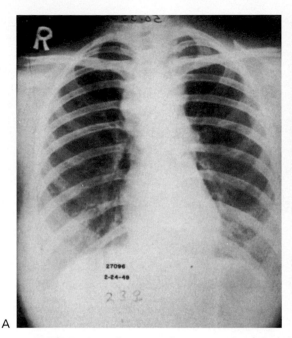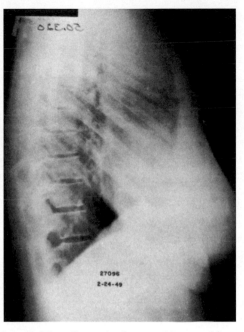

FIGURE 17.4. Thymoma. Posteroanterior **(A)** and lateral **(B)** radiographs from a 23-year-old woman with a malignant thymoma. On the posteroanterior view, the superior mediastinum is widened, while on the lateral view, the retrosternal air space is obliterated.

have Hodgkin's lymphoma while 15% to 25% have non-Hodgkin's lymphoma. Nodular sclerosing Hodgkin's lymphoma, the most common subtype of Hodgkin's lymphoma in women, has a unique predilection for the anterior mediastinum, especially the thymus (117). Two variants of non-Hodgkin's lymphoma—large B-cell lymphoma and lymphoblastic lymphoma—also primarily involve the anterior

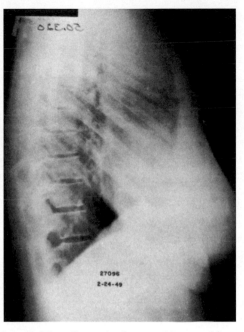

FIGURE 17.5. Mediastinal lymphoma. Posteroanterior radiograph from a patient with lymphocytic lymphoma demonstrating marked widening of the entire mediastinum.

mediastinum and are the most frequent primary mediastinal non-Hodgkin's lymphoma (117).

Patients with lymphomatous involvement of the mediastinum rarely present with isolated asymptomatic mediastinal disease. Usually they also have enlargement of peripheral lymph nodes, hepatosplenomegaly, constitutional symptoms, or cutaneous or retroperitoneal disease. The mediastinal lymph node enlargement secondary to lymphoma is usually bilateral but asymmetric. In most cases, the mass has a nodular contour that suggests lymph node enlargement. If the diagnosis cannot be made by biopsy of a peripheral or scalene node, then mediastinoscopy is recommended. Although the treatment in the past has included attempted surgical excision, radiotherapy and chemotherapy now appear to be the treatments of choice (117).

Germ Cell Tumors

These neoplasms, which include teratoma, seminoma, embryonal cell carcinoma, and choriocarcinoma, constitute the third most common tumors (following thymomas and lymphomas) occurring in the anterior mediastinum. These tumors develop from residual embryonal tissues which migrated from the branchial clefts. *Dermoid cysts* are germ cell tumors that consist of only epidermis and its appendages, while *teratomas* contain ectodermal, mesodermal, and endodermal derivatives. Although they are presumably present from birth, in the majority of cases they are discovered only in adolescence or early adulthood. About 20% of mediastinal teratomatous neoplasms are malignant, with malignancy much more common in male patients. More than 90% of these neoplasms are located in the anterior mediastinum, but a few are located in the middle or posterior mediastinum (118). Adenocarcinoma is the most common malignancy found in these tissues, but seminomas, choriocarcinomas, and embryonal carcinomas are also found. Mixed histologic patterns are common.

It is unusual for symptoms to be associated with these tumors if they are benign, but symptoms are common with malignant tumors (118). Tumors that grow large may give rise to shortness of breath, cough, or a sensation of pressure in the retrosternal area. Rarely, a cystic tumor becomes infected and spills its contents into the mediastinum or pleural cavity.

Radiographically, the majority of teratodermoid tumors are in the anterior mediastinum close to the origin of the major vessels from the heart. Benign lesions tend to be oval and smooth in contour, while malignant lesions tend to be lobulated. In rare cases a bone or tooth is visible radiographically in the mass, and this establishes the diagnosis.

Measurement of serum tumor markers, β-subunit human chorionic gonadotropin (HCG) and α-fetoprotein (AFP) is indispensable in the management of mediastinal germ cell tumors. Patients with benign teratoma are marker-negative; a significant elevation of HCG or AFP implies a malignant component of the tumor (118). The AFP is elevated in approximately 80% of malignant nonseminomatous germ cell tumors, while the HCG is elevated in 30%. Between 50% and 70% of patients with mediastinal testicular germ cell tumors will have elevated HCG or AFP. The diagnosis of malignant germ cell tumors can be made with fine needle aspiration or cutting-needle biopsy of the mass, but many oncologists would treat a mediastinal mass on the basis of elevated levels of the serum tumor markers.

Benign teratomatous tumors should be removed surgically, since they have a tendency toward malignant transformation and infection is common in cystic lesions. The recommended management of malignant teratomatous tumors is cisplatin-based chemotherapy followed by surgical removal of the residual tumor. Long-term survival with seminomas is now 60% to 80%, while long-term survival with nonseminomatous tumors is 60% (117).

Thyroid Masses

Intrathoracic goiter (Fig. 17.6) is the fourth most frequently seen anterior mediastinal mass, despite the fact that fewer than 3% of goiters at thyroidectomy extend into the thorax (109). Most intrathoracic thyroid masses arise from a lower pole or from the isthmus of the thyroid and extend into the anterior mediastinum in front of the trachea. Patients are usually asymptomatic, but if the trachea becomes compressed, stridor and respiratory distress may occur. More than half the patients will have associated thyromegaly with a nodular goiter, but hyperthyroidism is uncommon. The diagnosis may be made noninvasively with a CT scan of the mediastinum that demonstrates the thyroidal origin of the mass (119). The treatment should be surgical if symptoms are present and in most other cases (119). However, if the ^{131}I scan is positive and the patient is asymptomatic, observation may be the treatment of choice if the patient is a poor surgical candidate.

Parathyroid Masses

Parathyroid tumors are a rare cause of anterior mediastinal masses. They are usually small, encapsulated, benign lesions situated in the upper or middle portion of the anterior mediastinum. Since most of these tumors produce parathyroid hormone (PTH), the presence of signs and symptoms of

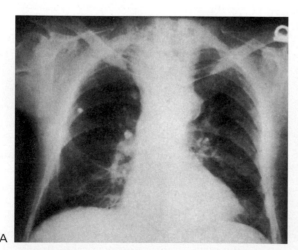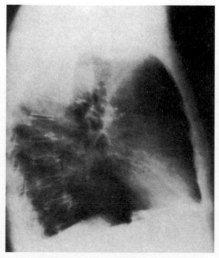

FIGURE 17.6. Intrathoracic goiter. Posteroanterior **(A)** and lateral **(B)** radiographs from a patient with intrathoracic goiter. The goiter is evident as a right paratracheal mass in the posteroanterior view and as an anterior superior mediastinal mass in the lateral view.

hyperparathyroidism allows one to make the diagnosis pre-operatively. It is difficult to identify the tumor preoperatively, but CT will demonstrate the lesion about 50% of the time, as will MRI. The best way to identify the location of this tumor is with ^{99m}Tc-sestamibi scintigraphy, which has a sensitivity of 88% to 100% (114). The treatment of choice is surgical excision.

Mesenchymal Tumors

The mesenchymal tumors (lipomas, fibromas, leiomyomas, lymphangiomas, hemangiomas, and mesotheliomas) account for fewer than 5% of mediastinal masses. Each tumor type has its malignant counterpart, and malignant changes occur in about 50% of these tumors (116). The majority of these tumors occur in the anterior mediastinum, with the exception of fibrosarcoma, which occurs primarily in the posterior mediastinum. The recommended treatment for all these tumors is surgical removal. In spite of treatment, malignant mesenchymal tumors are almost universally fatal (116).

Hernia Through Foramen of Morgagni

The foramina of Morgagni are small triangular deficiencies in the diaphragm between the muscle fibers originating from the sternum and the seventh rib. They are a few centimeters from the midline on each side. When the foramina of Morgagni are larger than normal, abdominal contents may herniate into the thorax. This herniation is into the anterior mediastinum and is usually right-sided, since the left foramen is protected by the pericardium. The diagnosis is easily established with thoracic CT. To avoid the possibility of obstruction, these hernias should be repaired surgically if they are large or if the bowel has herniated (120).

Mediastinal Masses Occurring Predominantly in the Middle Compartment

Giant Lymph Node Hyperplasia

This unusual condition, also known as Castleman's disease, usually presents as a solitary mass in the middle mediastinum, but sometimes it can occur in the anterior or posterior mediastinum. A distinctive microscopic appearance is present, with lymphoid follicles scattered widely throughout the mass instead of being confined to the peripheral cortical zones as in normal lymph nodes (120). Radiographically there is a solitary mass up to 10 cm in diameter with a smooth or lobulated contour. Giant lymph node hyperplasia itself is a benign condition, but it has the potential to evolve into frank lymphoma (120). Some patients with Castleman's disease also have associated immune defects. The treatment of choice is surgical excision.

Lymph Node Involvement in Granulomatous Mediastinitis

Granulomatous inflammation of the mediastinal lymph nodes (Fig. 17.7) is the most common cause of a middle mediastinal mass. This entity is discussed later in this chapter.

Metastatic Lymph Node Enlargement

Nearly 90% of tumors that develop in the middle mediastinum are malignant (116). Metastatic disease from the lungs, upper gastrointestinal tract, prostate, or kidney is the most common middle mediastinal neoplasm (Fig. 17.8). With metastatic disease, the bronchopulmonary nodes as well as the mediastinal nodes are almost invariably enlarged. When the primary lesion is in the lung, node enlargement is usually

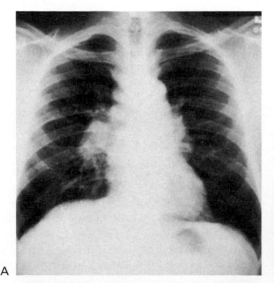
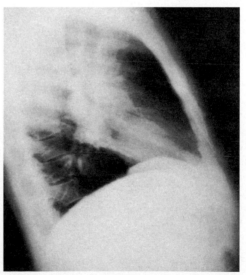

FIGURE 17.7. Mediastinal sarcoidosis. Posteroanterior **(A)** and lateral **(B)** radiographs from a 54-year-old patient with mediastinal sarcoidosis. Note that the lymph node enlargement is relatively symmetrical and involves both the bronchopulmonary and mediastinal lymph nodes.

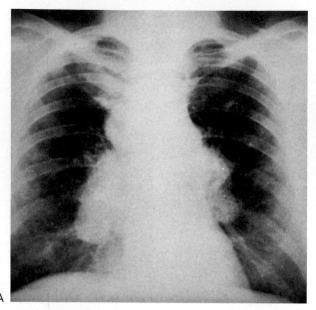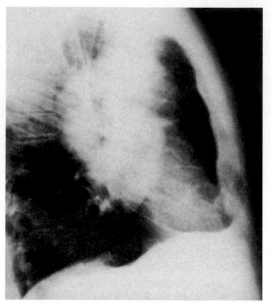

FIGURE 17.8. Metastatic lymph node enlargement. Posteroanterior **(A)** and lateral **(B)** radiographs from a patient with metastatic kidney carcinoma, demonstrating marked enlargement of both the mediastinal and bronchopulmonary nodes.

unilateral in the early stage. The majority of patients with metastatic disease to the mediastinum are symptomatic, with weight loss, retrosternal pain, fever, cough, or dyspnea. Symptoms secondary to involvement of other mediastinal structures, including the superior vena cava, the phrenic nerve, the recurrent laryngeal nerve, and the pericardium, are common. Treatment is dependent on the site of the primary tumor, but the prognosis is in general dismal.

Mesothelial Cysts

Mesothelial cysts, also called pericardial or pleuropericardial cysts, have a developmental origin and appear to result from sequestration of part of the pleuroperitoneal cavity by the developing diaphragm. They rarely cause symptoms and are usually discovered on screening chest radiographs. Their most common location by far is anteriorly in the right cardiophrenic angle (121). They may also occur in the left cardiophrenic angle, in the hilar region, and in the anterior mediastinum. Mesothelial cysts contain crystal-clear fluid and are at times called "spring water cysts" because of their contents. The diagnosis is strongly suggested by the CT and ultrasound. Aspiration of the lesion with demonstration of the clear fluid will establish the diagnosis. Once the diagnosis is established, resection is unnecessary since these cysts virtually never produce symptoms (121).

Bronchogenic Cysts

Bronchogenic cysts represent pinched-off buds of the primitive foregut or trachea and are lined with pseudostratified columnar epithelium. They occur paratracheally or adjacent

to the main carina and project into the posterior part of the middle mediastinum. Because they contain fluid, they have a relatively uniform density, a smooth border, and a round or teardrop configuration (as do pleuropericardial cysts). Esophageal endoscopic ultrasound is now the preferred imaging technique (122). Bronchogenic cysts frequently become symptomatic, and for this reason surgical removal is recommended (122).

Mediastinal Masses of Vascular Origin

Mediastinal masses of vascular origin are most frequently found in the middle mediastinum. However, it is important to consider this diagnosis with all mediastinal masses, since invasive procedures such as needle aspiration or biopsy or mediastinoscopy may have disastrous consequences if the lesion is vascular (Figs. 17.9 and 17.10). CT with contrast effectively demonstrates the vascular nature of the apparent mass.

Mediastinal Masses Situated Predominantly in the Posterior Compartment

Neurogenic Tumors

Neurogenic tumors are the most common cause of a posterior mediastinal mass (117). They are characteristically situated in the posterior mediastinum because they arise from the paravertebral sympathetic nerve trunk and the spinal nerves. Approximately 20% of neural tumors are malignant.

Neurogenic tumors may be divided into three groups: (a) tumors that arise from peripheral nerves (neurofibroma, neurofibrosarcoma, and neurilemoma); (b) tumors that arise from sympathetic ganglia (ganglioneuroma, neuroblastoma, and sympathicoblastoma); and (c) tumors that arise from paraganglionic cells (pheochromocytoma and chemodectoma). Chemodectoma is the only neurogenic tumor that shows no strong tendency to be located in the posterior mediastinum.

The highest incidence of neurogenic neoplasms is in the younger age group, but they may develop at any age. In von Recklinghausen's disease, mediastinal neurofibromas are associated with neurofibromas elsewhere in the body. The majority of patients with neurogenic tumors are asymptomatic, the tumors being discovered on screening radiographs. When symptoms are present, the most common is pain, presumably resulting from bony erosion. Radiographically, the tumors typically appear as round, dense, well-demarcated, solid-appearing masses in the posterior mediastinum in close association with a vertebral body. At times the ribs or vertebrae are eroded, with either benign or malignant lesions. A neurofibroma that originates in a nerve root within the spinal canal may be shaped like a dumbbell or hourglass, part being inside and part outside the spinal

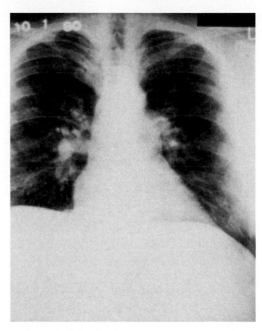

FIGURE 17.10. Enlarged pulmonary arteries. Posteroanterior radiograph from a 37-year-old man with primary pulmonary hypertension, demonstrating markedly enlarged pulmonary arteries that could be confused with a mediastinal mass.

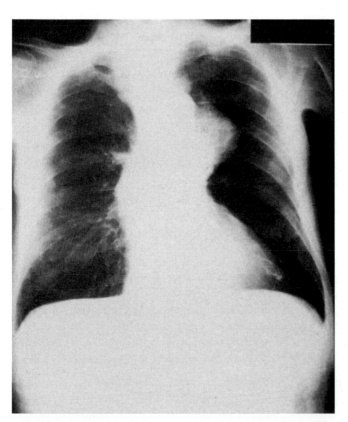

FIGURE 17.9. Aneurysm of ascending aorta. Posteroanterior radiograph demonstrating a mass in the superior left mediastinum. At aortography the mass proved to be an aneurysm of the ascending aorta. This case illustrates how deceiving vascular masses may be at times. In fact, this patient underwent needle aspiration of the mass before the correct diagnosis was established.

canal, with enlargement of the intervertebral foramen. Neurogenic tumors should be surgically removed because of their propensity to undergo malignant change (117). MRI should be performed preoperatively in all patients with suspected neurogenic tumors to definitely exclude intraspinal tumor extension.

Meningocele and Meningomyelocele

These are rare anomalies of the spinal canal in which the leptomeninges herniate through an intervertebral foramen. They are therefore located in the posterior mediastinum and are difficult to distinguish from neurogenic tumors. A meningocele contains only cerebrospinal fluid; a meningomyelocele contains nerve elements also. Myelography may be diagnostic; treatment is by excision.

Diseases of the Esophagus

The esophageal diseases described below produce masses in the posterior mediastinum.

Gastroenteric Cysts. These cysts are identical to bronchogenic cysts except that they are lined with esophageal, gastric, or small intestinal mucosa. They are located adjacent to the esophagus at any level in the posterior mediastinum. Most are found in infants less than one year of age, in whom they produce symptoms from tracheal or esophageal compression. Esophageal endoscopic ultrasound is now the preferred imaging technique (122). Since most are attached to the esophagus, the diagnosis is strongly suggested by a barium swallow that discloses a localized defect, covered with intact mucosa, in the esophageal lumen. Treatment is by surgical excision (121).

Esophageal Diverticula. Zenker's diverticulum originates between the transverse and oblique fibers of the inferior pharyngeal constrictor muscle (120). It may become large enough to be visible on a plain radiograph of the superior mediastinum. Frequently there is an air-fluid level. The diagnosis can be made with a barium swallow, and treatment is surgical. Diverticula arising from the lower third of the esophagus are almost always congenital. They present as round, cystlike structures to the right of the midline and just above the diaphragm (120). An air-fluid level is present in most cases. The diagnosis is established with a barium swallow, and surgical treatment is definitive.

Hiatal Hernia. In patients with hiatal hernia, the chest radiograph often shows abnormalities behind the heart and slightly to the right of the midline. Many times an air-fluid level is present. A barium swallow should be obtained in all patients with radiographic abnormalities in this area to rule out hiatal hernia (120).

Dilation. When the esophagus becomes dilated, it is apparent as a shadow projecting entirely to the right side of the mediastinum. Depending on the underlying cause of the dilation, an air-fluid level may be present or the entire esophagus may contain air. The diagnosis is made with a barium swallow.

Hernia Through the Foramen of Bochdalek
The Bochdalek hernia is the most common congenital diaphragmatic hernia, and at times it presents as a posterior mediastinal mass. Although any portion of the diaphragm may be absent, most defects are posterolateral on the left side and result from failure of the fetal pleuroperitoneal membrane to fuse. Since the defects are congenital, herniation is identified most frequently in children and only occasionally in adults. Any intraabdominal organ may herniate through these foramina. A definitive diagnosis can be established with CT. Only symptomatic hernias require surgical intervention (123).

Diseases of the Thoracic Spine
A wide variety of primary neoplasms of bone and cartilage may involve the thoracic spine and posterior rib cage. The majority of these lesions do not produce an extraosseous mass, but occasionally the major radiographic finding is a posterior mediastinal mass. Tuberculous and nontuberculous spondylitis are often associated with a paraspinal mass. This is most commonly manifested as a bilateral fusiform mass in the paravertebral zone, with its maximal diameter at the point of major bone destruction. Fractures of thoracic vertebral bodies may result in extraosseous hemorrhage and

the development of unilateral or bilateral paraspinal masses (120).

Extramedullary Hematopoiesis
This is a rare entity but should be kept in mind in any case of a paravertebral mass in a patient with severe anemia. Characteristically, extramedullary hematopoiesis is manifested as multiple paravertebral masses, smooth or lobulated in contour and of homogeneous density, either unilaterally or bilaterally. A presumptive diagnosis can usually be made on the basis of the radiographic appearance in patients with severe anemia and splenomegaly.

Mediastinitis

Acute Mediastinitis

Most cases of acute mediastinitis are either due to esophageal perforation or occur after median sternotomy for cardiac surgery. The diagnosis and management of patients with esophageal perforation have been discussed earlier in this chapter. Rupture or perforation of the trachea or bronchi can also lead to acute mediastinitis. Occasionally, acute mediastinitis results from direct extension of infection from adjacent soft tissues. Prognosis in acute mediastinitis is inversely related to how long it takes to establish the diagnosis. Therapy in all cases consists of immediate surgical drainage in conjunction with high doses of systemic broad-spectrum antibiotics.

Mediastinitis after Cardiac Surgery

The incidence of mediastinitis following median sternotomy is approximately 0.5% to 1% (124). The incidence appears to be higher in obese patients and patients with chronic obstructive lung disease. Most commonly the mediastinitis manifests itself between four and 30 days postoperatively and usually within two weeks of the original procedure. The most common presentation of patients with mediastinitis is wound drainage. Some will have a widened mediastinum on the chest radiograph; at times the patients may present with occult sepsis. The primary diagnostic procedure has been mediastinal needle aspiration, although computed tomography, indium-111 leukocyte scanning, and epicardial pacer wire cultures also appear to be useful (125). Treatment requires immediate drainage, debridement, and parenteral antibiotic therapy. Mortality is in the range of 15% (124).

Granulomatous Mediastinitis and Fibrosing Mediastinitis

These two conditions represent separate ends of a spectrum of chronic granulomatous inflammation of the mediastinum. The mediastinal lymph nodes participate in the primary phase of certain granulomatous infections of the lung. Tuberculosis and histoplasmosis are the most common causes of mediastinal granulomatous disease, but it can also be due to sarcoidosis (Fig. 17.7), silicosis, and other fungal diseases. In the vast majority of patients, the primary infections are relatively asymptomatic and the adenitis subsides spontaneously over a period of weeks to months without untoward incident. However, in some instances there may be considerable periadenitis, and eventually a mediastinal granuloma is formed when a cluster of caseating lymph nodes breaks down into a single mass, which then heals by fibrous encapsulation. The diameter of these mediastinal granulomas ranges from 4 to 10 cm. The thickness of the fibrous capsule, rather than the size of the mass, is the major determinant of structural and functional damage to contiguous organs. The reason that inflammation and fibrosis progress in some individuals but not in others is unknown (120).

In the spectrum from active granulomatous mediastinitis to burned-out mediastinal fibrosis, the former tends to be asymptomatic and to be discovered incidentally on chest roentgenography, while the latter is symptomatic either from a localized mass effect or as a result of the fibrotic process invading or compressing mediastinal structures. Clinical presentations include (a) the superior vena cava syndrome; (b) traction diverticula, disturbances of esophageal motility, or dysphagia from esophageal involvement; (c) obstruction of the trachea or major bronchi; (d) obstruction of the pulmonary artery or proximal pulmonary veins; or (e) involvement of the mediastinal nerves producing hoarseness due to compression of the recurrent laryngeal nerve, diaphragmatic paralysis due to phrenic nerve involvement, or Horner's syndrome from involvement of autonomic ganglions or nerves.

Although most cases of mediastinal fibrosis are thought to represent end stages of chronic granulomatous mediastinitis, there appear to be a few other situations in which this entity occurs. A small percentage of patients have an associated similar fibrotic process elsewhere, such as retroperitoneal fibrosis, pseudotumor of the orbit, Riedel's struma of the thyroid, or ligneous perityphlitis of the cecum. In more than 40 cases, sclerosing mediastinitis has occurred during treatment with methysergide, an antiseritonin drug used for the relief of migraine headaches. In all cases but one, regression occurred when the drug was withdrawn (126).

In most instances, surgical exploration is necessary to distinguish between benign and malignant causes for these clinical manifestations. Occasionally, dense calcification within the mass allows a definite diagnosis without operation. The chest radiograph with granulomatous mediastinitis usually demonstrates a localized mass, usually in the right paratracheal area. Subsequently, with the development of fibrosing mediastinitis, there is generalized widening of the superior portion of the mediastinum. CT may be helpful in demonstrating areas of impingement on mediastinal structures or other abnormalities not evident on plain radiographs (127). MRI is superior in assessing vascular patency without the need for contrast media (120).

Specific therapy for granulomatous mediastinitis or mediastinal fibrosis is generally not indicated. Antituberculous therapy should be initiated if smears or cultures are positive for tuberculosis. If histoplasmosis is demonstrated, amphotericin B need not be administered. Corticosteroids and radiotherapy do not appear to be useful in the treatment of mediastinal fibrosis (128). At the time of exploration for diagnosis, some surgeons advise removal of as much of the inflammatory or fibrous mass as possible, but the efficacy of this practice has not been demonstrated by a controlled clinical trial. Surgery to relieve the obstruction of an airway or a blood vessel is difficult technically but at times is successful (128).

Mediastinal Emphysema

Mediastinal emphysema (pneumomediastinum) is the presence of gas in the interstices of the mediastinum. The primary causes are (a) alveolar rupture with dissection of air into the mediastinum; (b) perforation or rupture of the esophagus, trachea, or main bronchi; and (c) dissection of air from the neck or the abdomen into the mediastinum.

If there is a local increase in alveolar pressure, the alveolus may rupture. Air then enters the interstitial space of the lungs, and if air dissects along interstitial spaces to the hilum and mediastinum, mediastinal emphysema is produced (129). If the air dissects peripherally and the visceral pleura ruptures, a pneumothorax is produced. With mediastinal emphysema, a pneumothorax can also be produced if the mediastinal pleura ruptures.

To produce the local increase in alveolar pressure, there usually needs to be airway disease plus some maneuver such as coughing, vomiting, sneezing, mechanical ventilation, or repeated Valsalva maneuvers to increase alveolar pressure. It follows that mediastinal emphysema is seen in asthmatics and in patients with diabetic ketoacidosis with hyperventilation and pernicious vomiting, and may also occur during childbirth (repeated Valsalva maneuvers), mechanical ventilation, scuba diving, and rapid ascents in airplanes. Pneumomediastinum has been reported in an individual who inhaled cocaine while his partner was applying positive ventilatory pressure (130).

The symptoms associated with pneumomediastinum range from none to severe. Typically, there is severe substernal chest pain with or without radiation into the neck and arms. The pain may be aggravated by respiration or swallowing. Physical examination usually reveals subcutaneous emphysema in the suprasternal notch. *Hamman's sign;* a crunching or clicking noise synchronous with the heartbeat and best heard in the left lateral decubitus position, is present in about 50% of cases. The diagnosis is confirmed by the radiographic demonstration of gas within the mediastinal tissues. In the posteroanterior projection, the mediastinal pleura is displaced laterally, creating a longitudinal line shadow parallel to the heart border and separated from the heart by gas (120).

Usually no treatment is required, but the mediastinal air will be absorbed faster if the patient inspires high concentrations of oxygen. On rare occasions, the mediastinal air can compress the veins in the mediastinum, impeding venous return and leading to hypotension. In such cases, surgical decompression of the mediastinum should be performed, usually through needle aspiration or mediastinotomy just above the suprasternal notch (131).

DISEASES OF THE CHEST WALL

Kyphoscoliosis

Kyphoscoliosis is a combination of excessive anteroposterior and lateral curvature of the thoracic spine. The abnormal curvature may be predominantly lateral (scoliosis) or posterior (kyphosis). Abnormalities of curvature are common, occurring in about 3% of the population. However, deformity of a sufficient degree to lead to symptoms and signs referable to the heart and lungs is rare, occurring in less than 3% of those with abnormal curvature.

Etiology

About 85% of the cases of scoliosis are idiopathic, that is, of no clear origin. Idiopathic scoliosis is classified into one of three types—infantile, juvenile, or adolescent—depending on the age at onset (132). Most cases fall into the adolescent class, in which the onset is between ages 10 and 14. In these patients the curvature increases rapidly in the fast-growth period. The ratio of females to males is 4:1. The second category of kyphoscoliosis is congenital. These cases are related either to abnormalities of the thoracic spine, such as hemivertebrae, or to various hereditary diseases in which deformity of the thoracic spine constitutes only a part of the clinical picture—neurofibromatosis, muscular dystrophy, Friedreich's ataxia, and several others. The third category is neuromuscular, in which kyphoscoliosis develops in response to asymmetrical neuromuscular diseases such as poliomyelitis.

Pathophysiology

The major pathophysiologic effects of severe kyphoscoliosis are restrictive lung disease and ventilation-perfusion imbalances that result in chronic alveolar hypoventilation, hypoxic vasoconstriction, and eventually pulmonary arterial hypertension and cor pulmonale. Pathologic studies of the lungs of patients with kyphoscoliosis and cor pulmonale reveal severe muscular hypertrophy of the pulmonary arter-

ies (133). The genesis of the pulmonary artery hypertension is thought to be chronic hypoxia secondary to regional inhomogeneity of ventilation and perfusion. Arterial hypoxemia may be present in some adolescents with severe kyphoscoliosis, but it becomes more prevalent as the age of the patient increases (134). Older patients with kyphoscoliosis also tend to develop an elevated $PaCO_2$. This elevation is thought to be related to the combination of the increased work of breathing secondary to the skeletal abnormality and the decreased functional capacity of the inspiratory muscles. Indeed, the PaO_2 and the $PaCO_2$ are much more closely correlated with the maximal transdiaphragmatic pressure than with the forced vital capacity or the degree of scoliosis (135).

As would be expected from the deformity of the chest wall, pulmonary function tests reveal a decreased vital capacity and total lung capacity and an increase in residual volume. Flow is reduced only in proportion to the reduction in vital capacity. In addition, the inspiratory muscle function is markedly impaired in patients with severe kyphoscoliosis, presumably from the mechanical disadvantages from the thoracoabdominal deformity.

In general, the degree of scoliosis correlates with the severity of the cardiopulmonary disease. The degree of scoliosis is best quantitated by using the Cobb method to calculate the angle of curvature (Fig. 17.11). In subjects with an angle of curvature less than 60°, there is seldom severe

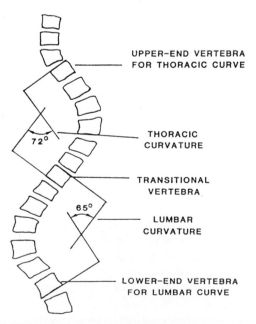

FIGURE 17.11. Cobb method of measuring scoliosis curves. First the "end vertebrae" of the curve are identified. These are the vertebrae that have the maximum tilting toward the curve to be measured. Then horizontal lines are drawn at the superior border of the superior-end vertebra and at the inferior border of the inferior-end vertebra. Then perpendicular lines are erected from each of the horizontal lines. The angle between the intersecting perpendicular lines is the angle of curvature.

ventilatory impairment or significant alteration of blood gases. Individuals with curvatures between 60° and 90° have an increasing frequency of severe ventilatory abnormalities, and most patients with curvatures exceeding 90° develop marked ventilatory abnormalities.

It should be emphasized that there are other factors in addition to the degree of scoliosis that are correlated with the reduction in the vital capacity. Patients with a greater number of vertebrae involved with the scoliosis, with a more cephalad location of the curve, and with loss of the normal thoracic kyphosis will have a greater reduction in the FVC for a given degree of scoliosis (136). Patients with kyphoscoliosis have a reduced work capacity. In one study of 79 patients with a mean Cobb angle of 45 ± 18.5°, the mean work capacity was 86% of predicted. The work capacity correlated better with the vital capacity than with the angle of scoliosis (137).

Clinical Picture

Patients with severe spinal deformity generally present with increasing exertional dyspnea and exercise intolerance. Eventually they may develop a rapidly deteriorating course characterized by recurrent respiratory infections, hypoxia, hypercapnia, and the development of pulmonary hypertension and right heart failure. There may be associated polycythemia secondary to hypoxemia. Respiratory failure rarely appears before the fourth decade. Some adults with severe kyphoscoliosis remain asymptomatic.

Treatment

Much effort has been devoted to restoring the normal curvature of the spine by either internal or external devices. In general, these manipulations result in more improvement in the cosmetic appearance of the patients than in their pulmonary function. Indeed, in one report of 14 patients with a mean age of 26 who underwent surgery, the mean vital capacity actually decreased by 0.21 L postoperatively (138). However, one report of 15 teenagers studied one year after corrective therapy demonstrated that the maximal inspiratory pressure increased by 14 cm H_2O and the peak expiratory flow rate increased by 32% (139). The earlier corrective actions are undertaken, the better the results. Once cardiorespiratory failure has developed, there is a high mortality from operative intervention.

It appears that patients with kyphoscoliosis and recurrent episodes of respiratory failure benefit from chronic nocturnal mechanical ventilation. Studies with substantial follow-up have demonstrated that chronic nocturnal ventilation with either custom-made cuirass negative-pressure ventilators or positive-pressure ventilators can significantly diminish the symptoms of dyspnea on exertion and the signs of cor pulmonale. In addition, the arterial PCO_2 falls markedly, the arterial PO_2 increases, and the pulmonary artery pressures fall (140). Therefore consideration of nocturnal ventilation should be given to all patients with kyphoscoliosis and recurrent respiratory failure. Recent studies have suggested that nasal continuous positive airway pressure (CPAP) with the machines used for treating sleep-disordered breathing is probably the initial therapy of choice (141,142).

Ankylosing Spondylitis

Ankylosing spondylitis is an inherited arthritic condition that ultimately immobilizes the spine. Ankylosis of the posterior intervertebral, costovertebral, and sacroiliac joints and ossification of the spinal ligaments and the margins of the intervertebral disks result in fixation of the thoracic cage. Accordingly, ventilation becomes almost entirely dependent on diaphragmatic movement. Since the diaphragm is the major contributor to ventilation normally, the fixation of the chest wall results in only minimal disability, and respiratory symptoms are uncommon. Patients with ankylosing spondylitis have a mild restrictive ventilatory dysfunction and a normal diffusing capacity. Blood gases remain nearly normal and the lungs are usually normal at autopsy, although some patients develop upper-lobe fibrosis (143).

Pectus Excavatum (Funnel Chest) and Pectus Carinatum (pigeon Breast)

With pectus excavatum, the lower portion of the sternum is displaced posteriorly. The anterior ribs are markedly bowed, which results in a depressed panel in the anterior chest. The intrathoracic structures may be displaced laterally, and this may cause the heart to appear enlarged when actually it is not. Pectus carinatum is the opposite of pectus excavatum, with the sternum protruding anteriorly. The most common cause of acquired pectus carinatum is congenital atrial or ventricular septal defects.

Approximately 50% of individuals with these cardiac defects have a pigeon breast. Severe prolonged childhood asthma is also associated with pectus carinatum. Symptoms referable to these conditions are mainly due to psychological embarrassment from the deformity. Respiratory symptoms are uncommon and pulmonary function tests are nearly normal. The general consensus is that surgical correction is seldom indicated, and then only to prevent psychological upset resulting from the cosmetic deformity (143), although there have been some reports which suggest that exercise tolerance improves after the deformity is corrected surgically (144).

Fractures of Single Ribs

Trauma to the chest is responsible for most rib fractures. Nevertheless, minimal stress can result in fracture of a single rib if the rib is diseased. Ribs affected with bone cysts or metastatic neoplasms may fracture during stresses so slight that they have been unrecognized by the patient. An apparently normal rib may be fractured with modest stress such as from coughing or a passionate embrace. Cough fractures of the ribs occur more often in women than in men and almost invariably involve the sixth to ninth ribs, most often the seventh, and usually in the posterior axillary line.

Typically, the patient with a fractured rib will complain of severe, well-localized chest pain with deep breathing, coughing, stooping, and lifting. Physical examination usually reveals point tenderness over the fractured rib and localization of the pain when pressure is applied over the sternum. Chest radiographs may demonstrate the fracture; however, with nondisplaced fractures, the chest x-ray film is frequently positive only after three to six weeks, when callus formation is established. Therefore the diagnosis should be made on the basis of the history and physical examination.

The treatment of fractured ribs has two goals: to alleviate the chest pain and to prevent secondary disease. The chest pain is probably best treated with systemic analgesics, although these must be administered carefully to patients with chronic obstructive pulmonary disease. Local relief may be provided by a local anesthetic injected at the fracture site or by an intercostal nerve block. Chest strapping to immobilize the ribs may be used, but in general it is not recommended because it is not very effective. The pain and tenderness tend to improve markedly within 10 days regardless of treatment, although some pain on inspiration or cough may persist for up to six months.

Fractures of Multiple Ribs

When multiple rib fractures are present, the chest wall may become unstable; this condition is designated *flail chest*. During inspiration, when the thorax normally expands in all directions, the negative intrapleural pressure will cause the unstable portion of the chest wall to draw in. Similarly, on expiration the unstable portion of the chest wall will move outward with the positive pleural pressure. Frequently the flail chest is not apparent within the first few hours of the injury on account of splinting. Flail chest generally results from fractures of three or more ribs in at least two locations. The major result of flail chest is to diminish the effectiveness of ventilation. The pain from the rib fractures, with the resultant splinting of the chest wall, further impairs ventilation. The major determinant of survival of patients with flail chest is the extent of the associated injuries.

The management of patients with flail chest is difficult and requires a great deal of skill and judgment. Patients with minimal degrees of instability require no ventilatory assistance, but should be observed carefully for the development of atelectasis or pulmonary infections related to the rib fractures. In patients with larger degrees of chest wall instability, mechanical ventilation must be considered. Hy-

poxia can usually be managed with increased concentrations of inspired oxygen. However, if a PaO_2 of 60 mm Hg cannot be maintained or if the $PaCO_2$ starts to increase, intubation and mechanical ventilation should be initiated (145). The mechanical ventilation provides internal fixation of the unstable chest wall. For optimal care, the patient should not be permitted to make an inspiratory effort, since the resulting negative intrapleural pressure would result in retraction of the mobile panel. Although one would expect that controlled ventilation would be necessary until the chest wall becomes fixed, mechanical ventilation can usually be discontinued within 14 days (145). This is probably related to the recovery of the underlying lung from its acute injuries. An alternative approach is to perform a thoracotomy and internally fixate the ribs. Patients treated in the latter fashion tend to have less time on the ventilator (3.9 versus 14 days) and less time in the hospital than do patients treated with intubation and ventilation (146).

DISEASES OF THE DIAPHRAGM

Unilateral Paralysis of the Diaphragm

Diaphragmatic paralysis results from interruption of the nerve supply (the phrenic nerve) to the diaphragm. The most common cause is nerve invasion from malignancy, usually a bronchogenic carcinoma. The second most common category of diaphragmatic paralysis is that for which no etiology can be detected. An increasingly common cause is open heart surgery. Injury to the phrenic nerve, almost always the left, occurs in approximately 20% of open heart surgery patients and is attributed to the use of cold cardioplegic solutions or stretching of the nerve. The paralysis disappears within 12 months in about two-thirds of patients (147). Benign causes of diaphragmatic paralysis include poliomyelitis, herpes zoster, Huntington's chorea, injuries or diseases of the cervical vertebrae, diphtheria, lead poisoning, tetanus antitoxin, measles, pulmonary infarction, pneumonia, mediastinitis, and pericarditis (148).

The diagnosis of unilateral paralysis of the diaphragm is suggested by finding an elevated hemidiaphragm on the chest roentgenogram. With diaphragmatic paralysis, the negative pleural pressure tends to pull the paralyzed diaphragm upward. Normally, the right diaphragmatic dome is on a plane approximately half an interspace above the left. In a review of 500 normal subjects by Felson (149), the right diaphragm was more than 3 cm higher than the left in 2%. However, the left diaphragm was at the same height or higher than the right in 9%. Confirmation of diaphragmatic paralysis is best established with the "sniff test." In this test the diaphragm is observed fluoroscopically as the patient sniffs. The normal diaphragm will move downward during the sniff maneuver as the diaphragmatic muscles contract. A paralyzed diaphragm will move paradoxically upward because of the negative pleural pressure (148). With a normal large breath, a paralyzed diaphragm may move downward because of the change in the configuration of the chest wall. The diagnosis of a paralyzed diaphragm can also be made with ultrasonography (150).

Patients with a paralyzed diaphragm may be asymptomatic or may complain of dyspnea on effort. Pulmonary function testing reveals that the vital capacity and the total lung capacity are reduced by about 25%. In addition, the maximal transdiaphragmatic pressure is reduced by about 50%, and the maximal inspiratory pressure is reduced by about 40% (151).

The management of patients with diaphragmatic paralysis depends on the likely diagnosis. For example, a hilar mass in conjunction with diaphragmatic paralysis suggests bronchogenic carcinoma and serves as an indication for bronchoscopy. In patients post–coronary artery surgery, the paralysis will usually resolve within one year. In asymptomatic patients with normal chest roentgenograms save for the diaphragmatic paralysis, probably no invasive procedures are warranted. In one report of 142 such patients, the diaphragmatic paralysis persisted in more than 90%, but over a mean follow-up period of nearly 10 years, only 4% developed intrathoracic malignancy (152).

Bilateral Paralysis or Paresis of the Diaphragm

The presence of bilateral diaphragmatic paralysis or severe paresis almost always causes severe morbidity in adults. The most common causes include high spinal cord injury, thoracic trauma (including cardiac surgery), multiple sclerosis, anterior horn cell disease, and muscular dystrophy.

Most patients with severe diaphragmatic weakness will present with hypercapnic respiratory failure, frequently complicated by cor pulmonale and right ventricular failure, atelectasis, and pneumonia. Most will have dyspnea at rest that is worse in the supine position. Anxiety, insomnia, and excessive daytime somnolence are common, as is morning headache. The characteristic physical finding is Hoover's sign, which is a paradoxical inward motion of the anterior abdominal wall on inspiration which is most readily detectable in the supine position. The chest roentgenogram usually shows elevation of both hemidiaphragms, and the respiratory excursion of the diaphragm is usually minimal or absent.

The degree of diaphragmatic weakness is best quantitated by measuring transdiaphragmatic pressures. Probably the best measure is the transdiaphragmatic pressure generated during a sniff maneuver. Normally, this pressure is greater than 98 cm H_2O, but in patients with diaphragmatic weakness the pressure may be less than 20 cm H_2O. The transdiaphragmatic pressures generated during the sniff maneuver appear to be more reproducible than the maximal transdiaphragmatic pressure at total lung capacity or functional re-

sidual capacity. In patients with severe diaphragmatic weakness, the forced vital capacity diminishes from the seated to the supine position. A decrease of more than 30% is suggestive of severe diaphragmatic weakness (153). The maximal inspiratory pressure at the mouth is also reduced proportional to the diaphragmatic weakness (153).

The clinical course of patients with bilateral diaphragmatic weakness (and accordingly, the treatment) depends on the underlying disease. There can be recovery of diaphragmatic function when the nerve injury is not permanent. A good example of such recovery is that which occurs in patients who have bilateral diaphragmatic paralysis after cardiac surgery (153). In such patients it may take six or more months for recovery to occur. In such cases nasal intermittent positive airway pressure at night may be helpful until recovery (153). Most patients with progressive neuromuscular disease eventually require mechanical ventilation to maintain adequate ventilation.

Diaphragmatic Pacing

This is one alternative that can be considered in patients in whom the primary problem is above the anterior horn cell and the phrenic nerve is intact—for example, a patient with a high cervical spinal cord lesion. Before pacing is seriously considered, one must document the functional integrity of the phrenic nerve. This can be done by measuring the velocity of conduction of an electrical pulse delivered percutaneously in the neck and recorded as the diaphragm action potential. This is best done by recording the diaphragmatic electromyelogram with an esophageal electrode and measuring the transdiaphragmatic pressure (154).

Once the functional integrity of the phrenic nerve has been demonstrated, consideration can be given to implanting a permanent diaphragmatic pacer. There are three different systems currently available, and each costs approximately $30,000. If continuous ventilation is required, bilateral pacers must be implanted, since one can stimulate a phrenic nerve continuously only for about 12 hours. It should be emphasized that even in centers with much experience with diaphragmatic pacing, the outcome is not always successful. In one series of 81 patients in whom diaphragmatic pacers were implanted, only 38 (47%) were fully successful in that no other method of ventilatory support was needed (155).

Eventration

Eventration is a congenital anomaly resulting from faulty muscular development of part or all of one or both diaphragms. The eventrated diaphragm consists of a thin membranous sheet attached peripherally to normal muscle at points of origin from the rib cage. Radiologically, eventration cannot be distinguished from diaphragmatic paralysis. However, a previously normal chest x-ray will rule out eventration. If the eventration is complete, consideration should be given to diaphragmatic plication. With this procedure, the redundant fibrous tissue is folded on itself and stitched laterally to the chest wall so that the dome becomes almost flat.

Hiccup

A hiccup is an involuntary spasm of the inspiratory muscles followed by an abrupt closure of the glottis, which is responsible for the characteristic sound. Hiccups are usually precipitated by irritation of the diaphragm. This is most commonly due to gastric distention or inflammation following rapid or excessive eating or drinking. Hiccups also occur in other conditions in which the vagus nerve is stimulated, such as inferior wall myocardial infarction, peritonitis, pleurisy, pericarditis, and mediastinitis. Hiccups may be troublesome in uremia, in which instance they are thought to have a central origin.

Although hiccups are usually of short duration and resolve spontaneously, long-continued hiccups can be a serious symptom and a manifestation of important disease. Engleman's treatment with granulated sugar is very effective and consists of having the patient swallow 1 teaspoon of ordinary white, granulated, dry sugar (156). If this does not work, the stomach can be decompressed with a nasogastric tube in conjunction with pharyngeal irritation. The next step is to administer chlorpromazine, 25 to 50 mg intravenously. If this works, the drug should be administered orally 10 to 20 mg every four to six hours for 10 days. In cases of intractable hiccups (daily hiccup present for at least six months), the administration of baclofen, an analogue of γ-amino-butyric acid at a dose of 10 mg t.i.d. will significantly reduce the severity of the hiccup and increase the percentage of the hiccup-free periods (157).

REFERENCES

1. Albertine KH, Wiener-Kronish JP, Roos RJ, et al. Structure, blood supply, and lymphatic vessels of the sheep's visceral pleura. *Am J Anat* 1982;165:277–294.
2. Albertine KH, Wiener-Kronish JP, Staub NC. The structure of the parietal pleura and its relationship to pleural liquid dynamics in sheep. *Anat Rec* 1984;208:401–409.
3. Negrini D, Townsley MI, Taylor AE. Hydraulic conductivity of the canine parietal pleura in vivo. *J Appl Physiol* 1990;69:438–442.
4. Bhattacharya J, Gropper MA, Staub NC. Interstitial fluid pressure gradient measured by micropuncture in excised dog lung. *J Appl Physiol* 1984;56:271–277.
5. Wiener-Kronish JP, Broaddus VC, Albertine KH, et al. Relationship of pleural effusions to increased permeability pulmonary edema in anesthetized sheep. *J Clin Invest* 1988;82:1422–1429.
6. Broaddus VC, Wiener-Kronish JP, Staub NC. Clearance of lung edema into the pleural space of volume-loaded, anesthetized sheep. *J Appl Physiol* 1990;68:2623–2630.
7. Wiener-Kronish JP, Matthay MA, Callen PW, et al. Relationship of pleural effusions to pulmonary hemodynamics in patients with congestive heart failure. *Am Rev Respir Dis* 1985;132:1253–1256.
8. Broaddus C, Staub NC. Pleural liquid and protein turnover in health and disease. *Semin Respir Med* 1987;9:7–12.
9. Light RW, Stansbury DW, Brown SE. The relationship between pleural pressures and changes in pulmonary function following therapeutic thoracentesis. *Am Rev Respir Dis* 1986;133:658–661.
10. McLoud TC, Flower CD. Imaging the pleura: sonography, CT, and MR imaging. *AJR* 1991;156:1145–1153.
11. Weiss JM, Spodick DH. Laterality of pleural effusions in chronic congestive heart failure. *Am J Cardiol* 1984;53:951.
12. Shinto RA, Light RW. The effects of diuresis upon the characteristics of pleural fluid in patients with congestive heart failure. *Am J Med* 1990;88:230–233.
13. Lieberman FL, Hidemura R, Peters RL, et al. Pathogenesis and treatment of hydrothorax complicating cirrhosis with ascites. *Ann Intern Med* 1966;64:341–351.
14. Gordon FD, Anastopoulos HT, Crenshaw W, et al. The successful treatment of symptomatic, refractory hepatic hydrothorax with transjugular intrahepatic portosystemic shunt. *Hepatology* 1997;25:1366–1369.
15. Mouroux J, Perrin C, Venissac N, et al. Management of pleural effusion of cirrhotic origin. *Chest* 1996;109:1093–1096.
16. Weiss JM, Spodick DH. Association of left pleural effusion with pericardial disease. *N Engl J Med* 1983;308:696–697.
17. Kinasewitz GT. Transudative effusions. *Eur Respir J* 1997;10:714–718.
18. Light RW. *Pleural diseases,* 3rd ed. Baltimore: Williams & Wilkins, 1995.
19. Di Bisceglie M, Paladini P, Voltolini L, et al. Videothoracoscopic obliteration of pleuroperitoneal fistula in continuous peritoneal dialysis. *Ann Thorac Surg* 1996;62:1509–1510.
20. Light RW, Girard WM, Jenkinson SG, et al. Parapneumonic effusions. *Am J Med* 1980;69:507–511.
21. Light RW. The management of parapneumonic effusion and empyema. *Curr Opin Pulm Med* 1998;4:227–229.
22. Morgenroth A, Pleuffer HP, Seelmann R, et al. Pleural penetration of ciprofloxacin in patients with empyema thoracis. *Chest* 1991;100:406–409.
23. Davies RJO, Traill ZC, Gleeson FV. Randomised controlled trial of intrapleural streptokinase in community acquired pleural infection. *Thorax* 1997;52:416–421.
24. Bouros D, Schiza S, Tzanakis N, et al. Intrapleural urokinase vs normal saline in the treatment of complicated parapneumonic effusions and empyema: a randomized, double-blind study. *Am J Respir Crit Care Med* 1999;159:37–42.
25. Wait MA, Sharma S, Hohn J, et al. A randomized trial of empyema therapy. *Chest* 1997;111:1548–1551.
26. Silen ML, Naunheim KS. Thoracoscopic approach to the management of empyema thoracis. Indications and results. *Chest Surg Clin N Am* 1996;6:491–499.
27. Mehta JB, Dutt A, Harvill L, et al. Epidemiology of extrapulmonary tuberculosis. *Chest* 1991;99:1134–1138.
28. Mlika-Cabanne N, Brauner M, Mugusi F, et al. Radiographic abnormalities in tuberculosis and risk of coexisting human immunodeficiency virus infection. *Am J Respir Crit Care Med* 1995;152:786–793.
29. Rossi GA, Balbi B, Manca FP. Tuberculous pleural effusions: evidence for selective presence of PPD-specific T-lymphocytes at site of inflammation in the early phase of the infection. *Am Rev Respir Dis* 1987;136:575–579.
30. Patiala J. Initial tuberculous pleuritis in the Finnish armed forces

in 1939–1945 with special reference to eventual post-pleuritic tuberculosis. *Acta Tuberc Scand Suppl* 1957;36:1–57.

31. Light RW. Closed needle biopsy of the pleura was important in its time, but should be relegated to the archives of medical history. *J Bronchol* 1998;5:332–336.

32. Valdes L, Alvarez D, San Jose E, et al. Tuberculous pleurisy: a study of 254 patients. *Arch Intern Med* 158:2017–2021, 1998.

33. Villena V, Lopez-Encuentra A, Echave-Sustaeta J, et al. Interferon-gamma in 388 immunocompromised and immunocompetent patients for diagnosing pleural tuberculosis. *Eur Respir J* 1996;9:2635–2639.

34. Querol JM, Minguez J, Garcia-Sanchez E, et al. Rapid diagnosis of pleural tuberculosis by polymerase chain reaction. *Am J Respir Crit Care Med* 1995;152;1977–1981.

35. Hillerdal G. Pulmonary aspergillus infection invading the pleura. *Thorax* 1981;36:745–751.

36. Lonky SA, Catanzaro A, Moser KM, et al. Acute coccidioidal pleural effusion. *Am Rev Respir Dis* 1976;114:681–688.

37. Cunningham RT, Einstein H. Coccidioidal pulmonary cavities with rupture. *J Thorac Cardiovasc Surg* 1982;84:172–177.

38. Conces DJ Jr, Vix VA, Tarver RD. Pleural cryptococcosis. *J Thorac Imaging* 1990;5:84–86.

39. Fine NL, Smith LR, Sheedy PF. Frequency of pleural effusions in mycoplasma and viral pneumonias. *N Engl J Med* 1970;282:790–793.

40. Drugs for parasitic infections. *Med Lett Drugs Ther* 1998;40:1–12.

41. Johnson RJ, Johnson JR. Paragonimiasis in Indochinese refugees. *Am Rev Respir Dis* 1983;128:534–538.

42. Wen H, New RRC, Craig PS. Diagnosis and treatment of human hydatidosis. *Br J Clin Pharmacol* 1993;35:565–574.

43. Cheng D-S, Rodriguez RM, Perkett EA, et al. Vascular endothelial growth factor in pleural fluid. *Chest* 1999;115:760–765.

44. Meyer P. Metastatic carcinoma of the pleura. *Thorax* 1966;21:437–443.

45. Light RW. Useful tests on the pleural fluid in the management of patients with pleural effusions. *Curr Opin Pulm Med* 1999;5:245–249.

46. Light RW, Erozan Y, Ball WC Jr. Cells in pleural fluid. *Arch Intern Med* 1973;132:854–860.

47. Poe RW, Israel RH, Utell MJ, et al. Sensitivity, specificity, and predictive values of closed pleural biopsy. *Arch Intern Med* 1984;144:325–328.

48. Hartman DL, Gaither JM, Kesler KA, et al. Comparison of insufflated talc under thoracoscopic guidance with standard tetracycline and bleomycin pleurodesis for control of malignant pleural effusions. *J Thorac Cardiovasc Surg* 1993;105:743–748.

49. Milanez Campos JR, Werebe EC, Vargas FS, et al. Respiratory failure due to insufflated talc. *Lancet* 1997;349:251–252.

50. Rehse DH, Aye RW, Florence MG. Respiratory failure following talc pleurodesis. *Am J Surg* 1999;177:437–40.

51. Walker-Renard, Vaughan LM, Sahn SA. Chemical pleurodesis for malignant pleural effusions. *Ann Intern Med* 1994;120:56–64.

52. Vargas FS, Wang N-S, Lee HM, et al. Effectiveness of bleomycin in comparison to tetracycline as pleural sclerosing agent in rabbits. *Chest* 1993;104:1582–1584.

53. Light RW, O'Hara VS, Moritz TE, et al. Intrapleural tetracycline for the prevention of recurrent spontaneous pneumothorax. *JAMA* 1990;264:2224–2230.

54. Vargas FS, Teixeira LR, Coelho IJC, et al. Distribution of pleural injectate: effect of volume of injectate and animal rotation. *Chest* 1994;106:2146–2149.

55. Putnam JB, Light RW, Rodriguez RM, et al. Randomized comparison of indwelling pleural catheter with doxycycline pleurodesis in the management of malignant pleural effusions. *Cancer* 1999;86:1992–1999.

56. Patz EF Jr, McAdams HP, Goodman PC, et al. Ambulatory sclerotherapy for malignant pleural effusions. *Radiology* 1996;199:133–135.

57. Light RW, Rodriguez RM. Factors predicting spontaneous pleurodesis in patients with indwelling pleural catheters. *Eur Respir J* 1998;12:238S.

58. Little AG, Kadowaki MH, Ferguson MK, et al. Pleuro-peritoneal shunting: alternative therapy for pleural effusions. *Ann Surg* 1988;208:443–450.

59. Herndon JE, Green MR, Chahinian AP, et al. Factors predictive of survival among 337 patients with mesothelioma treated between 1984 and 1994 by the Cancer and Leukemia Group B. *Chest* 1998;113:723–731.

60. De Pangher Manzini V, Brollo A, Franceschi S, et al. Prognostic factors of malignant mesothelioma of the pleura. *Cancer* 1993;72:410–417.

61. Boutin C, Rey F. Thoracoscopy in pleural malignant mesothelioma: a prospective study of 188 consecutive patients. Part 1: diagnosis. *Cancer* 1993;72:389–393.

62. Antman KH. Natural history and epidemiology of malignant mesothelioma. *Chest* 1993;103[Suppl 4]:373S–376S.

63. Brown RW, Clark GM, Tandon AK, et al. Multiple-marker immunohistochemical phenotypes distinguishing malignant pleural mesothelioma from pulmonary adenocarcinoma. *Hum Pathol* 1993;24:347–354.

64. Ruffie PA. Pleural mesothelioma. *Curr Opin Oncol* 1991;3:328–334.

65. Briselli M, Mark EJ, Dickersin GR. Solitary fibrous tumors of the pleura: Eight new cases and review of 360 cases in the literature. *Cancer* 1981;47:2678–2689.

66. Nador RG, Cesarman E, Chadburn A, et al. Primary effusion lymphoma: a distinct clinicopathologic entity associated with the Kaposi's sarcoma-associated herpes virus. *Blood* 1996;88:645–656.

67. Taniere P, Manai A, Charpentier R, et al. Pyothorax-associated lymphoma: relationship with Epstein-Barr virus, human herpes virus-8 and body cavity-based high grade lymphomas. *Eur Respir J* 1998;11:779–783.

68. Halla JT, Schrohenloher RE, Volanakis JE. Immune complexes and other laboratory features of pleural effusions. A comparison of rheumatoid arthritis, systemic lupus erythematosus and other disease. *Ann Intern Med* 1980;92:748–752.

69. Khare V, Baethge B, Lang S, et al. Antinuclear antibodies in pleural fluid. *Chest* 1994;106:866–871.

70. Chapman PT, O'Donnell JL, Moller PW. Rheumatoid pleural effusion: response to intrapleural corticosteroid. *Rheumatol* 1992;19:478–480.

71. Stein PD, Henry JW. Clinical characteristics of patients with acute pulmonary embolism stratified according to their presenting syndromes. *Chest* 1997;112:974–979.

72. Coche EE, Muller NL, Kim KI, et al. Acute pulmonary embolism: ancillary findings at spiral CT. *Radiology* 1998;207:753–758.

73. Johnson PT, Wechsler RJ, Salazar AM, et al. Spiral CT of acute pulmonary thromboembolism: evaluation of pleuroparenchymal abnormalities. *J Comput Assist Tomogr* 1999;23:369–373.

74. Lankisch PG, Groge M, Becher R. Pleural effusions: a new negative prognostic parameter for acute pancreatitis. *Am J Gastroenterol* 1994;89:1849–1851.

75. Rockey DC, Cello JP. Pancreaticopleural fistula. Report of 7 patients and review of the literature. *Medicine* 1990;69:332–344.

76. Sherr HP, Light RW, Merson MH, et al. Origin of pleural

fluid amylase in esophageal rupture. *Ann Intern Med* 1972;76: 985–986.

77. Bufkin BL, Miller JI Jr, Mansour KA. Esophageal perforation: emphasis on management. *Ann Thorac Surg* 1996;61: 1447–1451.

78. Voros D, Gouliamos A, Kotoulas G, et al. Percutaneous drainage of intra-abdominal abscesses using large lumen tubes under computed tomographic control *Eur J Surg* 1996;162:895–898.

79. Peng M-J, Vargas FS, Cukier A, et al. Postoperative pleural changes after coronary revascularization. Comparison between saphenous vein and internal mammary artery grafting. *Chest* 1992;101:327–330.

80. Rodriguez RM, Moyers JP, Rogers JT, et al. Incidence of pleural effusions 30 days post coronary artery bypass surgery. *Chest* 1998;114:387S.

81. Light RW, Rogers JT, Cheng D-S, et al. Large pleural effusions occurring after coronary artery bypass grafting. *Ann Intern Med* 1999;130:891–896.

82. Sadikot RT, Wheeler AP, Cheng DS, et al. Cytokines in Post-CABG pleural effusions. *Am J Respir Crit Care Med* 1999;159: 389A.

83. Light RW, George RB. Incidence and significance of pleural effusion after abdominal surgery. *Chest* 1976;69:621–626.

84. Medina LS, Siegel MJ, Bejarano PA, et al. Pediatric lung transplantation: radiographic-histologic correlation. *Radiology* 1993; 187:807–810.

85. Spizarny DL, Gross BH, McLoud T. Enlarging pleural effusion after liver transplantation. *J Thorac Imaging* 1993;8:85–87.

86. Uetsuji S, Komada Y, Kwon AH, et al. Prevention of pleural effusion after hepatectomy using fibrin sealant. *Int Surg* 1994; 79:135–137.

87. Edling JE, Bacon BR. Pleuropulmonary complications of endoscopic variceal sclerotherapy. *Chest* 1991;99:1252–1257.

88. Morelock SY, Sahn SA. Drugs and the pleura. Chest 1999;116: 212–221.

89. Epler GR, McLoud TC, Gaensler EA. Prevalence and incidence of benign asbestos pleural effusion in a working population. *JAMA* 1982;247:617–622.

90. Hillerdal G, Ozesmi M. Benign asbestos pleural effusion: 73 exudates in 60 patients. *Eur J Respir Dis* 1987;71:113–121.

91. Lemming R. Meigs' syndrome and pathogenesis of pleurisy and polyserositis. *Acta Med Scand* 1960;168:197–204.

92. Taylor JR, Ryu J, Colby TV, et al. Lymphangioleiomyomatosis: clinical course in 32 patients. *N Engl J Med* 1990;323: 1254–1260.

93. Kalassian KG, Doyle R, Kao P, et al. Lymphangioleiomyomatosis: New insights. *Am J Respir Crit Care Med* 1997;155: 1183–1186.

94. Berger HW, Rammohan G, Neff MS, et al. Uremic pleural effusion: study in 14 patients on chronic dialysis. *Ann Intern Med* 1975;82:362–364.

95. Coskun M, Boyvat F, Bozkurt B, et al. Thoracic CT findings in long-term hemodialysis patients. *Acta Radiol* 1998;40:181–186.

96. Light RW, Jenkinson SG, Minh VD, et al. Observations on pleural fluid pressures as fluid is withdrawn during thoracentesis. *Am Rev Respir Dis* 1980;121:799–804.

97. Stelzner TJ, King TE Jr, Antony VB, et al. The pleuropulmonary manifestations of postcardiac injury syndrome. *Chest* 1983; 84:383–388.

98. Nordkild P, Kromann-Andersen H, Stuve-Christensen E. Yellow nail syndrome—the triad of yellow nails, lymphedema and pleural effusions. *Acta Med Scand* 1986;219:221–227.

99. Nicholls AJ, Friend JAR, Legge JS. Sarcoid pleural effusion: three cases and review of the literature. *Thorax* 1980;35: 277–281.

100. Baron RL, Stark DD, McClennan BL, et al. Intrathoracic extension of retroperitoneal urine collections. *AJR* 1981;137:37–41.

101. Romero S, Martin C, Hernandez L, et al. Chylothorax in cirrhosis of the liver: analysis of its frequency and clinical characteristics. *Chest* 1998;114:154–159.

102. Murphy MC, Newman BM, Rodgers BM. Pleuroperitoneal shunts in the management of persistent chylothorax. *Ann Thorac Surg* 1989;48:195–200.

103. Hillerdal G. The pathogenesis of pleural plaques and pulmonary asbestosis: possibilities and impossibilities. *Eur J Respir Dis* 1980;61:129–138.

104. Wilson JM, Boren CH Jr, Peterson SR, et al. Traumatic hemothorax: is decortication necessary? *J Thorac Cardiovasc Surg* 1979;77:489–495.

105. Carrillo EH, Richardson JD. Thoracoscopy in the management of hemothorax and retained blood after trauma. *Curr Opin Pulm Med* 1998;4:243–246.

106. Light RW. Management of spontaneous pneumothorax. *Am Rev Respir Dis* 1993;148:245–248.

107. Bertrand PC, Regnard JF, Spaggiari L, et al. Immediate and long-term results after surgical treatment of primary spontaneous pneumothorax by VATS. *Ann Thorac Surg* 1996;61: 1641–1645.

108. Jones KW, Pietra GG, Sabiston DC Jr. Primary neoplasms and cysts of the mediastinum. In: Fishman AP, ed. *Pulmonary diseases and disorders.* New York: McGraw-Hill, 1980:1490.

109. Lyons HA, Calvy GL, Sammons BP. The diagnosis and classification of mediastinal masses. A study of 782 cases. *Ann Intern Med* 1959;51:897–932.

110. Brown LR, Aughenbaugh GL. Masses of the anterior mediastinum. CT and MR imaging. *AJR* 1991;157:1171–1180.

111. Morrissey B, Adams H, Gibbs AR, et al. Percutaneous needle biopsy of the mediastinum: review of 94 procedures. *Thorax* 1993;48:632–637.

112. Widstrom A, Schnurer L. The value of mediastinoscopy—experience of 374 cases. *J Otolaryngol* 1978;7:103–109.

113. Best LA, Munichor M, Ben-Shakhar M, et al. The contribution of anterior mediastinotomy in the diagnosis and evaluation of diseases of the mediastinum and lung. *Ann Thorac Surg* 1987; 43:78–81.

114. Strollo DDC, Rosado de Christenson ML, Jett JR. Primary mediastinal tumors. Part 1. Tumors of the anterior mediastinum. *Chest* 1997;112:511–522.

115. Gripp S, Hilgers K, Wurm R, et al. Thymoma. Prognostic factors and treatment outcome. *Cancer* 1998;83:1495–1503.

116. Wychulis AR, Payne WS, Clagett OF, et al. Surgical treatment of mediastinal tumors. A 40 year experience. *J Thorac Cardiovasc Surg* 1971;62:379–392.

117. Strollo DC, Rosado de Christenson ML, Jett JR. Primary mediastinal tumors. Part II. Tumors of the middle and posterior mediastinum. *Chest* 1997;112:1344–1357.

118. Nichols CR. Mediastinal germ cell tumors. Clinical features and biologic correlate. *Chest* 1991;99:472–479.

119. Wax MK, Briant TDR. The management of substernal goiter. *J Otolaryngol* 1992;21:165–170.

120. Fraser RS, Muller NL, Colman N, et al. Masses situated predominantly in the middle-posterior mediastinal compartment. In: *Diagnosis of diseases of the chest,* 4th ed. Philadelphia: WB Saunders, 1999:2738–2972.

121. Salyer DC, Salyer WR, Eggleston JC. Benign developmental cysts of the mediastinum. *Arch Pathol Lab Med* 1977;101: 136–139.

122. Cioffi U, Bonavina L, De Simone M, et al. Presentation and surgical management of bronchogenic and esophageal duplication cysts in adults. *Chest* 1998;113:1492–1496.

123. Shin MS, Mulligan SA, Baxley WA, et al. Bochdalek hernia of

diaphragm in the adult. Diagnosis by computed tomography. *Chest* 1987;92:1098–1101.

124. El Oakley R, Paul E, Wong PS, et al. Mediastinitis in patients undergoing cardiopulmonary bypass: risk analysis and midterm results. *J Cardiovasc Surg* 1997;38:595–600.

125. Browdie DA, Bernstein RW, Agnew R, et al. Diagnosis of poststernotomy infection: comparison of three means of assessment. *Ann Thorac Surg* 1991;51:290–292.

126. DuPont HL, Varco RL, Winchell CP. Chronic fibrous mediastinitis simulating pulmonic stenosis, associated with inflammatory pseudotumor of the orbit. *Am J Med* 1968;44:447–452.

127. Loyd JE, Tillman BF, Atkinson JB, et al. Mediastinal fibrosis complicating histoplasmosis. *Medicine* 1988;67:295–310.

128. Kalweit G, Huwer H, Straub U, et al. Mediastinal compression syndromes due to idiopathic fibrosing mediastinitis—Report of three cases and review of the literature. *Thorac Cardiovasc Surg* 1996;44:105–109.

129. Macklin MT, Macklin CC. Malignant interstitial emphysema of the lungs and mediastinum as an important occult complication in many respiratory diseases and other conditions: an interpretation of the clinical literature in the light of laboratory experiment. *Medicine* 1944;23:281–352.

130. Adrouny A, Magnusson P. Pneumopericardium from cocaine inhalation. *N Engl J Med* 1985;313:48–49.

131. Maunder RJ, Pierson DJ, Hudson LD. Subcutaneous and mediastinal emphysema. *Arch Intern Med* 1984;144:1447–1453.

132. Bergofsky EH, Turino GM, Fishman AP. Cardiorespiratory failure in kyphoscoliosis. *Medicine* 1959;38:263–317.

133. Fraser RS, Muller NL, Colman N, et al. Diseases of the diaphragm and chest wall. In: *Diagnosis of diseases of the chest,* 4th ed. Philadelphia: WB Saunders, 1999:2985–3042.

134. Kafer ER. Idiopathic scoliosis. Gas exchange and the age dependence of arterial blood gases. *J Clin Invest* 1976;58:825–833.

135. Lisboa C, Moreno R, Fava M, et al. Inspiratory muscle function in patients with severe kyphoscoliosis. *Am Rev Respir Dis* 1985;132:48–52.

136. Kearon C, Viviani G, Kirkley A, et al. Factors determining pulmonary function in adolescent idiopathic thoracic scoliosis. *Am Rev Respir Dis* 1993;148:288–294.

137. Kearon C, Viviani GR, Killian KJ. Factors influencing work capacity in adolescent idiopathic thoracic scoliosis. *Am Rev Respir Dis* 1993;148:295–303.

138. Wong CA, Cole AA, Watson L, et al. Pulmonary function before and after anterior spinal surgery in adults idiopathic scoliosis. *Thorax* 1999;51:534–536.

139. Cooper D, Rojas J, Mellins R, et al. Respiratory mechanics in adolescents with idiopathic scoliosis. *Am Rev Respir Dis* 1984;130:16–22.

140. Hoeppner V, Cockcroft D, Dosman J, et al. Nighttime ventilation improves respiratory failure in secondary kyphoscoliosis. *Am Rev Respir Dis* 1984;129:240–243.

141. Hill NS. Noninvasive ventilation. Does it work, for whom, and how? *Am Rev Respir Dis* 1993;147:1050–1055.

142. Leger P, Bedicam JM, Cornette A, et al. Nasal intermittent positive pressure ventilation. *Chest* 1994;105:100–105.

143. Lee-Chiong TL Jr. Pulmonary manifestations of ankylosing spondylitis and relapsing polychondritis. *Clin Chest Med* 1998;19:747–757.

144. Fonkalsrud EW, Bustorff-Silva J. Repair of pectus excavatum and carinatum in adults. *Am J Surg* 1999;177:121–124.

145. Shackford SR, Virgilio RW, Peters RM. Selective use of ventilator therapy in flail chest injury. *J Thorac Cardiovasc Surg* 1981;81:194–201.

146. Ahmed Z, Mohyuddin Z. Management of flail chest injury: internal fixation versus endotracheal intubation and ventilation. *J Thorac Cardiovasc Surg* 1995;110:1676–1680.

147. Efthimiou J, Butler J, Woodham C, et al. Diaphragm paralysis following cardiac surgery: role of phrenic nerve cold injury. *Ann Thorac Surg* 1991;52:1005–1008.

148. Gierada DS, Slone RM, Fleishman MJ. Imaging evaluation of the diaphragm. *Chest Surg Clin N Am* 1998;6:237–280.

149. Felson B. *Chest roentgenology.* Philadelphia. WB Saunders, 1973.

150. Gottesman E, McCool FD. Ultrasound evaluation of the paralyzed diaphragm. *Am J Respir Crit Care Med* 1997;155:1570–1574.

151. Lisboa C, Paré PD, Pertuze J, et al. Inspiratory muscle function in unilateral diaphragmatic paralysis. *Am Rev Respir Dis* 1986;134:488–492.

152. Piehler JM, Pairolero PC, Gracey DR, et al. Unexplained diaphragmatic paralysis: a harbinger of malignant disease? *J Thorac Cardiovasc Surg* 1982;84:861–864.

153. Mier-Jedrzejowica A, Brophy C, Moxham J, et al. Assessment of diaphragm weakness. *Am Rev Respir Dis* 1988;137:877–883.

154. Moxham J, Shneerson JM. Diaphragmatic pacing. *Am Rev Respir Dis* 1993;148:533–536.

155. Glenn WW, Phelps ML, Elefteriades JA, et al. Twenty years of experience in phrenic nerve stimulation to pace the diaphragm. *PACE* 1986;9:780–784.

156. Engleman EG, Lankton J, Lankton B. Granulated sugar as treatment for hiccups in conscious patients. *N Engl J Med* 1971;285:1489.

157. Ramirez FC, Graham DY. Treatment of intractable hiccup with baclofen. Results of a double-blind randomized, controlled, cross-over study. *Am J Gastroenterol* 1992;87:1789–1791.

18

SLEEP-RELATED BREATHING DISORDERS

RICHARD B. BERRY

SLEEP ARCHITECTURE

VENTILATION AND SLEEP

RESPIRATORY DEFINITIONS

SLEEP MONITORING
Multiple Sleep Latency Test

SLEEP DISORDERS CAUSING EXCESSIVE DAYTIME SLEEPINESS
Narcolepsy
Idiopathic Hypersomnia
Insufficient Sleep Syndrome
Periodic Limb Movement Disorder
Sleep Apnea Syndromes
Sleep and Asthma
Sleep and Chronic Obstructive Pulmonary Disease

In the last few decades there has been an explosion of knowledge about sleep and sleep disorders. Consequently, the topic of sleep disorders is much too broad to be covered in any detail in a single chapter. Therefore the goal of this chapter is to present the elements of sleep physiology and monitoring that are relevant to sleep-related breathing disorders and to discuss these disorders with an emphasis on the sleep apnea syndromes.

SLEEP ARCHITECTURE

Sleep is not a homogeneous state and therefore has been divided into sleep stages. This is relevant for the study of breathing during sleep, because each stage has a characteristic impact on respiration. Furthermore, disease processes frequently alter not only the total sleep time but also the relative amount of time spent in the various sleep stages.

Sleep is composed of non–rapid eye movement (NREM) sleep and rapid eye movement (REM) sleep. NREM sleep is further divided into stages 1 to 4. Stages 1 and 2 are referred to as light sleep and stages 3 and 4 as deep or slow-wave sleep. A given night of sleep is divided into periods of time called epochs (usually 30 seconds in duration). The predominant stage in a given epoch names that epoch. Staging is based on electroencephalographic (EEG), electrooculographic (EOG), that is, eye movement, and electromyographic (EMG) criteria (1–5).

While only central EEG electrodes (C_3 and C_4) are required to stage sleep, occipital leads (O_1 and O_2) are also commonly used (Fig. 18.1). The odd and even numbers refer to the left and right sides of the body, respectively. EEG recording for sleep monitoring is referential, with a given scalp electrode usually referenced to an electrode in the opposite mastoid area (A_1, A_2). The term *derivation* refers to the signal obtained from a pair of electrodes (e.g., C_4-A_1) amplified with a differential amplifier.

The EOG electrodes are positioned near the eyes. Because a potential difference exists across each eyeball (positive anterior and negative posterior), eye movements result in voltage changes that are detected in the EOG leads. Two EOG derivations (leads) are usually monitored on separate amplifier channels (ROC-A_1, LOC-A_2) where ROC and LOC are right and left outer canthus electrodes (see Fig. 18.1). One of the eye electrodes is placed slightly above the eye and the other below, so that vertical as well as horizontal movement may be detected. As eye movements are conjugate (same direction), both eyes move toward one electrode and away from the other. This causes out-of-phase deflections (one up, one down) in the two eye channels. In contrast, when high-voltage EEG activity is detected in the eye channels, the deflections are in phase. Surface EMG leads, usually in the chin area, detect electrical activity whose amplitude reflects the relative amount of muscle tone.

The awake EEG (Fig. 18.2) is characterized by low-amplitude, high-frequency activity, and rapid eye movements may occur. With the onset of drowsiness, the EEG reveals alpha waves (8 to 13 Hz), which are associated with eye closure and are best detected by electrodes in the occipital area. Slow eye movements (slow rolling eye movements)

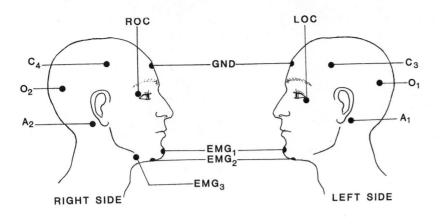

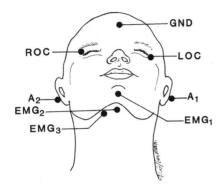

FIGURE 18.1. Electrode placement for EEG, EOG, and EMG leads. C_4, C_3 are the central EEG electrodes, O_2, O_1 are the occipital EEG electrodes, and A_2, A_1 are the mastoid electrodes. Even (odd) indices refer to the right (left) side of the body. ROC and LOC are the right and left outer canthus electrodes.

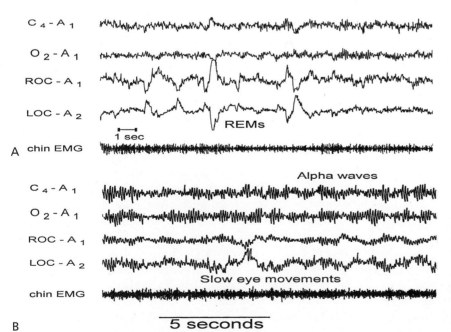

FIGURE 18.2. (A) Wakefulness (stage Wake) with the eyes open is characterized by low-voltage high-frequency EEG activity, rapid eye movements (REMs) and relatively high EMG activity. C_4-A_1 and O_2-A_1 are central and occipital EEG tracings, and ROC-A_1 and LOC-A_2 are right and left EOG tracings. **(B)** Drowsy wakefulness is illustrated. Prominent alpha activity is present throughout the EEG tracing, and slow eye movements are also seen.

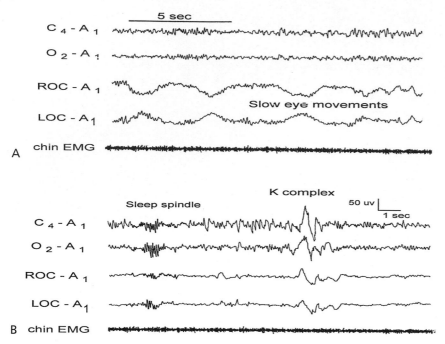

FIGURE 18.3. **(A)** Stage 1 sleep is characterized by low-voltage mixed-frequency EEG activity. Alpha-wave activity is present in less than 50% of the EEG tracings. Slow eye movements are present in the right and left EOG tracings (ROC-A_1,LOC-A_1). No sleep spindles or K complexes are present. **(B)** Stage 2 sleep is characterized by the presence of either sleep spindles or K complexes. Note that the K-complex activity results in deflections in the EOG leads that are in phase.

in the EOG tracings may also be present. The stage 1 EEG (Fig. 18.3) is characterized by low-voltage, mixed-frequency activity (3 to 7 Hz). Stage 1 is scored when less than 50% of an epoch contains alpha waves. Slow eye movements may also be present in stage 1 sleep. Stage 2 is characterized by the presence of either sleep spindles, which are bursts of 12 to 14 Hz activity, or K complexes, which are large-amplitude biphasic EEG deflections (see Fig. 18.3). To qualify as stage 2, less than 20% of an epoch may contain slow (delta) wave activity. Slow (delta) waves are high-amplitude broad waves. Delta EEG activity is usually defined as having a frequency less than 4 Hz. However, in scoring human sleep, the criteria for scoring slow (delta) wave activity are a frequency of 2 Hz or under (0.5 second duration) and a peak-to-peak amplitude at or over 75 μV. An epoch is scored as stage 3 when it contains 20% to 50% slow-wave EEG activity and as stage 4 when it consists of more than 50% slow-wave activity (Fig. 18.4). The chin EMG usually falls progressively on transition from wakefulness (stage Wake) to stage 4, but this is somewhat variable and depends on the amplifier gain. Stage REM is defined by the presence of rapid eye movements (REMs), which are relatively sharp deflections in the EOG tracings, low-voltage, mixed-frequency EEG activity (which may contain sawtooth waves), and relatively reduced muscle tone (see Fig. 18.4). "Relatively reduced" means that the EMG amplitude in REM is always equal to or lower than the lowest level recorded in NREM sleep. Note that a low-amplitude EEG pattern with EOG tracings showing REMs can occur with eyes-open wakefulness, but the muscle tone is higher than in REM sleep. More detailed discussions of the rules of sleep staging with examples are available (1–5).

There is a normal progression of sleep stages during the night (1–3), with sleep cycles composed of NREM followed by REM sleep. Periods of wakefulness may also be present during the night. Usually two to four cycles of stages 1 → 2 → 3 → 4 → 3 → 2 → REM of 70 to 120 minutes duration are present in the first portion of the night. The NREM cycles in the remainder of the night contain mainly stages 1 and 2. Thus, most stage 3 to 4 sleep occurs in the early part of the night. In contrast, episodes of REM sleep increase in duration in the later parts of the night, as does the REM density (the number of rapid eye movements per unit time).

Total sleep time (TST) is the total minutes of REM and NREM sleep. *Sleep period time* (SPT) equals TST plus any stage Wake that occurs after sleep onset but before the final awakening. The *sleep latency* is the time from lights-out (beginning of monitoring) to the onset of sleep. A sleep latency of more than 30 minutes is typical of patients complaining of difficulty falling asleep (insomnia). The *REM latency* is defined as the time from sleep onset until the first epoch of stage REM. A normal REM latency is around 90 minutes (70 to 120 minutes). *Sleep onset REM* refers to the appearance of REM sleep within 15 minutes of sleep onset. The time in bed (TIB) is the time from lights-out to lights-on. *Sleep efficiency* is defined as TST divided by TIB. It is customary to express the time spent in each stage (including the stage Wake present during the SPT) as a percentage of SPT. A young adult typically spends less than 5% of SPT in stage Wake, 5% to 10% in stage 1, 50% in stage 2, 20% to 30% in stages 3 and 4, and 20% to 25% in stage REM. A normal 60-year-old has a greater percentage of stage Wake

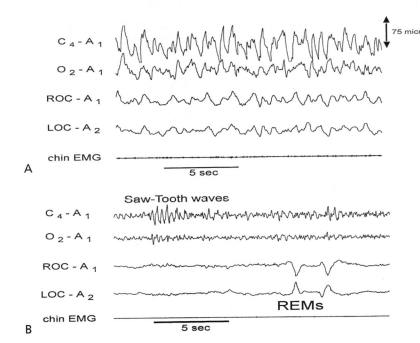

FIGURE 18.4. **(A)** Stage 4 sleep. More than 50% of the EEG tracings contain high-voltage, slow-wave activity which is also present in the EOG tracings. Note that the EMG activity has also decreased in this example. **(B)** Stage REM is characterized by low-voltage mixed-frequency activity that may contain bursts of sawtooth waves. The rapid eye movements (REMs) result in out-of-phase deflections in the right and left EOG leads (ROC-A_1 and LOC-A_2). The EMG level of activity is relatively reduced (at or below the lowest in NREM sleep).

and stage 1 sleep and reduced stage 3 and 4 sleep (less than 10%), but about the same percentage of stage REM (2).

An arousal is usually defined as an abrupt shift to a lighter stage of sleep or to an awakening which may be brief or may result in prolonged wakefulness (4,6). A task force of the American Sleep Disorders Association has proposed a set of rules for scoring arousals (6). An arousal is characterized by an abrupt shift in EEG frequency that may include theta (4 to 8 Hz), alpha, and/or frequencies greater than 16 Hz (but not spindles) lasting 3 seconds or longer. In NREM sleep an arousal can be scored without an increase in EMG amplitude. However, in REM sleep an increase in EMG amplitude is required, as well as an EEG frequency shift. The rationale for this rule is that bursts of alpha waves are common in REM sleep. This definition of arousal is somewhat restrictive, and the task force recognized that some EEG changes not meeting these criteria likely represent events of physiological significance. When sleep is filled with many brief arousals, it is not restorative. Thus daytime sleepiness can occur even if the TST (as scored by standard criteria) is not markedly shortened (7). Sleep interrupted by frequent arousals and stage shifts is said to be fragmented. One can define the *arousal index* as the number of arousals divided by the TST in hours. The upper limit of normal for the arousal index is not well defined but can be as high as 20 to 25 arousals per hour, especially in older individuals (8).

VENTILATION AND SLEEP

Respiratory drive is reduced during NREM sleep due to loss of the stimulatory effect of wakefulness ("the wakefulness stimulus") and decreases in chemosensitivity (9–11). There is a decrease in the ventilatory responses to hypoxia and hypercapnia. In most studies a further decrease in chemosensitivity has been present in stage REM. Stages 1 and 2 are often characterized by a periodic waxing and waning of tidal volume and respiratory rate. This is thought to be due to transition between the awake setpoint for P_{CO_2} and the sleep setpoint, which is somewhat higher (9–11). Stages 3 and 4 are characterized by a regular pattern of tidal volume and respiratory rate. Compared to awake values, ventilation is reduced by 1 to 2 L per minute, P_{CO_2} increased by 2 to 8 mm Hg, and P_{O_2} decreased by 5 to 10 mm Hg. While animal studies have consistently shown a fall in tidal volume and an increase in respiratory rate during NREM sleep, studies in humans are less consistent. Most studies have shown a reduction in minute ventilation associated with a decrease in tidal volume and either a decrease in respiratory rate or an increase not large enough to compensate for the fall in tidal volume (11–12). Upper-airway resistance increases during NREM sleep, and this acts as a resistive load on the ventilatory system (13). Functional residual capacity decreases during NREM sleep compared to wakefulness (14).

Ventilation during REM sleep is characterized by an irregular pattern of varying tidal volume and respiratory rate; short periods of central apnea may be seen. Skeletal muscle activity (intercostal muscles, etc.) is generally inhibited during all portions of REM sleep, and inspiration is dependent on persistent diaphragmatic activity. REM sleep is often characterized by a decrease in respiratory rib cage movement. Those portions of REM sleep containing bursts of rapid eye movements (REMs) are referred to as phasic REM (as opposed to tonic REM). During phasic REM, ventilation is irregular, with increases and decreases in tidal volume (15–16). Episodic decrements in inspiratory diaphragmatic and upper-airway muscle activity often occur during bursts of REMs and result in transient reductions in ventilation. As REM episodes are longer and the REM density is higher during the early morning, these REM periods are usually associated with the largest reductions in ventilation. One might expect that upper-airway resistance might be higher in REM than NREM sleep because of skeletal muscle hypotonia, but the mean upper-airway resistances are similar in normal subjects (13). The reduction in intercostal muscle activity during REM sleep is especially important in patients with diaphragmatic weakness or a mechanical disadvantage due to hyperinflation (chronic obstructive pulmonary disease or asthma) (17). Indeed, stage REM is usually the stage of sleep associated with the most severe hypoventilation and oxygen desaturation in patients with sleep-related respiratory disorders.

RESPIRATORY DEFINITIONS

An apnea is defined as the cessation of airflow at the nose and mouth for 10 seconds or longer. Obstructive sleep apnea (OSA) (Fig. 18.5) is present when there is continued respiratory effort (evidence of central respiratory drive such as chest and abdominal movement) during the absence of airflow. Central apneas are characterized by absence of both airflow and respiratory effort. Mixed apneas are those in which the initial portion of the apnea is central (no respiratory effort) and the remaining portion obstructive (respiratory effort present). Desaturations are usually defined as a fall in arterial oxygen saturation (SaO_2) of 4% or more from baseline. It is important to remember that the change in Po_2 associated with a 4% change in saturation depends critically on the initial Po_2 (position on the oxyhemoglobin saturation curve). The above definitions are arbitrary but widely used (4,18).

Periods of reduced tidal volume or airflow may also be associated with desaturations or sleep disturbance. These events are called *hypopneas* (see Figure 18.5). Definitions of hypopnea vary among clinicians (4,18,19). Some require only a reduction in airflow or tidal volume by between one-third and one-half of the baseline value, while others require that an associated drop in SaO_2 of 2% to 4% be present. Although hypopneas could be due to a fall in central drive (central hypopneas) or partial airway obstruction (obstructive hypopneas), such a separation is not always possible from routine measurements. Obstructive hypopneas are often associated with paradoxical movements of the chest and abdomen, although in some patients only more subtle changes in phase between chest and abdominal movements can be detected (20–21). The apnea index (or apnea-plus-hypopnea index) is defined as the number of events per hour of sleep (number of events per TST in hours). An alternate term for the apnea-plus-hypopnea index (AHI) is the respiratory disturbance index (RDI).

SLEEP MONITORING

The detailed monitoring of sleep is called polysomnography. All of the electrodes in Figure 18.1 are usually placed but only a portion are used at one time to detect the presence and stage of sleep. The others are available in case of electrode failure. A typical set (montage) might include (C_4-A_1, O_2-A_1, ROC-A_1, LOC-A_1, EMG_1-EMG_2). This montage uses a common mastoid electrode (A_1) as the reference. In general, the further apart electrodes are spaced, the greater the signal. An alternate method references the EOG leads to the contralateral mastoid (ROC-A_1, LOC-A_2). An EKG lead is also monitored to detect changes in cardiac rhythm. For more information on the technical aspects of recording sleep, the reader is referred to the references (1–5).

Airflow is usually detected qualitatively by using thermistors or thermocouples at the nose and mouth (4). Airflow across these devices changes their temperature and hence their resistance (thermistor) or voltage output (thermocouple). Unfortunately, these devices may not accurately reflect changes in either the magnitude or the time profile (shape) of airflow. Accurate measurements of airflow are possible with a pneumotachograph inserted into a face mask. Airflow is determined by measuring the pressure drop across this device (a fixed linear resistance). A more comfortable alternative that is gaining popularity is to measure nasal pressure using a small nasal cannula connected to a sensitive pressure

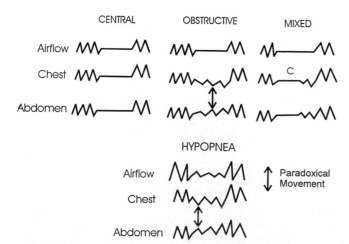

FIGURE 18.5. Schematic illustrations of apnea (obstructive, central, mixed) and hypopnea. Paradoxical movement of chest and abdominal movement may be seen in obstructive events. (Reprinted with permission from Berry RB. *Sleep medicine pearls.* Philadelphia: Hanley & Belfus, 1999.)

transducer (22). This measures the pressure drop across the resistance of the nasal inlet. While this is not a linear resistance, a much more accurate airflow tracing is obtained than with devices measuring temperature. Airflow can also be detected by using CO_2 measuring devices that detect the increased CO_2 content in exhaled gas. This method can be misleading, because small exhalations rich in CO_2 may occur during obstructive apneas despite the absence of inspiratory airflow. The resulting substantial fluctuations in CO_2 may give the appearance of significant airflow (4).

Respiratory effort is commonly monitored by devices that detect chest and abdominal movement (4,19–21). Such devices include impedance plethysmography, strain gauges, piezoelectric sensors, or respiratory inductance plethysmography (RIP). In RIP, the sum of signals from rib cage and abdominal bands can be calibrated to estimate tidal volume (21). In some obese individuals, respiratory effort during obstructive apnea does not result in easily discernible motion of the chest wall or abdomen. A more sensitive method for detecting respiratory effort employs measurement of esophageal pressure changes, which reflect changes in pleural pressure due to inspiratory muscle contraction (20). This method is not routinely used, although a small percentage of apneas will be misclassified as central on the basis of surface measurements of respiratory effort. Recently, many laboratories have been using small, fluid-filled catheters connected to a pressure transducer to detect esophageal pressure changes, rather than the more uncomfortable esophageal balloons.

Arterial oxygen saturation is continuously measured by pulse oximetry using ear or finger probes. One should note that the nadir of a desaturation associated with a respiratory event usually occurs after the event has ended. The delay is due to the circulation time to the sensing device as well as instrumental delay.

Leg movements are detected by monitoring leg electromyograms using surface electrodes placed over both the anterior tibialis muscles (leg EMGs). Periodic leg movements during sleep can cause sleep disturbance and result in symptoms that can mimic the sleep apnea syndromes (see later section). All of the parameters described above were traditionally recorded on a polygraph, which usually ran at a paper speed of 10 mm per second. This speed is not optimum for either respiratory or ECG recording but is commonly used to stage sleep. Today, many clinical sleep laboratories record directly on computer-based systems. This allows archiving of studies on optical disks or CD devices, thereby solving the costly problem of storing studies recorded on paper. Although sleep staging may be somewhat more difficult on a monitor screen compared to paper, tracings can be viewed using multiple time scales (virtual paper speeds), which facilitates identification of longer events or trends.

Multiple Sleep Latency Test

In addition to nocturnal polysomnography, daytime tests are used to document the degree of daytime sleepiness and detect sleep onset REM sleep (23). The multiple sleep latency test (MSLT) consists of four or five short naps, usually spaced across the day in two-hour intervals (for example, 8:00 A.M., 10:00 A.M., noon, 2:00 P.M., and 4:00 P.M.). Patients are given 20 minutes to fall asleep. If sleep occurs, patients are given another 15 minutes to reach REM sleep. Once REM sleep is reached or the period of time has run out, the test is terminated. The subject then gets out of bed until the next nap. The sleep latency (time from lights-out to initial sleep) and the presence or absence of REM sleep are determined. The standard MSLT criteria are shown in Table 18.1. It is important not to confuse the significance of a short *nocturnal* sleep latency (which is normal) with a short mean daytime sleep latency. For correct interpretation, the MSLT should always follow an all-night polysomnogram. A sleep diary documenting the pattern of sleep for one or two weeks before the test may also be useful. A modest self-imposed reduction in nocturnal sleep from eight to six hours can shorten the mean daytime sleep latency into the abnormal range (under 10 minutes) (24). Medications that affect sleep (especially REM sleep) such as stimulants, sedatives (ethanol), and tricyclic antidepressants should be withdrawn, if possible, for two weeks before testing.

In a variation of the MSLT termed the *maintenance of wakefulness test* (MWT), subjects are requested to stay awake in a dark, quiet room during multiple 20- or 40-minute periods while semirecumbent and monitored for sleep (25–26). Certain patients will have a short sleep latency on the MSLT but are able to stay awake for 40 minutes during the MWT. These tests may well measure different aspects of the same process. While the MSLT is considered the standard test for assessing daytime sleepiness, the MWT may be more sensitive for demonstrating an effect of treatment or evaluating a given patient's ability to function in the tasks of daily living. If the sleep latency on a 20-minute MWT is less than 11 minutes, the patient may have a difficult time performing tasks requiring attention (25).

TABLE 18.1. MULTIPLE SLEEP LATENCY CRITERIA

Mean Sleep Latency (min)	Severity of Sleepiness	Number of REM Periods in 5 Naps
<5	Severe	0–1 Normal
5–10	Moderate	≥2 Abnormal
10–15	Mild sleepiness (some normal subjects)	Causes: narcolepsy, OSA, prior REM deprivation, withdrawal of REM suppressant medications
>15	Normal	

SLEEP DISORDERS CAUSING EXCESSIVE DAYTIME SLEEPINESS

The revised International Classification of Sleep Disorders (ICSD) provides a scheme for classifying the full spectrum of sleep disorders (27). The reader is referred to this valuable reference, as this chapter will concentrate on the sleep apnea syndromes with only a brief discussion of several of the other sleep disorders which are associated with excessive daytime sleepiness (Table 18.2). One should not assume that every sleepy, snoring patient has sleep apnea. In addition, patients with sleep apnea can also have narcolepsy or periodic limb movements (PLMs) in sleep. Therefore the evaluation of every sleepy patient should include questions relevant to narcolepsy, PLMs, and depression as well as to sleep apnea. A careful history of medications and the use of ethanol, stimulants (including caffeine), and sedatives must be obtained. A recording of the patient's usual amount and pattern of sleep may also be instructive. Most sleep centers use a sleep log (diary) that the patient completes before coming for evaluation. A brief discussion of the first four nonrespiratory disorders listed in Table 18.2 will precede a discussion of sleep apnea.

Narcolepsy

Narcolepsy (28,29) is a syndrome associated with the tetrad of sleep attacks, cataplexy, hypnagogic hallucinations, and sleep paralysis. All four components of the narcolepsy tetrad are present in only 11% to 25% of cases. Unfortunately sleep attacks, sleep paralysis, and hypnogogic hallucinations can occur in other sleep disorders. Cataplexy is the only symptom specific to narcolepsy. Only when both daytime sleepiness and unequivocal cataplexy are present can a *clinical* diagnosis of narcolepsy be made with confidence. Unfortunately, the sleep attacks may be present for many years before cataplexy. In addition, cataplexy is often subtle and difficult to document. Narcolepsy without cataplexy can be diagnosed using the MSLT. However, the MSLT can be interpreted correctly only with the results of the preceding nocturnal polysomnogram and clinical history in mind.

TABLE 18.2. CONDITIONS PRESENTING WITH EXCESSIVE DAYTIME SLEEPINESS (EDS)

Sleep apnea syndromes (including the upper airway resistance syndrome)
Narcolepsy
Idiopathic hypersomnia
Insufficient sleep syndrome
Periodic limb movements in sleep
Posttraumatic hypersomnia
Psychiatric disorders (depression)
Drug and alcohol dependency
Circadian disorders (jet lag, shift work)

The attacks of sleepiness associated with narcolepsy usually begin in adolescence or early adulthood and can occur at any time of the day. After a brief nap the patient may awaken completely refreshed. Patients with narcolepsy may also complain of chronic sleepiness as well as discrete sleep attacks. Cataplexy refers to the sudden loss of muscle tone or strength following a period of high emotion such as surprise, laughter, or anger. The cataplectic attacks may vary from subtle weakness of an isolated muscle group (loss of facial muscle tone) to sudden paralysis of all skeletal muscles and postural collapse. Some prolonged episodes of cataplexy are also associated with hallucinations. Hypnagogic (sleep onset) and hypnopompic (at awakening) hallucinations are vivid, dreamlike experiences often associated with fear. Sleep paralysis also occurs at the transitions between wakefulness and sleep, and involves an inability to move, even though awake, that lasts from a few seconds to 20 minutes. Fortunately, respiration is usually not affected, although some patients complain of dyspnea during the paralysis episodes.

The polysomnographic hallmark of narcolepsy is sleep-onset stage REM (SOREM). Whereas the normal REM latency is about 90 minutes, patients with narcolepsy often have a REM latency of less than 15 minutes. However, only around 50% of patients with narcolepsy will have a short *nocturnal* REM latency on any given sleep study. The MSLT is very useful for supporting the diagnosis of narcolepsy because it allows for more opportunities to detect sleep-onset REM as well as to document daytime sleepiness. The standard criteria are a mean sleep latency of less than five minutes and two or more REM onsets in five nap opportunities. Over 80% of patients with narcolepsy will meet these diagnostic criteria. An occasional patient will have a sleep latency from five to 10 minutes with two or more SOREM periods. A negative MSLT does not rule out narcolepsy. In such cases, a firm diagnosis of narcolepsy would require that a history of both daytime sleepiness and unequivocal cataplexy be present. The MSLT should follow a night of polysomnography to document that the SOREM is not due to preceding REM deprivation (and to rule out other sleep pathology). Sleep-onset REM may also be seen in some patients with sleep apnea (which can reduce the amount of REM sleep), depression, schizophrenia, and following withdrawal of REM-suppressing medications. If sleep apnea is found on nocturnal polysomnography, the MSLT should be delayed until after the patient has been adequately treated for this problem for several weeks. For example, if obstructive sleep apnea is treated with nasal continuous positive airway pressure (CPAP), a repeat sleep study is ordered with the patient sleeping on CPAP (this documents treatment efficacy). An MSLT is then performed with the patient on CPAP. If the results of the MSLT meet the criteria for narcolepsy, a diagnosis of the combination of narcolepsy and OSA would be supported.

Narcolepsy occurs in about four of 10,000 people. In a national cooperative study of sleep disorders centers, narcolepsy was present in about 25% of the patients complaining of increased daytime sleepiness (30). In community sleep centers the percentage may be much lower, but narcolepsy is quite common in most practices. The cause of narcolepsy is unknown, but there appears to be a genetic predisposition to this disorder. Initial studies found that 80% to 95% of Caucasian or Japanese patients with classic narcolepsy were positive for the HLA-DR2 antigen. Unfortunately, 25% to 36% of the general population is positive for this antigen, and black narcoleptics are not usually HLA-DR2-positive. Recent studies have suggested that DQB1*0602 and DQA1*0102 are better markers of narcolepsy across all racial groups (31). However, cases of well-defined narcolepsy have been described which are negative for these alleles. The utility of genetic testing in diagnosing narcolepsy remains to be determined.

The treatment of excessive daytime sleepiness in narcolepsy usually includes the use of stimulants such as methylphenidate (Ritalin). Methylphenidate is started at a dose of 15 to 20 mg per day, divided into three or four doses. The drug is most effective if given before sleep attacks characteristically occur. Once a sleep attack is in progress, the best treatment is a short nap. Most patients are controlled on 15 to 60 mg per day. Modafinil, a promising new nonstimulant medication recently made available in the United States, appears to be effective and has fewer side effects than stimulants (32).

The attacks of cataplexy are effectively suppressed by tricyclic antidepressants in doses below those used for depression. Protriptyline (Vivactil) (15 to 30 mg per day in three divided doses) and imipramine (Tofranil) (75 mg per day) are the most commonly used agents. Selective serotonin reuptake inhibitors (fluoxetine) in antidepressant doses are also effective (fluoxetine 20 mg per day).

Idiopathic Hypersomnia

This syndrome was formerly called idiopathic central nervous system hypersomnolence. It is characterized by daytime somnolence but not cataplexy or sleep-onset REM (28). Unlike narcolepsy, the daytime naps are typically not refreshing, and the night sleep period can be unusually long in some patients. Polysomnography reveals no explanation for daytime sleepiness. MSLT shows a short sleep latency but no SOREM. A sleep diary of two weeks before the MSLT should rule out insufficient sleep as an explanation for the short sleep latency. These patients made up about 10% of all patients complaining of exessive daytime sleepiness (EDS) in a large cooperative study (30). Treatment with CNS stimulants is usually attempted but is less effective than with narcolepsy.

Insufficient Sleep Syndrome

Surprisingly, some patients have excessive daytime sleepiness simply due to an inadequate sleep period which is often self-enforced for societal reasons. The sleep need is genetic and cannot be shortened without impairment in daytime functioning. These patients typically sleep longer on weekends and report less daytime sleepiness (33). A sleep diary is essential in making this diagnosis. In addition, insufficient sleep will aggravate symptoms in other disorders such as narcolepsy.

Periodic Limb Movement Disorder

The syndrome of periodic limb movements (PLMs) (also known as periodic *leg* movements) consists of stereotypic periodic leg (or arm) movements during sleep that may or may not be associated with arousals (27,34). If enough arousals occur, sleep may be so fragmented that daytime sleepiness results. While about 10% to 12% of patients seen in sleep centers for insomnia complaints have PLMs as the etiology, only 2% to 3% of the patients presenting with excessive daytime sleepiness are found to have PLMs as the major cause of their sleepiness. Probably a much higher percentage of elderly patients have PLMs but no symptoms. Because narcoleptics frequently have PLMs, any patient with excessive daytime sleepiness and PLMs on a polysomnogram should be questioned carefully concerning narcoleptic manifestations. PLMs can also appear after withdrawal of anticonvulsants, benzodiazepines, barbiturates, or other hypnotics. Patients with sleep apnea on occasion exhibit a large increase in PLMs after treatment with nasal CPAP (35).

Patients with PLMs may or may not remember the awakenings during the night but almost never remember the leg movements. The movements usually consist of dorsiflexion of the foot at the ankle, extension of the big toe and partial flexion of the knee and hip. A small portion of the patients have the *restless leg syndrome* (RLS), which involves a creeping sensation in the legs associated with a desire to move them. Movement reduces the sensations, but they return with inactivity. These sensations commonly occur at bedtime. It is important to question patients about these sensations, because if a patient has RLS symptoms he or she frequently also has PLMs (80% or more).

The diagnosis of the PLM syndrome requires monitoring of leg EMGs. Leg movements may occur in one or both legs, and therefore monitoring of both legs is suggested (they can be monitored on one amplifier channel). Not all events are associated with arousals. Only movements leading to arousals are considered detrimental. Guidelines for monitoring and scoring leg movements (LMs) have been published (36). To be scored as a PLM (or part of a PLM sequence), an LM must occur during sleep, must not follow an arousal due to other events, and must occur in a group of four or more LMs separated by more than five seconds and less than 90 seconds (event onset to onset). The number of these events per hour of sleep (PLM index) and the number per hour of sleep followed by an arousal (PLM-arousal index) are used to diagnose the PLM syndrome. A PLM index greater than 5 is considered abnormal; 5 to 24, mild; 25 to 49, moderate; and 50 or more, severe (27). The true impact of this disorder is probably more accurately assessed by looking at the PLM-arousal index. Severe daytime sleepiness is usually associated with a PLM-arousal index greater than 25.

Treatment of the PLM syndrome is usually with carbidopa/levodopa 25mg/100mg started as half a pill at bedtime with another half-pill during the night if needed (34,37). The dose is slowly increased if needed until symptoms improve or to a maximum of three pills per night. Benzodiazepines, which suppress the arousals but not the PLMs, are an alternative treatment. The most commonly used agent is clonazepam 0.5 mg taken a half-hour before bedtime. The dose may be titrated upward to 1.5 mg. Other benzodiazepines with a shorter duration of action (triazolam, temazepam) may cause less morning grogginess. The restless leg syndrome is more difficult to treat than PLMs. Higher doses of carbidopa/levodopa may be required but may eventually induce an increase in symptoms (augmentation). A switch to other treatments such as dopamine agonists (pergolide, bromocriptine), narcotics or combination therapy may be needed (37).

Sleep Apnea Syndromes

The sleep apnea syndromes may be divided into the obstructive sleep apnea syndromes (OSAS) and the central sleep apnea syndromes (CSAS). While patients with OSA may have some central apneas, the diagnosis of CSA requires that a majority of apneas be central in nature. The CSAS is much less common than the OSAS, which composes more than 85% to 90% of all sleep apnea patients evaluated at most sleep centers. Patients with predominantly mixed apneas or repetitive hypopneas due to partial airway obstruction (19) behave like those with pure obstructive apneas and are considered to have the OSAS (38). Other associated disorders which can be considered subtypes of the OSAS include the obesity hypoventilation syndrome (OHS), the overlap syndrome (OSA and COPD), and the upper airway resistance syndrome (UARS). These syndromes will be discussed in the following sections.

Obstructive Sleep Apnea

The true incidence of OSA is unknown, but estimates of 1% to 4% have been quoted (38,39). Patients with the OSAS usually present with a complaint of EDS. They typically have a long history of snoring, and bedmates frequently report pauses in breathing terminated by snorts. A history of chronic nasal obstruction or congestion, hypertension, or recent weight gain preceding an exacerbation of daytime sleepiness is common. Other manifestations or associations include impotence, enuresis, and morning headaches (38).

Conditions known to predispose patients to sleep apnea include the male sex (18,39), increasing age (39), alcohol use (40), obesity (41), hypothyroidism (42), acromegaly (43), and hypnotic use (44). Recent studies have suggested that the OSAS may be more common in female subjects than was formerly suspected (39).

Symptoms and signs of right heart failure are present in a minority (10% to 15%) of cases (45). Physical examination frequently reveals nasal obstruction, a large tongue, retrognathia (posterior displacement of the mandible), a dependent soft palate, or a hypertrophied uvula. Many patients have a short, thick neck. In fact, neck circumference correlates better with the AHI than body weight. Up to 40% of patients in some sleep centers are not obese. Thyroid studies should be ordered if symptoms or signs of hypothyroidism are present. The majority of patients with OSAS do not have either polycythemia or evidence of CO_2 retention on arterial blood gas analysis. We reserve arterial blood gas analysis for patients who have low awake oxygen saturations or unexplained elevations in serum bicarbonate. In one study, the best clinical predictors of the presence of the OSAS were a history of snoring, a history of apnea/gasping, a large neck circumference, and the presence of hypertension (46). Interestingly, the presence of daytime sleepiness (a cardinal manifestation of OSA) was not a reliable predictor. It appears that many patients minimize or underestimate the severity of this symptom.

Polysomnography in the OSAS

Polysomnography of patients with OSAS reveals repetitive obstructive apneas and hypopneas (Fig. 18.6). Apneas are followed by resumption of airflow, which usually coincides with evidence of arousal and often movement. The nadir of oxygen saturation usually occurs after apnea termination. During the apnea, the chest and abdomen move in a paradoxical manner. The heart rate usually slows at the onset of apnea and then speeds up at apnea termination/arousal (47).

Because many totally asymptomatic elderly males may have a small amount of obstructive apnea, defining exact criteria for normality based on the apnea index (or apnea-plus-hypopnea index) is difficult (18,39). Although some have suggested that an apnea index greater than five per hour or 30 apneas per night should be considered abnormal, an apnea-plus-hypopnea index from 5 to 10 may be normal if symptoms are absent. A retrospective study (48) found an increase in mortality when the apnea index exceeded 20 per hour. An arbitrary but useful scheme is to consider a combined apnea-plus-hypopnea index less than 20 as mild, 20 to 40 as moderate, and greater than 40 as severe.

Occasionally a sleepy, snoring patient will have relatively few apneas or hypopneas when studied. In such cases, one must consider the effects of ethanol intake, sleep stage, and posture. If a patient abstains from his or her usual ethanol intake, this could reduce the severity of apnea. Patients with

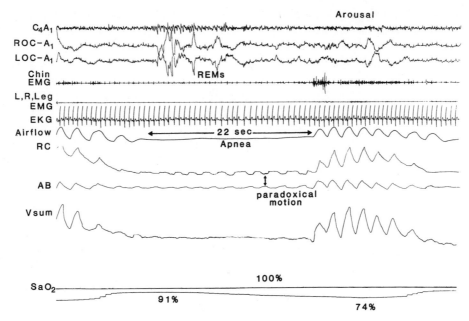

FIGURE 18.6. A complete polysomnographic tracing of an obstructive apnea during REM sleep. Note that the EEG and EMG change at apnea termination, signifying an arousal, and that the nadir of arterial oxygen saturation (SaO_2) occurs after the apnea has terminated.

mild-to-moderate apnea may also have positional apnea (AHI much greater in the supine position) or REM-related apnea (AHI much greater or present only in REM sleep). In these cases, the severity of OSA may be underestimated if small amounts of sleep in the supine position or REM sleep were recorded. Many sleep centers compute a separate AHI for NREM and REM sleep as well as the supine and lateral sleep positions to help identify patients with sleep-stage-specific or positional sleep apnea. Sleepy patients with a low AHI could also have the UARS, which is discussed in a section below. Finally, the presence of other sleep disorders such as PLMs, narcolepsy, idiopathic hypersomnia, and insufficient sleep must all be considered as possible explanations of the patient's sleepiness.

The degree of arterial oxygen desaturation in patients with OSA is not necessarily correlated with the apnea index and must also be considered in assessing the severity of disease. A study of the factors determining the severity of desaturation found that (a) a lower baseline Po_2, (b) a greater percentage of sleep time spent in apnea, and (c) a smaller expiratory reserve volume (functional residual capacity minus residual volume) all tended to produce more severe desaturation (49). This is consistent with the observation that patients with baseline hypoxemia due to obesity (with or without CO_2 retention) or superimposed chronic obstructive pulmonary disease tend to desaturate more rapidly during apnea.

Upper-Airway Obstruction—Pathophysiology

The pathophysiology of upper-airway obstruction is complex and still under active investigation. During normal breathing, upper-airway muscle activity maintains upper-airway patency despite negative intraluminal pressure and positive extraluminal pressure (the effects of gravity on the tissue surrounding the airway) (50–52). Upper-airway muscle activity is augmented by chemical stimuli (hypoxia and hypercapnia), mechanoreceptor stimuli (negative upper airway pressure) and brain-stem activation associated with wakefulness (the "wakefulness stimulus"). Negative intraluminal pressure augments the activity of upper-airway muscles via a brain-stem reflex when mucosal receptors in the upper airway are stimulated by negative pressure (50). Upper-airway muscles exhibit resting tone, referred to as tonic activity, and some have inspiratory increases in tone, referred to as phasic activity. For example, the genioglossus (tongue protruder) usually displays prominent phasic activity while the tensor palatini (a palate muscle) may not (53). With sleep onset, the wakefulness stimulus is lost and the negative pressure reflex is diminished. Thus within one or two breaths after sleep onset, upper-airway muscle activity generally decreases (54) and upper-airway resistance increases, even in normal subjects (13). With sustained sleep, the activity of the genioglossus may return to waking levels, but the activity of the palate muscles often remains below that during wakefulness (54). The major site of upper-airway narrowing in normal subjects appears to be in the retropalatal area (55).

The patency of the upper airway depends on extraluminal tissue/gravitation factors (the supine posture predisposes to narrowing), anatomical factors (airway size and shape), the amount of negative intraluminal pressure, as well as amount of upper-airway muscle activity. An additional important factor is tracheal traction, which describes the downward pull on upper-airway structures during inspiratory chest-wall expansion and the resulting passive dilation of the upper airway (56). During inspiration, the phasic activation of upper-airway muscles and the effects of tracheal traction help maintain upper-airway patency despite negative intraluminal pressure. In fact, upper-airway volume is actually smallest at end expiration, when muscle activity and tracheal traction are minimal (55). If the forces tending to close the airway exceed those maintaining airway patency, airway closure occurs.

In patients with OSA, an obstruction to airflow (extreme narrowing or closure) occurs during sleep at one or several locations in the upper airway (57). Studies of the upper airway in awake patients with OSA by cephalometric radiographs, computed tomography, acoustic reflection techniques, and magnetic resonance imaging have usually shown smaller than normal upper airways (55). These patients have an increased supraglottic resistance (58) and, unlike normal subjects, require a positive intraluminal pressure to prevent airway closure during sleep (59). Some patients have a bony abnormality, while in others a long soft palate, a large posteriorly placed tongue, increased fat deposition, or tissue edema may all play a role in narrowing the airway. The shape of the upper airway also differs, with the airway being most narrowed in the lateral dimension in OSA patients versus anterior-posteriorly in normal subjects. The lateral pharyngeal walls appear increased in thickness, although this is not explained by fat deposition. There is considerable overlap in *awake* airway size between normals and patients with OSA. However, airway size during wakefulness is influenced by both anatomy and upper-airway muscle activity. Studies have shown that during wakefulness, a higher-than-normal percentage of the maximal upper-airway muscle activity is required to preserve upper-airway patency in OSA patients compared to normal subjects (54), and that at sleep onset there is an abrupt and often a greater-than-normal fall in upper-airway muscle activity. However, again, considerable overlap between normal subjects and patients with OSA exists. While early theories of airway collapse focused on the balance between negative intraluminal pressure and dilating forces, recent studies have shown that negative intraluminal pressure is not required for airway closure (52). Airway collapse has been demonstrated endoscopically during central apnea. Indeed, upper-airway obstruction in patients with OSA usually begins when both ventilatory drive and upper-airway muscle activity are relatively reduced (60). Thus, our current understanding emphasizes susceptible upper-airway anatomy and a loss of upper-airway muscle activity as the key elements in upper-airway obstruction.

The postapnea ventilatory period may have consequences if the patient returns to sleep quickly. If the PCO_2 falls below a point called the "apneic threshold" (usually 0 to 2 mm Hg above the stable awake PCO_2 or 4 to 6 mm Hg below

the sleeping PCO_2 setpoint), then respiratory drive ceases, resulting in central apnea (61). This is thought to be the origin of the central portion of mixed apnea (62). When the upper airway is stabilized using nasal CPAP, both the central and obstructive components of mixed apnea are usually abolished.

Apnea Termination/Arousal
During obstructive apnea, the phasic activity of the genioglossus (and many other upper-airway muscles) and respiratory muscles progressively increases as the apneic period continues. However, the upper airway does not open. This may occur because increasingly negative intraluminal pressure maintains airway collapse. Upper-airway opening appears to occur only after arousal and a preferential large increase in upper-airway tone (51). The fact that arousal does not occur despite prolonged periods of apnea and arterial oxygen desaturation suggests that a defect in arousal mechanisms is present. The magnitude of the stimulus inducing respiratory arousal from NREM sleep appears to be related to the level of inspiratory effort (esophageal or supraglottic pressure), rather than the individual levels of PO_2 or PCO_2 stimulating ventilatory drive (63). Normal subjects arouse from mask occlusion at suction pressures of 20 to 30 cm H_2O, while patients with OSA may exert esophageal pressures more negative than 60 cm H_2O before awakening. The causes of impaired arousal in patients with OSA are unknown but are probably explained at least in part by the effects of chronic sleep fragmentation on arousal mechanisms. Respiratory-related arousal from REM sleep is even less well understood. Normal subjects arouse much more quickly from mask occlusion during REM than NREM sleep. In contrast, the longest apneas occur during REM sleep in patients with OSA.

Impaired Sleep and Daytime Sleepiness in the OSAS
The sleep architecture of patients with OSAS is impaired, with reduced amounts of REM and stage 3 and 4 sleep as well as frequent arousals and a reduced sleep efficiency. On daytime MSLT testing, a shortened sleep latency is usually noted. Two or more naps may contain REM sleep, suggesting REM deprivation. The first night of effective treatment of OSA with tracheostomy or nasal CPAP frequently results in long periods of stages 3, 4, and REM ("deep sleep and REM rebound"). A rapid improvement in daytime alertness is noted in many patients (64). The sleep latency on the MSLT after tracheostomy/nasal CPAP treatment usually improves, but not always to the normal range. In one study the MWT sleep latency improved from 18 to 32 minutes after treatment with nasal CPAP (65).

The exact causes of the excessive daytime somnolence in the OSAS are still under investigation. Sleep fragmentation is probably the most important factor, although hypoxemia may also play a role. In one study the apnea-plus-hypopnea index did not differ between a group of hypersomnolent and nonhypersomnolent patients with OSA (66). In another study, the respiratory arousal index (arousals related to respiratory events per hour of sleep) correlated best with the sleep latency on the MSLT (67). Measures of sleep fragmentation, such as the arousal frequency or alterations in sleep architecture (increased stage 1 and decreased stages 3 and 4), appear to be more abnormal in sleepy OSA patients (68). Cognitive impairment appears to be more severe in patients with sleep apnea who have hypoxemia (69).

OSAS and Daytime Hypercapnia

A small subset of patients with OSA are very obese and manifest daytime hypoventilation (increased P_{CO_2}). These patients, formerly called Pickwickian, are now said to have the obesity hypoventilation syndrome (OHS). Most (but not all) patients with this syndrome have severe OSA. Occasionally a patient will not have discrete apneas or hypopneas during sleep but will simply manifest hypoventilation during the day, which worsens during sleep. Most patients with sleep apnea have a normal daytime P_{CO_2} and P_{O_2} and normal ventilatory responses to hypercapnia and hypoxemia (70), although their responses to resistive loads may be reduced (71). Those with the OHS have reduced ventilatory responses to hypoxemia and hypercapnia (72,73) and have a lower compliance of the respiratory system compared to nonhypercapnic patients with equivalent obesity (74). With adequate treatment of sleep apnea, the daytime CO_2 retention will improve in some but not all OHS patients (75,76). This implies both acquired (reversible) and intrinsic dysfunction of ventilatory control.

The other group of OSAS patients that commonly have daytime CO_2 retention is the group with the overlap syndrome (COPD and OSA). While most patients with COPD do not retain CO_2 until the FEV_1 falls below 1 L, patients with the overlap syndrome develop hypercarbia at less severe levels of airflow obstruction. The CO_2 retention in this group may also improve with effective treatment of their OSA.

Upper Airway Resistance Syndrome

Recently there has been increased recognition of a group of patients with few discrete apneas and hypopneas but with recurrent brief arousals associated with increased upper airway resistance (77). These patients present with symptoms of excessive daytime sleepiness or fatigue. Some may have a history of snoring. They have evidence of a short sleep latency on the MSLT and improve when treated for upper-airway obstruction. The frequent arousals which cause daytime sleepiness are the result of increased respiratory effort during upper-airway narrowing. Since increased effort rather than a high upper-airway resistance is believed to trigger arousal (63), some have suggested that the events be termed RERAs (respiratory-effort-related arousals). Definitive diagnosis of the UARS requires demonstration of a high or progressive increase in supraglottic or esophageal pressure

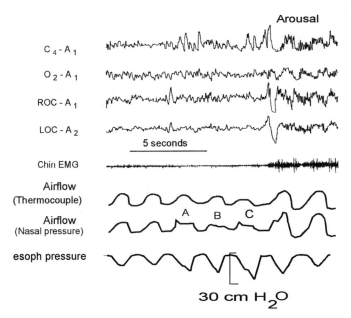

FIGURE 18.7. An example of a respiratory-effort-related arousal (RERA) in the upper airway resistance syndrome is shown here. Note that airflow by nasal pressure shows a flattened profile prior to arousal **(A,B,C)** while the thermocouple shows only a subtle decrease in amplitude. The reduction in airflow was not severe enough to be called an hypopnea. A crescendo increase in respiratory effort (esophageal pressure) precedes arousal. (Reprinted with permission from Berry RB. *Sleep medicine pearls.* Philadelphia: Hanley & Belfus, 1999.)

deflections preceding the brief arousals (Fig. 18.7). Routine airflow monitoring methods (thermistors) show that sometimes only subtle changes in airflow precede arousal. If a pneumotachograph or nasal pressure monitoring is used to detect airflow, a reduction in airflow and flattening of the airflow profile (a plateau) is noted to precede arousal. Simultaneous measurement of esophageal pressure shows that airflow is constant despite an increasing pressure gradient across the upper airway (airflow limitation). Some have suggested that detection of flattening of the airflow profile preceding arousal allows diagnosis without the need for esophageal pressure monitoring (22). In any case, repeated unexplained arousals in a sleepy patient should always raise the suspicion of the UARS. Currently there are no definitive guidelines on how to tabulate these events. Some have suggested that a RERA rate of 25–30 per hour is probably required to produce significant daytime sleepiness. The UARS or RERA syndrome really appears to represent one end of the spectrum of OSAS and responds to the same treatments as mild to moderate OSA. The syndrome illustrates the importance of frequent brief arousals in causing daytime sleepiness in the OSAS.

Cardiovascular Consequences of OSAS

The cardiovascular consequences of OSAS include episodic nocturnal pulmonary and systemic hypertension, cyclic variation in heart rate, increased afterload, and the potential for worsening coronary and cerebral ischemia (78). It is likely that much of the increase in mortality associated with OSA is due to the cardiovascular consequences of OSAS. Ongoing and future studies will hopefully better define these consequences.

Pulmonary arterial blood pressure rises during apneas and then falls when the oxygen saturation returns to normal after apnea (78,79). The main cause of these episodic increases in pulmonary arterial blood pressure is hypoxic vasoconstriction. Studies have suggested that *daytime* pulmonary hypertension (78) and right heart failure (45) are generally confined to OSA patients with daytime hypoxemia. Patients with OSA and daytime hypoxemia usually have either the OHS or a mixture of OSA and COPD. Therefore it is these groups that usually show evidence of cor pulmonale.

Systemic arterial blood pressure falls during sleep in *both* normal individuals and patients with essential hypertension. In contrast, an increase in systemic blood pressure is associated with each obstructive apnea/hypopnea in patients with OSA. There is a slow rise in blood pressure during the apnea and a steeper increase at the time of arousal (78). Studies have found that a large proportion of patients with sleep apnea have *daytime* hypertension (46), and a significant proportion of hypertensive patients have OSA (80). Does the association between hypertension and sleep apnea indicate causality or simply that both entities are due to other factors such as obesity (78)? This question remains unanswered. However, even if OSAS does not cause daytime hypertension, it may worsen the *consequences*. The lack of the normal nocturnal dip in blood pressure in hypertensive OSAS patients may predispose to a greater degree of left ventricular hypertrophy (81). Generally adequate treatment of OSAS patients with hypertension does not eliminate the necessity of medical treatment of daytime hypertension. However, in many patients daytime systemic hypertension is more easily and effectively controlled (82).

The most common change in cardiac rhythm in OSA is an exaggerated sinus arrhythmia. The heart rate usually slows during the initial part of apnea and then speeds up during the postapnea arousal. The increase in heart rate at arousal appears to be secondary to a combination of an increase in sympathetic tone and a reduction in vagal tone, with the reverse on the return to sleep (and the start of the next apnea)(47). Sinus bradycardia, heart block (all types), and atrial and ventricular arrhythmias may also be associated with sleep apnea (83). While many OSA patients have frequent PVCs during sleep, 24-hour monitoring often shows a reduction in PVC rate during sleep. Therefore, the presence of ventricular arrhythmias during sleep apnea does not necessarily imply causality. One study found little relationship between the PVC frequency and arterial oxygen saturation until the saturation fell below 60% (84).

Treatment of Obstructive Sleep Apnea

The treatment of OSA begins with an identification and elimination of exacerbating factors such as hypothyroidism and ethanol ingestion, as well as an examination of the patient's upper-airway anatomy. Surgical and medical therapies are discussed below, followed by general guidelines for selecting an appropriate treatment.

The gold standard of therapy for OSA has been tracheostomy (85). This bypasses the upper-airway obstruction and results in almost uniform abolition of obstructive apneas and symptoms. However, in addition to the psychological morbidity, the procedure has frequent complications, especially in patients with fat necks. Now that nasal CPAP is available, tracheostomy is usually reserved for severe cases not tolerating nasal CPAP. A less drastic surgical procedure is uvulopalatopharyngoplasty (UPPP). The uvula, portions of the soft palate, and redundant pharyngeal tissue are removed (86). If nasal obstruction is present, this is often repaired. Unfortunately UPPP significantly reduces the severity of apnea and desaturation in only about 40% to 50% of the patients (86,87). Often the AHI remains above 20 events per hour. UPPP is a very effective procedure for snoring. Several methods of evaluation of the upper airway while patients are awake or asleep have suggested that patients who have significant airway narrowing mainly in the retropalatal area are more likely to improve after UPPP (57). However, no method can predict with absolute certainty which patients will benefit from this surgery. Laser-assisted palatoplasty (LAP) and radiofrequency ablation (somnoplasty) are new methods of increasing the retropalatal airway. LAP may be performed without general anesthesia and is associated with less pain than traditional UPPP. These procedures are currently used mainly for snoring. All patients undergoing palatal surgery should be followed even if a postsurgical improvement occurs. The return of apnea can occur even if snoring is absent or less noisy.

Because of dissatisfaction with UPPP, several new surgical procedures have been developed to treat obstruction behind the tongue or in the lower pharynx (87,88). With anterior mandibular osteotomy, a window of bone where the genioglossus inserts on the mandible is cut and pulled anteriorly, which results in the tongue moving forward. This procedure is usually combined with a hyoid suspension in which the hyoid bone is pulled up and suspended from the mandible. If this fails, the next step is maxillary mandibular osteotomy (MMO). In this procedure the maxilla and mandible are moved forward and the orthodontic occlusion is preserved. Either tracheotomy or nasal CPAP is needed in the immediate postoperative period. This extensive procedure appears to be effective, but it is expensive and is available only at specialized centers.

Medical therapy should always include weight loss if the patient is obese. Some patients will have a significant improvement after moderate weight loss (89). Position therapy (elevation of the head or avoidance of the supine sleep position) may be effective in selected patients (90). Drug therapy with the nonsedating tricyclic antidepressant protriptyline and the selective serotonin reuptake inhibitors (SSRIs) fluoxetine and paroxetine have been demonstrated to lower the AHI in some patients (91). Up to 50% of patients must discontinue using protriptyline due to side effects (urinary retention, etc.). Fluoxetine and paroxetine may be better tolerated than protriptyline, but they have the potential to disturb sleep. All these drugs decrease the amount of REM sleep. However, they reduce the AHI in NREM sleep, presumably by augmenting upper-airway muscle activity secondary to increased serotonin at brain-stem motor nuclei innervating the affected muscles. The role, if any, of SSRIs in OSA treatment remains to be defined but, if useful, will probably be so in milder cases of OSA. Medroxyprogesterone (Provera) is a progestational agent with respiratory stimulant activity. Treatment with this drug appears to benefit patients with the OHS mainly by lowering the daytime P_{CO_2} with a subsequent improvement in the P_{O_2} (92). Little, if any, effect on the frequency of apnea has been demonstrated (93), although the severity of desaturation and the associated right heart failure may improve in some patients. Side effects include impotence, hair loss, and hyperglycemia. In general, nasal CPAP (or tracheostomy) rather than medroxyprogesterone is the treatment of choice for patients with OHS.

Nocturnal oxygen therapy has also been tried in patients with obstructive sleep apnea (94). Acute and chronic studies using continuous low-flow oxygen have usually found improved oxygenation and small increases in event duration. The frequency of respiratory events usually decreases only slightly or remains unchanged. Therefore it is not surprising that oxygen therapy does not improve the sleep latency on MSLT testing (95). No long-term studies have shown an improvement in morbidity or mortality with oxygen therapy. However, if the patient refuses or cannot tolerate more effective therapy, oxygen therapy may be tried to improve nocturnal oxygenation and therefore reduce cardiac sequelae. Sleep monitoring during oxygen administration is warranted before this therapy is prescribed to patients with sleep apnea, to document efficacy. Oxygen therapy can dramatically increase the amount of CO_2 retention during sleep in patients with both hypercapnic COPD and sleep apnea (96).

Medical therapy for OSA was revolutionized by the introduction of nasal CPAP by Sullivan and coworkers (97). With this method, a flow of pressurized room air via the nose maintains a positive pressure in the upper airway. Therefore airway closure is prevented by a "pneumatic splint." Although a nasal mask is most commonly used, an alternative device (nasal pillows) fits into the external nares, providing a seal. The amount of pressure needed to maintain airway patency is determined by a sleep study (nasal CPAP trial or titration) in which the level of CPAP is increased until apnea, hypopnea, desaturation, snoring, and respiratory effort arousals are prevented. Pressures in the range of 5 to 20 cm H_2O are commonly used. Usually higher CPAP pressures are needed during REM sleep or when the patient is supine. In patients with awake hypoxemia or severe obesity, hypoxemia may persist during sleep despite the reversal of upper-airway obstruction with nasal CPAP. This can be especially severe during the prolonged REM episodes (REM rebound) that occur on the first night of CPAP. In such cases, oxygen can be added (and may be needed on a regular basis during sleep in a few patients in addition to nasal CPAP). Due to economic constraints, many sleep laboratories use partial night or "split" studies (98). In such studies, the initial part of the night is used to document the presence and severity of sleep apnea and the second part of the night is a nasal CPAP trial. Such a strategy may be satisfactory in patients with clear-cut severe OSA, provided that the patients receive adequate education about nasal CPAP before bedtime and are allowed to become familiar with the equipment.

The main difficulty with nasal CPAP therapy is the problem with patient acceptance and compliance. Long-term compliance is at best around 40% to 60%. Common complaints include dryness of the nose/mouth, difficulty with the mask seal (or mask discomfort), claustrophobia (difficulty tolerating the pressure), and noise. Improvements in mask and machine design have been made in an attempt to reduce these problems (99). Recent innovations include bilevel positive pressure, in which different levels of pressure may be provided for inspiration (inspiratory positive airway pressure, IPAP) and expiration (expiratory positive airway pressure, EPAP). This potentially allows maintenance of airway patency with a lower level of pressure during expiration and therefore less discomfort and better tolerance (100). However, one study found no difference in compliance between a group of patients treated with CPAP and bilevel pressure (101). The usual bilevel pressure titration protocol is to use IPAP equals EPAP until apnea has been converted to hypopnea. Then IPAP is titrated upward until hypopnea/snoring have been abolished. Another advantage of bilevel pressure is that it allows application of pressure support ventilation noninvasively to treat hypoventilation. For example, if IPAP is at 15 cm H_2O and EPAP is at 5 cm H_2O, the system provides a pressure support of 10 cm H_2O. Another useful innovation to improve CPAP compliance is the "ramp" system. Positive pressure slowly increases to the preset goal over a set time interval. This allows patients to fall asleep on lower pressures and increases the tolerance to higher pressures. Humidification systems have also been introduced to reduce complaints of a dry upper airway. Devices that automatically titrate the amount of pressure needed to maintain airway patency ("smart CPAP") are now available. The mean pressure for a given night may be reduced, because less pressure may be needed during the side sleep position or during NREM sleep. There is some evidence that these devices may increase compliance.

They may also be useful in allowing a sleep lab to perform more CPAP titrations at the same time. Almost all modern CPAP devices now have a meter to record the hours the unit is run at pressure. This allows the physician an objective estimate of compliance.

Recently, there has been considerable interest in the use of oral appliances (OA) as a treatment for obstructive sleep apnea (102). These devices include tongue retaining devices (TRDs) which position the tongue anteriorly using a suction bulb and dental devices (Fig. 18.8) which work by moving the lower jaw (and hence the tongue) forward (103). Additional effects of dental devices may be a downward rotation of the mandible and traction on the palate via the palatoglossal muscle. One problem to date has been a lack of standardization with a large number of devices. Dental devices require the involvement of a qualified dentist to ensure that occlusal or temporomandibular joint problems do not occur. To date oral appliances appear most effective in patients with mild-to-moderate sleep apnea. In one study of patients successfully treated with both nasal CPAP and an oral appliance, the latter device was preferred (104). Oral appliances may also be tried in UPPP failures when nasal CPAP is refused (105).

With the different treatment modalities in mind, one can select an appropriate therapy depending on the severity of the patient's symptoms and the results of the polysomnogram (Table 18.3). Tracheostomy and nasal CPAP are the most uniformly effective treatments and, unlike UPPP, were associated with a reduction in mortality compared to no treatment in a retrospective study of a group of patients with moderate-to-severe OSA (48). However, these treatments may not be appropriate for milder cases of OSA or acceptable to all patients with moderate-to-severe OSA. In assessing the severity of disease one must consider the apnea-plus-hypopnea index, the severity of sleep fragmentation

TABLE 18.3. TREATMENTS FOR OBSTRUCTIVE SLEEP APNEA

Mild OSA/UARS	Moderate OSA	Severe OSA
Weight loss	Nasal CPAP/ bilevel pressure	Nasal CPAP/ bilevel pressure
Position therapy	Oral appliances	Tracheostomy
Oral appliances	UPPP	Maxillofacial surgery
UPPP	Maxillofacial surgery	UPPP[a]
Medications	Weight loss (adjunctive)	Oral appliances[a]
Nasal CPAP		Weight loss (adjunctive)

[a] Less commonly used but may be successful in some cases.
OSA, obstructive sleep apnea; UARS, upper airway resistance syndrome; UPPP, uvulopalatopharyngoplasty.

and arterial oxygen desaturation, the presence of significant arrhythmias during sleep, evidence of right heart failure, the severity of daytime sleepiness, and the impact on comorbid disease such as congestive heart failure. The patient's own estimate of the degree of daytime sleepiness is very unreliable. There is no substitute for good physician judgment. The significance of a mild degree of sleepiness in an elderly sedentary individual is entirely different from that in a commercial truck driver. Alternatively, an asymptomatic patient with moderate sleep apnea and severe hypertensive disease should probably be treated aggressively.

Persistent Daytime Sleepiness On Nasal CPAP

The practicing sleep physician is often presented with the difficult problem of how to evaluate a patient continuing to complain of daytime sleepiness after treatment with nasal CPAP. One must first consider problems with CPAP treatment. These include lack of compliance (not using CPAP

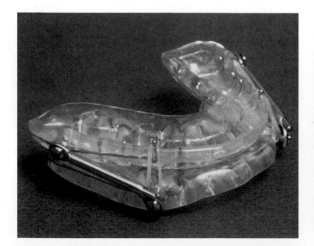
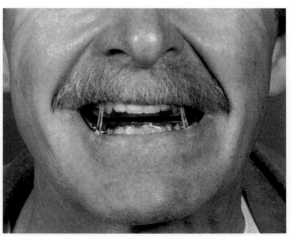

FIGURE 18.8. **A,** A typical oral appliance (Herbst) used to treat obstructive sleep apnea is illustrated. **B,** This appliance fits snugly over the upper and lower teeth. (Reprinted with permission from Berry RB. *Sleep medicine pearls.* Philadelphia: Hanley & Belfus, 1999.)

or using it for only part of the night), inadequate pressure, poor mask seal (therefore inadequate pressure), or an inadequate sleep period. Compliance can be checked by looking at the time meter on the CPAP machine or downloading information from machine memory on some of the newer models. A history of snoring while on CPAP or considerable weight gain suggests a higher prescription pressure may be needed.

If none of the above explanations is likely, one must consider other sleep pathology. Narcolepsy and periodic leg movements are not rare in patients with OSA. An all-night polysomnogram using CPAP and an MSLT (also using CPAP) should be performed (27). The polysomnogram would determine if the prescribed level of CPAP was adequate and if significant PLM-associated arousals were present. The MSLT will document that persistent daytime sleepiness is present and allow a diagnosis of other disorders. For example, a diagnosis of narcolepsy would be supported if the polysomnogram documented adequate sleep (including a normal amount of REM sleep) but the MSLT met the criteria for narcolepsy. In such cases, stimulant medications as well as nasal CPAP may be indicated.

Prognosis and Mortality in OSA/Risk of Automobile Accidents

Limited information has been available concerning the natural history of the OSAS or the effect of therapy. This is an important issue, as some patients with substantial sleep apnea are relatively asymptomatic. It may be difficult to insist that they undergo treatment if they lack evidence of apnea-induced arrhythmias or heart failure when the natural history of their disorder is still unclear. One retrospective study found an increase in mortality in patients with moderate to severe obstructive sleep apnea (apnea index greater than 20 per hour) and that both tracheostomy and nasal CPAP decreased both mortality and morbidity (48). While this study included a large group of patients, many were lost to follow-up and the precise cause of death was not presented. Indeed it may be impossible to perform a randomized placebo-controlled study of the effect of treatment on mortality. Therefore conclusive evidence of an increase in mortality in patients with obstructive sleep apnea is not available.

Another difficult issue is whether patients with OSA are fit to drive an automobile. Patients with OSA are at increased risk for automobile accidents (106,107). Those patients with a history of a recent automobile accident or episodes of falling asleep at the wheel are the group with the highest risk. State laws vary on the physician's responsibility to report patients with "impaired consciousness." The physician must balance such responsibilities with the patient's right for confidentiality. It seems prudent to instruct patients with OSA and severe sleepiness not to drive until adequate treatment has begun. It has been our practice to report only those patients with severe daytime sleepiness who do not adequately comply with therapy. The physician treating patients with OSA should consult his or her local physician organizations for standard-of-practice guidelines.

Central Sleep Apnea Syndromes and Cheyne-Stokes Breathing

A diagnosis of the central sleep apnea (CSA) syndrome requires that a majority of apneas be central in nature (108,109). Usually only 10% to 15% of sleep apnea patients in large series are classified as having CSA. One complicating factor is that CSA is a heterogeneous group of disorders, each having different clinical presentations and pathophysiology and requiring different therapy. In fact, the only common characteristic is apnea due to a loss of central respiratory drive during sleep. A convenient classification is to divide patients with CSA into groups with and without daytime CO_2 retention (108). The nonhypercapnic group is further divided into patients with idiopathic CSA and those with Cheyne-Stokes breathing (CSA-CSB).

Hypercapnic Central Sleep Apnea

Those patients with CSA and daytime hypoventilation usually have evidence of abnormalities in awake ventilatory control, neuromuscular weakness, or an abnormality in chest-wall compliance (kyphoscoliosis) (109). The defects in ventilatory control (central alveolar hypoventilation) may be primary or secondary to brain stem dysfunction (cerebrovascular infarction, neoplasm, or infection). Neuromuscular diseases include poliomyelitis (110), amyotrophic lateral sclerosis, diaphragmatic paralysis, and myopathies. These patients with CSA usually present with episodes of hypercapnic respiratory failure and cor pulmonale. Morning headaches and daytime sleepiness are common. Polysomnography reveals worsening hypoventilation during sleep and periods of central hypopnea and apnea. The degree of arterial oxygen desaturation tends to be rather severe, especially during REM sleep.

Treatment of this group of CSA patients (Table 18.4)

TABLE 18.4. POSSIBLE TREATMENTS FOR CENTRAL SLEEP APNEA

Hypercapnic CSA	Nonhypercapnic CSA
Oxygen (selected cases)	Idiopathic CSA
Diaphragmatic pacing (selected cases)	Hypnotics?
	Nasal CPAP
Negative pressure ventilation	Acetazolamide
Cuirass	
Body wrap	
Nasal bilevel positive pressure (noninvasive pressure support)	Cheyne-Stokes (CHF)
	Optimize CHF treatment
	Oxygen
Volume cycled ventilation (via mask or tracheostomy)	Nasal CPAP
	Theophylline?

CHF, congestive heart failure; CSA, central sleep apnea.

depends on the underlying disease. In those with central alveolar hypoventilation, respiratory stimulants may be tried but are rarely effective. Supplemental oxygen may prevent nocturnal desaturation and improve symptoms (111). A sleep study is required to demonstrate efficacy and to rule out a worsening of hypoventilation with oxygen therapy. If the respiratory muscles are intact, diaphragmatic pacing has been effective in some patients. Negative-pressure ventilation (112) can also be attempted. Unfortunately, these last two modes of therapy frequently tend to induce obstructive sleep apnea, because respiratory efforts are not coordinated with increases in upper-airway tone. Nocturnal positive-pressure ventilation, via a nasal/full face mask, oral lip seal, or tracheostomy, is probably the most effective therapy (113,114). If a mask is used, some positive-end expiratory pressure may be needed to maintain airway patency. In milder cases, bilevel positive pressure providing noninvasive pressure support ventilation may prove effective. In more severe cases, volume cycled ventilation is usually required. Mask ventilation requires that the patient be alert, able to mobilize secretions, and have intact reflexes to prevent aspiration.

Nonhypercapnic Central Sleep Apnea

The second group of patients with central sleep apnea have a normal or low daytime PCO_2. They manifest central apnea when their PCO_2 level falls below a level required to trigger ventilation during sleep. This "apneic threshold" varies between individuals but is usually 0 to 2 mmHg above the the resting *awake* PCO_2 level (61). These patients may present with complaints of disturbed sleep (awakenings, choking), insomnia, or excessive daytime sleepiness. Cor pulmonale and polycythemia are usually not present. This group can be further divided into those with idiopathic CSA and those with CSA associated with CSB.

In CSB there is a crescendo-decrescendo pattern of breathing (tidal volume and ventilatory drive) with central hypopnea or apnea at the nadir in ventilatory drive (Fig. 18.9). If arousal occurs after apnea in CSB, it is usually several breaths after event termination during maximal ventilatory effort. The delay in the nadir in arterial oxygen saturation following apnea termination is quite long in CSA-CSB associated with congestive heart failure. In idiopathic CSA there is an abrupt resumption of ventilatory effort at apnea termination, usually associated with an arousal. If repetitive central apneas occur, the periods of ventilation between the apneas tend to be much shorter than in CSA-CSB.

Idiopathic Central Sleep Apnea

Patients with this uncommon disorder are usually male (108) and are generally less obese than patients with OSA. Complaints of insomnia may be more prominent than in typical OSA. Polysomnography shows central apnea usually

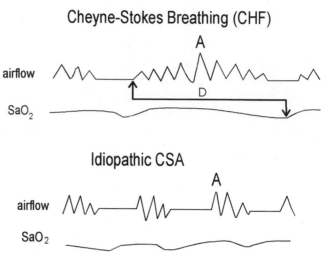

FIGURE 18.9. A schematic illustrating differences in the patterns of idiopathic central sleep apnea and central apnea associated with Cheyne-Stokes breathing (CSB) secondary to congestive heart failure. **(A)** marks the typical position of arousal and **(D)** illustrates the long delay between apnea termination and the nadir in arterial oxygen saturation that occurs in CSB associated with heart failure. (Redrawn with permission from Berry RB. *Sleep medicine pearls.* Philadelphia: Hanley & Belfus, 1999.)

in stage 1 or 2 sleep, often following arousals and awakenings. The associated desaturations are usually modest in severity, but the frequent arousals can cause severe sleep fragmentation. This group tends to have daytime hypocapnia and increased hypercapnic ventilatory responses (115). The sleeping PCO_2 also tends to be low and is believed to be close to the apneic threshold. Therefore even slight increases in ventilation (and reductions in PCO_2) may result in central apnea. Arousal plays an important role in initiating or perpetuating central apnea in these patients (116). Arousals precipitating apnea are typically associated with one or more large tidal volumes which lower the PCO_2 and increase the tendency for central apnea on the subsequent return to sleep. Indeed, arousal due to any cause may trigger a subsequent series of central apnea–arousal–central apnea events.

Several treatments have been tried for idiopathic CSA (see Table 18.4). Some have suggested that sedatives might be efficacious in this specific group of CSA patients by reducing arousal or minimizing the increase in ventilation associated with arousal. In fact, a small study found the benzodiazepine hypnotic triazolam was of modest benefit (117). Acetazolamide (Diamox) 250 mg given one hour before bedtime also proved effective in a group of patients with nonhypercapnic CSA, presumably by inducing metabolic acidosis (118). Application of a high flow of gas with increased carbon dioxide or increasing dead space also prevented central apnea in another study of patients with idiopathic CSA, presumably by raising the waking/sleeping PCO_2 (119). However, neither of these measures is clinically feasible. Issa and Sullivan found that nasal CPAP was efficacious in a group of patients with idiopathic CSA (120). Two explanations for the efficacy of nasal CPAP in this disorder are (a) CPAP prevents airway collapse and subsequent reflex central apnea, and (b) nasal CPAP is an expiratory load and induces mild increases in PCO_2. Further evidence for the concept that upper-airway collapse may be triggering central apnea in these patients is the observation that some patients develop central apnea only in the supine sleeping position. At present, there is little data about the long-term efficacy of any of the treatments listed above for this relatively rare group of patients. Treatment must be individualized. If medication is prescribed, a sleep study should document efficacy.

Cheyne-Stokes Breathing–associated CSA

The causes of CSA associated with CSB include congestive heart failure (CHF) (121,122) and neurological insults (123). Indeed, CSB secondary to CHF is the most common cause of central sleep apnea, with up to 40% of patients with significant CHF having CSB. CSB is more common during sleep stages 1 and 2. Patients with CSB have an underlying instability in ventilatory control, with oscillations in ventilation. Central hypopnea or apnea occurs when the PCO_2 approaches or falls below the apneic threshold. Instability is more likely with high controller gain (high ventilatory drive), feedback delay (increased circulation time), or an underdamped system (124). The traditional explanation for CSB in patients in heart failure was an increase in circulation time (low cardiac output) producing feedback delay in ventilatory control. However, one study found no difference in left ventricular ejection fraction or circulation time between groups of CHF patients with and without CSB (125). The major difference between the groups was that the patients with CSB had a lower daytime and sleeping PCO_2. The length of the cycle time (time from the start of one event until start of the next) was correlated with circulation time. Having a sleeping arterial PCO_2 near the apneic threshold may predispose to an instability in control (122). The reason for the lower PCO_2 is not known but could be related to pulmonary congestion, with stimulation of breathing by reflex mechanisms. Another study found that the presence of symptoms of nocturnal dyspnea or the presence of atrial fibrillation made CSB more likely (126). CSB results in periodic desaturations during sleep and sleep disturbance (arousals). Patients may complain of daytime sleepiness, and the hypoxemia and CSB may cause recurrent activation of the sympathetic nervous system. Thus CSB may have long-term adverse effects on cardiac function. One study found that the presence of CSB may signal a poor prognosis (127).

In CSA-CSB secondary to neurological insults, supplemental oxygen or theophylline has been reported to be effective (123). Possible treatments for CSA-CSB secondary to CHF are listed in Table 18.4. Medical treatment of heart failure, with improvement in cardiac function, may reduce the amount of CSB. Studies have also shown that the amount of CSB can be reduced and oxygenation improved in patients with CHF using theophylline (128), supplemental oxygen (129), and nasal CPAP (122,130). However, the potential for exacerbating arrhythmias has limited the use of theophylline. While oxygen can usually prevent desaturation, some patients will continue to have some CSB and sleep disturbance. The acute application of nasal CPAP may abolish CSB in a few patients; however, most will continue to have CSB. One approach is slowly to increase the level of nasal CPAP to around 10 cm H_2O as tolerated over several nights. When a group of patients with CSB secondary to heart failure were treated for three months using this approach, the frequency of central apnea and hypopnea fell from 43 to 15 events per hour, and both the left ventricular ejection fraction and symptoms of heart failure improved (130). Nasal CPAP is believed to improve CSB by reducing hypoxemia, inducing an increase in PCO_2, and improving cardiac function. The improvement in cardiac function is thought secondary to reductions in nocturnal sympathetic activity, improvements in oxygenation, and afterload reduction during nightly CPAP use (122). Unfortunately, not all patients with CSB and CHF may benefit or tolerate nasal CPAP (131). To date, nasal CPAP seems most useful in patients with coexistent upper-airway obstruction (see next section) or higher filling pressures. In the absence of long-term studies showing the superiority of any one treatment for CSB, the physician should treat each case on an individual basis, with a sleep study to document efficacy.

Congestive Heart Failure and Sleep

It is important for physicians to recognize that patients with CHF may have significant sleep-disordered breathing and arterial oxygen desaturations during sleep in the absence of daytime hypoxemia. One study found that almost 50% of patients with stable CHF had an AHI of over 20 per hour (132). Complaints of poor nocturnal sleep, frequent awakening, and daytime sleepiness may be erroneously assumed to be due to CHF alone. Sleep-disordered breathing may occur in CHF patients as (a) OSA, (b) CSA with CSB, (c) a combination of OSA and CSB (133).

When a group of patients with dilated cardiomyopathy and OSA were treated with nasal CPAP, not only were sleep quality and oxygen saturation improved, but the left ventricular ejection fraction during wakefulness increased significantly (134). The mechanisms by which nighttime nasal CPAP improves daytime cardiac function may include decreased activation of the sympathetic nervous system and decreased cardiac work during sleep.

Patients with heart failure and CSB may sometimes be mistakenly thought to have typical OSA. They may complain of daytime sleepiness and exhibit mixed obstructive apnea. If underlying CSB is not recognized, the sudden appearance of central apnea during CPAP titration may be

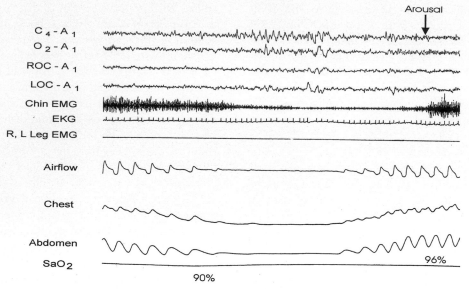

FIGURE 18.10. A polysomnographic tracing of a patient with cardiomyopathy and atrial fibrillation while on nasal CPAP of 10 cm H_2O. This level of CPAP eliminated upper-airway obstruction (on lower pressures a mixed apnea pattern was present), but central apnea with a Cheyne-Stokes breathing pattern persisted. Note that arousal occurred several breaths after termination of the central apnea. Higher levels of CPAP did not eliminate Cheyne-Stokes breathing in this patient.

quite confusing. These patients have upper-airway closure during the waxing period of respiratory effort in CSB. When nasal CPAP prevents upper-airway closure, a traditional pattern of CSA-CSB may emerge (Fig. 18.10). However, unlike typical mixed obstructive apnea, repetitive central apneas usually persist once upper-airway obstruction has been prevented. Three clues for the presence of CSB in the setting of mixed apnea (Fig. 18.11) are that the maximal breaths tend to occur several breaths after the apnea is broken (rather than immediately postapnea), the central component is long, and the nadir in oxygen saturation is markedly delayed (increased circulation time). Recognition that CSB

(as well as obstructive apnea) is present may direct attention to better treatment of congestive heart failure. In addition, the end point of nasal CPAP treatment may be unclear, as central apnea typically persists even with further increases in CPAP. In such cases, an empiric approach is to treat with nasal CPAP at a level around 10 cm H_2O (as outlined above) unless a higher CPAP level is needed to prevent airway obstruction.

Sleep and Asthma

Nocturnal asthma is a significant problem for both asthmatic patients and their physicians. In a large survey of asthmatics, 74% responded that they awoke from sleep at least one night each week with symptoms of asthma (135). The study of the effect of sleep on asthma has been complicated by the time-related rhythms in bronchomotor tone. In normal persons, the best pulmonary function occurs at 4:00 P.M. and the worst at 4:00 A.M. This fluctuation in airway function is even more dramatic in many asthmatics. Thus studies must consider the effects of the 24-hour clock as well as those of recumbency and sleep. It appears that sleep induces an independent worsening of lung function, although no sleep stage-specific effects have been documented (136). Arterial oxygen desaturation is usually mild and most severe during REM sleep. Polysomnography is not indicated unless sleep apnea is suspected. The simplest way to document a patient's predisposition for nocturnal asthma is to have the patient record a peak expiratory flow rate (PEFR) at bedtime, during nocturnal awakening, and

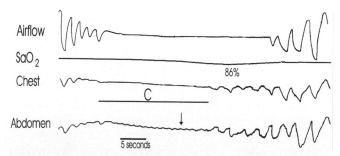

FIGURE 18.11. A mixed apnea in a patient with a cardiomyopathy and Cheyne-Stokes breathing. The nadir in arterial oxygen saturation shown here *precedes* apnea termination. This desaturation was actually related to the previous event. The long delay in the nadir in saturation is caused by a long circulation time. The central portion of the mixed apnea is marked by C. The small deflections in this portion (arrow) are secondary to cardiac pulsations.

in the morning. A detailed discussion of the pathophysiology of the nocturnal worsening of asthma is beyond the scope of this chapter and is available in the literature (137). Briefly, nocturnal falls in circulating epinephrine and corticosteroids and increases in histamine, vagal tone, and possibly increased leukotriene synthesis may be important. In patients with nocturnal asthma, the β-adrenergic receptor function decreases at night. In addition, a recent study suggests that patients with significant worsening of lung function at night have a circadian influx of effector cells into the lung. In those patients, a significant increase in neutrophils and eosinophils was noted in the bronchoalveolar lavage fluid at 4:00 A.M. (138).

The ideal treatment for nocturnal asthma would require bronchodilators with a long duration of action that do not disturb sleep. Salmeterol, a long-acting inhaled β-agonist, may be particularly useful in patients with nocturnal asthma. This medication could conceivably cause less central nervous system stimulation than oral sustained-action theophylline. However, a study comparing theophylline and salmeterol in nocturnal asthma (139) found no difference in patient preference and no clinically meaningful differences in sleep quality. While tolerance to the side effects of theophylline may develop in many patients, others may sleep better with salmeterol. If theophylline is used, the dosing should be arranged so that maximum serum levels occur at night (137). Long-acting oral β-agonists are also of potential benefit but also have the potential for sleep disturbance (140). Corticosteroid therapy can also decrease the nocturnal worsening of lung function (141). The timing as well as the dose appears to be important. Preliminary results suggest that a 3:00 P.M. steroid dose may be more efficacious than one in the morning or at bedtime in preventing the nocturnal worsening of lung function (142) and the influx of inflammatory cells into the lung. While asthmatics generally have a greater response to β-agonists than to anticholinergic medications, vagal tone is increased at night. Therefore, anticholinergics such as ipratropium bromide are of potential benefit in nocturnal asthma (143). A higher bedtime dose (four puffs) may be needed so that the duration of action is long enough to last for most of the night. There is also some preliminary evidence that medications blocking the synthesis or action of leukotrienes may benefit many patients with nocturnal asthma (144,145). If an asthmatic patient has obstructive sleep apnea, nasal CPAP may actually reduce asthmatic attacks (146). Snoring and recurrent upper-airway obstruction may be triggering mechanisms in these patients.

Sleep and Chronic Obstructive Pulmonary Disease

Some patients with COPD may have nocturnal desaturation without the cyclic apnea-desaturation-arousal pattern common in OSA. Others have considerable OSA as well as airway disease (the overlap syndrome). This latter group of patients may have particularly severe oxygen desaturation since their preapnea saturations may be quite low.

A typical pattern of nocturnal arterial oxygen saturation in a COPD patient (147–149) without substantial obstructive apnea includes (a) a fall in the baseline arterial oxygen saturation on transition from wakefulness to sleep, (b) small transient fluctuations in oxygen saturation (3% to 5%) during NREM sleep, and (c) larger drops in saturation during REM sleep (10% to 50%) that may last from several minutes to a half hour or more. One should recall that even normal persons have a small fall in P_{O_2} during sleep but, due to their position on the flat portion of the oxyhemoglobin saturation curve, little desaturation occurs. Conversely, patients with an awake P_{O_2} in the 55 to 60 mm Hg range (the steep portion of the curve) will have significant desaturation from small falls in P_{O_2}. It appears that in some COPD patients the fall in P_{O_2} with sleep is within the normal range (149) but desaturation is worse because of a lower baseline P_{O_2}. Patients with CO_2 retention or low awake P_{O_2} are more likely to exhibit severe desaturation (150).

The episodes of profound desaturation during stage REM are usually associated with periods of hypopnea in which tidal volume is reduced but respiratory rate is essentially unchanged (151). There is a reduction in pleural pressure swings in most cases, implying a reduction in central drive. However, one should note that during stage REM a loss of intercostal muscle tone makes the diaphragm less effective, especially in patients with hyperinflation, which places this muscle at a mechanical disadvantage. Thus, even if the neural output to the diaphragm was constant, less inspiratory pressure might be generated. The reduction in minute ventilation during hypopneas is thought to lead to alveolar hypoventilation, with a resulting increase in P_{CO_2} and fall in P_{O_2}. Some evidence (152) suggests that increases in ventilation-perfusion mismatch may also contribute to the dramatic REM-associated falls in the oxygen saturation. During stage REM, a loss of intercostal muscle tone is believed to decrease the functional residual capacity, and this may increase ventilation-perfusion mismatch.

Hypoxemia leads to pulmonary vasoconstriction and pulmonary hypertension. Some have hypothesized that prolonged nocturnal hypoxemia and pulmonary hypertension may lead to cor pulmonale in the absence of daytime desaturation (153). This interesting hypothesis remains unproven. It is known that patients with daytime hypoxemia (P_{O_2} under 55 mmHg) or borderline hypoxemia (55 to 60 mm Hg with evidence of cor pulmonale) will benefit from continuous oxygen therapy (154). The benefits of *nocturnal* oxygen treatment for COPD patients with daytime P_{O_2} above 60 mm Hg and nocturnal desaturation remain unproved. In such patients, nocturnal desaturation occurs most commonly in REM sleep. While REM sleep desaturation may be severe, the total duration of this type of desaturation typically lasts less than an hour per night. Is treatment of this type of desaturation beneficial? Nocturnal supplemental oxygen or room air was administered in a double-blind manner to a group of COPD patients with daytime PO_2 above 60 mm Hg and documented REM sleep desaturation. At three years the oxygen group showed nearly a 4 mm Hg decrease in daytime mean pulmonary pressure, while the room air group showed about a 4 mm Hg rise (155). However, no study has documented that supplemental nocturnal oxygen will decrease mortality or morbidity in this group of patients with nocturnal desaturations confined to REM sleep.

Nocturnal low-flow oxygen therapy prevents the episodes of nonapneic desaturation associated with COPD without markedly increasing the PCO_2 (96). The exception is COPD patients with significant obstructive sleep apnea in whom large increases in PCO_2 may occur. While oxygen therapy definitely improves the mortality and morbidity of patients with daytime hypoxemia (PO_2 under 55 mm Hg) the benefits of treatment of isolated nocturnal desaturation remain unproved. Until the clinical importance of isolated nocturnal desaturation in patients with COPD is clarified, widespread sleep monitoring in these patients cannot be justified except to rule out OSA (150). A possible exception is to document the need for nocturnal oxygen therapy when significant cor pulmonale is not explained by daytime arterial blood gas analysis (PO_2 over 60 mmHg). A sleep study may reveal unsuspected OSA or arterial oxygen desaturation that is worse than expected. If significant sleep apnea is present it should be treated (see below). In patients with nonapneic arterial oxygen desaturation, no firm guidelines exist concerning the amount of desaturation required to justify nocturnal administration of oxygen. Patients with evidence of cor pulmonale and a baseline sleeping saturation (NREM sleep) that remains below 85% for a majority of the night should probably be treated with nocturnal oxygen. This recommendation assumes that the other medical treatment for COPD has been optimized.

The sleep quality in patients with significant COPD is frequently poor. A shortened TST, low sleep efficiency, and frequent arousals are common. Many patients complain of coughing or difficult breathing during the night. Like asthmatics, the diurnal variation in pulmonary function may be exaggerated in these patients, and many patients have the greatest difficulty breathing in the early morning hours. There are conflicting data on whether the sleep quality of patients with COPD is improved by oxygen therapy (156,157). As with asthmatics, bronchodilators, while improving lung function, could potentially worsen sleep quality due to central stimulation. However, in one study, sustained-action theophylline improved early-morning spirometry and the oxygen saturation in NREM sleep without impairing sleep quality (158). If patients do complain of sleep disturbance with theophylline, the long-acting inhaled β-agonist salmeterol may be better tolerated. Inhaled ipratropium bromide at bedtime (four puffs) may also prove

useful. Many patients request hypnotics to improve sleep quality. The benzodiazepine triazolam (159) and the nonbenzodiazepine zolpidem both appear to increase sleep length without significantly worsening oxygenation (160). Caution is still advised. Sedatives of any type are contraindicated in hypercapnic or unstable patients.

The group of patients with both COPD and OSA (overlap syndrome) tend to have more severe cardiopulmonary sequelae than those with equivalent amounts of sleep apnea (161). Furthermore, these patients may continue to have impressive nocturnal desaturation during REM sleep even after treatment of obstructive apnea with a tracheostomy or nasal CPAP (162). Alternatively, oxygen alone rarely completely reverses the hypoxemia and may lead to considerable CO_2 retention and morning headache (96). One approach is to treat the OSA with nasal CPAP and then add oxygen as needed if nocturnal desaturation persists even though airway patency during sleep is restored (163).

REFERENCES

1. Rechtschaffen A, Kales A, eds. *A manual of standardized terminology techniques and scoring system for sleep stages of human sleep.* Los Angeles: Brain Information Service/Brain Research Institute, UCLA, 1968.
2. Williams RL, Karacan I, Hursch CJ. *Electroencephalography (EEG) of human sleep: clinical applications.* New York: John Wiley & Sons, 1974.
3. Carskadon MA, Rechtschaffen A. Monitoring and staging human sleep. In: Kryger MH, Roth T, Dement WC, eds. *Principles and practice of sleep medicine.* Philadelphia: WB Saunders Co., 1994:943–960.
4. West P, Kryger MH. Sleep and respiration: terminology and methodology *Clin Chest Med* 1985;4:691–712.
5. Berry RB. *Sleep Medicine Pearls.* Philadelphia: Hanley & Belfus, 1999.
6. ASDA Task Force. EEG arousals: Scoring rules and examples. *Sleep* 1992;15:173–184.
7. Downey R, Bonnet MH. Performance during frequent sleep disruption. *Sleep* 1987;10:354–363.
8. Mathur R, Douglas NJ. Frequency of EEG arousals from nocturnal sleep in normal subjects. *Sleep.* 1995;18:330–333.
9. Phillipson EA. Control of breathing during sleep. *Am Rev Respir Dis* 1978;118:909–937.
10. Douglas NJ. Control of ventilation during sleep. *Clin Chest Med* 1985;6:563–575.
11. Phillipson EA. Sleep disorders. In: Murray JF, Nadel JA, eds. *Textbook of respiratory medicine.* Philadelphia: WB Saunders, 1994:2301–2324.
12. Krieger J. Breathing during sleep in normal subjects. *Clin Chest Med* 1985;6:577–594.
13. Hudgel DW, Martin RJ, Johnson B, et al. Mechanics of the respiratory system and breathing pattern during sleep in normal humans. *J Appl Physiol* 1984;56:1–137.
14. Hudgel DW, Devadatta P. Decrease in functional residual capacity during sleep in normal humans. *J Appl Physiol* 1984;57:1319–1322.
15. Wiegand L, Zwillich CW, Wiegand D, et al. Changes in upper airway muscle activation and ventilation during phasic REM sleep in normal men. *J Appl Physiol* 1991;71:488–497.
16. Gould GA, Gugger M, Molloy J, et al. Breathing pattern and

eye movement density during REM sleep in humans. *Am Rev Respir Dis* 1988;138:874–877.

17. Tabachnik E, Muller NL, Bryan AC, et al. Changes in ventilation and chest wall mechanics during sleep in normal adolescents. *J Appl Physiol* 1981;51:557–564.

18. Block AJ, Boysen PG, Wynne JW, et al. Sleep apnea, hypopnea, and oxygen desaturation in normal subjects. A strong male predominance. *N Engl J Med* 1979;300:513–517.

19. Gould GA, Whyte KF, Rhind GB, et al. The sleep hypopnea syndrome. *Am Rev Respir Dis* 1988;137:895–898.

20. Staats BA, Bonekat HW, Harris CD, et al. Chest wall motion in sleep apnea. *Am Rev Respir Dis* 1984;130:59–63.

21. Tobin MJ, Cohn MA, Sackner MA. Breathing abnormalities during sleep. *Arch Intern Med* 1983;143:1221–1228.

22. Hosselet J, Norman RC, Ayappa I, et al. Detection of flow limitation with nasal cannula/pressure transducer system. *Am J Respir Crit Care Med* 1998;157:1461–1467.

23. American Sleep Disorders Association. The clinical use of the multiple sleep latency test. *Sleep* 1992;15:268–276.

24. Rosenthal L, Roehrs TA, Rosen A, et al. Level of sleepiness and total sleep time following various time in bed conditions. *Sleep* 1993;16:226–232.

25. Doghramji K, Mitler MM, Sangal RB, et al. A normative study of the maintenance of wakefulness test (MWT). *Electroencephalogr Clin Neurophysiol* 1997;103:554–562.

26. Sangal RB, Thomas L, Mitler MM. Maintenance of wakefulness test and multiple sleep latency test. *Chest* 1992;101:898–902.

27. American Sleep Disorders Association. International classification of sleep disorders, revised. *Diagnostic and coding manual.* Rochester, MN: American Sleep Disorders Association, 1997.

28. Aldrich MS. The clinical spectrum of narcolepsy and idiopathic hypersomnia. *Neurology* 1996;46:383–401.

29. Basetti C, Aldrich MS. Narcolepsy. *Neurolog Clin* 1996;14: 545–571.

30. Coleman RM, Roffwarg HP, Kennedy SJ, et al. Sleep-wake disorders based on a polysomnographic diagnosis—a national cooperative study. *JAMA* 1982;247:997–1003.

31. Mignot E, Lin X, Arrigoni J, et al. DQB1*0602 and DQA1*0102 are better markers than DR2 for narcolepsy in Caucasians and African-Americans. *Sleep* 1994;17:60–67.

32. US Modafinil in Narcolepsy Multicenter Study Group. Randomized trial of modafinil for the treatment of pathological somnolence in narcolepsy. *Ann Neurol* 1998;43:88–97.

33. Roehrs T, Zorick F, Sicklesteel J, et al. Excessive daytime sleepiness associated with insufficient sleep. *Sleep* 1983;6:319–325.

34. Monteplaisir J, Lapierre O, Warnes H, et al. The treatment of the restless leg syndrome with or without periodic leg movements in sleep. *Sleep* 1992;15:391–395.

35. Fry JM, Diphillip MA, Pressman MR. Periodic leg movements in sleep following treatment of obstructive sleep apnea with nasal CPAP. *Chest* 1989;96:89–91.

36. ASDA Atlas Task Force. Recording and scoring leg movements. *Sleep* 1993;16:749–759.

37. Trenkwalder C, Walters RS, Hening W. Periodic limb movements and restless leg syndrome. *Neurol Clin* 1996;14:629–650.

38. Strollo PJ Jr, Rogers RM. Obstructive sleep apnea. *N Engl J Med* 1996;334:99–104.

39. Young T, Palta M, Dempsey J, et al. The occurrence of sleep-disordered breathing among middle-aged adults. *N Engl J Med* 1993;328:1230–1235.

40. Block AJ, Hellard DW, Slayton PC. Effect of alcohol ingestion on breathing and oxygenation during sleep. *Am J Med* 1986; 80:595–600.

41. Harman E, Wynne JW, Block AJ, et al. Sleep-disordered breathing and oxygen desaturation in obese patients. *Chest* 1981;79: 256–260.

42. Rajagopal KR, Abbrecht PH, Derderian SS, et al. Obstructive sleep apnea in hypothyroidism. *Ann Intern Med* 1984;101: 491–494.

43. Mezon BJ, Maclean JP, Kryger MH. Sleep apnea in acromegaly. *Am J Med* 1980;69:615–618.

44. Dolly FR, Block AJ. Effect of flurazepam on sleep-disordered breathing and nocturnal oxygen desaturation in asymptomatic subjects. *Am J Med* 1982;73:239–243.

45. Bradley TD, Rutherford R, Grossman R, et al. Role of daytime hypoxemia in the pathogenesis of right heart failure in obstructive sleep apnea syndrome. *Am Rev Respir Dis* 1985;131: 835–839.

46. Flemons WW, Whitelaw, WA, Brant R, et al. Likelihood ratios for a sleep apnea clinical prediction rule. *Am J Respir Crit Care Med* 1994;150:1279–1285.

47. Weiss JW, Remsburg S, Garpestad E, et al. Hemodynamic consequences of obstructive sleep apnea. *Sleep* 1996;19:388–397.

48. He J, Kryger MH, Zorick FJ, et al. Mortality and apnea index in obstructive sleep apnea. *Chest* 1988;94:9–14.

49. Bradley TD, Martinez D, Rutherford R. Physiological determinants of nocturnal arterial oxygenation in patients with obstructive sleep apnea. *J Appl Physiol* 1985;59:1364–1368.

50. Horner RL. Motor control of pharyngeal musculature and implications for the pathogenesis of obstructive sleep apnea. *Sleep* 1996;19:827–853.

51. Remmers JE, Degroot WJ, Sauerland EK, et al. Pathogenesis of upper airway occlusion during sleep. *J Appl Physiol* 1978;44: 931–938.

52. Badr MS. Pathophysiology of upper airway obstruction during sleep. *Clin Chest Med* 1998;19:21–32.

53. Tangel DJ, Mezzanotte WS, Sandberg EJ, et al. Influences of NREM sleep on the activity of tonic versus inspiratory phasic muscles in normal men. *J Appl Physiol* 1992;73:1058–1066.

54. Mezzanotte WS, Tangel DJ, White DP. Influence of sleep onset on upper airway muscle activity in apnea patients versus normal controls. *Am J Respir Crit Care Med* 1996;153:1880–1887.

55. Schwab RJ. Upper airway imaging. *Clin Chest Med* 1998;19: 33–54.

56. Van de Graaff WB. Thoracic influence on upper airway patency. *J Appl Physiol* 1988;65:2124–2131.

57. Launois SH, Feroah TR, Campbell WN, et al. Site of pharyngeal narrowing predicts outcome of surgery for obstructive sleep apnea. *Am Rev Respir Dis* 1993;147:182–189.

58. Anch AM, Remmers JE, Bunce H III. Supraglottic resistance in normal subjects and patients with occlusive sleep apnea. *J Appl Physiol* 1982;53:1158–1163.

59. Gold AR, Schwartz AR. The pharyngeal critical pressure. *Chest* 1996;110:1077–1088.

60. Onal E, Lopata M, O'Connor T. Pathogenesis of apneas in hypersomnia–sleep apnea syndrome. *Am Rev Respir Dis* 1982; 125:167–174.

61. Dempsey JA, Skatrud JB. A sleep induced apneic threshold and it consequences. *Am Rev Respir Dis* 1986;133:1163–1170.

62. Iber C, Davies SF, Chapman RC, et al. A possible mechanism for mixed apnea in obstructive sleep apnea. *Chest* 1986;89: 800–805.

63. Berry RB, Gleeson K. Respiratory arousal from sleep: mechanisms and significance. *Sleep* 1997;20:654–675.

64. Rajagopal KR, Bennett LL, Dillard TA. Overnight nasal CPAP improves hypersomnolence in sleep apnea. *Chest* 1986;90: 172–176.

65. Poceta JS, Timms RM, Jeong D, et al. Maintenance of wakefulness test in obstructive sleep apnea syndrome. *Chest* 1992;101: 893–897.

66. Orr WC, Martin RJ, Imes NK, et al. Hypersomnolent and

nonhypersomnolent patients with upper airway obstruction during sleep. *Chest* 1979;75:418–422.

67. Roehrs T, Zorick F, Wittig R, et al. Predictors of objective level of daytime sleepiness in patients with sleep-related breathing disorders. *Chest* 1989;95:1202–1206.

68. Guilleminault C, Partinen M, Quera-Salva MA, et al. Determinants of daytime sleepiness in obstructive sleep apnea. *Chest* 1988;94:32–37.

69. Findley LJ, Barth JT, Powers DC, et al. Cognitive impairment in patients with obstructive sleep apnea and associated hypoxemia. *Chest* 1986;90:686–690.

70. Garay SM, Rapoport D, Sorkin B, et al. Regulation of ventilation in the obstructive sleep apnea syndrome. *Am Rev Respir Dis* 1981,124:451–457.

71. Rajagopal KR, Abbrecht PH, Tellis CJ. Control of breathing in obstructive sleep apnea. *Chest* 1984;85:174–180.

72. Zwillich CW, Sutton FD, Pierson DJ, et al. Decreased hypoxic ventilatory drive in the obesity-hypoventilation syndrome. *Am J Med* 1975;59:343–348.

73. Rochester DF, Enson Y. Current concepts in the pathogenesis of the obesity hypoventilation syndrome. *Am J Med* 1974;57:402–420.

74. Sharp JT. The chest wall and respiratory muscles in obesity, pregnancy, and ascites. In: Roussos C, Macklem PT, eds. *The thorax.* New York: Marcel Dekker, 1985:999–1016.

75. Rapoport DM, Garay SM, Epstein H, et al. Hypercapnia in the obstructive sleep apnea syndrome. *Chest* 1986;89:627–635.

76. Sullivan CE, Berthon-Jones M, Issa FG. Remission of severe obesity-hypoventilation syndrome after short-term treatment during sleep with nasal continuous positive airway pressure. *Am Rev Respir Dis* 1983;128:177–181.

77. Guilleminault C, Stoohs R, Clerk A, et al. Cause of excessive daytime sleepiness: the upper airway resistance syndrome. *Chest* 1993;104:781–787.

78. Shephard JW Jr. Hypertension, cardiac arrhythmias, myocardial infarction, and stroke in relation to obstructive sleep apnea. *Clin Chest Med* 1992;13:437–458.

79. Weitzenblum E, Krieger J, Apprill M, et al. Daytime pulmonary hypertension in patients with obstructive sleep apnea syndrome. *Am Rev Respir Dis* 1988;138:345–349.

80. Kales A, Bixler EO, Cadieux RJ, et al. Sleep apnea in a hypertensive population. *Lancet* 1984;2:1005–1008.

81. Verdecchia P, Schiallica G, Guerrier M, et al. Circadian blood pressure changes and left ventricular hypertrophy in essential hypertension. *Circulation* 1990;81:528–536.

82. Fletcher EC. Can treatment of sleep apnea syndrome prevent cardiovascular consequences? *Sleep* 1996;19:S67–S70.

83. Tilkian AG, Guilleminault C, Schroeder JS, et al. Sleep-induced apnea syndrome. Prevalence of cardiac arrhythmias and their reversal after tracheostomy. *Am J Med* 1977;63:348–358.

84. Shephard JW Jr, Garrison MW, Grither DA, et al. Relationship of ventricular ectopy to oxyhemoglobin desaturation in patients with obstructive sleep apnea. *Chest* 1985;88:335–340.

85. Guilleminault C, Simmons FB, Motta J, et al. Obstructive sleep apnea syndrome and tracheostomy—long term follow up and experience. *Arch Intern Med* 1982;126:14–20.

86. Fujita S, Conway W, Zorick F, et al. Surgical correction of anatomic abnormalities in obstructive sleep apnea syndrome: uvulopalatopharyngoplasty. *Otolaryngol Head Neck Surg* 1981; 89:923–934.

87. Sher AE, Schechtman KB, Piccirillo JF. The efficacy of surgical modification of the upper airway in adults with obstructive sleep apnea syndrome. *Sleep* 1996;19:156–177.

88. Riley RW, Powell NB, Guilleminault C. Maxillary, mandibular, and hyoid advancement for treatment of obstructive sleep apnea. *J Oral Maxillofac Surg* 1990;48:20–26.

89. Smith PL, Gold AR, Moyers DA, et al. Weight loss in mildly to moderately obese patients with obstructive sleep apnea. *Ann Intern Med* 1985;103:850–855.

90. Neill AM, Angus SM, Sajkov K, et al. Effects of sleep posture on upper airway stability in patients with obstructive sleep apnea. *Am J Respir Crit Care Med* 1997;155:199–204.

91. Hudgel DW, Thanakitcharu S. Pharmacologic treatment of sleep-disordered breathing. *Am J Resp Crit Care Med* 1998;158: 691–696.

92. Sutton FD, Zwillich CW, Creagh CE, et al. Progesterone for outpatient treatment of the Pickwickian syndrome. *Ann Intern Med* 1975;83:476–479.

93. Rajagopal KR, Abbrecht PH, Jabbari B. Effects of medroxyprogesterone acetate in obstructive sleep apnea. *Chest* 1996;90: 815–821.

94. Fletcher EC, Munafo D. Role of nocturnal oxygen therapy in obstructive sleep apnea. *Chest* 1990;98:1497–1504.

95. Smith PL, Haponik EF, Bleecker ER. The effects of oxygen in patients with sleep apnea. *Am Rev Respir Dis* 1984;130: 957–963.

96. Goldstein RS, Ramcharan V, Bowes G, et al. Effect of supplemental nocturnal oxygen on gas exchange in patients with severe obstructive lung disease. *N Engl J Med* 1984;310:425–429.

97. Sullivan CE, Issa FG, Berthon-Jones M, et al. Reversal of obstructive sleep apnoea by continuous positive airway pressure applied through the nares. *Lancet* 1981;1:862–865.

98. Sanders MH, Kern NB, Costantino JP, et al. Adequacy of prescribing positive airway pressure therapy by mask for sleep apnea on the basis of a partial-night trial. *Am Rev Respir Dis* 1993; 147:1169–1174.

99. Strollo PJ Jr, Saunders MH, Atwood CW. Positive pressure therapy. *Clin Chest Med* 1998;19:55–68.

100. Sanders MH, Kern N. Obstructive sleep apnea treated by independently adjusted inspiratory and expiratory positive airway pressures via nasal mask. *Chest* 1990;98:317–324.

101. Reeves-Hoché MK, Hudgel DW, Meck R, et al. Continuous versus bilevel positive airway pressure for obstructive sleep apnea. *Am J Resp Crit Care Med* 1995;151:443–449.

102. Schmidt-Nowara W, Lowe A, Wiegand L, et al. Oral appliances for the treatment of snoring and obstructive sleep apnea. A review. *Sleep* 1995;18:501–510.

103. Lowe AA. Dental devices for treatment of snoring and obstructive sleep apnea. In: Kryger M, Roth T, Dement W, eds, *Principles and practice of sleep medicine,* 2nd ed. Philadelphia: WB Saunders Co, 1994:722–735.

104. Ferguson KA, Ono T, Lowe AA, et al. A randomized crossover study of oral appliance vs nasal-continuous positive airway pressure in treatment of mild-moderate sleep apnea. *Chest* 1996; 109:1269–1275.

105. Millman RP, Rosenberg CL, Carlisle CC, et al. The efficacy of oral appliances in treatment of persistent sleep apnea after uvulopalatopharyngoplasty. *Chest* 1998;113:992–996.

106. Findley LJ, Unverzagt ME, Suratt PM. Automobile accidents involving patients with obstructive sleep apnea. *Am Rev Respir Dis* 1988;138:337–340.

107. American Thoracic Society. Official statement. Sleep apnea, sleepiness, and driving risk. *Am J Respir Crit Care Med* 1994; 150:1463–1473.

108. Bradley TD, McNicholas WT, Rutherford R, et al. Clinical and physiologic heterogeneity of the central sleep apnea syndrome. *Am Rev Respir Dis* 1986;134:217–221.

109. Phillipson EA. Hypoventilation syndromes. In: Murray JF, Nadel JA, eds. *Textbook of respiratory medicine.* Philadelphia: WB Saunders, 1994:2291–2300.

110. Hill R, Robbins AW, Messing R, et al. Sleep apnea syndrome after poliomyelitis. *Am Rev Respir Dis* 1983;127:129–131.

111. McNicholas WT, Carter JL, Rutherford R, et al. Beneficial effect of oxygen in primary alveolar hypoventilation with central sleep apnea. *Am Rev Respir Dis* 1982;125:773–775.
112. Hill NS. Clinical applications of body ventilators. *Chest* 1986; 90:897–905.
113. Unterborn JN, Hill NS. Options for mechanical ventilation in neuromuscular diseases. *Clin Chest Med* 1994;15:765–781.
114. Calman DM, Piper A, Sanders MH, et al. Nocturnal noninvasive positive pressure ventilatory assistance. *Chest* 1996;110:1581–1588.
115. Xie A, Rutherford R, Rankin F, et al. Hypocapnia and increased ventilatory responsiveness in patients with idiopathic central sleep apnea. *Am J Respir Crit Care Med* 1995;152:1950–1955.
116. Xie A, Wong B, Phillipson EA, et al. Interaction of hyperventilation and arousals in the pathogenesis of idiopathic central sleep apnea. *Am J Respir Crit Care Med* 1994;250:489–495.
117. Bonnet MH, Dexter JR, Arand DL. The effect of triazolam on arousal and respiration in central sleep apnea patients. *Sleep* 1990;13:31–41.
118. Debacker WA, Verbracken J, Willemen M, et al. Central apnea index decreases after prolonged treatment with acetazolamide. *Am J Resp Crit Care Med* 1995;151:87–91.
119. Xie A, Rankin F, Rutherford R, et al. Effects of inhaled CO_2 and added dead space of idiopathic central sleep apnea. *J Appl Physiol* 1997;82:918–926.
120. Issa FG, Sullivan CE. Reversal of central sleep apnea using nasal CPAP. *Chest* 1986;90:165–171.
121. Findley LJ, Zwillich CW, Ancoli-Israel S, et al. Cheyne-Stokes breathing during sleep in patients with left ventricular heart failure. *South Med J* 1985;78:11–15.
122. Naughton MT, Bradley TD. Sleep apnea in congestive heart failure. *Clin Chest Med* 1998;19:99–113.
123. Nachtman A, Siebler M, Rose G, et al. Cheyne-Stokes respiration in ischemic stroke. *Neurology* 1995;45:820–821.
124. Khoo MC. Periodic breathing. In: Crystal RB, West JB, eds. *The lung.* New York: Raven Press, Ltd., 1991:1419–1431.
125. Naughton M, Benard D, Tam A, et al. Role of hyperventilation in the pathogenesis of central sleep apneas in patients with congestive heart failure. *Am Rev Respir Dis* 1993;1498:330–338.
126. Blackshear JL, Kaplan J, Thompson RC, et al. Nocturnal dyspnea and atrial fibrillation predict Cheyne-Stokes respiration in patients with congestive heart failure. *Arch Intern Med* 1995; 155:1297–1302.
127. Hanly PJ, Zuberi-Khokar NS. Increased mortality associated with Cheyne-Stokes respiration in patients with congestive heart failure. *Am J Respir Crit Care Med* 1996;153:272–276.
128. Javaheri S, Parker TJ, Wexler L, et al. Effect of theophylline on sleep disordered breathing in heart failure. *N Engl J Med* 1996;335:562–567.
129. Hanly PJ, Millar TW, Steljes DG, et al. The effect of oxygen of respiration and sleep in patients with congestive heart failure. *Ann Intern Med* 1989;111:777–782.
130. Naughton MT, Liu PP, Benard DC, et al. Treatment of congestive heart failure and Cheyne-Stokes respiration during sleep by continuous positive airway pressure. *Am J Respir Crit Care Med* 1995;151:92–97.
131. Davies RJ, Harrington KJ, Ormedrod OJM, et al. Nasal continuous positive airway pressure in chronic heart failure with sleep-disordered breathing. *Am Rev Respir Dis* 1993;147:630–634.
132. Javaheri S, Parker TJ, Wexler L, et al. Occult sleep-disordered breathing in stable congestive heart failure. *Ann Intern Med* 1995;122:487–492.
133. Dowdell WT, Javaheri S, Mcginnis W. Cheyne-Stokes respiration presenting as sleep apnea syndrome. *Am Rev Respir Dis* 1990;141:871–879.
134. Malone S, Liu PP, Holloway R, et al. Obstructive sleep apnea in patients with dilated cardiomyopathy: effects of continuous positive airway pressure. *Lancet* 1991;338:1480–1484.
135. Turner-Warwick M. Epidemiology of nocturnal asthma. *Am J Med* 1988;85:6–8.
136. Ballard RD, Saathoff MC, Patel DK, et al. Effect of sleep on nocturnal bronchoconstriction and ventilatory patterns in asthmatics. *J Appl Physiol* 1989;67:243–249.
137. Martin RJ, Banks-Schlegel S. Chronobiology of Asthma. *Am J Respir Crit Care Med* 1998;158:1002–1007.
138. Martin RJ, Cicutto LC, Smith HR, et al. Airways inflammation in nocturnal asthma. *Am Rev Respir Dis* 1991;143:351–357.
139. Selby C, Engleman HM, Fitzpatrick MF, et al. Inhaled salmeterol or oral theophylline in nocturnal asthma? *Am J Respir Crit Care Med* 1997;155:104–108.
140. Stewart IC, Rhind GB, Power JT, et al. Effect of sustained release terbutaline on symptoms and sleep quality in patients with nocturnal asthma. *Thorax* 1987;42:797–800.
141. Beam WR, Ballard RD, Martin RJ. Spectrum of corticosteroid sensitivity in nocturnal asthma. *Am Rev Respir Dis* 1992;145:1082–1086.
142. Beam WR, Weiner DE, Martin RJ. Timing of prednisone and alterations of airways inflammation in nocturnal asthma. *Am Rev Respir Dis* 1992;146:1524–1536.
143. Coe CI, Barnes PJ. Reduction of nocturnal asthma by an inhaled anticholinergic drug. *Chest* 1986;90:485–488.
144. Wenzel SE, Trudeau JB, Kaminsky DA, et al. Effect of 5-lipoxygenase inhibition on bronchoconstriction and airways inflammation in nocturnal asthma. *Am J Respir Crit Care Med* 1995;152:897–905.
145. Spector SL, Smith LJ, Glass M, et al. Effects of 6 weeks of therapy with oral doses of ICI204.219 a leukotriene D4 receptor antagonist in subjects with bronchial asthma. *Am J Respir Crit Care Med* 1994;150:618–623.
146. Chan CS, Woolcock AJ, Sullivan CE. Nocturnal asthma: role of snoring and obstructive sleep apnea. *Am Rev Respir Dis* 1988;137:1502–1504.
147. Douglas NJ. Sleep in patients with chronic obstructive pulmonary disease. *Clin Chest Med* 1998;19;115–125.
148. Fletcher EC. Sleep, breathing, and oxyhemoglobin saturation in chronic lung disease. In: Fletcher EC, ed. *Abnormalities of respiration during sleep.* Orlando, FL: Grune & Stratton, 1986:155–179.
149. Catterall JR, Douglas NJ, Calverley PMA, et al. Transient hypoxemia during sleep is not a sleep apnea syndrome. *Am Rev Respir Dis* 1983;128:24–29.
150. Connaughton JJ, Catterall JR, Elton RA, et al. Do sleep studies contribute to the management of patients with severe chronic obstructive pulmonary disease? *Am Rev Respir Dis* 1988;138:341–344.
151. Hudgel DW, Martin RJ, Capehart M, et al. Contribution of hypoventilation to sleep oxygen desaturation in chronic obstructive pulmonary disease. *J Appl Physiol* 1983;55:669–677.
152. Fletcher EC, Gray BA, Levin DC. Nonapneic mechanisms of arterial oxygen desaturation during rapid-eye-movements sleep. *J Appl Physiol* 1983;54:632–639.
153. Block AJ, Boysen PG, Wynne JW, et al. The origins of cor pulmonale: a hypothesis. *Chest* 1979;300:513–517.
154. Nocturnal Oxygen Therapy Trial Group. Continuous or nocturnal oxygen therapy in hypoxemic chronic obstructive lung disease. *Ann Intern Med* 1980;93:391–398.
155. Fletcher EC, Luckett RA, Goodnight-White S, et al. A double blind trial of nocturnal supplemental oxygen for sleep desaturation in patients with chronic obstructive pulmonary disease and a daytime PO_2 above 60 mmHg. *Am Rev Respir Dis* 1992;145:1070–1076.
156. Calverley PMA, Brezinova V, Douglas NJ, et al. The effect of

oxygenation on sleep quality in chronic bronchitis and emphysema. *Am Rev Respir Dis* 1982;126:206–210.

157. Fleetham J, West P, Mezon B, et al. Sleep, arousals, and oxygen desaturation in chronic obstructive pulmonary disease. The effect of oxygen therapy. *Am Rev Respir Dis* 1982;125:429–433.

158. Berry RB, Desa MM, Branum JP, et al. Effect of theophylline on sleep and sleep-disordered breathing in patients with chronic obstructive pulmonary disease. *Am Rev Respir Dis* 1991;143:245–250.

159. Timms RM, Dawson A, Hajdukovic R, et al. Effect of triazolam on sleep and arterial oxygen saturation in patients with chronic obstructive pulmonary disease. *Arch Intern Med* 1988;148:2159–2163.

160. Girault C, Muir JF, Mihaltan F, et al. Effects of repeated administration of zolpidem on sleep, diurnal and nocturnal respiratory function, vigilance, and physical performance in patients with COPD. *Chest* 1996;110:1203–1211.

161. Fletcher EC, Schaaf JW, Miller J, et al. Long-term cardiopulmonary sequelae in patients with sleep apnea and chronic lung disease. *Am Rev Respir Dis* 1987;135:525–533.

162. Fletcher EC, Brown DL. Nocturnal oxyhemoglobin desaturation following tracheostomy for obstructive sleep apnea. *Am J Med* 1985;79:35–42.

163. Sampol G, Sagales MT, Rocca A, et al. Nasal continuous positive airway pressure with supplemental oxygen in coexistent sleep apnea–hypopnea syndrome and severe chronic obstructive pulmonary disease. *Eur Resp J* 1996;9:111–116.

19

PULMONARY AND CRITICAL CARE PROBLEMS IN THE ELDERLY

E. WESLEY ELY

INTRODUCTION

MECHANICAL VENTILATION IN THE ELDERLY
Recent Cohorts of Elderly Patients on Mechanical Ventilation
Weaning in the Elderly
Conclusions Regarding Mechanical Ventilation in the Elderly

ETHICAL DECISIONS RELATED TO THE INSTITUTION AND WITHDRAWAL OF MECHANICAL VENTILATION
Quality End-of-Life Care and Patients' Preferences
Futility and Withdrawal of Care

PREOPERATIVE PULMONARY EVALUATION IN THE ELDERLY

INTRODUCTION

As physicians in the 21st century, we are faced with striking changes in the demographics of those for whom we will devote our energy and time. Adults over the age of 85 are the most rapidly growing segment of our population, and their number is currently estimated at 4 million. This number is expected to double by the year 2030 (1), and by the year 2050 there will be an estimated 15.3 million persons in this age group (2). Over the next 20 years, those above 65 will account for over a fifth of our population. Among people older than 65, 12% have chronic lung disease (3), and these people are at particularly high risk for experiencing serious health complications (4). The rate of hospitalization for pneumonia in the subgroup of elderly who have chronic lung disease, for example, is two to seven times higher than for their counterparts without coexistent pulmonary disease (5,6).

Because of the increasing population of elderly patients in our society, issues pertinent to geriatrics are increasingly important to all health professionals who manage patients with pulmonary diseases. This chapter represents a new addition to this textbook and a sign of the priority that we as clinicians will need to place on this topic. Rather than cover the numerous aspects of care that are unique to the elderly, we have chosen three especially challenging topics:

1. Mechanical ventilation in the elderly;
2. Ethical decisions related to the institution and withdrawal of mechanical ventilation (note: another chapter in this book will cover additional aspects of ethics in pulmonary and critical care medicine);
3. Preoperative pulmonary evaluation in the elderly.

MECHANICAL VENTILATION IN THE ELDERLY

U.S. health care expenditures for persons over the age of 65 are currently $1,740 billion (38% of total expenditures). By 2030, this amount is estimated to become $15,970 billion (74% of total). One approach to decreasing health care costs might be to limit or ration the intensive care provided to the aged in order to conserve resources (7–10). Indeed, recent data have demonstrated that elderly do receive less aggressive management for some medical illnesses (11). Data from the SUPPORT investigators have shown that age (especially above 70 to 75) has great importance on the intensity of care given to patients (12–14) (Figs. 19.1 and 19.2). In addition, both physician and patient preferences for cardiopulmonary resuscitation influence hospital resource consumption (15). There are surprisingly few "expert consensus" reports regarding the decision to treat seniors with mechanical ventilation (MV). One publication from the Office of Technology Assessment (16) discussed very reasonable perspectives, but few data were presented and opinions were divided as to whether or not age should be a major determinant in the use of MV.

Age has been considered an important prognostic indicator of hospital outcome (9,17), but many prior investigations of MV have been limited by their retrospective design and the absence of adjustment for confounding factors such as severity of illness (18–20). Among 22 published reports (Table 19.1) (18–38) which included age-specific data on mechanically ventilated elderly patients, the authors' conclusions were divided regarding whether age influences outcome. Seventeen of these studies were restricted to mechani-

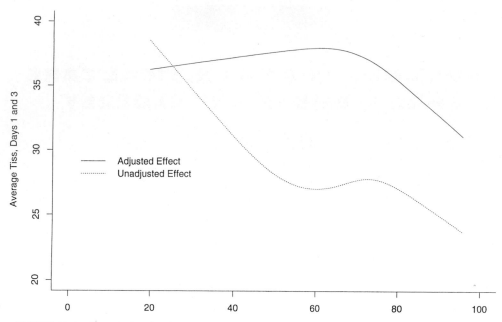

FIGURE 19.1. The relationship between patient age and the intensity of care delivered to patients enrolled in the SUPPORT trial is depicted as patient age (x axis) versus average Therapeutic Intervention Scoring System (TISS) on days 1 and 3 (y axis). TISS is a valid and reliable method of measuring resource use in cohorts of patients. The dotted line is unadjusted TISS, while the solid line represents the TISS scores after adjustment for severity of illness and functional status. While it is apparent that overall intensity of care dropped off at around the age of 70, the reasons for this remain an important area for future research. (Reprinted with permission from Hamel MB, Philips RS, Teno JM, et al. Seriously ill hospitalized adults: do we spend less on older patients? *J Am Geriatr Soc* 1996;44:1043–1048.)

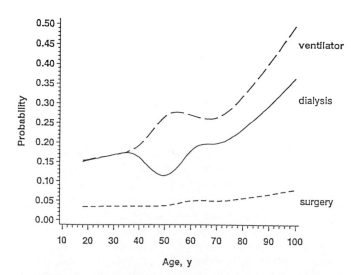

FIGURE 19.2. The relationship between patient age and the adjusted probability of a decision to withhold each life-sustaining treatment by study day 30 in the SUPPORT investigation. (Reprinted with permission from Hamel MB, Teno JM, Goldman L, et al. Patient age and decisions to withhold life-sustaining treatments from seriously ill, hospitalized adults. *Ann Intern Med* 1999; 130:116–125.)

cally ventilated patients (18–21,25,26,28,31,33–38), and only five of them had prospective design (21,24,25,37,38). Of the latter, four concluded that age had an important effect on the outcome (21,24,37,38) while one concluded that age did not matter in outcome of mechanically ventilated patients (25). The diversity of the design and conclusions of these investigations have only served to fuel the controversy over the role of age on outcomes from MV.

Recent Cohorts of Elderly Patients on Mechanical Ventilation

We analyzed a prospectively followed cohort of mechanically ventilated patients to determine whether age had an independent impact upon the outcomes of patients treated with MV (39). Patients of 75 years or over remained on the mechanical ventilator a median of four days (interquartile ranges, two to nine) versus six days (three to 11) for patients under 75 years (p = 0.14). Using the time it took to pass a daily screen of weaning parameters as a marker of recovery from respiratory failure, elderly patients passed the daily screen earlier than younger patients (risk ratio 1.58 [95% confidence interval, 1.13 to 2.22], p = 0.03) (Figure 19.3). The ICU cost of care was lower ($12,822 [$9,821 to

TABLE 19.1. INVESTIGATIONS DESCRIBING OUTCOMES AFTER MECHANICAL VENTILATION IN THE ELDERLY

Author/Year/Reference	Elderly (N) & Definition		Design of Study	Inclusion Criteria	Hospital Mortality (%)	Multivariate Analysis	Severity Adjustment	Age Influences Outcome[b]
Nunn, 1979, 27	15	>75	Prospective	ICU[a]	73	No	No	Yes
Campion, 1981, 22	565	≥75	Retrospective	ICU/CCU	16	No	No	No
Fedullo, 1983, 23	84	≥70	Retrospective	MICU only	39	No	No	No
Witek, 1985, 24	51	>70	Prospective	ICU[a]	51	No	No	Yes
McLean, 1985, 25	49	≥75	Prospective	ICU[a]	43	No	No	No
Elpern, 1989, 26	95	≥60	Retrospective	ICU ≥ 3 days[a]	66	No	No	Yes
Tran, 1990, 27	92	>70	Retrospective	MICU only	46	No	No	Yes
O'Donnell, 1991, 28	17	>70	Retrospective	ICU[a]	59	No	No	No
Pesau, 1992, 29	99	≥70	Retrospective	ICU	60	Yes	Yes	No
Gracey, 1992, 30	496	>65	Retrospective	ICU[a]	46	No	No	Yes
Chelluri, 1992, 31	34	≥85	Retrospective	MICU only[a]	38	No	No	No
Stauffer, 1993, 32	118	>70	Retrospective	ICU[a]	62	Yes	No	Yes
Swinburne, 1993, 33	282	≥80	Retrospective	ICU[a]	69	No	No	No
Cohen, 1993, 34	109	≥80	Retrospective	ICU ≥ 3 days[a]	62	No	No	Yes
Papadakis, 1993, 35	138	≥70	Retrospective	ICU[a]	76	Yes	Yes	Yes
Dardaine, 1995, 36	110	≥70	Retrospective	ICU[a]	38	No	No	No
Cohen, 1995, 18	21,342	≥70	Retrospective	ICU[a]	59	No	No	Yes
Steiner, 1997, 37	40	>65	Prospective	ICU/Stroke Pts[a]	32 at 2 mo	Yes	No	Yes
Kurek, 1997, 20	3,256	≥70	Retrospective	Tracheostomy[a]	64	No	No	Yes
Zilberberg, 1998, 38	31	>65	Prospective	MICU[a]	74	Yes	Yes	Yes
Kurek, 1998, 20	4,101	≥75	Retrospective	ICU[a]	55	No	No	Yes
Ely, 1998 (current report), 39	63	≥75	Prospective	MICU/CCU[a]	39	Yes	Yes	No

[a] Investigations including only mechanically ventilated patients.
[b] Indicates the predominant conclusion of the authors as to whether or not age is independently important.

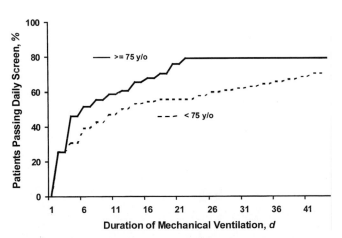

FIGURE 19.3. Kaplan-Meier analysis of the days on mechanical ventilation versus the rate of recovery of respiratory failure (using the percent passing a daily screen of weaning parameters as a surrogate marker of "recovery") after adjustment for sex, race, and severity of illness at baseline using a modified APACHE II score which excluded age. Using Cox proportional-hazards analysis to compare the proportions of patients who passed the daily screen in each group, elderly patients passed the daily screen earlier than younger patients (risk ratio 1.58 [95% confidence interval, 1.13 to 2.22], p = 0.03). The solid line indicates patients over 75 years old; dashed line indicates patients under 75 years old. (Ely EW, Evans GW, Liaponik EF. Mechanical ventilation in a cohort of elderly patients admitted to an intensive care unit. *Ann Intern Med* 1999;131:96–104, with permission.)

$26,313] versus $19,316 [$9,699 to $39,950]) in older patients (p = 0.03). Median hospital costs tended to be lower in the older group, though not significantly so ($21,292 versus $29,049, p = 0.17). Using multivariate logistic regression analysis to adjust for race, gender, and severity of illness, patient age of 75 or over was predictive of approximately one day less on the ventilator, but this was not statistically significant (95% confidence interval, − 2.8 to 1.2). Multivariate analyses also confirmed that ICU and hospital LOS were not different after adjustment (p > 0.1), but ICU and hospital costs were lower in the elderly (p = 0.02). In-hospital mortality among the elderly was 38% versus 39% among younger patients (p = 0.98), and Cox proportional-hazards analysis confirmed that there was no difference in survival between the two groups (Figure 19.4) (relative risk for older patients = 0.82, 95% confidence interval 0.52 to 1.29) (39).

Data were recently reported from 1,638 patients in the Mechanical Ventilation International Study Group (40). In this observational cohort, it was noted that despite a higher severity of illness, the 254 patients over the age of 75 spent significantly less time on mechanical ventilation than did the 1,355 patients under 75 years old (14 ± 23 vs. 21 ± 110, p = 0.02).

Among elderly patients requiring MV, there is usually a higher proportion of women (39), a finding consistent with the well-established demographics of aging. Kollef and colleagues (41) reported that female patients spent longer on

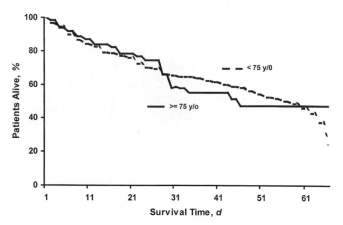

FIGURE 19.4. Kaplan-Meier analysis showed the survival time of patients on a log scale. After adjustment for the severity of illness at baseline as measured by the modified APACHE II score, sex and race, Cox proportional-hazards analysis showed that there was no difference in survival between those 75 years or older and those under 75 years old (relative risk for older patients = 0.82, 95% confidence intervals 0.52 to 1.29, p = 0.78). The solid line indicates patients over 75 years old; dashed line indicates patients under 75 years old. (Ely EW, Evans GW, Liaponik EF. Mechanical ventilation in a cohort of elderly patients admitted to an intensive care unit. *Ann Intern Med* 1999;131:96–104, with permission.)

MV (p = 0.056), but we detected no gender differences in the rate of recovery of respiratory failure or length of stay on MV. Because of general limitations in access to basic health care for women (42) and differences among physicians in their practice styles (including the vigor of their approaches to liberation from the ventilator), further prospective analyses of gender differences in outcomes from MV are needed. We believe that the care of elderly women will represent a major future priority of critical care medicine.

Weaning in the Elderly

Specific age-related decisions regarding the management of weaning from mechanical ventilation have been poorly studied. Gender, body habitus, and age are appropriate considerations which may affect outcome from mechanical ventilation. Female gender, smaller endotracheal tube size (under 7 mm), and age over 70 have been associated with an elevated f/VT ratio (43,44), and it may be appropriate to adjust the "passing" threshold for this measurement in these instances (Figure 19.5). However, these age-related modifications of ventilator weaning parameters will require further prospective study prior to firm recommendations.

In just the past five years, over 500 articles have been written on weaning from mechanical ventilation, yet few have focused on the elderly population. In elderly as well as younger patients, one of the most important concepts to arise from recent prospective, randomized controlled trials (RCTs) in adults is that conventional "weaning" may unne-

cessarily delay extubation of patients who have recovered from respiratory failure (45,46). With increasing recognition of the complications of MV and growing attention to resources consumed during the care of elderly patients with respiratory failure, a change in this clinical paradigm of "weaning" is warranted. In its place, evidence supports the concept of aggressive liberation from MV (46–49). That is, the rapid identification of patients who have recovered from respiratory failure is more important than any manipulation of MV in an attempt to accelerate this recovery.

Because of the increased likelihood of comorbid illnesses in elderly patients, it will be important to develop a routine approach to those elderly who have a difficult time weaning from mechanical ventilation. Special factors which are important considerations in weaning failure patients (with comments specific for the elderly in parentheses) are summarized in the Table 19.2 mnemonic, which is entitled "WHEANS NOT": reactive airways disease or chronic obstructive pulmonary disease (COPD) (which is often unrecognized in elderly patients until an episode of pneumonia); cardiac diseases such as ischemic disease, congestive heart failure, and even uncontrolled hypertension contributing to pulmonary edema (diastolic dysfunction due to a stiff ventricle may be an unrecognized organ dysfunction present in elderly); metabolic disturbances such as electrolyte disturbances or metabolic alkalosis; uncontrolled anxiety or pain; ongoing aspiration and secretion problems (pharyngeal dysfunction and an increased incidence of delirium make this problematic in the elderly); neuromuscular disorders, including prior use of neuromuscular blockers or diaphragm dysfunction; ongoing sepsis or other infections such as

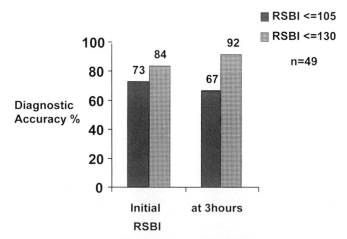

FIGURE 19.5. The diagnostic accuracy of the rapid-shallow-breathing index (RSBI) in 49 patients over the age of 70 who were being weaned from mechanical ventilation. The highest accuracy of the RSBI in these patients was obtained by using a cutoff of 130 breaths per liter per minute at a delayed (three hour) time point. (Adapted with permission from Krieger BP, Isber J, Breitenbucher A, et al. Serial measurements of the rapid-shallow-breathing index as a predictor of weaning outcome in elderly medical patients. *Chest* 1997;112:1029–1034.)

TABLE 19.2. "WHEANS NOT"

This mnemonic is not meant to be all inclusive, but rather as an aid in considering the possible reasons why a patient might have difficulty being liberated from mechanical ventilation:

- **Wh**eezes
- **He**art disease, Hypertension
- **E**lectrolytes
- **A**nxiety, **A**irway abnormalities and **A**spiration, **A**lkalosis (metabolic)
- **N**euromuscular Disease (including diaphragm dysfunction and prior use of **N**euromuscular blockers)
- **S**epsis, **S**edation
- **N**utrition (over- and underfeeding)
- **O**piates, **O**besity
- **T**hyroid Disease

pneumonia (in which age is a strong independent risk factor for mortality); malnutrition or overfeeding with carbohydrates; sedation imbalance with overutilization of narcotics or sedative/hypnotics (elderly patients are particularly prone to the effects of benzodiazepines and narcotics); obesity and the need to be elevated in the bed to utilize gravity to help maintain tidal volume (perhaps even more important in frail elderly and obese short women); and lastly hypothyroidism (which is common in the aging population). While this list is long, it is imperative that any clinician caring for mechanically ventilated elderly patients be aware of these commonly found reasons for failure to wean.

Conclusions Regarding Mechanical Ventilation in the Elderly

In view of current uncertainties in physician decision-making regarding the use of MV in the elderly, major pitfalls should be recognized and avoided. These include the premature application of predictive equations (34) or anecdotal experiences. Further prospective investigations are needed in order to define "physiological age" and to determine whether or not it is truly more important than chronological age (16,50). In the absence of validated measures of "physiological age," the current observations suggest that an overreliance on chronological age is inappropriate. By using multivariate analysis to adjust for severity of illness and other variables, we found that the elderly (over 75 years old) spent an amount of time on the mechanical ventilator comparable to younger patients but had a lower cost of ICU and in-hospital care. These outcomes are not explained by differences in mortality, since both groups had similar survival rates. Accordingly, the decision to use MV should not be based upon age alone, and the appropriate use of ventilatory support in the elderly requires further prospective evaluation.

ETHICAL DECISIONS RELATED TO THE INSTITUTION AND WITHDRAWAL OF MECHANICAL VENTILATION

There is widespread belief that many patients do not want aggressive care at the end of life. Moreover, 78% of health care professionals feel that the treatments they offer to patients are often overly burdensome (51). In fact, more consistency in our attempts to obtain patients' preferences for do-not-resuscitate (DNR) orders might reduce the expense and burden of aggressive medical care in the elderly. While appropriate end-of-life care and patient preferences are being considered by some investigators (52,53), relatively little is taught to most physicians in most medical schools or residency programs regarding this topic. Hamel and co-workers (14) recently reported data from the SUPPORT study which showed that physician error rates in approximating patients' preferences for mechanical ventilation increased from 36% at ages under 50 to 79% at ages over 80. Furthermore, SUPPORT data also show that predicting death is very difficult for most illnesses (54). At a time point of only seven days before death, experienced physicians prospectively estimated that 50% of patients with congestive heart failure, chronic obstructive pulmonary disease, and cirrhosis would live for six months. For patients with acute respiratory failure and multiple organ dysfunction syndrome, the same physicians estimated that 20% of the patients would live for six months, when in actuality they lived for only seven days (54).

Quality End-Of-Life Care and Patients' Preferences

Considering the difficulty in estimating prognosis and the frequent misunderstanding and lack of communication between patients, families, and physicians, it is little wonder that we commonly err in establishing the appropriate end-of-life care plan for our critically ill patients (13,14,54–56). In order to increase the quality of end-of-life care for our patients, it would be helpful to know what components of care patients consider most important. Singer and coworkers (57) recently sought to identify and describe elements of quality end-of-life care from patients' perspectives using in-depth, open-ended, face-to-face interviews. This study showed that the following five domains of quality of end-of-life care were considered the most important by patients:

1. Receiving adequate pain and symptom management;
2. Avoiding inappropriate prolongation of death;
3. Achieving a sense of control;
4. Relieving burden;
5. Strengthening relationships with loved ones.

Regarding the first priority, it seems obvious that physicians ought to prioritize adequate pain and symptom management. In the SUPPORT project, four of 10 family interviews reported serious pain (moderate to severe pain most or all of the time) during the last three days of life (58). They did not report (nor were they asked) whether the pain was "adequately relieved." Physicians need to learn more and become appropriately aggressive in the use of sedatives and analgesics to relieve suffering in dying patients. The second priority—avoiding inappropriate prolongation of dying—has to do with patients' decisions to limit aggressive life support. Most patients say that they would prefer to forgo life-sustaining treatment if their quality of life after the treatment would be severely impaired (59,60). Lo and Johnson (61) discussed four reasons to limit treatment which included futility, patient refusal of therapy, excessive costs, and unacceptable quality of life. After careful consideration of these important concerns, clinical decisions to limit treatment will, it is hoped, avoid unnecessary prolongation of death while providing compassionate terminal care. It is imperative that physicians and other health care professionals have discussions with patients and their families to determine their preferences for life-sustaining therapy and the options of ICU care versus palliative care in the event of a life-threatening illness.

Many patients feel that DNR orders and advance directives help to achieve a sense of control over the possibility of dying in an unwanted environment such as the ICU (13,56). While patients prefer to participate actively in determining their "code status," they often get confused by the precise treatment options (57). In addition, once an acute illness occurs, the presence of associated delirium makes it very difficult to establish the patient's preferences with certainty if they are not already known. For these reasons, a surrogate decision-maker for elderly persons should be established in advance.

The last two priorities listed by patients—relieving burden and strengthening relationships—seem to go hand in hand. Patients are often most worried about becoming a burden to their loved ones. This psychosocial burden includes the mental hardships, financial burdens, and time-intensive obligations placed on family members who care for their dying loved ones. Involving patients' loved ones in decisions about end-of-life care and treatment may lead to improved outcomes for everyone involved. In fact, the dying process frequently offers important opportunities for growth, intimacy, reconciliation, and closure of relationships (62).

Futility and Withdrawal of Care

In the course of caring for our critically ill patients, it may become apparent to the patient, the family, or the health care professionals that further intervention would not be of benefit. While focus on the above-outlined list of objectives is warranted, it is not always clear what constitutes a futile intervention. To aid in this complicated ethical dilemma, we refer the reader to the recent report of the Council on Ethical and Judicial Affairs of the American Medical Association (63). It is fair to say, however, that a strict definition of "futility" is difficult due to the fact that each determination is dependent on people's values, which vary greatly. Therefore, the AMA recommends a standardized "fair process" rather than a strict definition of futility. As much as possible, physicians should base futility decisions on factors such as clinical efficacy of treatments, likelihood of mortality, and subsequent quality-of-life considerations rather than on chronological age alone (39,61,63).

In order to determine the frequency of withdrawal of life support in our country, a national survey of every American postgraduate training program with significant clinical exposure to critical care medicine was recently conducted (64). Prendergast and Luce (64) reviewed information on 6,303 ICU-related deaths which occurred under the following circumstances: 26% (range 4% to 79%) received full ICU care including failed cardiopulmonary resuscitation (CPR), 24% (range 0% to 83%) received full ICU care without CPR, 14% (range 0% to 67%) had life support withheld, and 36% (the single largest group with a range across ICUs of 0% to 79%) had life support actively withdrawn. While there was a wide variation in the practice pattern of the different ICUs, the authors concluded that limitation of life support prior to death is a common practice in our teaching ICUs across the country. The variable circumstances in the methods of withdrawal of life support in our ICUs does not seem to be explained by ICU, hospital type, mortality rates, or number of admissions per year (64–66). While there is no recognized standard of practice in this important area of medicine, it is increasingly common for institutions to track their own end-of-life practices and even to rank the "quality" of the dying experience.

PREOPERATIVE PULMONARY EVALUATION IN THE ELDERLY

Physicians are commonly asked to perform "preoperative evaluations" on elderly patients scheduled for either elective or emergent surgical procedures. Furthermore, they are also asked to comment on the likelihood of postoperative pulmonary complications. While there are well-defined assessment tools to determine the perioperative risk factors for cardiac complications (67), the development of pulmonary complications has been studied less extensively. In reality, the development of pulmonary complications is at least as common (if not more so) than cardiac complications (68). Elderly patients tend to have more surgical procedures. Over half of all malignancies occur in patients over 65 years old, and the primary treatment of many of these is surgery (69,70). In addition, there are an increasing number of elderly patients receiving coronary artery bypass grafting surgery (71). This section of the chapter will focus on the preoperative pulmonary evaluation, with special focus on the role of age in these assessments.

Postoperative pulmonary complications have been reported to prolong the hospital stay by an average of one to two weeks (68). One inherent difficulty in interpreting these data is that studies vary widely in their criteria for postoperative pulmonary complications—including definitions ranging from atelectasis or bronchospasm to postoperative pneumonia or acute respiratory distress syndrome (68). Postoperative "respiratory failure" may be defined as the inability to be extubated 48 hours after surgery, but some have considered it only if the patients were not liberated by day 5 (72). The in-hospital mortality rate for those with postoperative respiratory failure is around 40%, versus 5% for those without respiratory failure (72).

Potential patient-related risk factors for the development of postoperative pulmonary complications include smoking, general health status, age, obesity, chronic obstructive pulmonary disease (COPD), neurological status, cardiovascular status, and fluid or intravascular volume status. Procedure-related risk factors include the site of the incision (thorax versus upper or lower abdomen), length of surgery, and the type of anesthesia. The risk of pulmonary complications increases as the incision approaches the diaphragm, with upper-abdominal and thoracic procedures carrying the greatest risk (10% to 40%) (68). With the exceptions of neurological (73,74) and head and neck procedures (73), pulmonary complications are rare following procedures outside the thorax and abdomen. The incidence and unadjusted

relative risk of pulmonary complications in association with many of these factors are summarized in Table 19.3, which was adapted from an excellent review by Smetana (68).

The independent importance of age in the development of postoperative pulmonary complications has not been studied in a manner which would control for coexisting conditions. In fact, according to the American Society of Anesthesia (ASA) class stratification scheme, the perioperative mortality for ASA classes II through V is the same for all ages (75). In an investigation of patients of 80 years old or over (n = 500), ASA Class II had a 30-day mortality of less than 1%, and for the entire cohort the 30-day mortality rate was only 6.2% (76). There are no data to support the notion that age-related changes in lung function increase postoperative pulmonary complications in those without chronic pulmonary disease. Even among those with severe COPD, age was not shown to be an independent risk factor for pulmonary complications (77,78). Much like the situation with mechanical ventilation discussed previously, chronological age is less predictive of pulmonary complications following surgery than coexisting conditions. Therefore advanced age alone is not a reason to withhold surgery.

A carefully performed history and physical examination are the most important aspects of preoperative consultations. Asking the patient about his or her ability to ambulate, details regarding the presence and character of cough, and any recent changes in the level of dyspnea are key factors to include in the history. As summarized in Table 19.3, the presence of chronic obstructive pulmonary disease increases

TABLE 19.3. POTENTIAL RISK FACTORS FOR POSTOPERATIVE PULMONARY COMPLICATIONS

Potential Risk Factor	Type of Surgery	Incidence of Pulmonary Complications		Unadjusted Relative Risk
Patient-Related		When Factor was Present	When Factor was Absent	Associated with Risk Factor
Smoking	Coronary bypass	39	11	3.4
	Abdominal	15–46	6–21	1.4–4.3
ASA Class >II	Unselected	26	16	1.7
	Thoracic or abdominal	26–44	13–18	1.5–3.2
Age >70 yr	Unselected	9–17	4–9	1.9–2.4
	Thoracic or abdominal	17–22	12–21	0.9–1.9
Obesity	Unselected	11	9	1.3
	Thoracic or abdominal	19–36	17–27	0.8–1.7
COPD	Unselected	6–26	2–8	2.7–3.6
	Thoracic or abdominal	18	4	4.7
Procedure-Related				
Surgery >3 hr	Unselected	10–53	3–15	1.6–5.2
	Thoracic or abdominal	40	11	3.6
General anesthesia	Unselected	8–19	0–17	1.2–∞
	Thoracic, abdominal, vascular	28–32	11–12	2.2–3.0
Use of pancuronium	Unselected	17	5	3.2

ASA, American Society of Anesthesia; COPD, chronic obstructive pulmonary disease.
Adapted with permission from Smetana GW. Preoperative pulmonary evaluation. *N Engl J Med* 1999;340:937–934.

the risk of postoperative pulmonary complications by about three to five times. Many patients who have significant obstruction remain undiagnosed at the time of preoperative evaluation. Guidelines for using the clinical examination to diagnose airflow limitation could be summarized as follows (79–81):

- No single item or combination of items from the clinical examination rules out airflow limitation.
- The best finding associated with decreased likelihood of airflow limitation is a history of never having smoked cigarettes (especially in patients without a history of wheezing and without wheezing on examination).
- Wheezing noted on physical examination is the most potent predictor of airflow limitation, and patients with obstructive airflow limitation are 36 times more likely to have wheezing than are patients without this problem (i.e., likelihood ratio of 36) (79,81).
- Other findings associated with increased likelihood of airflow limitation are barrel chest, a positive match test (81,82), hyperresonance, a forced expiratory time of nine seconds or more (80,83), and a subxyphoid apical impulse.

Considering that the presence of underlying COPD is probably the largest risk factor for the development of postoperative pulmonary complication (see Table 19.3), it would be prudent for physicians to detect this disease in patients not yet diagnosed. Two validated bedside maneuvers which can be performed to detect unrecognized pulmonary dysfunction include the match test and the forced expiratory time (FET). To perform the match test, the clinician holds a burning match 10 cm from the patient's widely open mouth. If the match is still burning after the forced expiration, the test result is positive. The inability to extinguish a match held 10 cm from the open mouth is associated with a moderate increase in the likelihood of airway obstruction (likelihood ratio = 7.1) (81,82). The FET (80,83) is performed by asking the patient to take a deep breath and *forcefully* exhale until no more air can be expelled. During this maneuver, the patient must keep his or her mouth and glottis fully open as if yawning. While the patient is performing the FET, the clinician listens over the larynx or lower trachea with a stethoscope and records the duration of audible airflow. When the longest expiratory time of a patient is chosen, a result less than six seconds was associated with a modest decrease in the likelihood of airflow limitation (likelihood ratio = 0.45); a result greater than nine seconds was associated with an increase in the likelihood of having a FEV_1/FVC of 70% or less, a level suggesting the diagnosis of airflow limitation (likelihood ratio = 4.8). The FET provided less diagnostic information in patients younger than 60 years (e.g., in those under 60 the likelihood ratio for FET at or over eight seconds was 2.32) (83). Since the peak expiratory flow rate may add to other helpful predictors, such as the years of cigarette smoking and wheezing,

some may choose to have the patient perform a peak expiratory flow measurement with a Wright peak flow meter. Clinicians' ability to diagnose airflow limitation clinically is variable, but it seems to improve as the severity of the disorder increases.

The utility of routine preoperative pulmonary function tests (PFTs) remains controversial. Not all candidates for lung resection or other surgical procedures need to undergo PFTs. Rather, these tests should be performed selectively in patients who demonstrate significant risks for adverse outcome (as outlined above). The American College of Physicians position paper (84) recommends spirometry in the following groups of patients: those with a history of tobacco use or dyspnea who are undergoing coronary artery or upper abdominal surgery, patients with unexplained shortness of breath undergoing head and neck, orthopedic, or lower-abdominal surgery, and all patients who are to receive lung resection. While these may be prudent recommendations, it is worth noting that many of the 22 early studies of preoperative spirometry are felt to be methodologically flawed (85), and that more recent investigations have shown variable predictive results of PFTs (68). In the several studies including both clinical findings and PFTs, the history and physical examination have been found to be better predictors of pulmonary complications than PFTs (68).

Regarding risk indexes developed to predict postoperative pulmonary complications, Epstein and colleagues (86) developed a cardiopulmonary risk index for lung resection patients which included pulmonary risk factors including obesity, smoking, productive cough, diffuse wheezing or rhonchi, an FEV_1/FVC ratio of less than 70%, and a P_aCO_2 greater than 45 mm Hg (known as a modified Goldman index). Those with half of these risk factors were over 10 times more likely to develop pulmonary complications than were those with fewer risk factors. While potentially helpful, this index has not been validated by other investigators and has not been studied in patients undergoing abdominal surgery. It also requires the incorporation of routine preoperative arterial blood gas and PFT analysis. In general, it is not necessary to perform arterial blood gas analysis unless the patient's pulse oximetry readings are borderline to low and/or the clinician suspects significant obstructive lung disease of acid/base disturbances. In the future, other investigators will need to devise schemes for preoperative risk assessment for pulmonary complications, which might not require preoperative PFTs (87). Both thoracic and abdominal surgical procedures will also need to be incorporated into these investigations. On the other hand, risk stratification, which does not incorporate PFTs and arterial blood gas analysis, might be greatly hampered by the inability appropriately to stratify the degree of chronic pulmonary disease. In Table 19.4 (which was constructed using variable levels of evidence-based observations from the literature), there are several preoperative, intraoperative, and postoperative sugges-

TABLE 19.4. RISK REDUCTION STRATEGIES TO REDUCE POSTOPERATIVE PULMONARY COMPLICATIONS

Preoperative
Encourage cessation of cigarette smoking for at least 8 weeks
Treat airflow obstruction in patients with chronic obstructive pulmonary disease or asthma
Administer antibiotics and delay surgery if respiratory infection is present
Begin patient education regarding lung-expansion maneuvers

Intraoperative
Limit duration of surgery to less than 3 hours if possible
Use spinal or epidural anesthesia
Avoid use of pancuronium
Use laparoscopic procedures when possible
Substitute less ambitious procedure for upper abdominal or thoracic surgery when possible

Postoperative
Use deep-breathing exercises or incentive spirometry
Use continuous positive airway pressure
Use epidural analgesia
Use intercostal nerve blocks

Adapted with permission from Smetana GW. Preoperative pulmonary evaluation. *N Engl J Med* 1999;340:937–934.

tions which seem prudent to help reduce the risk of postoperative pulmonary complications (68).

REFERENCES

1. US Bureau of the Census. *Current population reports, special studies, P23–190. Sixty-five plus in the United States.* Washington, DC: U.S. Printing Office, 1996.
2. Randall T. Demographers ponder the aging of the aged and await unprecedented looming elder boom. *JAMA* 1993;269:2331–2332.
3. Assessing adult vaccination status at age 50 years. *MMWR Morb Mortal Wkly Rep* 1995;44:561–563.
4. Chan ED, Welsh CH. Geriatric respiratory medicine. *Chest* 1998;114:1704–1733.
5. Ohmit SE, Monto AS. Influenza vaccine effectiveness in preventing hospitalization among the elderly during influenza type A and type B seasons. *Int J Epidemiol* 1995;24:1240–1248.
6. Nichol KL, Baken L, Nelson A. Relation between influenza vaccination and outpatient visits, hospitalization, and mortality in elderly patients with chronic lung disease. *Ann Intern Med* 1999;130:397–403.
7. Shaw AB. Age as a basis for healthcare rationing. Support for agist policies. *Drugs Aging* 1996;9:403–405.
8. Baltussen R, Leidl R, Ament A. The impact of age on cost-effectiveness ratios and its control in decision making. *Health Econ* 1996;5:227–239.
9. Sage WM, Hurst CR, Silverman JF, et al. Intensive care for the elderly: outcome of elective and nonelective admissions. *J Am Geriatr Soc* 1987;35:312–318.
10. Singer PA. Rationing, patient preferences, and cost of care at the end of life. *Arch Intern Med* 1992;152:478–480.
11. Giugliano RP, Camargo CA, Lloyd-Jones DM, et al. Elderly patients receive less aggressive medical and invasive management of unstable angina. *Arch Intern Med* 1998;158:1113–1120.
12. Hamel MB, Philips RS, Teno JM, et al. Seriously ill hospitalized adults: do we spend less on older patients? *J Am Geriatr Soc* 1996;44:1043–1048.
13. Hakim RB, Teno JM, Harrell FE, et al. Factors associated with do-not-resuscitate orders: patients' preferences, prognoses, and physicians' judgments. SUPPORT investigators. The study to understand prognoses and preferences for outcome and risks of treatments. *Ann Intern Med* 1996;125:284–293.
14. Hamel MB, Teno JM, Goldman L, et al. Patient age and decisions to withhold life-sustaining treatments from seriously ill, hospitalized adults. *Ann Intern Med* 1999;130:116–125.
15. Teno JM, Hakim RB, Knaus WA, et al. Preferences for cardiopulmonary resuscitation: physician-patient agreement and hospital resource use. SUPPORT investigators. *J Gen Intern Med* 1995;10:179–186.
16. Goldberg AI. Life-sustaining technology and the elderly. Prolonged mechanical ventilation factors influencing the treatment decision. *Chest* 1988;94:1277–1282.
17. Knaus WA, Draper EA, Wagner DP, et al. An evaluation of outcome from intensive care in major medical centers. *Ann Intern Med* 1986;104:410–418.
18. Cohen IL, Lambrinos J. Investigating the impact of age on outcome of mechanical ventilation using a population of 41,848 patients from a statewide database. *Chest* 1995;107:1673–1680.
19. Kurek CJ, Cohen IL, Lambrinos J, et al. Clinical and economic outcome of patients undergoing tracheostomy for prolonged mechanical ventilation in New York state during 1993: analysis of 6,353 cases under diagnosis-related group 483. *Crit Care Med* 1997;25:983–988.
20. Kurek CJ, Dewar D, Lambrinos J, et al. Clinical and economic outcome of mechanically ventilated patients in New York state during 1993. *Chest* 1998;114:214–222.
21. Nunn JF, Milledge JS, Singaraya J. Survival of patients ventilated in an intensive therapy unit. *Br Med J* 1979;1:1525–1527.
22. Campion EW, Mulley AG, Goldstein RL, et al. Medical intensive care for the elderly. A study of current use, costs, and outcomes. *JAMA* 1981;246:2052–2056.
23. Fedullo AJ, Swinburne AJ. Relationship of patient age to cost and survival in a medical ICU. *Crit Care Med* 1983;11:155–159.
24. Witek TJ, Schachter EN, Dean NL, et al. Mechanically assisted ventilation in a community hospital: immediate outcome, hospital charges, and follow-up of patients. *Arch Intern Med* 1985;145:235–239.
25. McLean RF, McIntosh JD, Kung GY, et al. Outcome of respiratory intensive care for the elderly. *Crit Care Med* 1985;13:625–629.
26. Elpern EH, Larson R, Douglass P, et al. Long-term outcomes for elderly survivors of prolonged ventilator assistance. *Chest* 1989;96:1120–1124.
27. Tran DD, Groeneveld AB, van der Meulen J, et al. Age, chronic disease, sepsis, organ system failure, and mortality in a medical intensive care unit. *Crit Care Med* 1990;18:474–479.
28. O'Donnell A, Bohner B. Outcome in patients requiring prolonged mechanical ventilation: Three year experience. *Chest* 1991;100:29S.
29. Pesau B, Falger S, Berger E, et al. Influence of age on outcome of mechanically ventilated patients in an intensive care unit. *Crit Care Med* 1992;20:489–492.
30. Gracey DR, Naessens JM, Krishan I, et al. Hospital and posthospital survival in patients mechanically ventilated for more than 29 days. *Chest* 1992;101:211–214.
31. Chelluri L, Pinsky MR, Grenvik AN. Outcome of intensive care of the "oldest-old" critically ill patients. *Crit Care Med* 1992;20:757–761.
32. Stauffer JL, Fayter NA, Graves B, et al. Survival following me-

chanical ventilation for acute respiratory failure in adult men. *Chest* 1993;104:1222–1229.

33. Swinburne AJ, Fedullo AJ, Bixby K, et al. Respiratory failure in the elderly. Analysis of outcome after treatment with mechanical ventilation. *Arch Intern Med* 1993;153:1657–1662.

34. Cohen IL, Lambrinos J, Fein IA. Mechanical ventilation for the elderly patient in intensive care. Incremental changes and benefits. *JAMA* 1993;269:1025–1029.

35. Papadakis MA, Lee KK, Browner WS, et al. Prognosis of mechanically ventilated patients. *West J Med* 1993;159:659–664.

36. Dardaine V, Constans T, Lasfargues G, et al. Outcome of elderly patients requiring ventilatory support in intensive care. *Aging* 1995;7:221–227.

37. Steiner T, Mendoza G, De GM, et al. Prognosis of stroke patients requiring mechanical ventilation in a neurological critical care unit. *Stroke* 1997;28:711–715.

38. Zilberberg MD, Epstein SK. Acute lung injury in the medical ICU. Comorbid conditions, age, etiology, and hospital outcome. *Am J Respir Crit Care Med* 1998;157:1159–1164.

39. Ely EW, Evans GW, Haponik EF. Mechanical ventilation in a cohort of elderly patients admitted to an intensive care unit. *Ann Intern Med* 1999;131:96–104.

40. Antonelli M, Conti G, Rocco M, et al. A comparison of noninvasive positive-pressure ventilation and conventional mechanical ventilation in patients with acute respiratory failure. *N Engl J Med* 1998;339:429–435.

41. Kollef MH, O'Brien JD, Silver P. The impact of gender on outcome from mechanical ventilation. *Chest* 1997;111:434–441.

42. Yuen EJ, Gonnella JS, Louis DZ, et al. Severity-adjusted differences in hospital utilization by gender. *Am J Med Qual* 1995;10:76–80.

43. Epstein SK, Ciubotaru RL. Influence of gender and endotracheal tube size on preextubation breathing pattern. *Am J Respir Crit Care Med* 1997;154:1647–1652.

44. Krieger BP, Isber J, Breitenbucher A, et al. Serial measurements of the rapid-shallow-breathing index as a predictor of weaning outcome in elderly medical patients. *Chest* 1997;112:1029–1034.

45. Weinberger SE, Weiss JW. Weaning from ventilatory support. *N Engl J Med* 1995;332:388–389.

46. Ely EW, Baker AM, Dunagan DP, et al. Effect on the duration of mechanical ventilation of identifying patients capable of breathing spontaneously. *N Engl J Med* 1996;335:1864–1869.

47. Manthous CA, Schmidt GA, Hall JB. Liberation from mechanical ventilation: a decade of progress. *Chest* 1998;114:886–901.

48. Hall JB, Wood LD. Liberation of the patient from mechanical ventilation. *JAMA* 1987;257:1621–1628.

49. Esteban A, Frutos F, Tobin MJ, et al. A comparison of four methods of weaning patients from mechanical ventilation. *N Engl J Med* 1995;332:345–350.

50. Boult C, Dowd B, McCaffrey D, et al. Screening elders for risk of hospital admission. *J Am Geriatr Soc* 1993;41:811–817.

51. Solomon MZ, O'Donnell L, Jennings B, et al. Decisions near the end of life: professional views on life-sustaining treatments. *Am J Public Health* 1993;83:14–23.

52. Council on Ethical and Judicial Affairs, AMA. Decisions near the end of life. *JAMA* 1992;268:1859–1860.

53. Hofmann JC, Wenger NS, Davis RB, et al. Patient preferences for communication with physicians about end-of-life decisions. *Ann Intern Med* 1997;127:1–12.

54. Lynn J, Harrell FE, Cohn F, et al. Prognoses of seriously ill hospitalized patients on the days before death: implications for patient care and public policy. *New Horiz* 1997;5:56–61.

55. Seckler AB, Meier DE, Mulvihill M, et al. Substituted judgement:

how accurate are proxy predictions? *Ann Intern Med* 1997;115:92–98.

56. Teno JM, Lynn J. Putting advanced-care planning into action. *J Clin Ethics* 1996;7:205–213.

57. Singer PA, Martin DK, Merrijoy K. Quality end-of-life-care: patients' perspectives. *JAMA* 1999;281:163–168.

58. Lynn J, Teno JM, Phillips RS, et al. Perceptions by family members of the dying experience of older and seriously ill patients. *Ann Intern Med* 1997;126:97–106.

59. Murphy DJ, Burrows D, Santilli S, et al. The influence of the probability of survival on patients' preferences regarding cardiopulmonary resuscitation. *N Engl J Med* 1994;330:545–549.

60. Gerety MB, Chiodo LK, Kanten DB, et al. Medical treatment preferences of nursing home residents: relationship to function and concordance with surrogate decision-makers. *J Am Geriatr Soc* 1993;41:953–960.

61. Lo B, Johnson AR. Clinical decisions to limit treatment. *Ann Intern Med* 1980;93:764–768.

62. Byock, I. *Dying well: peace and possibilities at the end of life.* New York: Riverhead Books, 1997.

63. Council on Ethical and Judicial Affairs, AMA. Medical futility in end-of-life care: report of the council on ethical and judicial affairs. *JAMA* 1999;281:937–941.

64. Prendergast TJ, Luce JM. A national survey of end-of-life care for critically ill patients. *Am J Respir Crit Care Med* 1998;158:1163–1167.

65. Campbell ML, Bizek KS, Thill M. Patient responses during rapid terminal weaning from mechanical ventilation: a prospective study. *Crit Care Med* 1999;27:73–77.

66. Faber-Langendoen K. The clinical management of dying patients receiving mechanical ventilation. *Chest* 1994;106:880–888.

67. Goldman L, Caldera DL, Nussbaum SR, et al. Multifactorial index of cardiac risk in noncardiac surgical procedures. *N Engl J Med* 1977;297:845–850.

68. Smetana GW. Preoperative pulmonary evaluation. *N Engl J Med* 1999;340:937–944.

69. Berger DH, Roslyn JJ. Cancer surgery in the elderly. *Clin Geriatr Med* 1997;13:119–141.

70. Fong Y, Blumgart LH, Fortner JG, et al. Pancreatic or liver resection for malignancy is safe and effective for the elderly. *Ann Surg* 1995;122:426–437.

71. Harris WO, Mock MB, Orszulak TA, et al. Use of coronary artery bypass surgical procedure and coronary angioplasty in treatment of coronary artery disease: changes during a 10-year period at Mayo Clinic Rochester. *Mayo Clin Proc* 1996;71:927–935.

72. Money SR, Rice K, Crockett D, et al. Risk of respiratory failure after repair of thoracoabdominal aortic aneurysms. *Am J Surg* 1994;168:152–155.

73. Daley J, Khuri SF, Henderson W, et al. Risk adjustment of the postoperative morbidity rate for the comparative assessment of the quality of surgical care: results of the national veterans affairs surgical risk study. *J Am Coll Cardiol* 1997;185:328–340.

74. Ely EW, Namen AM, Tatter S, et al. Impact of a ventilator weaning protocol in neurosurgical patients: a randomized, controlled trial. *Am J Respir Crit Care Med* 1999;159:A370.

75. Marx GF, Mateo CV, Orkin LR. Computer analysis of postanesthetic deaths. *Anesthesiology* 1973;39:54–58.

76. Djokovic JL, Hedley-Whyte J. Prediction of outcome of surgery and anesthesia in patients over 80. *JAMA* 1979;242:2301–2306.

77. Kroenke K, Lawrence VA, Theroux JF, et al. Operative risk in patients with severe obstructive pulmonary disease. *Arch Intern Med* 1992;152:967–971.

78. Wong D, Weber EC, Schell MJ, et al. Factors associated with postoperative pulmonary complications in patients with severe

chronic obstructive pulmonary disease. *Anesth Analg* 1995;80: 276–284.

79. Holleman DR, Simel DL. Does the clinical examination predict airflow limitation? *JAMA* 1995;273:313–319.

80. Holleman DR, Simel DL, Goldberg JS. Diagnosis of obstructive airways disease from the clinical examination. *J Gen Intern Med* 1993;8:63–68.

81. Badgett RG, Tanaka DJ, Hunt DK, et al. Can moderate chronic obstructive pulmonary disease be diagnosed by historical and physical findings alone? *Am J Med* 1993;94:188–196.

82. Marks A, Bocles J. The match test and its significance. *South Med J* 1960;53:1211–1216.

83. Schapira RM, Schapira MM, Funahashi A, et al. The value of the forced expiratory time in the physical diagnosis of obstructive airways disease. *JAMA* 1993;270:731–736.

84. American College of Physicians. Preoperative pulmonary function testing. *Ann Intern Med* 1990;112:793–794.

85. Lawrence VA, Page CP, Harris GD. Preoperative spirometry before abdominal operations: a critical appraisal of its predictive value. *Arch Intern Med* 1989;149:280–285.

86. Epstein SK, Faling LJ, Daly BD, et al. Predicting complications after pulmonary resection: preoperative exercise testing vs a multifactorial cardiopulmonary risk index. *Chest* 1993;104:694–700.

87. Lawrence VA, Dhanda R, Hilsenbeck SG, et al. Risk of pulmonary complications after elective abdominal surgery. *Chest* 1996; 110:744–750.

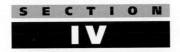

THE CRITICALLY ILL PATIENT

ADMINISTRATIVE, NUTRITIONAL, AND ETHICAL PRINCIPLES FOR THE MANAGEMENT OF CRITICALLY ILL PATIENTS

ANNETTE STRALOVICH-ROMANI
C. KEES MAHUTTE
MICHAEL A. MATTHAY
JOHN M. LUCE

ADMINISTRATION
Criteria for Admission and Discharge
Quality Assurance
Other Administrative Responsibilities

NUTRITION IN CRITICAL ILLNESS AND INJURY
Fuel Utilization During Critical Illness
Nutritional Assessment
Nutritional Requirements
Goals of Nutritional Support

Role of the Gut
Nutrition Support Modalities
Conclusions

ETHICAL PRINCIPLES
Medical Decision-Making
Informed Consent
Foregoing Life-Sustaining Therapy
How Deaths Are Managed
Future Management of Death

This chapter provides information regarding administrative, nutritional, and ethical principles that are important in managing critically ill patients. The initial section on administrative responsibilities is intended to emphasize those clinical issues that are important for directors of intensive care units. The second section regarding nutritional management provides guidelines for providing nutritional supplementation to both medical and surgical critically ill patients. Considerable progress has been made in nutritional treatment for critically ill patients in the last 10 years, and this chapter reviews some of this progress in detail. The final section considers the ethical principles that should guide management of critically ill patients, including the decision to withhold and withdraw life support when further medical care appears futile. Important communication among the physicians, nurses, respiratory therapists, and family members is essential for compassionate, ethically guided care of the critically ill patient.

ADMINISTRATION

The medical care director of an intensive care unit must have both short- and long-term objectives to monitor the performance of the critical care unit in several major areas. An organized plan to ensure uniform guidelines for admission and discharge, quality assurance, as well as guidelines for control of infection and nutritional replacement are important. In addition, there should be a system for regular communication with the nursing director of the intensive care unit as well as the critical care members of the respiratory therapy team that helps provide care to critically ill patients. Furthermore, there must be an ongoing emphasis on strategies to prevent, recognize, and treat complications that may occur in critically ill patients.

Criteria for Admission and Discharge

There are no rigid published guidelines for the criteria that mandate admission or discharge to any individual intensive care unit. However, in each hospital, depending on the particular expertise and focus of the intensive care unit, there should be some general guidelines regarding the monitoring and treatment that an intensive care unit can and should provide. If there are intermediate care units in which monitoring is available, then the primary responsibility of the critical care unit is to provide treatment for patients who have respiratory insufficiency, cardiac insufficiency, or serious infection. An intensive care unit may also, of course, provide careful monitoring and supportive treatment for a variety of patients who have neurologic abnormalities. The decision to admit a patient to the intensive care unit should represent a recognition on both the part of the admitting physician as well as critical care physicians that the patient is likely to benefit from monitoring or treatment in the critical care unit. In some instances, admission to the intensive care unit is needed to institute a diagnostic work-up that is required to determine the etiology of the patient's illness. For example, patients with cryptogenic shock may require a variety of diagnostic procedures that can be carried out in the intensive care unit along with initial treatment modalities.

The decision to discharge a patient from the intensive care unit usually represents a recognition that the primary critical care problem has resolved to a sufficient degree that further monitoring and treatment in an intensive care unit is no longer required. A hospital's capacity to discharge a patient from the critical care unit is determined in part by the monitoring available outside the unit. In some cases, telemetry on medical floors makes it possible to discharge patients with a variety of cardiac abnormalities that otherwise could not be safely discharged from the intensive care unit. In addition, intermediate care units can provide a level of monitoring that allows patients to be discharged from a high level intensive care unit. In some hospitals, monitoring of some high-risk patients postoperatively is required at least for 12 to 24 hours to ensure that the patients are hemodynamically stable and that they do not develop postoperative respiratory failure.

There should be some guidelines established among both the medical and nursing staff regarding the usual responsibilities of the intensive care unit and general guidelines for appropriate criteria for admission and discharge from the intensive care unit.

Quality Assurance

Quality assurance is a standard requirement of all hospitals in order to ensure that there is a system for recognizing and preventing complications. The intensive care unit is an environment in which complications occur more frequently, partly because the patients are critically ill, and partly because invasive procedures are often needed to diagnose and treat the patient's medical problems. The last chapter of this critical care section considers how to prevent, recognize, and treat common nonpulmonary complications in the intensive care unit. There also are recent review articles that consider these issues in detail. There needs to be a regular monthly meeting of the medical and nursing staff to review complications that might have been preventable. For example, complications occurring from the insertion of central lines, including infection and acute complications

associated with insertion of lines, need to be documented and carefully monitored. In addition, there should be a monthly morbidity and mortality conference to review the charts and post-mortem examinations, when available, of patients who have died and patients who have suffered major complications.

Other Administrative Responsibilities

The administration of the intensive care unit also requires that there be uniform guidelines for nutritional management, as discussed in the next section. Guidelines for infection control, particularly outbreaks of resistant organisms such as nafcillin-resistant *Staphylococcus aureus* or vancomycin-resistant *Enterococcus,* should be established. Methods to control infection and prevent spread of nosocomial infection should be reviewed carefully by the medical director with the nursing staff. Finally, as discussed in the last section of this chapter, there needs to be a careful monitoring of critically ill patients for whom continuing critical care is considered futile. As discussed in the final section of this chapter, withdrawal of life support has become the most common mechanism by which patients die in the intensive care unit, largely because of increasing recognition of the limitations of supportive care for some patients. Several clinical studies to help guide ethical management of critically ill patients are now available.

NUTRITION IN CRITICAL ILLNESS AND INJURY

Malnutrition is recognized as a complication of critical illness. The prevention of malnutrition or its detection and subsequent treatment are important goals in the care of critically ill patients. Critical illness and injury precipitate a hypercatabolic and hypermetabolic response triggered by the release of catecholamines, glucocorticoids, inflammatory cytokines, and other inflammatory products. The metabolic hallmarks of stress or injury include increased energy expenditure, anorexia, impaired immune function, and rapid weight loss associated with significant loss of skeletal muscle mass. Besides impairing wound healing and immune function, malnutrition can have deleterious effects on respiratory function by decreasing respiratory muscle strength and ventilatory drive, and impairing lung defenses.

Nutrition is an integral component of critical care medicine. Identifying patients who will benefit from nutrition intervention will lead to cost-effective and beneficial outcomes. Gaining a better understanding of the metabolic response to stress or injury will allow for the proper determination of nutrient requirements and the provision of appropriate nutrition support regimens.

Enteral nutrition is the preferred modality of nutrition support because it is cost-effective and has beneficial clinical

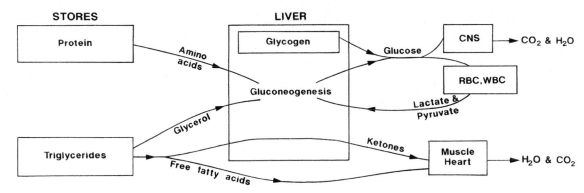

FIGURE 20.1. Major metabolic pathways. During stress, amino acids are used to produce glucose, and fats are used for energy, but the elevated glucose level suppresses ketone production. During nonstressed starvation, ketones are present and supply a substantial portion of the brain's energy.

outcomes. Perhaps the most striking clinical benefit of enteral nutrition therapy is preservation of the gastrointestinal tract. Disruption of the gastrointestinal barrier is a common occurrence during critical illness and the therapies provided. Early initiation of enteral nutrition helps to support the gastrointestinal tract during critical illness. In addition, the fortification of enteral formulas with specific nutrients that may play a role in the maintenance of GI integrity and immune function is being investigated.

Complications can occur with either enteral or parenteral nutrition. However, with careful monitoring along with new knowledge and technical advances, patient safety and tolerance to nutritional therapy have significantly improved.

Fuel Utilization During Critical Illness

Injury caused by burns, trauma, or sepsis evokes increases in both metabolic and catabolic rates. Even in the presence of inadequate intake, these hormone-mediated responses ensure the delivery of abundant glucose, obtained primarily via gluconeogenesis from endogenous proteins, to the sites of injury. Teleologically, one might argue that these metabolic and catabolic responses enhance survival. Both afferent nerve signals and cytokines (e.g., interleukin-1 [IL-1], tumor necrosis factor [TNF]) originating at the site of injury act on the hypothalamus, which in turn activates the sympathetic nervous system and pituitary gland (1). Consequent increases in norepinephrine, epinephrine, cortisol, glucagon, and insulin ensue. Infusion of cortisol, glucagon, and epinephrine into normal subjects elicits the same metabolic stress responses as are seen in critical illness, including the increased levels of insulin (2). The overriding influence of the counterregulatory hormones—cortisol, glucagon, and epinephrine—stimulates gluconeogenesis, glycogenolysis, lipolysis, and proteolysis. As a result, circulating levels of glucose are increased. Substrate cycling (turnover) of carbohydrates, proteins, and fats all increase (Fig. 20.1).

To better understand the changes that occur during the hypermetabolic hypercatabolic state of stress, the hypometabolic catabolic state of nonstressed starvation is discussed first (Table 20.1).

Nonstressed Starvation

The normal body contains substantial caloric reserves (3). Of these reserves, the oxidative metabolism of fat yields considerably more energy than that of protein or glucose (Table 20.2). During the initial phase of nonstressed starva-

TABLE 20.1. NONSTRESSED STARVATION AND THE HYPERMETABOLIC HYPERCATABOLIC STRESS RESPONSE

	Starvation	Stress
Metabolic rate	↓	↑
Urinary nitrogen losses	↓	↑
Insulin	↓	↑ (resistance)
Counterregulatory hormones[a]	Normal	↑
Ketones	↑	Absent
Glucose	Normal	↑
Gluconeogenesis	Present	↑
Glycogenolysis	↑	↑
Lipolysis	↑	↑
Proteolysis	↓	↑
Primary fuel sources	Fat	Fat

[a] Glucagon, cortisol, catecholamines.

TABLE 20.2. NORMAL CALORIC STORES IN A 70-KG MAN

Fuel	kg	kcal/g[a]	Calories (kcal)
Fat	15	9.3	140,000
Muscle protein	6	4.4	26,000
Glycogen	0.26	4.2	1,000
Total			167,000

[a] Energy from the body's oxidative metabolism of fat, protein, and carbohydrates (3.7 kcal/g for glucose).

tion (lasting a few days), glycogen stores are broken down to provide the glucose necessary for the brain, erythrocytes, white blood cells, and renal medulla. Glycogen stores are soon depleted because they are small (containing about 1,000 kcal), and the brain alone requires 100 to 150 g of glucose per day, and in addition, the blood cells require about 40 g per day (3). Insulin levels are low to facilitate mobilization of carbohydrate, fat, and protein for energy. Because glycogen is depleted within 48 to 72 hours, fat gradually becomes the major caloric source, providing about 85% of the total required calories from free fatty acids or ketones (produced in the liver). The remaining 15% of calories, required by the glucose-dependent tissues (brain, blood cells, and renal medulla) is obtained from glucose. Most of this glucose is derived from gluconeogenesis of amino acids, and only a small portion of the glucose is derived from gluconeogenesis of glycerol. Within a few days, the brain adapts to the utilization of ketone bodies, which thereafter may supply 50% to 80% of the brain's energy needs. Brain utilization of ketones spares the breakdown of protein that would otherwise be required for gluconeogenesis. In addition, the metabolic rate may also decrease by 20% to 40% below basal levels. Thus, urinary nitrogen excretion (indicating protein breakdown), which increases from about 10 g per day in the equilibrium state prior to the fast to about 12 g per day in the initial days of the fast, may, with prolonged fasting, decrease to about 3 g per day. Despite these adaptive processes and total potential energy stores in a 70-kg man of approximately 170,000 kcal, death typically occurs in about 2 months (Table 20.2).

Glucose Metabolism During Stress

During the stressed state of critical illness, carbohydrate metabolism is characterized by hyperglycemia, which in turn induces a relative hyperinsulinemia. However, because of the predominance of the counterregulatory hormones (glucagon, cortisol, catecholamines), the glucose levels are higher than expected for a given insulin level, leading to the so-called insulin resistance of critical illness. The high glucose levels fuel the cells involved in the reparative processes. These cells are the white blood cells, macrophages, and fibroblasts, all of which require glucose to generate energy via the glycolytic pathway. Because the hyperglycemia of critical illness may be beneficial, it is usually recommended that glucose not be tightly controlled with insulin, even though there is some evidence that insulin infusion can decrease protein catabolism (4). The necessity for frequent glucose sampling (to monitor for hypoglycemia) and the risk of causing lipogenesis (with consequent increases in carbon dioxide production) temper the enthusiasm for insulin administration. Consequently, glucose values of 200 to 250 mg/mL are generally tolerated during critical illness.

During very severe stresses, such as those induced by burns, glucose utilization and turnover increase (from nor-

mal value of less than 2 mg/kg per min) and maximally may reach 5 to 7 mg/kg per min (5). Because glycogen stores are rapidly depleted, these quantities of glucose are primarily obtained from gluconeogenesis, which occurs in the liver (typically more than 75%) and kidney (less than 25%). The major gluconeogenic precursors are lactate, pyruvate, glycerol, and some amino acids, such as alanine and glutamine. Lactate and pyruvate, resulting from glycolysis of glucose by the red blood and phagocytic cells, are used as substrates for gluconeogenesis in the liver. The newly produced glucose is then again transferred to the peripheral tissues where it is needed, and where it is incompletely oxidized via glycolysis to lactate (Cori cycle). Increased rates of lactate cycling via the Cori cycle occur in trauma, sepsis, and burns (6) (Fig. 20.2). Glycerol, derived from fat, may also be metabolized to glucose. During nonstressed starvation glycerol accounts for only a small portion of total glucose production (about 3%); during sepsis the amount of glucose produced from glycerol may reach 20% (7). However, most of the glucose derived from gluconeogenesis originates from degradation of muscle protein. Alanine is the major amino acid precursor in this pathway (Fig. 20.3). The alanine used for gluconeogenesis is derived from two sources: direct release of alanine from muscle and conversion of glutamine (released from muscle) to alanine in the gastrointestinal tract. Alanine and pyruvate (from glycolysis and protein breakdown) are then again converted to glucose via the glucose-alanine cycle. In the stressed patient, the exogenous infusion of glucose (up to 6 mg/kg per min) only partially suppresses gluconeogenesis, and a portion of the infused glucose is metabolized to glycogen and fat (8). Glucose infusions exceeding 6 mg/kg per min result in a respiratory quotient above 1, indicating net lipogenesis (9). Since

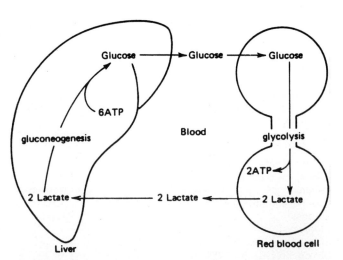

FIGURE 20.2. The Cori cycle. Glucose carbons shuttle potential energy between the liver and anaerobically metabolizing cells. Energy ultimately derives from lipid. (From Devlin T (ed). *Textbook of Biochemistry.* New York, John Wiley & Sons, 1982; with permission.)

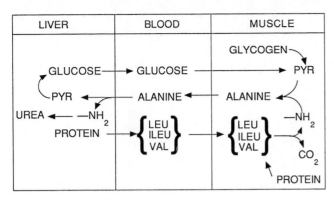

FIGURE 20.3. The glucose-alanine cycle. (From Felig P, Wahren J: Amino acid metabolism in exercising man. *J Clin Invest* 1971; 50:2703–2714, with permission.)

these amounts of glucose (6 mg/kg per min) also do not suppress protein breakdown, glucose alone cannot meet the nutritional requirements in critically ill patients. The overriding stimulation for glucose production appears to derive from several factors: a decreased level of pyruvate dehydrogenase activity, an increase in the glucagon-to-insulin ratio, and an elevation of plasma catecholamine levels (10).

In summary, during stress, hyperglycemia satisfies the increased peripheral glucose demands. The hyperglycemia is the result of incomplete glucose oxidation (glycolysis in phagocytic cells and insulin resistance in other tissues) and increased glucose synthesis. The latter uses amino acid, pyruvate, and lactate substrates.

Fat Metabolism During Stress

Fat becomes the preferred oxidative fuel in the hypermetabolic patient (1,11). This shift from glucose to fat oxidation decreases the muscle proteolysis that would otherwise occur. In contrast to the situation during nonstressed starvation, the increased turnover of fat persists even when exogenous glucose is infused (7,11). Despite this increase in lipolysis, the concentration of free fatty acids is generally not significantly increased, whereas the triglyceride and glycerol concentrations are increased (1,11). Oxidation of free fatty acids may provide 70% to 90% of the total energy needs. However, in septic or injured patients, the elevated glucose levels suppress the conversion of free fatty acids to ketones in proportion to the severity of the insult (12). Thus, in contrast to prolonged nonstressed starvation, during the stressed state, ketone production is inadequate to meet the energy needs of the brain. Therefore, the brain's energy requirements (about 100 to 150 g of glucose per day) must be satisfied via gluconeogenesis fueled (in part) by protein degradation. (It takes about 200 g of protein to make 100 g of glucose.)

In summary, fat is the preferred oxidative fuel in the stressed patient. Ketone production is decreased and is insufficient to meet the brain's energy demands (necessitating proteolysis to provide glucose).

Protein Metabolism During Stress

Under normal equilibrium conditions, protein degradation is balanced by protein synthesis. After a few days of starvation in normal man, the initial catabolic response diminishes and protein sparing occurs. In contrast, with burns, trauma, or sepsis, protein catabolism far exceeds synthesis. In addition, in contrast to nonstressed starvation, during stress the administration of glucose alone does not suppress the proteolysis that occurs (8). Similarly, administration of fat alone does not suppress proteolysis. Protein sparing is optimal when either a combination of carbohydrate and protein or fat and protein is administered (13,14). Protein requirements range from 1 to 1.5 g/kg per day, and excessive protein administration (more than 2 g/kg per day) neither prevents endogenous protein catabolism nor leads to enhanced protein synthesis (15). During the stress response, only about 20% of the muscle protein that is broken down is used directly for energy generation. The remainder enters the liver and is used for gluconeogenesis or synthesis of acute-phase reactant proteins (e.g., C-reactive protein, fibrinogen, $_{-1}$-antitrypsin). As mentioned, glucose is required by the brain and phagocytic cells involved in the reparative processes. The synthesis of acute-phase reactant proteins enhances immune function, coagulation, and antiprotease activity and thereby may enhance survival. The muscle proteolysis occurs because of an increase in stress hormones (e.g., catecholamines, glucagon, and cortisol) as well as cytokines, including IL-1 (16). In the liver, the amino acids not used directly in gluconeogenesis or acute-phase reactant protein production are deaminated to yield pyruvate (used in gluconeogenesis) and an amino group. The latter is eventually excreted as urea, resulting in increased urinary nitrogen excretion. In the critically ill patient, muscle mass and protein losses may be substantial (Fig. 20.4). To appreciate the magnitude of these losses, 30 g of muscle mass contains 6.25 g of protein, which when fully catabolized leads to 1 g of urinary nitrogen excretion. Daily urinary nitrogen excretion may range from 20 to 40 g with burns and 20 to 30 g with trauma or sepsis. Therefore, a loss of 30 g of urinary nitrogen each day corresponds to a loss of 0.9 kg of muscle per day. Such a loss leads to severe life-threatening protein malnutrition within 1 to 2 weeks.

In summary, during critical illness increased proteolysis of skeletal muscle occurs. The resultant amino acids are used to produce glucose (via gluconeogenesis) and acute-phase reactant proteins. Massive protein losses (measured by urinary nitrogen excretion) may be incurred rapidly, with catastrophic consequences.

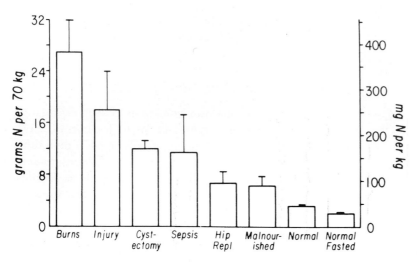

FIGURE 20.4. Total nitrogen excretion during 5% dextrose infusion in injured, septic, burned, or malnourished patients and normal subjects. Mean + SD. (From Elwyn DH: Protein metabolism and requirements in the critically ill patient. *Crit Care Clin* 1987; 3:57–69, with permission.)

Nutritional Assessment

Malnutrition is recognized as a major contributor to the development of morbidity and mortality of hospitalized patients (17). Many hospitalized patients are malnourished at the time of admission and nutritional status tends to decline with length of stay; therefore, it is imperative to intervene before nutritional depletion becomes more significant.

The evaluation of nutritional status is a vital step in formulating nutritional care plans for patients. The nutritional assessment process is used to identify those patients who have preexisting malnutrition or who are at risk for nutritional compromise. One of the greatest challenges for clinicians, however, is to assess body composition and function because there is no gold standard for identifying malnutrition. No single parameter has proven to be useful in all patients. An ideal test for nutritional assessment should be highly sensitive and specific, be unaffected by factors unrelated to nutrition, and correlate with response to nutritional repletion (18). Unfortunately, most markers of malnutrition lack specificity and sensitivity; therefore, until improved methods of identifying malnutrition are developed, it is necessary to perform a comprehensive assessment that includes carefully selected objective parameters, nutritionally focused physical examination, and other subjective parameters. However, in daily clinical practice, the nutritional assessment process must center around assessment parameters that are clinically relevant, easy to obtain, and cost effective (19).

When evaluating nutritional status, it is important to obtain subjective data from the medical history that may bear relevance on the patient's nutritional well-being. For example, acute or chronic illnesses, medications (e.g., immunosuppressive agents, corticosteroids), psychosocial history, diagnostic tests and procedures, and surgeries or other treatment modalities (e.g., chemotherapy, radiation therapy) may be factors that significantly impact on nutritional status (20,21). A thorough nutritional history should also be completed and include weight and appetite changes, diet information, bowel habits, chewing and swallowing abilities, and activity level (22). Another widely accepted nutritional assessment tool is the subjective global assessment (SGA). The SGA relies on history of weight and dietary change, persistent gastrointestinal symptoms, functional capacity, effects of disease on nutritional requirements, and physical appearance (19).

Careful observation of physical appearance adds a dimension to the evaluation of nutritional adequacy. Severe wasting of lean body mass and subcutaneous fat stores are signs of frank malnutrition. The physical examination should also focus on edema, dermatitis, and overt signs of vitamin and mineral deficiencies (e.g., alopecia, cheilosis, glossitis, stomatitis, bleeding gums, bruising, visual changes, rickets) (23,24).

Anthropometry can be used to obtain objective parameters for assessment of nutritional status. Body weight is one of the best general parameters for establishing the diagnosis of malnutrition; however, it provides only a crude evaluation of overall fat and muscle stores. Usual body weight, rather than ideal body weight, is a much more useful nutritional assessment parameter in the ill population. Loss of 5% of body weight in one month or greater than 10% of body weight in the 6 months preceding admission most certainly signifies nutritional depletion. When assessing the weight status of a critically ill patient, exercise caution as to what weight is being used, because weights generally are obscured by fluid shifts; therefore, they are unreliable. Dry weights are more ideal for determining nutritional status and nutrient requirements, and monitoring response to nutritional therapy.

Skinfold measurements, although rarely used in the clinical setting, are indirect methods of measuring somatic protein and subcutaneous fat. These measurements have limited utility in the critical care setting because of edema and fluid shifts. Skinfold measurements tend to have more merit in the outpatient arena, when nutritional status is being serially evaluated over time, or in the pediatric population, to assess growth.

One of the more recent techniques for analysis of body composition is bioelectrical impedence (BIA). BIA is based on the principle that lean tissue has a higher electrical conductivity and a lower impedance relative to water because of its greater electrolyte content (19,25). However, because BIA is considered to be unreliable in the presence of fever, edema, obesity, and electrolyte abnormalities, it is unlikely to be a useful assessment tool in the intensive care setting.

Various serum protein levels have been used in assessment of nutritional status. Albumin, transferrin, thyroxine-binding prealbumin, and retinol-binding protein are most commonly used in the clinical setting (Table 20.3). Serum albumin is best evaluated at admission because levels rarely show nutritionally relevant changes during hospitalization owing to its long half-life (18 to 20 days). The advantages of albumin as an assessment parameter are that it is an inexpensive laboratory measurement, it is useful with long-term assessments, and it is a valuable prognostic indicator of morbidity and mortality. Serum albumin levels dramatically decrease, however, with metabolic stress and injury owing to a combination of factors, including downregulation of the genes for albumin synthesis by tumor necrosis factor (TNF) and interleukin-1 (Il-1), increased degradation, increased transcapillary losses, and specific disease state (liver failure). Albumin levels may change quickly as a result of nonnutritional factors, and respond slowly even with adequate nutrition support. In fact, plasma albumin levels will not increase in stressed patients until the inflammatory response remits. Therefore, little credence should be given to albumin as a marker of nutritional status or response to nutritional therapy during a period of metabolic stress (19,22,26). Because of their shorter half lives and smaller protein pools, transferrin, prealbumin, and retinol binding protein have been touted as better markers of nutritional status (Table 20.3). However, like albumin, these constitutive proteins decrease independently of nutritional status during critical illness because of the preferential production of acute phase reactants over the synthesis of visceral proteins. It should not be assumed, therefore, that decreased levels of serum proteins are caused solely by malnutrition. Normal patterns of hepatic protein synthesis and degradation are altered during critical illness, making evaluation difficult.

Nutritional Requirements

Energy Requirements

The amount of energy required is a function of resting needs (those required to complete daily metabolic work), with adjustments added for activity, specific dynamic action of food, healing, repair of nutritional deficits, painful stimuli, and any catabolic insult such as trauma, sepsis, and surgery (11). Several methods exist to determine energy requirements, such as predictive equations, nomograms, and indirect calorimetry.

Predictive Equations

Predictive equations are most often estimated using the Harris-Benedict equation, which represents resting energy expenditure and then is multiplied by stress factors ranging from 1.2 to 2.0, depending on the clinical condition of the patient (Table 20.4). The utility of this formula in critically ill patients is limited because this equation was developed

TABLE 20.3. SERUM PROTEINS FOR NUTRITIONAL ASSESSMENT

Serum Protein	Half-life	Normal Range	Comments
Albumin	20 Days	3.5–5.0 g/dL	Large body pool; reliable indicator of morbidity and mortality; reflects chronic vs acute protein depletion; responds slowly to changes in nutritional status; decreased levels with fluid overload, malabsorptive states, stress (sepsis, burns, trauma, postoperative states); disease process (liver failure, congestive heart failure); increased levels with anabolic agents, dehydration, and infusion of albumin, fresh frozen plasma and whole blood
Transferrin	8–10 Days	200–400 mg/dL	Smaller body pool; sensitive to changes in nutritional status; calculated from total iron binding capacity; decreased with chronic infection, stress, uremia, iron overdose, overhydration, liver failure; increased levels with pregnancy, iron deficiency, hypoxia, hepatitis, dehydration, estrogens
Prealbumin (Transthyretin)	2–3 Days	15–40 mg/dL	Rapid turnover rate; small body pool; responds quickly with changes in nutritional status; decreased levels with stress, inflammation, surgery, liver disease; increased levels with renal dysfunction
Retinol-binding Protein	8–10 Hours	2.7–7.6 mg/dL	Highly sensitive to changes in nutritional status; decreased levels (same as prealbumin) as well as vitamin A deficiency; increased levels with renal dysfunction and vitamin A supplementation

TABLE 20.4. HARRIS-BENEDICT EQUATION FOR ESTIMATING ENERGY REQUIREMENT

Men: Resting energy expenditure (REE) = 66.5 + 13.75 × (W) + 5 × (H) − 6.76 × (A)
Women: Resting energy expenditure (REE) = 655 + 9.56 × (W) + 1.85 × (H) − 4.68 (A)
W = Weight (kg)
H = Height (cm)
A = Age (years)

TABLE 20.6. THE FICK EQUATION FOR DETERMINING ENERGY EXPENDITURE

Resting Energy Expenditure = CO × Hgb × (Sao_2 − $Smvo_2$) × 105
CO = Cardiac output (L/min)
Hgb = Hemoglobin (g/dL)
Sao_2 = Arterial oxygenation saturation percentage
$Smvo_2$ = Mixed venous oxygenation percentage

from data on normal volunteers. Ireton-Jones developed a predictive equation to estimate energy expenditure in both ventilator-dependent and spontaneously breathing hospitalized patients based on statistical analysis of measurements using indirect calorimetry (Table 20.5) (28,29).

Indirect Calorimetry

A more accurate method to calculate energy expenditure, especially in the complex and rapidly changing setting of critical illness, is indirect calorimetry. This method can be carried out at the bedside using portable machines that are costly and require trained personnel to operate. The premise of indirect calorimetry is that it calculates energy expenditure by measurement of respiratory gas exchange, specifically the measurement of oxygen consumption (VO_2), carbon dioxide production (Vco_2), and minute ventilation (VE). Caloric needs are quantified based on the measurements of VO_2 and Vco_2 and the application of the Weir equation (28–31).

$$Energy\ expenditure = [(VO_2)\ (3.941) + (Vco_2)\ (1.11) \times 1,440 \quad [Eq.\ 20.1]$$

When measured energy expenditure is obtained from indirect calorimetry, some clinicians add a factor of 10% to 20% to account for 24-hour variability (32). Besides determining energy expenditure, respiratory quotient (RQ) can also be obtained, which is helpful in guiding caloric and carbohydrate therapy (RQ = Vco_2/VO_2). RQ values from carbohydrate, fat, and protein are 1.0, 0.7, and 0.8, respectively. An RQ exceeding 1.0 suggests either excessive caloric and or carbohydrate overfeeding, which can result in increased

CO_2 production, increased work of breathing, and unwanted net fat synthesis (28). The one major limitation to using indirect calorimetry is that the measurement becomes unreliable when the oxygen setting (Fio_2) on the ventilator is greater than 50%.

Fick Equation

When high ventilator settings preclude indirect calorimetry, the cardiovascular Fick equation is an option for determining energy requirements, provided the patient has a pulmonary artery catheter (Table 20.6).

Protein Requirements

The goal of protein provision is to minimize the degree of net nitrogen loss. Protein must be continually replenished because protein reserves do not exist in the body. Under normal circumstances the recommended daily intake of protein is approximately 0.8 gm of protein per kg body weight (Table 20.7). In critical illness, the proper provision of protein is crucial because it is the most important macronutrient with stress or injury (Table 20.7). Protein requirements are high with trauma, sepsis, and the demands for healing of burns, necrotizing fasciitis, and other types of large

TABLE 20.5. IRETON-JONES PREDICTIVE EQUATION FOR ENERGY EXPENDITURE IN VENTILATED PATIENTS

Energy expenditure = 1,784 − 11 (A) + 5 (W) + 244 (G) + 239 (T) + 804 (B)
A = Age (years)
W = Weight (kg)
G = Gender (female = 0; male = 1)
T = Diagnosis of trauma (absent = 0; present = 1)
B = Diagnosis of burn (absent = 0; present = 1)

TABLE 20.7. ESTIMATING PROTEIN REQUIREMENTS

	Normal Renal Function
Maintenance	0.8–1.2 gm of protein/kg per day
Moderate stress	1.3–1.5 gm of protein/kg per day
Severe stress	1.5–2.0 gm of protein/kg per day
	Renal Failure
Nondialyzed	0.8–1.2 gm of protein/kg per day
Hemodialyzed (may be adjusted based on frequency of dialysis)	1.0–1.4 gm of protein/kg per day
CAPD/CAVHD/CVVHD	1.3–1.7 gm of protein/kg per day
Hepatic failure	Begin at 1.0 gm of protein/kg per day, increase as tolerated to 1.5–2.0 gm of protein/kg per day
Hepatic failure with encephalopathy	0.6–0.8 gm of protein/kg per day (no less than 40 gm per day)

wounds. In some disease states, such as renal failure and hepatic encephalopathy, protein requirements may be reduced (Table 20.7).

Nitrogen Balance

Assessing protein requirements for patients can pose quite a challenge because protein metabolism changes during the various phases of critical illness, injury, and recovery. Nitrogen balance, when correctly measured and calculated, remains the best available marker of the effects of acute nutrition intervention. In fact, nitrogen balance is the single nutritional parameter associated most consistently with improved outcomes. Nitrogen balance determines the amount of protein required to maintain nitrogen equilibrium by assessing urinary nitrogen losses (33,34). Urinary nitrogen losses following injury and illness tend to parallel the increased energy expenditure with increased degree of stress. The magnitude of nitrogen loss varies with the severity of disease (35). Protein requirements and efficacy of nutrition therapies may be determined from the nitrogen balance calculation. Nitrogen balance is equal to nitrogen intake minus urinary nitrogen output plus obligatory losses from skin, stool, and respiration, ranging from 2 to 4 g per day.

$$\text{Nitrogen balance (g)} = (\text{protein intake}/6.25)$$
$$- (\text{urinary urea nitrogen} + 2\text{--}4) \quad [\text{Eq. 20.2}]$$

When there are excessive losses of nitrogen from severe diarrhea, fistula drainage, burn exudate, ostomy output, wounds, or pleural drainage, total nitrogen content should be determined if practical.

A positive nitrogen balance correlates with net protein synthesis (anabolic state) and suggests adequacy of nutritional support. A negative nitrogen balance, on the other hand, indicates that the rate of protein breakdown exceeds the rate of protein synthesis (catabolic state); therefore, it requires adjustments in the nutritional support regimen (33). Positive or even neutral nitrogen balance may be difficult to achieve in critically ill patients because of the effects of catabolic hormones, medications, bed rest, fever, and infection. The goal of nutrition support, therefore, is to offset the degree of catabolism rather than to achieve positive balance. Once the source of stress is resolved, an anabolic state can be attainable.

A nitrogen balance study should only be completed after the patient has been on a relatively constant protein and energy intake for 3 days, thus allowing the urea cycle and gluconeogenic enzymes to adjust to protein intake. Urine should be kept on ice during the collection and analyzed within 4 hours to prevent loss of urea owing to bacterial conversion to ammonia.

The major limitation of using a standard nitrogen balance study in critically ill patients is that a creatinine clearance greater than 50 mL/min is required for accurate interpretation (24). When renal function is impaired nitrogen balance can be calculated using urea kinetic modeling (6). Nitrogen balance studies are usually invalid with liver failure because of decreased urea production.

Goals of Nutritional Support

Nutrition support is paramount in maintaining the patient's nutritional status during a period of critical illness. Preservation and restoration of lean body mass are the primary objectives of nutritional therapy (26). Additionally, specialized nutrition support to provide substrates (macronutrients and micronutrients) for improving immune function, facilitating wound and tissue repair, and supporting hepatic protein synthesis remain major goals for the management of the critically ill and injured patient (34). Of course, the overall goal of nutrition therapy is to reduce morbidity and mortality, and optimize clinical outcomes to minimize cost and the length of stay in the hospital.

Nutritional Support of Ventilator-Dependent Patients

Patients requiring ventilatory support need adequate nutrition to maintain the integrity of their respiratory systems. Ventilator-dependent patients are prone to respiratory infections, especially when nutritional depletion is aggravated by hypercatabolic states such as sepsis, burns, or trauma (36). Catabolism of the respiratory musculature, edema formation from hypoalbuminemia, compromised immune function, decreased surfactant production, prolonged intubation, and decreased repair of epithelial surfaces are all deleterious effects that malnutrition plays on respiratory function (37).

Electrolyte abnormalities, particularly hypophosphatemia, can impact on respiratory function as well. Low serum phosphorus levels can lead to respiratory muscle weakness. Additionally, hypophosphatemia can result in decreased levels of 2,3-diphosphoglycerate in red blood cells, which can lead to increased oxyhemoglobin affinity and decreased oxygen delivery to tissues (36).

When designing the nutrition support prescription for ventilator-dependent patients, it is important to examine the proportion of carbohydrate, fat, and protein. Although there are no definitive recommendations, a well-balanced fuel mix comprised of 30% to 40% of total calories as fat, 40% to 50% of total calories as carbohydrate, and 20% to 25% of total calories as protein is advised. The effect of protein and nitrogen intake on ventilatory drive is controversial. Adequate protein provision is essential for the repletion of lean body mass. One of the major goals of nutritional therapy is to prevent hypercapnia associated with overfeeding. Excessive caloric or carbohydrate administration may cause increased CO_2 production. The substitution of fat as a metabolic fuel may be beneficial when carbohydrate limits have been reached (28). However, increased CO_2

production is primarily related to the total calories administered rather than to the specific carbohydrate:fat calorie ratio (38). Ongoing nutritional assessments and evaluations of clinical status is necessary with adjustments in total caloric intake and manipulation of nutrient substrate mixtures as needed to improve nutritional status and to facilitate weaning from mechanical ventilation.

Role of the Gut

Besides its role in digestion and absorption, the GI tract has the distinct property of maintaining barrier function and normal bacterial flora of the intestine. Gastrointestinal tissues require direct contact with nutrients to support cell replication and to undergo the numerous metabolic and immunologic functions required for successful adaptation to stress (39). There are nonspecific defense mechanisms (peristalsis, mucus, gastric acid, bile salts, desquamation, microflora) that work in concert with immunological defenses to maintain the function of the gut barrier. However, the single most important influence on intestinal structure and function are luminal nutrients (39–41).

An integral component of mucosal immunity, besides the epithelial cells that line the GI tract, is the presence of gut-associated lymphoid tissue (GALT). It is estimated that 25% of the intestinal mucosa is lymphoid tissue and that 70% to 80% of all immunologic-secreting cells are located within the intestine. Interestingly, this makes the digestive tract one of the largest immune organs within the body (40). Secretory IGA (sIGA) is the prominent immunoglobulin in the intestine, and it is believed to inhibit bacterial colonization by curtailing adherence of pathogenic microorganisms to the epithelium. Furthermore, sIGA provides protection from antigens that have invaded the enterocytes (41).

Alteration of intestinal structure and function may lead to barrier dysfunction of the gut. Impaired immunity, malabsorption, motility disorders, and bacterial translocation are all contributing factors to the breakdown of the gut barrier during critical illness (41).

Intestinal injury or atrophy can potentially lead to a quantitative reduction in GALT, in addition to a decreased production of secretory IGA, both of which can have deleterious immunologic effects (41). The malabsorption that typically occurs in critically ill patients can result from bowel wall edema, mucosal atrophy, and impaired mesenteric blood flow. Furthermore, reduced intestinal secretions, causing abdominal distention and dysmotility, and narcotic-induced ileus contribute to altered GI motility in critical illness.

Failure of the intestine to exclude toxic substances, particularly bacteria and their products, may result in bacterial translocation (41). The term bacterial translocation implies the migration of gut bacteria or bacterial byproducts from the bowel lumen to the bloodstream or lymphatic system (35). Maintenance of the epithelial lining of the GI tract is of utmost importance in preventing gut barrier dysfunction. The physiochemical presence of nutrients in the intestinal lumen is vital in preserving the integrity of mucosal immune function. Absence of luminal nutrient stimulation, therefore, may lead to gut atrophy, which could result in bacterial translocation. Although bacterial translocation has been implicated in the pathogenesis of multisystem organ failure based on animal models in critical illness, there is lack of evidence for bacterial translocation in humans. It is believed, however, that the integrity of intestinal immunity, particularly during a period of physiologic stress, is helpful in preventing infectious complications and may avert the development of multisystem organ failure in the critically ill.

Gut Fuels

Over the past few decades much attention has focused on the use of specific nutrients and growth factors in maintaining GI integrity, improving immune function, and preventing the profound lean tissue dissolution associated with critical illness. Glutamine, fiber, arginine, peptides, Omega-3 fatty acids, and antioxidants have all been touted to have salutary effects on intestinal integrity and immunity and possibly alter the metabolic response to stress or injury.

Glutamine is the most abundant amino acid in plasma. Normally considered to be a nonessential amino acid, recent studies have shown that glutamine is conditionally essential in critical illness (43). During catabolic states, glutamine is preferentially consumed and oxidized by intestinal mucosa in place of glucose (43). Glutamine plays a major role in maintaining intestinal metabolism, structure, and function; decreasing mucosal injury; and preventing bacterial translocation. Supplemental glutamine may also preserve gut glutathione levels during ischemia and reperfusion, which may lessen the associated intestinal injury (41).

Recent research has shown that dietary fiber has diverse functions in both the upper and lower GI tract (Table 20.8). Dietary fiber is classified as either insoluble or soluble based on chemical structure. Besides the functions of fiber listed in Table 20.8, the most pronounced effect of fiber is the colonic fermentation of dietary residue to short-chain fatty

TABLE 20.8. FUNCTIONS OF FIBER

Function	Soluble	Insoluble
Increased water-holding capacity (increased stool weight)	Yes	Yes
Delayed gastric emptying	Yes	No
Hypocholesterolemic effects	Yes	No
Decreased rate of glucose absorption	Yes	No
Short-chain fatty acid production (bacterial fermentation)	Yes	No
Protection against bacterial translocation in gut	Yes	Yes

acids (acetate, butyrate, propionate) (44). Short-chain fatty acids are rapidly absorbed by the intestinal mucosa and are readily metabolized by the intestinal epithelium and the liver. The most desirable effect of the short-chain fatty acids, however, is the trophic effect it exerts on the entire intestinal tract (44,45).

The use of peptide-based diets is beneficial in the critically ill patient with impaired GI absorption. Compared with amino acid diets, peptide diets have been shown to decrease gut permeability by maintaining better intestinal blood flow and protecting intestinal integrity, as well as stimulating greater release of gut hormones and growth factors. Peptides also attenuate hypoalbuminemic diarrhea by excessive protein loss and increasing absorption of protein precursors (46,47).

Arginine is another specific nutrient that has had purported immune-enhancing and wound-healing properties (34). Omega-3 fatty acids may enhance the immune system and to have antiinflammatory properties. There is some discussion that the benefit of antioxidants in inflammatory processes such as ARDS is increasing. At this time, however, there are no specific recommendations for supplementation. Finally, a number of anabolic agents have been investigated for their potential to attenuate the catabolic response, to promote wound healing, and to support the growth and integrity of the GI tract (34).

Although clinical studies on the gut fuels mentioned in the preceding are promising, further human studies are needed to substantiate claims made on these specialized nutrients before their routine clinical use is advocated.

Nutrition Support Modalities

Enteral Nutrition

Because of the development of more sophisticated enteral products and feeding techniques, along with all the known clinical benefits of enteral feeding, there is growing use of enteral nutrition support in the critical care setting. There is increasing evidence that enteral delivery through the GI tract provides significant benefits to the critically ill patient. Enteral nutrition minimizes many of the inimical responses of the GI tract to critical illness or injury (41). It is favored over parenteral nutrition because some studies have shown that there is a significantly lower incidence of septic complications in patients fed enterally than in those fed parenterally (35). Enteral alimentation is also more physiologic and cost effective.

Timing may be crucial when it comes to instituting enteral alimentation in critically ill or injured patients. Preferably, enteral feeding tubes should be placed within 48 hours of admission to the ICU. Administration of enteral nutrition into the small bowel 8 to 12 hours following surgery is being practiced widely, and with good success, because peristalsis is often well maintained in the small bowel post-

operatively. Bowel sounds should not be used to indicate feasibility of enteral alimentation, but rather to indicate the adequacy of gastric emptying. Although gastric and colonic motility are impaired in most critically ill patients, small bowel motility and absorption are usually intact.

The most important features associated with the early administration of enteral nutrition appear to be the minimization of gut atrophy, decreased incidence of sepsis, enhanced immunocompetence, and blunted hypermetabolic response to stress (41). The role of pharmacomodulation of the gut has also received increased attention. Pathologic conditions and unavoidable iatrogenic disorders that affect gut function may be able to be managed with drug therapy (e.g., octreotide, propofol, 5-hydroxytryptamine-3, erythromycin, naloxone), so that the simplest level of enteral feeding may be used (48).

Technological advances in enteral feeding have significantly influenced the practice of enteral nutrition support. Improvements in placement procedures, enteral feeding devices, and nutritional products have allowed enteral nutrition to be provided to patients who previously would not have been candidates for enteral alimentation.

New Clinical Applications for Enteral Nutrition

Several clinical conditions now deemed appropriate for enteral nutrition support deserve mention. The use of enteral feeding in fistula management is becoming more widespread. The ability to enterally feed is contingent on the site and extent of usable intestine for feeding. To avoid reflux, it is necessary to feed 40 cm distal to the fistula. Spontaneous closure rates comparable to TPN have been reported (43).

Enteral feeding is used in conjunction with parenteral nutrition in short bowel syndrome. Minimal infusion of enteral nutrition has been shown to foster intestinal adaptation and rehabilitation. Utilization of alternative substrates (e.g., glutamine, fiber, growth hormone) may be important contributors for successful adaptation.

A new alternative for providing nutrition support to the patient with acute pancreatitis has been jejunal feedings placed either nasojejunally or with an operative jejunostomy. Because the cephalic and gastric phases of digestion are bypassed, there is decreased pancreatic stimulation allowing for the safe and efficacious administration of enteral nutrition.

Another area in which the efficacy of enteral feeding warrants in-depth investigation is in patients undergoing bone marrow transplantation. Restoration of the GI mucosa following chemotherapy and radiation therapy, prevention of bacterial translocation (especially in an immunocompromised patient), maintenance of normal immune responses, smoother transition to oral feeding, and cost could all conceivably be beneficial in this patient population.

Tube Types and Location

The administration of enteral nutrition is generally accomplished by using nasoenteric feeding tubes inserted into the stomach, duodenum, or jejunum. Nasoenteric feeding tubes are the most frequently used because of the ease of placement and the decreased cost and risk to the patient in comparison to a tube requiring surgical insertion (49). Using small-bore feeding tubes over the traditional nasogastric tubes (salem sumps) is preferred because there is less risk of tracheoesophageal fistula and aspiration and they are more comfortable for the patient. The downside to using the small feeding tubes is that they are prone to collapse and clogging, making it difficult to check for feeding residuals.

In critically ill patients, transpyloric feedings are believed to be better tolerated and have fewer infectious complications owing to aspiration than gastric feedings. Many bedside placement techniques for passage of weighted tubes beyond the pylorus in patients in the intensive care unit are available and usually successful. The right lateral decubitus position with auscultation can be used to track the tube into the small intestine (50). However, if the aforementioned method is unsuccessful, then endoscopically or fluoroscopically guided tube placement may be indicated. Prokinetic drugs can also help facilitate tube positioning. Radiographic confirmation is necessary before initiating the enteral feeding regimen on placement of the feeding tube.

Methods of Delivery. Enteral nutrition can be delivered by either bolus, intermittent or continuous feeding. Bolus feeding is the rapid infusion of a large volume of enteral formula over a short period of time (51). Frequent GI complications (e.g., diarrhea, nausea, vomiting, aspiration, distention) are associated with this method of administration. Intermittent feeding using either gravity drip or an infusion pump is the delivery of a moderate to large volume of enteral formula over a defined period, usually from 1 to 16 hours (51). Continuous tube feeding is the infusion of a small amount of enteral formula over 24 hours using an infusion pump (51). In critically ill patients and with small bowel feedings, the continuous delivery method is essential. Continuous feedings are better tolerated than bolus or intermittent feedings and are associated with reduced incidence of high gastric residuals, gastroesophageal reflux, and aspiration.

Formula Composition
There are numerous commercially available enteral products that differ in composition and proportion of nutrients as well as cost. All formulas contain the macronutrients carbohydrate, fat, protein, water, and the micronutrients, vitamins, minerals, trace elements, and electrolytes (Table 20.9). Polymeric formulas contain intact nutrients and require normal digestion and absorption. Lactose-free mixtures are the basic feeding formulation because a majority of patients have genetic or acquired lactase deficiency (50). Osmolality of these formulas can be isotonic or hypertonic (300 to 800 mOsm/kg of water). Caloric density varies from 1.0 to 2.0 kcal/mL with 40% to 55% of total calories from carbohydrate, 12% to 20% from protein, and 30% to 50% from fat. Fats are provided as long-chain triglycerides (LCTs) and medium-chain triglycerides (MCTs).

Oligomeric and monomeric formulas are classified as elemental and semielemental/peptide-based formulas. They contain one or more partially digested macronutrients and are reserved for patients with compromised GI function

TABLE 20.9. CLASSIFICATION OF ENTERAL FORMULAS

Category	Subcategory	Comments
Polymeric	Blenderized	Real food; requires normal digestion and absorption; lactose and lactose-free; isotonic; nutritionally complete
	Standard	Intact nutrients; lactose free; low residue; isotonic; nutritionally complete; requires normal digestion and absorption
	High nitrogen	Intact nutrients; lactose-free; isotonic; protein > 15% of total kcal; nutritionally complete; requires normal digestion and absorption
	Fiber-enriched	Intact nutrients; lactose-free; isotonic; soluble and insoluble fiber; regulation of bowel function; nutritionally complete; requires normal digestion and absorption
	Calorically dense	Intact nutrients, 1.5–2.0 kcal/mL; high osmolality; use with fluid restriction; lactose-free; nutritionally complete; requires normal digestion and absorption
	Disease specific	Intact nutrients; protein, fat, and carbohydrate source varies depending on disease state formula designed for; electrolyte content and osmolality vary; require normal digestion and absorption; expensive; efficacy controversial
Oligomeric (partially hydrolyzed)		Hydrolyzed protein; ditripeptides, free amino acids; fat semielemental content varies (3%–40% of total kcal); lactose free; osmolality varies (250–700 mOsm/kg); nutritionally complete; digestion required; limited absorptive surface of GI tract
Monomeric (elemental/chemically-defined)		Free amino acids; lactose free; fat varies (1%–15% of total kcal); high osmolality; may include glutamine; nutritionally complete; minimal digestion required; limited absorptive surface of GI tract
Modular		Individual nutrient (carbohydrate, fat, protein) modules; used to modify preexisting commercial formula to increase nutrient density or to make unique formula; requires normal digestion and absorption

(e.g., critical illness, pancreatic or bile salt deficiencies, intestinal atrophy, short bowel syndrome, and IBD) (52). Caloric density is usually 1.0 kcal/mL. The elemental diets have a much higher osmolality than the semielemental diets. Protein is supplied as crystalline amino acids (monmeric/elemental) or as hydrolyzed whey, casein, or lactalbumin (oligomeric/semielemental). These formulas are considered low fat and may contain a high proportion of fat in the form of MCT (52). The efficacy of elemental diets has been controversial for several years.

Modular formulas are composed of individual nutrient modules (fat, protein, carbohydrate) to produce a unique formula customized to meet the specific needs of the patient. Typically, modular components are used to modify a preexisting commercial formula to add caloric or protein density.

Widespread use of enteral feeding and an expanding knowledge of specific disease processes has led to an explosion in the development of disease specific formulas (50). These formulas have been designed for specific organ failure, metabolic dysfunction, or immunomodulation. Given the cost and questionable efficacy of these specialized formulas, they should be used judiciously. Detailed formula descriptions, clinical indications, and possible benefits are beyond the scope of this chapter (53).

Formula Selection

Enteral formula selection should be based on the patient's digestive and absorptive capacity, organ function, specific nutrient needs, tolerances, allergies, and should take into account the formula composition and total calories. Attention must also be given to fluid requirements, vitamin and mineral needs, and osmolality. The quantity of water in enteral formulas is often described as water content or moisture content. Most enteral formulas contain water in the general range of 700 to 900 mL per 1,000 mL of enteral formula. The general rule of thumb is to provide 30 mL water per kg body weight, or as clinical status permits. When provided in sufficient volume, most nutritionally complete products contain adequate vitamins and minerals to meet all of the US recommended dietary intake (RDI). If the volume of enteral formula given is inadequate to provide the RDI, a daily multivitamin and mineral supplement is warranted unless contraindicated because of disease states that may reduce requirements of some micronutrients (53).

The osmolality of enteral formulas can directly affect a patient's GI tolerance to the formula. Generally, isotonic formulas (270 to 320 mOsm/kg) are well tolerated and do not need to be diluted for administration. Hypertonic feedings (>500 mOsm) may be initiated at half-strength (diluted 1 : 1 with water) in patients who are critically ill, have GI atrophy from prolonged gut disuse, have undergone intestinal resections, or who have a history of diarrhea, malabsorption, or prior tube feeding intolerance to decrease the risk of osmotic diarrhea (35).

Initiation and advancement of enteral feedings will vary with the method of administration. Bolus feedings are generally administered over several minutes and are best tolerated when given at less than 60 mL/min (e.g., 240 mL of formula every 3 hours over at least 3 min) (54). Intermittent feedings are generally better received if a maximum of 200 to 300 mL of formula is delivered over a 30- to 60-minute period every 4 to 6 hours. Continuous feedings are introduced at 10 to 30 mL/hour and advanced in 10- to 20-mL increments every 8 to 12 hours until the goal flow rate is attained. In patients who are critically ill, who have not been fed for an extended period of time, and those who are receiving calorie-dense or high osmolality enteral formulas, conservative initiation and advancement rates are highly advised (e.g., 10-mL increments every 12 to 24 hours) (54).

Complications

Complications associated with enteral feeding may be avoided and managed with appropriate monitoring. The major goal of monitoring is to minimze the complications of enteral therapy and to maintain the patency of the small-bore feeding tube. An assessment of GI tolerance (i.e., nausea, vomiting, abdominal discomfort and distention, stool pattern) is mandatory when a patient is on enteral nutrition support. Hydration status and laboratory data must also be evaluated when a patient is being enterally fed. Preventive measures should be taken to minimize the risk of aspiration. Keeping the head of bed elevated at a 30- to 45-degree angle and checking for tube feeding residuals are recommended to lessen the potential for aspiration (54). With continuous feeding residuals should be checked every 4 hours and should not exceed 200 mL. In the critically ill patient residuals are considered to be high at greater than 120 mL. If the patient has a cuffed tracheostomy, the cuff can be deflated 2 hours after bolus feedings; for continuous feeds, the cuff may be deflated only when necessary to prevent tracheal complications (55). Routine flushing of feeding tubes with 30 to 60 mL of water every 4 to 6 hours helps to extend the life span of the small tubes.

Enteral nutrition is a safe means of delivering nutritional support. However, complications arise with this modality of feeding. There are three types of complications: mechanical, gastrointestinal, and metabolic. Mechanical complications of nasoenteric tube feedings include tube obstruction, displacement, or dislodgement; nasopharyngeal irritation; and gastric rupture. Obstruction or clogging of the tube occurs most frequently from inadequate crushing of medications and from formula residue adhering to the lumen of the tube (55). Giving liquid medications (elixirs, suspensions) rather than pills or syrups may help to avoid clogging of tubes. Flushing with water, as previously described, helps to maintain patency of feeding tubes. Following proper procedures for feeding tube placement and verifying tube position helps to avoid the complication of tube displacement. By using small soft tubes, lubricating tubes for insertion, and maintaining good hygiene of the mouth and nares, greater patient comfort is achieved.

The most common complications of tube feedings are gastrointestinal, including diarrhea, nausea, vomiting, constipation, delayed gastric emptying, and GI bleeding (56). Diarrhea is the most common cause of GI intolerance. The major causes of formula-related diarrhea are rapid infusion rate, formula characteristics (e.g., hypertonic, low fiber or residue, high fat), and bacterial contamination (54). Medications (e.g., sorbitol-containing elixirs, antibiotics, laxatives, magnesium, and phosphorus supplements), pancreatic insufficiency, fecal impaction, and pathogenic bacteria (*Clostridium difficile*) can all be non–formula-related causes of diarrhea in the tube-fed patient (54). The type of tube feeding formula is rarely the source of diarrhea, and it is not necessary to stop the feeding until the cause is identified (35). Treatment of diarrhea is contingent on the etiology. Antimotility agents (e.g., lomotil, immodium, paregoric, deoderized tincture of opium) can be used in the treatment of diarrhea provided stool cultures are negative for an infectious etiology (54).

High gastric residuals from delayed emptying can result from high-fat and high-fiber formulas, rapid infusion rate, high osmolality formulas, disease state (diabetic gastroparesis), elevated intracranial pressure, sepsis, and medications including narcotics. As previously discussed, checking feeding residuals is an essential component of the monitoring process. If patients have persistently high residuals, giving prokinetic drugs or placing the feeding tube in the small bowel should help alleviate the problem. When checking for residuals during small bowel feedings, essentially there should be no residuals obtained. If residuals are obtained, then chances are the feeding tube has relocated to the stomach and verification of tube placement is warranted.

Constipation can result from low fiber or residue formulas, inadequate water or fluid intake, inactivity, decreased bowel motility, and medications such as phosphate binders, narcotics, and calcium-channel antagonists. Neuromuscular blocking agents do not paralyze gut smooth muscle but may slow bowel motility via anticholinergic actions (54). Adequate hydration, fiber-enriched formulas, stool softeners, and bowel motility agents are helpful in improving constipation (54). Monitoring the stool pattern of the patient is also important for prevention of fecal impaction.

Metabolic complications that occur during enteral nutrition therapy are similar to those developed during parenteral nutrition but are generally less severe (57). The metabolic disturbances most frequently seen include hyperglycemia, dehydration, and electrolyte imbalances, such as hyper-hypophosphatemia, hyper-hyponatremia, hyper-hypokalemia. Hyperglycemia is common in patients who are diabetic, have poor glucose utilization owing to insulin resistance from stress (e.g., trauma, sepsis), or are on diabetogenic medications such as corticosteroids (57). Urine and blood glucose should be monitored at periodic intervals in all pa-

tients who receive enteral feeding. For optimal nutrient substrate utilization blood glucose levels should be less than or equal to 200 mg/dL. Insulin administration is required in patients with persistently elevated blood glucose levels. Subcutaneous administration of insulin is poorly absorbed in critically ill patients with circulatory problems; therefore, an insulin infusion is required for the treatment of hyperglycemia.

Repleting malnourished patients can result in the intracellular uptake of phosphorous, potassium, and magnesium as anabolism is stimulated, causing decreased serum levels of these electrolytes (54). These electrolytes should be closely monitored for refeeding shifts, and replaced as needed. Thiamine supplementation is also needed in the malnourished patient (54). For a comprehensive list of the complications associated with enteral nutrition therapy, along with prevention and treatment strategies, the reader is referred elsewhere (58).

Parenteral Nutrition

Parenteral nutrition is the intravenous administration of a hypertonic solution of carbohydrate, fat, protein, electrolytes, vitamins, minerals, and fluid. Although enteral nutrition support is the preferred modality of nutritional therapy, PN is an important technique for nutrient provision in patients who have absolute gut failure, such as short bowel syndrome, small bowel obstruction, and fistulas not amenable to enteral feeding. In addition, PN should be initiated in any critically ill patient not tolerating full enteral nutrition support within 5 to 7 days. Guidelines for indications and appropriateness of use for PN have been established by the American Society for Parenteral and Enteral Nutrition (59).

The administration of parenteral nutrition is dependent on the osmolarity of the nutrient solution, anticipated duration of therapy, nutrient requirements, and the need for fluid restriction. The dextrose concentration, however, is the limiting factor for the route of venous access. A central line is necessary when infusing dextrose concentrations greater than 10%, whereas parenteral nutrition solutions with dextrose concentrations less than 10% can be administered peripherally. Because of the large fluid load generally needed to adequately meet a patient's nutrient goals, peripheral parenteral nutrition (PPN) is not usually feasible in the critical care setting.

Formula Composition

Carbohydrate is the primary energy source in a parenteral nutrition solution. Dextrose monohydrate is the carbohydrate source yielding 3.4 calories per gram, and ranging in concentration from 5% to 70%. The most frequently used dextrose concentrations for critically ill patients are 20% and 25%. The quantity of carbohydrate, however, is based on the patient's caloric requirement, optimal fuel balance, and glucose oxidation rate (i.e., hepatic oxidative capacity).

Administration of no greater than 4 to 6 mg dextrose/kg per min per 24-hour period is recommended for optimal oxidation and prevention of fat synthesis (lipogenesis). Excessive carbohydrate provision is also associated with hepatic dysfunction and increased carbon dioxide production.

Crystalline amino acids are the form in which protein is currently added to the PN admixture, and are classified as either standard or modified preparations (60). The standard amino acid solutions contain a balance of nonessential and essential amino acids tailored to the normal serum amino acid profile. Concentrations range from 3% to 15% and are 4.0 calories per gram.

The modified amino acid formulas contain a blend of amino acids designed to meet disease- or age-specific requirements (60). Standard amino acid solutions are glutamine free. Recent studies have shown that glutamine-enriched parenteral nutrition solutions sustain better gut mass than parenteral nutrition alone; however, parenteral nutrition preparations with glutamine stimulate the gut less effectively than do enteral formulations. In the future, the use of intravenous dipeptides as the nitrogen source in parenteral nutrition solutions may increase. Preliminary data have indicated that these agents have the same capacity to spare nitrogen and support serum protein synthesis as free amino acids in catabolic patients. Additionally, the dipeptides have the advantage of being more soluble and stable in aqueous solutions than amino acids (61). Further studies are required, however, before recommending their use in the clinical setting.

Intravenous fat is an aqueous dispersion containing soybean or safflower oil, egg yolk phospholipid (an emulsifier), and glycerin to achieve isotonicity. Long-chain fatty acid emulsions are currently the only commercially available IV fat. They are available as either 10%, 20%, or 30% emulsions. Maintenance essential fatty acids (EFA) requirements can be met by providing 4% to 10% of the total calories as fat (2% to 4% as linoleic acid). The 10% lipid emulsion provides 1.1 kcal/mL; 20% provides 2.0 kcal/mL; 30% provides 3.0 kcal/mL. IV fat is contraindicated in patients with the following: disturbances in normal fat metabolism (i.e., pathologic hyperlipidemia, triglyceride levels at upper limit of normal laboratory values greater than or equal to 400 to 500 mg/dL), lipid nephrosis when accompanied by hyperlipidemia, and severe egg allergy because egg yolk phospholipids are used in emulsification. Intravenous fat infusions in patients with pancreatitis of etiologies other than hypertriglyceridemia are not contraindicated. The recommended infusion rate varies depending on the lipid concentrations. For the 10% emulsion, a minimum of 8 hours and a minimum of 12 hours for the 20% emulsion is suggested. Propofol is in 10% intravenous fat providing 1.1 kcal/mL. Attention must be given to those patients who are on TPN with lipids and on propofol. Because of the dose of propofol that is being administered, occasionally intravenous fat needs to be discontinued to avoid the excessive provision of fat or total calories. Propofol infusion can be associated with hypertriglyceridemia, so serum triglycerides need to be closely monitored.

Electrolyte requirements in patients receiving parenteral nutrition are patient-specific and influenced by nutritional status. Organ function, acid-base balance, medications, and gastrointestinal losses will also influence the electrolyte adjustments that are needed in the PN solution to maintain electrolyte homeostasis (60). In stable patients, acid-base balance can, for the most part, be maintained by adding equal amounts of chloride and acetate (i.e., 1:1 ratio). However, in patients with acid-base disturbances, the acetate, which is metabolized to bicarbonate, and the chloride need to be adjusted in an effort to help correct the abnormality. For example, in patients with a significant metabolic alkalosis, the acetate should be minimized and the chloride maximized. Alternately, in patients with severe metabolic acidosis, the chloride should be minimized and the acetate maximized. Vitamins and trace elements are added to PN solutions in doses consistent with the American Medical Association Nutrition Advisory Group's recommendations (Table 20.10) (60). Adult multivitamin preparations do not contain vitamin K; therefore, supplementation is necessary on a weekly basis (10 mg vitamin K can be administered by IV infusion in the PN solution, subcutaneously, or intramuscularly). Iron is absent in the multitrace element preparation owing to the fear of anaphylaxis, but iron can be given as iron dextran either in the PN formula or intramuscularly. Copper and manganese are excreted via biliary excretion. Requirements for both are diminished with cholestatic liver failure to avoid potential toxicities from the hepatic deposition and elevated CNS levels of these trace elements. Consequently, supplementation of copper and manganese should be discontinued if baseline total bilirubin is three times the upper limit of normal or if total bilirubin triples from baseline value. This can be achieved by deleting the multitrace

TABLE 20.10. SUGGESTED VITAMIN AND MINERAL INTAKE FOR PARENTERAL NUTRITION

Vitamin A	3300 IU
Vitamin D	200 IU
Vitamin E	100 mg
Folic acid	400 mcg
Niacin	40 mg
Riboflavin	3.6 mg
Thiamine	3.0 mg
Pyridoxine (Vitamin B$_6$)	4.0 mg
Vitamin B$_{12}$	5.0 mcg
Pantothenic acid	15.0 mg
Biotin	60 mcg
Zinc	2.5–4.0 mg
Copper	0.5–1.5 mg
Chromium	10.0–15.0 mcg
Manganese	0.15–0.8 mg

elements from the PN solution and separately adding back zinc, chromium, and selenium.

Initiation and Advancement

Parenteral nutrition therapy should be initiated at a slow rate (e.g., 30 to 40 mL/hour), using the final concentration planned for therapy and advanced as glucose tolerance permits until the nutrient needs of a patient are met. In critically ill patients, advancement of parenteral nutrition should be conservative (e.g., increased 20 mL every 24 hours until the goal rate is attained). The slow advancement in rate helps with metabolic tolerance in the setting of metabolic disturbances such as hyperglycemia and hypertriglyceridemia. Because dextrose concentration is limited with peripheral parenteral nutrition (5% or 10% dextrose), it may be initiated at the same rate as peripheral IV fluids.

Monitoring

Monitoring guidelines for PN are essential for the successful administration and tolerance of parenteral nutrition support. Blood glucose monitoring via finger sticks every 4 to 6 hours (more frequently in the ICU) is indicated until the infusion rate has stabilized. Serum glucose should be maintained under 200 mg/dL for optimal nutrient substrate utilization. Serum triglycerides should be checked approximately 6 hours after the completion of the intravenous fat infusion to assess the patient's lipid clearing capacity, especially in the face of hyperglycemia and steroid therapy. Serum triglyceride levels should be less than or equal to 500 mg/dL. Monitoring electrolytes to assure adequate hydration, renal function, and need for supplementation or restriction is mandatory. Finally, liver function should be .periodically monitored to detect hepatic dysfunction related to parenteral nutrition therapy.

Complications

There are several complications that may occur when using parenteral nutrition support, including mechanical, metabolic, infectious, and hepatic complications. Pneumothorax is the most common mechanical complication associated with parenteral nutrition. Others include thrombus, catheter occlusion, and air embolus. The infectious complications seen with parenteral nutrition are typically catheter related. Of the metabolic complications, hyperglycemia is the most prevalent. Risk factors for hyperglycemia include metabolic stress, medications, obesity, diabetes, and excess calories or carbohydrates (62). Insulin administration may be warranted to lower blood glucose levels, especially in the critically ill patient. Malnourished patients are prone to refeeding shifts (as discussed in the enteral section of this chapter) with parenteral nutrition therapy. For an extensive list of the metabolic complications of parenteral nutrition and suggestions for prevention and treatment, the reader is referred to a major text on parenteral nutrition (63).

Hepatobiliary abnormalities have been identified in pa-tients on total parenteral nutrition who have no underlying liver disease. Elevated transaminases, alkaline phosphatase, and bilirubin concentrations may occur days to weeks after initiation of parenteral nutrition (62). Enzyme levels may return to normal while a patient is on parenteral nutrition, but almost always normalize when parenteral nutrition is discontinued (62). Steatosis (fatty liver) is the most frequent hepatic derangement that occurs with PN. High glucose infusions, exceeding 4 to 6 mg dextrose/kg per min, is the primary etiologic agent in the production of fatty liver (64). The excessive provision of intravenous fat can also result in fatty infiltration of the liver. Other proposed etiologies of steatosis are toxins and specific nutritional deficiencies, such as carnitine, essential fatty acids, and protein malnutrition, which cause decreased apoprotein synthesis resulting in impaired hepatic triglyceride transport (64,65).

The possible causes of cholestasis include lack of enteral stimulation, bacterial sepsis, endogenous recycling of lithocholic acid, and molybdenum deficiency (64–66). Gallbladder stasis (biliary sludging) is felt to be the primary cause of parenteral nutrition-associated biliary disease. Stimulating gallbladder contractility with enteral feedings usually reverses this process. Several recommendations exist for the management and prevention of parenteral nutrition-induced hepatic dysfunction, including use of the GI tract whenever possible, avoidance of overfeeding, provision of a well-balanced fuel mix, cycling of the parenteral nutrition regimen, consideration of carnitine and glutamine supplementation, and work-up of alternative causes such as hepatitis, biliary, obstruction, hepatotoxic drugs, and sepsis (65).

Conclusions

Nutrition is of vital importance in maintaining nutritional status during a period of critical illness. Appropriate delivery of nutrition support in critical illness is contingent on a thorough understanding of the metabolic response to stress and injury. Stress metabolism, driven by the counterregulatory hormones, is characterized by increased energy expenditure and profound protein catabolism that results in rapid deterioration of nutritional status. The loss of body protein can lead to delayed wound healing and tissue repair, immunosuppression, and loss of muscle strength (an effect that can impede weaning from mechanical ventilation). Because many of the routine nutritional assessment parameters are invalid with critical illness, assessment of nutritional status is difficult. The accurate determination of energy and protein requirements is paramount in delivering proper nutrition support. Measurement of energy expenditure using indirect calorimetry and nitrogen balance studies is recommended in some patients because it can guide nutrition and metabolic management of critically ill patients.

Enteral nutrition therapy is the preferred modality of nutrition support because of the significant benefits on the gastrointestinal tract, particularly during a period of critical illness or injury. Alimentation via the enteral route preserves gut barrier integrity, physiologic function, and cell mass, and prevents bacterial translocation. Initiation of early postoperative or early-injury feeding can maintain intestinal mass and barrier function, decrease infection rates, improve immune function and wound healing, blunt the hypermetabolic response to stress, and perhaps improve patient outcome. Although enteral nourishment is the optimal route of nutrient administration, at times it is not medically feasible or well tolerated. Under these circumstances total parenteral nutrition is indicated; however, every effort should be made to switch to enteral feeding in critically ill patients when possible.

ETHICAL PRINCIPLES

Medical ethics is a set of moral principles that govern the behavior of physicians and other health professionals. As discussed by Beauchamp and Childress, one principle of medical ethics is autonomy: respect for the patient's capacity of self-determination and exercise of personal, informed choice (67). Another is nonmaleficence: the obligation not to harm intentionally. A third principle is beneficence: the provision of benefit, which generally is defined as something that promotes well-being. A fourth is distributive justice: the fair, equitable, and appropriate distribution of medical resources in society.

The first three ethical principles outlined in the preceding paragraph are the foundation of the fiduciary relationship that characterizes the practice of medicine. Under the unwritten terms of this relationship, physicians are expected to serve the best interests of their patients, particularly as the patients define these interests (68,69). The fiduciary relationship is based on trust: Patients, who are relatively helpless because of their underlying illnesses and limited familiarity with various treatments, rely on physicians, who are relatively powerful because of their concurrent health and superior knowledge of medicine, to care for them.

Medical Decision-Making

Some previously competent patients remain so throughout a critical illness; and therefore, they can participate in medical decisions. However, when patients are incompetent to begin with or are unable to communicate because they are comatose or sedated, their surrogates may become involved in the decision-making process. The proper role for surrogates is to represent patients' interests and previously expressed wishes; surrogates are less helpful in decision-making when they represent their own interests or speak only from their own points of view. When family members disagree among themselves about patients' interests and wishes, they should be asked to designate spokespersons who can represent the group if such spokespersons have not already been selected

by the patients. Physicians who work with surrogates of this sort can reach decisions more rapidly than with entire families.

Ideal surrogates are those who have been designated by patients before or during their critical illness to make medical decisions in the event of incapacity. In California and some other states, such surrogates may be granted what is called a "durable power of attorney" for health care (70). Proxy directives of this sort are legally binding so long as patient interests are being protected. They are more helpful than living wills and other instructional directives, most of which are either too broadly or too narrowly drawn (71).

When surrogates are not available, critical care physicians must rely on other sources of information in determining their patients' wishes. Among these sources are the patients' primary physicians, if they have already discussed issues such as resuscitation with the patients. These physicians should be called on to articulate their patients' wishes even if they are not supervising their care in the ICU. Critical care nurses frequently have explored these issues with patients at the bedside while the patients were lucid, and they too should be consulted. So, should clergy members who either knew the patients before hospitalization or have come to know them in the hospital.

When surrogates are not available and other sources of information are inadequate, physicians have two options. One is to ask the courts to appoint conservators to help preserve the autonomy of their patients. This approach is cumbersome and time-consuming, and conservators usually prefer that physicians make medical decisions anyway. Alternatively, and especially when urgent decisions must be made, physicians may decide what is in their patients' best interests and use beneficence to justify this strategy.

Although decisions based on what physicians consider their patients' best interests may be ethically acceptable, it must be stressed that the principles of beneficence—or medical paternalism, as some would have it—and autonomy frequently conflict in the ICU. This seems inevitable, given the realities of critical care practice, but physicians still should remind themselves of the great personal authority they exercise. Whenever appropriate, they should review their decisions either with colleagues or with members of biomedical ethics committees (72,73).

Informed Consent

The ethical principle of autonomy is contained in the concept of informed consent. This may be defined as the voluntary acceptance of physician recommendations by competent patients or surrogates who have been provided with sufficient truthful information regarding risks, benefits, and alternatives and who adequately indicate their comprehension of this information (67). Consent may be implied rather than informed in emergency situations wherein physicians are obligated to provide medically necessary treatment when patients or surrogates have not expressed their wishes or cannot do so (74). The rationale for treatment in such situations is that patients or surrogates would consent if they could and that harm would result from delaying care.

Informed consent is called for especially when patients are given innovative treatments or are recruited for research. Physicians frequently are tempted to try new therapies in critically ill patients either on a one-time basis or as part of ongoing trials. This is ethically supportable only after consent has been obtained from patients or surrogates or, when consent cannot be obtained, when the treatments are known to be safe and of great potential value. In keeping with the fiduciary relationship, physician obligation is to present-day patients; such patients should not be experimented on solely because future patients might benefit from what has happened to them.

Foregoing Life-Sustaining Therapy

Although the fiduciary relationship remains vital to medical practice in the ICU, interpretation of the phrase "best interests of their patients" on the part of physicians has changed over time. Intensive care units proliferated in the United States and other developed countries during and after the 1950s alongside the advances in scientific knowledge, improvements in artificial ventilation, the introduction of cardiac monitoring, and the need for prolonged support following complex surgeries. For most of their history, ICUs have reported death rates of from 10% to 20%, depending on the types of patients treated therein (75,76). Furthermore, until recently, most of the patients who have died in the ICU did so despite full life support, including attempted cardiopulmonary resuscitation (CPR). The wishes of patients and their surrogates regarding support have rarely been solicited, in our experience, and do-not-resuscitate (DNR) orders have seldom been used to limit treatment. This practice has been consonant with the belief, held by health professionals and the public alike, that the ICU and its technologies have the obligation to preserve life whenever possible regardless of the human and economic costs.

In recent years, however, the obligation of the ICU has been challenged, just as its expenses have been scrutinized. For example, clinical research has revealed that many patients, including those with severe respiratory failure and such underlying conditions as advanced hematological malignancies, rarely leave the ICU alive or do so only after prolonged pain and suffering (77). Furthermore, these and other survivors of critical illness frequently die shortly after being transferred out of the ICU, thereby minimizing its apparent benefits (78). As the clinical limitations of intensive care have become recognized, physicians and hospital administrators have questioned whether the economic resources used to finance ICUs should be used for other, more beneficial medical purposes, especially in our era of capitation and managed care. And although patients and their surrogates seldom pay the ICU bill directly, they nevertheless have come to question the value of intensive care in all instances and to seek ways to refuse it if they so desire.

The right of patients and their surrogates to refuse treatment and have it withdrawn, over the objections of physicians and hospitals if necessary, was first legally affirmed on a state level in the cases of Karen Ann Quinlan in 1976 and Joseph Barber in 1983. In the case of Nancy Cruzan in 1990, the US Supreme Court reaffirmed this right on the part of patients who can participate in medical decisions but allowed states to require evidence of patients' wishes regarding life support if the patients are incapable of decision-making. The federal Patient Self-Determination Act of 1991 was passed to encourage the expression of patients' wishes by requiring that health care facilities ask admitted patients if they have advance directives and help them prepare such directives if they do not (79).

Although the Patient Self-Determination Act and the legal cases that preceded it support patient and surrogate autonomy, more recent cases have involved physicians and hospitals that seek to restrain autonomy. For example, in the case of Helen Wanglie in 1991, the Hennepin County Medical Center asked a district court to replace a surrogate because he insisted on continued mechanical ventilation for his wife, a therapy Mrs. Wanglie's physicians considered not beneficial because it would not heal her lungs or end her unconsciousness. Similarly, in the case of Catherine Gilgunn, the Massachusetts General Hospital and several of its physicians were sued for writing a DNR order for and removing mechanical ventilation from Mrs. Gilgunn over the objections of her daughter. In 1995, a Suffolk County Superior Court jury absolved the physicians and hospital of liability, apparently because they believed that further treatment was futile despite the possibility that Mrs. Gilgunn might have wanted to be kept alive (79).

In parallel with these legal cases from *Quinlan* to *Gilgunn*, presidential commissions, individual authors, institutional ethics committees, and professional societies have supported patient and surrogate autonomy while also spelling out circumstances in which futile care should be foregone (80–85). At the same time, the advent of medical cost-consciousness related to managed care has restrained the application of therapies that merely prolong death with little hope of long-term cure (86). The legal, ethical, and economic consensus that has resulted from these developments has in turn reinforced a trend toward the limitation of ineffective treatments that is currently reflected in the changing nature of death in the ICU. Whereas critically ill patients previously died despite full support and attempted CPR, such patients are more likely to die today during the withholding and withdrawal of life support with DNR orders in place. Thus, physicians with the implicit or explicit approval of the hospitals in which they practice, increasingly have become involved in managing death in the ICU, just as they manage cardiovascular decompensation and respiratory failure.

How Deaths Are Managed

The first major observational study of how critically ill patients die was conducted over the academic year 1987–1988 in two medical-surgical ICUs at hospitals affiliated with the University of California, San Francisco (UCSF) (87). During the 1-year period, 224 (13%) of the 1,719 patients admitted to the ICUs died. Of the 224 patients who died, 114 (51%) did so after a decision had been made to limit treatment; 22 patients had life support, including CPR, withheld, and 92 had life support withdrawn. Of the 114 patients who were not supported, 89 died in the ICU, and 15 died after they were transferred to other areas of the hospitals with the provision that they would not be readmitted to the ICU if they decompensated. None of the 114 patients received attempted CPR, and DNR orders were written for 109 of them.

Over the academic year 1992–1993, 5 years after the first study, a similar investigation was conducted in the same medical-surgical ICUs affiliated with UCSF (88). During this second period, 200 (13%) of the 1,711 patients admitted to the ICUs died, the same proportion as previously. A decision was made to withhold or withdraw life support from 179 (90%) of the 200 patients who died, compared with 51% in the first study. Life support was withheld from 27 of the 179 patients and withdrawn from 140 of them in the second study; 12 patients had CPR only withheld. Of the 179 patients, 162 died in the ICU and 17 died after transfer. None of the 179 patients received attempted CPR, and most had DNR orders.

To determine the generalizability of these observations, the directors of all American postgraduate training programs in critical care medicine were contacted and asked to categorize prospectively all patients who died in their ICUs over a 6-month period in 1994 and 1995 into one of five mutually exclusive categories. The national survey of end-of-life care that resulted from this effort involved 131 ICUs from 110 institutions in 38 states (89). A total of 74,502 patients were admitted to these ICUs during the 6-month study period, 6,303 of whom died (9% mortality in the units). Of the 6,303 patients who died, 1,544 (20%) did so despite full ICU support including attempted CPR, 1,430 (24%) did so after receiving full support but not attempted CPR, 794 (14%) had life support withheld, 2,139 (36%) had life support withdrawn, and 393 (6%) were brain dead. Thus, of the 5,910 patients who died in the ICU and were not brain dead, 4,366 (74%) received less than full support. This percentage probably would have been higher had patients who died shortly after being transferred out of the ICU with no provision for readmission been included.

One striking finding of the national survey was the wide variation in end-of-life care: The range of proportions of

death preceded by failed CPR, DNR status, and withholding or withdrawal of life support was 4% to 79%, 0% to 83%, 0% to 67%, and 0% to 79%, respectively. This variation could not be explained by the types of ICUs (medical, surgical, medical-surgical, neurosciences, and other), hospital types (university, community, public, veterans, and other), or the geographic regions of the hospitals. However, a pattern was observed in the two states with strict legal standards for care limitation by surrogates. Thus, ICUs in New York and Missouri had lower proportions of deaths preceded by withdrawal of support than did the entire mid-Atlantic and Midwest regions in which these states are located.

Although the national survey did not demonstrate changes in ICU deaths over time, it did suggest that limits to life support have become so commonplace in the United States as to represent a *de facto* standard of end-of-life care for critically ill patients. This suggestion is reinforced by other studies that document changes in terminal care management at other institutions (90–95). Nevertheless, the extreme variation in the categories of ICU death in all these studies underscores the absence of a true consensual approach to end-of-life care. A first step in creating consensus would be for all hospitals to track their own end-of-life practices. A second would be for critical care specialists to develop guidelines for limiting treatment, as is presently being done.

Future Management of Death

It is likely that critical care specialists will care for most, if not all ICU patients in the future. Kollef and Kollef and Ward have reported that intensivists are more likely to limit treatment when appropriate, and other studies have demonstrated that "closed" units in which such specialists direct care are associated with better risk-adjusted mortality, shorter length of stay, and more appropriate use of resources (96–98). Given that death has been and remains commonplace in ICUs (the mortality rate was 9% in the national end-of-life care study), the specialists who will care for critically ill patients in the future must become specialists in the management of death in the ICU if they have not already become proficient in this area.

To help manage death, intensivists must learn how death is managed in ICUs and whether it is managed well. The Study to Understand Prognoses and Preferences for Outcomes and Risks of Treatment (SUPPORT) suggested that physicians do not communicate adequately with patients and surrogates and that patients suffer greatly as they die, at least in the ICUs studied (99). Further research is needed to determine whether the SUPPORT findings are generalizable and, if they are not, what measures are useful in improving the quality of death. From such research should come practice guidelines to accompany current recommendations regarding compassionate care (100). In fact, one recent article provides excellent guidelines for the pharmacologic and clinical management of withdrawal of life support in critically ill patients (101).

In addition to research, critical care specialists require clinical training in death management. In particular, better education in how to prognosticate for ICU patients and how to access and use the large data sets that increasingly make prognostication a scientific process are called for. Training also is needed in communication and conflict resolution, skills that commonly are called for with our patients and their surrogates. Finally, a curriculum in death management for intensivists that befits the changing nature of death in the ICU should be developed.

REFERENCES

1. Goldstein SA, Elwyn DH. The effects of injury and sepsis on fuel utilization. *Annu Rev Nutr* 1989;9:445–473.
2. Bessey PQ, Watters J, Aoki TT, et al. Combined hormone infusion stimulates the metabolic response to injury. *Ann Surg* 1984;200:264–281.
3. Cahill GF Jr. Starvation in man. *N Engl J Med* 1970;282:668–675.
4. Woolfson AMJ, Heatly RV, Allison SP. Insulin to inhibit protein catabolism after injury. *N Engl J Med* 1979;300:14–17.
5. Wolfe RR, Herndon DN, Jahoor F, et al. Effect of severe burn injury on substrate cycling by glucose and fatty acids. *N Engl J Med* 1987;317:403–408.
6. Clowes GHA, Randall HT, Cha JC. Amino acid and energy metabolism in septic and traumatized patients. *JPEN* 1980;4:195–205.
7. Jeevanadam M, Grote-Holman AE, Chikenji T, et al. Effects of glucose on fuel utilization and turnover in normal and injured man. *Crit Care Med* 1990;18:125–135.
8. Long CL, Kinney JM, Geiger JW. Nonsuppressibility of gluconeogenesis by glucose in septic patients. *Metabolism* 1976;25:193–201.
9. Burke JF, Wolfe RR, Mullany CJ, et al. Glucose requirements following burn injury: parameters of optimal glucose infusion and possible hepatic and respiratory abnormalities following excessive glucose intake. *Ann Surg* 1979;190:274–285.
10. Vary TC, Siegel JH, Nakatani T, et al. Regulation of glucose metabolism by altered pyruvate dehydrogenase activity in sepsis. *JPEN* 1986;10:351–355.
11. Nordenstrom J, Carpentier YA, Askanazi IE, et al. Free fatty acid mobilization and oxidation during total parenteral nutrition in trauma and infection. *Ann Surg* 1983;198:725–735.
12. Birkhahn RH, Long CL, Fitkin DL, et al. A comparison of the effects of skeletal trauma and surgery on ketosis of starvation in man. *J Trauma* 1981;21:513–518.
13. Elwyn DH, Gump FE, Iles M, et al. Protein and energy sparing of glucose added in hypocaloric amounts to peripheral infusions of amino acids. *Metabolism* 1978;27:325–331.
14. Yamazaki K, Maiz A, Sobrado J, et al. Hypocaloric lipid emulsions and amino acid metabolism in injured rats. *JPEN* 1984;8:360–366.
15. Shaw JHF, Wildbore M, Wolfe RR. An integrated analysis of glucose, fat, and protein metabolism in severely traumatized patients: studies in the basal state and the response to total parenteral nutrition. *Ann Surg* 1987;209:66–72.
16. Baracos V, Rodemann HP, Dinarello, et al. Stimulation of mus-cle protein degradation and prostaglandin E$_2$ release by leukocyte pyrogen (interleukin-1). *N Engl J Med* 1983;308:553–558.
17. Mullen JL, Buzby, GP, Matthews DC, et al. Reduction of operative morbidity and mortality by combined pre-operative nutrition support. *Ann Surg* 1980;192:604–613.
18. Buzby GP, Mullen JL. Nutritional assessment. In Rombeau J, Caldwell MD, eds. *Clinical nutrition.* Philadelphia: Saunders, 1984:127–148.
19. Shronts EP, Fish JA, Pesce-Hammond K. Nutritional assessment. In Souba WW, Kohn-Keeth C, Mueller C, et al, eds. *The A.S.P.E.N nutrition support practice manual.* Silver Spring, MD: A.S.P.E.N., 1998.
20. A.S.P.E.N. Standards for nutrition support: hospitalized patients. *Nutr Clin Pract* 1995;10(6):208–218.
21. Ireton-Jones CS, Hasse JM. Comprehensive nutritional assessment: the dietitian's contribution to the team effort. *Nutrition* 1992;8(2):75–81.
22. Hopkins B. Assessment of nutritional status. In Gottshclich MM, Matarese LE, Shronts EP, eds. *Nutrition support dietetics core curriculum,* 2nd ed. Silver Spring, MD: A.S.P.E.N., 1993.
23. Lang CE, Shutte CV. Nutrition assessment: adult patient. In Lang CE, ed. *Nutrition support in critical care.* Rockville, MD: Aspen Publishers, 1982:61–91.
24. Grant A, DeHoog S, eds. Biochemical assessment. In *Nutritional Assessment and Support.* Seattle, WA: 1985:35–73.
25. Lipman TO. Nutritional assessment. *Curr Opin Gastroenterol* 1991;7:271–276.
26. Haider M, Sanbober HQ. Assessment of protein-calorie malnutrition. *Clin Chem* 1984;30(8):1286–1299.
27. Sax HC, Souba WW. Nutritional goals and macronutrient requirements. In Souba WW, Kohn-Keeth C, Mueller C, et al, eds. *The A.S.P.E.N. nutrition support practice manual.* Silver Spring, MD: A.S.P.E.N., 1998.
28. Ireton-Jones CS, Borman KR, Turner WW. Nutrition considerations in the management of ventilator-dependent patients. *Nutr Clin Pract* 1993;8:60–64.
29. Ireton-Jones CS, Jones JD. Should predictive equations or indirect calorimetry be used to design nutrition support regimens? Predictive equations should be used. *Nutr Clin Pract* 19(Suppl):228.
30. McClave SA, Snider HL. Use of indirect calorimetry in clinical nutrition. *Nutr Clin Pract* 1992;7:208–221.
31. Feurer I, Mullen JL. Bedside measurement of resting energy expenditure and respiratory quotient via indirect calorimetry. *Nutr Clin Pract* 1986;43–49.
32. Porter C, Cohen N. Indirect calorimetry in critically ill patients: role of the clinical dietitian in interpreting results. *J Am Diet Assoc* 1996;96:49–57.
33. Konstantinides FN. Nitrogen balance studies in clinical nutrition. *Nutr Clin Pract* 1992;7:231–238.
34. Barton RG. Nutrition support in critical illness. *Nutr Clin Pract* 1994;9:127–139.
35. Trujillo EB, Robinson MK, Jacobs DO. Critical illness. In Souba WW, Kohn-Keeth C, Mueller C, et al, eds. *The A.S.P.E.N. nutrition support practice manual.* Silver Spring, MD: A.S.P.E.N., 1998.
36. Spector N. Nutritional support of the ventilator-dependent patient. *Nursing Clin N Am* 1989;24(2):407–413.
37. Schwartz DB. Pulmonary failure. In Gottschlich MM, Matarese LE, Shronts EP, eds. *Nutrition support core curriculum.* 2nd ed. Silver Spring, MD: A.S.P.E.N., 1993.
38. Talpers SS, Romberger DJ, Bunce SB, et al. Nutritionally associated increased carbon dioxide production: excess total calories vs. high proportion of carbohydrate calories. *Chest* 1992;102:551–555.

39. Lord LM, Sax HC. The role of the gut in critical illness. *AACN Clin Issues* 1994;9(4):450–458.

40. Langkamp-Henken B, Glezer JA, Kudsk KA. Immunologic structure and function of the gastrointestinal tract. *Nutr Clin Pract* 1992;7:100–108.

41. Thompson JS. The intestinal response to critical illness. *Am J Gastroenterol* 1995;90(2):190–200.

42. Albanese CT, Smith SD, Watkins S, et al. Effect of secretory IgA on transepithelial passage of bacteria across the intact ileum in vitro. *J Am Coll Surg* 1994;179:679–688.

43. Stralovich A. Gastrointestinal and pancreatic disease. In Gottschlich MM, Matarese LE, Shronts EP, eds. *Nutrition support core curriculum.* 2nd ed. Silver Spring, MD: A.S.P.E.N., 1993.

44. Palacio JC, Rombeau JL. Dietary fiber: a brief review and potential application to enteral nutrition. *Nutr Clin Pract* 1990;5:99–106.

45. Rombeau JL, Kripke SA. Metabolic and intestinal effects of short-chain fatty acids. *JPEN* 1990;14(5)(Suppl):181S–185S.

46. Brinson RB, Hanumanthu SK, Pitts WM. A reappraisal of the peptide-based enteral formulas: clinical applications. *Nutr Clin Pract* 1989;4:211–217.

47. Zaloga GP. Physiological effects of peptide-based enteral formulas. *Nutr Clin Pract* 1990;5:231–237.

48. Bloss CS. Pharmacomodulation of the gut: implications for the enterally fed patient. *Nutr Clin Pract* 1998;13:201–214.

49. Schwartz DB. Enteral therapy. In Lang CE, ed. *Nutrition support in critcal care.* Rockville, MD: Aspen Publishers, 1982:93–111.

50. American Gastroenterological Association Patient Care Committee. American Gastroenterological Association technical review on tube feeding for enteral nutrition. *Gastroenterol* 1995;108(4):1282–1301.

51. DeLegge MH, Rhodes BM. Continuous versus intermittent feedings: slow and steady or fast and furious? *Support Line* 1998;20(5):11–15.

52. Olree K, Vitello J, Sullivan J, et al. Enteral Formulations. In Souba WW, Kohn-Keeth C, Mueller C, et al, eds. *The A.S.P.E.N. nutrition support practice manual.* Silver Spring, MD: A.S.P.E.N., 1998.

53. Evans MA, Shronts EP. Intestinal fuels: glutamine, short-chain fatty acids, and dietary fiber. *J Am Diet Assoc* 1992;92:1239–1246, 1249.

54. Lord L, Trumbore L, Zaloga G. Enteral nutrition implementation and management. In Souba WW, Kohn-Keeth C, Mueller C, et al, eds. *The A.S.P.E.N. nutrition support practice manual.* Silver Spring, MD: A.S.P.E.N., 1998.

55. Breach CL, Saldanha LG. Tube feeding complications. Part II: mechanical. *Nutr Support Serv* 1088;8(5):28–32.

56. Breach CL, Saldanha LG. Tube feeding complications. Part I: gastrointestinal. *Nutr Support Serv* 1988;8(30):15–19.

57. Breach CL, Saldanha LG. Tube feeding complications. Part III: metabolic. *Nutr Support Serv* 1988;8(6):16–19.

58. Ideno KT. Enteral nutrition. In Gottschlich MM, Matarese LE, Shronts EP, eds. *Nutrition support dietetics core curriculum.* 2nd ed. Silver Spring, MD: A.S.P.E.N., 1993.

59. A.S.P.E.N. Board of Directors. Guidelines for the use of parenteral and enteral nutrition in adult and pediatric patients. *JPEN* 1993;17(Suppl):1SA–52SA.

60. Strausberg KM. Parenteral nutrition admixture. In Souba WW, Kohn-Keeth C, Mueller C, et al, eds. *The A.S.P.E.N. nutrition support practice manual.* Silver Spring, MD: A.S.P.E.N., 1998.

61. Vazquez JA, Hannelore D, Adibi SA. Dipeptides in parenteral nutrition: from basic science to clinial applications. *Nutr Clin Pract* 1993;8:95–105.

62. Skipper A, Millikan KW. Parenteral nutrition implementation and management. In Souba WW, Kohn-Keeth C, Mueller C, et al, eds. *The A.S.P.E.N nutrition support practice manual.* Silver Spring, MD: A.S.P.E.N., 1998.

63. Rombeau JL, Rolandelli RR, eds. *Parenteral nutrition.* Philadelphia: Saunders, 1998.

64. Fisher RL. Hepatobiliary abnormalities associated with total parenteral nutrition. *Gastroenterol Clin N Am* 1989;18(3):645–661.

65. Sax HC, Bower RH. Hepatic complications of total parenteral nutrition. *JPEN* 1988;12(6):615–618.

66. Freund HR. Abnormalities of liver function and hepatic damage associated with total parenteral nutrition. *Nutrition* 1991;7(1):1–5.

67. Beauchamp TL, Childress JF. *Principles of biomedical ethics,* 4th ed. New York: Oxford University Press, 1994.

68. Luce JM. Ethical principles in critical care. *JAMA* 1990;213:696–700.

69. Luce JM. Conflicts over ethical principles in the intensive care unit. *Crit Care Med* 1992;20:313–315.

70. Steinbrook R, Lo B. Decision making for incompetent patients by designated proxy. *N Engl J Med* 1984;310:1598–1601.

71. Raffin TA. Value of the living will. *Chest* 1986;90:444–446.

72. Rosner F. Hospital medical ethics committee. a review of their development. *JAMA* 1985;255:2693–3697.

73. Brennan TA. Ethics committees and decisions to limit care in the experience at the Massachusetts General Hospital. *JAMA* 1988;260:803–807.

74. Lidz CW, Meisel A, Osterweis M, et al. Barriers to informed consent. *Ann Intern Med* 1983;99:539–543.

75. Thibault GE, Mulley AG, Barnett GO, et al. Medical intensive care: indications, interventions, and outcomes. *N Engl J Med* 1980;302:938–942.

76. Knaus WA, Draper EA, Wagner DP, et al. An evaluation of outcome from intensive care in major medical centers. *Ann Intern Med* 1986;104:410–418.

77. Rubenfeld GD, Crawford SW. Withdrawing life support from mechanically ventilated recipients of bone marrow transplants: a case for evidence-based guidelines. *Ann Intern Med* 1996;125:625–633.

78. Seneff MG, Wagner DP, Wagner RP, et al. Hospital and 1-year survival of patients admitted to intensive care units with acute exacerbation of chronic obstructive pulmonary disease. *JAMA* 1995;274:1852–1857.

79. Luce JM. Withholding and withdrawal of life support from critically ill patients. *West J Med* 1997;167:411–416.

80. President's Commission for the Study of Ethical Problems in Medicine and Biomedical and Behavioral Research. Deciding to forego life-sustaining treatment: a report on the ethical, medical, and legal issues in treatment decisions. Washington, DC: Government Printing Office, 1983.

81. Ruark JE, Raffin TA, Stanford University Medical Center Committee on Ethics. Initiating and withdrawing life support: principles and practice in adult medicine. *N Engl J Med* 1988;318:25–30.

82. Council on Ethical and Judicial Affairs, American Medical Association. Decisions near the end of life. *JAMA* 1992;267:2229–2233.

83. American Thoracic Society. Withholding and withdrawing life-sustaining therapy. *Am Rev Respir Dis* 1991;144:726–731.

84. Task Force on Ethics of the Society of Critical Care Medicine. Consensus report on the ethics of foregoing life-sustaining treatments in the critically ill. *Crit Care Med* 1990;18:1435–1439.

85. Council on Ethical and Judicial Affairs, American Medical Association. Medical futility in end-of-life care: report of the Council on Ethical and Judicial Affairs. *JAMA* 1999;281:937–941.

86. Cher DJ, Lenert LA. Method of Medicare reimbursement and

the rate of potentially ineffective care of critically ill patients. *JAMA* 1997;278:1001–1007.

87. Smedira NG, Evans BH, Grais LS, et al. Withholding and withdrawal of life support from the critically ill. *N Engl J Med* 1990; 322:309–315.

88. Prendergast TJ, Luce JM. Increasing incidence of withholding and withdrawal of life support from the critically ill. *Am J Respir Crit Care Med* 1997;155:15–20.

89. Prendergast TJ, Claessens MT, Luce JM. A national survey of end-of-life care for critically ill patients. *Am J Respir Crit Care Med* 1998;158:1163–1167.

90. Eidelman LA, Jakobson KJ, Pizov R, et al. Foregoing life-sustaining treatment in an Israeli ICU. *Int Care Med* 1998;24: 162–166.

91. Keenan SP, Busche KD, Chen LM, et al. A retrospective review of a large cohort of patients undergoing the process of withholding and withdrawal of life support. *Crit Care Med* 1997;25: 1324–1331.

92. Turner JS, Michell WL, Morgan CJ, et al. Limitation of life support: frequency and practice in a London and a Cape Town intensive care unit. *Int Care Med* 1996;22:1020–1025.

93. Koch KA, Rodeffer HD, Wears RL. Changing patterns of terminal care management in an intensive care unit. *Crit Care Med* 1994;22:233–243.

94. Vernon DD, Dean JM, Timmons OD, et al. Modes of death in the pediatric intensive care unit: withdrawal and limitation of supportive care. *Crit Care Med* 1993;21:1798–1802.

95. Vincent JL, Parquier JN, Preiser JC, et al. Terminal events in the intensive care unit: review of 258 fatal cases in one year. *Crit Care Med* 1989;17:530–533.

96. Kollef MH. Private attending physician status and the withdrawal of life-sustaining interventions in a medical intensive care unit population. *Crit Care Med* 1996;24:968–975.

97. Kollef MH, Ward S. The influence of access to a private attending physician on the withdrawal of life-sustaining therapies in the intensive care unit. *Crit Care Med* 1999;27:2125–2132.

98. Carson SS, Stocking C, Podsadecki T, et al. Effects of organizational change in the medical intensive care unit of a teaching hospital: a comparison of 'open' and 'closed' formats. *JAMA* 1996;276:322–328.

99. Desbiens NA, Wu AW, Broste SK, et al. Pain and satisfaction with pain control in seriously ill hospitalized adults: findings from the SUPPORT research investigations. *Crit Care Med* 1996;24:1953–1961.

100. Brody H, Campbell ML, Faber-Langendoen K, et al. Withdrawing intensive life-sustaining treatment—recommendations for compassionate clinical management. *N Engl J Med* 1997;336: 652–657.

101. Truog RD, Burns JP, Mitchelle, et al. Pharmacologic paralysis and withdrawal of mechanical ventilation in the intensive care unit. N Engl J Med 2000;342:508–512.

GENERAL PRINCIPLES OF MANAGING THE PATIENT WITH RESPIRATORY FAILURE

JAMES A. FRANK
DAVID SCHWARTZ
BRIAN M. DANIEL
ROBERT M. JASMER
MICHAEL A. MATTHAY

ASSESSMENT OF SEVERE RESPIRATORY DYSFUNCTION
Clinical Evaluation
General Laboratory Evaluation
Arterial Blood Gases
Acid-Base Abnormalities
Measurement of Lung Function
Calculation of Respiratory Variables

TREATMENT MODALITIES
Supplemental Oxygen
Noninvasive Ventilation for Acute Respiratory Failure
Airway Management
Mechanical Ventilation
Weaning from Mechanical Ventilation
Emergencies in the Ventilated Patient

RESPIRATORY MONITORING

This chapter reviews the assessment of respiratory failure in severely ill patients and describes the major elements of supportive care and monitoring available in intensive care units.

ASSESSMENT OF SEVERE RESPIRATORY DYSFUNCTION

This section considers the clinical and laboratory evaluation of patients with acute respiratory failure.

Clinical Evaluation

The course of acute respiratory failure may evolve slowly over a period of days, or rapidly, in minutes to a few hours. The clinical manifestations and the ways in which they are perceived by the patient vary, depending on the nature of the process itself and on its course. In most instances, the symptomatic hallmark of acute respiratory failure is dyspnea. However, the presence of this symptom, as with any subjective manifestation of disease, requires that the patient be sufficiently alert to be aware of the sensation and be able to convey that awareness to observers. For example, patients who have taken overdoses of sedative-hypnotic drugs or narcotic agents, even if awake, may not be dyspneic in the presence of marked gas exchange abnormalities. Also, dyspnea tends to be more intense when it develops rapidly. When respiratory failure develops more slowly, dyspnea may appear at first only with exertion or with assumption of the supine position (orthopnea), but as the process becomes more severe the dyspnea becomes constant and may even be present at rest. Patients with chronic airways obstruction commonly have chronic dyspnea; in these patients, minor changes from the baseline level of dyspnea may represent a major worsening of gas exchange. Progressive hypoxemia, hypercarbia, or both may blunt the sensation of dyspnea and occasionally result in a misleading symptomatic assessment. In spite of its frequency as a symptom, dyspnea is poorly defined and difficult to quantify and correlates very poorly with the severity of respiratory failure (1). For these reasons, more objective assessments are important in evaluating dyspneic patients. Other symptoms such as cough, sputum production, and chest pain are important manifestations of processes that may be associated with respiratory failure but are less helpful than dyspnea as an indicator of respiratory dysfunction.

In addition to the symptoms that are frequently directly

associated with respiratory or cardiac disease, other, less specific, subjective manifestations may be important. Patients with progressive hypoxemia or hypercarbia may have alterations in mental function, including headache, visual disturbances, memory loss, confusion, insomnia, hallucinations, and even transient loss of consciousness.

The physical examination may also provide important information in patients with respiratory failure. Perhaps the most important evaluation rests on a general assessment of the severity of illness based on the patient's appearance, including the degree of apparent respiratory distress and the patient's mental status. Both of these assessments help guide the initial approach to management by indicating the degree of cooperation that can be anticipated. Cyanosis, especially central cyanosis, is helpful as an indication of hypoxemia but it may not be detectable. The respiratory rate, although influenced by a large number of factors, may serve as an indicator of the severity of respiratory distress, and measuring the respiratory rate also can be used as a monitoring technique to judge the response to therapy. As described for the symptom of dyspnea, however, tachypnea may not be present in patients whose ventilatory drive is blunted.

The degree of respiratory failure may also be estimated by noting the patient's ability to speak. Severely distressed patients are able to speak only a few words at a time. As the respiratory failure becomes less severe, longer phrases and sentences are possible. Stridorous breathing represents an important finding that suggests severe upper airway obstruction. An inability to phonate may be associated with marked obstruction at the larynx or above. Retraction of the sternum and supraclavicular, suprasternal, and intercostal spaces constitutes evidence of respiratory distress and increased resistance to lung inflation, generally caused by airways obstruction or an infiltrative process. These findings have been correlated with the severity of airways obstruction in patients with asthma and with pneumonia in children (2,3). The decrease in arterial systolic blood pressure that occurs with inspiration (pulsus paradoxus) also correlates with the severity of airways obstruction, especially in asthma (4). Changes in the magnitude of the pulsus paradoxus can also be used to evaluate the response to therapy.

Examination of the lungs does not provide sufficient information concerning the severity of respiratory dysfunction but may be helpful in determining the cause of respiratory failure. The findings associated with specific processes are discussed in Chapter 5, Chest Imaging, but several points are worth emphasizing. First, although wheezing is the characteristic feature of severe airways obstruction, the absence of wheezing may be an even more important finding. In patients with very severe airways obstruction, air flow may be so reduced as to be inadequate to produce the turbulence required for wheezing. Second, unilateral absence of breath sounds in a patient with respiratory distress may be associated with pneumothorax or mucus plugging of a main bronchus. Physical findings suggestive of pneumothorax are es-

pecially important in a mechanically ventilated patient because of the greater likelihood of a tension pneumothorax. Subcutaneous emphysema and a systolic "crunch" heard with systole (Hamman's sign) indicate pneumomediastinum with or without pneumothorax. The finding of digital clubbing in a person with respiratory failure suggests a chronic process. This finding may be helpful, for example, in distinguishing chronic interstitial fibrosis in which clubbing is common from a diffuse infiltrative process caused by an acute infection or left ventricular failure. It is important to search for evidence of heart failure, although in patients who are critically ill the physical examination may not be suggestive of left ventricular failure when it is present (5). The presence of right ventricular failure often implies a chronic pulmonary process usually with longstanding hypoxemia. On the other hand, left ventricular failure with consequent pulmonary edema may be the cause of the respiratory failure, either alone or superimposed on lung disease.

General Laboratory Evaluation

Routine hematologic and blood chemistry studies have limited relevance in assessing patients with respiratory failure, although clues to the acuity or chronicity of the process may be provided. An elevated hemoglobin level with a high hematocrit implies the presence of chronic hypoxemia, which leads to secondary polycythemia.

Hypercarbia may be inferred to be chronic if the plasma bicarbonate concentration is increased. Renal compensation for respiratory acidosis requires several days to occur; hence, increases in bicarbonate concentration do not occur as a result of acute respiratory failure of short duration (6). Patients who have longstanding elevations in arterial carbon dioxide tension ($PaCO_2$) are also likely to be hypochloremic and hypokalemic. These abnormalities tend to be more marked in patients who have been taking diuretics or glucocorticoids. Hypokalemia and hypophosphatemia may be associated with weakness of the respiratory muscles that on occasion can lead to respiratory failure or can complicate underlying lung disease (7,8). These electrolyte abnormalities can also be a cause for difficulties in weaning a patient from mechanical ventilation.

As with the physical examination of the chest, the chest radiograph cannot assist in quantifying the severity of respiratory dysfunction. It is, however, often very valuable in determining the etiology of the respiratory disorder and it is an essential component of the initial evaluation. Likewise, the electrocardiogram is essential to detect arrhythmias, myocardial ischemia or infarction, and cardiac chamber enlargement.

Arterial Blood Gases

The single most useful test in evaluating the severity of respiratory dysfunction is the measurement of arterial blood gas tensions (PaO_2, $PaCO_2$) and pH. This provides an indication of the status of integrated cardiorespiratory function and acid-base balance. Although these measurements are not specific for the kind of abnormality present, they provide valuable physiologic information in patients with severe dysfunction. This section focuses on the interpretation of arterial blood gas and pH values in the assessment of severely ill patients and discusses how these interpretations can be used to infer the pathophysiology of respiratory failure and to guide the general approach to treatment.

Hypoxemia

The mechanisms by which clinically significant reductions in PaO_2 are produced include alveolar hypoventilation ($PaCO_2$ greater than 40 mm Hg), mismatching of ventilation to perfusion, and right-to-left intrapulmonary or intracardiac shunting of blood. It is important to identify the physiologic basis for hypoxemia to provide insight regarding the pathologic process causing the hypoxemia. If hypoxemia is caused only by hypoventilation, this implies that the lung itself is normal and that the only necessary therapeutic goal is improved ventilation. This type of hypoxemia is characterized by a normal alveolar-to-arterial PO_2 difference (PAO_2-PaO_2). The PAO_2-PaO_2 can be determined using the alveolar gas equation to calculate PAO_2 and measuring PaO_2. In young patients breathing room air, the difference should not be greater than 10 mm Hg, and may increase to 16 mm Hg in older persons (9). With an increased fractional concentration of oxygen in inspired gas (FIO_2) sufficient to cause a PAO_2 of 200 mm Hg or greater, the PAO_2-PaO_2 should not be greater than 40 mm Hg.

The distinction between ventilation-perfusion mismatching and shunting can be made by measuring the response to administration of 100% O_2. The PaO_2 increases normally to values of nearly 600 mm Hg if the hypoxemia is owing purely to mismatching, whereas with a shunt the increase may be markedly reduced depending on the magnitude of the shunt flow (Fig. 21.1). The approach to treatment of acute respiratory failure varies considerably depending on whether the hypoxemia is caused primarily by shunting or ventilation-perfusion mismatching. With ventilation-perfusion mismatching, relatively small amounts of supplemental oxygen can increase the PaO_2 sufficiently, whereas with shunting mechanical ventilation is much more likely to be necessary.

Hypercapnia

Alveolar hypoventilation is the only mechanism by which hypercapnia occurs. The amount of alveolar ventilation necessary to eliminate CO_2 and maintain a normal $PaCO_2$ varies depending on carbon dioxide production. Also, alveolar ventilation will in turn be influenced by the amount of wasted ventilation, as discussed in Chapter 4, The Respira-

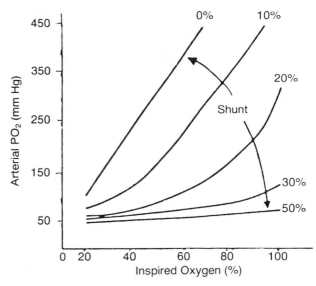

FIGURE 21.1. The relationship between inspired oxygen concentration and arterial PO_2 for lungs with varying degrees of shunt. The increase in PO_2 is small for lungs with large shunts. (From Dantzker DR. Gas exchange in ARDS. *Clin Chest Med* 1982;3: 57–62.)

tory History and Physical Examination. Thus, hypercapnia can occur because of increased production of CO_2, a decrease in minute ventilation, or an increase in wasted ventilation, or a combination of all three mechanisms.

The relationship between $PaCO_2$ and plasma bicarbonate concentrations (HCO_3^-) determine the arterial pH, as shown in the Henderson-Hasselbalch equation. The relationship between $PaCO_2$ and arterial pH varies, however, depending on the time during which the $PaCO_2$ has increased. Thus, by examining the relationships among $PaCO_2$, arterial pH, and HCO_3^-, the acuity or chronicity of the carbon dioxide elevation can usually be determined (Fig. 21.2). Acute increases in $PaCO_2$ are accompanied by only small increases in HCO_3^-, and arterial pH changes in a nearly linear fashion with $PaCO_2$. For every 1 mm Hg change in $PaCO_2$ the pH changes by approximately 0.008 in the opposite direction (10). An acute rise in $PaCO_2$ from 40 mm Hg to 60 mm Hg would be expected to cause a decrease in arterial pH to 7.24. Over a period of 1 to 3 days, however, renal conservation of bicarbonate causes the HCO_3^- to increase and therefore buffers the pH change. Thus, for a given change in $PaCO_2$, the change in pH is much less than when the change occurs slowly. Obviously, the therapeutic implications of an acute versus a chronic change in $PaCO_2$ makes this an important distinction.

Acid-Base Abnormalities

In addition to respiratory acidosis, other acid-base disorders such as metabolic acidosis, metabolic alkalosis, and respiratory alkalosis are important problems in some patients with

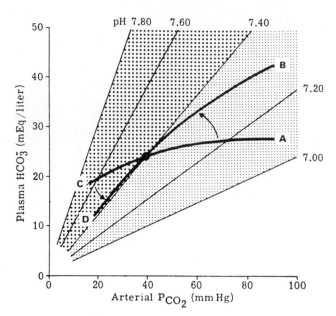

FIGURE 21.2. Effects of acute and chronic variations in Pa_{CO_2} on plasma Hco_3^- and pH. The line connecting points *A* and *C* represents the effects of an acute change in Pa_{CO_2} to a value above or below 40 mm Hg. Renal compensation over time results in a shift of the relationship to that represented by the line connecting points *B* and *D*, as indicated by the arrows. (From Murray JF. *The normal lung.* Philadelphia: Saunders, 1976:224.)

acute respiratory dysfunction. One of the several causes of metabolic acidosis is an imbalance between oxygen delivery and metabolic oxygen needs, which can lead to anaerobic metabolism and lactic acid production. In patients with severe respiratory disorders, such as severe asthma, this imbalance may occur because the work of breathing increases the demand for oxygen in the presence of hypoxia caused by the lung disease. Metabolic acidosis in this setting is a particularly ominous finding, suggesting that rapid deterioration is imminent and that prompt therapeutic interventions are necessary (11).

Both respiratory and metabolic alkalosis have important nonrespiratory effects in critically ill patients. Alkalosis may predispose to arrhythmias, decreases cardiac output, and reduces the threshold for seizures (12). Hypocapnia per se with or without alkalosis reduces cerebral blood flow and may depress the level of consciousness (13). For these reasons, alkalosis should be recognized as an important acid-base disturbance and corrective measures should be taken.

Measurement of Lung Function

The lung function studies that can be used in severely ill patients are rather limited. Depending on the nature and severity of the illness and the patient's ability to cooperate, one may measure vital capacity ($\dot{V}C$), timed forced expiratory volume (FEV_1), peak expiratory flow rate (PEFR), and maximal inspiratory pressure (MIP). The $\dot{V}C$ is the maximal volume of air that can be exhaled after maximal inspiration and provides an indication of the patient's ventilatory capability. Because the $\dot{V}C$ is influenced by the respiratory neuromuscular system, the chest wall, the elastic properties of the lung, and the caliber of the airways, it cannot be used to identify specific abnormalities. Nevertheless, it is particularly helpful in assessing and observing patients with neuromuscular illness and in evaluating patients being ventilated mechanically to determine if it is feasible to consider weaning from the ventilator. The minimal acceptable $\dot{V}C$ in most instances is 10 to 15 mL/kg body weight. This value must, however, be interpreted in light of the patient's clinical condition.

Measurement of MIP provides some of the same information as the $\dot{V}C$ and it is influenced by most of the same factors. However, the ability to generate an acceptable inspiratory pressure, less than -20 cm H_2O, does not necessarily imply that the $\dot{V}C$ will be acceptable.

The timed forced expiratory volume, which is usually expressed as the FEV_1 over the forced vital capacity (FVC), is used to measure the severity of airways obstruction in patients with asthma or chronic airways obstruction. The measurement may not be possible in severely obstructed patients who have marked tachypnea; the maneuver may even transiently worsen airways obstruction. However, the FEV_1 provides the best objective indicator of the degree of airways obstruction and, when measured serially, the response to therapy. Absolute FEV_1 values of less than 0.75 L or less than 25% of the predicted value are commonly associated with increased Pa_{CO_2} values (14).

Measurement of the peak expiratory flow rate (PEFR) provides information similar to the FEV_1 in patients with airways obstruction. The PEFR has the distinct advantage, however, of not requiring a full inhalation followed by a full forced exhalation. It is measured by having the patient slowly inhale and then blow a short forced puff through the flowmeter, a maneuver similar to a cough. Values below 60 L/min indicate severe obstruction.

Calculation of Respiratory Variables

A number of equations and calculations are helpful in the assessment of respiratory function. The use of these equations is discussed later in the chapter in the section that considers specific cases of acute respiratory failure. Descriptions of the physiologic principles involved with the equations were presented in the preceding section. Representative normal values for selected cardiorespiratory variables are listed in Table 21.1.

Equations Related to Arterial Carbon Dioxide Tension

Pa_{CO_2} is related directly to carbon dioxide production ($\dot{V}_{CO_2}$ in milliliters per minute $\dot{V}_{CO_2}$) and inversely to alve-

TABLE 21.1. REPRESENTATIVE NORMAL VALUES FOR SELECTED RESPIRATORY AND HEMODYNAMIC VALUES

Variable	Normal
Pa_{O_2}	95 mm Hg
Pa_{CO_2}	40 mm Hg
pH (arterial)	7.40
$P(A-a)_{O_2}$	<10 mm Hg
O_2 saturation	98%
Ca_{O_2}	19.8 mL/100 mL
Pv_{O_2}	40 mm Hg
VO_2	240 mL/min
Vco_2 i	192 mL/min
R	0.8
Respiratory rate	12
$\dot{V}E$	6 L/min
$\dot{V}D$	150 mL
$\dot{V}T$	450 mL
VD/VT	0.33
Q_t	5 L/min
Q_s/Q_t	7%
PVR	50–150 dyn $\times$ s/cm^5
SVR	800–1200 dyn $\times$ s/cm^5

olar ventilation ($\dot{V}A$, in L/min $\dot{V}A$) as follows:

$$Pa_{CO_2} = \frac{K \dot{V}_{CO_2}}{\dot{V}A}$$

in which the K is a constant.

The VA is the difference between the tidal volume ($\dot{V}T$ in liters) and the wasted or dead-space ventilation ($\dot{V}D$) multiplied by the respiratory rate (F, in breaths/min):

$$\dot{V}A = (\dot{V}T - \dot{V}D) \times F$$

Total minute ventilation ($\dot{V}E$) in L/min is the product of VT and F:

$$\dot{V}E = \dot{V}T \times F$$

From these three equations, it is evident that the factors determining the Pa_{CO_2} are $\dot{V}T$, $\dot{V}D$, F, and $\dot{V}_{CO_2}$.

The volume of dead-space or wasted ventilation can be calculated from a modification of the Bohr equation.

$$\dot{V}D = \frac{Pa_{CO_2} - Pe_{CO_2} \times \dot{V}T}{Pa_{CO_2}}$$

in which the Pe_{CO_2} is the partial pressure of carbon dioxide in mixed expired air. The $\dot{V}D$ so derived is commonly expressed as a fraction of $\dot{V}T$. Normal values for the VD/VT are 0.30 to 0.35.

Equations Related To Oxygenation

The partial pressure of oxygen in the alveolus (PA_{O_2}) can be calculated from the alveolar gas equation as follows:

$$PA_{O_2} = FI_{O_2} (P_b - 47 \text{ mm Hg}) - Pa_{CO_2}/R$$

in which R is the respiratory exchange ratio ($\dot{V}_{CO_2}/\dot{V}_{O_2}$), P_b is barometric pressure, and 47 is the partial pressure of water vapor in millimeters of mercury in fully saturated air at body temperature. The value of R is usually assumed to be 0.8. Having calculated the PA_{O_2}, the $P(A-a)_{O_2}$ can then be determined, enabling a quantitative assessment of the degree of hypoxemia and the mechanisms responsible for it. For example, a normal $P(A-a)_{O_2}$ indicates that hypoxemia is secondary to alveolar hypoventilation alone. On the other hand, an increased $P(A-a)_{O_2}$ indicates either an intrapulmonary or intracardiac right-to-left shunt or mismatching of ventilation and perfusion. Oxygen consumption ($\dot{V}_{O_2}$, in L/min—$\dot{V}_{O_2}$) can be estimated fairly accurately from the relationship:

$$\dot{V}_{O_2} = (FI_{O_2} - Fe_{O_2}) \times \dot{V}E$$

in which the Fe_{O_2} is the fractional concentration of oxygen in expired air.

TREATMENT MODALITIES

Supplemental Oxygen

The administration of supplemental oxygen is frequently necessary in patients with any cardiorespiratory disorder that results in arterial hypoxemia or in which hypoxemia may be expected. The decision to use an external device as opposed to an endotracheal tube depends on the quantity of oxygen needed and the potential consequences of failure to provide oxygen should the external device be malpositioned. Generally speaking, it is not prudent to rely on external oxygen delivery devices for patients with hypoxemia sufficient to require an FI_{O_2} of 0.7 or greater, or who could be expected to suffer serious consequences should the device not be positioned properly.

There are a variety of types of external oxygen delivery systems that can be used to provide supplemental oxygen. The choice of a particular device depends on at least four factors: (*a*) the amount of oxygen needed; (*b*) the need for precise control of the FI_{O_2}; (*c*) the need for humidification; and (*d*) the patient's comfort. Nasal prongs are the simplest and most comfortable delivery device. However, the FI_{O_2} provided cannot be quantitated reliably and humidification is poor. Open face masks or face tents provide a high flow of well-humidified gas with a moderately reliable FI_{O_2} usually set by a venturi device in a humidifier-mixer. Tight-fitting face masks provide higher concentrations of oxygen, and if a reservoir bag is added, even higher concentrations of oxygen, perhaps up to an FI_{O_2} of 0.8 to 0.9 can be provided for short periods. The FI_{O_2} is controlled most precisely by the venturi mask, which uses a calibrated venturi device in the delivery line to provide high flows of gas containing 24%, 28%, 35%, or 40% oxygen (15). This sort of mask is used for patients with chronic airways obstruction and chronic hypercapnia in whom high oxygen concentrations may cause further alveolar hypoventilation.

Noninvasive Ventilation for Acute Respiratory Failure

Background and Rationale for the Use of Noninvasive Ventilation

Noninvasive positive pressure ventilation (NIPPV) refers to techniques that provide alveolar ventilation without an artificial airway in place. Although positive pressure ventilation with a translaryngeal endotracheal or tracheostomy tube constitutes the standard of care for patients with acute respiratory failure who require ventilatory support, there are disadvantages to this method of ventilation, including tracheal injury, the need for sedation, inability to swallow or talk, and increased risk of infections such as pneumonia and sinusitis (16). Noninvasive ventilation overcomes some of these disadvantages, and in selected patients, NIPPV has the potential to provide ventilatory assistance with fewer complications than endotracheal intubation.

During noninvasive ventilation, air enters the nose, mouth, or both by way of a nasal mask, mouthpiece, or face mask, which is connected to a positive pressure ventilator. Regardless of the type of mask used, proper fit is crucial to minimize air leaks and enhance patient compliance. Almost any ventilator mode that can be used with an endotracheal tube in place can be administered noninvasively, but one of the advantages of NIPPV is that certain modes can be administered with small, portable devices rather than a standard mechanical ventilator. The most frequently used modes of noninvasive ventilation are pressure support ventilation, discussed in detail later in this chapter, and biphasic

positive airway pressure (biphasic PAP). With biphasic PAP, the patient receives alternating cycles of airflow at two preset pressures, the highest during inhalation (Fig. 21.3). Some devices sense both airflow and airway pressure and alternate between the two preset pressures through the respiratory cycle. Others alternate between the two pressures based on a preset inspiratory and expiratory time. Continuous positive airway pressure (CPAP) differs from noninvasive ventilation in that it provides minimal ventilatory assistance.

Noninvasive ventilation has the potential to provide effective ventilation for acute respiratory failure, especially hypercapnic respiratory failure, while avoiding some of the complications of mechanical ventilation and endotracheal intubation. However, the results of randomized, controlled studies have been mixed (17,18). Patient selection is clearly the most important issue when considering noninvasive ventilation for acute respiratory failure. Unfortunately, the patients who benefit from noninvasive ventilation seem to represent a minority of all patients with respiratory failure; thus, it is difficult to make broad conclusions concerning applicability of this treatment modality.

Important advantages of noninvasive ventilation include increased patient comfort, maintenance of airway defenses, ability to eat and speak, and avoidance of the complications associated with endotracheal intubation, such as nosocomial pneumonia and upper airway trauma (16). The disadvantages include the need for a motivated, cooperative patient and decreased ability to suction secretions from the airway, a problem that can lead to mucus plugging and respiratory compromise. In a recently reported case series of 158 patients, the complications related to noninvasive ventilation included facial skin necrosis in 13%, gastric distension requiring insertion of a nasogastric tube in 2%, nosocomial pneumonia in 1%, and unilateral lung hyperinflation in

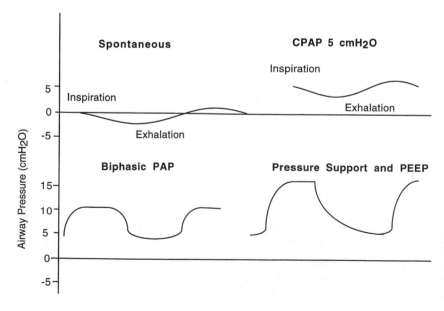

FIGURE 21.3. Pressure in the large airways during various forms of noninvasive ventilation and during pressure support ventilation. During spontaneous breathing, without any ventilatory assistance, airway pressures oscillate around zero and reflect similar changes in pleural pressures. Delivery of continuous positive airway pressure (CPAP) of 5 cm H_2O via a nasal or face mask results in an increase in airway pressure such that inspiratory and expiratory swings oscillate around 5 cmH_2O. During noninvasive biphasic positive airway pressure ventilation, inspiratory and expiratory pressures are set by the clinician. In this example, the settings are 10 cmH_2O inspiratory pressure and 5 cmH_2O expiratory pressure. A similar mode of ventilation is pressure support ventilation, which can be administered invasively or noninvasively. In this example, the settings are pressure support of 10 cmH_2O and positive end expiratory pressure (PEEP) of 5 cmH_2O.

1% in patients ventilated with a face mask (19). There are conflicting results as to whether noninvasive ventilation requires excessive time on the part of caregivers (20,21). The mode of providing noninvasive ventilation and the type of interface (nasal or mouthpiece or face mask) has not seemed to significantly affect the results. Several studies have used pressure-limited ventilation in the form of pressure-support ventilation, whereas others have used volume-cycled ventilators (20,22–35). Pressure-support ventilation provides better control of mask leaks and, at least in one study, was better tolerated than volume cycled ventilation (28). These modes of ventilation are discussed in detail later in this chapter. Additionally, most studies have utilized nasal masks because they add less dead space and permit oral intake and speech to continue, although most patients with acute respiratory failure are mouth breathers, possibly leading to decreased efficacy of nasal masks compared to face masks (29,30).

In the past several years, there have been an increasing number of studies focusing on the use of noninvasive ventilation for acute respiratory failure as a primary therapy. Although controversial, increased interest in noninvasive ventilation for acute respiratory failure has been attributed to the successful adaptation of CPAP masks, initially designed to treat obstructive sleep apnea, for use in noninvasive ventilation in selected patients with chronic hypercapnic respiratory failure (29–40).

Several prospective, randomized trials of noninvasive ventilation as a primary treatment for acute respiratory failure have been published in recent years (41–47). Entry diagnoses, ventilator modes and the masks that were used in these studies varied. The endpoints of these studies were not uniform, but usually included the number of patients who avoided endotracheal intubation and had evidence of improved gas exchange during the trial of noninvasive ventilation. All but one of these studies required respiratory acidosis as one of the entry criteria. Thus, more is known about the utility of noninvasive ventilation for acute hypercapnic respiratory failure rather than for acute hypoxemic respiratory failure. This is not surprising because noninvasive ventilation is believed to work primarily by improving alveolar ventilation. In a randomized study that assessed the use of noninvasive ventilation in hypoxemic respiratory failure, Antonelli et al. studied 64 patients with adult respiratory distress syndrome (ARDS), atelectasis, pneumonia, trauma, or aspiration (43). These investigators found that oxygenation improved equally in the group randomized to noninvasive ventilation compared to the control group who underwent endotracheal intubation followed by mechanical ventilation, and that significantly fewer infectious complications occurred in the noninvasive ventilation group. These findings need to be confirmed in other studies before noninvasive ventilation can be recommended as an effective treatment for acute hypoxemic respiratory failure (43a).

Because the results of these studies have been mixed, there are no clear guidelines for the clinical use of noninvasive ventilation for acute respiratory failure. Reasons for variation in the findings between studies include different patients and clinical settings, different types of noninvasive ventilatory modes and interfaces, different definitions of success and failure, and different treatment of the control groups.

Patient Selection for NIPPV

Patient selection is critical to the success of noninvasive ventilation. Noninvasive ventilation requires cooperative and alert patients who can protect their airway and are hemodynamically stable. Patients must also be able to synchronize their breathing with the ventilator. Patients with a rapidly reversible process (preferably within 48 hours) appear to derive the greatest benefit from noninvasive ventilation. Some selection guidelines for the use of noninvasive ventilation for acute respiratory failure are provided in Table 21.2.

Successful treatment with noninvasive ventilation is associated with an increase in arterial pH and decrease in $PaCO_2$ as early as 1 hour after treatment has begun. Furthermore, the response to noninvasive ventilation can usually be predicted by the level of acidosis before initiating ventilation (25,48) . In one study of 18 patients, a pH greater than 7.30 at 2 hours predicted success of noninvasive ventilation with a positive predictive value of 92% (25). Ambrosino et al. reported that baseline pH was the only significant factor in a retrospective multivariate analysis to assess which of many variables predicted successful treatment with noninvasive ventilation (48,48a). The mean baseline pH in the group of patients in whom noninvasive ventilation was successful was 7.28 versus 7.22 in those in whom it was unsuccessful. Thus, it appears that arterial pH at baseline and 2 hours after initiation of noninvasive ventilation are currently the best methods to identify responders.

Potential Mechanisms of Action

In acute respiratory failure, the precise mechanisms that explain how noninvasive ventilation improves gas exchange and symptoms are not fully known, although relief of inspi-

TABLE 21.2. GUIDELINES FOR THE USE OF NONINVASIVE VENTILATION FOR ACUTE RESPIRATORY FAILURE

Acute respiratory failure with at least two: acute respiratory acidosis, respiratory distress, or accessory muscle use
Baseline arterial pH >7.22
Hemodynamically stable
No evidence of upper airway obstruction
Absence of excessive secretions
Rapidly reversible (<48 hours) cause of respiratory failure
Awake, cooperative patient

ratory muscle fatigue is thought to play a primary role (22,29,49). In one study, Brochard et al. measured transdiaphragmatic pressure and electromyographic activity in 11 patients with acute respiratory failure owing to decompensated chronic obstructive pulmonary disease (22). During treatment with noninvasive ventilation, there were significant reductions in transdiaphragmatic pressure and the pressure-time product for the diaphragm (calculated as the product of the mean transdiaphragmatic-diaphragmatic pressure and the duration of inspiration), indices of inspiratory muscle activity. In addition, the mean amplitude of the averaged diaphragmatic electromyographic signal decreased by 44% with noninvasive ventilation. These findings suggest the possibility that treatment with noninvasive ventilation reduces inspiratory muscle effort. Diaz et al. examined the effects of noninvasive ventilation on both pulmonary gas exchange and hemodynamics during acute exacerbation of chronic obstructive pulmonary disease (50). Measurements were taken in 10 patients while breathing spontaneously. After 15 and 30 minutes of noninvasive ventilation in the pressure support mode with positive end-expiratory pressure, and 15 minutes after withdrawal of noninvasive ventilation, arterial oxygen levels increased and carbon dioxide levels decreased significantly. Importantly, respiratory rate decreased significantly during noninvasive ventilation and the tidal volume increased significantly. The cardiac output decreased with no effect on mixed venous oxygenation. No significant changes in ventilation-perfusion mismatching were detected. These investigators concluded that the primary mechanism by which noninvasive ventilation improves gas exchange in acute hypercapnic respiratory failure is related to improvement in alveolar ventilation rather than ventilation-perfusion matching. The clinical corollary is that monitoring of the patient's breathing pattern during noninvasive ventilation can be useful in determining whether or not a patient is responding to noninvasive ventilation; responders will breathe more slowly and with larger tidal volumes than nonresponders, leading to an increase in their arterial pH and a decrease in their arterial carbon dioxide level.

Another possible mechanism to explain the improvement in symptoms and gas exchange with noninvasive ventilation in acute respiratory failure includes a decrease in the work of breathing by overcoming the effect of intrinsic positive end-expiratory pressure (PEEP) on the inspiratory muscles (49,51).

Future studies will focus on determining the specific patient populations who would most benefit from NIPPV, evaluating the optimal mode and mask for providing noninvasive ventilation, and its potential impact on outcomes such as cost-effectiveness.

Airway Management

Definitive, unambiguous indications for endotracheal intubation that apply to all situations are difficult to define.

TABLE 21.3. INDICATIONS FOR ENDOTRACHEAL INTUBATION AND MECHANICAL VENTILATION

Hypoxemia despite supplemental oxygen administration (PO_2 <60 mm Hg)
Alveolar hypoventilation resulting hypercapnia and respiratory acidosis (pH <7.25)
Altered mental status and inability to protect the airway from aspiration
Hemodynamic instability/shock or cardiopulmonary arrest
Flow limiting obstruction of the upper airway
Requirement of heavy sedation or general anesthesia for completion of a procedure such as endoscopy
Copious secretions with the inability to cough and clear the airway
Postoperative patients in whom maintenance of adequate gas exchange requires excessive energy expenditure (e.g., following cardiac, thoracic, or upper abdominal surgery)
Major trauma

However, the decision to proceed to endotracheal intubation is often based on more subjective criteria and observation of the patient's clinical course. Regardless of the situation, the potential reversibility of the patient's underlying disorder must be considered to determine if endotracheal intubation is appropriate. Table 21.3 lists the most common indications for endotracheal intubation and mechanical ventilation.

Endotracheal tubes may be passed through either the mouth or the nose. The oral route has the advantage of accepting a larger-diameter tube and is easier to use under emergency circumstances. Because direct laryngoscopy is required, sedation and often muscle relaxing agents are needed. Nonemergent tube placement in a spontaneously ventilating patient may be accomplished via the nose without direct visualization of the vocal cords; however, nasotracheal intubation may be facilitated by direct visualization of the larynx with a fiberoptic bronchoscope, especially in difficult cases such as when the neck is immobilized. A fiberoptic bronchoscope can also be used to guide the endotracheal tube via the oral route. Topical anesthesia is usually necessary for bronchoscope-guided intubation, but usually only small doses of systemic agents are required. Intubation should be performed only by physicians experienced with the procedure who are familiar with the pharmacological agents that may be necessary, such as intravenous anesthetics and muscle relaxing agents.

Nasal endotracheal tubes have certain advantages over oral endotracheal tubes: They are generally more comfortable for the patient, oral hygiene can be better maintained, and the tube is less likely to become dislodged (52). The most important disadvantage of nasotracheal intubation is the increased risk of sinusitis (52). Nasal tubes also have the disadvantage of being more difficult to suction through compared to oral tubes because usually they are smaller in diameter. The effective lumen may be further narrowed by

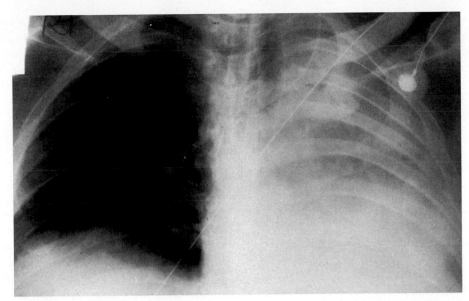

FIGURE 21.4. An anterior-posterior chest radiograph of a recently intubated patient. Note that the tip of the endotracheal tube is in the right main stem bronchus, resulting in atelectasis of the left lung.

compression or kinking within the nose or nasopharynx. In addition, bronchoscopy may be difficult or impossible through a small nasal tube. There is currently no consensus on which route is best (53). Clinical practice varies with institution.

Immediately after the tube is placed, the lungs should be auscultated to determine if air is entering both hemithoraces. Because of the relatively obtuse angle of the right main bronchus, positioning of the tip of the tube in the right main airway is quite common (Fig. 21.4). If the tube seems to be in good position by auscultation, it should be taped securely in place. The position should then be confirmed by a chest radiograph.

All endotracheal tubes should be fitted with a bonded high-volume, low-pressure cuff that will occlude the trachea around the tube, enabling positive-pressure ventilation and minimizing aspiration of oropharyngeal contents. Care should be taken to avoid overinflation of the cuff. An overinflated cuff (greater than 20 mm Hg) may cause pressure necrosis of the adjacent tracheal mucosa and predispose to development of a tracheoesophageal fistula or subsequent tracheal stenosis (54,55).

Endotracheal tubes can be left in place for long periods of time in patients who continue to require mechanical ventilation or airway protection. There is no absolute time limit for endotracheal intubation beyond which tracheostomy is indicated and no evidence to date to suggest that tracheostomy results in fewer airway complications, or shortens the duration of mechanical ventilation (56). Tracheostomy may be necessary, however, because of complications such as infection or soft tissue necrosis in the upper air passages,

including the nose. Occasionally, tracheostomy facilitates removal of secretions more effectively than an endotracheal tube. In addition, patients may find a tracheostomy more comfortable and may be able to eat and talk with a tracheostomy tube in place (57); talking is made possible by attaching a Passey-Muir valve to a specialized tracheostomy tube. When complete separation of the airway from the oropharynx is indicated, a tracheostomy tube with a Blum-Singer valve can be used to allow patients to phonate.

In recent years, bedside percutaneous dilational tracheostomy has become increasingly popular. With this technique, critical care physicians can quickly and safely place a tracheostomy tube without transporting the patient to the operating room. Although still under investigation, this technique is relatively simple and may be associated with fewer complications than traditional tracheostomy (58–61).

Because endotracheal and tracheostomy tubes bypass the normal humidifying mechanisms in the upper airway, all inspired gas must be fully humidified. Removal of pulmonary secretions using a suction catheter should be done at regular intervals as determined by the volume of secretions present. Sterile technique must be used for suctioning. Likewise, all gas delivery circuits in direct communication with the airway should be sterile when connected. Replacement of ventilator circuit tubing and inline suction catheters is commonly performed on a weekly basis; however, recent randomized controlled studies showed no increase in nosocomial pneumonia or duration of mechanical ventilation when these were not routinely changed (62–64).

It is important to realize that once an endotracheal tube is in place, complete responsibility for the airway rests with the individuals caring for the patient. The patient can no longer humidify inspired air, cough effectively, or defend the lower airways against airborne microorganisms. Perhaps more important, he or she cannot call for help or unblock the tube should it become obstructed. For all of these reasons, in addition to the gravity of the illness for which the airway tube was inserted, patients with an artificial airway should nearly always be managed in a critical care unit.

Mechanical Ventilation

Through the use of mechanical ventilation, patients who have severe derangement of gas exchange not corrected with less invasive supportive measures may be temporarily supported until the underlying disease process has resolved. Less commonly, the need for mechanical ventilation may be long term, as in patients with chronic, progressive neuromuscular disease. This section discusses the indications for intubation and mechanical ventilation, reviews the basic features of modern mechanical ventilators, and discusses the most commonly used modes of mechanical ventilation. Strategies of mechanical ventilation in certain clinical situations are reviewed.

Indications for Mechanical Ventilation

Typical indications for mechanical ventilation are listed in Table 21.3; however, there is no substitute for skilled clinical assessment of disease severity, response to therapy and the potential role of less invasive supportive measures. The most common clinical situations in which mechanical ventilation is necessary include alveolar hypoventilation with severe respiratory acidosis (Chapter 22, Acute Hypercapnic Respiratory Failure: Neuromuscular and Obstructive Diseases) and hypoxemia owing to intrapulmonary shunting of blood wherein noninvasive modalities cannot provide a sufficiently high F_{IO_2} (Chapter 23, Acute Hypoxemic Respiratory Failure: Pulmonary Edema and Acute Lung Injury).

Features of Mechanical Ventilators

Modern mechanical ventilators are equipped with several important features to provide support in a variety of respiratory disorders. Most essential is the capacity to deliver a wide range of tidal volumes with an adjustable frequency and an accurate, adjustable F_{IO_2}. Ventilator-delivered breaths are provided spontaneously at a predetermined rate or in response to a patient's inspiratory effort. Controls to adjust inspiratory flow rate and the wave form, inspiratory to expiratory time ratio and inspiratory pressure limit are also necessary. Alarms to alert the clinician to low exhaled tidal volume, high and low inspiratory pressure, and reduction in F_{IO_2} are provided. Temperature and humidity of inspired gas are controlled.

A flow-limiting valve in the expiratory limb of the ventilator circuit allows titration of end-expiratory pressure. In addition to pressure sensing capability, most ventilators monitor airflow to allow for biphasic or continuous positive airway pressure (CPAP) in spontaneously breathing patients.

Commonly Used Modes of Mechanical Ventilation

The most basic feature used to categorize modes of mechanical ventilation is the mechanism determining the transition from the inspiratory phase to the expiratory phase. Specifically, the inspiratory phase may be limited by a preset volume as in volume-cycled ventilation, or by a preset maximal inspiratory pressure as in pressure-cycled ventilation. The major disadvantage of conventional pressure-cycled ventilation is that a tidal volume and therefore minute ventilation cannot be guaranteed. For this reason, volume cycled modes of ventilation are most commonly used.

Volume-Cycled Ventilation
The oldest and most basic of volume-cycled modes is controlled mechanical ventilation (CMV). During CMV, the ventilator, regardless of patient effort, delivers a preset number of breaths of a specified tidal volume. Ventilators also provide an assist mode in which the patient's inspiratory effort triggers the machine to deliver a predetermined tidal volume breath. More precisely, these two modalities are combined as assist-control (AC) ventilation; the ventilator delivers a breath with every inspiratory effort and a preset minimum number of breaths if the patient's respiratory rate falls below the set rate (Fig. 21.5). Because tidal volume and respiratory rate are set, minimum minute ventilation is predetermined.

The disadvantages of volume-AC ventilation include the potential for hyperinflation and resultant lung injury when the respiratory rate is high and insufficient time is allowed for exhalation. This breath stacking can result in high alveolar pressure and intrinsic positive-end-expiratory pressure (see the following), which increases the risk of pneumothorax, pneumomediastinum, and hypotension from decreased cardiac output. Additionally, patients are more likely to develop a respiratory alkalosis because every inspiratory effort results in the delivery of a full-size breath.

In the late 1970s, an alternative mode of volume-cycled ventilation was introduced with the goal of minimizing the risk of hyperinflation and respiratory alkalosis—intermittent mandatory ventilation (IMV). IMV is similar to AC in that a preset number of breaths of a set tidal volume are delivered to the patient each minute. The difference from AC is that the patient may take additional, *unassisted* breaths. The inspired air for these additional breaths comes from a reservoir in parallel with the primary ventilator circuit. Essentially, all ventilators in use today provide synchro-

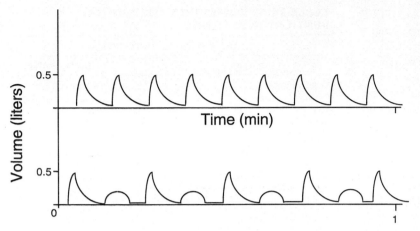

FIGURE 21.5. A comparison of two volume-cycled modes of mechanical ventilation. The upper graph compares volume versus time for a patient being ventilated with assist-control ventilation. Tidal volume is set to 500 mL and the rate is set at 5. The patient is making nine respiratory efforts per minute. The lower graph is for a patient being ventilated with synchronized-intermittent-mandatory-ventilation with a set rate of 5. The patient is making nine respiratory efforts per minute.

nized IMV (SIMV) where the ventilator attempts to synchronize the machine breaths to the patient's intrinsic respiratory rate rather than evenly spacing the breaths over each minute. SIMV, one of the most commonly used modes of ventilation in medical and surgical patients, is usually combined with pressure-support ventilation in clinical practice (65). In selected patients, SIMV with pressure support may be more comfortable and efficient compared with IMV or AC (66).

The main disadvantage of SIMV is that the clinician may overestimate the amount of support the patient is receiving resulting in patient fatigue; patients may be less likely to develop respiratory alkalosis in part because the work of breathing is actually increased compared to AC (67). Therefore, SIMV has no advantage over AC in patients with a high work of breathing (68).

Pressure-Cycled Ventilation

Pressure-cycled ventilation differs from volume-cycled ventilation in that pressure and time rather than volume determine the transition from inspiration to exhalation. Pressure controlled (PC) ventilation, otherwise analogous to AC ventilation, has the main disadvantage of not ensuring a predetermined minute ventilation. The clinician sets the frequency, maximum inspiratory pressure, end expiratory pressure and the inspiration to exhalation (I : E) ratio. *Inverse ratio ventilation* (IRV), occasionally used in patients with very low thoracic compliance, is PC ventilation with an increased inspiratory time such that I : E is 2 : 1 rather than the more physiologic 1 : 2 or lower. IRV can also be administered by adding an inspiratory pause to volume-cycled ventilation. This mode theoretically allows a greater percentage of alveoli to open and participate in gas exchange while avoiding high peak airway pressures in select patients with a low thoracic compliance owing to ARDS (69). However, because IRV actually increases mean airway pressure without consistent improvement in oxygenation, this mode has

been largely replaced with low tidal volume, volume-cycled ventilation in these patients (70,71).

Pressure Support Ventilation

Pressure support (PS) ventilation is a type of pressure- and flow-cycled ventilation in which spontaneous inspiratory efforts are rewarded with high airflow until a preset inspiratory pressure is reached, usually in the range of 5–20 cmH$_2$O. When the airflow required to maintain this pressure decreases by 25%, the onset of exhalation, inspiratory support from the ventilator stops until the next patient-triggered breath (Fig. 21.5). This mode of ventilation can be used alone in a spontaneously breathing patient, or in combination with SIMV to provide additional support to the patient's spontaneous breaths. PS ventilation is also commonly used to wean patients from mechanical ventilation, as discussed later in this chapter. The main advantage of PS ventilation is that the patient has more control over inspiratory time and tidal volume, resulting in a more physiologic respiratory cycle (72).

Positive-End-Expiratory Pressure

Positive-end-expiratory pressure (PEEP) may be added to any mode of mechanical ventilation and is produced with an adjustable valve in the expiratory limb of the ventilator circuit. By increasing distending pressure across the walls of the airways and alveoli, PEEP increases the volume of gas in the lung at end exhalation (functional residual capacity). This counteracts the alveolar collapse or microatelectasis characteristic of conditions producing pulmonary edema and low thoracic compliance like ARDS. Also termed *alveolar recruitment,* the result is decreased intrapulmonary shunting of blood and improved Pa$_{O_2}$, often allowing the use of lower FI$_{O_2}$.

The benefits of applied PEEP in patients with respiratory failure due to obstructive airways disease are less clear. These patients commonly develop *intrinsic* PEEP or *auto*-PEEP as a result of small airway obstruction and gas trapping, a condition made worse by insufficient expiratory time. Applied PEEP may actually contribute to this phenomenon. Prospective studies in this patient group have found that applied PEEP raises already high airway and alveolar pressures and may contribute to hyperinflation (73,74). Available data from the few published prospective trials, however, are inconsistent (75). MacIntyre et al. found that PEEP applied to a level of 85% of measured intrinsic PEEP in COPD patients resulted in decreased work of breathing and lower intrinsic PEEP (76).

Hemodynamic Effects of PEEP

Because intrathoracic pressure is increased, PEEP can have hemodynamic consequences; however, the effect in a given patient is unpredictable. This uncertainty results from only partial and varying transmission of applied PEEP to transmural capillary pressure and from differing effects on the right and left heart.

Increased intrathoracic pressure from applied PEEP decreases venous return to the right heart and may compromise cardiac output, particularly in patients with poor right-ventricular function or with volume depletion (77–79). In addition, PEEP increases right-ventricle afterload while preventing a compensatory increase in preload, resulting in decreased cardiac output (80,81). The decrease in cardiac output may actually decrease oxygen delivery to tissues despite an increased PaO_2. Conversely, increased intrathoracic pressure can augment left-ventricular emptying in systole and decrease left-ventricle afterload, resulting in increased cardiac output (79). The hemodynamic effects of PEEP become more pronounced in patients with low thoracic compliance because a greater fraction of the applied pressure is transmitted to the alveoli, resulting in larger changes in transmural capillary pressure.

Determination of the optimal level of PEEP, can be difficult. However, levels in the range of 5–20 cmH_2O are commonly used. Benefits to oxygenation provided by increased PEEP must be balanced against a decrease in cardiac output and the effect of PEEP on dynamic airway pressure.

Mechanical Ventilation Strategies

"Conventional" mechanical ventilation refers to the traditional standard ventilator settings targeted at maintaining normal blood pH and arterial blood gasses. Table 21.4 shows typical initial ventilator settings targeted at this goal. An emerging strategy for mechanical ventilation is *protective ventilation*. For patients with obstructive lung disease, this refers to the prevention of high airway pressures and hyperinflation with its associated complications (82). In this context, protective ventilation would include ventilation with low PEEP, lower tidal volumes, and longer exhalation times

TABLE 21.4. COMMONLY USED INITIAL VENTILATOR SETTINGS

Volume-Cycled Ventilation	
Parameter	**Initial Setting**
Tidal volume	6–10 mL/kg
Repiratory rate	10–20 breaths/min
FiO_2	1.0
PEEP	5–10 cmH_2O
Waveform	Decelerating[b]
Inspiratory flow	60–100 L/min[b]
PIP limit[a]	45–50 cmH_2O
Pressure support (SIMV mode)	5–20 cmH_2O

Pressure-Cycled Ventilation	
Parameter	**Initial Setting**
Respiratory rate	10–20 breaths/min
FiO_2	1.0
PIP	25–35 cmH_2O
PEEP	5–10 cmH_2O
I:E	1:2

FiO_2 = Fraction of inspired oxygen.
PIP = Peak inspiratory pressure.
SIMV = Synchronized intermittent mandatory ventilation.
I:E = Inspiratory to expiratory time ratio.
[a] Alarm setting. Other available alarms include low inspiratory pressure (ventilator disconnected from patient), low minute ventilation (inadequate spontaneous tidal volume or respiratory rate), low exhaled tidal volume (air leak in circuit), and apnea alarm.
[b] Using a square waveform or increasing the inspiratory flow rate results in an effective decrease in inspiratory time (decreased I:E) and usually a higher peak inspiratory pressure. Expiratory time is increased.

(e.g., square waveform, increased inspiratory flow rate). Although hyperinflation is minimized, alveolar ventilation is also decreased. This results in increased $PaCO_2$, a concept known as *permissive hypercapnia* (83). In the subset of patients with severe obstructive lung disease, a protective ventilation strategy may result in fewer ventilator related complications and may reduce mortality (82,84). However, the resultant hypercapnea can contribute to patient agitation, resulting in the need for more sedation. The associated acidosis may also require treatment with sodium bicarbonate.

Patients with decreased thoracic compliance and pulmonary edema are prone to regional atelectasis, increased shunt fraction, and hypoxemia, features that are characteristic of ARDS. The cyclic collapse and re-expansion of these lung regions may contribute to further lung injury. A strategy of protective ventilation aimed at preventing minimizing the effects of high airway pressures and cyclic re-expansion of alveoli, has been termed the *open lung approach*—"open lung" refers to increased alveolar recruitment and the prevention of cyclic opening and closing of alveoli. Optimal ventilation with a lung protective strategy is discussed in Chapter 23, Acute Hypoxemic Respiratory Failure: Pulmonary Edema and Acute Lung Injury.

Other Modes of Mechanical Ventilation

Although not commonly used, there are less conventional modes of ventilation that are occasionally used in critically ill patients with respiratory failure. These are briefly reviewed.

Pressure-Regulated-Volume-Controlled Ventilation

Pressure-regulated-volume-controlled ventilation (PRVC) is a newer mode of ventilation in which the clinician sets a minimum tidal volume, respiratory rate, and inspiratory time. The ventilator delivers the set tidal volume at the lowest possible pressure within the inspiratory time. The amount of support provided by the ventilator is variable; if the patient can generate the target tidal volume spontaneously, the ventilator provides no assistance. PRVC produces lower peak inspiratory pressures and in neonates may decrease the risk of barotrauma-associated complications (85,86). However, definitive data are not yet available.

Variable Pressure-Support and Volume-Support Ventilation

This is another, newer mode of ventilation roughly analogous to PS. The main difference from a conventional PS mode is that the clinician sets a minimum *minute volume*. The ventilator monitors tidal volume and variable PS is applied to generate volumes that will meet the minute volume goal. As in conventional PS ventilation, the patient sets the respiratory rate. The putative advantages of this type of proportional assist ventilation include patient comfort and lower peak airway pressures (87).

Airway Pressure Release Ventilation

This mode is analogous to CPAP or biphasic positive airway pressure ventilation. Here, a preset, continuous pressure is periodically released for a single breath. The goal is to limit peak airway pressures without compromising ventilation or hemodynamics to the same degree as volume-cycled ventilation. Data to support these claims are lacking; small, prospective studies have demonstrated that these goals are not consistently achieved (88,89).

High-Frequency Oscillatory Ventilation

This mode differs from all of those described in the preceding. In high-frequency oscillatory ventilation, a very small tidal volume, smaller than the anatomic dead space, is delivered at a very high frequency (60–100 or more per minute) (90,91). This strategy, now more commonly used in neonates with respiratory distress syndrome, avoids high peak inspiratory pressures and may result in lower mean airway pressures than conventional volume-cycled ventilation (92,93). If mean airway pressure is lower, the transalveolar pressure may be lower, particularly when respiratory system compliance is low. Theoretically, this strategy may result in a lower incidence of barotrauma-associated clinical sequelae

of conventional mechanical ventilation. A second type of high frequency ventilation is *jet ventilation*. This can be accomplished with a small-diameter catheter passed into the trachea through the larynx, or through the cricothyroid membrane in emergency situations. Oxygen is delivered with high-pressure pulses at a frequency of 100 or more per minute. Exhalation is passive. Neither tidal volume nor airway pressure can be precisely regulated, but peak airway pressures are generally lower than with conventional modes of ventilation (94). Alveolar ventilation and oxygenation are comparable to conventional mechanical ventilation (95). Alveolar pressures may not be lower than with conventional modes because mean airway pressure may not accurately reflect alveolar pressure (96).

Weaning from Mechanical Ventilation

Discontinuation of mechanical ventilation can be a rapid process, such as following a surgical procedure; however, in many cases, the withdrawal of mechanical ventilation must be more gradual. This process is referred to as weaning. This section discusses clinical criteria to initiate weaning, weaning techniques, and the use of standardized weaning protocols.

Weaning Criteria

Patients who are being mechanically ventilated should be frequently evaluated to determine if their lung function has sufficiently improved to enable discontinuation of mechanical ventilation and subsequent removal of the endotracheal tube. When a patient recovering from respiratory failure meets basic clinical criteria for weaning, a trial of spontaneous ventilation should be attempted (Table 21.5). This is accomplished by setting the ventilator to a CPAP of 5 cmH$_2$O with pressure support of 0–5 cmH$_2$O, or by connecting the endotracheal tube to a T-piece (discussed in the following) for 30 minutes to 2 hours or more. Although the ideal duration of a spontaneous breathing trial is not known, recent evidence supports the hypothesis that short trials are as predictive as longer trials (97). If the patient tolerates this trial of spontaneous breathing, mechanical ventilation may be safely discontinued (98). Depending on the nature of the underlying disorder and other clinical variables, some physicians prefer to see more than one successful trial of spontaneous breathing prior to discontinuing mechanical ventilation. In the subset of patients who fail this initial trial, weaning is necessary. The initiation, technique, and duration of weaning may vary considerably depending on the nature of the underlying disorder. In one recent prospective study, approximately 41% of the time that patients remained on mechanical ventilation was attributable to weaning (65).

Of the specific criteria used to assess readiness for a spontaneous breathing trial and to predict successful extubation

TABLE 21.5. GUIDELINES FOR IDENTIFYING CANDIDATES FOR WEANING AND DISCONTINUATION OF MECHANICAL VENTILATION

General
Resolution of the underlying disorder
Appropriate mental status, wakefulness, and strength to cooperate with weaning
Hemodynamic stability and discontinuation of vasopressors
Adequate nutritional status and repletion of electrolytes (potassium, calcium, magnesium, phosphorus)
Absence of upper airway obstruction or edema

	Minimal Weaning Criteria	
	Minimum	Normal (Not Ventilated)
FIO_2	<0.6	0.21
PaO_2/FIO_2	>240	>450
Vital capacity	>10 mL/kg	60–80 mL/kg
Tidal volume (VT)	>300 mL	450 mL
Minute ventilation (VE)	<10 L/min	6 L/min
MVV	>twice VE	>10 times VE
MIP	< −20 cmH$_2$O	< −100 cmH$_2$O
Respiratory rate/VT (RSBI)	<105	<30

MVV = maximal voluntary ventilation
MIP = maximal inspiratory pressure
RSBI = rapid shallow breathing index

listed in Table 21.5, perhaps the most reliable are the Rapid Shallow Breathing Index (RSBI) and the maximal inspiratory pressure (MIP) (99,100). RSBI as described by Yang and Tobin in 1991 is the respiratory rate divided by the tidal volume in liters while the patient breathes spontaneously. A threshold value of 105 was found to be most predictive. MIP is measured by the respiratory therapist and is simply the greatest negative pressure the patient can generate during spontaneous inhalation. A threshold value of negative 20 cmH$_2$O is most predictive. These variables have been found to be very sensitive for identifying medical patients likely to fail removal of mechanical ventilation (RSBI sensitivity = 0.97, negative predictive value 95%, and MIP sensitivity = 1.0, negative predictive value 100%). These variables perform less well in predicting which patients will succeed (RSBI specificity = 0.64, positive predictive value 73% and MIP specificity = 0.11, positive predictive value 53%), but unlike other more detailed indices used to predict weaning success, RSBI and MIP have the advantage of being easy to determine at the bedside (99,101). The use of these criteria to predict weaning success or failure does not obviate the need to perform weaning trials; some patients require re-intubation or mechanical ventilation despite meeting established weaning criteria. Likewise, some patients do not meet criteria, but still tolerate liberation from the ventilator. Therefore, a patient should prove him- or herself unweanable by direct testing rather than through the use of bedside criteria alone.

Discontinuation of mechanical ventilation and removal of an endotracheal tube should be considered separate decisions because the indications for each are not necessarily the same (Table 21.2). Most notably, neurologic abnormalities, especially a diminished level of consciousness, contribute to a delay in extubation in up to one-third of medical and surgical patients intubated for at least 48 hours. Alteration in mental status is often attributable to sepsis, liver failure, or other metabolic abnormalities as opposed to a primary neurologic disease (102).

Weaning Techniques

Three basic weaning strategies are used in clinical practice today: pressure support (PS) ventilation weaning, T-piece weaning, and intermittent mandatory ventilation (IMV) weaning. Recent studies have compared these strategies and shown that there are clinically important differences among them. Each technique is described followed by a discussion of the differences.

Pressure Support Weaning

When weaning with pressure support, the ventilator is changed to a PS mode, usually 5 to 20 cmH$_2$O, and the level of support is decreased as rapidly as is tolerated by the patient until a minimal level is reached. Generally, decrements of 2 to 5 cmH$_2$O are attempted in one or two daily adjustments. Based on clinical criteria such as RSBI, arterial, or mixed venous blood gasses, as well as patient comfort and overall clinical trajectory, the decision is then made to discontinue mechanical ventilation (103,104).

The most important disadvantage to PS weaning is the tendency to overestimate the amount of work the patient is doing. The amount of PS needed to overcome resistance in the ventilator circuit and other contributors to inspiratory load may indeed be less than 5 cmH$_2$O. Therefore, the level of ventilatory assistance received while on PS may occasionally exceed the patient's reserve, resulting in failure of extubation despite acceptable indices on a low level of PS. For this reason, some clinicians occasionally order a trial of spontaneous ventilation without PS prior to discontinuing mechanical ventilation, even for patients receiving PS as low as 5 cmH$_2$O.

The main potential advantages of PS weaning include a shorter duration of weaning and increased patient comfort compared to IMV because the patient determines the respiratory rate and breath size (105,106). However, one recent study found no difference in patient comfort when PS was compared with SIMV weaning (107). Another advantage is that, unlike T-piece weaning, all monitors and alarms remain active during PS weaning.

T-Piece Weaning

This mode of weaning is the most direct and is analogous to a spontaneous breathing trial. When the patient meets minimal weaning criteria, the endotracheal tube is attached to a T-piece such that one of the two remaining limbs of the T is connected to the ventilator, which supplies fresh air. The third limb is left open to allow for exhalation. T-piece weaning can be performed in single or multiple short daily trials. For patients with a high probability of weaning success, the trial may be as short as 30 minutes—for most patients, once daily trials of 2 or more hours duration are used. A recent randomized trial including medical and surgical patients showed that more than one 2-hour weaning trial per day did not result in more rapid weaning or result in a higher rate of weaning success compared to a single daily trial (108).

The primary disadvantage of this method of weaning is that apnea, low minute ventilation, and airway pressure alarms are disabled. Consequently, close visual monitoring is required. The most important advantage of T-piece weaning is the more accurate approximation of postextubation breathing. This results in more rapid recognition of patients able to tolerate discontinuation of mechanical ventilation and faster weaning compared to IMV and certain PS weaning protocols (105,108).

As an alternative to T-piece weaning, some centers have begun using CPAP for both spontaneous breathing trials and weaning (109). CPAP allows for alarms to remain active and may actually better approximate post extubation breathing. This is because during T-piece weaning (airway pressure approximately 0 cmH$_2$O), the patient may have to assume an increased inspiratory load resulting from resistance in the ventilator tubing and endotracheal tube and potentially increased intrinsic PEEP (in patients with obstructive airways disease) (110,111). Differences between CPAP and T-piece are subtle and may not be clinically important (112); however, CPAP can be continued noninvasively after extubation.

IMV Weaning

IMV is discussed in detail earlier in this chapter. Its use in weaning from mechanical ventilation is straightforward; the number of machine breaths is gradually decreased by one or more per day until the patient tolerates only four to five assisted breaths per minute for several hours. One of the disadvantages of this method of weaning is that the work of breathing required for the unassisted breaths can be high. This is largely owing to the resistance to airflow in the ventilator circuit. This additional work of breathing may not be appreciated by the clinician and can result in patient fatigue. For this reason, IMV weaning is often combined with a low level of pressure support (5 cmH$_2$O) such that the unassisted breaths are augmented by PS ventilation (66); however, this variable level of ventilatory support does not necessarily decrease work of breathing, partly because the muscles of respiration contract to the same degree regardless of the level of extrinsic support when the amount of assistance is variable (107,113).

Comparison of Weaning Techniques

Two recent prospective, randomized studies comparing these three weaning techniques in medical and surgical patients failing initial attempts at spontaneous breathing have shown that IMV weaning is up to three times slower than either T-piece or PS weaning without a difference in eventual success rates. This results in fewer days of assisted ventilation in patients weaned with T-piece or PS (105,108). Differences between T-piece and PS are subtle; therefore, it is important to consider the exact protocols used in these studies when comparing these strategies. For example, duration of weaning with PS is related to the rapidity with which the level of support is decreased. Based on current data, it is reasonable to consider all three weaning techniques equal with respect to eventual weaning success, but T-piece and PS weaning are faster than IMV because the patient's ability to tolerate spontaneous breathing is recognized earlier.

Weaning Protocols

Based on the results of prospective, randomized trials, the use of respiratory therapist or nurse directed weaning protocols has become popular. This type of protocol requires daily evaluation of readiness for weaning using the criteria in Table 21.5. If the patient meets the minimum criteria, the patient is given a spontaneous breathing trial (generally CPAP 5 cmH$_2$O or T-piece). The physician is notified if the patient tolerates the trial in order to make the final decision to proceed to extubation. Studies have confirmed that protocol-directed weaning results in more rapid liberation from mechanical ventilation without an increase in reintubation rates (114,115).

Emergencies in the Ventilated Patient

Patients who are being mechanically ventilated are subject to many potentially disastrous events related to malfunction of the ventilator or artificial airway. Further, the patient's underlying disorder may increase the risk of certain life-threatening complications, such as pneumothorax. Because such occurrences may be rapidly fatal, it is important that personnel caring for critically ill patients develop a routine for assessment and management of these situations.

The most frequent indication that a problem has developed is that the patient is no longer being ventilated. This may be manifested by patient distress, by sounding of the high pressure limit or low tidal volume alarm, or by sudden hemodynamic changes in the patient. The problems that should be suspected when the high pressure limit is exceeded include obstruction of the endotracheal or tracheostomy tube by kinking, mucus, or blood clot, obstruction in the patient's airways, or pneumothorax. Occasionally, migration of the tip of the tube into a mainstream bronchus (usually the right) causes the high pressure limit to be exceeded, but this is usually not so dramatic an occurrence (Fig. 21.4). When the high pressure limit is exceeded and the patient is not being ventilated adequately, the first step is to disconnect the patient from the ventilator and begin hand ventilation with an anesthesia bag using an FIO_2 of 1.0. At nearly the same time as bagging begins, the artificial airway should be checked for position and for evidence of external obstruction such as kinking between the ventilator tubing connection and the nose, mouth, or hypopharynx. If there is no external obstruction, the tube position seems correct, and compression of the bag is still difficult, the next step should be to pass a suction catheter through the tube to check its patency and to remove mucus plugs or blood clots that may be causing the problem. Assuming the suction catheter can be passed, failure of these maneuvers to relieve the apparent obstruction indicates that the problem is within the thorax and may be caused by major airway obstruction that was not removed by suctioning, sudden severe peripheral airways obstruction, or pneumothorax. These can usually be distinguished from one another by a rapid physical examination of the chest. Tracheal obstruction is manifested by the finding of no or markedly reduced entry of air into the lungs. Main bronchial obstruction is usually indicated by the absence of entry of air into the lung distal to the obstruction, causing a rocking motion of the chest with the affected side not expanding with inspiration and the unobstructed side being overinflated. Peripheral airways obstruction may be suspected from the patient's history and is usually indicated by wheezing, although with severe bronchoconstriction there may be little air movement and thus little or no wheezing. Nearly always, a pneumothorax that occurs in a patient being ventilated mechanically quickly becomes a tension pneumothorax. This is signaled not only by difficulty with ventilation but by a reduction in systemic arterial blood pressure and an increase in central venous pressure. In addition, examination of the chest shows no entry of air on the affected side, but in contrast to the findings of mainstem bronchial obstruction, the affected side is hyperinflated and hyperresonant to percussion. If the clinical situation allows, a chest roentgenogram allows a definitive diagnosis; often, however, there is not sufficient time and a presumption of pneumothorax must be acted on (Fig 21.6).

Management of each of these situations is obviously different. Vigorous chest physical therapy and suctioning of the airway usually removes obstructing mucus plugs or clots. Occasionally, emergency fiberoptic bronchoscopy may be necessary, as in the case of total lung atelectasis or to inspect the airway for obstruction. Occasionally, a bloodclot or mucus plug can act as a ball-valve in the airway allowing passage of a suction catheter, but quickly reoccluding the airway when the catheter is removed. Therefore, if other causes of high airway pressure have been reasonably excluded, consideration should be given to replacing the artificial airway.

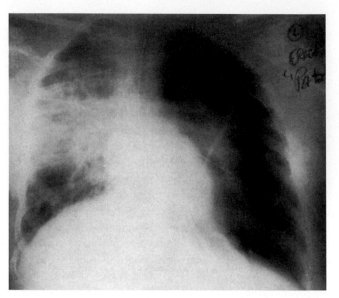

FIGURE 21.6. Anterior-posterior chest radiograph showing a large left pneumothorax in a patient who was being mechanically ventilated for the acute respiratory distress syndrome.

A tension pneumothorax requires prompt intervention to reduce the intrathoracic pressure. In an emergency situation, a 14-gauge needle can be placed in the second anterior intercostal space. This serves to relieve the tension with prompt restoration of the hemodynamic status and the ability to ventilate the patient. After the needle is inserted, a chest tube should always be placed. Even if the diagnosis of pneumothorax was mistaken, a chest tube must be placed because of the high probability of lung puncture with the needle.

When inadequate ventilation is noted and the high pressure limit is not being exceeded, the possible problems to be considered are leaks in the ventilator tubing or around the cuff of the artificial airway, ventilator malfunction, or a tracheoesophageal fistula. Again, the first step is to disconnect the ventilator and begin manual ventilation using an FIO_2 of 1.0. At the same time, the position of the tube and the inflation of the cuff should be checked. If the external pilot balloon is deflated, more air should be added. Leaks around the cuff may be indicated by air escaping from the mouth with each ventilator inflation. The leaks may be caused by breaks in the cuff itself or in the external pilot balloon. Occasionally, an endotracheal tube may have migrated too high in the airway with the cuff at the level of the vocal cords or higher, causing air to leak around the cuff. For this reason, visual inspection of the mouth and pharynx is warranted. If the cuff itself is leaking, the tube must be replaced. With some kinds of tubes, the outer balloon may be replaced without changing the tube. Leaks may also be caused by enlargement of the trachea at the site of the cuff because of the pressure on the tracheal wall. If this is the origin of the leak, the problem may be solved by adding air to the cuff within the trachea. If air is added, care should be taken in general to not exceed a measured intracuff pressure of 20 to 25 mm Hg, especially in patients with systemic hypotension, because this may compromise tracheal perfusion and lead to necrosis (54,55).

Tracheal dilation is often the precursor of a much more serious problem—formation of a tracheoesophageal fistula. This can usually be prevented by maintaining the intracuff pressures less than 20 to 25 mm Hg (54). When a fistula does develop, however, it is often catastrophic. Patients with fistulas can sometimes be managed temporarily by placing the tube at a lower level in the trachea with the cuff below the fistula. Definitive management is surgical correction of the fistula.

RESPIRATORY MONITORING

This section considers a wide range of techniques for monitoring the respiratory status in critically ill patients with respiratory failure. Recently, there has been increasing interest in developing noninvasive methods for monitoring important physiologic variables with the goal of reducing the risk and expense of invasive measurements whenever possible.

Respiratory monitoring should always include the measurement of respiratory rate and, depending on the patient's clinical condition, measurement of the arterial pH, PaO_2, and $PaCO_2$. The respiratory rate can be measured and recorded automatically in nonintubated, spontaneously ventilating patients with impedance devices to which alarms can be attached. In patients who are intubated and spontaneously breathing, respiratory rates and tidal volume can be monitored with a pneumotachograph. Other approaches include the use of a respiratory inductance plethysmograph (RIP) to monitor lung volume by recording the inductance change in wire coils applied to the abdomen and rib cage. RIP has been used to measure tidal volume in both normal subjects and those with respiratory disease (116). This method may be useful for the early detection of respiratory failure in patients in critical care units, but further study of its sensitivity and clinical value is needed.

Because respiratory muscle fatigue has been recognized as an important contributing factor in many patients with acute respiratory failure, attempts have been made to monitor respiratory muscle function (117,118). In one study, investigators demonstrated that a fall in the ratio of high- to low-frequency power over the diaphragm often preceded clinical manifestations of impending respiratory failure in recently weaned patients. The change in the power ratio preceded the development of tachypnea, altered breathing patterns (respiratory alternans and abdominal paradox), and

the increase in $PaCO_2$ (Fig. 21.7) (119). It is possible that monitoring respiratory muscle EMG signals may become clinically useful to follow patients with early respiratory failure or to aid in assessing patients during weaning with spontaneous breathing trials on a T-piece or CPAP.

In patients who are mechanically ventilated, it is mandatory to monitor the respiratory rate, exhaled tidal volume, and airway pressure. An acute decrease in airway pressure indicates a leak in the system or a disconnection of the ventilator tubing from the endotracheal tube. Therefore, a low-pressure alarm system is essential. Acute increases in airway pressure may indicate simply the need for suctioning of the endotracheal tube or a change in chest wall compliance because the patient is agitated or in pain. On the other hand, acute increases in airway pressure may herald a more serious problem such as pneumothorax, lobar atelectasis, malposition of the endotracheal tube in the right mainstem bronchus, or acute bronchospasm. Patients with severe airway obstruction have elevated peak airway pressures during gas flow but normal plateau pressures (measured by occluding outflow on the ventilator momentarily) during no flow (120). The effects of inhaled bronchodilator therapy can be followed sequentially in patients with an increase in the peak-plateau pressure difference (greater than 10 cmH$_2$O).

Recently, the interruptor technique has been adapted to determine the mechanical properties of the respiratory system in patients. Flow, volume, and tracheal pressure have been measured through a series of brief (1.5-sec) interruptions of expiratory flow in patients to determine passive flow resistances as well as elastance of the total respiratory system. This method is yet another approach to assess respiratory compliance. The limitations of the method are that lung volume cannot be directly assessed and the chest wall needs to be relaxed (121).

Another approach to measuring mechanical function and work of breathing has been developed. The work of breathing can be estimated by simultaneous recording of pressure changes and flow over time. Work (expressed in kg-m) is obtained by integration of power (pressure times flow in kg/m per sec) over time. Work can be analyzed as either total respiratory work (lung and chest wall) by using transthoracic pressure differences (airway opening minus atmosphere) or only work done to move the lungs and produce air flow by using transpulmonary pressures (airway-esophageal balloon pressures). The inspiratory work of breathing during assisted mechanical ventilation has been measured and evidence has been presented that, even with the assist control mode of ventilation, patients may exert considerable respiratory muscle work (122).

There are a number of additional monitoring techniques but their clinical value is uncertain. Breath-by-breath measurements of respiratory system compliance and both volume-pressure and volume-flow relationships can be made. Also, mass spectrometer systems are available to measure FIO_2 and exhaled carbon dioxide and oxygen. These mea-

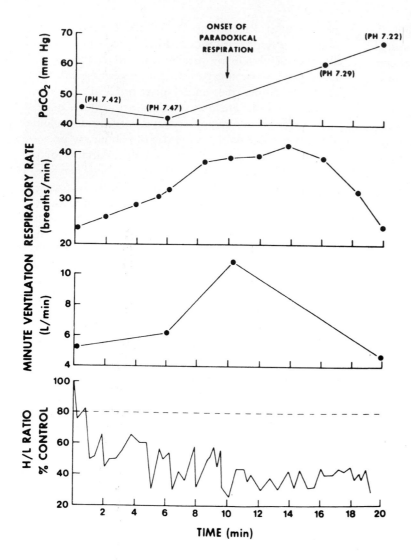

FIGURE 21.7. Sequence of changes in a patient during a 20-min attempt to discontinue mechanical ventilation. The initial change was a fall in the ratio of high- to low-frequency power of the respiratory muscles as detected by surface electromyography. After the change in high :low ratio, there was a progressive rise in respiratory rate and an initial respiratory alkalosis. After the onset of paradoxic respiration, minute ventilation progressively decreased and hypercapnia and res[ho]piratory acidosis developed. Thus, the fall in high:low ratio may be a useful predictor of diaphragmatic fatigue that precedes clinical evidence of impending res[ho]piratory failure. (From Cohen CA, Zagelbaum G, Gross D, et al. Clinical manifestations of inspiratory muscle fatigue. *Am J Med* 1982;73:308–316.)

surements of exhaled gases, especially the Pe_{CO_2}, may provide an early indicator of changes in alveolar ventilation but their utility in a critical care unit has not been clearly demonstrated. In some patients with respiratory failure, however, measurement of expired gas Pe_{CO_2} concentration is useful for calculation of the dead space fraction. Measurements of the dead space fraction can be used to assess the physiologic basis for respiratory failure. Physiologic dead space may be elevated in patients with pulmonary vascular disease, chronic obstructive lung disease, necrotizing pneumonitis, or the ARDS. A dead space fraction greater than 0.55 often correlates with major difficulty in weaning a patient from mechanical ventilation because the required minute ventilation and work of breathing are excessive.

Measurement of CO_2 production can also be useful in determining an etiology for persistent hypercapnic respiratory failure. For example, elevated CO_2 production has been associated with excessive caloric and carbohydrate nutritional therapy, thus making it difficult for the patient to be weaned from mechanical ventilation (123).

Monitoring of arterial oxygen and carbon dioxide tensions can be most accurately accomplished with direct arterial blood gas sampling. There are indwelling catheter electrodes now available for continuous intraarterial measurement of Pa_{O_2}, Pa_{CO_2}, and pH. They have some technical limitations, and their superiority over more conventional periodic blood sampling from an indwelling arterial line has not been proved. In addition, there is a fiberoptic pulmonary artery catheter for continuous measurement of oxyhemoglobin saturation in the mixed venous blood. The clinical value of these devices remains to be definitively established (124).

Transcutaneous PO_2 and PCO_2 measurements are noninvasive methods that use heated skin electrodes and provide indirect reflections of Pa_{O_2} and Pa_{CO_2}. They have been useful in infants but are not as clinically valuable in adults. A more useful noninvasive approach is pulse oximetry, which measures oxygen saturation in arterialized blood in a finger tip (125). Pulse oximetry is an advance from the prior technique of using ear oximetry, which required preparation of the site and calibration. Pulse oximetry, unlike transcutaneous PO_2 and PCO_2 measurements, does not require skin preparation or rotation to a new site. Under conditions of poor perfusion from local vasoconstriction or a low cardiac output, both methods may become inaccurate (126). The pulse oximeter can be very useful, particularly when weaning patients from mechanical ventilation, evaluating oxygen saturation during sleep, and performing procedures such as bronchoscopy and gastroscopy. Monitoring of pulmonary and systemic hemodynamics may be important in some patients with acute respiratory failure and hemodynamic instability (127). This issue is covered elsewhere in this volume.

REFERENCES

1. Wasserman K. Exercise testing in the dyspneic patient. The chairman's postconference reflections. *Am Rev Resp Dis* 1984; 129(Suppl):1–2.
2. McFadden ER, Kiser R, De Groot WJ. Acute bronchial asthma: relations between clinical and physiologic manifestations. *N Engl J Med* 1973;288:221–225.
3. Leventhal JM. Clinical predictors of pneumonia as a guide to ordering chest roentgenograms. *Clin Pediatr* 1982;21:730–734.
4. Rebuck AS, Pengelly LD. Development of pulsus paradoxus in the presence of airways obstruction. *N Engl J Med* 1973;288: 66–69.
5. Connors AF Jr, McCaffree DR, Gray BA. Evaluation of right-heart catheterization in the critically ill patient without acute myocardial infarction. *N Engl J Med* 1983;308:263–267.
6. Brackett NC Jr, Wingo CF, Muren O, et al. Acid-base response to chronic hypercapnia in man. *N Engl J Med* 1969;280: 124–130.
7. Sperelakis N. Pathophysiology of skeletal muscle and effect of some hormones. In Roussos C, Macklem PT, eds. *The thorax.* New York: Marcel Dekker, 1985:115–140.
8. Newman JH, Neff TA, Zipporin P. Acute respiratory failure associated with hypophosphatemia. *N Engl J Med* 1977;296: 1101–1103.
9. Mellemgaard K. The alveolar-arterial oxygen difference: its size and components in normal man. *Acta Physiol Scand* 1967;67: 10–20.
10. Brackett NC Jr, Cohen JJ, Schwartz WB. Carbon dioxide titration curve of normal man. Effect of increasing degrees of acute hypercapnia on acid-base equilibrium. *N Engl J Med* 1965;272: 6–12.
11. Appel D, Rubenstein R, Schrager K, et al. Lactic acidosis in severe asthma. *Am J Med* 1983;75:580–584.
12. Kilburn KH. Shock, seizures and coma with alkalosis during mechanical ventilation. *Ann Int Med* 1966;66:977–984.
13. Ketty SS, Schmidt CF. The effects of altered arterial tensions of carbon dioxide and oxygen on cerebral blood flow and cerebral oxygen consumption of normal young men. *J Clin Invest* 1948; 27:484–492.
14. Rebuck AS, Read J. Assessment and management of severe asthma. *Am J Med* 1971;51:788–798.
15. O'Donohue WJ Jr, Baker JP. Controlled low-flow oxygen in the management of acute respiratory failure. *Chest* 1973;63: 818–821.
16. McCulloch TM, Bishop MJ. Complications of translaryngeal intubation. *Clin Chest Med* 1991;12:507–521.
17. Jasmer RM, Luce JM, Matthay MA. Noninvasive positive pressure ventilation for acute respiratory failure: underutilized or overrated? *Chest* 1997;111:1672–1678.
18. Baumel MJ, Schwab RJ, Collman RG. Noninvasive ventilation for exacerbations of chronic obstructive pulmonary disease. *N Engl J Med* 1996;334:735–736.
19. Meduri GU, Turner RE, Abou-Shala N, et al. Noninvasive positive pressure ventilation via face mask. First-line intervention in patients with acute hypercapnic and hypoxemic respiratory failure. *Chest* 1996;109:179–193.
20. Chevrolet JC, Jolliet P, Abajo B, et al. Nasal positive pressure ventilation in patients with acute respiratory failure. Difficult and time-consuming procedure for nurses. *Chest* 1991;100: 775–782.
21. Patrick W, Webster K, Ludwig L, et al. Noninvasive positive-pressure ventilation in acute respiratory distress without prior chronic respiratory failure. *Am J Respir Crit Care Med* 1996; 153:1005–1011.
22. Brochard L, Isabey D, Piquet J, et al. Reversal of acute exacerbations of chronic obstructive lung disease by inspiratory assistance with a face mask. *N Engl J Med* 1990;323:1523–1530.
23. Pennock BE, Crawshaw L, Kaplan PD. Noninvasive nasal mask ventilation for acute respiratory failure. Institution of a new therapeutic technology for routine use. *Chest* 1994;105: 441–444.
24. Meduri GU, Conoscenti CC, Menashe P, et al. Noninvasive face mask ventilation in patients with acute respiratory failure. *Chest* 1989;95:865–870.
25. Meduri GU, Abou-Shala N, Fox RC, et al. Noninvasive face mask mechanical ventilation in patients with acute hypercapnic respiratory failure. *Chest* 1991;100:445–454.
26. Benhamou D, Girault C, Faure C, et al. Nasal mask ventilation in acute respiratory failure. Experience in elderly patients. *Chest* 1992;102:912–917.
27. Marino W. Intermittent volume cycled mechanical ventilation via nasal mask in patients with respiratory failure due to COPD. *Chest* 1991;99:681–684.
28. Vitacca F, Rubini K, Foglio S, et al. Non-invasive modalities of positive pressure ventilation. *Int Care Med* 1993;19:450–455.
29. Carrey Z, Gottfried SB, Levy RD. Ventilatory muscle support in respiratory failure with nasal positive pressure ventilation. *Chest* 1990;97:150–158.
30. Criner GJ, Travaline JM, Brennan KJ, et al. Efficacy of a new full face mask for noninvasive positive pressure ventilation. *Chest* 1994;106:1109–1115.
31. Sullivan CE, Issa FG, Berthon-Jones M, et al. Reversal of obstructive sleep apnoea by continuous positive airway pressure applied through the nares. *Lancet* 1981;1:862–865.
32. DiMarco AF, Connors AF, Altose MD. Management of chronic alveolar hypoventilation with nasal positive pressure breathing. *Chest* 1987;92:952–954.
33. Ellis ER, Grunstein RR, Chan S, et al. Noninvasive ventilatory support during sleep improves respiratory failure in kyphoscoliosis. *Chest* 1988;94:811–815.
34. Goldstein RS, Molotiu N, Skrastins R, et al. Reversal of sleep-induced hypoventilation and chronic respiratory failure by nocturnal negative pressure ventilation in patients with restrictive ventilatory impairment. *Am Rev Respir Dis* 1987;135: 1049–1055.
35. Bach JR, Alba A, Mosher R, et al. Intermittent positive pressure ventilation via nasal access in the management of respiratory insufficiency. *Chest* 1987;92:168–170.
36. Carroll N, Branthwaite MA. Control of nocturnal hypoventilation by nasal intermittent positive pressure ventilation. *Thorax* 1988;43:349–353.
37. Bach JR, Alba AS. Management of chronic alveolar hypoventilation by nasal ventilation. *Chest* 1990;97:52–57.
38. Kerby GR, Mayer LS, Pingleton SK. Nocturnal positive pressure

ventilation via nasal mask. *Am Rev Respir Dis* 1987;135: 738–740.

39. Leger P, Jennequin J, Gerard M, et al. Home positive pressure ventilation via nasal mask for patients with neuromusculoskeletal disorders. *Eur Respir J* 1989;7(Suppl):640s–644s.

40. Waldhorn RE. Nocturnal nasal intermittent positive pressure ventilation with bi-level positive airway pressure (BiPAP) in respiratory failure. *Chest* 1992;101:516–521.

41. Bott J, Carroll MP, Conway JH, et al. Randomised controlled trial of nasal ventilation in acute ventilatory failure due to chronic obstructive airways disease. *Lancet* 1993;341: 1555–1557.

42. Brochard L, Mancebo J, Wysocki M, et al. Noninvasive ventilation for acute exacerbations of chronic obstructive pulmonary disease. *N Engl J Med* 1995;333:817–822.

43. Antonelli M, Conti G, Rocco M, et al. A comparison of noninvasive positive-pressure ventilation and conventional mechanical ventilation in patients with acute respiratory failure. *N Engl J Med* 1998;339:429–435.

43a. Antonelli M, Conti G, Bufi M, et al. Noninvasive ventilation for treatment of acute respiratory failure in patients undergoing solid organ transplantation: a randomized trial. *JAMA* 2000; 283:235–241.

44. Kramer N, Meyer TJ, Meharg J, et al. Randomized, prospective trial of noninvasive positive pressure ventilation in acute respiratory failure. *Am J Respir Crit Care Med* 1995;151:1799–1806.

45. Mehta S, Jay GD, Woolard RH, et al. Randomized, prospective trial of bilevel versus continuous positive airway pressure in acute pulmonary edema. *Crit Care Med* 1997;25:620–628.

46. Wood KA, Lewis L, Von Harz B, et al. The use of noninvasive positive pressure ventilation in the emergency department: results of a randomized clinical trial. *Chest* 1998;113:1339–1346.

47. Wysocki M, Tric L, Wolff MA, et al. Noninvasive pressure support ventilation in patients with acute respiratory failure. A randomized comparison with conventional therapy. *Chest* 1995; 107:761–768.

48. Ambrosino N, Foglio K, Rubini F, et al. Non-invasive mechanical ventilation in acute respiratory failure due to chronic obstructive pulmonary disease: correlates for success. *Thorax* 1995; 50:755–757.

48a. Anton A, Gruell R, Gomez J, et al. Predicting the result of noninvasive ventilation in severe acute exacerbations of patients with chronic air flow limitation. *Chest* 2000;112:828–833.

49. Appendini L, Patessio A, Zanaboni S, et al. Physiologic effects of positive end-expiratory pressure and mask pressure support during exacerbations of chronic obstructive pulmonary disease. *Am J Respir Crit Care Med* 1994;149:1069–1076.

50. Diaz O, Iglesia R, Ferrer M, et al. Effects of noninvasive ventilation on pulmonary gas exchange and hemodynamics during acute hypercapnic exacerbations of chronic obstructive pulmonary disease. *Am J Respir Crit Care Med* 1997;156:1840–1845.

51. Aldrich TK, Hendler JM, Vizioli LD, et al. Intrinsic positive end-expiratory pressure in ambulatory patients with airways obstruction. *Am Rev Respir Dis* 1993;147:845–849.

52. Bach A, Boehrer H, Schmidt H, et al. Nosocomial sinusitis in ventilated patients. Nasotracheal versus orotracheal intubation. *Anaesthesia* 1992;47:335–339.

53. Depoix JP, Malbezin S, Videcoq M, et al. Oral intubation v. nasal intubation in adult cardiac surgery. *Br J Anaes* 1987;59: 167–169.

54. Schwartz D, Matthay M, Cohen N. Death and other complications of mechanical ventilation. *Anesthesiology* 1995;82: 367–376.

55. Stauffer J, Silvestri R. Complications of endotracheal intubation, tracheostomy and artificial airways. *Respir Care* 1982;27: 417–434.

56. Maziak DE, Meade MO, Todd TR. The timing of tracheotomy: a systematic review. *Chest* 1998;114:605–609.

57. Heffner J, Miller K, Sahn S. Tracheostomy in the intensive care unit. *Chest* 1986;90:269–274, 430–436.

58. Stoeckli SJ, Breitbach T, Schmid S. A clinical and histologic comparison of percutaneous dilational versus conventional surgical tracheostomy. *Laryngoscope* 1997;107:1643–1646.

59. Petros S, Engelmann L. Percutaneous dilatational tracheostomy in a medical ICU. *Int Care Med* 1997;23:630–634.

60. Van Natta TL, Morris JA Jr, Eddy VA, et al. Elective bedside surgery in critically injured patients is safe and cost-effective. *Ann Surgery* 1998;227:24–26, 618–624.

61. van Heurn LW, Goei R, de Ploeg I, et al. Late complications of percutaneous dilatational tracheotomy. *Chest* 1996;110: 1572–1576.

62. Kollef MH, Shapiro SD, Fraser VJ, et al. Mechanical ventilation with or without 7-day circuit changes. A randomized controlled trial. *Annals of Internal Medicine* 1995;123:168–174.

63. Kollef MH, Prentice D, Shapiro SD, et al. Mechanical ventilation with or without daily changes of in-line suction catheters. *Am J Respir Crit Care Med* 1997;156:466–472.

64. Fink JB, Krause SA, Barrett L, et al. Extending ventilator circuit change interval beyond 2 days reduces the likelihood of ventilator-associated pneumonia. *Chest* 1998;113:405–411.

65. Esteban A, Alia I, Ibanez J, et al. Modes of mechanical ventilation and weaning. A national survey of Spanish hospitals. The Spanish Lung Failure Collaborative Group. *Chest* 1994;106: 1188–1193.

66. Shelledy DC, Rau JL, Thomas-Goodfellow L. A comparison of the effects of assist-control, SIMV, and SIMV with pressure support on ventilation, oxygen consumption, and ventilatory equivalent. *Heart Lung* 1995;24:67–75.

67. Hudson LD, Hurlow RS, Craig KC, et al. Does intermittent mandatory ventilation correct respiratory alkalosis in patients receiving assisted mechanical ventilation? *Am Rev Respir Dis* 1985;132:1071–1074.

68. Leung P, Jubran A, Tobin MJ. Comparison of assisted ventilator modes on triggering, patient effort, and dyspnea. *Am J Respir Crit Care Med* 1997;155:1940–1948.

69. Armstrong BW Jr, MacIntyre NR. Pressure-controlled, inverse ratio ventilation that avoids air trapping in the adult respiratory distress syndrome. *Crit Care Med* 1995;23:279–285.

70. Mercat A, Titiriga M, Anguel N, et al. Inverse ratio ventilation (I/E = 2/1) in acute respiratory distress syndrome: a six-hour controlled study. *Am J Respir Crit Care Med* 1997;155: 1637–1642.

71. Lessard MR, Guerot E, Lorino H, et al. Effects of pressure-controlled with different I:E ratios versus volume-controlled ventilation on respiratory mechanics, gas exchange, and hemodynamics in patients with adult respiratory distress syndrome. *Anesthesiology* 1994;80:983–991.

72. Dekel B, Segal E, Perel A. Pressure support ventilation. *Arch Int Med* 1996;156:369–373.

73. Tuxen DV. Detrimental effects of positive end-expiratory pressure during controlled mechanical ventilation of patients with severe airflow obstruction. *Am Rev Respir Dis* 1989;140:5–9.

74. Ranieri VM, Giuliani R, Cinnella G, et al. Physiologic effects of positive end-expiratory pressure in patients with chronic obstructive pulmonary disease during acute ventilatory failure and controlled mechanical ventilation. *Am Rev Respir Dis* 1993;147: 5–13.

75. Guerin C, LeMasson S, de Varax R, et al. Small airway closure and positive end-expiratory pressure in mechanically ventilated patients with chronic obstructive pulmonary disease. *Am J Respir Crit Care Med* 1997;155:1949–1956.

76. MacIntyre NR, Cheng KC, McConnell R. Applied PEEP dur-

ing pressure support reduces the inspiratory threshold load of intrinsic PEEP. *Chest* 1997;111:188–193.

77. Huemer G, Kolev N, Kurz A, et al. Influence of positive end-expiratory pressure on right and left ventricular performance assessed by Doppler two-dimensional echocardiography. *Chest* 1994;106:67–73.

78. Cheatham ML, Nelson LD, Chang MC, et al. Right ventricular end-diastolic volume index as a predictor of preload status in patients on positive end-expiratory pressure (see comments). *Crit Care Med* 1998;26:1801–1806.

79. Schuster S, Erbel R, Weilemann LS, et al. Hemodynamics during PEEP ventilation in patients with severe left ventricular failure studied by transesophageal echocardiography. *Chest* 1990;97:1181–1189.

80. Jardin F, Brun-Ney D, Hardy A, et al. Combined thermodilution and two-dimensional echocardiographic evaluation of right ventricular function during respiratory support with PEEP. *Chest* 1991;99:162–168.

81. Dhainaut JF, Bricard C, Monsallier FJ, et al. Left ventricular contractility using isovolumic phase indices during PEEP in ARDS patients. *Crit Care Med* 1982;10:631–635.

82. Tuxen DV, Williams TJ, Scheinkestel CD, et al. Use of a measurement of pulmonary hyperinflation to control the level of mechanical ventilation in patients with acute severe asthma. *Am Rev Respir Dis* 1992;146:1136–1142.

83. Darioli R, Perret C. Mechanical controlled hypoventilation in status asthmaticus. *Am Rev Respir Dis* 1984;129:385–387.

84. Williams TJ, Tuxen DV, Scheinkestel CD, et al. Risk factors for morbidity in mechanically ventilated patients with acute severe asthma. *Am Rev Respir Dis* 1992;146:607–615.

85. Alvarez A, Subirana M, Benito S. Decelerating flow ventilation effects in acute respiratory failure. *J Crit Care* 1998;13:21–25.

86. Piotrowski A, Sobala W, Kawczynski P. Patient-initiated, pressure-regulated, volume-controlled ventilation compared with intermittent mandatory ventilation in neonates: a prospective, randomised study. *Int Care Med* 1997;23:975–981.

87. Younes M, Puddy A, Roberts D, et al. Proportional assist ventilation. Results of an initial clinical trial. *Am Rev Respir Dis* 1992;145:121–129.

88. Cane RD, Peruzzi WT, Shapiro BA. Airway pressure release ventilation in severe acute respiratory failure. *Chest* 1991;100:460–463.

89. Davis K Jr, Johnson DJ, Branson RD, et al. Airway pressure release ventilation. *Arch Surg* 1993;128:1348–1352.

90. Abu-Dbai J, Flatau E, Lev A, et al. The use of conventional ventilators for high frequency positive pressure ventilation. *Crit Care Med* 1983;11:356–358.

91. El-Baz N, Faber LP, Doolas A. Combined high-frequency ventilation for management of terminal respiratory failure: a new technique. *Anesthesia Analgesia* 1983;62:39–49.

92. Gerstmann DR, Minton SD, Stoddard RA, et al. The Provo multicenter early high-frequency oscillatory ventilation trial: improved pulmonary and clinical outcome in respiratory distress syndrome. *Pediatrics* 1996;98:1044–1057.

93. Rettwitz-Volk W, Veldman A, Roth B, et al. A prospective, randomized, multicenter trial of high-frequency oscillatory ventilation compared with conventional ventilation in preterm infants with respiratory distress syndrome receiving surfactant. *J Pediatr* 1998;132:249–254.

94. Keszler M, Modanlou HD, Brudno DS, et al. Multicenter controlled clinical trial of high-frequency jet ventilation in preterm infants with uncomplicated respiratory distress syndrome. *Pediatrics* 1997;100:593–599.

95. Schuster DP, Klain M, Snyder JV. Comparison of high frequency jet ventilation to conventional ventilation during severe acute respiratory failure in humans. *Crit Care Med* 1982;10:625–630.

96. Valta P, Corbeil C, Chasse M, et al. Mean airway pressure as an index of mean alveolar pressure. *Am J Respir Crit Care Med* 1996;153:1825–1830.

97. Esteban I, Alia M, Tobin J et al. Effect of spontaneous breathing trial duration on outcome of attempts to discontinue mechanical ventilation. Spanish Lung Failure Collaborative Group. *Am J Respir Crit Care Med* 1999;159:512–518.

98. Esteban A, Alia I, Gordo F, et al. Extubation outcome after spontaneous breathing trials with T-tube or pressure support ventilation. The Spanish Lung Failure Collaborative Group. [Published erratum appears in *Am J Respir Crit Care Med* 1997; 156(6):2028.] *Am J Respir Crit Care Med* 1997;156:459–465.

99. Yang KL, Tobin MJ. A prospective study of indexes predicting the outcome of trials of weaning from mechanical ventilation. *N Engl J Med* 1991;324:1445–1450.

100. Epstein SK. Etiology of extubation failure and the predictive value of the rapid shallow breathing index. *Am J Respir Crit Care Med* 1995;152:545–549.

101. Vassilakopoulos S, Zakynthinos S, Roussos C. The tension-time index and the frequency-tidal volume ratio are the major pathophysiologic determinants of weaning failure and success. *Am J Respir Crit Care Med* 1998;158:378–385.

102. Kelly BJ, Matthay MA. Prevalence and severity of neurologic dysfunction in critically ill patients. *Chest* 1993;104:1818–1824.

103. Jubran A, Mathru M, Dries D, et al. Continuous recordings of mixed venous oxygen saturation during weaning from mechanical ventilation and the ramifications thereof. *Am J Respir Crit Care Med* 1998;158:1763–1769.

104. Bouley H, Froman R, Shah H. The experience of dyspnea during weaning. *Heart Lung* 1992;21:471–476.

105. Brochard L, Rauss A, Benito S, et al. Comparison of three methods of gradual withdrawal from ventilatory support during weaning from mechanical ventilation. *Am J Respir Crit Care Med* 1994;150:896–903.

106. MacIntyre NR. Respiratory function during pressure support ventilation. *Chest* 1986;89:677–683.

107. Knebel R, Janson-Bjerklie SL, Malley JD, et al. Comparison of breathing comfort during weaning with two ventilatory modes. *Am J Respir Crit Care Med* 1994;149:14–18.

108. Esteban A, Frutos F, Tobin MJ, et al. A comparison of four methods of weaning patients from mechanical ventilation. Spanish Lung Failure Collaborative Group. *N Engl J Med* 1995; 332:345–350.

109. Robertson J, Hamilton PA. Randomised trial of elective continuous positive airway pressure (CPAP) compared with rescue CPAP after extubation. *Arch Dis Child Fetal Neonatal Ed* 1998; 79:F58–60.

110. Petrof J, Legare M, Goldberg P, et al. Continuous positive airway pressure reduces work of breathing and dyspnea during weaning from mechanical ventilation in severe chronic obstructive pulmonary disease. *Am Rev Respir Dis* 1990;141:281–289.

111. Appendini L, Purro A, Patessio A, et al. Partitioning of inspiratory muscle workload and pressure assistance in ventilator-dependent COPD patients. *Am J Respir Crit Care Med* 1996;154:1301–1309.

112. Bailey R, Jones RM, Kelleher AA. The role of continuous positive airway pressure during weaning from mechanical ventilation in cardiac surgical patients. *Anaesthesia* 1995;50:677–681.

113. Sassoon S, Del Rosario N, Fei R, et al. Influence of pressure- and flow-triggered synchronous intermittent mandatory ventila-

tion on inspiratory muscle work. *Crit Care Med* 1994;22: 1933–1941.

114. Kollef H, Shapiro SD, Silver P, et al. A randomized, controlled trial of protocol-directed versus physician-directed weaning from mechanical ventilation. *Crit Care Med* 1997;25:567–574.

115. Ely W, Baker AM, Dunagan DP, et al. Effect on the duration of mechanical ventilation of identifying patients capable of breathing spontaneously. *N Engl J Med* 1996;335:1864–1869.

116. Sackner JD, Nixon AJ, Davis B, et al. Noninvasive measurement of ventilation during exercise using a respiratory inductive plethysmograph. *Am Rev Respir Dis* 1981;122:867–871.

117. Dantzker DR, Tobin MJ. Monitoring respiratory muscle function. *Respir Care* 1985;30:422–431.

118. Roussos CS, Macklem PT. Diaphragmatic fatigue in man. *J Appl Physiol* 1977;43:189–197.

119. Cohen CA, Zagelbaum G, Gross D, et al. Clinical manifestations of inspiratory muscle fatigue. *Am J Med* 1982;73: 308–316.

120. Bone RC. Monitoring ventilatory mechanics in acute respiratory failure. *Respir Care* 1983;28:597–604.

121. Gottfried SB, Higgs BD, Rossi A, et al. Interrupter technique for measurement of respiratory mechanics in anesthetized humans. *J Appl Physiol* 1985;59:647–652.

122. Marini JJ, Rodriguez RM, Lamb V. Bedside elimination of the inspiratory work of breathing during mechanical ventilation. *Chest* 1986;89:56–63.

123. Pierson DJ. Weaning from mechanical ventilation in acute respiratory failure: concepts, indications, and techniques. *Respir Care* 1983;28:646–662.

124. Boutros AR, Lee C. Value of continuous monitoring of mixed venous blood oxygen saturation in the management of critically ill patients. *Crit Care Med* 1986;14:132–135.

125. Fanconi S, Doherty P, Edmonds J, et al. Pulse oximetry in pediatric intensive care comparison with measure saturations and transcutaneous oxygen tension. *J Pediatr* 1985;107: 362–366.

126. Barker SJ, Tremper KK, Gamel DM. A clinical comparison of transcutaneous P_{O_2} and pulse oximetry in the operating room. *Anesth Analg* 1986;65:805–808.

127. Matthay MA, Chatterjee K. Bedside pulmonary artery catheterization. *Ann Intern Med* 1988;109:826–834.

ACUTE HYPERCAPNIC RESPIRATORY FAILURE: NEUROMUSCULAR AND OBSTRUCTIVE DISEASES

MICHAEL A. MATTHAY
KAMRAN ATABAI

NEUROMUSCULAR ETIOLOGIES OF RESPIRATORY FAILURE

DRUG OVERDOSES

CHEST WALL ABNORMALITIES AS A CAUSE OF ACUTE RESPIRATORY FAILURE

UPPER AIRWAY OBSTRUCTION

CHRONIC OBSTRUCTIVE AIRWAYS DISEASE

RESPIRATORY FAILURE IN ASTHMA

This chapter considers the causes of acute respiratory failure that are primarily associated with inadequate alveolar ventilation, which often results in arterial hypercapnia and acute respiratory acidosis. These patients usually have abnormal oxygenation because of ventilation and perfusion mismatch in the lung. However, the primary cause of respiratory failure is usually associated with inadequate alveolar ventilation and carbon dioxide excretion, either from: (*a*) inadequate central ventilatory drive; (*b*) insufficient neuromuscular transmission of the respiratory drive; or (*c*) lung disease with obstructive airway disease and the need for a high work of breathing.

NEUROMUSCULAR ETIOLOGIES OF RESPIRATORY FAILURE

There are numerous causes of acute respiratory failure from neuromuscular disorders. These include the Guillain-Barré syndrome, myasthenia gravis, botulism, poliomyelitis, heavy metal intoxication, organic phosphate poisoning, and, rarely, administration of aminoglycoside antibiotics. Severe electrolyte disorders such as hypokalemia and hypophosphatemia may also be associated with muscle weakness sufficient to cause or worsen acute respiratory failure. Respiratory failure also may be worsened by the use of neuromuscular blocking agents in critically ill patients (1). There are, of course, a variety of congenital and acquired neuromuscular diseases that may be associated with progressive respiratory failure. Acute respiratory failure may also follow injury to the spinal cord, if the lesion is at a high enough level to affect function of the phrenic nerve (2).

Acute respiratory failure is the most life-threatening complication of the Guillain-Barré syndrome. In most large series, approximately 20% to 37% of patients with Guillain-Barré syndrome require mechanical ventilation (3,4). The average duration of mechanical ventilation is 4 to 6 weeks but the range is quite variable (7 days to 93 days in one series) (3,4,4a). Characteristically, patients who require mechanical ventilation have a forced vital capacity less than 4 to 5 mL/kg body weight, are progressively unable to handle oral secretions, have a poor cough, and develop hypoventilation. In addition, lobar atelectasis and pneumonia may occur (3,5). The basic pathophysiology stems from a combination of inadequate neuromuscular strength leading to alveolar hypoventilation, low tidal volume breathing, and diffuse atelectasis. Although this form of acute respiratory failure can be classified as primarily hypercapnic respiratory failure, it is frequently accompanied by a widened alveolar-arterial oxygen gradient secondary to atelectasis and pneumonia.

Patients who develop Guillain-Barré syndrome should be closely monitored with frequent measurements of vital capacity, arterial blood gases, and careful clinical evaluation of their ability to cough and protect their airway. Initial monitoring in a critical care unit is usually desirable so that immediate respiratory support can be provided if the patient's respiratory status deteriorates. Treatment for Guillain-Barré syndrome has been mainly supportive with mechanical ventilation, intravenous fluids, and nutritional support. In addition, the use of prophylactic subcutaneous heparin is recommended (3). Careful attention to psychosocial issues is very important in managing Guillain-Barré patients in the intensive care unit (5,6).

A prospective controlled study of 245 patients reported that plasmapheresis was superior to conventional, supportive therapy in hastening recovery of muscle strength (7). If plasmapheresis was started before the patient required mechanical ventilation, the median time on the ventilator was 9 days versus 23 days in the control group. There was less clear-cut benefit of plasmapheresis in shortening the duration of mechanical ventilation if the patient already required ventilation. Although the study was not blinded, the basic beneficial effects of plasmapheresis in this syndrome seem to have been well established (8). Presumably, the process of plasmapheresis removes a circulating factor from the plasma that is important in the pathogenesis of acute paralysis. Intravenous immunoglobulin therapy provides a less cumbersome, more accessible alternative to plasmapheresis, although the possibility of a higher relapse rate has been raised (9). A recent randomized trial of 150 patients compared the benefits of plasmapheresis and intravenous immunoglobulin. At 4 weeks, the intravenous immunoglobulin group had more improvement in functional class (53% versus 34%), with shorter time to improvement (27 versus 41 days), less need for intubation (27% versus 41%), and less time on mechanical ventilation (15 versus 22 days) (10). A trial comparing intravenous immunoglobulin, plasmapheresis, or plasmapheresis followed by intravenous immunoglobulin, found no significant difference at 4 weeks in ventilatory dependence, disability grade improvement, or time required for independent walking in the three study arms (11). Several smaller studies have reported favorable

results with combined treatment modalities such as selective immunoglobulin adsorption followed by extracorporeal elimination or intravenous immunoglobulin combined with high-dose methylprednisolone (9).

Myasthenia gravis may result in acute respiratory failure at any time during the clinical course of the disease. Some patients present with acute respiratory failure, others develop respiratory failure at some point during the course of their illness, whereas other patients may develop the need for mechanical ventilation following thymectomy. The muscle weakness caused by the disease results in a decrease in vital capacity and consequent inadequate alveolar ventilation with the associated risks of atelectasis and secondary pneumonia. Frequent monitoring of the vital capacity is useful, but should not substitute for clinical evaluation of the patient's degree of weakness and ability to protect the airway, as well as measurement of arterial blood gases. In trying to assess the need for postoperative mechanical ventilation in patients undergoing thymectomy, investigators in one study found that four risk factors were particularly helpful in predicting the need for mechanical ventilation: duration of myasthenia gravis, history of chronic respiratory disease, pyridostigmine dosage greater than 750 mg per day, and a preoperative vital capacity of less than 2.9 L (12). Management of patients who require mechanical ventilation with myasthenia gravis is primarily supportive unless the respiratory failure is complicated by secondary pneumonia. Treatment with anticholinesterase agents are useful for improving muscle strength. Corticosteroids and plasmapheresis have been effective in treating acute exacerbations in many patients with myasthenia gravis (13,14). In the only trial comparing intravenous immunoglobulin therapy with plasmapharesis in the treatment of 87 patients with

TABLE 22.1. CLINICAL DESCRIPTION OF RESPIRATORY FAILURE IN DERANGEMENTS OF THE THORAX

	Respiratory Failure		Clinical Course	Secretions, Atelectasis, Pneumonia[a]
Category	Incidence	Severity[a]		
Mechanical				
Scoliosis	Common	+++	Slow	NL+
Obesity-hypoventilation	Common	+++	Periodic	NL or ↑
Fibrothorax	Common	+++	Slow	NL
Thoracoplasty	Common	+++	Slow	NL or ↑
Ankylosing spondylitis	Rare	+	Slow	NL
Neuromascular				
Postpoliomyelitis	Common	+++	Slow	↑
Amyotrophic lateral sclerosis	Common	+++	Fast	↑
Muscular dystrophies	Common	+	Slow	↑
Spinal cord injury	Common	++	Slow	↑
Multiple sclerosis	Uncommon	+	Slow	↑
Myasthenia gravis	Common	+++	Periodic	↑

[a] +, Dyspnea on exertion; ++, dyspnea, mild hypoxemia, and hypercapnia only; +++, severe hypoventilation; NL, normal lungs; ↑, increased incidence.
Source: Bergofsky EH. Respiratory failure in disorders of the thoracic cage. *Am Rev Respir Dis* 1979; 119:643–649.

acute myasthenia gravis exacerbations, there were no significant differences in improvement in the myasthenic muscle score at day 15 between the two groups. The response to intravenous immunoglobulin, however, is slower than to therapeutic plasmapheresis (15).

The other etiologies of acute neuromuscular failure require supportive treatment similar to that described for Guillain-Barré syndrome and myasthenia gravis (Table 22.1). For patients who have a neuromuscular etiology for their acute respiratory failure, weaning from mechanical ventilation must be performed gradually.

Unilateral or bilateral impairment of diaphragm function may also lead to acute respiratory failure (17). The diaphragm is the principal muscle of inspiration, being almost totally responsible for inspiration during quiet breathing. Weakness or paralysis of both hemidiaphragms is most likely to be associated with chronic neuromuscular disease, but it may also occur as an isolated abnormality and with spinal cord trauma. In addition, the phrenic nerves may be interrupted inadvertently during surgical procedures in the neck or thorax such as coronary artery bypass (18). Clinically, paradoxical or inward movement of the abdominal wall during spontaneous inspiration in the supine posture may be overlooked, and it is therefore necessary to use fluoroscopy or ultrasound to demonstrate paradoxical movement of the diaphragm with spontaneous inspiration. Additional evaluation with transdiaphragmatic pressure measurements and phrenic nerve conduction studies may be necessary (19). Ventilatory support by pacing of the diaphragm has been used in a number of patients with trauma or infarction of the cervical cord above C2 when it was certain that the lower motor neurons of the phrenic nerve were viable (19).

DRUG OVERDOSES

Drug overdoses are a common cause of acute respiratory failure, usually through direct depression of respiratory drive. Cardiopulmonary complications of drug overdose occur commonly and may include hypotension, arrhythmias, and central nervous system (CNS) dysfunction, including status epilepticus. This section focuses primarily on acute respiratory failure that may occur in drug-overdosed patients.

Overdoses with narcotics and sedative hypnotics may result in the need for mechanical ventilation. Most patients who require intubation and mechanical ventilation from drug overdoses do not develop primary pulmonary complications. Their need for mechanical ventilation is usually related to a depression of central ventilatory drive, which recovers as the drug is removed from the circulation. The decision to intubate and ventilate patients with drug overdose is based on clinical evaluation of the patient including mental status, hemodynamic stability, and the ability of the

patient to protect the airway. As a general rule, it is preferable to intubate patients with known drug overdoses who have a decrease in mental function, even if their arterial blood gases remain acceptable.

Acute respiratory failure secondary to intrinsic lung disease does occur in some patients following drug overdose and may become the primary clinical problem in the management of the patient (20). Certain drugs have been specifically implicated as causing acute lung injury, presumably through a direct toxic effect on the lung parenchyma. In patients overdosed on these drugs, pulmonary edema may occur from an increase in lung vascular permeability, resulting in protein-rich edema fluid collecting in the interstitium and air spaces of the lung, even in the absence of elevated pulmonary microvascular pressures. In many of these cases the lung injury is further complicated by gastric aspiration leading to diffuse and severe lung injury with secondary pulmonary and pleural space infections (21).

Heroin is one of the most common drugs implicated in acute respiratory failure and causes both direct suppression of central respiratory drive and intrinsic lung damage. Heroin and other narcotics can cause noncardiogenic pulmonary edema. The pathophysiology of narcotic-induced pulmonary edema is not well established. Possible mechanisms include a direct toxic effect, an acute hypoxic insult to the alveolar capillary membrane, an allergic/hypersensitivity response, or a neurogenic response to a CNS insult. Heroin overdose is complicated by gastric aspiration in up to one-half of cases (22).

Tricyclic antidepressants are another common cause of drug overdoses and can cause severe pulmonary complications. Tricyclics can induce both cardiogenic and noncardiogenic pulmonary edema, as well aspiration induced lung injury (23). In one large series examining 82 consecutive patients with tricyclic overdose, 80% had a widened alveolar-arterial oxygen difference at initial presentation, 75% required mechanical ventilation for an average of 46 hours, and 25% had evidence of aspiration of activated charcoal. Forty percent of these patients developed abnormal chest radiographs within 48 hours. The severity of the chest radiograph abnormality correlated with the mean blood levels of tricyclics (20). Both chronic and acute ingestions of salicylates can cause noncardiogenic pulmonary resulting in acute respiratory failure (24). In addition, aspirin-sensitive asthmatics may suffer acute respiratory failure and death from aggravated bronchospasm secondary to aspirin ingestion (25).

The management of the patient with drug overdose begins with the collection of any clues as to specific drug and dose ingested. In general, the patient's history of specific ingested drugs may not be reliable. Medication containers and samples of drugs or substances, if they can be obtained, are helpful in the emergency department. Gastric contents, urine, and blood may also be collected for toxicologic examination. Initial treatment of the drug overdose patient in the emergency room includes attempts to remove any unabsorbed drug with emesis or gastric lavage. Activated charcoal can be used to bind and prevent absorption of some drugs that were not removed by emesis or by lavage, as well as helping to remove some drugs that undergo intrahepatic recirculation. Further discussion of these issues is available in other texts (26). Definitive management of drug-induced respiratory failure is primarily supportive, with meticulous attention to secondary complications of infection and mechanical ventilation.

CHEST WALL ABNORMALITIES AS A CAUSE OF ACUTE RESPIRATORY FAILURE

Traumatic injury to the chest wall with subsequent rib fractures is the most frequent cause of acute respiratory failure in this category. This type of injury is usually associated with pain that prevents full lung inflation and results in atelectasis and occasionally alveolar hypoventilation. If multiple ribs are fractured in multiple locations, lung inflation may be limited because of the loss of normal chest wall rigidity and a subsequent paradoxical motion of the involved area (flail chest). Underlying injury to the lung contributes to abnormalities of gas exchange. Some patients can be managed without intubation and mechanical ventilation, depending on the severity of their injury and associated pulmonary dysfunction, as indicated by arterial blood gas tensions (Chapter 21, General Principles of Managing the Patient with Respiratory Failure). The primary indications for placement of an endotracheal tube and mechanical ventilation are deteriorating gas exchange, particularly hypoxemia, and a requirement for large doses of narcotic agents to control pain (27).

Chronic deformities of the chest wall or marked pleural disease may also result in acute respiratory failure, although in these situations the pathophysiologic alterations are more complex than in acute injuries to the chest wall because they involve chronic parenchymal and pulmonary vascular abnormalities as well (28). These abnormalities include ventilation-perfusion mismatching owing to airway closure when lung volumes are reduced by a deformed thoracic cage, incapability to cough, malfunction or acquired defect of the respiratory center in conjunction with increased work of breathing, and excessive blood volume and fluid retention that aggravate the work of breathing and ventilation-perfusion mismatch.

Table 22.1 includes a list of clinical conditions that can best be described as mechanical causes of respiratory failure. These conditions include scoliosis, severe obesity, fibrothorax, thoracoplasty, and ankylosing spondylitis. The incidence of respiratory failure, its clinical course, and associated problems are indicated in Table 22.1 (28).

Many of the disorders that affect the chest wall are associated with chronic respiratory failure that may be accompanied by chronic alveolar hypoventilation and hypoxemia, which in turn may lead to chronic pulmonary hypertension. Thus, some patients who present with acute respiratory failure may also have associated cor pulmonale with signs and symptoms of right heart failure in association with moderate to severe pulmonary hypertension. The pulmonary hypertension may also be related to mechanical compression of portions of the pulmonary circulation. There are some data suggesting that there is a relationship between pulmonary arterial pressures and the angle of spinal deformity in patients with scoliosis (28).

Treatment for acute respiratory failure in patients with chest wall abnormalities described in Table 22.1 must be directed toward reversing hypoxemia and improving alveolar ventilation. There is some evidence that hyperinflation with positive-pressure breathing devices or incentive spirometers may be useful in improving lung inflation and oxygenation. In many cases, acute respiratory failure occurs because of the development of an associated lung infection (28).

Endotracheal intubation and mechanical ventilation may be necessary to reverse acute deteriorations in blood gases as well as to help clear pulmonary secretions. Mechanical ventilation may also be necessary in patients with the obesity-hypoventilation syndrome in whom central respiratory drive is inadequate to maintain ventilation. Treatment of right heart failure can best be accomplished by improving oxygenation. In general, digitalis has not been shown to be of benefit in right heart failure alone (28a).

There are other mechanical causes of acute respiratory failure that should be remembered. These include tension pneumothorax, severe ascites, and metabolic disorders such as hypothyroidism. In addition, chest wall or pleural abnormalities may contribute to respiratory failure in patients who have a primary pulmonary etiology for their respiratory distress. For example, patients with acute exacerbations of chronic obstructive lung disease may have their respiratory failure worsened by ascites, obesity, or an endocrine disorder such as hypothyroidism. Similarly, patients with primary chest wall or pleural disease may develop secondary parenchyma abnormalities such as pneumonia or pulmonary edema that, in the presence of their underlying chest wall abnormality, leads to acute respiratory failure. Thus, acute respiratory failure can often be attributed to multiple factors.

UPPER AIRWAY OBSTRUCTION

There are many possible causes of upper airway obstruction that may lead to acute respiratory failure and the need for emergency treatment. In children, croup and epiglottitis are the most common causes of upper airway obstruction. Acute epiglottitis also occurs in adults. In addition, upper airway obstruction may be the result of obstructing tumors in the base of the tongue, the larynx, or in the hypopharynx. Acute upper airway obstruction may also occur from aspirated liquid or food contents or any foreign object that becomes lodged in the airway. In some massively obese patients, obstruction of the upper airway may occur when the patient is supine.

Management of acute upper airway obstruction requires an understanding of the pathogenesis of the disorder. In patients who have severe carbon dioxide retention or apnea, emergency endotracheal intubation must be carried out. If oral intubation is not possible, an emergency crycothyroidotomy or tracheostomy should be done. In patients with progressive upper airway obstruction, as may occur in acute epiglottitis, a number of studies have shown that early intubation in a controlled setting with a skilled anesthesiologist present is the best treatment. In some patients with tumors causing upper airway obstruction, temporizing measures such as treatment with helium-oxygen mixtures have been reported to preclude the need for intubation while the patient is receiving radiation therapy, chemotherapy, and corticosteroids to reduce the size of the tumor (29). Pulmonary edema may complicate upper airway obstruction in both children and adults (30). The mechanism for the formation of pulmonary edema after upper airway obstruction and pulmonary edema has been recently elucidated. In an analysis of three cases of severe postobstructive pulmonary edema, the ratios of pulmonary edema protein to plasma total protein was on average 0.42, indicating a hydrostatic mechanism for edema fluid formation (31).

CHRONIC OBSTRUCTIVE AIRWAYS DISEASE

In contrast to disorders that primarily involve alveoli, acute respiratory failure in patients with chronic airways obstruction is characterized by an increase in arterial carbon dioxide tension as well as a mild to moderate decrease in arterial oxygenation. The pathogenesis of the hypoxemia is mainly dependent on mismatching of ventilation and perfusion (32). This is a consequence of the anatomic abnormalities described previously. In addition, superimposed conditions such as pneumonia, atelectasis, or left ventricular failure cause hypoxemia because of intrapulmonary right-to-left shunting of blood.

The mechanisms of impaired CO_2 elimination are more complex but also relate in part to mismatching of ventilation to perfusion (33). Unless there is severe airways obstruction, reductions in ventilation to some alveoli can be offset by increased ventilation to other alveoli. However, with increasing airways obstruction, this compensatory mechanism is not sufficient to cope with the overall reduction in alveolar ventilation. At least three important factors also play a role in compounding the effects of airways obstruction. First, because of the increased work of breathing in the presence of hypoxia, the respiratory muscles may become fatigued

and unable to maintain the necessary level of minute ventilation (33). Second, also related to the increased work of breathing, CO_2 production is increased (34). Finally, there may be a decrease in central ventilatory drive, partly genetic and partly acquired (35–37). Also, either hypercarbia or hypoxemia, or both, may depress central respiratory drive, thus leading to further hypoventilation. In patients with acute decompensation, administration of oxygen leads to further hypercapnia. This may be partly owing to a decrease in ventilatory drive from the loss of hypoxic stimulus, although some studies have suggested that an increase in alveolar dead space associated with oxygen therapy may be primarily responsible (38).

Chronic obstructive airways disease is generally regarded as an inexorably, albeit slowly, progressive disorder (39). Patients may have symptoms of cough and sputum production for many years. As the airways obstruction progresses, however, patients become more vulnerable to what in persons with normal lungs would be minor insults. Although acute respiratory failure may be a consequence of severe progressive airways obstruction, first episodes are generally precipitated by some complicating disorder. Most commonly, the precipitating problem is a lower respiratory tract infection, either bronchitis or pneumonia (40). The inflammation resulting from the infection, together with increased mucus production, causes further airways narrowing. If pneumonia is present, the alveolar filling causes shunting of blood and worsens lung mechanics. As a result, a vicious cycle may be initiated in which the acute process superimposed on chronic airways disease results in further increases in airways resistance, worsening of gas exchange with both increases in $PaCO_2$ and decreases in PaO_2 and increased work of breathing. As a consequence of increasing demands placed on respiratory muscles at a time when oxygen delivery is reduced, muscle fatigue ensues. The increased work of breathing also increases CO_2 production, as does fever if present, thereby presenting the lungs with an increased load of CO_2 that they are incapable of eliminating. This results in a progressively increasing $PaCO_2$ and decreasing PaO_2 unless the cycle is interrupted.

A number of other processes in addition to infection may also be involved, either alone or in combination, in producing acute respiratory failure. These include left ventricular failure, pneumothorax, pulmonary embolism, and worsening of the airways obstruction in response to inhaled irritants.

As the abnormalities of gas exchange become more severe, the function of other organs, especially the heart and CNS, may be affected. With regard to the heart, these effects may be manifested as arrhythmias, ischemia, heart failure, or actual myocardial infarction. CNS effects include alterations in behavior, reduction in level of consciousness, coma, seizures, or myoclonus. Obviously, either cardiovascular or CNS effects could have a major adverse influence on the course of respiratory failure and themselves become a part of the progressive downward spiral.

The symptoms associated with respiratory failure in patients with chronic airways obstruction usually represent an exacerbation of the baseline symptoms. Most patients with airways obstruction have cough and sputum production. Acute lower respiratory tract infections generally increase these symptoms and are often associated with an increase in the volume of sputum. However, as airways obstruction increases, the ability to clear mucus from the lungs may decrease. Thus, a report of a decrease in sputum production associated with other symptoms may also be indicative of worsening clinical status.

In some patients cardiovascular complaints may predominate. These include palpitations, orthopnea, paroxysmal nocturnal dyspnea, ankle swelling, and chest pain. Complaints related to CNS dysfunction may also be prominent. Headache, visual problems, sleep disturbances, memory loss, and behavioral alterations may be reported. In some patients these may be of sufficient severity to obscure the respiratory symptoms.

Findings on physical examination may be quite helpful and provide an important context in which to evaluate the more objective measurements, such as blood gas tensions. Of the physical findings, the general appearance of the patient is very important. A patient who appears reasonably

well and is alert and able to cooperate with therapy obviously represents quite a different management problem than the patient who is confused, combative, stuporous, or comatose, even though both patients may have the same blood gas and pH values. Alterations in behavior or level of consciousness may not be caused by the abnormal blood gas tensions per se, but could be related to drugs or other factors; however, the implications for treatment are the same. In addition to providing information concerning the lung disease per se, the physical examination should be targeted to detect disorders that may have precipitated the acute deterioration, for example, left ventricular failure. At least in the acute setting, the degree of pulsus paradoxus correlates with the severity of airways obstruction. Chest examination may or may not be helpful. Most patients with acute exacerbations of chronic airways obstruction have supraclavicular and intercostal space retractions. The chest is usually hyperinflated and tympanitic with very limited diaphragmatic excursion. Breath sounds commonly are markedly diminished. Wheezing may or may not be heard.

The chest film may simply show the classic changes of longstanding obstructive lung disease (Fig. 22.1). However, there may also be evidence for pneumonia, left ventricular failure, or pneumothorax that was not evident on physical examination. The electrocardiogram is less often helpful, but it is important if it shows right atrial or right ventricular

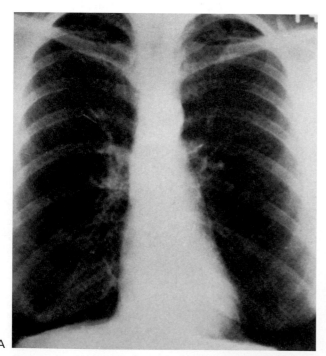
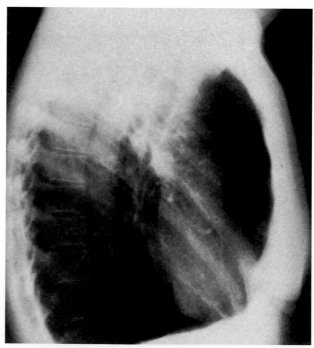

FIGURE 22.1. Posterior-anterior (**A**) and lateral (**B**) chest roentgenograms of a 62-year-old woman with advanced chronic obstructive pulmonary disease, mainly emphysema, showing low, flattened diaphragms, large retrosternal airspace, vertically oriented heart, and hyperlucency of peripheral lung fields. (From Hinshaw HC, Murray JF: Chronic bronchitis and emphysema. In Hinshaw HC, Murray JF [eds]: *Diseases of the Chest.* Philadelphia, WB Saunders, 1980, p. 578.)

enlargement, an arrhythmia, or evidence of left ventricular disease. Routine blood studies may provide evidence of other processes but, except for the hematocrit, do not relate to lung disease. Patients who have been hypoxemic for long periods of time, unless other factors supervene, will have secondary polycythemia (41). This finding gives some indication of the duration of the hypoxemia.

Of all the assessments that can be made, measurements of arterial PO_2, PCO_2 and pH are the most important. Serial measurements of PaO_2, $PaCO_2$, and pH are much more helpful than a single determination and can indicate success or failure of initial therapy. Blood gas and pH values taken together with the general status of the patient often determine the necessary intensity of supportive measures, particularly whether or not endotracheal intubation and mechanical ventilation will be necessary. Nearly all patients with chronic airways obstruction have some degree of hypoxemia and some have CO_2 retention when they are at their functional baseline. As noted, chronicity of hypoxemia may be attested to by polycythemia and, in addition, by findings of pulmonary hypertension with or without right ventricular failure. A single measurement of $PaCO_2$ without a prior baseline value may be very difficult to interpret; hence, the clinical context is important. An elevated plasma bicarbonate concentration is an indication that an elevated $PaCO_2$ has been present for a sufficiently long period of time to allow metabolic compensation.

Direct measurements of air flow are often difficult to obtain in severely ill patients and may not be useful. If feasible, measurements of FEV_1 and FVC may be helpful in evaluating response to therapy.

Effective management of acute respiratory failure in patients with chronic airways obstruction requires a critical care unit. The approach to treatment should always be directed to providing supportive care while treating the specific processes, such as lower respiratory tract infection that precipitated the acute deterioration.

The major supportive intervention necessary in this setting is provision of supplemental oxygen. Because the pathophysiologic mechanism by which hypoxemia develops is mismatching of ventilation to perfusion, increases in PaO_2 usually are easily achieved by administration of low concentrations of oxygen. The concern with overadministration of oxygen causing an increase in $PaCO_2$ has been well described and is a potential problem in patients who have a chronically elevated $PaCO_2$ (38,42). This concern, however, should not deter oxygen administration. The basic principle should be to administer the lowest amount of oxygen necessary to increase PaO_2 to approximately 60 mm Hg. Frequently, this can be achieved using nasal prongs or cannulae with flows of 1 to 2 L/min. Occasionally, higher flows are needed (Fig. 22.2). The FIO_2 delivered by devices such as nasal prongs varies considerably depending on the patient's minute ventilation. Although this does not usually present a problem, more precise control of the FIO_2 can be provided by a mask

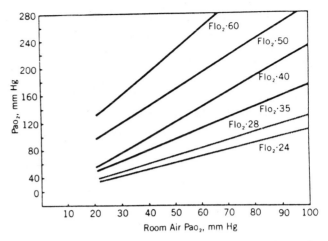

FIGURE 22.2. The relationship of PaO_2 to FIO_2 administered to patients with COPD. Each line gives the expected arterial oxygen tension for the FIO_2 administered. These lines were obtained in a study of patients with acute respiratory failure and stable patients with COPD. (From Bone RC: Treatment of respiratory failure due to advanced chronic obstructive lung disease. *Arch Intern Med* 140:1019, 1980. Copyright 1980, American Medical Association.)

that uses a venturi device through which a high flow of oxygen is delivered that entrains sufficient room air to produce the desired FIO_2. The disadvantages of the venturi delivery device are that the inspired gas is usually poorly humidified and the mask interferes with talking and eating.

Regardless of the oxygen delivery system, arterial blood gas tension must be measured soon after oxygen therapy is begun. The goal as cited is to increase the PaO_2 to 60 mm Hg (i.e., 90% hemoglobin saturation) without undue effects on $PaCO_2$. Blood gas measurements should be made thereafter as frequently as the clinical circumstances dictate. In this situation, because of the concern with the interactions of PaO_2 and $PaCO_2$, noninvasive oximetric monitoring of oxyhemoglobin saturation alone is not sufficient. Because reductions in PaO_2 below the target value of 60 mm Hg cause reduction in saturation to less than 90%, monitoring of oxyhemoglobin saturation may complement direct measurements of PaO_2 and $PaCO_2$.

In the majority of patients, provision of supplemental oxygen is the only supportive therapy needed. In some, however, endotracheal intubation and mechanical ventilation are required. Precise criteria for intubation and mechanical ventilation are difficult to define and commonly involve subjective as well as objective assessments. Hypoxemia per se is usually not in itself an indication for intubation because of the relative ease with which PaO_2 can be increased with supplemental oxygen provided by external devices. The major indication for ventilatory assistance is a poorly compensated acute respiratory acidosis. This may be apparent at the time of initial evaluation and dictate prompt institution of mechanical ventilation. Commonly, however, the need for ventilatory assistance is indicated by the failure of the patient to improve, or worsening with conservative management. This determination is made through careful monitoring of the response to oxygen administration as well as an assessment of other variables such as respiratory distress, fatigue, mental status, and ability to cooperate with conservative management.

In appropriately selected patients, noninvasive ventilation may reverse the acute respiratory decompensation and allow the patient to avoid endotracheal intubation. Noninvasive positive pressure ventilation utilizes a face mask, mouthpiece, or nasal mask to deliver oxygen from a positive pressure ventilator. Although clinical trials have had mixed results, a significant proportion of patients benefit from noninvasive ventilation while avoiding the potential complications of endotracheal intubation. A more extensive discussion of this subject can be found in Chapter 21, General Principles of Managing the Patient with Respiratory Failure.

When endotracheal intubation is necessary, mechanical ventilation should be accomplished using a volume-cycled ventilator and IPPV rather than IMV. The use of IPPV enables resting of the respiratory muscles. Respiratory muscle fatigue presumably plays a major role in the need for mechanical ventilation in this setting. Tidal volume should be set approximately 5–8 mL/kg body weight. Assuming that the patient is awake, he or she determines the respiratory rate. Given the tachypnea that is common in such patients, sedation is often necessary to enable an optimum ventilatory pattern. Ideally, the rate should be relatively slow, providing sufficient time for full exhalation of the previous breath to avoid stacking breaths with a consequent further increase in functional residual capacity. A long inspiratory time also is desirable to improve the distribution of inspired gas. As a general rule, positive end-expiratory pressure (PEEP) should not be used. The effect of PEEP would be to further increase the already greatly enlarged functional residual capacity and cause further overdistention of the lungs. In patients with airways obstruction an auto-PEEP effect may occur because of the occurrence of airway closure prior to full exhalation (43). Because the patient is now being mechanically ventilated there should no longer be concern with the overadministration of oxygen, and the FIO_2 should be sufficient to maintain a PaO_2 over 60 mm Hg.

Within 10 to 20 minutes of beginning mechanical ventilation, arterial blood gases should be measured. Because many patients with acute respiratory failure and chronic airways obstruction have had CO_2 retention for days, months, or years, metabolic compensation has occurred. This compensation generally is insufficient in the setting of an acute deterioration but is appropriate for the baseline $PaCO_2$. When mechanical ventilation is applied, the $PaCO_2$ generally can be decreased very quickly and, if it is reduced well below the patient's baseline to a normal value of 40 mm Hg, the patient will be left with an uncompensated, sometimes profound, metabolic alkalosis. Alkalosis has a

number of potential adverse effects including depression of cardiac output, increasing the risk of both supraventricular and ventricular arrhythmias, depressing the level of consciousness, and causing seizures (44). Because of the concern with alkalosis, the adequacy of mechanical ventilation should be determined not by $PaCO_2$ but by pH. The $PaCO_2$ should be maintained at a level that keeps the pH no higher than 7.45 to 7.50, and preferably close to a pH of 7.40. Also, because of chronic increases in $PaCO_2$, patients are commonly deficient in potassium and chloride. A reduction in plasma bicarbonate concentration does not occur until sufficient chloride has been given (45).

Weaning patients with chronic airways obstruction from mechanical ventilation can present a difficult problem. Implicit in the decision to intubate and ventilate is the assumption that there is a reversible factor contributing to the acute deterioration and that treatment will restore the patient to baseline status. Thus, mechanical ventilation supports the patient until specific therapy has had its effect, although resting the muscles of respiration may be of value in itself. Given this assumption, weaning efforts should begin as soon as the reversible component has been improved. In the case of left ventricular failure, for example, this may occur quite rapidly in response to diuresis. On the other hand, if pneumonia caused the acute deterioration, improvement may be slow.

A number of criteria have been developed as predictors of ability to be weaned. Unfortunately, these criteria are rarely applicable to patients with chronic airways obstruction who may not have been able to perform at the levels indicated by the criteria for many years. For this reason assessment of ability to be weaned in this setting is more subjective (46). Measurements such as VC and MIP can be made, but low values should not be assumed to predict failure. The patient should be alert and psychologically prepared for weaning. Serum electrolyte concentrations, especially potassium, phosphate, calcium and magnesium, should be optimum and the patient should be hemodynamically stable.

In general, prior to beginning the process of weaning the PaO_2, $PaCO_2$ and pH should be maintained approximately at their baseline values, if known. Thus, patients may be mildly hypoxemic, hypercapnic, and acidemic. The technique of weaning is somewhat controversial, with some clinicians favoring spontaneous breathing on a T-piece and others favoring the use of IMV with progressively decreasing ventilatory rates. The use of a T-piece trial offers the advantage of being able to determine fairly quickly if a patient is ready to be extubated, whereas IMV may delay this determination. In addition, because IMV uses spontaneous as well as machine-generated breaths, this form of weaning may be associated with increasing respiratory muscle fatigue. If the patient ventilates adequately via a T-piece for 1 or 2 hours without a deterioration in arterial blood gas tension, usually the endotracheal tube can be removed. Longer periods of spontaneous breathing (especially through a small endotracheal tube less than 7 mm in diameter), because of the resistance of the tube, may cause respiratory muscle fatigue. Though several different approaches to weaning from mechanical ventilation may be equally effective (47), there is some evidence that intermittent CPAP or T-piece trials are perhaps the most effective. In a recent trial, 138 patients who were considered difficult to wean were divided into four weaning strategies: intermittent mandatory ventilation, pressure support, intermittent daily trials of spontaneous ventilation, or one daily trial of spontaneous breathing with a T-piece or CPAP. Patients in the spontaneous breathing trial arms were weaned at a median of three days, whereas the median duration was four and five days for the pressure support and IMV groups, respectively (48). A more comprehensive discussion of weaning techniques can be found in Chapter 21, General Principles of Managing the Patient with Respiratory Failure.

In managing patients with acute respiratory failure and chronic airways obstruction, important and difficult ethical issues may be raised. As stated previously, in undertaking mechanical ventilatory support it is assumed that the respiratory failure has a reversible component. This may not be the case. The respiratory failure may simply represent the end stage of a disease that is known to be inexorably progressive. Providing mechanical ventilation for a patient who has no reversible component usually means that the patient will not be able to be weaned successfully. Under ideal circumstances the patient and his or her physician will have had the opportunity to discuss the outlook for the illness prior to acute deterioration, and the patient can make an informed decision regarding the use of mechanical ventilation. Such a patient may decide that ventilation should be undertaken on the chance that there is a reversible component. If facilities are available, the patient may also choose chronic ventilatory support. Given the multiplicity of disorders commonly present in these sorts of patients, chronic mechanical ventilation is usually a very unattractive option even if available. Patients who are being ventilated mechanically may also elect to have this support discontinued. In the face of previously reviewed difficulties in predicting weanability, abrupt discontinuation of support may not mean death. If mechanical ventilation is not undertaken or is discontinued, vigorous treatment can still be provided but, in addition, particular attention should be paid to the patient's comfort (Chapter 21, General Principles of Managing the Patient with Respiratory Failure).

Survival rates for acute respiratory failure in patients with chronic airways obstruction have been surprisingly similar in several studies, ranging from 58% to 79%. Not surprisingly, 24-month survival has been much lower, from 35% to 72% (49).

In addition to the supportive care described in this section, treatment of the airways obstruction and the precipitating disorder must be prompt and vigorous. Although there is controversy concerning the use of bronchodilators in patients with chronic airways obstruction, it should always be assumed that there is a reversible component. Inhaled β-adrenergic agonists such as albuterol, metaproterenol, and terbutaline should be used at intervals of 2 to 4 hours at the beginning of treatment and decreased in frequency if adverse reactions are encountered. They can be administered directly via a nebulizer drive by a compressed gas source or through a mechanical ventilator. With either of these devices the amount of drug actually delivered is difficult to quantify; thus, the dose given should be limited mainly by side effects. Inhaled ipratropium has also been shown to be useful for bonchodilation and perhaps for reducing the volume of secretions (50).

Metered dose inhalation is a simpler and usually equally effective route for delivery of these agents. Intravenous theophylline may also be of benefit, although less than inhaled β-agonists. The loading dose of aminophylline in patients who have not been taking the drug is 5 to 6 mg/kg. Maintenance doses in patients with severe airways obstruction, some of whom may have heart failure, should be 0.3 to 0.5 mg/kg per min (50,51). After 18 to 24 hours, a serum theophylline concentration should be measured and the infusion rate adjusted appropriately. The concentration should be approximately 15 mg/mL, with 20 mg/mL the usual threshold for toxicity. Theophylline has been shown to increase the strength of respiratory muscles, but in one study the dose needed to achieve this effect required concentrations that were toxic (52). Also, one study suggested that theophylline was of minimal benefit in treating acute respiratory failure in COPD, if the patient was already treated with β-agonists, antibiotics, and corticosteroids (53).

The benefit of systemic corticosteroids in COPD exacerbations are not as well established as for acute asthmatic attacks (54). A recent double-blind placebo controlled randomized clinical trial compared high dose systemic corticosteroids (2- and 8-week regimes) or placebo in 271 patients hospitalized for COPD exacerbations. All patients received a 1-week course of antibiotics as well as inhaled β-agonists, ipratropium, and glucorticoids for the duration of follow-up (6 months). The patients in the corticosteroid treatment arm had significantly shorter hospital stays, significantly less treatment failures at 1 and 3 months, and a small improvement in FEV_1. There was no advantage to the longer course of systemic corticosteroids. At 6 months, the three arms had no significant differences in rates of death, intubation, readmission, or treatment intensification (55).

Antimicrobial drugs are given commonly and are of obvious value if there is a bacterial bronchitis or pneumonia (56). The routine use of antibiotics in COPD exacerbations also appear to be of benefit (56a). The choice of agents should be guided initially by the results of sputum Gram stains. If Gram stains and cultures do not provide guidance, empiric therapy with amoxacillin, trimethoprim-sulfameth-oxazole, or doxycycline may be used.

RESPIRATORY FAILURE IN ASTHMA

Asthma prevalence and mortality has been on the rise in the United States and worldwide (57,57a). Most deaths occur in asthmatics from status asthmaticus. Acute airways obstruction in asthma results in increased resistance to air flow during inspiration (especially expiration), and this leads to air trapping and overinflation of the lung (58). Because the air flow obstruction is not uniform, the distribution of inspired air is uneven, causing mismatching of ventilation to perfusion. This results in hypoxemia and an increase in wasted ventilation (59,60). The hyperinflation serves to maintain airway patency, but as functional residual capacity (FRC) increases and approaches the predicted normal total lung capacity (TLC), a greater change in transpulmonary pressure is required to produce an adequate tidal volume. This, together with the rise in airways resistance, markedly increases the work of breathing. As a consequence of these abnormalities, in severe airways obstruction there is an increased O_2 demand caused by the increased work of breathing at the same time that hypoxemia may result from mismatching of ventilation to perfusion. Moreover, the increases in wasted ventilation and in CO_2 production require a greater minute ventilation, which can be achieved only by imposing an additional workload on the respiratory muscles. Because of the hyperinflation, the intercostal, accessory, and diaphragmatic muscles are forced to work at a considerable mechanical disadvantage (61). At some point, if the airways obstruction is not corrected, the system fails and CO_2 retention occurs. In addition, as the O_2 demands of the respiratory muscles begin to outstrip the supply of O_2 anaerobic metabolism results with subsequent metabolic (lactic) acidosis. Because there is no possibility for respiratory compensation, the pH rapidly decreases. Metabolic acidosis in this setting must be dealt with promptly or rapid deterioration will occur.

Assessment of the severity of an asthmatic episode is of obvious importance in determining the approach to management of the patient. Although the vast majority of asthma attacks are treated entirely on an outpatient basis, it is essential that both the patient and medical personnel be aware of when more intensive treatment is needed. Several groups of investigators have identified factors of importance in deciding which patients with asthma require hospital admission (62–64). However, the utility and accuracy of numerical indices derived from such data have been questioned (65,66). Thus, both objective and subjective individualized patient assessment determines the severity of an asthmatic

TABLE 22.2. IMPORTANT FACTORS IN ASSESSING SEVERITY OF ACUTE ASTHMA

1. History of prior hospitalization for asthma
2. History of prior or current corticosteroid therapy
3. Patient's subjective sense of severity of attack
4. Failure to respond to usual treatment (i.e., persistent wheezing despite bronchodilator therapy)
5. Duration of attack
6. Patient too distressed to talk
7. Silent chest (i.e., minimal breath sounds)
8. Disturbances in mental status
9. Systemic hypertension, tachycardia >110/min
10. Cardiac arrhythmias
11. Cyanosis
12. Prominent accessory muscle use
13. Pulsus paradoxus >10 mm Hg
14. Mediastinal emphysema, pneumothorax
15. FEV <1.0 L
16. Acute respiratory acidosis or arterial Pa_{O_2} <60 on room air

episode. Factors that should be taken into account in such evaluations are listed in Table 22.2.

The history is of major importance in assessing the severity of a given asthmatic episode and provides information that influences the interpretation of the more objective physiologic data. Patients who have a history of having severe attacks tend to continue to have severe attacks. Thus, information from the patient or from the medical record that he or she has previously required hospitalization increases concern for the current episode. The duration of the current attack is also important, because the mechanism of airway obstruction changes as the attack persists. Early it is mainly smooth muscle spasm, whereas later it is mucous plugging and edema. Spasm can resolve within minutes, but days may be required to improve obstruction that is caused by edema and plugging.

Patients with acute asthmatic episodes are nearly always tachypneic and tachycardic, either of which correlates well with the degree of airway obstruction. The amount of pulsus paradoxus does, however, correlate with greater degrees of obstruction (67). Therefore, this finding can be used both to indicate severity and to judge response to therapy. The intensity of wheezing cannot be used to infer the amount of airways obstruction, although prolongation of the expiratory phase varies roughly with obstruction. The absence of wheezing in a patient who by all other indicators has asthma is an ominous finding, indicating that air flow is so reduced that there is not sufficient turbulence to cause wheezing. Unilateral absence of wheezing may be the result of a pneumothorax or mucus plug in a large airway and likewise is indicative of a very serious clinical problem. Although not specific, abnormalities in mental status are important in patients with severe airways obstruction. Such findings may be the result of hypoxia or CO_2 retention or be unrelated to the asthma per se but influence management by interfering with patient cooperation.

Although an understanding of the alterations in pulmonary function is necessary to conceptualize the pathophysiology of asthma, in clinical practice the only measurements that can be made routinely are the FEV_1, PEF, and FVC. Of these, the PEF is the most easily obtained because it does not require a full forced exhalation but rather a short forced puff similar to a cough after a full inhalation. Severe obstruction is indicated by a peak flow of less than 100 L/min. This has been shown to correspond to an FEV_1 of less than 0.7 L (68).

The FEV_1 is more difficult to measure because it requires a full inspiration followed by a full forced exhalation, maneuvers that a severe asthmatic may not be able to perform because of dyspnea and that in some patients actually worsens the obstruction (69). Nevertheless, the FEV_1 is the most direct measurement of air flow and correlates well with other variables and clinical outcomes. Nowak and associates found that an FEV_1 of less than 1 L or 20% of the predicted value was associated with a poor bronchodilator response, the need for hospitalization, and the likelihood of relapse (68). Similar findings were reported by Kelsen and coworkers (64). Several investigators have related the FEV_1 to PaO_2 and $PaCO_2$ and have demonstrated that in general, in acute asthma, CO_2 retentions begins to occur at an FEV_1 of approximately 750 mL or 25% of the predicted value (70,71). An increase in $PaCO_2$ is a direct consequence of the airways obstruction with limited ventilatory capability in the face of increased CO_2 production. Because mild degrees of acute airways obstruction are usually associated with a lower than normal $PaCO_2$ the finding of a value in the range of 40 mm Hg should be viewed with concern.

Although there is a tendency for the PaO_2 to decrease with decreasing values of FEV_1 the relationship is not as predictable as with $PaCO_2$ (72). Nearly all patients with any degree of airways obstruction have some degree of arterial hypoxemia. Values of less than 50 mm Hg are distinctly unusual, however, and suggest that factors in addition to airways obstruction are playing a role.

Acute hypoventilation results in a reduction in arterial pH of about 0.008 pH unit for every 1 mm Hg increase in $PaCO_2$; thus, an increase in $PaCO_2$ from 40 to 60 mm Hg would result in a pH of 7.25. A reduction in pH that is in excess of the change in $PaCO_2$ indicates the presence of a metabolic as well as respiratory acidosis. As discussed previously, metabolic acidosis in this setting is owing to an imbalance between the supply and consumption of O_2 by the respiratory muscles plus perhaps a reduction in clearance of lactate from blood. The finding of metabolic acidosis in a patient with severe asthma is perhaps the single most ominous finding of all (73).

Chest radiographs should be obtained routinely in patients with severe asthma. The most common finding is overinflation of the lungs, but occasionally pneumonia, pneumomediastinum, pneumothorax, or atelectasis from mucous plugging of larger airways may be found. Electro-cardiograms should also be obtained, especially in older patients. The common abnormalities include P-pulmonale, right ventricular strain, and right axis deviation, all of which may be reversible. Much less commonly, changes indicative of ischemia or arrhythmias may be encountered (74). The treatment modalities employed in severe asthma are directed both toward support of the patient and reversal of the airways obstruction. Supplemental oxygen is an essential supportive measure that should be instituted in all patients with acute airways obstruction. Because there is no concern with depression of ventilatory drive by oxygen in most patients with asthma, the choice of an oxygen delivery system should mainly be dictated by patient comfort. For example, face masks that fit tightly may not be tolerated, and humidification of the inspired gas mixture, although desirable, may stimulate more bronchoconstriction. Normal saline is less likely to produce this effect than distilled water. In addition, heated humidification is preferable.

It can be difficult to determine when to institute mechanical ventilation in severe asthma. There are no uniformly applicable criteria that can guide the decision and, as with the general assessment, both subjective and objective criteria should be used (75). Generally, mechanical ventilation should not be undertaken before the patient has been given maximal bronchodilator therapy even though marked abnormalities of gas exchange may be present. Exceptions to this generalization include the presence of significant mental status changes, life-threatening cardiac arrhythmias, electro-cardiographic evidence of myocardial ischemia, or a history of previous severe asthmatic episodes requiring mechanical ventilation (75).

Patients who continue to deteriorate in the face of aggressive, in-hospital management generally require mechanical ventilation. This is indicated by increasing respiratory acidosis often accompanied by metabolic acidosis. Hypoxemia in itself, because it can be managed effectively with supplemental O_2, is rarely an indication for mechanical ventilation.

Placement of an endotracheal tube should be done semielectively rather than waiting until the patient is in extremis. A nasotracheal intubation using adequate topical anesthesia may be performed in an awake patient after preoxygenation. Because there are irritant receptors in the larynx and trachea, the process of endotracheal intubation may provoke increased bronchoconstriction. This response is mediated by the parasympathetic nervous system and may be reduced by premedication with atropine or topical lidocaine in the pharynx and larynx. In most patients, orotracheal intubation with sedation and paralysis is necessary.

Once control of the airway is achieved, sedation is generally necessary. Mechanical ventilation should be provided with a volume-cycled ventilator. At least early in the course, the ventilatory mode should be IPPV rather than IMV. This allows the respiratory muscles to rest completely. Tidal volume should usually be in the range of 5–6 mL/kg body weight. Because the FRC is markedly increased, positive end-expiratory pressure, which further increases the FRC, should not be used, although the auto-PEEP phenomenon is common.

Appropriate adjustment of the ratio of inspiration to expiration is the most difficult aspect of mechanical ventilation in the setting of severe airways obstruction. An interplay of four factors is involved: (*a*) marked slowing of the expiratory flow because of the airways obstruction; (*b*) dyspnea and tachypnea; (*c*) the need for a minute ventilation that will reduce the $PaCO_2$; and (*d*) the desirability of a slow inspiratory time to minimize peak airway pressures and enable optimum distribution of the inspired gas. Because of the reduction in expiratory flow, a relatively long expiratory time is needed. If expiratory time is too short, further air trapping occurs. To avoid this, either the inspiratory time can be shortened or the tidal volume reduced, neither of which is desirable. Thus, it is generally preferable to sedate the patient until apnea is produced so that a slow ventilatory rate can be used, thereby allowing both a slower inspiratory flow and a longer expiratory time. In addition to a narcotic or diazepam, muscle relaxants may be necessary. Pancuronium or vecuronium are the muscle relaxants of choice because curare, succinylcholine, and atracurium cause release of histamine, but these agents can be associated with prolonged neuromuscular blockade and myopathy; therefore, their use should be minimized (76).

One study reported excellent results with controlled hypoventilation with hyperoxic mixtures in mechanically ventilated patients (77). In this study, the authors did not allow peak airway pressures to exceed 50 cm H_2O and thus allowed the patients to be hypercapnic but well oxygenated. Alveolar hypoventilation was maintained for hours or even up to 4 days until airway obstruction was relieved and the hypercapnia resolved. There were no deaths with this approach, which contrasts with prior studies (Table 22.3).

During the course of mechanical ventilation, in addition

to following PaO_2, $PaCO_2$, and pH, the peak and mean airway pressures should be noted because they provide a rough indication of the inspiratory flow resistance. With mechanical ventilation, PaO_2 and $PaCO_2$ generally can be brought into the normal range quite promptly; however, weaning cannot begin until the airways obstruction remits. This is indicated by a reduction in peak inspiratory pressure, a spontaneous maximum inspiratory force of at least -30 cm H_2O, and a vital capacity of at least 15 mL/kg body weight. If these are achieved, weaning can usually proceed using either conventional T-piece trials with spontaneous ventilation or IMV with a progressively decreasing frequency of mechanical breaths.

The principles for the use of bronchodilator agents apply equally in mild, moderate, and severe asthma. As discussed previously, however, one of the clinical features that serves to define severe asthma is a failure to respond promptly to the usual bronchodilators. In spite of the poor early response to bronchodilators in patients with severe asthma, these agents together with corticosteroids remain the keystone of treatment. In severe asthma, both theophylline and β-adrenergic agonists can be given in doses as guided by blood concentrations (theophylline) or toxicity (β-adrenergic agents and theophylline). In at least two studies, this approach was substantiated as providing more bronchodilation than either agent given alone in maximal doses, although in a third trial inhaled isoproterenol proved to have as much effect alone as when combined with aminophylline (78).

β-adrenergic agonists may be administered orally, by inhalation, subcutaneously, or intravenously. However, there is substantial evidence that when given by inhalation there is a much more favorable ratio between benefit and untoward effects (79,80). Frequently, because of limitation of inspiratory flow, use of a metered dose inhaler is not adequate to deliver the aerosol. Placing a spacer or reservoir between the inhaler and the mouth may enable more effective use of the metered dose inhaler. The usual doses are, for metaproterenol solution, 15 mg (0.3 mL of 5% solution), for albuterol, 2.5 mg (0.5 to 1 mL of 0.5% solution), and for terbutaline, 1.5 to 2.5 mg. Normal saline is added to the drug to make a total volume of 2.5 to 3 mL. Using standard nebulizers, this volume should be completely aerosolized in 10 to 15 minutes. It should be realized that nebulization is continuous with most compressed gas or driven systems, but only the portion of the nebulized drug that is inhaled constitutes an effective dose; thus, the doses listed herein are substantially greater than the doses delivered.

Aerosolized agents have an onset of action within minutes and the effect of a single dose peaks at 30 to 60 minutes. The duration of effect is 4 to 6 hours following a single dose. In treating severe episodes of asthma, inhalation of a B_2-selective agent should be given nearly continuously during the first hour unless toxicity develops as indicated by cardiac arrhythmia or intolerable tremor. During the next

TABLE 22.3. PROGNOSIS IN PATIENTS REQUIRING MECHANICAL VENTILATION IN STATUS ASTHMATICUS

Study	Year	Episodes (n)	Deaths	Mortality (%)
Riding and Ambiavagar	1967	26	4	15
Iisalo et al.	1969	29	4	14
Lissac et al.	1971	19	4	21
Sheehy et al.	1972	22	2	9
Scoggin et al.	1977	21	8	38
Cornil et al.	1977	58	6	10
Westerman et al.	1979	42	4	9.5
Webb et al.	1979	20	7	35
Picado et al.	1983	26	6	23
Darioli et al.	1983	34	0	0

Source: Darioli R, Perrec C. Mechanical controlled hypoventilation in status asthmaticus. *Am Rev Respir Dis* 1994;129:385–387.

several hours, inhalation can be given at hourly intervals with close monitoring for toxicity. As the airways obstruction improves, the dosing interval can be increased to 4 to 6 hours, and metered dose inhalers can be used. In asthmatics who require endotracheal intubation and mechanical ventilation, the drug can be delivered using an in-line nebulizer in the inspiratory limb of the ventilator circuit. Longer-acting β-adrenergic agonists may also prove to be of some value by inhalation, although the delay in the onset of their action may limit their utility in the acute setting (81).

The use of theophylline was discussed the preceding section on COPD and acute respiratory failure. It should be noted, however, that the factors that tend to alter the pharmacokinetics of theophylline (such as pneumonia, heart failure, and severe airways obstruction) are more likely to be present in severe asthma than in milder forms. Because of the severity of the process and perhaps because of coexisting diseases it is more difficult to determine if a given occurrence (cardiac arrhythmia, seizure) is owing to theophylline. For these reasons the use of theophylline in severe asthma must be monitored closely using measurements of serum concentration of the drug.

Treatment with corticosteroids is essential therapy in severe asthma. In patients who do not respond promptly to initial bronchodilator therapy, treatment with a systemic, generally intravenous, corticosteroid should be instituted (82). This does not obligate the patient to a long course of corticosteroids nor cause him or her to be steroid dependent. Because the peak effect occurs no sooner than 4 to 6 hours after intravenous administration, it is best to give the initial dose early in the course of treatment and reevaluate the need for continuation at a later time. There appears to be a dose–response relationship between increasing doses of methylprednisolone (15, 40, and 125 mg, all given three times a day) and FEV_1 (83). Given that the adverse effects of even high doses of corticosteroids are minimal if the duration of administration is short, it is probably better to err on the side of giving too much of the drug than too little. Based on the scant data that are available, a dose of methylprednisolone in the range of 60 to 120 mg given intravenously at 6- to 8-hour intervals for 48 to 72 hours represents a reasonable initial approach to corticosteroid administration in patients with severe asthma. Higher doses should be used in patients who have been taking corticosteroids prior to being seen or who are taking other drugs, such as barbiturates, phenytoin, or rifampin, that accelerate the metabolism of corticosteroids (84). The dose can be reduced rapidly to maintenance doses given orally or discontinued altogether in patients who respond promptly.

Aerosols of corticosteroids, although effective in maintenance therapy, have no demonstrated role in management of the severe attack. However, patients who have asthma and are being mechanically ventilated for other reasons can be given agents such as beclomethasone via the endotracheal tube.

Because both airway smooth muscle and mucociliary function are modulated by the parasympathetic nervous system with stimulation causing both bronchoconstriction and an increase in mucous production, it is logical to assume that antimuscarinic agents such as atropine might be of benefit in asthma. Although the benefit of adding of anticholinergic therapy to maximal β-agonist therapy has not been well studied in critically ill patients, numerous clinical trials comparing combination therapy versus β-agonist treatment have produced conflicting results. A pooled analysis of three large double-blind, randomized control trials involving 1,064 patients treated in the emergency room showed that the combination treatment group had a small improvement in FEV_1 at 45 and 90 minutes, and require less treatment and hospitalization (85). A more recent meta-analysis also demonstrated improvements in lung function and rates of hospitalization (85a).

Antimicrobial agents are of questionable value in the routine management of acute asthmatic episodes (84). However, antimicrobial therapy is clearly indicated in patients who have bacterial pneumonia as seen on chest radiographs and supported by the presence of bacteria and polymorphonuclear leukocytes in a Gram-stained sputum smear. Antimicrobial agents should also be used in patients with severe asthma and bacterial bronchitis. Other strategies used in severe asthma exacerbations and supported by some clinical data include the use of helium-oxygen mixtures or intravenous magnesium sulfate. In general, mucolytic agents are of little use in severe asthma. General anesthesia with inhalational agents has been used in the treatment of refractory asthma for a number of years. Halothane, because it possesses inherent bronchodilating properties, was frequently used (88). Isofluorance has now been substituted for halothane when an inhalational anesthetic is used. These inhalational agents can antagonize the effects on smooth muscle of acetylcholine and histamine as well as reducing antigen-induced bronchospasm in dogs. In addition to the pharmacologic effects of the anesthetic agent, general anesthesia may allow more effective mechanical ventilation, although this objective can also be achieved in the vast majority of instances by proper use of sedatives and muscle relaxants in patients who are already being ventilated mechanically.

REFERENCES

1. Segredo V, Caldwell JE, Matthay MA, et al. Persistent paralysis in critically ill patients after long-term administration of vecuronium. *N Engl J Med* 1992;327:524–528.
2. Luce JM. Medical management of spinal cord injury. *Crit Care Med* 1985;13:126–131.
3. Moore P, James O. Guillain-Barré syndrome: incidence, management and outcome of major complications. *Crit Care Med* 1981; 9:549–555.
4. Gracey D, McMichan JC, Divertie MB, et al. Respiratory failure in Guillain-Barré syndrome. *Mayo Clin Proc* 1982;57:742–746.
4a. Melillo EM, Sethi JM, Mohsenin V. Guillian-Barré Syndrome:

rehabilitation outcome and recent developments. *Yale J Biol and Med* 1998;71:383–389.

5. Eisendrath SJ, Matthay MA, Dunkel J, et al. Guillain-Barré syndrome: psychosocial aspects of management. *Psychosomatics* 1983;24:465–475.

6. Henschel EO. The Guillain-Barré syndrome: a personal experience. *Anesthesiology* 1977;47:228–231.

7. Guillain-Barré Syndrome Study Group. Plasmapheresis and acute Guillain-Barré syndrome. *Neurology* 1985;35:1096–1104.

8. Dyck PJ, Kurtzke JF. Plasmapheresis in Guillain-Barré syndrome. *Neurology* 1985;35:1105–1107.

9. Sater RA, Rostami A. Treatment of Guillain-Barré syndrome with intravenous immunoglobulin. *Neurology* 1998;51(Suppl 5):S9–S15.

10. Van Der Meche FGA, Schmitz PIM, and the Dutch Guillain-Barré Study Group. A randomized trial comparing intravenous immune globulin and plasma exchange in Guillain-Barré syndrome. *N Engl J Med* 1992;326:1123–1129.

11. Plasma Exchange/Sandoglobulin Guillain-Barré Syndrome Trial Group. Randomized trial of plasma exchange, intravenous immunoglobulin, and combined treatments in Guillain-Barré syndrome. *Lancet* 1997;349:225–230.

12. Leventhal SR, Orkin FK, Hirsh RA. Prediction of the need for postoperative mechanical ventilation in myasthenia gravis. *Anesthesiology* 1980;53:26–30.

13. Grob D. Acute neuromuscular disorders. *Med Clin N Am* 1981;65:189–207.

14. Dou PL, Lindstrom JM, Cassel LK, et al. Plasmapheresis and immunosuppressive drug therapy in myasthenia gravis. *N Engl J Med* 1977;297:1134–1139.

15. Gadjos P, Chevret S, Calir B, et al. Clinical trial of plasma exchange and high-dose intravenous immunoglobulin in myasthenia gravis. *Ann Neurol* 1997;41:789–796.

16. Keys PA, Blume RP. Therapeutic strategies for myasthenia gravis. *Ann Pharm Therapy* 1991;25:1101–1108.

17. Mickell JJ, Kook SO, Siewers RD, et al. Clinical implications of postoperative unilateral phrenic nerve paralysis. *J Thorac Cardiovasc Surg* 1978;75:297–304.

18. Wilcox P, Baile E, Hards J, et al. Phrenic nerve function and its relationship to atelectasis after coronary artery by pass surgery. *Chest* 1988;93:693–698.

19. Glenn WW, Hogan JF, Luke JS, et al. Ventilatory support by pacing of the conditioned diaphragm in quadriplegia. *N Engl J Med* 1984;310:1150–1155.

20. Roy TM, Ossorio MA, Cipolla LM, et al. Pulmonary complications after tricyclic antidepressant overdose. *Chest* 1989;96:852–856.

21. Bynum LJ, Pierce AK Pulmonary aspiration of gastric contents. *Am Rev Respir Dis* 1976;114:1129–1136.

22. Rosenow EC. Drug-induced pulmonary disease. In Murray JF, Naydel JA. *Textbook of respiratory medicine,* 2nd ed. Philadelphia: Saunders, 1994:2117–2144.

23. Rosenow EC, Myers JL, Swensen SJ, et al. Drug-induced pulmonary disease an update. *Chest* 1992;102:239–250.

24. Heffner JE, Sahn SA. Salicylate-induced pulmonary edema. *Ann Intern Med* 1981;95:405–409.

25. Picado C, Castillo JA, Montserrat JM et al. Aspirin intolerance as precipitating factor of life-threatening attacks of asthma requiring mechanical ventilation. *Eur Resp J* 1989;2:127–129.

26. Corbridge TC, Murray P. Toxicology in adults. In Hall JB, Schmidt GA, Wood LDH, eds. *Principles of Critical Care Medicine.* New York: McGraw Hill, 1998:1473–1519.

27. Mayberry JC, Trunkey DD. The fractured rib in chest wall trauma. *Chest Surgery Clinics of North America* 1997;7:234–261.

28. Bergofsky EH. Respiratory failure in disorders of the thoracic cage. *Am Rev Respir Dis* 1979;119:643–669.

28a.Polic S, Rumboldt Z, Dujic Z, et al. Role of digoxin in right ventricular failure due to chronic core pulmonale. *Int J Clin Pharm Research* 1990;10:153–162.

29. Curtis JL, Mahlmeister M, Fink J, et al. Helium-oxygen gas therapy: use and availability for the emergency treatment of inoperable airway obstruction. *Chest* 1986;90:455–457.

30. Tami T, Chu F, Wildes T, et al. Pulmonary edema and acute upper airway obstruction. *Laryngoscope* 1986;96:506–509.

31. Kallet RH, Daniel BM, Gropper M, et al. Acute pulmonary edema following upper airway obstruction: case reports and brief review. *Resp Care* 1998;43(6):476–480.

32. Wagner PD, Dantzker DR, Dueck R, et al. Ventilation-perfusion inequality in chronic obstructive pulmonary disease. *J Clin Invest* 1977;59:203–216.

33. Roussos C, Moxham J. Respiratory muscle fatigue. In Roussos C, Macklem PT, eds. *The thorax.* New York: Marcel Dekker, 1985:829–870.

34. Roussos C. Ventilatory failure and respiratory muscle. In Roussos C, Macklem PT, eds. *The thorax.* New York: Marcel Dekker, 1985:1253–1279.

35. Anthonisen NR, Cherniack RM. Ventilatory control in lung disease. In Roussos C, Macklem PT, eds. *The thorax.* New York: Marcel Dekker, 1985:965–987.

36. Mountain R, Zwillich C, Weil JV. Hypoventilation in obstructive lung disease. *N Engl J Med* 1978;10:521–525.

37. Broadovsky D, McDonnell JA, Cherniack RM. The respiratory response to carbon dioxide in health and in emphysema. *J Clin Invest* 1960;39:724–729.

38. Aubier M, Murciano D, Fournier M, et al. Central respiratory drive in acute respiratory failure of patients with chronic obstructive lung disease. *Am Rev Respir Dis* 1980;122:191–199.

39. Burrows B, Earle RH. Course and prognosis of chronic obstructive pulmonary disease. *N Engl J Med* 1969;280:397–404.

40. Gump DW, Phillips CA, Forsyth BR, et al. Role of infection in chronic bronchitis. *Am Rev Respir Dis* 1976;113:465–470.

41. Murray JF. Classification of polycythemic disorders with comments on the diagnostic value of arterial blood oxygen analysis. *Ann Intern Med* 1966;64:892–903.

42. Campbell EJM. The management of acute respiraty failure in chronic bronchitis and emphysema. *Am Rev Respir Dis* 1967;95:626–639.

43. Pepe P, Marini JJ. Occult positive end-expiratory pressure in mechanically ventilated patients with airflow obstruction: the auto-PEEP effect. *Am Rev Respir Dis* 1982;126:166–170.

44. Kilburn KH. Shock, seizures and coma with alkalosis during mechanical ventilation. *Ann Intern Med* 1966;66:977–984.

45. Kassires JP, Berkman PM, Lawrence DR, et al. The critical role of chloride in the correction of hypokalemic alkalosis in man. *Am J Med* 1965;38:172–189.

46. Petty TL. Acute respiratory failure in COPD. In Petty TL, ed. *Chronic obstructive pulmonary disease.* New York: Marcel Dekker, 1978:163–180.

47. Weinberger SF, Weiss JW. Weaning from ventilatory support. *N Engl J Med* 1995;332:388–389.

48. Esteban A, Frutos F, Tobin MJ, et al. A comparison of four methods of weaning patients from mechanical ventilation. *N Engl J Med* 1995;332:345–350.

49. Martin TR, Lewis S, Albert RK. The prognosis of patients with chronic obstructive pulmonary disease after hospitalization for acute respiratory failure. *Chest* 1982;82:310–314.

50. Ferguson GT, Cherniack RM. Management of chronic obstructive lung disease. *N Engl J Med* 1993;328:1017–1022.

51. Weinberger M, Hendeles L, Ahrens R. Pharmacologic management of reversible obstructive lung disease. *Med Clin N Am* 1980;65:579–591.

52. Dimarco A, Nochomovits M, Dimarco M, et al. Comparative

effect of aminophylline on diaphragm and cardiac contractility. *Am Rev Respir Dis* 1985;132:800–805.

53. Rice K, Leatherman JW, Duane PG, et al. Aminophylline for acute exacerbations of chronic obstructive pulmonary disease. *Ann Intern Med* 1987;107:305–309.

54. Albert RK, Martin TR, Lewis SW. Controlled clinical trial of methylprednisolone in patients with chronic bronchitis and acute respiratory insufficiency. *Ann Intern Med* 1980;92:753–758.

55. Niedwoehner DE, Erbland ML, Deupree RH, et al. Effect of systemic glucocorticoids on exacerbations of chronic obstructive pulmonary disease. *N Engl J Med* 1999;340:1941–1947.

56. Towes GB. Use of antibiotics in patients with chronic obstructive pulmonary disease. *Semin Respir Med* 1986;8:165–170.

56a. Saint S, Bent S, Vittinghoff W, et al. Antibiotics in chronic obstructive disease exacerbations. *JAMA* 1995;273:957–960.

57. Barret TE, Strom BL. Inhaled beta-adrenergic receptor agonists in asthma: more harm than good? *Am J Respir Crit Care Med* 1995;151:574–577.

57a. Grant EN, Wagner R, Weiss KB. Observations on emerging patterns of asthma in our society. *J Aller Clin Immun* 1999;104:51–59.

58. Woolcock AJ, Read J. Lung volume in exacerbations of asthma. *Am J Med* 1966;41:259–264.

59. Rubinfeld AR, Wagner PD, West JB. Gas exchange during acute experimental canine asthma. *Am Rev Respir Dis* 1978;118:525–536.

60. Wagner PD, Dantzker DR, Iacovoni WC, et al. Ventilation perfusion inequality in asymptomatic asthma. *Am Rev Respir Dis* 1978;118:511–524.

61. Martin J, Powell E, Shore S, et al. The role of respiratory muscles in the hyperinflation of bronchial asthma. *Am Rev Respir Dis* 1980;121:441–447.

62. Banner AS, Shah RS, Addington WW. Rapid prediction of need for hospitalization in acute asthma. *JAMA* 1976;235:1337–1338.

63. Fischl MA, Pitchenik A, Gardner LB. An index predicting relapse and need for hospitalization in patients with acute bronchial asthma. *N Engl J Med* 1981;305:783–789.

64. Kelsen SG, Kelsen DP, Fleezer RF, et al. Emergency room assessment and treatment of patients with acute asthma. *Am J Med* 1978;64:622–628.

65. Centor RM, Yarbrough B, Wood JP. Inability to predict relapse in bronchial asthma. *N Engl J Med* 1984;310:577–580.

66. Rose CC, Murphy JG, Schwartz JS. Performance of an index predicting the response of patients with acute bronchial asthma to intensive emergency department treatment. *N Engl J Med* 1984;310:573–577.

67. Rebuck AS, Pengelly LD. Development of pulsus paradoxus in the presence of airway obstruction. *N Engl J Med* 1973;288:66–69.

68. Nowak RM, Pensler MJ, Sarkar DD, et al. Comparison of peak expiratory flow and FEV$_1$ admission criteria for acute bronchial asthma. *Ann Emerg Med* 1982;11:64–69.

69. Nadel JA, Tierney DF. Effect of a previous deep inspiration on airway resistance in man. *J Appl Physiol* 1961;16:401–407.

70. Rees HA, Millar JS, Wood KW. A study of the clinical course and arterial blood gas tensions of patients in status asthmaticus. *Q J Med* 1968;148:541–561.

71. Tai E, Read J. Blood gas tensions in bronchial asthma. *Lancet* 1967;1:644–646.

72. Fanta CH, Rossing TH, McFadden ER Jr. Emergency room treatment of asthma. *Am J Med* 1982;72:416–422.

73. Appel D, Rubenstein R, Schrager K, et al. Lactic acidosis in severe asthma. *Am J Med* 1983;75:580–584.

74. Molfino NA, Nannini LJ, Martelli AN, et al. Respiratory arrest in near-fatal asthma. *N Engl J Med* 1991;324:285–288.

75. FitzGerald JM, Hargreave FE. The assessment and management of acute life-threatening asthma. *Chest* 1989;95(4):888–894.

76. Bellomo R, McLaughlin P, Tai E, et al. Asthma requiring mechanical ventilation a low morbidity approach. *Chest* 1994;5(3):891–896.

77. Darioli R, Perret C. Mechanical controlled hypoventilation in status asthmaticus. *Am Rev Respir Dis* 1984;129:385–387.

78. Rossing TH, Fanta CH, McFadden ER Jr. Medical Housestaff of the Peter Bent Brigham Hospital: a controlled trial of single versus combined drug therapy in the treatment of acute episodes of asthma. *Am Rev Respir Dis* 1981;123:190–194.

79. Wolfe JD, Tashkin DP, Calvarese B, et al. Bronchodilator effects of terbutaline and aminophylline alone and in combination in asthmatic patients. *N Engl J Med* 1978;298:363–367.

80. Larsson S, Svedmyr N. Bronchodilating effect and side effects of beta-adrenoceptor stimulants by different routes of administration (tablets, metered aerosol, and combinations thereof. *Am Rev Respir Dis* 1977;116:861–869.

81. Pearlman DS, Chervinsky P, Laforce C, et al. A comparison of salmeterol with albuterol in the treatment of mild to moderate asthma. *N Engl J Med* 1992;327:1420–1425.

82. King TE, Chang SW. Corticosteroid therapy in the management of asthma. *Semin Respir Med* 1987;8:387–399.

83. Haskell RJ, Wong BM, Hansen JE. A double-bind, randomized clinical trial of methylprednisolone in status asthmaticus. *Arch Intern Med* 1983;143:1324–1327.

84. Cook JL. Infection in asthma. *Semin Respir Med* 1987;8:259–263.

85. Lanes SF, Garret JE, Wentworth CE, et al. The effect of adding ipratropium bromide to salbutamol in the treatment of acute asthma a pooled analysis of three trials. *Chest* 1998;114:365–372.

85a. Rodrigo G, Rodrigo C, Burschtin O. A meta-analysis of the effects of ipratropium bromide in adults with acute asthma. *Am J Med* 1999;107:363–370.

86. Kass JE, Terregino CA. The effect of heliox in acute asthma: a randomized controlled trial. *Chest* 1999;116:296–300.

87. Gluckman TJ, Corbridge T. Management of respiratory failure in patients with asthma. *Curr Opinion Pulm Med* 2000;6:79–85.

88. O'Rourke PP, Crone PK. Halothane in status asthmaticus. *Crit Care Med* 1982;10:341–343.

23

ACUTE HYPOXEMIC RESPIRATORY FAILURE: PULMONARY EDEMA AND ACUTE LUNG INJURY

LORRAINE B. WARE
MICHAEL A. MATTHAY

INTRODUCTION

PHYSIOLOGIC AND STRUCTURAL ASPECTS OF FLUID EXCHANGE IN THE LUNG

HIGH-PRESSURE CARDIOGENIC PULMONARY EDEMA
Implications for Treatment of High-Pressure Cardiogenic Pulmonary Edema

INCREASED-PERMEABILITY PULMONARY EDEMA (ACUTE LUNG INJURY AND ARDS)
Implications for Treatment of Increased-Permeability Edema and ARDS

INTRODUCTION

This chapter will consider the causes of acute respiratory failure that are primarily associated with severe hypoxemia. In the majority of these patients, the defect in oxygenation is due to filling of the distal air spaces of the lung with edema fluid, blood, or purulent exudate. Microatelectasis may also contribute to the hypoxemia. The physiologic basis for the hypoxemia includes both ventilation to perfusion mismatch and right-to-left intrapulmonary shunting through fluid-filled or collapsed alveoli. Although alveolar filling may be caused by a variety of disorders, this chapter focuses on cardiogenic and noncardiogenic pulmonary edema (clinical acute lung injury), the most common causes of acute hypoxemic respiratory failure.

Two types of pulmonary edema occur in humans: (a) high-pressure edema (usually cardiogenic), and (b) edema secondary to increased permeability of the lung microvascular endothelium and/or the alveolar epithelium. The correct diagnosis and appropriate treatment of both kinds of pulmonary edema require a good understanding of the normal physiology of fluid exchange in the microcirculation of the lung. In addition, familiarity with the structures that surround the fluid-exchanging vessels is essential to understanding how and where edema fluid accumulates in the lung.

This discussion of pulmonary edema is divided into three sections. The first part briefly reviews transvascular fluid and protein movement in the normal lung. This first section also considers the influence of the lung structure on the distribution and removal of normal and excessive quantities of fluid. The second part of the chapter describes the interstitial and alveolar phases of high-pressure (cardiogenic) pulmonary edema. The chapter concludes with experimental and clinical examples to illustrate the fundamental physiologic abnormalities that characterize increased-permeability edema. This final section also briefly reviews the common clinical disorders that have been associated with increased-permeability edema, also called acute lung injury or acute respiratory distress syndrome (ALI/ARDS). Principles of therapy for ALI/ARDS are considered in this chapter, although the general principles for the treatment of acute respiratory failure with mechanical ventilation are discussed in Chapter 21, General Principles of Managing the Patient with Respiratory Failure, and hemodynamic assessment and management are considered in detail in Chapter 25, Managing the Patient with Hemodynamic Insufficiency, Shock, and Multiple Organ Failure.

PHYSIOLOGIC AND STRUCTURAL ASPECTS OF FLUID EXCHANGE IN THE LUNG

In the normal lung, as in all other organs, there is a net outward movement of fluid from the vascular to the interstitial space. This fluid is removed by lymphatics, which under normal conditions prevent excess fluid from accumulating in the interstitial space of the lung (1). The factors that determine the quantity of fluid that leaves the vascular space are included in the Starling equation for filtration of fluid across a semipermeable membrane (2). A simplified version of the equation is:

$$Q = K\left[(Pmv - Ppmv) - (\pi mv - \pi pmv)\right]$$

where Q is the net transvascular flow of fluid, K describes quantitatively the permeability of the membrane, Pmv is the hydrostatic pressure in the lumen of the microvessels, and $Ppmv$ is the hydrostatic pressure in the perimicrovascular interstitial space. The term πmv is the plasma protein osmotic pressure in the circulation, and πpmv is the protein osmotic pressure in the perimicrovascular compartment. This equation is applicable to the microcirculation of the lung, because normal pulmonary capillary permeability allows some water and solutes (electrolytes) to leave the circulation but restricts the movement of larger molecules such as plasma proteins. Thus the net transvascular filtration of fluid (Q) into the interstitium of the lung depends on the net difference between hydrostatic and protein osmotic pressures, as well as on the permeability of the capillary membrane.

Most evidence suggests that under normal circumstances the hydrostatic pressure in the perimicrovascular interstitial space ($Ppmv$) is close to alveolar pressure, which is approximately zero, or atmospheric pressure (3). Thus the main hydrostatic force for fluid filtration in the lung is the hydrostatic pressure within the capillaries (Pmv). The absolute value for hydrostatic pressure in the lung microcirculation increases from the top to the bottom of the lung (4). Hydrostatic pressure in the microvessels also varies along the length of the pre- to postcapillary vessels, depending on the resistance of the vessels (5). Hydrostatic pressure also depends on whether the vessel is in a zone 1, 2, or 3 condition (see also Chapter 2, Mechanics of Ventilation). Clinically, it has generally been assumed that the average value for Pmv in the lung is roughly equal to left atrial pressure. However, some investigators have estimated that Pmv is probably closer to left atrial pressure plus about one-half of the differ-

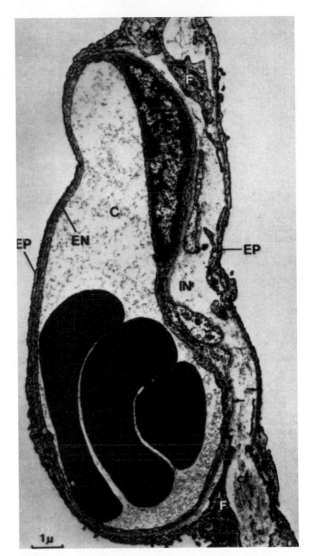

FIGURE 23.1. Electron micrograph of an alveolar capillary (C) cross-section from human lung. Blood cells are suspended in the interalveolar septum between two alveolar spaces. The alveolar epithelium (EP) is the barrier that separates the air spaces from the interstitium (IN). The endothelium (EN) separates the vascular space from the interstitium. Fluid and protein exchange probably occurs through small gaps between the endothelial cells in the alveolar capillaries. Connective tissue fibers are found in the interstitium, where the basal laminae (arrows) of the epithelium and endothelium are separated. (F) fibroblast. (From Fishman AP, Renkin E. *Pulmonary edema.* Bethesda, MD: American Physiological Society, 1979:4, with permission.)

TABLE 23.1. STARLING EQUATION

$$\dot{Q} = K[(Pmv - Ppmv) - (\pi mv - \pi pmv)]$$

Transvascular fluid flow = permeability fluid flux × [hydrostatic pressure − protein osmotic pressure]. Then, substituting estimated values for the variables under normal conditions:

$$\dot{Q} = K[(10 - 0) - (25 - 19)]$$
$$\dot{Q} = K[10 - 6] = K \times 4.$$

1. Net calculated transvascular fluid flow ($\dot{Q}$) is positive from the capillary lumen into the perimicrovascular interstitial space.
2. Note that the protein osmotic pressure gradient normally opposes fluid filtration out of the vessels. If the gradient were abolished, i.e., if protein osmotic pressure were assumed to be equal on both sides of the capillary, then the calculated transvascular fluid flow would more than double.
3. Also, if permeability (K) increases, there are two apparent effects: (a) transvascular fluid flux increases, even at normal hydrostatic pressures, and (b) the protein osmotic pressure difference across the capillary membrane decreases as proteins leak into the interstitium, further increasing transvascular fluid flux.

ence between mean pulmonary artery pressure and left atrial pressure (6). Thus pulmonary artery wedge pressure measurements of left atrial pressure remain the most reliable clinical indicator of hydrostatic pressure in the microcirculation of the lung, but the precapillary or pulmonary arterial pressure may also contribute to fluid filtration under some conditions (7).

Protein osmotic pressure in the circulation (πmv) is higher than protein osmotic pressure in the perimicrovascular interstitial space (πpmv). This gradient is maintained because the normal permeability of the capillary endothelial junctions allows only a small quantity of protein to flow out of the circulation into the interstitial space of the lung. Thus the sum of protein osmotic pressures normally favors fluid absorption into the circulation and thereby partially offsets the net hydrostatic force that causes fluid to leave the vascular space. In Table 23.1 we have estimated a value for each of the Starling forces and then calculated a value for net fluid filtration (Q) that is consistent with experimental studies of transvascular fluid movement in the normal lung (8).

Most of the available evidence indicates that the primary site for fluid exchange in the lung is in the microcirculation of the alveolar vessels (see Chapter 2, Mechanics of Ventilation, for a definition of alveolar versus extra-alveolar vessels). Anatomically, the microvessels in humans have no media or adventitia, and thus their walls are thinner than those of larger vessels (9). However, a number of experimental studies have shown that some liquid probably also leaks from small arterioles and venules that are located at the corners of alveolar wall junctions (10,11). Figure 23.1 shows an alveolar vessel (capillary) in the lung, surrounded by an interstitial space. In the normal lung, fluid and protein leakage is believed to occur through small gaps between the capillary endothelial cells (3,12).

Fluid that is filtered into the alveolar interstitial space normally does not enter the alveoli, because the alveolar epithelium is composed of very tight junctions (Fig. 23.1) that prevent fluid and protein from entering the alveolar air spaces (12–14). Rather, once the filtered fluid enters the alveolar interstitial space, it moves proximally toward the peribronchial and perivascular space in the extra-alveolar interstitium (15). Since interstitial pressure in the extra-alveolar space is negative relative to the alveolar interstitial space, the loose connective tissue space acts as a sump to drain fluid from the alveolar wall interstitium (16-18). Under ordinary conditions the lymphatics ultimately remove all the filtered fluid and return it to the systemic circulation (Fig. 23.2). It has been estimated that about 10 to 20 mL of fluid per hour is filtered in the lung and removed by the lymphatics in normal humans (19).

Since surface tension in the normal alveolus is low, it is thought that surface tension has a minimal effect on interstitial pressure around alveolar vessels and thus little effect on normal fluid balance in the lung. However, if surface tension were high, then perimicrovascular interstitial hydrostatic pressure (*Ppmv*) could become more negative and thereby increase the transvascular pressure gradient for movement of fluid from the alveolar vessels or the extra-alveolar corner vessels into the interstitial space (see Table 23.1). A deficiency of surfactant could lead to high surface tension and possibly favor the development of pulmonary edema (20,21). Clinically, abnormal or inactivated surfactant may

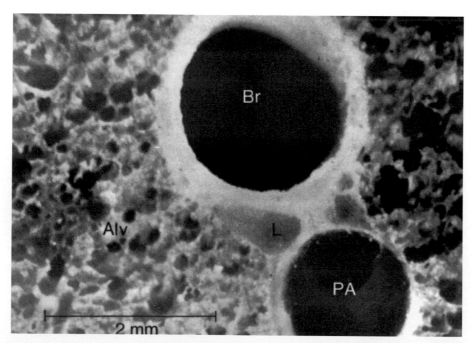

FIGURE 23.2. A photomicrograph from a sheep lung frozen at normal inflation pressure. The bronchus (Br), lymphatic (L), and partially blood-filled pulmonary artery (PA) are surrounded by loose connective tissue. This is the extra-alveolar interstitial space. The alveolar ducts and alveoli (Alv) surround the bronchovascular sheath. The lymphatics drain fluid that is filtered from the capillaries, and return this fluid to the systemic circulation.

contribute to the extent of pulmonary edema in some patients (22).

In summary, there is a constant flow of fluid through the interstitium of the lungs. Small amounts of fluid leak from the alveolar and some extra-alveolar vessels into the perimicrovascular interstitial space. This fluid does not enter the alveolar space because of the high resistance of the normally tight alveolar epithelium. The filtered fluid moves to the extra-alveolar interstitial space, where lymphatics remove it from the lung.

For experimental purposes, lung lymph flow can be collected from some species (sheep, goats, or dogs) to study the normal physiology of fluid and protein balance in the lung as well as to learn how the lung responds to pathologic conditions (8,15). The quantity of lung lymph flow can be used to estimate the quantity of fluid leaving the vascular space in the lung; the protein concentration of the lymph can be measured to determine the amount of protein leaving the microcirculation and thereby to evaluate the permeability of the pulmonary microvascular barrier (23). Several investigators have studied lung lymph flow in animal models in an effort better to understand the pathogenesis of the various kinds of pulmonary edema (24–26).

As stated, pulmonary edema is caused by high pressure, increased permeability, or both. In the next section, high-pressure edema is examined, with an emphasis on correlating the clinical features with the physiologic abnormalities.

HIGH-PRESSURE CARDIOGENIC PULMONARY EDEMA

According to the Starling equation, when hydrostatic pressure increases in the microcirculation, the rate of transvascular fluid filtration rises. The clinical counterpart of this physiologic principle occurs in humans when there is a rise in left atrial pressure, usually as a result of left ventricular failure. This increased left atrial pressure is transmitted to the microcirculation of the lung, resulting in an increase in transvascular fluid flow into the interstitium of the lung. With a small increase in left atrial pressure (to 14 to 20 mm Hg), most patients experience only a mild degree of dyspnea. The chest radiograph usually demonstrates prominent interlobular septae (Kerley B lines) consistent with pulmonary edema confined to the interstitium (Fig. 23.3). Histologically, mild elevations of left atrial pressure lead to interstitial edema in the alveolar septae and in the extraalveolar spaces in the loose connective tissue around the bronchovascular sheath. Figure 23.4 illustrates the prominent perivascular fluid cuffs in this phase of interstitial pulmonary edema.

As left atrial pressure acutely rises above 25 to 30 mm Hg, the capacity of the interstitial space in the lung and the pumping ability of the lymphatics to clear fluid are usually exceeded, and the edema fluid breaks through the

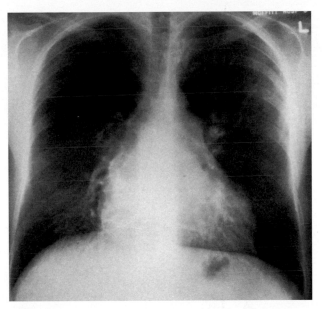

FIGURE 23.3. A posterior-anterior chest radiograph from a patient with interstitial pulmonary edema secondary to left ventricular heart failure. Pulmonary capillary wedge pressure was measured at 20 mm Hg. The arrow in the left upper lobe indicates prominent vascular markings. The arrows in the right lower lobe draw attention to prominent Kerley B lines, which indicate fluid-filled interlobular septae.

alveolar epithelium and begins to flood the alveolar air spaces (1). The development of arterial hypoxemia has been shown experimentally to correlate with alveolar flooding (27).

High-pressure cardiogenic edema has been well studied in experimental animals by using samples of lung lymph to quantify the amount of fluid leaving the vascular space and the protein content of that fluid (8,15). As left atrial pressure is increased by placing an inflatable balloon in the left atrium, lung lymph flow rises and the concentration of protein declines (Fig. 23.5). This indicates, as the Starling equation predicts, that transvascular flow of water and solutes into the interstitium of the lung is increasing. Since the permeability of the capillary endothelium remains normal, the fluid leaving the circulation has a low protein content, resulting in a fall in the lymph to plasma protein ratio.

During the early, interstitial phase of high-pressure pulmonary edema, the lung has at least three safety factors that function to protect against alveolar flooding. First, lung lymph flow increases, clearing some of the edema fluid from the lung as shown in Figure 23.5. Second, the concentration of protein in the perimicrovascular interstitial space falls, since there is an increase in water and solutes entering the interstitial space surrounding the alveolar vessels. This decrease in perimicrovascular protein concentration leads to an increase in the protein osmotic pressure difference between the plasma and the interstitial fluid ($\pi mv - \pi pmv$). This results in an increased protein osmotic force to absorb

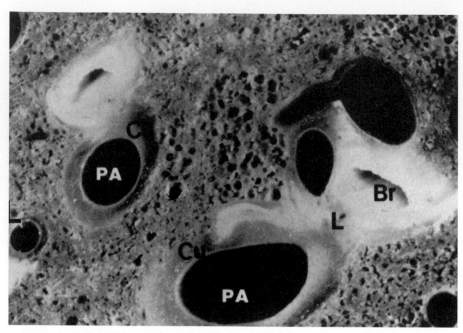

FIGURE 23.4. Photograph of a frozen sheep lung. In this experimental study, left atrial pressure was elevated to 20 cm H_2O for four hours. The result is interstitial pulmonary edema with perivascular fluid cuffs (Cu) around pulmonary arteries (PA) and small airways (Br). There are some lymphatics (L) visible in the fluid cuffs also.

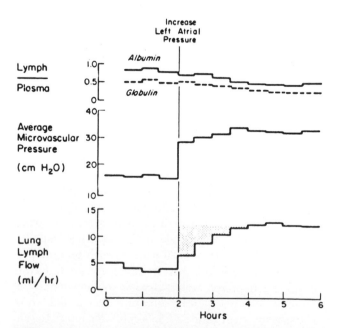

FIGURE 23.5. The time course of a sheep experiment in which left atrial pressure was elevated after a two-hour stable baseline period. Note that with left atrial hypertension, the lung lymph flow rises sharply and the lymph:plasma protein concentrations fall. This is typical of high-pressure pulmonary edema. (From Erdmann AJ III, Vaughn TR, Brigham KL, et al. Effect of increased vascular pressure on lung fluid balance in unanesthetized sheep. *Circ Res* 1975;37:271–284. With permission of the American Heart Association, Inc.)

fluid back into the circulation. It has been estimated that this increased protein osmotic pressure difference offsets about one-half of the rise in transvascular fluid filtration that can occur from a rise in hydrostatic pressure alone (15). In fact, patients with low plasma protein concentrations are likely to develop clinical pulmonary edema at lower levels of left atrial pressure elevation than those with normal plasma protein concentrations (28). The third safety factor against alveolar flooding is the capacity of the interstitial space in the lung to accommodate approximately 500 mL of edema fluid in the bronchovascular cuffs (Fig. 23.4) (15).

When the capacity of the interstitial space is exceeded, the interstitial edema fluid moves through the visceral pleura and causes pleural effusions (29,30). These effusions are primarily related to the elevation of left atrial pressure and the magnitude of pulmonary edema, as demonstrated by studies in patients with congestive heart failure (31,32) or in experimental studies of hydrostatic pulmonary edema (33) or increased-permeability pulmonary edema (34).

When the capacity of the interstitial space is exceeded, the edema fluid also breaks through the alveolar epithelium and fills the air spaces by bulk flow. Samples of edema fluid in experimental animals have demonstrated that the initial sample of high-pressure cardiogenic pulmonary edema flow is low in protein content relative to the plasma protein (less than 65%) (23). Sampling of undiluted alveolar fluid using a tracheal suction catheter wedged in a distal airway is a useful diagnostic test to separate patients with high-pressure pulmonary edema from those with an increased-permeability edema since the latter group of patients have an alveolar fluid to plasma protein ratio of 75% or greater, providing the edema fluid is sampled before resolution has occurred and alveolar liquid reabsorption has begun (35–38).

Both *in vivo* and *in vitro* work has shown that resolution or clearance of edema from the air spaces of the lung depends on active sodium transport across the alveolar epithelial barrier. The primary site of sodium reabsorption is through epithelial sodium channels located on the apical membrane of alveolar epithelial type II cells (39–41). Sodium is then actively extruded into the interstitial space via the NaK-ATPase located on the basolateral membrane of type II cells. Water follows passively, predominantly through water channels, the aquaporins, found on alveolar epithelial type I cells (42,43). Alveolar fluid is removed even in the face of a rising alveolar edema protein concentration in excess of the plasma protein concentration (44–47). Interestingly, in experimental studies in a variety of species, including humans, β-adrenergic agonist therapy increases sodium transport, resulting in a marked increase in the clearance of alveolar liquid (48–54).

Clinically, high-pressure cardiogenic edema is the most common form of pulmonary edema. Measurement of elevated pulmonary arterial wedge pressures with a pulmonary artery catheter helps to confirm that the pulmonary edema is from high pressure when the etiology of the pulmonary edema cannot be established on clinical grounds alone (55–57). Use of noninvasive techniques such as two-dimensional echocardiography to measure left ventricular contractility and ejection fraction is also extremely helpful. The underlying cause is usually left ventricular failure from ischemic heart disease, aortic or mitral valve disease, or a cardiomyopathy. Occasionally, patients with normal cardiac function develop high-pressure pulmonary edema from fluid overload. In addition, some noncardiogenic causes of pulmonary edema may be complicated by an element of high pressure in the pulmonary circulation (58).

Implications for Treatment of High-Pressure Cardiogenic Pulmonary Edema

Effective therapy for high-pressure pulmonary edema depends on lowering left atrial pressure and thus decreasing the driving force ($Pmv - Ppmv$) responsible for increased filtration of fluid into the extravascular space. A reduction in left atrial filling pressure (preload) can be accomplished by decreasing venous filling of the heart. Osler's classic method for treatment of cardiogenic pulmonary edema is based on this principle of decreasing venous return to the heart by sitting the patient upright and using rotating tourniquets on the extremities to impede blood return to the heart (59).

For more than 50 years, morphine sulfate has been known to be effective in treating cardiogenic pulmonary edema. Part of the beneficial effect of morphine depends on a reduction in preload to the heart because it causes systemic venodilation (60). Venodilators such as sublingual, topical, or intravenous nitroglycerin are also effective in reducing venous return and left ventricular preload (61). More potent agents such as sodium nitroprusside can rapidly decrease venous return (62). Nitroprusside also reduces systemic blood pressure, reducing the afterload (resistance) on the left ventricle, which may result in better cardiac function with a subsequent lowering of left atrial filling pressures, particularly if cardiac insufficiency is complicated by systemic hypertension (63). Potent diuretics such as furosemide lower left atrial filling pressure by decreasing systemic venous tone (when given intravenously) and inducing diuresis of the expanded extracellular volume (61,64).

Finally, agents that improve myocardial contractility can lower cardiac filling pressures. Acutely, this can be accomplished with inotropic vasopressors such as dopamine or dobutamine given in low doses (65,66). In patients with chronic congestive heart failure and pulmonary congestion, digitalis augments myocardial contractility and thereby decreases left atrial and left ventricular filling pressures (67).

Patients with acute cardiogenic pulmonary edema and severe respiratory distress often generate very negative pleural pressures in an effort to maintain adequate alveolar ventilation. These negative pleural pressures may increase left ventricular transmural pressure and thus increase left ventricular afterload (68). Patients with acute pulmonary edema also are more susceptible to respiratory muscle fatigue (69,70). It is not surprising, therefore, that some patients with acute cardiogenic pulmonary edema develop refractory hypoxemia and hypercapnia, even with adequate supplemental oxygen and appropriate pharmacologic therapy. These more seriously ill patients usually require tracheal intubation and positive pressure mechanical ventilation to achieve adequate arterial oxygenation and adequate alveolar ventilation, although recently some patients have been treated successfully with noninvasive positive pressure ventilation (see Chapter 21, General Principles of Managing the Patient with Respiratory Failure). Institution of positive pressure ventilation in patients with acute cardiogenic pulmonary edema usually results in prompt improvement in oxygenation and sometimes in cardiac output as well. The improved oxygenation is due to better lung inflation, with improved matching of ventilation and perfusion. An improvement in left ventricular function may occur because of at least four possible factors: (a) improved arterial oxygen saturation and hence better myocardial oxygen supply; (b) reduction in the extreme pleural pressure swings present with spontaneous ventilation, and hence reduction in afterload on the left ventricle; (c) less workload on the failing heart because the work of breathing (and the oxygen needed to perform it) has been assumed by a mechanical ventilator; (d) reduction in atrial filling pressure (preload) because positive pressure ventilation decreases venous return to the heart.

INCREASED-PERMEABILITY PULMONARY EDEMA (ACUTE LUNG INJURY AND ARDS)

The Starling equation predicts that a change in permeability of the microvascular membrane (*K*) will result in a marked increase in the amount of fluid and protein leaving the vascular space. Pulmonary edema of this type should have a high protein content because a more permeable vascular membrane does not have a normal capacity to restrict the outward movement of larger molecules such as plasma proteins. Results of clinical and experimental studies demonstrate that this is exactly what happens in most types of noncardiogenic pulmonary edema (24,25,46,71,72).

Increased-permeability pulmonary edema usually develops in the setting of an acute lung injury. The acute lung injury syndrome of poor oxygenation, dense pulmonary infiltrates, and decreased lung compliance was first described by Petty and Ashbaugh in 1971 and termed the adult respiratory distress syndrome (73). A more specific definition that requires quantitative scoring of the physiologic and radiographic abnormalities to determine whether the acute lung injury is mild, moderate, or severe ARDS was proposed in 1988 (74). This lung injury score also takes into account the presence of absence of nonpulmonary organ failure and the associated clinical disorder, since prognosis depends on these factors as well as the extent of acute lung injury (75,76). In 1994, a simplified definition was proposed by a North American European Consensus Conference for what is now termed the acute (rather than adult) respiratory distress syndrome (77). Using this definition, ARDS is defined as the acute onset of bilateral infiltrates indistinguishable from cardiogenic pulmonary edema, with an inspired to arterial oxygen ratio of less than 200, and no clinical evidence of left atrial hypertension. A less severe form of ARDS, termed acute lung injury (ALI) was defined similarly to ARDS but with an inspired to arterial oxygen ratio of less than 300. These new consensus definitions for ALI and ARDS are widely used and have improved standardization of clinical trials. However, they fail to take into account the underlying cause of acute lung injury and the presence or absence of multiorgan failure, both factors which can influence outcome (78–82).

The list of clinical disorders associated with the development of ALI/ARDS is impressively long (Table 23.2) (83,84). The acute lung injury can occur via either the blood (sepsis, fat embolism) or the airways (liquid aspiration, pulmonary infections). In some clinical disorders, such as drug overdose or acute pancreatitis, the route of lung injury is not known. Because of this heterogeneity of causes and clinical manifestations of ALI/ARDS and the lack of standardized definitions prior to 1994, the incidence of ALI/ARDS has been difficult to quantify. One estimate places the incidence at 150,000 cases of ALI/ARDS in the United States annu-

TABLE 23.2. CLINICAL DISORDERS ASSOCIATED WITH ARDS

Sepsis
Trauma
  Fat emboli
  Lung contusion
  Nonthoracic trauma
Liquid aspiration
  Gastric contents
  Fresh and salt water (drowning)
  Hydrocarbon fluids
Drug-associated
  Heroin
  Methadone
  Propoxyphene
  Barbiturates
  Colchicine
  Ethchlorvynol
  Aspirin
  Hydrochlorothiazide
Inhaled toxins
  Smoke
  Oxygen (high concentration)
  Corrosive chemicals
  (NO_2, Cl_2, NH_3, phosgene)
Shock of any etiology
Hematologic disorders
  Massive blood transfusion
  Disseminated intravascular coagulation
Metabolic
  Acute pancreatitis
  Uremia
Miscellaneous
  Lymphangiography
  Reexpansion pulmonary edema
  Increased intracranial pressure
  Postcardiopulmonary bypass
  Eclampsia
  Air emboli
  Amniotic fluid embolism
  Ascent to high altitude
Primary pneumonias
  Viral
  Bacterial
  Mycobacterium
  Tuberculosis
  Fungal
  Pneumocystis carinii

ally, however, prospective epidemiologic studies are needed to determine the current incidence of ALI/ARDS (85,86).

Overall mortality in ALI/ARDS has been exceedingly high, from 50% to 70%, partly because of associated multiorgan failure as well as uncontrolled or recurrent infection (76,78,79,82). Two recent studies suggest that mortality from ALI/ARDS may be decreasing (87,88). The reasons for this decline are unclear but are perhaps related to better supportive care of critically ill patients or better management of sepsis. Although the lung appears to be the primary target organ for failure in ALI/ARDS, a number of studies have shown that mortality in ALI/ARDS is closely related to multiorgan failure, uncontrolled infection, and chronic medical diseases such as liver failure that are associated with ALI/ARDS (74–76,89). In fact, mortality seems to be directly caused by respiratory failure alone in less than 20% of ARDS cases, although most patients die with severe respiratory failure (76). Sepsis appears to be the most important cause of both early and late mortality (76,89).

The principal clinical manifestations of ALI/ARDS are similar, regardless of what the associated clinical condition may be. The typical findings are (a) severe hypoxemia, unresponsive to low-flow oxygen and due to intrapulmonary right-to-left shunting of blood through fluid-filled and atelectatic alveoli (90); (b) bilateral, fluffy infiltrates on the chest radiograph, indistinguishable from cardiogenic pulmonary edema (Fig. 23.6); and (c) a decrease in the static lung compliance. Clinically, this change in the mechanical properties of the lungs is manifested by the high ventilatory pressures that are required to deliver an adequate tidal volume.

In the acute phase of permeability pulmonary edema and respiratory failure, the densities on the chest radiograph result from a combination of interstitial and alveolar edema in addition to a variable degree of atelectasis. Typically, the lung volumes are reduced because of a change in the mechanical properties of the lung. A reduction in vital capacity and functional residual capacity and an increase in lung compliance occur for three main reasons: (a) edema fluid in the air spaces displaces air, decreasing gas volumes; (b) edema in peribronchovascular interstitial spaces causes airways to narrow or close, which results in atelectasis (see Fig. 23.4); and (c) there may be a reduction in surfactant (secondary to alveolar epithelial injury), which could increase surface tension and thereby decrease lung compliance (91–93).

Histologically, in this acute phase of lung injury there is widespread interstitial and alveolar edema, with an abun-

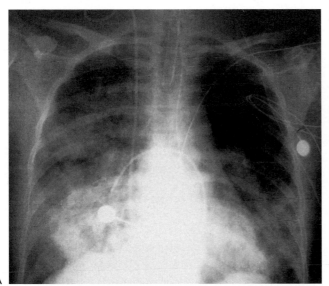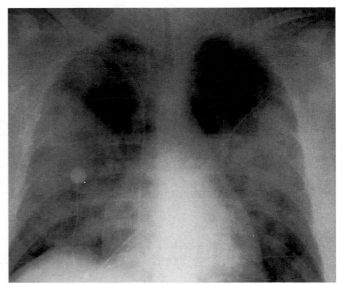

A   B

FIGURE 23.6. **(A)** Anterior-posterior chest radiograph from a 40-year-old man with acute respiratory failure from gastric aspiration. Note that the endotracheal tube is in good position. The pulmonary artery line, inserted through the right internal jugular vein, passes through the superior vena cava, right atrium, right ventricle, and main pulmonary artery, and terminates in a branch of pulmonary artery in the right lower lobe. The wedge pressure was 2 mm Hg. The radiographic pattern indicates a typical location for pulmonary aspiration into dependent segments of the left lower lobe, right lower lobe, and right upper lobe. Before tracheal intubation, this patient's PaO$_2$ was 55 mm Hg on an FiO$_2$ of 0.9. The fluffy bilateral infiltrates progressed to involve all lung zones within three days. However, the patient ultimately recovered after two weeks of treatment with antibiotics and mechanical ventilation with PEEP. **(B)** Anterior-posterior chest radiograph from a 55-year-old man who developed noncardiogenic pulmonary edema from Gram-negative sepsis. The pulmonary artery line was inserted through the right subclavian vein and terminated in a posterior branch (visible on a lateral chest film) of the right pulmonary artery. The cardiac silhouette appears slightly enlarged, but the wedge pressure was 4 mm Hg and the cardiac output was high (consistent with sepsis). The PaO$_2$ was 45 mm Hg on an FiO$_2$ of 0.90 prior to ventilation with positive pressure. The patient's acute respiratory failure and sepsis were successfully treated and the FiO$_2$ was lowered to 0.50 with 15 cm H$_2$O of PEEP within two days. Subsequently the patient did not improve, and he ultimately developed recurrent sepsis and died with severe ARDS.

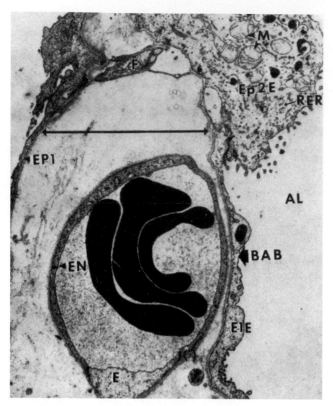

FIGURE 23.7. Electron micrograph of an alveolar capillary in the interalveolar septum between alveolar spaces (AL) from a patient with ARDS. The interstitial space is widened by edema fluid (arrows), and the capillary endothelium has normal areas (EN) and swollen, abnormal areas (E). Some of the alveolar epithelium is normal (EP1), whereas other type 1 and 2 cells are swollen (E1E and Ep2E). The damaged type 2 cell shows degenerative features, with swollen mitochondria (M) and degranulating rough endoplasmic reticulum (RER). There is a fibrocyte (F) that anchors the epithelial basement membrane. (From Fishman AP, Renkin E. *Pulmonary edema.* Bethesda, MD: American Physiological Society: 103, with permission.)

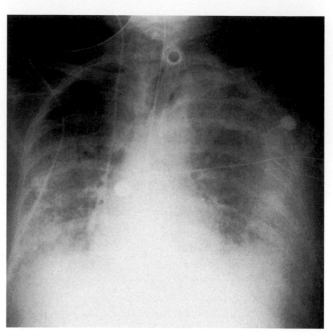

FIGURE 23.8. Anterior-posterior chest radiograph of a 42-year-old woman being ventilated through a cuffed tracheostomy tube. Her respiratory failure had begun three weeks previously when she developed ARDS from severe acute pancreatitis. Note the diffuse ground-glass appearance of the lung fields. At this point in her clinical course she had noncompliant lungs that required very high airway pressures to provide an adequate tidal volume. She died of persistent respiratory failure one week after this chest radiograph was taken. Postmortem examination of the lungs revealed extensive interstitial fibrosis and hyaline membranes.

dance of polymorphonuclear leukocytes, erythrocytes, macrophages, cell debris, plasma proteins, and strands of fibrin. Electron microscopy studies have shown injury to the capillary endothelium and denuding of the alveolar epithelium (Fig. 23.7) (94). If the patient survives the acute phase of the lung injury, the pulmonary edema may resolve and the patient may completely recover normal lung function over a few months (95,96).

However, some patients with ARDS progress from the acute lung injury to a subacute phase over seven to 14 days, during which time they still require mechanical ventilation with high airway pressures and high fractions of inspired oxygen, and may have worsening pulmonary hypertension (Fig. 23.8) (97). These patients develop fibrosis and capillary obliteration in the lungs, a condition which is termed fibrosing alveolitis (94,98). It is not clear why some patients successfully repair their injured lungs and recover, whereas progressive fibrosis and even bullae develop in the lungs

of others (Fig. 23.9). The development of fibrosis and the resultant reduced lung compliance predispose patients to develop barotrauma, which may manifest as pneumothoraces, pneumomediastinum, and subcutaneous emphysema (Fig. 23.10) (99,100). The role of secondary lung injury from oxygen toxicity has been difficult to quantify experimentally or even to estimate clinically (98,101,102).

Numerous experimental and clinical studies have been done during the last 15 years to determine the mechanisms of acute lung injury in noncardiogenic pulmonary edema. Since many disorders are associated with ARDS, the cause of the increased-permeability edema may depend on the specific associated etiology. For example, neutrophils have been implicated as a major factor in lung injury from sepsis and microembolism (103,104). Complement activation in sepsis may play a role in activating white blood cells to release toxic enzymes (e.g., neutral proteases) that could increase endothelial permeability in the lung (105). One study showed that neutrophil elastolytic activity in air spaces is very high in half of ARDS patients (106). However, some investigators have shown that neither white blood cells nor complement are necessary for some kinds of permeability pulmonary edema (107,108). Also, other investigators have implicated the fibrinogen and coagulation system in the

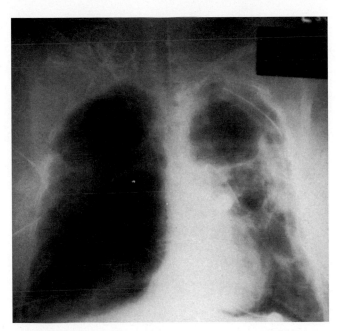

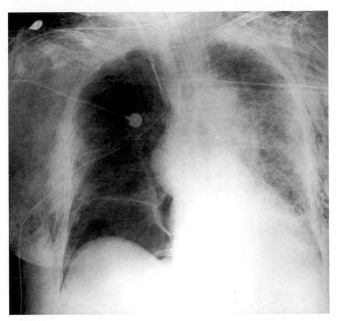

FIGURE 23.9. Anterior-posterior chest radiograph of a 36-year-old woman who had developed ARDS from Gram-negative sepsis six weeks prior to this chest film. Her clinical course was characterized by persistent respiratory failure and ventilator dependence. Her chest radiograph initially showed noncardiogenic pulmonary edema with fluffy infiltrates (as in Fig. 23.6B). About two weeks following the development of ARDS from sepsis, her chest radiograph showed a diffuse ground-glass appearance (as in Fig. 23.6) and her lungs became very noncompliant. Finally, five weeks following the onset of ARDS she developed bilateral bullae in the upper and lower lung zones and required multiple chest tubes to drain recurrent pneumothoraces. She died two days after this chest film was taken. At postmortem examination her lungs showed large bullae with extensive loss of lung tissue. She had no prior history of smoking and her chest film was normal prior to the onset of sepsis and ARDS.

FIGURE 23.10. Anteroposterior chest radiograph of a 42-year-old woman who developed severe ARDS from aspiration of gastric contents. This radiograph was taken 10 days into her course. Note the severe barotrauma, with bilateral chest tubes, pneumomediastinum and severe subcutaneous emphysema.

pathogenesis of acute lung injury (109,110). The possible role of proinflammatory cytokines, such as tumor necrosis factor, interleukin-1, or interleukin-8, in mediating pulmonary and systemic lung injury from sepsis has been studied in experimental and clinical studies (104,111,112). Recently, the role of oxidants in mediating acute lung injury has also been explored. There are several reviews which summarize much of the progress that has been made in unraveling the mechanisms of acute lung injury (89,104,113–115). Further research in the next few years probably will result in more specific information about the basic causes of acute lung injury.

An in-depth discussion of each of the associated causes of ALI/ARDS is not possible in this chapter. However, the two most common clinical disorders associated with the development of ARDS—gastric aspiration and sepsis—are considered below.

The acute respiratory failure that can follow gastric aspiration is a good example of ALI/ARDS resulting from direct injury to the alveolar epithelium and air spaces of the lung

(see Fig. 23.6A). Aspiration of gastric contents injures the lung if the pH is less than 2.5, even if the volume of aspirated fluid is small as 50 mL (116). The aspirated, acidic fluid acutely causes an increase in the permeability of the alveolar epithelium and the rapid development of pulmonary edema (117). The severe hypoxemia that occurs after massive gastric aspiration has been attributed to a combination of pulmonary edema and the atelectasis resulting from alterations of surfactant activity and subsequent closure of small airways (118). In fact, mortality in patients with ALI/ARDS secondary to gastric aspiration can be predicted in part by the severity of the arterial hypoxemia in relation to the alveolar oxygen tension (the $PaO_2:PAO_2$ ratio). If the $PaO_2:PAO_2$ is less than 0.50 immediately after gastric aspiration, the mortality rate is 50%, compared with 14% in patients with a ratio of greater than 0.50 (119). The ultimate outcome in patients with ALI/ARDS from gastric aspiration is also influenced by the delayed development of secondary bacterial lung infections with aerobic and anaerobic bacteria (120).

While massive gastric aspiration is a good illustration of acute respiratory failure from direct injury to the alveolar epithelium, systemic sepsis is an example of ALI/ARDS that develops from injury to the endothelium of the pulmonary microcirculation (see Fig. 23.6B). Clinical studies have shown that acute lung injury develops in about 60% of patients with sepsis syndrome, and about 25% to 35% of these patients develop severe acute lung injury (ARDS)

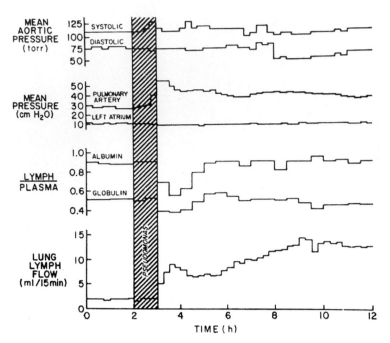

FIGURE 23.11. Effects of infusion of *Pseudomonas aeruginosa* on lung vascular pressures, lymph flow, and lymph:-plasma protein concentration in an unanesthetized sheep. Note that the lymph flow rises steeply several hours after the infusion of *Pseudomonas* organism, indicating that the capillary leak of protein-rich fluid occurs a few hours after the septic insult. (Reproduced from Brigham KL, Woolverton WC, Blake LH, et al. Increased sheep lung vascular permeability caused by *Pseudomonas* bacteria. *J Clin Invest* 1974;54:792–804, by copyright permission of the American Society for Clinical Investigation.)

(121,122). The mortality from ARDS secondary to sepsis ranges from 60% to 90% (75,122,123).

Studies in experimental animals have provided important information regarding the early phase of acute lung injury from sepsis. Brigham and associates (24,124,125) demonstrated that when sheep are given either *Pseudomonas* organisms or *Escherichia coli* endotoxin intravenously, lung lymph flow increases markedly. In these studies, the increase in lymph flow is associated with a high lymph to plasma protein ratio and a dramatic rise in lymph protein transport (Fig. 23.11). The increased lung lymph flow cannot be accounted for exclusively by a change in hydrostatic or protein osmotic pressures in the microcirculation of the lung and therefore must be due partly to an increase in lung vascular permeability. Histologic examination of the sheep lungs in this early phase shows interstitial edema with perivascular fluid cuffs, as seen in the interstitial phase of high-pressure pulmonary edema (see Fig. 23.4). The next phase of pulmonary edema is for the edema fluid to flood into the air spaces, although recent experimental studies have shown that the alveolar epithelium is more resistant than the lung endothelium to the injurious effects of *E. coli* endotoxin (126).

Clinically, the early phase of increased-permeability pulmonary edema from sepsis with interstitial edema is often not recognized (127). This is partly due to the lack of sensitive clinical indicators of a mild increase in extravascular lung water. The chest radiograph, for example, may not show edema until there is a 30% increase in lung water content (128,129). Also, major arterial blood gas abnormalities do not usually develop until edema fluid enters the air spaces, when there is a dramatic decrease in arterial oxygenation secondary to both ventilation-perfusion mismatch and right-to-left shunting of blood through fluid-filled alveoli (27,90).

Clinical studies of patients with permeability pulmonary edema from sepsis have shown that the pulmonary edema fluid has a high protein concentration (75% to 100%) compared with the plasma protein level (35,36,46,72). In addition, measurements of cardiac filling pressures with a pulmonary artery catheter usually demonstrate normal or even low pressures (71). Both these findings add further support to the concept that pulmonary edema from sepsis occurs because of an increase in permeability of the vascular endothelium and perhaps the alveolar epithelium as well.

Implications for Treatment of Increased-Permeability Edema and Ards

Ideal treatment for patients with increased-permeability edema would be an agent that could restore the abnormal vascular permeability of the pulmonary microcirculation and the alveolar epithelium to its normal state. This would prevent additional leakage of protein-rich fluid into the interstitium and alveoli of the lung. Unfortunately, no such agent is available at present. Although corticosteroids and antioxidant agents have been shown experimentally to modestly ameliorate acute lung injury if they are given before or immediately after the injury occurs, clinical studies have demonstrated no benefit of glucocorticoids or antioxidants for treatment of sepsis-induced ARDS (115).

At present, the best approach to therapy of ARDS is to identify and treat, if possible, the precipitating cause of the acute respiratory failure. The most treatable causes of ARDS are sepsis, respiratory infections, and shock. In many cases, such as smoke inhalation, trauma, and gastric aspiration, the injury has already occurred when the patient is first seen. In other cases, such as acute pancreatitis or viral pneumonia, the cause of the ARDS cannot be easily controlled. Supportive care for patients with ALI/ARDS is also critically important and should include adequate nutrition, identification, treatment and prevention of nosocomial infection, and prevention of thromboemboli and gastrointestinal bleeding (130).

The diagnosis of noncardiogenic pulmonary edema may need to be confirmed by measuring the vascular filling pressures in the pulmonary circulation to be certain that the pulmonary edema is not of cardiogenic origin (56). A pulmonary arterial catheter can be passed percutaneously into the pulmonary artery via the internal jugular, subclavian, femoral, or antecubital vein. As described in Chapter 25, Managing the Patient with Hemodynamic Insufficiency, Shock, and Multiple Organ Failure, the pulmonary artery wedge pressure usually reflects the left atrial filling pressure. Normal or low pressures (less than 12 mm Hg) indicate that the pulmonary edema is from a noncardiogenic cause. Occasionally, patients with pulmonary edema primarily from increased permeability also have an element of fluid overload with mildly elevated wedge pressures (131). As the Starling equation predicts, an increase in hydrostatic pressure (Pmv) in the face of increased vascular permeability (K) will result in an exponential rise in transvascular fluid flux (19,131–133). These patients may benefit from treatment (such as diuretics) that decreases left atrial filling pressures to a normal range.

Since most patients with ARDS have severe pulmonary edema and poorly compliant lungs, they usually experience respiratory muscle fatigue from the hypoxemia and the increased work of breathing. Mechanical ventilation with positive pressure is usually necessary to improve oxygenation and stabilize alveolar ventilation in patients with ARDS. Positive end–expiratory pressure (PEEP) in the range of 5 to 15 cm H_2O improves oxygenation further by inflating poorly ventilated alveoli and thereby decreasing the amount of venous admixture (or intrapulmonary shunting) in the lung (131). PEEP usually permits the fraction of inspired oxygen to be lowered, thus reducing the risk of superimposed oxygen toxicity to the lungs.

PEEP does not, however, alter the course of the primary lung injury. It does not, for example, reduce extravascular lung water content in pulmonary edema (134,135). High levels of PEEP (greater than 10 cm H_2O) usually cause a reduction in cardiac output (131). This reduction in cardiac output may result in an even higher arterial PaO_2. This improved oxygenation with a declining cardiac output results from either decreased blood flow to poorly ventilated lung regions or a longer time for oxygen diffusion in edematous lung units when pulmonary blood flow is reduced. Clinically, a reduction in cardiac output from PEEP may interfere with overall oxygen transport even if the arterial

oxygen tension is adequate. Careful monitoring of the effects of PEEP on cardiac output and perfusion to vital organs (brain, kidney) may be helpful in patients with ALI/ARDS and a low-output syndrome (131). Although some investigators have recommended adjusting the PEEP level in each patient based on a pressure volume curve to maximize alveolar recruitment, this approach cannot be recommended until it is studied in a large multicenter clinical trial (136).

The appropriate mode of mechanical ventilation for patients with ALI/ARDS has been controversial since the syndrome was first described. In the past, high tidal volumes of 12 to 15 mL per kg were routinely advocated to maintain normal levels of alveolar ventilation in the setting of decreased lung compliance. However, experimental evidence has been accumulating to suggest that ventilation with high tidal volumes and pressures may be injurious to the lung, and may worsen or prolong a preexisting lung injury (137–139). For this reason, several clinical trials of low tidal volume ventilation for ALI/ARDS have recently been completed. Although initial small trials were discouraging (140,141), a recently completed NIH-sponsored multicenter trial in 861 patients of 6 mL per kg versus 12 mL per kg tidal volume showed a 22% reduction in ALI/ARDS mortality with the low-tidal-volume approach (142). Since ventilation with low tidal volumes frequently causes alveolar hypoventilation and respiratory acidosis, patients must be carefully monitored and profound acidosis should be treated with bicarbonate administration.

In the future, other modalities of therapy for ALI/ARDS may be helpful, including surfactant replacement (143), monoclonal antibody treatment for sepsis (144), and modulation of pulmonary vascular tone (145), although recent experience with these approaches has not been encouraging (146–148). Manipulation of cytokine balance and antioxidant therapy may also have a role in the future, but clinical studies are lacking. It is also possible that efforts directed at accelerating recovery from acute lung injury may offer more long-term promise for effective therapy (149–152).

REFERENCES

1. Staub NC. Pulmonary edema. *Physiol Rev* 1974;54:678–811.
2. Starling EH. On the absorption of fluids from the connective tissue spaces. *J Physiol* 1986;19:312–326.
3. Staub NC. The pathogenesis of pulmonary edema. *Prog Cardiovasc Dis* 1980;23:53–80.
4. Blake LH, Staub NC. Pulmonary vascular transport in sheep. A mathematical model. *Microvasc Res* 1976;12:197–220.
5. Bhattacharya J, Staub NC. Direct measurement of microvascular pressure in the isolated, perfused dog lung. *Microvasc Res* 1979;17[Part 2]:586.
6. Gaar KA, Taylor AE, Owens LJ. Pulmonary capillary pressure and filtration coefficient in the isolated perfused lung. *Am J Physiol* 1967;213:910–914.
7. Brigham KL. Mechanisms of acute lung injury. *Clin Chest Med* 1982;3:9–24.
8. Erdmann JA, Vaughn TRJ, Brigham KL, et al. Effect of in-

creased vascular pressure on lung fluid balance in unanesthetized sheep. *Circ Res* 1975;37:271–284.

9. Reid I, Meyrick B. Microcirculation: definition and organization at tissue level. *Ann N Y Acad Sci* 1982;384:3–20.

10. Bo G, Hauge A, Nicolayson G. Alveolar pressure and lung volume as determinants of net transvascular fluid filtration. *J Appl Physiol* 1977;42:476–482.

11. Albert RK, Lakshminarayan S, Kirk W, et al. Lung inflation can cause pulmonary edema in zone I of in situ dog lungs. *J Appl Physiol* 1980;49:815–819.

12. Schneeberger-Keeley EE, Karnovscy MJ. The ultrastructural basis of alveolar capillary membrane permeability to peroxidase used as a tracer. *J Cell Biol* 1968;37:781–793.

13. Gorin AB, Stewart PA. Differential permeability of endothelial and epithelial barriers to albumin flux. *J Appl Physiol* 1979;47:1315–1324.

14. Taylor AE, Gaar KAJ. Estimation of equivalent pore radii of pulmonary capillary and alveolar membranes. *Am J Physiol* 1970;218:1133–1140.

15. Gee MH, Havil AM. The relationship between pulmonary perivascular cuff fluid and lung lymph in dogs with edema. *Microvasc Res* 1978;19:209–216.

16. Howell JBL, Permutt S, Proctor DF, et al. Effect of inflation of the lung on different parts of the pulmonary vascular bed. *J Appl Physiol* 1961;16:71.

17. Gee MH, William DO. Effect of lung inflation on perivascular cuff fluid volume in isolated dog lung lobes. *Microvasc Res* 1979;17:192–201.

18. Goshy M, Lai-Fook SJ, Hyatt RE. Perivascular pressure measurements by wick-catheter technique in isolated dog lobes. *J Appl Physiol* 1979;46:950–955.

19. Staub NC. Pulmonary edema. Physiologic approaches to management. *Chest* 1978;74:559–564.

20. Albert RK, Lakshminarayan S, Hildebrandt J, et al. Increased surface tension favors pulmonary edema formation in anesthetized dogs' lungs. *J Clin Invest* 1979;63:1015.

21. Raj U. Alveolar liquid pressure measured by micropuncture in isolated lungs of mature and immature fetal rabbits. *J Clin Invest* 1987;79:1579–1588.

22. Gregory TJ. Surfactant chemical composition and biophysical activity in acute respiratory distress syndrome. *J Clin Invest* 1991;88:1976–1981.

23. Vreim CE, Snashall PD, Demling RH, et al. Lung lymph and free interstitial fluid protein composition in sheep with edema. *Am J Physiol* 1976;230:1650–1653.

24. Brigham KL, Woolverton WC, Blake LH, et al. Increased sheep lung vascular permeability caused by Pseudomonas bacteremia. *J Clin Invest* 1974;54:792–804.

25. Ohkuda K, Nakahara K, Weidner WJ, et al. Lung fluid exchange after uneven pulmonary artery obstruction in sheep. *Circ Res* 1978;43:152–161.

26. Jayr C, Matthay MA. Alveolar and lung liquid clearance in the absence of pulmonary blood flow in sheep. *J Appl Physiol* 1991;71:1679–1687.

27. Bongard F, Matthay MA, Mackeasie RC, et al. Morphologic and physiologic correlates of increased extravascular lung water. *Surgery* 1984;96:395–403.

28. DaLuz PL, Shubia H, Weil MH. Pulmonary edema related to changes in colloid osmotic and pulmonary artery pressure in patients after acute myocardial infarction. *Circulation* 1975;51:350–357.

29. Aberle DR, Wiener-Kronish JP, Webb RW, et al. Hydrostatic versus increased permeability pulmonary edema: diagnosis based on radiographic criteria in critically ill patients. *Radiology* 1988;168:73–79.

30. Wiener-Kronish JP, Matthay MA. Pleural effusions associated with hydrostatic and increased permeability pulmonary edema. *Chest* 1988;93:852–858.

31. Wiener-Kronish JP, Matthay MA, Collen PE, et al. Relationship of pulmonary hemodynamics to pleural effusions in patients with heart failure. *Am Rev Respir Dis* 1988;132:1253–1256.

32. Wiener-Kronish JP, Goldstein R, Matthay RA, et al. Chronic pulmonary arterial and right atrial hypertension are not associated with pleural effusions. *Chest* 1987;92:967–970.

33. Broaddus VC, Wiener-Kronish JP, Staub NC. Removal of pleural liquid and protein by lymphatics in awake sheep. *J Appl Physiol* 1990;64:384–390.

34. Wiener-Kronish JP, Broaddus VC, Albertine K, et al. The relationship of pleural effusions to increased permeability pulmonary edema in anesthetized sheep. *J Clin Invest* 1988;82:1422–1429.

35. Fein A, Grossman RF, Jones JG, et al. The value of edema fluid protein measurements in patients with pulmonary edema. *Am J Med* 1979;67:32–38.

36. Matthay MA, Eschenbacher WL, Goetzl E. Elevated concentration of leukotriene D4 in the pulmonary edema fluid of patients with the adult respiratory distress syndrome. *J Clin Immunol* 1984;4:479–483.

37. Matthay MA, Landolt CC, Staub NC. Differential liquid and protein clearance from the alveoli of anesthetized sheep. *J Appl Physiol* 1982;53:96–104.

38. Verghese GM, Ware LB, Matthay BA, et al. Alveolar epithelial fluid transport and the resolution of clinically severe hydrostatic pulmonary edema. *J Appl Physiol* 1999;87:1301–1312.

39. Basset G, Crone C, Saumon G. Significance of active ion transport in transalveolar water absorption: a study on isolated rat lung. *J Physiol* 1987;384:311–324.

40. Goodman BE, Fleisher RS, Crandall ED. Evidence for active sodium transport by cultured monolayers of pulmonary alveolar epithelial cells. *Am J Physiol* 1982;245:C78–C83.

41. Matalon S, Benos DJ, Jackson RM. Biophysical and molecular properties of amiloride-inhibitable sodium channels in alveolar epithelial cells. *Am J Physiol* 1996;271:L1-L22.

42. Dobbs LG, Gonzalez R, Matthay MA, et al. Highly water-permeable type I alveolar epithelial cells confer high water permeability between the airspace and vasculature in rat lung. *Proc Natl Acad Sci* 1998;95:2991–2996.

43. Matthay MA, Folkesson HG, Verkman AS. Salt and water transport across alveolar and distal airway epithelia in the adult lung. *Am J Physiol* 1996;270:L487–L503.

44. Matthay MA, Berthiaume Y, Staub NC. Long-term clearance of liquid and protein from the lungs of unanesthetized sheep. *J Appl Physiol* 1985;59:928–934.

45. Goodman BE, Brown JE, Crandall EP. Regulation of transport across pulmonary alveolar epithelial cell monolayers. *J Appl Physiol* 1984;57:703–710.

46. Matthay MA, Wiener-Kronish JP. Intact epithelial barrier function is critical for the resolution of alveolar edema in humans. *Am Rev Respir Dis* 1990;142:1250–1257.

47. Effros RM, Hacker A, Silverman P, et al. Protein concentrations have little effect on reabsorption of fluid from isolated rat lungs. *J Appl Physiol* 1991;70:416–422.

48. Berthiaume Y, Staub NC, Matthay MA. Beta-adrenergic agonists increase lung liquid clearance in anesthetized sheep. *J Clin Invest* 1987;79:335–343.

49. Berthiaume Y, Broaddus VC, Gropper MA, et al. Alveolar liquid and protein clearance from normal dog lungs. *J Appl Physiol* 1988;65:585–593.

50. Garat C, Carter E, Matthay M. New in situ mouse model to quantify alveolar epithelial fluid clearance. *J Appl Physiol* 1998;84:1763–1767.

51. Crandall ED, Heming TA, Palombo RL, et al. Effects of terbu-

taline on sodium transport in isolated perfused rat lung. *J Appl Physiol* 1986;60:289–294.

52. Maron MB. Doe-response relationship between plasma epinephrine concentration and alveolar liquid clearance in dogs. *J Appl Physiol* 1998;85:1702–1707.

53. Jayr C, Garat C, Meignan M, et al. Alveolar liquid and protein clearance in anesthetized, ventilated rats. *J Appl Physiol* 1994; 76:2626–2642.

54. Sakuma T, Folkesson HG, Suzuki S, et al. Beta-adrenergic agonist stimulated alveolar fluid clearance in ex vivo human and rat lungs. *Am J Respir Crit Care Med* 1997;155:506–512.

55. Swan HJC, Ganz W, Forrester J, et al. Catheterization of the heart in man with use of a flow directed balloon-tipped catheter. *N Engl J Med* 1970;283:447–451.

56. Conners AF, McCaffree RD, Gray BA Evaluation of right heart catheterization in the critically ill patient without acute myocardial infarction. *N Engl J Med* 1983;308:263–267.

57. Matthay MA, Chatterjee K. Bedside catheterization of the pulmonary artery: risks versus benefits. *Ann Intern Med* 1988;109: 826–834.

58. Unger KM, Shibel EM, Moser KM. Detection of left ventricular failure in patients with the adult respiratory distress syndrome. *Chest* 1975;67:8–13.

59. Osler W. *The principles and practice of medicine.* New York: D Appleton and Co., 1927.

60. Lee G, De Maria A, Amsterdam EA, et al. Comparative effects of morphine, meperidine, and pentazocine on cardiocirculatory dynamics in patients with acute myocardial infarction. *Am J Med* 1976;60:949–955.

61. Parmley WW, Chatterjee MB. *Cardiology.* Philadelphia: J. B. Lippincott and Co., 1988.

62. Packer M. Do vasodilators prolong life in heart failure. *N Engl J Med* 1987;316:1471–1473.

63. Cohn JN. Physiologic basis for vasodilator therapy for heart failure. *Am J Med* 1981;71:135–139.

64. Biddle TL, Ju PN. Effect of furosemide on hemodynamics and lung water in acute pulmonary edema secondary to myocardial infarction. *Am J Cardiol* 1979;43:86–90.

65. Goldstein RA, Passamani ER, Roberts R. A comparison of digoxin and dobutamine in patients with acute infarction and cardiac failure. *N Engl J Med* 1980;303:846–850.

66. Gray R, Shah PK, Singh B, et al. Low cardiac output states after open heart surgery. *Chest* 1981;80:16–22.

67. Arnold SB, Byrd RC, Meister W. Long-term digitalis therapy improves left ventricular function in heart failure. *N Engl J Med* 1980;303:1443–1448.

68. Buda AJ, Pinsky MR, Ingels NBJ, et al. Effect of intrathoracic pressure on left ventricular performance. *N Engl J Med* 1979; 301:453–459.

69. Macklem PT. Respiratory muscles: the vital pump. *Chest* 1980; 78:753–758.

70. Aubier M, Trippenback T, Roussos C. Respiratory muscle fatigue during cardiogenic shock. *J Appl Physiol* 1981;51: 499–508.

71. Anderson RR, Holliday RL, Driedger AA. Documentation of pulmonary capillary permeability in the adult respiratory distress syndrome accompanying human sepsis. *Am Rev Respir Dis* 1979; 119:869–877.

72. Ware LB, Matthay MA. Maximal alveolar epithelial fluid clearance in clinical acute lung injury: an excellent predictor of survival and the duration of mechanical ventilation. *Am J Respir Crit Care Med* 1999;159:A694.

73. Petty TL, Ashbaugh DG. The adult respiratory distress syndrome. *Chest* 1971;60:233–239.

74. Murray JF, Matthay MA, Luce JM, et al. An expanded definition of the adult respiratory distress syndrome. *Am Rev Respir Dis* 1988;138:720–723.

75. Rubin DB, Wiener-Kronish JP, Murray JF, et al. Elevated von-Willebrand factor antigen is an early plasma predictor of impending acute lung injury and death in non-pulmonary sepsis syndrome. *J Clin Invest* 1990;86:474–480.

76. Montgomery AB, Stager MA, Carrico CJ, et al. Causes of mortality in patients with the adult respiratory distress syndrome. *Am Rev Respir Dis* 1985;132:485–489.

77. Bernard GR, Artigas A, Brigham KL, et al. The American-European Consensus Conference on ARDS. Definitions, mechanisms, relevant outcomes, and clinical trial coordination. *Am J Respir Crit Care Med* 1994;149:818–824.

78. Doyle RL, Szaflarski N, Modin GW, et al. Identification of patients with acute lung injury. Predictors of mortality. *Am J Respir Crit Care Med* 1995;152:1818–1824.

79. Zilberberg MD, Epstein SK. Acute lung injury in the medical ICU. Comorbid conditions, age, etiology and hospital outcome. *Am J Respir Crit Care Med* 1998;157:1159–1164.

80. Sloane PJ, Gee MH, Gottlieb JE, et al. A multicenter registry of patients with acute respiratory distress syndrome. *Am Rev Respir Dis* 1992;146:419–426.

81. Baumann WR, Jung RC, Koss M, et al. Incidence and mortality of adult respiratory distress syndrome: A prospective analysis from a large metropolitan hospital. *Crit Care Med* 1986;14: 1–4.

82. Monchi M, Bellenfant F, Cariou A, et al. Early predictive factors of survival in the acute respiratory distress syndrome. A multivariate analysis. *Am J Respir Crit Care Med* 1998;158: 1076–1081.

83. Pepe PE, Potkin RT, Reus DJ, et al. Clinical predictors of the adult respiratory distress syndrome. *Am J Surg* 1982;144: 124–130.

84. Fowler AA, Hamman RF, Good JT, et al. Adult respiratory distress syndrome: risks with common predispositions. *Ann Intern Med* 1983;98:593–597.

85. Murray JF. Mechanisms of acute respiratory failure. *Am Rev Respir Dis* 1977;115:1071–1078.

86. Villar J, Slutsky AS. The incidence of the adult respiratory distress syndrome. *Am Rev Resp Dis* 1989;140:814–816.

87. Abel SJC, Finney SJ, Brett SJ, et al. Reduced mortality in association with the acute respiratory distress syndrome. *Thorax* 1998; 53:292–294.

88. Milberg JA, Davis DR, Steinberg KP, et al. Improved survival of patients with acute respiratory distress syndrome (ARDS): 1983–1993. *JAMA* 1995;273:306–309.

89. Bell RC, Coalson J, Smith JD, et al. Multiple organ failure and infection in the adult respiratory distress syndrome. *Ann Intern Med* 1983;99:293–298.

90. Dantzker DR, Brook CJ, Dehart P, et al. Ventilation-perfusion distributions in adult respiratory distress syndrome. *Am Rev Respir Dis* 1979;120:1039–1052.

91. Said SI, Avery ME, Davis RK, et al. Pulmonary surface activity in induced pulmonary edema. *J Clin Invest* 1965;44:458–464.

92. Hallman M, Spragg R, Harrell JH, et al. Evidence of lung surfactant abnormality in respiratory failure. A study of bronchoalveolar lavage phospholipids, surface activity, phospholipase activity, and plasma myoinositol. *J Clin Invest* 1982;70: 673–683.

93. Gregory TJ, Longmore WJ, Moxley MA, et al. Surfactant chemical composition and biophysical activity in acute respiratory distress syndrome. *J Clin Invest* 1991;88:1976–1981.

94. Bachofen M, Weibel ER. Alterations of the gas exchange apparatus in adult respiratory insufficiency associated with septicemia. *Am Rev Respir Dis* 1977;116:589–615.

95. Elliott CG, Morris AH, Cengiz M. Pulmonary function and

exercise gas exchange in survivors of adult respiratory distress syndrome. *Am Rev Respir Dis* 1981;123:492–495.

96. Lakshminarayan S, Stanford RE, Petty TL. Prognosis after recovery from adult respiratory distress syndrome. *Am Rev Respir Dis* 1976;113:7–16.

97. Zapol WM, Snider MT. Pulmonary hypertension in severe acute respiratory failure. *N Engl J Med* 1977;296:476–480.

98. Nash G, Blennerhassett JB, Pontoppidan H. Pulmonary lesions associated with oxygen therapy and artificial ventilation. *N Engl J Med* 1981;276:368–374.

99. Gammon RB, Shin MS, Groves RHJ, et al. Clinical risk factors for pulmonary barotrauma: a multivariate analysis. *Am J Respir Crit Care Med* 1995;152:1235–1240.

100. Schnapp LM, Chin DP, Szaflarski N, et al. Frequency and importance of barotrauma in 100 patients with acute lung injury. *Crit Care Med* 1995;23:272–278.

101. Pratt PC, Vollmer RT, Shelburne JD, et al. Pulmonary morphology in a multihospital collaborative extracorporeal membrane oxygenation project. I. Light microscopy. *Am J Pathol* 1979;85:210–228.

102. Witschi HR, Haschek WM, Klein-Szanto AJR, et al. Potentiation of diffuse lung damage by oxygen: determining variables. *Am Rev Respir Dis* 1981;123:98.

103. Rinaldo J. Mediation of ARDS by leukocytes. *Chest* 1986;89:590–593.

104. Pittet JF, Mackersie RC, Martin TR, et al. Biological markers of acute lung injury: prognostic and pathogenetic significance. *Am J Respir Crit Care Med* 1997;155:1187–1205.

105. Stevens JH, O'Hanley P, Shapiro JM, et al. Effects of anti-C5a antibodies on the adult respiratory distress syndrome in septic primates. *J Clin Invest* 1986;77:1812–1816.

106. Lee CT, Fein AM, Lippmann M, et al. Elastolytic activity in pulmonary lavage fluid from patients with adult respiratory distress syndrome. *N Engl J Med* 1981;304:192–196.

107. Maunder RJ, Hackman RC, Riff E, et al. Occurrence of the adult respiratory distress syndrome in neutropenic patients. *Am Rev Respir Dis* 1986;133:313–316.

108. Rinaldo JE, Borovetz H. Deterioration of oxygenation and abnormal lung microvascular permeability during resolution of leukopenia in patients with diffuse lung injury. *Am Rev Respir Dis* 1985;131:579–583.

109. Haynes JB, Hyers TM, Giclas PC, et al. Elevated fibrinogen degradation products in the adult respiratory distress syndrome. *Am Rev Respir Dis* 1980;122:841–847.

110. Malik AB, Vander Zee H. Mechanism of pulmonary edema induced by microembolism in dogs. *Circ Res* 1978;42:72–79.

111. Tracey KJ, Fong Y, Hesse DG, et al. Anti-cachectin/TNF monoclonal antibodies prevent septic shock during lethal bacteremia. *Nature* 1987;330:662–664.

112. Miller EJ, Cohen AB, Nagao S, et al. Elevated levels of NAP-1/Interleukin-8 are present in the airspaces of patients with the adult respiratory distress syndrome and are associated with increased mortality. *Am Rev Respir Dis* 1992;146:427–432.

113. Ware LB, Matthay MA. The acute respiratory distress syndrome. *N Engl J Med* 2000;342:1334–1349.

114. Wiedemann H, Matthay RA, Matthay MA, eds. *Acute lung injury. Critical care clinics.* Philadelphia: WB Saunders, 1986.

115. Luce JM, Montgomery AB, Marks JD, et al. Ineffectiveness of high-dose methylprednisolone in preventing parenchymal lung injury and improving mortality in patients with septic shock. *Am Rev Respir Dis* 1988;138:62–68.

116. Cameron JL, Zuidema GD. Aspiration pneumonia. Magnitude and frequency of the problem. *JAMA* 1972;219:1194–1196.

117. Jones JG, Grossman RF, Beny M, et al. Alveolar-capillary membrane permeability. *Am Rev Respir Dis* 1979;120:339–410.

118. Wynne JW, Modell JH. Respiratory aspiration of stomach contents. *Ann Intern Med* 1977;87:466–474.

119. Bynum LJ, Pierce AK. Pulmonary aspiration of gastric contents. *Am Rev Respir Dis* 1976;114:1129–1136.

120. Bartlett JG, Gorback SL, Finegold SM. The bacteriology of aspiration pneumonia. *Am J Med* 1974;56:202–208.

121. Kaplan RL, Sahn SA, Petty TL. Incidence and outcome of the respiratory distress syndrome in Gram-negative sepsis. *Arch Intern Med* 1979;139:867–869.

122. Weinberg PF, Matthay MA, Webster RO, et al. Biologically active products of complement and acute lung injury in patients with the sepsis syndrome. *Am Rev Respir Dis* 1984;130:791–796.

123. Hechtman HB, Lonergan EA, Shepro D. Platelet and leukocyte lung interactions in patients with respiratory failure. *Surgery* 1978;83:155–163.

124. Brigham KL, Meyrick B. Endotoxin and lung injury. *Am Rev Respir Dis* 1986;133:913–927.

125. Brigham KL, Bowers RE, Haynes J. Increased lung vascular permeability caused by E. coli endotoxin. *Circ Res* 1979;45:292–297.

126. Wiener-Kronish JP, Albertine KH, Matthay MA. Differential responses of the endothelial and epithelial barrier of the lung in sheep to E. coli endotoxin. *J Clin Invest* 1991;88:864–875.

127. Staub NC. Conference report on a workshop on the measurement of lung water. *Crit Care Med* 1980;8:752–759.

128. Pistolesi M, Guintini C. Assessment of extravascular lung water. *Radiol Clin North Am* 1978;16:551–574.

129. Noble WH, Kay JC, Obdrzalek J. Lung mechanics in hypervolemic pulmonary edema. *J Appl Physiol* 1975;38:681–687.

130. Saint S, Matthay MA. Risk reduction in the intensive care unit. *Am J Med* 1998;105:515–523.

131. Broaddus VC, Berthiaume Y, Biondi J, et al. Management of pulmonary hemodynamics in patients with the adult respiratory distress syndrome. *J Intensive Care Med* 1987;2:190–213.

132. Ohkuda K, Nakahara K, Binder A, et al. Venous air emboli in sheep: reversible increase in lung microvascular permeability. *J Appl Physiol* 1981;51:887–894.

133. Prewitt RM, McCarthy J, Wood LDH. Treatment of acute low pressure pulmonary edema in dogs. *J Clin Invest* 1981;67:409–418.

134. Demling RH, Staub NC, Edmunds LHJ. Effect of end-expiratory airway pressure on accumulation of extravascular lung water. *J Appl Physiol* 1975;38:907–912.

135. Hopewell PC, Murray JF. Effects of continuous positive pressure ventilation in experimental pulmonary edema. *J Appl Physiol* 1976;40:568–574.

136. Amato MB, Barbas CS, Medeiros DM, et al. Effect of a protective-ventilation strategy on mortality in the acute respiratory distress syndrome. *N Engl J Med* 1998;338:347–354.

137. Tremblay L, Valenza F, Ribeiro SP, et al. Injurious ventilatory strategies increase cytokines and c-fos mRNA expression in an isolated rat lung model. *J Clin Invest* 1997;99:944–952.

138. Corbridge TC, Wood LDH, Crawford GP, et al. Adverse effects of large tidal volumes and low PEEP in canine acid aspiration. *Am Rev Respir Dis* 1990;142:311–315.

139. Dreyfuss D, Basset G, Soler P, et al. Intermittent positive-pressure hyperventilation with high inflation pressures produces pulmonary microvascular injury in rats. *Am Rev Respir Dis* 1985;132:880–884.

140. Stewart TE, Meade MO, Cook DJ, et al. Evaluation of a ventilation strategy to prevent barotrauma in patients at high risk for acute respiratory distress syndrome. *N Engl J Med* 1998;338:355–361.

141. Brochard L, Roudot-Thoroval F, Roupie E, et al. Tidal volume reduction for prevention of ventilator-induced lung injury in

acute respiratory distress syndrome. *Am J Respir Crit Care Med* 1998;158:1831–1838.

142. The Acute Respiratory Distress Syndrome Network. Ventilation with lower tidal volumes as compared with traditional tidal volumes for acute lung injury and the acute respiratory distress syndrome. *N Engl J Med* 2000;342:1301–1308.

143. Merritt TA, Hallman M, Bloom BT, et al. Prophylactic treatment of very premature infants with human surfactant. *N Engl J Med* 1986;315:785–789.

144. Baumgartner JD, McCutchan JA, Melle GV, et al. Prevention of Gram-negative shock and death in surgical patients by antibody to core glycolipid. *Lancet* 1985;2:59–63.

145. Rossaint R, Falke KJ, Lopez F, et al. Inhaled nitric oxide for the adult respiratory distress syndrome. *N Engl J Med* 1993; 328:399–405.

146. Anzueto A, Baughman RP, Guntupalli KK, et al. Aerosolized surfactant in adults with sepsis-induced acute respiratory distress syndrome. *N Engl J Med* 1996;334:1417–1421.

147. Dellinger RP, Zimmerman JL, Taylor RW. Effects of inhaled nitric oxide in patients with acute respiratory distress syndrome. Results of a randomized phase II trial. *Crit Care Med* 1998;26: 15–23.

148. Payen D, Vallet B, the Genoa Group. Results of the French prospective multicentric randomized double-blind placebo-controlled trial on inhaled nitric oxide (NO) in ARDS. *Intensive Care Med* 2000; in press.

149. Matthay MA. Function of the alveolar epithelial barrier under pathologic conditions. *Chest* 1994;105[Suppl]:67S–74S.

150. Bitterman P. Pathogenesis of fibrosis in acute lung injury. *Am J Med* 1992;6A[Suppl]:6S–39S.

151. Wortel CH, Doerschuk CM. Neutrophils and neutrophil-endothelial cell adhesion in adult respiratory distress syndrome. *New Horiz* 1993;1:631–637.

152. Berthiaume Y, Lesur O, Dagenais A. Treatment of adult respiratory distress syndrome: plea for rescue therapy of the alveolar epithelium. *Thorax* 1999;54:150–160.

24

THORACIC TRAUMA, SURGERY, AND PERIOPERATIVE MANAGEMENT

MICHAEL W. OWENS
MUHAMMAD S. CHAUDRY
JANE M. EGGERSTEDT
LOU M. SMITH

CARDIOPULMONARY EFFECTS OF ANESTHESIA
Respiratory Effects
Cardiovascular Effects
General versus Regional Anesthesia

POSTOPERATIVE ANALGESIA

SURGICAL INCISION SITE AND DIAPHRAGMATIC FUNCTION

POSTOPERATIVE PULMONARY COMPLICATIONS
Postoperative Atelectasis and Hypoxemia
Prevention and Treatment of Atelectasis

PREOPERATIVE PULMONARY FUNCTION TESTING
Smoking in the Preoperative Period
Perioperative Aspiration

POSTOPERATIVE PNEUMONIA

SURGICAL CONSIDERATIONS IN THE ELDERLY

SURGICAL CONSIDERATIONS IN THE PATIENT WITH COPD

SURGICAL CONSIDERATIONS IN THE ASTHMATIC PATIENT

EVALUATION OF SUITABILITY FOR LUNG RESECTION
Predicting Postoperative Pulmonary Function and
    Complications
Cardiac Considerations for Lung Resection and General
    Surgery
Surgical Risk in Patients with Angina

CHEST TRAUMA
Diagnostic and Therapeutic Modalities
Injuries to the Chest Wall
Injuries to the Pulmonary Parenchyma
Injuries to the Diaphragm
Injuries to the Mediastinum

FAT EMBOLISM SYNDROME

The introduction of modern, safe anesthesia and improved operative techniques have dramatically reduced the incidence of complications of surgery. In spite of these vast improvements, pulmonary complications remain a significant cause of morbidity and increased health care expenditure. Prediction of the probability of developing postoperative complications is important clinically and has been the subject of debate for most of the 20th century. Several preoperative tests and composite classification systems have been devised, but the perfect preoperative indicator of operative morbidity remains elusive.

CARDIOPULMONARY EFFECTS OF ANESTHESIA

Respiratory Effects

Virtually every aspect of general anesthesia contributes negatively to pulmonary physiology. Most anesthetic agents de-

press the central ventilatory response to hypercapnia and hypoxemia and cause a decrease in tidal volume. There is also an increase in dead space due to the decreased minute ventilation (1). Other significant effects on the respiratory system include a reduction in muscle tone and upward movement of the diaphragm, causing a decrease in functional residual capacity (FRC) by about 15% to 20% (2). Most patients undergoing general anesthesia develop atelectasis in the dependent portions of their lungs, resulting in an increase in the shunt fraction (3,4).

The use of a high FIO_2 during the induction of anesthesia has been shown to have a role in the formation of atelectasis. In one study, atelectasis was three times more common with 100% oxygen compared to 30% (5). In another study, it was found that inflation of the lungs to vital capacity (an inflation pressure of 40 cm of water) at the end of the operation was effective in decreasing atelectasis in patients breathing 30% oxygen but not in subjects who received 100% oxygen during induction of anesthesia (6,7). These observations indicate that absorption of oxygen in lung units with decreased ventilation causes atelectasis formation during general anesthesia. However, when oxygen is mixed with a poorly absorbed gas such as nitrogen, the alveolar units remain stable and atelectasis is less likely. Intraoperative administration of positive end–expiratory pressure (PEEP) may also decrease the severity of atelectasis (8).

Intubation of the trachea can cause a reversible bronchoconstriction and an increase in airway resistance. Respiratory resistance after tracheal intubation has been shown to be lower when propofol is used as an induction agent as compared to etomidate or thiopental (9).

Many anesthesiologists have preferred to use halothane for patients with known asthma. Halothane and isoflurane are known to decrease bronchial smooth-muscle tone and airway resistance (10). More recently, sevoflurane has been shown to have more bronchodilator effects than halothane, isoflurane, or thiopental–nitrous oxide anesthesia (11).

Some studies have suggested an increased incidence of postoperative respiratory complications in patients who have had a recent upper respiratory infection. Elective surgery should be postponed for a few weeks after a viral respiratory infection (12,13).

Cardiovascular Effects

All inhalational anesthetic agents are myocardial depressants. Halothane has a marked depressant effect and also causes a reduction in heart rate. Isoflurane causes minimal myocardial depression but has a marked vasodilator effect that results in tachycardia. The effects of enflurane on myocardial contractility and heart rate are intermediate between those of halothane and isoflurane (14). Nitrous oxide tends to cause less myocardial depression and also has intrinsic sympathomimetic effects.

Among the intravenous induction agents, barbiturates are myocardial depressants compared to the narcotic agents. Morphine sulfate can cause histamine release, resulting in bronchospasm and hypotension. The newer sedative agents, fentanyl, sufentanil, and alfentanil, are preferred agents in patients with underlying heart disease. Ketamine and etomidate also have fewer adverse hemodynamic consequences than morphine and barbiturates (15).

General versus Regional Anesthesia

Epidural anesthesia has been advocated as an alternative in high-risk patients with underlying lung or heart disease, but comparisons have shown conflicting outcomes. During epidural anesthesia there is a reduction in expiratory flow rate and FRC; however, the effects on central ventilatory drive are negligible.

The hemodynamic effects of regional anesthesia are more pronounced. Vasodilation occurs as a result of sympathetic blockade and may result in significant hypotension (15,16).

In addition, all the local anesthetic agents used in regional anesthesia can cause a dose-dependent myocardial depression. In most studies, use of regional techniques has not been shown to decrease mortality when compared to general anesthesia (17,18); however, there may be a role for regional anesthesia in selected populations (19). Use of regional anesthesia has been reported to result in a decrease in postoperative confusion in elderly patients undergoing general surgery (20). Graft patency rates may be higher in vascular surgery patients operated on under regional anesthesia (21). However, current data does not support routine use of regional anesthesia for high-risk surgical patients. This decision is the prerogative of the attending anesthesiologist, based upon the patient's general hemodynamic and respiratory status.

POSTOPERATIVE ANALGESIA

It is felt that pain contributes to postoperative complications by preventing adequate lung inflation. It has been suggested that patients who are pain-free will have an earlier recovery of their pulmonary function and a decreased incidence of atelectasis and hypoxemia. In addition to systemic narcotic analgesics administered by medical personnel, patient-controlled parenteral analgesia systems have gained widespread acceptance in recent years (22).

Epidural administration of local anesthetics and narcotic agents has been studied extensively (23–25). In a recent meta-analysis of postoperative analgesic therapies, the authors found a significant decrease in the incidence of atelectasis when epidural opioids or local anesthetics were administered compared to systemic opioids (26). Epidural administration of local anesthetics was also associated with improved oxygenation, lower overall incidence of pulmonary infections, and respiratory complications, when compared to systemic opioids.

Intercostal nerve blockade, intrapleural administration of local anesthetics, and wound infiltration have also been described (26–28). There is some evidence that intercostal nerve blockade may also help decrease the incidence of respiratory complications in patients undergoing upper abdominal surgery. Intercostal nerve blockade may be a useful option for patients in whom epidural analgesia cannot be achieved or is otherwise contraindicated (27). Intrapleural infusion of local anesthetics has been described for postoperative analgesia after cholecystectomy and thoracotomy, resulting in improved pain control, better pulmonary function, and a decreased incidence of respiratory complications. Epidural, intercostal, and intrapleural therapies appear to be superior to systemic opioid administration for postoperative analgesia. Such therapy should be strongly considered following upper-abdominal surgery or thoracotomy.

SURGICAL INCISION SITE AND DIAPHRAGMATIC FUNCTION

In the normal awake subject, the diaphragm is the predominant inspiratory muscle. The intercostal and other accessory muscles assume a more central role during the first few days after surgery. This results in rapid, shallow breathing with small tidal volumes (29). Upper-abdominal surgery results in a higher incidence of diaphragmatic dysfunction compared to lower-abdominal incisions (30). Reflex inhibition of diaphragmatic motor activity resulting from the handling of abdominal viscera and the parietal peritoneum is one of the proposed mechanisms of diaphragmatic dysfunction (31).

Recently, a large prospective study on 994 patients was done to assess the role of the surgical incision site in perioperative hypoxemia. The results showed that hypoxemia (SaO_2 below 90%) during the early postoperative period was closely related to operative site. Patients who had thoracoabdominal incisions had a 52% incidence of hypoxemia, compared to a 38% incidence in those who underwent abdominal surgery. Only 7% of the patients who underwent elective superficial plastic surgery developed significant hypoxemia (32). In another study, subcostal incisions were reported to be associated with a lower rate of postoperative pulmonary complications than midline incisions (33). Transverse abdominal incisions are associated with the lowest pulmonary complication rate.

Laparoscopic surgery has been promoted as an alternative to conventional laparotomy because of shorter hospital stay, decreased postoperative pain, and early ambulation. There is some evidence that laparoscopic surgery may result in a lower incidence of postoperative respiratory complications (34–36). Video-assisted thoracoscopic surgery (VATS) is also known to cause lesser postoperative pain and impairment of pulmonary function compared to standard thoracotomy techniques (37–39).

POSTOPERATIVE PULMONARY COMPLICATIONS

Estimates of postoperative pulmonary complications (POPC) have varied depending on the patient population studied, the procedure performed, and the criteria used to define a POPC. The overall incidence of POPC in the general population is approximately 5%, but is below 1% for nonabdominal, nonthoracic procedures (40). Patients undergoing major vascular, upper-abdominal, and thoracic surgery are at higher risk and constitute a special group, and postoperative pulmonary complications are reported to occur in up to half of these patients (41–45).

Most pulmonary abnormalities after surgery are minor and self-limited. These include minor postoperative atelectasis, bronchospasm, hypoxemia, dyspnea, and cough. Major complications include postoperative pneumonia, lobar atelectasis, and aspiration and ventilatory failure, and are infrequent. Death and prolonged ventilator dependence are rare even among patients with severe COPD (45,46).

Postoperative Atelectasis and Hypoxemia

The major cause of postoperative hypoxemia is the formation of atelectasis resulting in areas of low V/Q (ventilation/perfusion) ratio. Other causes include hypoventilation, pulmonary edema, thromboembolism, and bronchial obstruction by retained secretions (Table 24.1). Residual anesthesia, pain, and immobilization also contribute to hypoxemia (2).

The anesthetic and surgical factors outlined above result in a decreased FRC. In individuals with no underlying lung disease, PaO_2 may decrease to 80% of baseline value. The FEV_1 and FVC also decrease to approximately two-thirds of the preoperative levels after low-risk lower-abdominal surgery (47). These decrements in lung function are more severe after upper-abdominal surgery (48). In up to 33% of patients, atelectasis can persist up to the third or fourth postoperative day. The extent of atelectasis has a direct correlation with the severity of postoperative hypoxemia, and an inverse relationship with the decrease in FEV_1 and FVC.

The volume of the lung at which small dependent airways begin to collapse is called the *closing volume*. In normal healthy patients, the closing volume is below FRC, so that the airways remain open during tidal breathing. The closing volume begins to increase with age and approaches the FRC in patients over 65 years of age. Patients with COPD, obesity, or a history of smoking have higher closing volumes. Even a small decrease in the FRC in these patients leads to dependent airway closure, placing them at very high risk for the formation of atelectasis (2,49). Patients given 100% oxygen during surgery and the immediate postoperative period tend to have a higher incidence of atelectasis, probably due to resorption of oxygen in areas of decreased ventilation, as noted above (5,6).

TABLE 24.1. COMMON MECHANISMS OF POSTOPERATIVE HYPOXEMIA

Atelectasis
  Microatelectasis
  Segmental or lobar atelectasis
Hypoventilation
  Residual anesthetic
  Narcotic analgesics
  Pain with splinting
Pulmonary edema
Venous thromboembolism
Bronchial mucous plugging

Atelectasis in the dorsal and basal lung regions has been demonstrated by CT scan in virtually 100% of patients undergoing abdominal surgery (4). These regions are generally well perfused and blood shunts through the airless lung units. In a great majority of patients, atelectasis is asymptomatic and resolves spontaneously. However among high-risk patient groups, atelectasis may be persistent, and pneumonia can result from retained secretions in collapsed lung units (47).

Prevention and Treatment of Atelectasis

The main objective of postoperative chest physiotherapy is to restore the FRC to preoperative levels as soon as possible. Earlier forms were aimed at the removal of mucus plugs from airways using deep coughing and forced expiratory maneuvers. However, the production of large volumes of sputum does not address the main mechanism of atelectasis. It has also been postulated that physiotherapy may be harmful to some patients in the early perioperative period (50).

In current practice, lung inflation is usually accomplished by deep-breathing exercises. The aim is to keep the lungs inflated to total lung capacity (TLC), or close to it, for as long as possible. Several different therapies and regimens have been explored. In a nationwide survey of the usage of lung expansion devices, incentive spirometry was found to be used most frequently. It was prescribed in over 95% of all U.S. hospitals (51). The advantages of incentive spirometry include its low cost and ease of administration. Chest physiotherapy (CPT) is more expensive because of the need for skilled therapists to administer it. Modern CPT includes deep-breathing and coughing exercises, percussion, vibration, postural drainage, and humidification. Other forms of therapy aimed at atelactasis prevention have included CPAP (continuous positive airway pressure), PEEP, PEP (positive expiratory pressure), inspiratory resistance and positive expiratory pressure (IR-PEP), intermittent positive pressure breathing (IPPB), and blow bottles. Several studies have compared these treatments. Although the results are conflicting, it is becoming clear that no single therapy is more effective than the others (52–58).

Although conflict exists about the best method of treatment, convincing evidence has shown that some form of therapy is better than none. In a randomized study, Celli and colleagues compared the incidence of postoperative pulmonary complications in patients who were treated with incentive spirometry, IPPB, deep-breathing exercises, or no treatment. The incidence of pulmonary complications in the treatment groups was 21% to 22%, but was 48% in the group that received no treatment (41). Preoperative respiratory rehabilitation has also been reported to improve postoperative outcomes (59). Stacked inspiratory spirometry is a newer technique that has been shown to reduce shunt fraction in the post–coronary artery bypass graft (CABG) population (60).

Fiber-optic removal of mucus plugs has been described, but seems to have no advantage when compared to other less invasive therapies (61). Marini and colleagues studied fiber-optic bronchoscopy versus CPT in acute lobar collapse and found no significant difference in outcome between the two treatment groups if an air bronchogram was present (62). Therefore, in acute lobar collapse, combined CPT and bronchodilation are the most effective and bronchoscopy cannot be advocated as initial therapy. In atelectasis refractory to conventional therapy, bronchoscopy may be useful, especially if air bronchograms are not seen. A reexpansion technique utilizing a balloon cuffed bronchoscope with air-insufflation has been described (63) but is not generally recommended.

PREOPERATIVE PULMONARY FUNCTION TESTING

Pulmonary function testing is commonly prescribed as part of the preoperative workup in patients who are suspected of having pulmonary disease. Such testing usually involves the measurement of expiratory flow rates. The patient exhales maximally from TLC to residual volume, and the volume recorded is termed FVC. In addition to the FVC, the other indices derived from this expiratory effort include the FEV_1, the FEV_1/FVC ratio, and the average forced expiratory flow from 25% to 75% of the FVC ($FEF_{25-75\%}$). The $FEF_{25-75\%}$ is a sensitive indicator of obstruction of the small airways (64).

The role of preoperative spirometry in evaluating the lung resection candidate is discussed in the section on lung resection. Spirometry has not been shown to predict accurately postoperative complications in patients undergoing upper-abdominal surgery (65–72). In upper-abdominal surgery, spirometry should be ordered in patients who are heavy smokers and have symptoms of chronic bronchitis that would place them at a higher risk of developing postoperative complications. Spirometry may be useful in identifying patients who are likely to need more intensive perioperative respiratory therapy.

The incidence of POPC in patients undergoing lower-abdominal surgery is low. It is even lower in patients undergoing orthopedic or urologic procedures. Preoperative spirometric testing is not routinely indicated in these population groups (73–77).

Smoking in the Preoperative Period

Cigarette smoking has been identified as a risk factor for postoperative pulmonary complications in several studies (78–83). The benefits of smoking cessation in promoting healthful living and preventing disease are well known. In an effort to reduce the risk of postoperative complications, many physicians recommend smoking cessation prior to surgery. The role of short-term smoking cessation prior to surgery in preventing complications is unclear. In one study of postoperative complications following upper-abdominal or thoracic surgery, the incidence of postoperative pulmonary complications in current smokers was almost twice that of past smokers and five times that of subjects who had never smoked (81).

In a study of 200 consecutive patients undergoing coronary artery bypass surgery, the risks for postoperative complications was reported to be four times higher in those who stopped smoking within eight weeks prior to surgery compared to those who had given up smoking for more than eight weeks prior to surgery (82). In another study, patients who were able to reduce their cigarette smoking prior to surgery had a seven times higher risk of developing postoperative complications compared to smokers who were unable to reduce their cigarette consumption (81). It appears that patients should give up smoking at least eight weeks prior to surgery for the most beneficial outcome. Short-term preoperative smoking cessation may be beneficial by causing a reduction in blood carbon monoxide levels; however, heavy smokers may experience a nicotine withdrawal in the perioperative period that can have harmful effects (80–83).

Perioperative Aspiration

Clinically significant aspiration of gastric contents is an uncommon but feared perioperative complication. Initially described by Mendelson in obstetric patients, the syndrome has been reported in patients undergoing all types of surgery (84). Modern anesthetic techniques and mandatory overnight preoperative fasting have decreased the incidence of aspiration. The incidence of aspiration in the surgical population has varied from study to study, varying from 0.2 to two per 10,000 cases, with an associated mortality rate of two to three per 100,000 anesthetic cases. A decrease in mortality has been seen over the past two decades (85,86).

It is estimated that the minimum amount of gastric contents needed to cause significant changes is about 0.4 mL per kg. The cutoff for gastric pH below which aspiration pneumonitis can occur is approximately 2.5 to 3.5 (84,87).

Risk factors for aspiration include the extremes of age (the very young and the elderly), pregnancy, obesity, intestinal obstruction, esophageal disorders, decreased gastric motility, depressed levels of consciousness, emergency surgery, and recent oral intake. The only factors that have been independently associated with aspiration are emergency surgery and poor preoperative physical status. In one large study, all the deaths attributed to aspiration occurred in patients with American Society of Anesthesiologists (ASA) class 4 preoperative risk category or higher (86). The periods

during an operation when aspiration is most likely to occur are during laryngoscopy and tracheal extubation (84,86).

Signs and symptoms of aspiration of gastric contents include cough, hypoxemia, and wheezing. Complications include pneumonitis, respiratory failure requiring mechanical ventilation, and death. Fortunately, the incidence of serious complications is very low. Patients who do not develop any symptoms within two hours of a witnessed aspiration are very unlikely to develop complications and can be safely monitored in a non-ICU setting. Those who develop respiratory symptoms or a new infiltrate on chest radiograph within two hours of a witnessed aspiration have a high incidence of respiratory complications and should be closely monitored.

A number of pharmacologic agents, including antacids, H-2 blockers, prokinetic agents, antimuscarinic agents, and proton pump inhibitors have been used preoperatively to reduce the incidence of complications. The goal has been to keep the gastric pH above 2.5 and the volume of gastric aspirate prior to induction below 25 mL. Cricoid pressure is also a very effective measure to reduce the incidence of aspiration during endotracheal intubation (87). H-2 blockers and proton pump inhibitors are effective in increasing gastric pH but do not decrease gastric volume. Pirenzepine, which is an antimuscarinic agent, has been shown to decrease gastric volume (88–93). In obstetric and pediatric cases, preoperative use of H-2 antagonists or prokinetic agents is commonly practiced. Whether such treatment should be offered to all patients undergoing surgery is controversial.

Treatment of aspiration pneumonitis is mainly supportive and includes the CPT measures outlined above. As much of the aspirated material should be coughed up and/or suctioned as possible. Bronchoscopic removal is possible in some cases, but is not routinely helpful. Steroids do not help after aspiration occurs. Antibiotics are useful only for secondary infections.

POSTOPERATIVE PNEUMONIA

The surgical patient is at risk for various nosocomial infections including urinary tract infections, surgical wound infections, and pneumonia. Pneumonia is the leading fatal postoperative nosocomial infection. Malnutrition and poor general medical condition constitute important risk factors for postoperative pneumonia in addition to other risk factors for postoperative pulmonary complications outlined in Table 24.2.

In one study of surgical patients, the incidence of postoperative pneumonia was 50% in malnourished patients versus 15% for patients with normal nutritional status (94,95). The organisms responsible for postoperative pneumonia are

TABLE 24.2. RISK FACTORS FOR POSTOPERATIVE PULMONARY COMPLICATIONS

Age over 70 years
Past or current smoking
Major surgery
   Upper gastrointestinal incisions
   Thoracic and thoracoabdominal operations
Emergency surgery
Coronary artery bypass grafting in COPD
Prolonged operations (more than 120 minutes)
General anesthesia involving muscle relaxants
Chronic obstructive lung disease
MI within past year
Chronic heart failure
Malnutrition

different from those of community-acquired pneumonia. A large proportion of postoperative pneumonias are caused by Gram-negative organisms, including *Pseudomonas, Klebsiella, E. coli, Proteus* and *Enterobacter* species. *Staphylococcus aureus* is also an important and frequent cause of ventilator-associated pneumonia.

Postoperative pneumonia is associated with a 50% mortality, increasing to 80% in pneumonias caused by *Pseudomonas* species. Diagnosis of postoperative pneumonia requires a high index of clinical suspicion. Sputum Gram stains and tracheal aspirates are often nonspecific and the positive predictive value of a positive isolate is low. Invasive diagnostic methods such as bronchoalveolar lavage (BAL) and/or protected specimen brushing (PSB) with quantitative cultures may be helpful for accurate diagnosis, but often these studies are not available and empirical antibiotic therapy is prescribed. The antibiotic regimen used should provide broad-spectrum coverage, including anti-Pseudomonal coverage in severely ill patients, since hospital-acquired pneumonia is polymicrobial in up to 40% of cases. Those who have pneumonia secondary to aspiration should also be treated for anaerobic and staphylococcal infection. Staphylococcal coverage should be considered in patients with diabetes, renal failure, head trauma, and coma (96).

SURGICAL CONSIDERATIONS IN THE ELDERLY

The elderly constitute the most rapidly increasing segment of the population, and this trend is expected to continue for the next several years. Older patients tend to have multiple medical problems simultaneously, complicating clinical decision-making. More than half a million elderly patients require major abdominal or thoracic surgery every year. They also have a higher incidence of cancers that require

surgical therapy. Assessment of surgical risk in the elderly is often an important task of the internist or pulmonologist. Many studies have suggested that operative mortality is increased in the elderly. The age threshold for increased risk of complications varies from study to study, but is probably about 70 to 75 years.

Age-related changes in pulmonary function include a decrease in elastic recoil of the lungs, which can result in an increased functional residual capacity and a decreased vital capacity. The airways tend to lose their elasticity, and hence closing volumes are increased. Arterial oxygen tension is also decreased associated with an increased alveolar-arterial oxygen gradient due to small airway closure during tidal breathing (97).

Successful surgery has been reported for patients older than 100 years, and surgery should not be denied solely because of age (99). Preoperative evaluation of the elderly patient for major surgery should include a careful assessment for evidence of preexisting pulmonary or cardiac disease. Preoperative spirometry may be helpful in identifying and treating high-risk patients. An additional noninvasive way of assessing pulmonary risk in elderly patients is bicycle ergometry. In a study reported by Gerson and colleagues patients who were unable to exercise to a heart rate greater than 99 beats per minute had a 22% incidence of cardiopulmonary complications, compared to a complication rate of 3% in those who were able to achieve that level of activity (98).

SURGICAL CONSIDERATIONS IN THE PATIENT WITH COPD

Patients with severe COPD have an increased risk of complications after major surgery. A decreased FEV_1 has been identified as an independent risk factor for postoperative pulmonary complications. Kroenke and colleagues studied a group of patients with severe COPD who underwent major abdominal and thoracic surgery excluding lung resection surgery (45). POPCs occurred in 29% of 107 patients. The incidence of complications was strongly associated with ASA class and the type and duration of surgery. Most of the patients did not experience a life-threatening complication. There were six deaths for the entire group, most of which occurred in the patients undergoing CABG. Three of these were due to cardiac causes and three were due to multiple causes, but respiratory failure was a contributing factor. Hence the overall mortality was 6% and the mortality attributable to COPD was 3%. The mortality in non-CABG patients was only 1.3%, suggesting that patients undergoing operations not involving lung resection should not be denied an operation because of the severity of their lung disease. Patients who have severe COPD have a tendency for a worse outcome in CABG operations secondary to coexisting

TABLE 24.3. PREPARING FOR ELECTIVE SURGERY IN PATIENTS WITH MODERATE TO SEVERE COPD

Clinical evaluation including a full medical history and examination

Evaluation of severity of respiratory symptoms such as cough, wheezing, etc. Surgery should be postponed in patients who have a URI or active symptoms.

Objective assessment of the severity of obstruction with ABG, spirometry/PFTs; treat reversible component with steroids prior to surgery if possible.

Detailed medication review. Discontinue β-blockers; these can worsen bronchospasm even if used as eyedrops.

Physical therapy consultation for instruction in postural drainage, deep breathing, incentive spirometry, etc. Chest physiotherapy should start preoperatively and should continue until patient is ambulatory.

Prescribe bronchodilator therapy in the perioperative period for patients who have evidence of bronchospasm.

Theophylline may improve pulmonary function; however, data is insufficient to recommend routine use of aminophylline infusions during the perioperative period.

Steroid-dependent patients should receive stress-dose steroids in the perioperative period.

DVT prophylaxis should be practiced in all patients.

ABG, arterial blood gas; DVT, deep vein thrombosis; URI, upper respiratory infection.

heart disease and other medical illnesses (45,46,100). Perioperative management of the patient with COPD is outlined in Table 24.3.

SURGICAL CONSIDERATIONS IN THE ASTHMATIC PATIENT

In a recent prospective study of 706 asthmatic patients undergoing surgery, the risk for perioperative bronchospasm was 2% (101). While refractory bronchospasm leading to respiratory failure is rare (101,102), those patients who have been recently hospitalized for asthma or required an emergency room or office visit within 30 days preceding surgery are at much greater risk of developing a significant exacerbation in the perioperative period (101). Operations associated with a higher incidence of bronchospasm include bronchoscopy and oropharyngeal instrumentation such as gastroscopy and ENT surgery. Mediastinoscopy can also provoke bronchospasm by reflex mechanisms.

Elective surgery should be postponed for a few weeks in patients who have had a recent asthma attack. All bronchodilators used preoperatively should be continued during the postoperative period. Intravenous aminophylline can be used in patients who are unable to take their oral medication, although inhaled bronchodilators are more efficacious. Inhaled steroids should be continued. Patients who are on systemic steroid medication should be given stress-dose steroids in the perioperative period to prevent adrenal insufficiency. Humidified air and oxygen should be used in the

perioperative period. Regional anesthesia may be an option for patients who have significant bronchospasm despite optimal medical therapy.

EVALUATION OF SUITABILITY FOR LUNG RESECTION

While spirometry has not been shown to be a good predictor of pulmonary complications in patients undergoing nonresectional thoracic or abdominal surgery, it has a definite role in evaluating patients for lung resection. The predicted postoperative FEV_1 has been shown to correlate significantly with postoperative complications (73).

While evaluating fitness for lung resection, the possibility of a pneumonectomy should always be considered. Patients who are deemed to be unfit for a pneumonectomy should be offered less aggressive surgical options such as VATS or nonsurgical therapy, rather than open thoracotomy.

In the past, patients were excluded from surgery if they did not meet the fitness criteria outlined in the Table 24.4 (65,66,73,76,103,104). There are varying recommendations as to the lowest acceptable value of the postoperative percent predicted FEV_1 and DLCO by different authors. Markos and associates found a mortality rate of 50% if the predicted postoperative FEV_1 was less than 40%. Predicted postoperative DLCO below 40% of the predicted value was associated with a 33% mortality rate (105).

Predicting Postoperative Pulmonary Function and Complications

Ventilation And Perfusion Lung Scanning

The contribution of each lung to pulmonary function can be assessed by quantitative ventilation and perfusion lung scans. After intravenous injection of technetium-99m labeled macroaggregates of albumin, images are obtained with a gamma camera linked to a computer. The counts are then recorded over each hemithorax from an anterior and posterior view, and the sum of these is divided by the total counts from both lungs to determine the contribution of each lung to overall perfusion. Standard oblique views can also be obtained to assess the contribution of each individual lobe to lung perfusion. Predicted postoperative FEV_1 is then measured as follows:

TABLE 24.4. CONTRAINDICATIONS TO LUNG RESECTION

Hypercarbia more than 45 mm HG at rest or exercise.

FEV_1 less than 2 L, FVC below 2 L and MVV less than 50% of the predicted value for patients undergoing pneumonectomy.

FEV_1 less than 1.5 L in those in whom a lobectomy is required.

Predicted postoperative FEV_1 below 800 mL determined preoperatively by spirometry and quantitative perfusion scans.

Predicted postoperative FEV_1 = Preoperative FEV_1 × (1-fractional contribution of the affected lung or lobe)

Calculation of predicted postoperative FEV_1 can also be performed by using preoperative PFT data and the number of bronchopulmonary segments to be removed (103). If it is assumed that each of the 19 bronchopulmonary segments contributes equally to ventilatory function, each segment would account for 5.26 percent of pulmonary function. Hence a right pneumonectomy is assumed to cause a loss of 55% of pulmonary function, while a left pneumonectomy would cause a loss of approximately 45% of lung function. Based on these assumptions, the predicted postoperative function can be calculated by the formula:

$$\text{Predicted postoperative } FEV_1 = \text{preoperative } FEV_1 \times [1 - (S \times 5.26/100)],$$

Where S is the number of segments to be resected

Exercise Testing

Several studies have evaluated the usefulness of preoperative exercise testing for predicting the incidence of postoperative complications (106–113). Whether exercise testing is superior to measurement of predicted postoperative lung function is controversial. There are studies to support both approaches, but neither method has been shown to be superior to the other. Exercise testing is attractive because exercise capacity is not dependent on lung function alone. It also measures hemodynamic performance and peripheral tissue oxygen utilization.

The exercise protocol used by most centers involves a graded increase in workload using a bicycle ergometer. Gas exchange is monitored and analyzed along with EKG monitoring, pulse oximetry, and frequent blood pressure monitoring. Some centers routinely use invasive blood pressure monitoring devices. Exercise is stopped when the patient develops limiting symptoms. The data is analyzed and the maximum oxygen consumption (VO_2max) is then calculated.

Most studies have reported a strong correlation between decreased exercise capacity and the frequency of cardiopulmonary complications. However, the threshold VO_2max for identifying high-risk patients has been difficult to define. In the study done by Smith and coworkers, patients who achieved a VO_2max above 20 mL per kg per minute had only a 10% incidence of postoperative complications, while all of the patients with a VO_2max below 15 mL per kg per minute suffered postoperative complications (107). In another study by Morice and coworkers, two out of the six patients with a VO_2max above 15 mL per kg per minute had postoperative complications after lung resection. Patients who had a VO_2max below 15 mL per kg per minute were not offered lung resection in that study (109). Most centers offer lung resection to patients if their VO_2max is above 15 mL per kg per minute and there are no other contraindications to surgery. The VO_2max has not been shown to correlate with spirometric measurements of pulmonary function (107).

Predicted postoperative maximal oxygen consumption (VO_2max-ppo) can be estimated with the use of preoperative pulmonary perfusion scans and exercise testing in a manner similar to prediction of postoperative FEV_1 and DLCO. A VO_2max-ppo below 10 mL/kg/minute was associated with a 100% mortality in a study by Bolliger and colleagues (108). In another study, eight out of nine patients who had a VO_2max below 60% of the predicted value suffered postoperative pulmonary complications, including three deaths (112).

Invasive cardiopulmonary exercise testing has also been employed to determine lung resectability. In a study by Olsen and colleagues, patients who tolerated lung resection poorly were found to have a lower cardiac index, oxygen delivery, and oxygen consumption compared to patients who tolerated resection well (114). A pulmonary vascular resistance (PVR) greater than 190 dyne.sec.cm has been proposed as a contraindication to lung resection by Fee and associates (113). However, in the study by Olsen and colleagues, PVR was not significantly different between the patients who tolerated lung resection and those who were classified as intolerant (114).

Epstein and coworkers have devised a cardiopulmonary risk index (CPRI) by combining a modified Goldman Index and six factors that have been shown to be associated with increased postoperative pulmonary complications (Table 24.5). These risk factors include obesity, cigarette smoking, productive cough within five days prior to surgery, diffuse ronchi or wheezing on physical examination, FEV_1/FVC under 70% and a $PaCO_2$ over 45 mm Hg. The total possible score for the pulmonary index is 6. The Goldman Index was modified by using an echocardiographic or radionuclide estimation of cardiac ejection fraction, and points were assigned for each of the four classes described by Goldman. The combined CPRI had a total possible score of 10. In a series of 42 patients undergoing lung resection, Epstein and coworkers observed that a CPRI score greater than 4 was associated with a 73% incidence of postoperative cardiopulmonary complications, versus 11% when the score was less

TABLE 24.5. CARDIOPULMONARY RISK INDEX

Variable	Points
Obesity (body mass index > 27 kg/m²)	1
Cigarette Smoking (within eight weeks of surgery)	1
Productive cough within five days	1
Diffuse wheezing or ronchi within five days of surgery	1
FEV_1/FVC < 70%	1
$PaCO_2$ > 45 mm Hg	1
Total	6

than 4. The CPRI was shown to have a sensitivity of 73%, a specificity of 89%, a positive predictive value of 79%, and a negative predictive value of 98%. The predictive value of CPRI is improved if it is combined with exercise testing using cycle ergometry (115,116). In a recent prospective study of 180 patients undergoing lung resection, the CPRI had an overall sensitivity of 23% and a specificity of 80% for predicting postoperative complications. In patients undergoing pneumonectomy, the sensitivity was improved to 44% and the specificity was 100% (117). The CPRI cannot be recommended as a screening test for all patients undergoing lung resection. It may be of value for the evaluation of elderly lung resection candidates who are likely to have a high prevalence of cardiac or pulmonary diseases.

Cardiac Considerations for Lung Resection and General Surgery

A large number of patients with chronic obstructive lung disease also have cardiovascular disease that contributes significantly to postoperative morbidity and mortality. Goldman and colleagues devised a multifactorial cardiac risk index to predict operative morbidity in unselected patients over the age of 40 years (118) (Table 24.6). This Goldman Index was based on a prospective study of 1,001 consecutive

TABLE 24.6. GOLDMAN MULTIFACTORIAL RISK INDEX

	Points
History	
Age >70 years	5
MI within six months	10
Physical	
JVD or S3 gallop*	11
Significant valvular aortic stenosis	3
Electrocardiogram	
Rhythm other than sinus or PACs on preoperative EKG	7
More than 5 PVCs per minute at any time prior to surgery	7
Poor general medical status	3
$PO_2 < 60$ or $PCO_2 > 50$ mm Hg	
K + < 3.0 or HCO3 < 20 meq/L	
BUN > 50 or creatinine > 3 mg/dL	
Abnormal SGOT, chronic liver disease	
Bedridden due to noncardiac disease	
Operation	
Intrathoracic, intraperitoneal, aortic surgery	3
Emergency surgery	4
Total points	53

Class 1, 0–5 points; Class 2, 6–12 points; Class 3, 13–25 points; Class 4, > 26 points**; PAC, premature atrial contraction; PVC, premature ventricular contraction.
* In CPRI described by Epstein et al. (116) LVEF < 40% was also included.
** In CPRI, Goldman Class 1, 1 point; Class 2, 2 points; Class 3, 3 points; Class 4, 4 points.

patients undergoing noncardiac surgery. The study identified nine risk factors that were associated with increased cardiac complications. Scores were assigned to each risk factor after multivariate analyses. The patients were assigned four risk categories according to their total score. This index provides clinicians with a simple way of assessing and modifying cardiac risk. It has been found to be reproducible and has been validated in several studies.

Surgical Risk in Patients with Angina

The Goldman Index does not address surgical risk in patients with angina pectoris. Patients with stable angina as their only risk factor are at low cardiac risk during noncardiac surgery. Patients with unstable angina are at significantly increased risk, and coronary revascularization should be considered prior to major surgery. For patients with myocardial infarction (MI) within the past six months, it is best to delay elective surgery. However, operations can be safely performed within four to six weeks after an MI if a delay is potentially dangerous. Patients who undergo successful revascularization following an MI can also undergo surgery four to six weeks after their MI.

It has been shown that beta-blockers in the perioperative period significantly reduce the risk of myocardial infarction and cardiac death, so that perioperative beta-blockers should be considered unless they are contraindicated (119).

CHEST TRAUMA

In spite of the implementation of a standardized assessment and management program for care of trauma patients, development of designated regional trauma centers, intensive training of paramedical personnel, and advances in the fields of trauma surgery and critical care medicine, trauma remains one of the five most common causes of death in the United States (120). Nearly 150,000 deaths occur in the United States yearly from trauma, and twice as many patients are left permanently disabled each year. The economic impact of trauma therapy is equally staggering, costing over fifty billion dollars per year (121).

Injuries to the chest occur in approximately 60% of all victims with multisystem injuries, and very often represent the most life-threatening component of the injury complex. For this reason, physicians caring for these patients should be trained in standardized Advanced Trauma Life Support (ATLS) assessment and procedures (122). Application of ATLS principles couples the initiation of the ABCs (Airway, Breathing, Circulation) of general resuscitation with the rapid initial assessment of the trauma patient, or primary survey (Table 24.7). The purpose of the primary survey is rapid identification and treatment of immediately life-threatening injuries. The vast majority of these injuries involve structures located within the chest cavity. Following

TABLE 24.7. INITIAL SURVEY OF THORACIC INJURIES

Primary Survey—Assessment of Immediately Life-Threatening Injuries
  Airway obstruction
  Tension pneumothorax
  Open pneumothorax
  Massive hemothorax
  Flail chest
  Cardiac tamponade

Secondary Survey—Assessment of Potentially Life-Threatening Injuries
  Simple pneumothorax
  Hemothorax
  Pulmonary contusion
  Traumatic aortic rupture
  Tracheobronchial disruption
  Esophageal disruption
  Traumatic diaphragmatic injury
  Blunt cardiac injury
  Penetrating wounds traversing the mediastinum

stabilization of these injuries, a secondary survey is performed. This is a full examination of the patient, assessing injuries in all systems and identifying specifically those that are deemed potentially life-threatening. Use of these ATLS management methods has greatly decreased morbidity and mortality in victims of trauma.

Diagnostic and Therapeutic Modalities

Radiologic Studies

In all patients with polytrauma, chest radiography is a vital diagnostic tool. This study should be done early in the course of the patient's care, after general resuscitation measures and the primary survey are completed. The great majority of chest radiographs obtained in this early care setting are portable anterior/posterior views and are taken with the patient in a supine position. Patient position combined with body habitus and the presence of emergency transport equipment (e.g., cervical collar) may limit the clinician's ability to interpret this initial film, and this should be taken into account when evaluating abnormalities. Evaluation of the initial chest radiograph should be done in a systematic manner (e.g., bony skeleton, soft tissues, pleural spaces, lungs, mediastinum, diaphragm) so that no abnormality is overlooked. Repeat chest radiographs should be done following any procedures such as endotracheal intubation, central venous line placement, or chest tube insertion, or if technical aspects of the initial film prevent adequate interpretation.

Thoracic Bony Skeleton

Detection of rib fractures is important in that they may be associated with other significant injuries within the chest.

They also indicate the need for pain control to help prevent secondary complications such as atelectasis and pneumonia. If clinical examination leads to the suspicion that a rib fracture is present, the patient should be treated for one even without radiologic confirmation, since they are not always evident on the chest film. The single best and most cost-effective test for detection of rib fractures is an upright posterior/anterior chest radiograph in full inspiration. In the vast majority of chest trauma cases, this will be a repeat film and not the initial chest radiograph performed, and will be done only after more critical studies and therapeutic procedures are completed. Occasionally, more specific views may be indicated for fractures of ribs 1 to 3 and 9 to 12, since fractures in these areas have a greater chance of association with significant underlying injuries (123,124). These additional films should be obtained only after full stabilization of the patient (125). When looking for rib fractures, the clinician should look particularly at the area of the anterior and posterior axillary lines, since it is in these areas of curvature that most rib fractures occur with anterior chest compression injuries.

Sternal fractures are uncommon and their detection is difficult. The best radiologic study for evaluation is a lateral chest radiograph using a horizontal beam. The presence of a sternal fracture is often associated with more significant soft-tissue injury beneath, particularly cardiac or pulmonary contusion. The clinician should be alert to the possibility of these injuries.

Since a significant amount of force is required for fracture of the scapula, the clinician should always be suspicious of more severe damage to vital intrathoracic structures if one is seen. A large percent of scapular fractures are missed on initial evaluation of the chest radiograph. More sensitive studies such as computerized tomography may be needed for diagnosis. Vertebral fractures often produce a paravertebral hematoma, a finding that commonly obscures the normal intrathoracic vascular structures and widens the mediastinal shadow on initial chest radiograph. This may lead many clinicians to suspect a major vascular injury. If suspected from the initial chest radiograph, a repeat chest radiograph that is overpenetrated can often be useful in determining the existence of vertebral injuries (126). If vertebral injury is noted or suspected, more sensitive diagnostic studies such as computerized tomography would be indicated.

Computerized Tomography And Magnetic Resonance Imaging

Computerized tomography (CT) of the chest is a much more sensitive study for identifying intrathoracic injuries than the supine AP chest radiograph, but it requires patient transport, is more time-consuming and costly, and requires more expertise for appropriate interpretation. If deemed necessary for evaluation of the chest in a trauma patient, this study should never be done until the secondary survey is completed. Information obtained from a chest CT study in this initial phase of patient care infrequently alters management. In specific instances, a CT may provide valuable information not noted on the admission chest radiograph (e.g., a small pneumothorax in a patient requiring positive pressure ventilation) (126). In some centers, CT is used prior to aortography to evaluate the patient with a widened mediastinal shadow and possible aortic transection. Some believe that this is a very valuable diagnostic step, since absence of a mediastinal hematoma eliminates the need for aortography (127–129). Others believe that a CT study for aortic transection is excessively time-consuming and has an unacceptably high false-negative rate (130). Until these controversies are sorted out, it is safe to say that at the majority of medical facilities, any suspicion of aortic transection should be immediately studied with the single most definitive test for this problem—aortography. Use of CT may prove more valuable later in the course of the trauma patient's care to evaluate abnormalities such as retained hemothorax, loculated empyema, pulmonary contusion, and intrapulmonary hematoma (130).

Magnetic Resonance Imaging (MRI) also provides more detail than plain radiographs, but like CT is virtually never indicated in the acute trauma setting for evaluation of the chest (126). It may prove helpful in a limited number of cases later in the course of the trauma patient's management for identification of residual abnormalities within the chest.

Ultrasound/Echocardiography/Aortography

Transthoracic ultrasound in acute chest trauma has proven less than ideal as a diagnostic modality with one exception: a good view of the pericardial space can be obtained using the subxiphoid view, thus allowing rapid diagnosis of intrapericardial fluid. This technology can be done rapidly and reliably by physicians with limited training. Several series have shown that this study has excellent sensitivity at centers in which it is used regularly (129).

Transesophageal echocardiography (TEE) has been used successfully for the diagnosis of acute dissection of the ascending aorta, but its value in the diagnosis of traumatic aortic transection has been questionable (129). Some centers report a significant number of false-negative studies. Also, this study requires specially trained personnel and is time-consuming. TEE is not presently a valuable diagnostic tool for diagnosis in acute chest trauma.

Aortography has long been considered the gold standard for diagnosis of acute aortic transection and remains so in the opinion of many. Except for this and for diagnosis of trauma to the brachiocephalic vessels, arteriography has very little value in acute chest trauma.

Bronchoscopy

Flexible fiber-optic bronchoscopy can be a very valuable diagnostic tool in chest trauma. The clinician should have a low threshold for its use in chest trauma patients presenting with any of the signs of major tracheobronchial injury (131) or airway foreign bodies (130). The procedure can be done in the emergency department, the operating room, or the intensive care unit, and is particularly easy in patients who have already been endotracheally intubated for airway control. One caveat that should not be overlooked in the intubated patient is the fact that the entire airway of a patient suspected of having a tracheobronchial injury should be visualized, not merely the portion visible distal to the endotracheal tube (132). This may require a coordinated effort by several personnel so that airway control is maintained. The endotracheal tube can be backed out over the fiber-optic bronchoscope up to the level of the vocal cords while the upper portion of the trachea is viewed, and then the endotracheal tube can be safely reinserted over the bronchoscope.

Rigid bronchoscopy may be required in the chest trauma patient presenting with massive hemoptysis, and in some cases of tracheobronchial injury (131). This procedure must be done in the operating room and is performed for localization of the source of bleeding prior to thoracotomy.

Tube Thoracostomy

Chest tube insertion is the most frequent therapeutic procedure performed for blunt and penetrating chest trauma and is a mainstay in the management of pneumothorax and hemothorax. Adequate chest tube size and proper intrathoracic placement are two important features in successful evacuation of a fluid collection within the chest cavity. A list of the indications for tube thoracostomy in the setting of chest trauma is given in Table 24.8. Though a common therapeutic procedure in chest trauma, it is associated with a complication rate of over 30% in some series. Proper technique is neccessary when inserting a chest tube (133).

Thoracoscopy

Over the past decade, video-assisted technology has been found increasingly applicable in patients suffering from

TABLE 24.8. INDICATIONS FOR TUBE THORACOSTOMY IN THORACIC TRAUMA

Simple pneumothorax associated with any chest trauma
Tension pneumothorax
Pneumothorax increasing in size
Pneumothorax in any unstable patient
Bilateral pneumothorax
Hemothorax or hemopneumothorax
Pneumothorax in an intubated, ventilated patient (including those about to undergo general anesthesia)
Open pneumothorax ("sucking" chest wound) in association with application of sterile occlusive dressing over the chest wall defect

chest trauma. It has been used as a diagnostic tool to identify and primarily control sources of bleeding within the chest in hemodynamically stable patients (134). Even when the site of bleeding cannot be readily controlled with these minimally invasive methods, limited thoracotomy plus thoracoscopic visualization can be used to approach the bleeding site (135,136). Thoracoscopic methods have also been used for identification and repair of diaphragmatic injuries (136). This minimally invasive technology is most commonly used later in the course of the trauma patient's care, for evacuation of retained hemothoraces (137–139), and in selected patients who develop an empyema after chest injury. One important management point to be observed is patient respiratory stability during a thoracoscopic procedure. Patients undergoing video-assisted thoracoscopic procedures must be able to tolerate single-lung ventilation while positioned in a lateral decubitus position on the operating table. This places the ventilated lung in a dependent position and may not be tolerated well by patients whose ventilatory status is marginal (134). Also, for this procedure, exchange of a standard endotracheal tube for a double-lumen tube is commonly required. This maneuver alone may be risky in marginally stable patients. Trauma patients who are difficult to oxygenate and/or ventilate due to massive pulmonary contusion, adult respiratory distress syndrome, pulmonary edema, or other conditions are not likely to tolerate the positioning and ventilatory settings required to perform a thorough thoracoscopic examination of the chest.

Thoracotomy

Thoracotomy is indicated in a small percentage of chest trauma patients in whom the injury is not adequately managed by other means such as tube thoracostomy (140). Large hemothorax and persistent hemorrhage are two common indications for exploration of the chest (Table 24.9).

Indications for thoracotomy in the emergency department are few. The best survival data for emergency department thoracotomy is found in patients who have sustained penetrating trauma to the chest and have vital signs detected at the scene of the injury but experience loss of vital signs

en route to the hospital or in the emergency department (141). Those who have sustained blunt chest injury and have no vital signs at the scene have been shown to derive virtually no benefit from thoracotomy in the emergency department and are not considered candidates for this procedure. It should be emphasized that emergency department thoracotomy should only be performed by qualified physicians with appropriate surgical training.

Injuries to the Chest Wall

Sternal Fractures

Motor vehicle crashes and more recently the mandatory use of seat belts have increased the incidence of sternal fracture. The classic scenario is that of a patient whose anterior chest wall strikes the steering wheel. Less common mechanisms are direct blows to the sternum or hyperflexion of the thoracic spine. These fractures are most common in women, patients over the age of 50, and those using shoulder restraints (142). The signs and symptoms are anterior chest pain, overlying tenderness, ecchymosis, crepitus, swelling, and/or deformity. Although some sternal fractures are evident on plain chest radiographs, a lateral film of the sternum is the best diagnostic tool. The upper and mid-portions of the sternum are the most prone to fracture.

Treatment is initially directed toward associated injuries, reported in approximately half of patients, with rib fractures, long bone fractures, and head injury reported in 40%, 25%, and 18% respectively (143,144). There is considerable controversy regarding whether or not sternal fractures are a hallmark for underlying cardiac injuries. Electrocardiogram and radionucleide abnormalities have been demonstrated in over half of the patients who present with sternal fracture, but the incidence of blunt cardiac injury does not seem to exceed that of the multiply injured population (145–150). Certainly, the possibility of blunt cardiac injury should receive consideration and investigation in patients with sternal fracture and a history of high-energy mechanism of injury and in those with hemodynamic instability. Therapy of sternal fracture is nearly always limited to pain relief and avoidance of excessive motion. Only patients with grossly displaced sternal fragments and severe pain need operative fixation (Figure 24.1). Patients with isolated sternal fracture can often be managed on an outpatient basis.

Rib Fractures

The most commonly encountered bony injury to the chest is a rib fracture, although the exact incidence is unknown. This diagnosis should be suspected in any patient with a blunt mechanism of injury who complains of chest pain and tenderness, particularly if there is an overlying abrasion or contusion. Motor vehicle crashes account for the majority of rib fractures; the incidence is not significantly reduced

TABLE 24.9. INDICATIONS FOR THORACOTOMY IN THORACIC TRAUMA

Operating Room Thoracotomy
  Initial evacuation of 1500 mL of blood or more from thoracostomy tube
  Persistent hemorrhage (>250 mL/hr for two to four hrs)
  Failure of tube thoracostomy with enlarging hemothorax
  Hemodynamic instability despite adequate rescuscitation

Emergency Department Thoracotomy
  Penetrating injury with trauma arrest en route to or in the emergency department

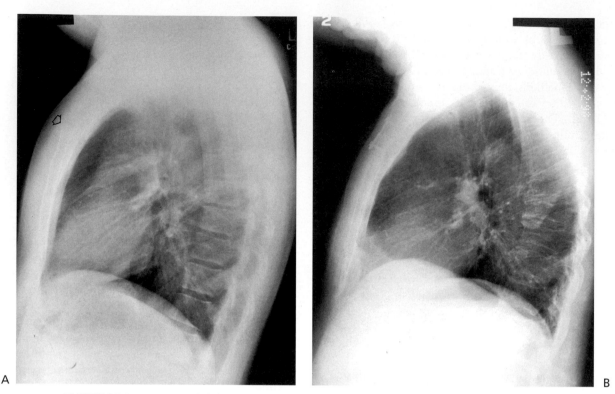

A

B

FIGURE 24.1. A, B, Sternal dislocation. This sternal dislocation required repair due to nonunion and chronic pain.

by use of seat belts (151). Penetrating trauma to the chest is not a common cause of rib fracture. In the conscious patient, careful physical examination will detect most rib fractures; however, Trunkey noted that 50% of rib fractures are not readily apparent on the initial anterior-posterior chest films routinely obtained in trauma patients (152,153) (Figure 24.2). In unconscious and severely injured patients, rib fractures are more difficult to detect. Rib detail films may aid in confirming a clinical suspicion based on mechanism of injury and physical examination. The treatment of rib fractures is primarily directed at pain relief, maintenance of effective pulmonary function, and prevention of complications. The optimal method of accomplishing these goals is dependent on a variety of factors which include the severity of injury to the chest, overall injury severity, patient factors such as age and medical condition, and the clinical modalities which are available within the treatment facility.

Patients who have one or two rib fractures, are in good medical condition, and have no other major injuries or complications can often be managed as outpatients with oral analgesia. The use of rib belts for additional analgesia remains controversial. There is at least one clinical study that indicates rib belts relieve pain without significantly impairing chest wall mechanics (154). However, in general, rib belts are disfavored due to the concept that restricted chest wall motion leads to atelectasis and other complications such as pneumonia. There is no major support in the litera-

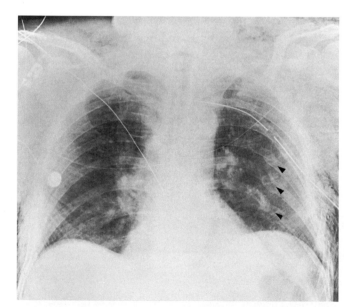

FIGURE 24.2. Multiple rib fractures. Multiple rib fractures with subcutaneous emphysema can be seen. Greater than three rib fractures correlates with an increased overall severity of injury score. Outpatient treatment is inadvisable.

ture for these ideas as they specifically relate to rib belts, and further study is needed. If a patient is to be treated as an outpatient, adequate pain relief and education regarding cough, deep breathing, and general pulmonary toilet are essential. The patient should also clearly understand the signs and symptoms that would necessitate a return to the hospital (dyspnea, tachypnea, persistent pain, fever, yellow sputum).

Three or more rib fractures or flail segments are indications of a greater overall injury severity, both inside and outside the chest cavity (155). Of particular note is that pneumothorax, hemothorax, and lung parenchymal and intraabdominal injuries are more common. These patients should be treated initially in the hospital. Also, individuals should be hospitalized who are elderly or pediatric, multiply injured, medically complicated, in a questionable state of health, or have inadequate pain control with oral analgesics. Complications occur in one-third of these patients. Predicting the need for ICU care and mechanical ventilation is challenging, and outpatient management is risky (156,157). The Respiratory Therapy Service should be involved with the patient and physician to establish an individualized program for maintaining pulmonary toilet and function. Pain management must also be individualized. There is no consensus on the best modality, although success has been reported with oral and IV narcotics, patient-controlled analgesia (PCA), intrapleural catheters, and intermittent and continuous epidural catheters. For nonintubated patients with mid to lower chest wall injuries involving multiple ribs, there is some evidence that continuous epidural management is superior to PCA and intrapleural catheters in maintaining tidal volume, vital capacity and maximum inspiratory pressure, and pain relief (158,159).

Special consideration should be given to patients with fractures of the first and second ribs. A fracture at this level indicates a high level of kinetic injury and is associated with a higher incidence of injury to the aorta and great vessels, as well as intraabdominal and intracranial structures. Investigations of these areas should be undertaken on a selective basis. Many of these patients will require inpatient observation to rule out other injuries.

In summary, rib fractures are a common sequela of trauma. Although simple fractures can be treated as an outpatient, rib fractures are a predictor for severe injury and often require hospitalization, not only for the treatment of pain and maintenance of adequate pulmonary function, but for the treatment of complications of nonchest injuries. Previous research indicates that half of these patients will require operative or ICU care (160).

Flail Chest

Flail chest is a multiple injury pattern of the chest wall that results in paradoxical motion of the hemithorax with breathing. The injured segment moves inward during inspi-

ration and outward during expiration. Usually flail chest results from the fractures of three or more ribs in two locations, typically posteriorly and laterally or anteriorly and laterally, but it may also result from a combination of fractures of the ribs and costal cartilages and/or sternum. Flail chest may not be diagnosed initially in patients who arrive intubated by prehospital personnel and may be suspected only after chest radiographs or during weaning from the ventilator. Flail chest is diagnosed by physical examination and may be confirmed radiographically.

As with rib fracture alone, treatment of flail chest is supportive. Pulmonary function abnormalities seen in flail chest include decreases in the vital capacity, total static lung compliance, maximum inspiratory force, and arterial oxygenation, and increases in airway resistance and the work of breathing. This pathophysiology is related to pain, splinting, abnormal chest wall mechanics, and in many cases, underlying pulmonary contusion.

Management concepts have changed through the years. Until the 1950s, emphasis was placed on external stabilization of the chest wall using a variety of operative and nonoperative techniques. In 1956, Avery, Morch, and Benson advocated internal stabilization of the chest wall with volume-control ventilators (161). More recently, Richardson and Shackford have demonstrated that adequate analgesia and aggressive pulmonary toilet reduce morbidity and hospital stay without a need for mechanical ventilation (157,162).

Even with these measures, a significant number of patients will require ventilator assistance. Factors associated with a greater need for mechanical ventilation are the overall injury severity, particularly injuries to the head, multiple long-bone fractures and truncal injuries requiring operation, blood transfusions in the first 24 hours, and shock on admission (163). Also affecting outcome adversely are age greater than 50 years, bilateral flail segments, the presence of a hemothorax and/or pneumothorax requiring a chest tube, and underlying pulmonary contusion. Patients involved in a motorcycle accident, pedestrians hit by automobiles, and fall victims also have a poorer prognosis (164).

Intubation is recommended for individuals with tachypnea (respiratory rate greater than 40 breaths per minute), tidal volumes of less than 10cc per kg, hypoxemia (PaO_2 less than 60 mm Hg on an FIO_2 of greater than 50%) and/or hypercapnea ($PaCO_2$ of over 50 mm Hg in patients with no history of COPD), and in patients whose associated injuries necessitate intubation. Extubation criteria are similar to those used in other ventilated patients. Adequate unassisted tidal volume and respiratory rates of 30 or less suggest that the chest wall has stabilized sufficiently to allow extubation.

In rare circumstances, patients require operative stabilization of the chest wall. Although criteria are not strictly established, paradoxical motion of the chest wall that prevents weaning from the ventilator and severe chest wall deformity with greater than 5 cm depression are accepted indications. Patients who are ventilated principally for severe pulmonary contusion have not been shown to benefit from chest wall stabilization. Patients who require thoracotomy for other traumatic indications (persistent air leak, diaphragmatic rupture, retained hemothorax, etc.) should also receive chest wall stabilization. Thomas and colleagues showed shortened duration of mechanical ventilation, improved pain control, and improved anatomic healing with early stabilization (165).

Long-term pulmonary disability exists in approximately 60% of patients recovering from a flail chest. All of the following complications have been documented: chest wall pain and deformity, dyspnea on exertion varying from months to lifetime, decreased minute ventilation, and mild restrictive pulmonary disease (166,167). Despite modern improvements in care, the mortality rate remains high (10% to 35%). Death is principally due to associated injuries and sepsis (164,168).

Pneumothorax

Pneumothorax is a common sequela of both blunt and penetrating chest trauma. The three types of pneumothorax seen in trauma victims are simple, open, and tension.

Simple pneumothorax most commonly occurs when air escapes from the visceral pleural surface of the lung. As the space within the thorax fills with air, the lung parenchyma collapses. If the lung injury is small, it may be rapidly sealed by platelets in the low-pressure setting of the lung. Mechanisms of lung injury include penetrating objects and missiles, iatrogenic causes such as central lines and bronchoscopic biopsy, and rib fractures. Blunt rupture of blebs and lung parenchyma may occur with high-kinetic energy transmission across the chest wall, such as in motor vehicle crashes and falls. Patients complain of shortness of breath and have decreased breath sounds and tympany to percussion in the affected hemithorax.

In the setting of trauma, it is neither necessary nor advisable to await a chest radiograph prior to instituting therapy. Initial treatment can be with a large-bore needle in the second intercostal space or a chest tube. If needle decompression is elected, chest tube placement should follow expeditiously. Except in iatrogenic trauma, use of needle-catheter drainage system is not recommended due to the high incidence of reaccumulation and concomitant presence of blood within the chest cavity. Chest tubes for trauma should be placed in the fourth or fifth intercostal space laterally and directed posteriorly. Since up to 25% of patients have pleural symphysis, chest tube placement should always be performed by or with the supervision of an experienced physician. A 32F-40F size tube will prevent inadequate evacuation of air and blood secondary to clots within the tube. Careful attention should be directed to ascertaining that all of the holes in the chest tube are within the thoracic cavity. Sturdy stitches (usually size 0, 1, or 2) should secure the tube to the skin and underlying fascia. Chest tubes

should be placed on suction of approximately 20 cm H_2O. A chest radiograph should be obtained after the tube is placed to assess for expansion of the lung and chest tube position.

A question often asked is whether a trauma patient can be treated for pneumothorax without a chest tube. There is little scientific data regarding this matter. In general, most experienced physicians would recommend this therapy only under the following circumstances: (a) the pneumothorax is unilateral and small (less than 20% of the volume of the hemithorax); (b) there is no associated hemothorax or detectable air leak; (c) there are no other major injuries; (d) the patient can understand worsening signs and symptoms and ask for assistance; (e) there is no requirement for positive pressure ventilation or anesthetic; (f) the patient requires no further transfer by ground or air; (g) an individual who can urgently place a chest tube is present in the hospital; and (h) the patient is largely asymptomatic. When in doubt, the placement of a chest tube is the safer option. If management without a chest tube is elected, a second chest radiograph should be obtained within four to six hours to be certain that the pneumothorax is not increasing in size. Any worsening of symptoms should result in prompt insertion of a chest tube.

An open pneumothorax occurs when there is an opening in the chest wall that exceeds two-thirds the diameter of the trachea. This creates a "sucking wound" that allows ingress and egress of air and blood. In the prehospital setting, the wound should be covered with an occlusive gauze and taped on three sides only. A completely occlusive dressing taped on four sides may convert the open pneumothorax to a tension pneumothorax. In the emergency room setting, a chest tube should be expeditiously placed and a fully occlusive bandage applied after the placement. The chest tube should not be introduced through the area of injury. Most of these wounds should proceed to the operating room for debridement and closure. Smaller wounds can be successfully managed in the emergency room setting. A chest radiograph should be obtained after chest tube placement to check for adequate expansion of the lung, evacuation of air and blood, location of the tube, and concomitant injuries to other organs within the thorax.

A tension pneumothorax occurs when air escapes from the lungs and/or mediastinal structures, or less commonly, enters from the outside, and fills the hemithorax. Not only does the lung collapse, but a continued accumulation of air will shift the mediastinum to the opposite hemithorax. If untreated, it will kink the vena cava and impede venous return to the heart. If the preload to the heart becomes sufficiently reduced, hypotension and cardiac arrest will occur. Tension pneumothorax should be suspected in patients with either blunt or penetrating chest injury and hypotension. Tension pneumothorax often presents with absent breath sounds, tympany to percussion, deviation of the trachea, neck vein distention, pulsus paradoxus, and/or worsening tachycardia, but these symptoms can be absent or difficult to detect. Additionally, the symptoms may mimic pericardial tamponade. If a tension pneumothorax is suspected, the patient should undergo an immediate large-bore needle decompression in the second intercostal space, followed by prompt chest tube placement. One should never wait for a chest radiograph when there is high clinical suspicion of tension pneumothorax.

Hemothorax

Hemothorax simply means blood within the pleural cavity. It is seen with both penetrating and blunt trauma. In penetrating trauma, there is nearly always associated trauma to the chest wall, lungs, great vessels, heart, or intraabdominal contents such as spleen or liver with an associated diaphragmatic injury. Blunt trauma produces hemothorax via injuries to the chest wall, particularly rib fractures with associated intercostal artery bleeding, lacerations to the lung due to rib punctures and/or shear forces on the pulmonary parenchyma, and tearing of adhesions between the visceral and parietal pleura. Great-vessel injury is also seen with blunt injuries, particularly aortic injury.

Patients with isolated hemothorax and blood loss of less than 250 mL will present with few symptoms. Generally, these hemothoraces are detected by blunting of the costophrenic angle on chest film. Patients with a greater blood loss present with all or a combination of the following signs and symptoms: chest pain, tachypnea, tachycardia, decreased or absent breath sounds, dullness to percussion, pallor, hypotension, and cardiovascular collapse. Shift of the mediastinum is also possible with hemothorax, but is less common than with tension pneumothorax (Figure 24.3).

Initial treatment for hemothorax is with a tube thoracostomy. Thoracentesis is not indicated. Eighty-five percent of patients with hemothorax can be successfully managed with chest tube alone. Large-size tubes, such as a 36 or 40F, placed in the fifth intercostal space and directed posteriorly, will most effectively evacuate blood and are less likely to clot. If a large hemothorax is suspected, it may be beneficial to use an evacuation device with autotransfusion capability. The amount of blood collected should be serially monitored.

If over 800 mL of blood is collected with insertion of the chest tube, it is defined as a massive hemothorax. Only 10% to 15% of patients requiring a chest tube progress to operative intervention, but this is a high-risk group. Early surgical consultation is mandatory. Criteria for operative intervention varies somewhat from surgeon to surgeon, but nearly all surgeons will operate if the chest tube output within the first hour after injury exceeds 1.5 L, or is over 250 mL per hr thereafter.

Approximately 5% of patients presenting with hemothorax will develop the complication of a clotted hemothorax. Small, clotted hemothoraces that do not become infected

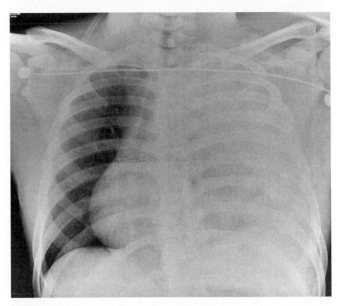

FIGURE 24.3. Hemothorax. This patient has a massive left hemothorax with mediastinal shift. A missile can be seen in the left hemothorax. Chest tube placement, volume resuscitation, and prompt surgical consultation are needed.

will resolve on their own without significant pulmonary sequela. If chest tubes do not successfully drain large blood clots within the chest cavity, the patient may develop an empyema or have trapping and fibrosis of a significant portion of the lung. A clotted hemothorax should be operatively evacuated if 25% or greater lung volume is lost on chest film or if signs of infection, such as fever and leukocytosis, develop. Timing of evacuation of a clotted hemothorax remains controversial. Generally, if a decision is made prior to one week, many patients can undergo an evacuation using the video-assisted thoracoscope. After one week, the patient is more likely to need a formal thoracotomy, resulting in increased morbidity and prolongation of the hospital stay (169).

Injuries to the Pulmonary Parenchyma

Pulmonary Contusion

Pulmonary contusion is a common finding after trauma, seen in about 20% of adult patients with multiple injuries (170). Pulmonary contusion is more common in children due to increased compliance of the chest wall (171). Motor vehicle accidents, falls, and penetrating injuries are the most common causes for pulmonary contusion in civilian settings. In a military setting, pulmonary contusions often result from high-velocity missiles and blast injuries from explosives.

There are three basic components in the pathophysiology of pulmonary contusion:

1. *The spalling effect.* This describes the shearing or burst effect that occurs at a gas/liquid interface with a dissipation of an applied force. In the lung, for example, the impact of the pulmonary parenchyma against the chest wall leads to a disruption of alveoli.
2. *The inertial effect.* The low-density alveolar tissues are stripped from the hilum as they accelerate at different rates.
3. *The implosion effect.* Gas bubbles rebound and overexpand after the shock wave passes.

Injury to the lung results from the actual transmission of mechanical forces from the chest wall; increased tissue pressure and tearing of tissues; direct laceration to the lung by ribs or penetrating objects; bleeding into uninvolved lungs; increased mucus production with decreased clearance; and decreased production of surfactant leading to alveolar collapse (172). On the microscopic level, animal models reveal interstitial hemorrhage initially, followed by edema within one to two hours of injury. This progresses in 24 hours to alveoli filled with protein, red cells, inflammatory cells, and fibrin deposits, and loss of architecture. At 48 hours these processes are worsened, and cellular debris, granules from type II alveolar cells, macrophages, and neutrophils are also present. Lymphatics are dilated and filled with protein. Edema is massive. Healing with minimal scarring is present at seven to 10 days (173,174).

This pathology is manifested clinically as hypoxemia, hypercarbia, and increased work of breathing. Ventilation/perfusion mismatch, intrapulmonary shunt, increased lung water and loss of compliance can lead to respiratory failure. Chest radiograph anomalies may not be present until four to six hours after the injury and may underestimate the degree of damage (175,176) (Figure 24.4). Computerized tomography of the lungs reveals the presence and extent of injury earlier and more accurately. Wagner and Jamieson have demonstrated that consolidation of 28% or more of the air spaces was 100% predictive of the need for mechanical ventilation. Chest CT, however, is not always practical in the multiply injured patient (176). Clinical decisions based on the mechanism of injury and examination of the patient may be required.

Treatment is primarily supportive. Supplemental oxygen, including mechanical ventilation, is the mainstay of therapy. The mode of ventilation must be tailored to the patient, but protective strategies that avoid overdistention of the uninvolved lung are recommended. Patients with severe unilateral disease and significant V/Q mismatch and intrapulmonary shunting may benefit from dual lung ventilation and/or nitric oxide therapy (177). Extracorporeal membrane oxygenation is not usually practical, as significant bleeding may occur within the lung or from associated injuries. In extreme cases lobectomy may be necessary. Excellent pulmonary toilet is also needed. In addition to cough, deep breathing, and postural drainage, pain management is required to optimize patient effort. Intravenous bolus or patient-controlled intrapleural and epidural analgesia all have a potential role in pain management. Except in the smallest of contusions, patients should be initially cared for with continuous cardiovascular monitoring and pulse oximetry in an ICU.

Several controversies exist in the management of pulmonary contusion. The most often investigated is fluid resuscitation. Overzealous fluid administration has been shown to be deleterious in animal models. However, in humans, there is no evidence that volume restriction or use of diuretic therapy has a positive impact on outcome (178). The current recommendation is that fluids should be given based upon the need for adequate hydration and perfusion of vital

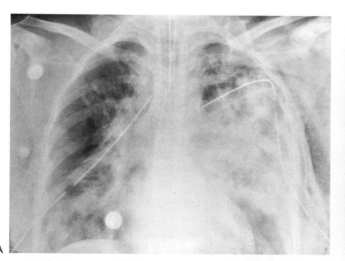
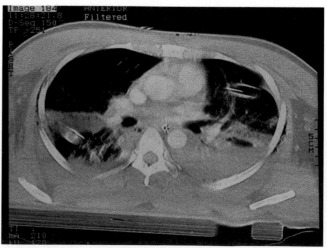

A   B

FIGURE 24.4. A, B, Pulmonary contusion. Chest radiograph and CT scan of a patient with blunt chest injury. Pulmonary contusions are often more evident on CT scans than on plain films.

organs. Fluid restriction and diuretics should be used only in patients with volume overload. A second controversy regarding fluids is use of colloid instead of crystalloid to avoid increased lung water, pulmonary edema, and the potential sequelae of these factors in lung injury. There is no strong evidence to support the use of colloids over crystalloids in resuscitation of patients with pulmonary contusion (178–181). Controversy also exists regarding the use of corticosteroids in pulmonary contusion. Animal models have shown both diminution of hypoxemia and decrease in lesion size (182). In humans, Svennevig and colleagues showed a decrease in pulmonary vascular resistance with high-dose steroids, but no change in clinical outcomes (183). Currently, the use of steroids is not recommended.

Generally, the pulmonary derangements associated with pulmonary contusion will resolve in less than a week, but problems with systemic immune response, ARDS, and secondary nosocomial pneumonia are not uncommon. Morbidity and mortality are related to injury severity scores, the severity of lung injury, and the development of complications. Long-term morbidity for recovered patients includes the possibility of decreased FRC and oxygenation, disabling dyspnea, and pulmonary fibrosis (184).

Pulmonary Hematoma

Pulmonary hematoma is a discrete collection of blood contained within the pulmonary parenchyma. This rather uncommon finding usually follows pulmonary contusion and laceration from blunt or penetrating injury (130). On initial radiologic studies, pulmonary hematoma is masked by the manifestations of the pulmonary contusion. It is usually later in the patient's course, after clearing of the acute pulmonary injury, that it becomes visible, often seen as a discrete density or mass within the lung tissue. Occasionally, if the original pulmonary parenchymal injury involved small airway structures in addition to pulmonary vessels, the loculation may have an air-fluid level or may present as a posttraumatic pneumatocele. Spontaneous resolution of these posttraumatic collections generally takes about five to six weeks, and unless infection or air leak develops, or evidence of continued hemorrhage exists, observation is continued and management is nonoperative. In cases where resolution has not occurred within five to six weeks, further investigation is warranted (185). Ideally, prior available chest radiographs would be helpful in revealing an abnormality that existed prior to the injury. Additional studies helpful in differentiating a persistent hematoma from some other type of lung lesion are CT and MRI (186). These have been used by some centers to follow residual posttraumatic masses and avoid surgical intervention. More commonly, when resolution of the mass lesion has not occurred in the anticipated time period, surgical excision of the lesion is performed.

Pulmonary Laceration And Air Embolization

Pulmonary laceration occurs more often after penetrating trauma but is also associated with blunt injury. In blunt trauma cases, it may result from direct penetration by fractured ribs or may occur from shear forces exerted upon the lung tissue during severe chest compression followed by sudden decompression (187). In these situations, both intrapulmonary vessels and airways can be torn, resulting in hemothorax, pneumothorax, or a combination of the two. Since perfusion pressure within the lungs is low and the injured vessel's caliber is small, bleeding is generally self-contained. Radiologic identification of a pulmonary laceration on plain chest radiography is often difficult, since its presence may be masked by the picture of contusion. CT is a much more exacting study for the delineation of pulmonary lacerations (187). Surgical intervention is required in about 5% of patients for either persistent bleeding or unresolved air leak.

While the vast majority of pulmonary lacerations are successfully treated with tube thoracostomy or with a thoracoscopic or surgical procedure, a few sustain potentially lethal air embolization. Left-sided air embolization is by far the more dangerous and potentially lethal form. Lung injuries involving adjacent bronchi and pulmonary venous structures can cause a bronchopulmonary venous fistula, setting the stage for air entry into the left heart and systemic arterial circulation. While air can travel to any end organ, the greatest risk for morbidity and mortality occurs with embolization to the coronary or cerebral circulation. Less than one milliliter of air in a critical vessel like the left anterior descending coronary artery is necessary to cause ventricular fibrillation and death. With regard to the cerebral circulation, symptoms of air embolization include dizziness, headache, and visual disturbance. Clinical manifestations can occur suddenly, and include loss of consciousness, focal seizures or convulsions, and a variety of neurologic deficits. Air may be visible in the retinal vessels on ophthalmologic examination.

Right-sided air embolization is most common in relation to accidental infusion from intravenous therapy. In cases of lung or chest wall trauma, air can enter via injured bronchial or intercostal veins or the superior vena cava or its major tributaries. In the majority of cases, a moderately large amount of right-sided air can be tolerated, although rapid infusion can affect the ability of the patient to tolerate air in the right-sided circulation. Large amounts of right-sided air (5 to 8 mL per kg) can be fatal. A secondary complication of right-sided air embolization is paradoxical embolization. Patients having any type of potential right-to-left shunt are at risk for this complication. This includes patients with a patent foramen ovale (15% to 25% of the population) or other types of congenital intracardiac defects and those who develop a intrapulmonary right-to-left shunt within injured lung tissue as a result of the trauma they experience. In paradoxical embolization, air can traverse the intracardiac defect or intrapulmonary shunt, enter the left side of the heart, and then travel to critical coronary or cerebral arteries. These patients are subject to the same risks as those patients who have primary systemic arterial air embolization (188).

It must be remembered that iatrogenic air embolization can easily occur in the trauma setting. Significant amounts of air can be infused into the systemic veins during hasty initiation of fluid resuscitation therapy. More importantly, vigorous positive pressure ventilation in patients with lung contusion or laceration may increase the likelihood of air embolization by forcing air through lacerated bronchial structures into adjacent injured pulmonary vessels. If clinical findings suggest systemic air embolism, the single best diagnostic study is TEE (189). The diagnosis can be made quickly and accurately since air bubbles are easily visible in the cardiac chambers. At times, the diagnosis is made when thoracotomy is performed.

Treatment of systemic air embolism includes maintenance of adequate intravascular volume, appropriate use of cardiotonic agents to sustain adequate systemic blood pressure, and judicious management of mechanical ventilation. Use of low tidal volume, decreased PEEP, and in some cases high-frequency jet ventilation may greatly reduce the detrimental hemodynamic consequences associated with systemic air embolization (189). Using TEE for continuous observation of cardiac function while adjusting pharmacologic agents or ventilatory modes can be very useful.

Injuries to the Diaphragm

Traumatic rupture of the diaphragm is seen with increasing frequency. Ten percent to 15% of patients with lower chest/upper abdomen–penetrating trauma and up to 5% of hospitalized victims of motor vehicle crashes will have a diaphragmatic injury (190–192).

The diagnosis of a ruptured hemidiaphragm is not always an easy one to make, particularly if there is no radiologic abnormality on chest film and the patient has no obvious need for thoracic or abdominal operation. The diagnosis is most frequently made on the left side, but that does not necessarily mean that it is more frequent on the left side. Most commonly, symptoms are due to associated injuries of the chest or abdominal cavity. Patients may present with dyspnea, orthopnea, and chest or abdominal pain. If gastric dilatation with obstruction occurs, the patient may have severe respiratory distress with ipsilateral lung collapse and symptoms that mimic tension pneumothorax. Patients may also be entirely asymptomatic. Physical signs of rupture include absence of breath sounds over the left hemithorax, displacement of the cardiac dullness to the right, presence of bowel sounds in the left chest, diminished left chest wall excursion, and cardiac and respiratory dysfunction. In the classic case of diaphragmatic rupture, the diagnosis can be made by a chest radiograph which shows an elevated left diaphragm and coiling of the nasogastric tube in the left chest. One may also see the curvilinear shadows of other abdominal viscera such as colon or small bowel in the thorax. The accuracy of the chest radiograph in the diagnosis of diaphragmatic rupture has been quoted to be from 13% to 94% (193) (Figure 24.5). Although it is impossible to know the accuracy of chest film, it is obvious that the potential for missed injury is significant. Therefore a high index of suspicion should prompt further testing. Additional studies which have proved useful in making the diagnosis are upper gastrointestinal contrast studies, barium enema, ultrasonography, computed tomographic scans, radioisotopic scintigraphy, magnetic resonance imaging, fluoroscopy, thoracoscopy, and laparoscopy and diagnostic peritoneal lavage (DPL). Generally, DPL is used to diagnose injury in penetrating wounds and the positive red cell count is dropped to 20,000 instead of 100,000. None of the modalities are foolproof. In general, one should consult with the radiologists and surgeons in your own hospital to determine the modality with which they are experiencing the most success in making an accurate diagnosis. The estimated incidence of missed injury is 12% to 60% (194–197).

Discovery of a diaphragmatic injury should prompt expeditious surgical consultation. Most surgeons will approach acute ruptures via a celiotomy. If there has been a significant delay in diagnosis of months to years, most will approach the herniation through the chest. There is, however, disagreement as to the best approach.

Morbidity and mortality are most often due to associated injuries. Mortality rates vary in the literature from 4.3% to 41%, with blunt injuries causing a higher mortality. Morbidity associated with diaphragmatic injury and repair includes: atelectasis, pneumonia, respiratory failure, systemic sepsis, failed repair, empyema, diaphragmatic paresis or paralysis, strangulation of visceral structures within the herniation, and lung and liver abscesses. The overall incidence of complications is 40% to 60%. Diaphragmatic injury is rarely an isolated event. Prevention of morbidity and mortality demands careful attention to the overall condition of the patient and care of associated injuries in addition to prompt and proper repair.

Injuries to the Mediastinum

Esophageal Injury

The course of the esophagus includes the neck, thorax, and abdomen. This discussion will be principally confined to injuries below the neck.

The exact incidence of trauma to the esophagus is unknown. The most common causes are penetrating wounds to the back, neck, and chest, and iatrogenic instrumentation. Blunt trauma rarely produces esophageal injury; the overall incidence is less than 0.1% in motor vehicle crashes. Accidental insufflation of pressurized air through the mouth

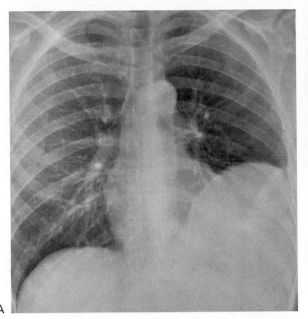
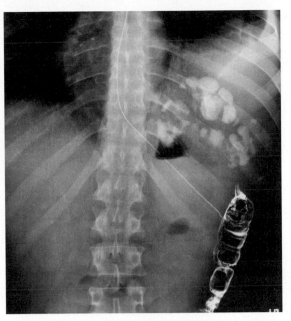

FIGURE 24.5. A, B, Diaphragmatic rupture. This patient has an elevated left hemidiaphragm after receiving blunt chest trauma. Diaphragmatic rupture should always be ruled out in such cases. The injury was not diagnosed in the acute setting, but was later discovered when the patient underwent a barium enema.

during resuscitation is another rare mechanism of injury. Because of the close anatomic relationship of the esophagus and trachea, both penetrating and blunt injuries may have associated tracheal injury.

Following injury to the esophagus, air and secretions escape into the mediastinum and cause extensive chemical and bacterial mediastinal contamination. Symptoms at presentation range from none to critical sepsis, depending on the size and layer of penetration of the wound, associated injuries, and the time frame of development. The most common symptom is pain in the chest or epigastrium. Other potential signs and symptoms include fever, hoarseness, dysphagia, subcutaneous emphysema, mediastinal crunch, splinting of the chest wall, respiratory distress, and shock. Abdominal pain and rigidity usually herald perforation at the esophagogastric junction rather than in the chest.

Diagnosis can be suspected by history, physical examination, and chest radiograph. Typical radiographic findings are mediastinal emphysema, hydrothorax, pneumothorax, and/or widening of the mediastinum (Figure 24.6). There may be increased space between the vertebral bodies and the trachea. In rare cases, the chest film may be without anomaly or anomalies may be attributable to concomitant injuries. For this reason, esophagrams should be performed on patients with transthoracic missile injuries near the mediastinum and stab wounds. In rare cases, esophagrams may be falsely negative. In patients in whom there is a high index of suspicion with a negative esophagram or in those whose condition does not technically permit esophagography, esophageal endoscopy is an accurate diagnostic alternative.

As soon as the diagnosis is suspected, treatment should begin. The general recommendations for any esophageal perforation are suspension of all oral intake, placement of a nasogastric tube with continuous suction, and antibiotic administration. Antibiotics should cover mouth flora (Gram

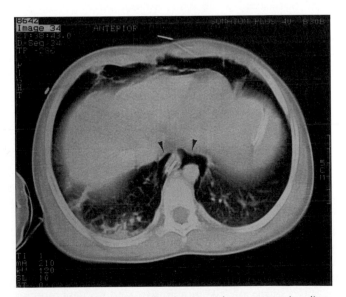

FIGURE 24.6. Pneumomediastinum and pneumopericardium. The CT scan demonstrates obvious air in the mediastinum and pericardium in a patient who suffered blunt chest trauma. Air in these locations can be easily missed on chest radiographs. Its presence should alert the physician to the possibility of esophageal and/or tracheobronchial injury, and warrants further study of these structures.

positives and anaerobes) and possible Gram-negative contaminants from penetrating wounds. If hydrothorax or pneumothorax is present, a chest tube is inserted. Surgical consultation should be made at the earliest possible juncture, as the morbidity and mortality associated with this injury increases with time to operation. Mortality ranges from 9% to 25% in various series (198).

Tracheal And Bronchial Disruption

Traumatic disruption of the tracheobronchial tree is an uncommon but potentially life-threatening injury resulting from either blunt or penetrating trauma. In civilian populations, it is most commonly associated with blunt injury, occurring in about 1% of cases (131,132). Its infrequency is related to the large amount of thoracic bony protection surrounding the major airway structures. Nearly 80% of patients in which this injury occurs expire before they reach a hospital. Of the remaining patients who reach the hospital alive, about 30% do not survive. Factors believed to contribute to these high mortality rates include anatomic location and degree of injury, severity of associated injuries, and asphyxia (199).

In cases of penetrating injury, the nature of the disruption depends upon the trajectory and force of the penetrating weapon or object. Much more controversy exists about the exact nature of the injury mechanism in cases resulting from blunt trauma. A number of factors are said to contribute, including rapid deceleration, torsion of the tracheobronchial tree, anterior-posterior compression between sternum and vertebral column, "splaying" of the major bronchi from the trachea laterally when anterior-posterior compression occurs, and in cases where trauma occurs just after deep inspiration and closure of the glottis, a barotrauma or "blowout" type of injury (200). More than 80% of these injuries occur within 2.5 cm of the carina (199). Injuries in this region vary from simple linear lacerations to complex stellate disruptions (131,200) or even complete transection. Distal (lobar or segmental) bronchial injuries occur even more uncommonly and are usually associated with extensive pulmonary parenchymal damage.

Disruption of the tracheobronchial tree can produce a constellation of early manifestations, some of which can be extremely subtle. Tracheobronchial injuries are most obvious when they communicate with the pleural space and produce findings that include a large pneumothorax, extensive and progressive subcutaneous and mediastinal emphysema with dyspnea and hypoxemia, persistent pneumothorax or air leak in spite of functioning thoracostomy tube, or failure of the affected lung to reexpand with appropriate thoracostomy drainage (131,199). Hemoptysis occurs in about 20% of cases (199). While airway injuries communicating with the pleural space are rather obvious, injuries that are contained by surrounding peribronchial tissues and pleura often present with more subtle findings. Patients may

present with a small initial leak of air into the pleural space or, more commonly, into the mediastinal tissues. Shortly after the leak occurs, the injury site is sealed by the surrounding tissues or clot. Hemoptysis in these cases is rare. Since air dissects predominantly into the peribronchial and mediastinal tissue planes in these cases, subcutaneous emphysema is the most common finding on a chest radiograph. Other associated findings may include pneumomediastinum, pneumothorax, and rib fractures. A subtle yet very reliable early finding on a plain chest radiograph is emphysema in the deep soft tissues of the neck (199).

Prior to the undertaking of any further diagnostic procedures, establishment of a stable airway and adequate gas exchange is of prime importance. If endotracheal intubation and positive pressure ventilation are required for management, these must be done with great caution and with attention to the location of the injury. Imprudent placement of an endotracheal tube or vigorous positive pressure ventilation may worsen the condition of the patient by enlarging a laceration or reopening one that has sealed. Positive pressure ventilation may increase an already existing ventilation/perfusion mismatch, since a large percent of each delivered breath will preferentially exit the injury site, leaving the uninjured lung underventilated. To secure satisfactory airway control in some cases, it may be necessary to direct the endotracheal tube into the uninjured bronchus or use a double-lumen endotracheal tube (201). In cases in which standard techniques of intubation may be difficult or dangerous, it may be prudent to position the endotracheal tube under direct vision by inserting it over a flexible fiber-optic bronchoscope. Also, in cases where the laceration is in the trachea or carina, an alternate mode of mechanical ventilation such as high-frequency ventilation may be useful.

For diagnosis of tracheobronchial injuries, the single best study is bronchoscopy (131,200,202). While most clinicians prefer the ease and ready availability of flexible fiberoptic bronchoscopy, rigid bronchoscopy is also useful in experienced hands. In cases where the leak is large or patient stability is in question, this procedure should be performed in the operating room so that thoracotomy can be immediately performed if needed. Bronchoscopy is performed to identify the existence, location, and extent of a laceration. It can be done quickly but must include the entire tracheobronchial tree, including the portion proximal to the distal tip of the endotracheal tube. The method for doing this has previously been described. In some cases, repeat bronchoscopy is needed to establish or confirm diagnosis (131). Bronchography is not indicated for patients with acute injuries (199).

After the extent and location of the injury have been identified it is best to proceed with early surgical repair in the vast majority of cases. Only a few exceptions allow for nonoperative management of these injuries in the acute set-

TABLE 24.10. INDICATIONS FOR NONOPERATIVE MANAGEMENT OF TRACHEOBRONCHIAL DISRUPTION

Tracheobronchial injury involves one-third or less of the circumference of the affected lumen

PLUS

Complete resolution of any accompanying pneumothorax and full reexpansion of the affected lung after tube thoracostomy

PLUS

No residual air leak

ting (199) and these are listed in Table 24.10. When surgical repair is done, the approach to most tracheobronchial injuries is a posterolateral incision through the right thorax at the fourth intercostal space. This allows for access to the entire right mainstem bronchus, the carina, and virtually all of the intrathoracic trachea. Injuries to the left mainstem bronchus distal to the carina are repaired through the left chest (131,200). Whenever possible, the anastamosis is reenforced externally with a pleural or intercostal muscle flap and is then tested for residual leak prior to closure of the chest. Critical care management postoperatively must be directed at avoiding prolonged intubation and positive pressure ventilation so that disruption of the anastamosis does not occur (131).

When tracheobronchial injury is missed in the acute setting, fibrous scarring occurs at the site over time, usually resulting in stricture formation (132). If left untreated, this complication leads to persistent atelectasis of the lung parenchyma distal to the stricture or recurrent infection secondary to retained secretions in the affected area, with the ultimate development of a bronchiectatic picture (200). Complete evaluation of pulmonary anatomy and functional status should be performed before undertaking surgery in these cases, since, depending on the degree of airway injury and the amount of damaged distal lung parenchyma, the operative procedure may range from tracheobronchial repair to distal lung resection such as lobectomy or pneumonectomy. If repair is attempted more than six months after injury, it is unlikely that the patients will have improvement in pulmonary function.

Finally, tracheoesophageal fistulae can result from thoracic trauma, but are extremely rare (200). Certainly, a penetrating injury directed toward the posterior mediastinum can result in injury to both structures. In cases of blunt trauma, the tracheobronchial injury likely occurs in one of the ways previously mentioned; the adjacent esophagus is also ruptured. If an esophageal injury is suspected in association with a tracheobronchial injury, esophagoscopy is warranted in addition to bronchoscopy (203). Once a fistula is discovered, airway protection is of primary importance, with placement of an endotracheal tube distal to the injury

site so that aspiration of gastric contents can be prevented. Endoscopic examination and barium swallow are indicated, followed by early surgical repair (204). If early operative intervention is done, both structures can be treated with local debridement and primary repair. If surgery is done at a later time, a more complex esophageal repair may be needed.

FAT EMBOLISM SYNDROME

First described by Zenker in 1861, fat embolism syndrome (FES) is still one of the least well defined entities in trauma. A variety of traumatic and nontraumatic conditions are associated with FES (205) (Table 24.11). In the trauma patient, FES is most commonly found in patients with fractures of the long bones and pelvis. The clinical prevalence of FES in these patients is 0.25% to 10% (206–208).

The pathophysiology of FES is poorly understood. There are two prevalent hypotheses:

1. The mechanical hypothesis suggests that disruption of intramedullary veins allows fat to gain access to the pul-

TABLE 24.11. CLINICAL SETTINGS FOR FAT EMBOLISM

Trauma
  Lower-extremity long-bone fractures
  Pelvic fractures
  Child abuse with or without fractures
  Blast concussion
  Liver contusion
  Severe burns
  Massive soft tissue injury

Surgery
  Total joint replacement
  Intramedullary nailing of femoral shaft
  Closed femoral osteotomy
  Femoral elongation
  Spinal fusion
  Liposuction
  Bone marrow transplant
  Renal transplant

Nonsurgical
  External cardiac massage
  Lipid emulsions in intravenous feedings
  Intraosseous venography
  Acute pancreatitis
  Carbon tetrachloride poisoning
  Prolonged corticosteroid therapy
  Fatty liver secondary to alcohol
  Acute osteomyelitis
  Bone infarction in sickle cell disease
  Epilepsy
  Diabetes mellitus
  Extracorporeal circulation
  Severe infection, especially clostridial species
  High altitude

monary and cardiac circulation. Echocardiography studies performed during intramedullary nailing demonstrate fat emboli to the heart. However, true FES was not demonstrated in most of these patients (209). In addition, fat can be detected in the bronchoalveolar lavage fluid (BALF) of patients with FES (210). However, Aoki and colleagues demonstrated fat in the BALF of patients who underwent intramedullary nailing and did not clinically progress to FES (211). Thus a purely mechanical etiology of FES seems unlikely.

2. The physiochemical hypothesis states that fracture sites produce chemical mediators that change intravascular lipid solubility, causing coalescence into fat globules and pulmonary embolism. Related is the hypothesis that free fatty acids produce mediators leading to FES (212,213).

FES is a clinical syndrome classically characterized by respiratory insufficiency, thrombocytopenia with petechiae, and deteriorating mental status. Respiratory insufficiency typically presents as tachypnea and hypoxemia. Classic locations of petechiae are the axilla, chest, root of the neck, and conjunctiva. Retinal emboli may also be visible on fundoscopic exam. Mental status changes may include restlessness, disorientation, stupor, or coma (214). Tachycardia, fever, and anemia may also develop. Peak incidence of FES is 24 to 48 hours after injury, with a range of six to 72 hours. Since trauma patients are prone to a variety of mechanisms producing respiratory insufficiency, the diagnosis of FES relies on the exclusion of other causes and an appropriate clinical setting. FES can coexist with ARDS, pulmonary contusion, and aspiration pneumonitis. No specific laboratory or radiographic test is pathognomic. Yoshida and colleagues have shown that MRI can be useful in the detection of fat emboli in the cerebrum, cerebellum, and brainstem. However, transport and monitoring of patients, the frequent presence of ferromagnetic materials in fracture patients, expense, and time consumption render MRI impractical (215). Fat globules may be detected in the blood, sputum, BALF, urine, and/or cerebrospinal fluid; however, the diagnosis of fat embolism is based on the history, clinical signs of pulmonary, cerebral, and cutaneous manifestations, and hypoxemia in the absence of other disorders.

Treatment is largely directed at prevention and supportive measures: adequate oxygenation, fracture splinting or fixation, judiciously administered fluids with avoidance of excessive hydration, and avoidance of unnecessary transport of the patient. FES has been treated with a variety of agents, including ethanol, heparin, hypertonic glucose, and corticosteroids. There are no prospective controlled studies to support any of these interventions. Timing and type of fixation of fractures are currently under scrutiny, but currently it does not appear that the type of fixation plays a major role in the development of FES. In most cases, FES is a self-limited process. Pulmonary function will return to normal if the patient has adequate oxygenation, and severe compli-

cations such as ARDS do not develop. Long-term morbidity, when present, is usually in the form of cerebral neurological deficits (216,217). The mortality rate from complicated FES is 5% to 15%.

REFERENCES

1. Stoelting RK. Inhaled anesthetics. In *Pharmacology and physiology in anesthetic practice.* Philadelphia: JB Lippincott, 1987: 35–68.
2. Scweieger I, Gamulin Z, Suter PM. Lung function during anesthesia and respiratory insufficiency in the postoperative period. *Acta Anaesthesiol Scand* 1989;33:527–534.
3. Wahbe RWM. Perioperative functional residual capacity. *Can J Anaesth* 1991;38:384–400.
4. Strandberg A, Tokics L, Brismar B, et al. Atelactasis during anaesthesia and in the postoperative period. *Acta Anaesthesiol Scand* 1986;30:154–158.
5. Rothen HU, Sporre B, Engberg G, et al. Prevention of atelactasis during general anaesthesia. *Lancet* 1995;345:1387–1391.
6. Rothen HU, Sporre B, Engberg G, et al. Influence of gas composition on recurrence of atelactasis after a reexpansion maneuver during general anesthesia. *Anesthesiology* 1995;82:832–842.
7. Magnusson L, Zemgulis V, Tenling A, et al. Use of a vital capacity maneuver to prevent atelactasis after cardiopulmonary bypass—an experimental study. *Anesthesiology* 1998;88: 134–142.
8. Marven SL, Elliott CG, Tocino I, et al. Positive end expiratory pressure following coronary artery bypass grafting. *Chest* 1986; 90:537–541.
9. Eames W, Rooke G, Wu R, et al. Comparison of the effects of etomidate, propofol and thiopental on respiratory resistance after tracheal intubation. *Anesthsiology* 1996;84:1307–1311.
10. Hirshman CA, Edelstein G, Peetz S, et al. Mechanism of action of inhalational anesthesia on airways. *Anesthesiology* 1982;56: 107–111.
11. Rooke G, Choi J, Bishop M. The effects of isoflurane, halothane, sevoflurane and thiopental/nitrous oxide on respiratory system resistance after tracheal intubation. *Anesthesiology* 1997; 86:1294–1299.
12. Tait AR, Knight PR. Intraoperative respiratory complications in patients with upper respiratory tract infections. *Can J Anaesth* 1987;34:300–303.
13. Fennelly ME, Hall GM. Anesthesia and upper respiratory tract infections—a nonexistent hazard? [Editorial]. *Br J Anaesth* 1990;64:535–536.
14. Pavlin EG. Cardiopulmonary pharmacology. In Miller RD, ed. *Anesthesia,* 3rd ed. New York: Churchill Livingstone, 1990: 105–134.
15. Sykes L, Bowe E. Cardiorespiratory effects of anesthesia. *Clin Chest Med* 1993;14:211–226.
16. Cousins MJ, Bromage PR. Epidural neural blockade. In Cousins MJ, ed. *Neural blockade in clinical anesthesia and pain management.* 3rd ed. Philadelphia: JB Lippincott, 1988:253–360.
17. Valentin N, Lomholt B, Jensen S, et al. Spinal or general anesthesia for surgery of the fractured hip? *Br J Anaesth* 1986;58: 284–291.
18. Davis FM, Woolner DF, Frampton C, et al. Prospective multicenter trial of mortality following general or spinal anaesthesia for hip fracture surgery in the elderly. *Br J Anaesth* 1987;59: 1080–1088.
19. Yeager MP, Glass DD, Neff RK, et al. Epidural anesthesia and analgesia in high risk surgical patients. *Anesthesiology* 1987;66: 729–736.
20. Chung F, Meier R, Lautenschlager E, et al. General or spinal

anesthesia: which is better in the elderly? *Anesthesiology* 1987; 67:422–427.

21. Christopherson R, Beattie C, Frank SM, et al. The perioperative ischemia randomized anesthesia trial study group: perioperative morbidity in patients randomized to epidural or general anesthesia for lower extremity vascular surgery. *Anesthesiology* 1993;79: 422–434.

22. Lutz LJ, Lamer TJ. Management of postoperative pain: review of current techniques and methods. *Mayo Clin Proc* 1990;65: 584–596.

23. Jayr C, Thomas H, Rey A, et al. Postoperative pulmonary complications: epidural analgesia using bupivacaine and opioids versus parenteral opioids. *Anesthesiology* 1993;78:666–76.

24. Hendloin H, Lahtinen J, Lansimies E, et al. The effect of thoracic epidural analgesia on respiratory function after cholecystectomy. *Acta Anaesthesiol Scan* 1987;31:645–651.

25. Cuschieri RJ, Morran CG, Howie JC, et al. Postoperative pain and pulmonary complications: comparison of three analgesic regimens. *Br J Surg* 1985;72:495–498.

26. Ballantyne JC, Carr CB, De Ferranti S, et al. The comparative effects of postoperative analgesic therapies on pulmonary outcome: cumulative meta-analyses of randomized controlled trials. *Anesth Analg* 1998;86:598–612.

27. Engberg G, Wiklund L. Pulmonary complications after upper abdominal surgery: their prevention with intercostal blocks. *Acta Anaesthesiol Scand* 1988;32:1–9.

28. Kaiser AM, Zollinger A, Lorezi DD, et al. Prospective randomized comparison of extrapleural versus epidural analgesia for postthoracotomy pain. *Ann Thorac Surg* 1998;66:367–372.

29. Ford GT, Whitelaw WA, Rosenal TW, et al. Diaphragm function after upper abdominal surgery in humans. *Am Rev Resp Dis* 1983;127:431–436.

30. Dureuil B, Cantineau JP, Desmonts JM. Effects of upper or lower abdominal surgery on diaphragmatic function. *Br J Anaesth* 1987;59:1230–1235.

31. Prabhakar NR, Marek W, Loeschcke HH. Altered breathing patterns elicited by stimulation of abdominal visceral afferents. *J Appl Physiol* 1985;58:1755–1760.

32. Xue FS, Li BW, Zhang GS, et al. The influence of surgical sites on early postoperative hypoxemia in adults undergoing elective surgery. *Anesth Analg* 1999;88:213–219.

33. Vaughan RW, Wise L. Choice of abdominal operative incision in the obese patients: a study using blood gas measurements. *Ann Surg* 1975;181:829–835.

34. Frazee R, Roberts J, Okeson G, et al. Open versus laparoscopic cholecystectomy: a comparison of postoperative pulmonary function. *Ann Surg* 1991;213:651–653.

35. Grace PA, Quereshi A, Colenian J, et al. Reduced postoperative hospitalization after laparoscopic cholecystectomy. *Br J Surg* 1991;78:160–162.

36. Meyers WA, Southern Surgeons Club. A prospective analysis of 1518 laparoscopic cholecystectomies. *N Engl J Med* 1991; 324:1073–1078.

37. Mack MJ, Aronoff RJ, Acuff TE, et al. Present role of thoracoscopy in the diagnosis and treatment of diseases of the chest. *Ann Thorac Surg* 1992;54:403–409.

38. Landrenau RJ, Hazelrigg SR, Ferson PF, et al. Thoracoscopic resection of 85 pulmonary lesions. *Ann Thorac Surg* 1992;54: 415–420.

39. Daniel TM, Kern JA, Tribble CJ, et al. Thoracoscopic surgery for diseases of the lung and pleura. *Ann Surg* 1993;217: 566–575.

40. Pederson T, Eliasen K, Henriksen E. A prospective study of risk factors and cardiopulmonary complications associated with anaesthesia and surgery: risk indicators of cardiopulmonary morbidity. *Acta Anaesthesiol Scand* 1990;34:144–155.

41. Celli BR, Rodriguez KS, Snider GL. A controlled trial of intermittent positive pressure breathing, incentive spirometry and deep breathing exercises in preventing pulmonary complications after abdominal surgery. *Am Rev Respir Dis* 1984;130:12–15.

42. Svensson L, Hess KR, Coselli JS, et al. A prospective study of respiratory failure after high risk surgery on the thoracoabdominal aorta. *J Vasc Surg* 1991;14:271–282.

43. Vodinh J, Bonnet F, Touboul C, et al. Risk factors for postoperative pulmonary complications after vascular surgery. *Surgery* 1989;105:360–365.

44. Roukema JA, Carol EJ, Prins JG. The prevalence of pulmonary complications after upper abdominal surgery in patients with noncompromised pulmonary status. *Arch Surg* 1988;123: 30–34.

45. Kroenke K, Lawrence VA, Theroux JF, et al. Operative risk in patients with severe obstructive pulmonary disease. *Arch Intern Med* 1992;152:967–971.

46. Wong DH, Weber EC, Schell MJ, et al. Factors associated with postoperative pulmonary complications in patients with severe chronic obstructive pulmonary disease. *Anesth Analg* 1995;80: 276–284.

47. Lindberg P, Gunnarsson L, Tokics L, et al. Atelactasis and lung function in the postoperative period. *Acta Anaesthesiol Scand* 1992;36:546–553.

48. Christensen EF, Schultz P, Jensen OV, et al. Postoperative pulmonary complications and lung function in high risk patients: a comparison of three physiotherapy regimens after upper abdominal surgery in general anesthesia. *Acta Anaesthesiol Scand* 1991;35:97–104.

49. Strandberg A, Brismar B, Lundquist H, et al. Constitutional factors promoting development of atelactasis during anaesthesia. *Acta Anaesthesiol Scand* 1987;31:21–24.

50. Selsby DS. Chest physiotherapy may be harmful in some patients. *Br Med J* 1989;3`8:541–542.

51. O'Donohue WJ. National survey of the usage of lung expansion modalities for the prevention and treatment of postoperative atelactasis following abdominal and thoracic surgery. *Chest* 1985;87:76–80.

52. Tan AKW. Incentive spirometry for tracheostomy and laryngectomy patients. *J Otolaryngol* 1995;24:292–294.

53. Warren CPW, Grimwood M. Pulmonary disorders and physiotherapy in patients who undergo cholecystectomy. *Can J Surg* 1980;23:4:384–386.

54. Iverson LI, Ecker RR, Fox HE, et al. A comparative study of IPPB, the incentive spirometer, and blow bottles: the prevention of atelactasis following cardiac surgery. *Ann Thorac Surg* 1978; 25:197–200.

55. Ingwersen UM, Larsen RK, Bertelsen MT, et al. Three different mask physiotherapy regimens for prevention of postoperative pulmonary complications after heart and pulmonary surgery. *Intensive Care Med* 1993;19:294–298.

56. Hall JC, Tarala R, Harris J, et al. Incentive spirometry versus routine chest physiotherapy for prevention of pulmonary complications after abdominal surgery. *Lancet* 1991;337:953–956.

57. Jung R, Wight J, Nusser R, et al. Comparison of three methods of respiratory care following upper abdominal surgery. *Chest* 1980;78:31–35.

58. Oikkonen M, Karjalainen K, Kahara V, et al. Comparison of incentive spirometry and intermittent positive pressure breathing after coronary artery bypass graft. *Chest* 1991;99:60–65.

59. Nomori H, Kobayashi R, Fuyuno G, et al. Preoperative respiratory muscle training—assessment in thoracic surgery patients with special reference to postoperative pulmonary complications. *Chest* 1994;105:1782–1787.

60. Strider D, Turner D, Egloff MB, et al. Stacked inspiratory spi-

rometry reduces pulmonary shunt in patients after coronary artery bypass. *Chest* 1994;106:391–395.

61. Jaworsky A, Goldberg SK, Walkenstein MD, et al. Utility of immediate postlobectomy fiberoptic bronchoscopy in preventing atelactasis. *Chest* 1988;94:38–43.

62. Marini JJ, Pierson DJ, Hudson LD. Acute lobar atelactasis: a prospective comparison of fiberoptic bronchoscopy and respiratory therapy. *Am Rev Resp Dis* 1979;119:971–978.

63. Harada K, Matsuda T, Saoyama N, et al. Reexpansion of refractory atelactasis using a bronchofiberscope with a balloon cuff. *Chest* 1983;84:725–728.

64. Lung function testing: selection of reference values and interpretative strategies. *Am Rev Respir Dis* 1991;144:1202–1218.

65. Gaensler EA, Cugell DW, Lindgren I, et al. The role of pulmonary insufficiency in mortality and invalidism following surgery for pulmonary tuberculosis. *J Thorac Cardiovasc Surg* 1955;29: 163–187.

66. Keagy BA, Schorlemmer GR, Murray GF, et al. Correlation of preoperative pulmonary function testing with clinical course in patients after pneumonectomy. *Ann Thorac Surg* 1983;36: 253–257.

67. Latimer RG, Dickman M, Day WC, et al. Ventilatory patterns and pulmonary complications after upper abdominal surgery determined by preoperative and postoperative computerized spirometry and blood gas analysis. *Am J Surg* 1971;122:622–632.

68. Stein M, Koota GM, Simon M, et al. Pulmonary evaluation of surgical patients. *JAMA* 1962;181:765–770.

69. Stein M, Cassara EL. Preoperative pulmonary evaluation and therapy for surgical patients. *JAMA* 1970;211:787–790.

70. Appleberg M, Gordon L, FaHi LP. Preoperative pulmonary evaluation of surgical patients using vitalograph. *Br J Surg* 1974; 61:57–59.

71. Fan ST, Lau WY, Yip WC. Prediction of postoperative pulmonary complications in esophago gastric cancer surgery. *Br J Surg* 1987;74:408–410.

72. Sugamuchi K, Matsuzaki K, Matsuura H, et al. Evaluation of surgical treatment of carcinoma of esophagus in the elderly. Twenty years experience. *Br J Surg* 1985;72:28–30.

73. Zibrak JD, O'Donnell CR, Marton K. Indications for pulmonary function testing. *Ann Intern Med* 1990;112:763–771.

74. Gass GD, Olsen GN. Clinical significance of pulmonary function tests. *Chest* 1986;89:127–135.

75. Lawrence VA, Page CP, Harris GA. Preoperative spirometry before abdominal operations. *Arch Intern Med* 1989;149: 280–285.

76. Milledge JS, Nunn JF. Criteria of fitness for anesthesia in patients with chronic obstructive lung disease. *Br Med J* 1975;3: 670–673.

77. Cain HD, Stevens PM, Adaniya R. Preoperative pulmonary function and complications after cardiovascular surgery. *Chest* 1979;76:130–135.

78. Fielding JE. Smoking: health effects and control [First of two parts]. *N Engl J Med* 1985;313:491–498.

79. Fielding JE. Smoking: health effects and control [Second of two parts]. *N Engl J Med* 1985;313:555–561.

80. Brooks-Brunn JA. Predictors of postoperative pulmonary complications following abdominal surgery. *Chest* 1997;111: 564–571.

81. Bluman LG, Mosca L, Newman N, et al. Preoperative smoking habits and postoperative pulmonary complications. *Chest* 1998; 113:4:883–889.

82. Warner MA, Offord KP, Warner ME, et al. Role of preoperative cessation of smoking and other factors in postoperative pulmonary complications: a blinded prospective study of coronary artery bypass patients. *Mayo Clin Proc* 1989;64:609–616.

83. Pearce AC, Jones RM. Smoking and anesthesia: preoperative

abstinence and perioperative morbidity. *Anesthesiology* 1984;61: 576–584.

84. Mendelson CL. Aspiration of stomach contents into lungs during obstetric anesthesia. *Am J Obstet Gynecol* 1946;53:196–205.

85. Olsson GL, Hallen B, Hambreas-Jonzon K. Aspiration during anaesthesia: a computer aided study of 185,358 Anaesthetics. *Acta Anaesthesiol Scand* 1986;30:84–92.

86. Warner MA, Warner ME, Weber JG. Clinical significance of pulmonary aspiration during the perioperative period. *Anesthesiology* 1993;78:56–62.

87. Sellick BA. Cricoid pressure to control regurgitation of stomach contents during induction of anesthesia. *Lancet* 1961;2: 404–406.

88. Orr DA, Bill KM, Gillon KRW, et al. Effects of omeprazole, with and without metclopramide, in elective obstetric anaesthesia. *Anaesthesia* 1993;48:114–119.

89. Manchikanti L, Colliver JA, Marrero TC, et al. Assessment of age related acid aspiration risk factors in pediatric, adult and geriatric patients. *Anesth Analg* 1985;64:11–17.

90. Levack ID, Bowie RA, Braid DP, et al. Comparison of the effects of two dose schedules of oral omeprazole with oral ranitidine on gastric pH and volume in patients undergoing elective surgery. *Br J Anaesth* 1996;76:567–569.

91. Maekawa N, Nishina K, Mikawa K, et al. Comparison of pirenzipine, ranitidine and pirenzipine-ranitidine combination for preoperative gastric fluid acidity and volume in children. *Br J Anaesth* 1998;80:53–57.

92. Salmenpera M, Kortilla K, Kalima T. Reduction of the risk of acid pulmonary aspiration in anesthitized patients after cimetidine premedication. *Acta Anaesthesiol Scand* 1980;24:25–30.

93. Wingtin LNG, Glomaud D, Hardy F, et al. Omeprazole for prophylaxis in elective surgery. *Anaesthesia* 1990;45:436–438.

94. Windsor JA, Hill GL. Risk factors for postoperative pneumonia—the importance of protein depletion. *Ann Surg* 1988; 209–214.

95. Garibaldi RA, Britt MR, Coleman ML, et al. Risk factors for postoperative pneumonia. *Am J Med* 1981;70:677–680.

96. Campbell GD Jr, Neiderman MS, Broughton WA, et al. ATS consensus committee. Hospital acquired pneumonia in adults: diagnosis, assessment of severity, initial antimicrobial therapy and preventive strategies. *Am J Respir Crit Care Med* 1995;153: 1711.

97. Chan ED, Welsh CH. Geriatric respiratory medicine. *Chest* 1998;114:1704–1733.

98. Gerson M, Hurst JM, Hertzberg VS, et al. Prediction of cardiac and pulmonary complications related to elective abdominal and noncardiac thoracic surgery in geriatric patients. *Am J Med* 1990;88:101–107.

99. Ishida T, Yokoyama H, Kaneko S, et al. Long term results of operation for non-small cell lung cancer in the elderly. *Ann Thorac Surg* 1990;50:919–922.

100. Samuels LE, Kaufman MS, Morris RJ, et al. Coronary artery bypass grafting in patients with COPD. *Chest* 1998;113: 378–382.

101. Warner DO, Warner MO, Barnes RD, et al. Perioperative respiratory complications in patients with asthma. *Anesthesiology* 1996;85:460–467.

102. Olsson GL. Bronchospasm during anesthesia. A computer aided incidence study of 136,929 patients. *Acta Anaesthesiol Scand* 1987;31:244–252.

103. Kearney DJ, Lee TH, Reilly JJ, et al. Assessment of operative risk in patients undergoing lung resection-importance of predicted pulmonary function. *Chest* 1994;105:753–759.

104. Olsen GN, Block AJ, Swenson EW, et al. Pulmonary function evaluation of the lung resection candidate: a prospective study. *Am Rev Resp Dis* 1975;111:379–387.

105. Markos J, Mullan BP, Hillman DR, et al. Preoperative assessment as a predictor of mortality and morbidity after lung resection. *Am Rev Resp Dis* 1989;139:901–910.

106. Holden DA, Rice TW, Stelmach K, et al. Exercise testing, 6 minute walk test and stair climb in the evaluation of patients at high risk for pulmonary resection. *Chest* 1992;102:1774–1779.

107. Smith TP, Kinasewitz GT, Tucker WY, et al. Exercise capacity as a predictor of post-thoracotomy morbidity. *Am Rev Resp Dis* 1984;129:730–734.

108. Bolliger CT, Wyser C, Roser H, et al. Lung scanning and exercise testing for the prediction of postoperative performance in lung resection candidates at increased risk for complications. *Chest* 1995;108:341–348.

109. Morice RC, Peters EJ, Ryan MB, et al. Exercise testing in the evaluation of patients at high risk for complications from lung resection. *Chest* 1992;101:356–361.

110. Olsen GN, Bolton JWR, Weiman DS, et al. Stair climbing as an exercise test to predict the postoperative complications of lung resection. *Chest* 1991;99:587–590.

111. Olsen GN. The evolving role of exercise testing prior to lung resection. *Chest* 1989;95:218–225.

112. Bolliger CT, Jordan P, Soler M, et al. Exercise capacity as a predictor of postoperative complications in lung resection candidates. *Am J Respir Crit Care Med* 1995;151:1472–1480.

113. Fee JH, Holmes EC, Gerwirtz HS, et al. Role of pulmonary resistance measurement in preoperative evaluation of candidates for lung resection. *J Thorac Cardiovasc Surg* 1975;75:519–524.

114. Olsen GN, Weiman DS, Bolton JWR, et al. Submaximal invasive exercise testing and quantitative lung scanning in the evaluation for tolerance of lung resection. *Chest* 1989;95:267–273.

115. Epstein SK, Faling LJ, Daly BDT, et al. Predicting pulmonary complications after pulmonary resection—preoperative exercise testing vs a multifactorial cardiopulmonary risk index. *Chest* 1993;104:694–700.

116. Epstein SK, Faling J, Daly BDT, et al. Inability to perform bicycle ergometry predicts increased morbidity and mortality after lung resection. *Chest* 1995;107:311–316.

117. Melendez J, Carlon VA. Cardiopulmonary risk index does not predict complications after thoracic surgery. *Chest* 1998;114: 69–75.

118. Goldman L, Caldera DL, Nussbaum JM, et al. Multifactorial index of cardiac risk in noncardiac surgical procedures. *N Engl J Med* 1977;297:845–850.

119. Palda VA, Detsky AS. Perioperative assessment and management of risk from coronary artery disease. *Ann Intern Med* 1997; 127:313–328.

120. Tortella BJ, Trunkey DD. Trauma care systems. *Trauma Q* 1984;11:17–24.

121. Bone L, Bucholz R. The management of fractures in the patient with multiple trauma. *J Bone Joint Surg AM* 1986;68:945–949.

122. American College of Surgeons Committee on Trauma. Course overview: the purpose, history and concepts of the ATLS program for doctors. In: *Advanced trauma life support for doctors: instructor course manual.* Chicago: The American College of Surgeons, 1997:9–19.

123. Yee ES, Thomas AN, Goodman, PC. Isolated first rib fracture: Clinical significance after blunt chest trauma. *Ann Thorac Surg* 1981;32:278–283.

124. Phillips EM, Rogers WF, Gaspar MR. First rib fractures: incidence of vascular injury and indications for angiography. *Surgery* 1981;89:42–47.

125. Thompson BM, Finger W, Tonsfeldt D, et al. Rib radiographs for trauma: useful or wasteful? *Ann Emerg Med* 1986;15: 261–265.

126. Chan O, Hiorns M. Chest trauma. *Eur J Radiol* 1996;23: 23–34.

127. Mirvis SE, Bidwell, JK, Buddemeyer EU, et al. Value of chest radiography in excluding traumatic aortic rupture. *Radiology* 1987;163:487–493.

128. Richardson P, Mirvis SE, Scorpio R, et al. Value of CT in determining the need for angiography when findings of mediastinal hemorrhage on chest radiographs are equivocal. *Am J Radiol* 1991;156:273–279.

129. Madayag MA, Kirshenbaum KJ, Nadimpalli SR, et al. Thoracic aortic trauma: role of dynamic CT. *Radiology* 1991;179: 853–855.

130. Boyd AD, Glassman LR. Trauma to the lung. *Chest Surg Clin North Am* 1997;7:263–284.

131. Huh J, Milliken JC, Chen JC. Management of tracheobronchial injuries following blunt and penetrating trauma. *Am Surg* 1997; 63:896–899.

132. Pembroke AP, Klineberg P, Johnson DC. Traumatic tracheal disruption—diagnostic difficulties. *Anaesth Intensive Care* 1995;23:206–207.

133. Etoch SW, Bar-Natan MF, Miller FB, et al. Tube thoracostomy: factors related to complications. *Arch Surg* 1995;130:521–526.

134. Graeber GM, Jones DR. The role of thoracoscopy in thoracic trauma. *Ann Thorac Surg* 1993;56:646–648.

135. Abolhoda A, Livingston DH, Donahoo JS, et al. Diagnostic and therapeutic video assisted thoracic surgery (VATS) following chest trauma. *Eur J Cardiothorac Surg* 1997;12:356–360.

136. Wong MS, Tsoi EK, Henderson VJ, et al. Videothoracoscopy: an effective method for evaluating and managing thoracic trauma patients. *Surg Endosc* 1996;10:118–121.

137. Coselli JS, Mattox KL, Beall AC. Reevaluation of early evacuation of clotted hemothorax. *Am J Surg* 1984;148:786–790.

138. Heniford BT, Carrillo EH, Spain DA, et al. The role of thoracoscopy in the management of retained thoracic collections after trauma. *Ann Thorac Surg* 1997;63:940–943.

139. Meyer DM, Jessen ME, Wait MA, et al. Early evacuation of traumatic retained hemothoraces using thoracoscopy: a prospective, randomized trial. *Ann Thorac Surg* 1997;64:1396–1401.

140. Richardson JD. Indications for thoracotomy in thoracic trauma. *Curr Surg* 1985;Sept-Oct42:361–364.

141. Cogbill TH, Moore EE, Millikan JS, et al. Rationale for selective application of emergency department thoracotomy in trauma. *J Trauma* 1983;23:453–458.

142. Richardson DJ, Spain DA. Injury to the lung and pleura. In Mattox EE, Feliciano DV, Moore EE, eds. *Trauma*, 3rd ed. Stamford CT: Appleton and Lange, 2000:523–542.

143. Buckman R, Troskin SZ, Slancbaum L, et al. The significant of stable patients with sternal fracture. *SGIO* 1987;164:261–265.

144. Wojcik JB, Morgan AS. Sternal fracture the natural history. *Ann Emerg Med* 1988;17:912–914.

145. Buckman R, Troskin SZ, Slancbaum L, et al. The significance of stable patients with sternal fracture. *SGO* 1987;164:261–265.

146. Harley DP, Mena I. Cardiac and vascular sequelae of sternal fractures. *J Trauma* 1986;26:553–555.

147. Brookes JG, Dunn RJ, Rogers IR. Sternal fractures, a retrospective analysis of 272 cases. *J Trauma* 1993;35:46–54.

148. Hills MW, Delprado AM, Deane SA. Sternal fractures: associated injuries and management. *J Trauma* 1993;35:55–60.

149. Jackson M, Walker WS. Isolated sternal fractures, a benign injury. *Injury* 1992;23:535–536.

150. Garzon AA, Seltzer B, Carlson KE. Pathophysiology of crushed chest injury. *Ann Surg* 1968;168:128–136.

151. Newman RJ, Jones IS. A prospective study of 413 consecutive car occupants with chest injuries. *J Trauma* 1984;24:129–135.

152. Pate JW. Chest wall injuries. *Surgical Clin North Am* 1989;69: 59–70.

153. Trunkey DD. Cervicothoracic trauma. In: Blaisdell FW, Trunkey DD, eds. *Trauma Management,* Vol. 3. New York: Thieme, 1986:14.

154. Quick G. A randomized clinical trial of rib belts for simple fractures. *Am J Emerg Med* 1990;8:277–281.

155. Lee RB, Bass SM. Three or more rib fractures as an indicator for transfer to a level I trauma center: a population based study. *J Trauma* 1990;30:689–694.

156. Ziegler DW, Agarwahl NN. The morbidity and mortality of rib fractures. *J Trauma* 1994;37:975–979.

157. Richardson JD, Adams L, Flint LM. Selective management of flail chest and pulmonary contusion. *Ann Surg* 1992;196:481–487.

158. Luchette FA, Radafsharsm SM, Kaiser R, et al. A prospective evaluation of epidural vs intrapleural catheters for analgesia in chest wall trauma. *J Trauma* 1994;39:865–870.

159. Mackersie RC, Karaginnes TG, Hoyt DB, et al. Prospective evaluation of epidural and intravenous administration of fentanyl for pain control and restoration of ventilatory function following multiple rib fractures. *J Trauma* 1991;31:443–451.

160. Ziegler DW, Agarwahl NN. The morbidity and mortality of rib fractures. *J Trauma* 1994;37:975–979.

161. Avery EE, Morch ET, Benson DW. Critically crushed chest. A new method of treatment with continuous mechanical hyperventilation to produce alkalotic apnea in internal pneumatic stabilization. *J Thorac Cardiovasc Surg* 1956;32:291–302.

162. Shackford SR, Virgilio RW, Peters RM. Selective use of ventilatory in flail chest injury. *J Thorac Cardiovasc Surg* 1981;81:194–201.

163. Freedland M, Wilson RF, Bender JS, et al. The management of flail chest injury: factors affecting outcome. *J Trauma* 1990;30:1460–1468.

164. Voggenreiter G, Newdeck S, Aufmkolh M, et al. Operative chest wall stabilization and flail chest. Outcomes of patients with and without pulmonary contusion. *J Am Coll Surg* 1998;187:130–138.

165. Thomas AN, Blaisdell FW, Lewis FR Jr, et al. Operative stabilization for flail chest with blunt trauma. *J Thorac Cardiovasc Surg* 1978;75:793–801.

166. Landercasper J, Cogbill TH, Lindesmith LA. Long term disability after flail chest injury. *J Trauma* 1984;24:410–414.

167. Beal SL, Oreskovich MR. Long term disability associated with flail chest injury. *Am J Surg* 1985;150:324–326.

168. Schaal MA, Fischer, RP, Perry JF. The unchanged mortality of flail chest injuries. *J Trauma* 1979;19:492–496.

169. Richardson JD, Miller FB. Injuries to the lungs and pleura. In: Feliciano D, Moore EE, Mattox K, eds. *Trauma* 3rd ed. Stamford, CT: Appleton and Lange, 1996:398–399.

170. Cohn, SM. Pulmonary contusion: a review of the clinical entity. *J Trauma* 1997;42:973–979.

171. Pecklet MH, Newman KD, Eichelberger MR, et al. Thoracic trauma in children, an indicator of increased mortality. *J Pediatr Surg* 1990;25:961–966.

172. Fulton RL, Peter ET. The progressive nature of pulmonary contusion. *Surgery* 1970;67:499–506.

173. Casley-Smith JR, Eckert P, Foldia-Borcsok E. The fine structure of pulmonary contusion and the effects of various drugs. *Br J Exp Pathol* 1976;57:487–496.

174. Alfano GS, Hale HW. Pulmonary contusion. *J Trauma* 1965;5:647–658.

175. Schield HH, Strunk H, Webber W. et al. Pulmonary contusion: CT vs plain radiograms. *J Comput Assist Tomogr* 1979;13:417–420.

176. Wagner RB, Jamieson PM. Pulmonary contusion: evaluation and classification by computed tomography. *Surg Clin North Am* 1989;69:31–40.

177. Johannigman JA, Campbell RS, Davis K Jr, et al. Combined differential lung ventilation and inhaled nitric oxide therapy in the management of unilateral pulmonary contusion. *J Trauma* 1997;42:108–111.

178. Johnson JA, Cogbill TH, Winga ER. Determinence of outcome after pulmonary contusion. *J Trauma* 1986;26:695–697.

179. Dodek PM, Rice TW, Bonsignore MR, et al. Effects of plasmapheresis and hypoproteinemia on lung liquid conductance in awake sheep. *Circ Res* 1986;58:269–280.

180. Bongard FS, Lewis FR. Crystalloid resuscitation of patients with pulmonary contusion. *Am J Surg* 1984;148:145–151.

181. Hoff SJ, Shotts SD, Eddy VA, et al. Outcome of isolated pulmonary contusion in blunt trauma patients. *Am Surg* 1994;60:138–142.

182. Foranz JL, Richardson JD, Grover FL, et al. Effect of methylprednisolone sodium succinate on experimental pulmonary contusion. *J Thorac Cardiovasc Surg* 1974;68:842–844.

183. Svennevig JL, Bugge-Asperheimb, Vaage J, et al. Corticosteroids in the treatment of blunt injury of the chest. *Br J Accid Surg* 1984;16:80–84.

184. Kishikawa M, Yoshioka T, Shimazu T, et al. Pulmonary contusion causes long term respiratory dysfunction with decreased functional residual capacity. *J Trauma* 1991;31:1203–1210.

185. Mathai M, Byrd RP Jr, Roy TM. The posttraumatic pulmonary mass. *J Tenn Med Assoc* 1996;89:41–42.

186. Takahashi N, Murakami J, Murayama S, et al. MR evaluation of intrapulmonary hematoma. *J Comput Assist Tomogr* 1995;19:125–127.

187. Hollister M, Stern EJ, Steinberg KP. Type 2 pulmonary laceration: a marker of blunt high-energy injury to the lung. *Am J Radiol* 1995;165:1126.

188. Thomas AN, Stephens BG. Air embolism: a cause of morbidity and death after penetrating chest trauma. *J Trauma* 1974;14:633–638.

189. Saada M, Goarin J-P, Riou B, et al. Systemic gas embolism complicating pulmonary contusion: diagnosis and management using transesophageal echocardiography. *Am J Respir Crit Care Med* 1995;152:812–815.

190. Rodrigus-Morales G, Rodrigus A, Shatney CH. Acute rupture of the diaphragm and blunt trauma: analysis of 60 patients. *J Trauma* 1986;26:438–444.

191. Voeller GR, Reisser JR, Fabian TC, et al. Blunt diaphragm injuries: A five year experience. *Am Surg* 1990:56:28–31.

192. Brandt ML, Luks FI, Spigland NA, et al. Diaphragmatic injury in children. *J Trauma* 1992;32:298–301.

193. Ascensio JA, Demetriades D, Rodrigus A. Injury to the diaphragm. In: Feliciano D, Moore EE, Mattox K, eds. *Trauma,* 3rd ed. Stamford, CT: Appleton and Lange, 1996:471.

194. Guth AA, Pachter HL, Kim U. Pitfalls in the diagnosis of blunt diaphagmatic trauma. *Am J Surg* 1995;170:5–9.

195. Shah R, Sabanathan S, Mearns AJ, et al. Traumatic rupture of the diaphragm. *Ann Thorac Surg* 1995;60:1444–1449.

196. Estrera AS, Platt MR, Mills LJ. Traumatic injuries of the diaphragm. *Chest* 1979;75:306–313.

197. Puffer P, Gaebler M. Traumatic diaphragmatic rupture in a forensic medicine autopsy symbol. *Beitr Gerichtl Med* 1991;49:149–152.

198. Symbas PN. Injury to the esophagus, trachea and bronchus. In: Feliciano D, Moore EE, Mattox K, eds. *Trauma.* Stamford, CT: Appleton and Lange, 1998.

199. Halttunen PE, Kostianen SA, Meurala HG. Bronchial rupture caused by blunt chest trauma. *Scand J Thorac Cardiovasc Surg* 1984;18:141–144.

200. Amauchi W, Birolini D, Branco PD, et al. Injuries to the tracheobronchial tree in closed trauma. *Thorax* 1983;38:923–928.

201. Wu M-H, Tseng Y-L, Lin M-Y, et al. Surgical results of 23 patients with tracheobronchial injuries. *Respirology* 1997;2:127–130.

202. Matsumoto K, Noguchi T, Ishikawa R, et al. The surgical treatment of lung lacerations and major bronchial disruptions caused by blunt thoracic trauma. *Surg Today* 1998;28:162–166.

203. Rupprecht H, Rumenapf G, Petermann H, et al. Transthoracic bronchial intubation in a case of main bronchus disruption. *J Trauma* 1996;41:895–898.

204. Feliciano DV. The diagnostic and therapeutic approach to chest trauma. *Semin Thorac Cardiovasc Surg* 1992;4:156–162.

205. Johnson MJ, Lucas GL. Fat embolism syndrome. *Orthopaedics* 1996;19:41–44.

206. Peltier LF. Fat embolism, a current concept. *Clin Orthop* 1969; 66:241–253.

207. Eddy A, Rice C, Carrico C. Fat embolism syndrome: monitoring and management. *J Crit Care* 1987;2:24–27.

208. Muller C, Rahn B, Pfister U, et al. The incidence, pathogenesis, diagnosis and treatment of fat embolism. *Orthop Rev* 1994;23: 107–117.

209. Pell ACH, Christi J, Keating J, et al. The detection of fat embolism by transesophageal echocardiography during reamed intramedullary nailing. *J Bone Joint Surg* 1993;75:921–925.

210. Chastre J, Fagon JY, Soler P, et al. Bronchoalveolar lavage for rapid diagnosis of fat embolism syndrome in trauma patients. *Ann Intern Med* 1990;113:583–588.

211. Aoki OBN, Kazui S, Masateru S, et al. Evaluation of potential fat emboli during placement of intramedullary nails after orthopaedic fractures. *Chest* 1998;113:178–181.

212. Fonte DA, Hausberger FX. Pulmonary free fatty acids in experimental fat embolism. *J Trauma* 1971;11:668–672.

213. Gossing HR, Pellegrini VD Jr. Fat embolism syndrome: a review of the pathophysiology and physiologic basis of treatment. *Clin Orthop* 1982;165:68–82.

214. Bulger EM, Smith DG, Maier RV, et al. Fat embolism syndrome: a ten year review. *Arch Surg* 1997;132:435–439.

215. Yoshida A, Okada Y, Nagata Y, et al. Assessment of cerebral fat embolism by magnetic resonance imaging in the acute stage. *J Trauma* 1996;40:437–440.

216. Moylan JA, Birnbaum M, Katz A, et al. Fat emboli syndrome. *J Trauma* 1976;16:341–347.

217. Jacobson DM, Terrance CF, Reinmuth OM. The neurologic manifestations of fat embolisms. *Neurology* 1986;36:847–851.

25

MANAGING THE PATIENT WITH HEMODYNAMIC INSUFFICIENCY, SHOCK, AND MULTIPLE ORGAN FAILURE

MICHAEL A. MATTHAY
PAUL M. DORINSKY

CARDIOVASCULAR MONITORING
Systemic Arterial Catheterization
Pulmonary Artery Catheterization

PULMONARY ARTERY CATHETERIZATION: CLINICAL INDICATIONS
Acute Cardiogenic Pulmonary Edema
Acute Noncardiogenic Pulmonary Edema
Shock

Management of Patients after Cardiac and Major Vascular Surgery

HOW TO DETERMINE THE PHYSIOLOGIC BASIS FOR SHOCK

MULTIPLE ORGAN FAILURE
Definition and Epidemiology
Pathogenesis
Management of the Patient with Multiple Organ Failure
Early Recognition and Prevention of Multiple Organ Failure

This chapter will initially focus on (a) the methods available for the diagnosis and monitoring of hemodynamic insufficiency in critically ill patients, (b) the indications for invasive hemodynamic monitoring in critically ill patients, and (c) the basic principles of determining the etiology of shock. The second half of the chapter considers multiple organ failure in critically ill patients, with a particular focus on sepsis.

CARDIOVASCULAR MONITORING

In this section, techniques for monitoring the hemodynamic and respiratory status of critically ill patients with respiratory failure are discussed. In the last three decades, many invasive techniques for monitoring the systemic and pulmonary circulation have been developed. However, there has been increasing interest in developing noninvasive methods for monitoring important physiologic variables with the goal of reducing the risk and expense of invasive measurements whenever possible.

Systemic Arterial Catheterization

Systemic arterial catheters are widely used in a variety of critically ill patients. They are most useful for monitoring systemic arterial blood pressure in patients who are hemodynamically unstable, including patients with severe, uncontrolled hypertension as well as patients with hypotension and clinical shock. In addition, systemic arterial catheters are useful as a means of obtaining repeated blood samples from patients, thus obviating the need for repeated percutaneous venous or arterial puncture. In general, systemic arterial catheters are well tolerated, although there are a few important concerns regarding insertion technique and complications that need to be remembered.

Insertion Techniques for Systemic Arterial Catheters

Peripheral arterial cannulation is accomplished most frequently by percutaneous insertion of a No. 18 or 20 gauge catheter using sterile technique. When percutaneous insertion is not possible, a surgical cutdown may be necessary. The radial artery is usually chosen because of its accessibility and because there is generally good collateral circulation via the ulnar artery. Prior to insertion, the status of this collateral circulation should be assessed with an Allen's test. With this test, both the ulnar and radial arteries are occluded by pressure at the wrist; after the hand becomes pale and cool, releasing only the ulnar artery occlusion should restore adequate circulation within five seconds. The femoral, dorsales pedis, and brachial arteries may also be cannulated. Femoral arterial catheterization has not been associated with any increased risk of complication compared with that of the radial artery, providing that the catheters are inserted with sterile technique percutaneously (1).

Complications of Systemic Arterial Catheters

Infection and ischemia are the most important major complications that may occur from systemic arterial catheterization. Ischemia may occur secondary to either thrombosis with local occlusion, or distal embolization. In one large prospective study, a 4% incidence of catheter-related septicemia and an 18% incidence of local infection (defined by semiquantitative culture of the catheter tip) were found (2). The risk factors favoring infection include insertion by surgical cutdown rather than percutaneously, duration of cannulation exceeding four days, and inflammation at the catheter site (2). Infection may originate in the transducer or fluid-delivery apparatus. One prospective study indicated that catheter-related infection can be decreased markedly if a continuous flush device is located immediately distal to the transducer apparatus rather than close to the insertion site (3). This eliminates a long proximal static fluid column between the transducer and flush intake. With this design and careful sterile precautions at the blood-sampling stop-cock, the incidence of catheter-related septicemia was reduced to less than 1%.

Clinically significant thrombosis or embolism is rare. In over 12,000 consecutive placements of arterial lines (including radial, brachial, and/or dorsalis pedis arteries), necrosis of the fingers or toes occurred in only 15 (0.2%) (4). Similarly, in another study, only 3 (0.6%) of 531 patients required emergency thrombectomies for distal ischemia (5). The clinical risk factors for acute distal ischemia include systemic hypotension, severe peripheral vascular disease, and the use of vasopressor drugs. Even though clinically important ischemia is rare, reversible subclinical arterial occlusion or reduced flow is common, with up to 24% of arteries still occluded one week after catheter removal (6). The risk factors for such occlusion include larger catheter size (18 versus 20 gauge), smaller wrist size (women and children), repeated attempts before successful cannulation, and duration of cannulation (risk increases after three to four days). Ulnar refill time determined by the Allen's test prior to insertion is also of some predictive value. As mentioned, a palmar blush due to filling via the ulnar artery should appear within five seconds. If 15 seconds is used as an acceptable upper limit, then distal ischemia is more frequent (approximately 10%) (7).

Once the catheter is placed, distal perfusion should be assessed at least daily by noting any changes in skin color, temperature, or capillary refill time. If the arterial pressure tracing becomes persistently dampened, or if blood-drawing is difficult, thrombus formation on the catheter tip is likely and the catheters should be removed, since the risk of occlusion is high (8).

Pulmonary Artery Catheterization

The availability of bedside pulmonary artery catheterization has had a major impact on the management of critically ill patients. There are numerous clinical conditions for which pulmonary artery catheterization has been accepted as useful (1). These include shock associated with acute myocardial infarction, sepsis, or major trauma, acute respiratory failure from cardiogenic or noncardiogenic pulmonary edema, and management of patients following cardiac or major vascular surgery. However, there has been increasing concern that clinicians need to be better informed regarding the risk and potential benefits of pulmonary artery catheterization (9–11). The clinical literature contains numerous examples of how incorrect information may be conveyed from pulmonary arterial pressure measurements when physicians and nurses are not sufficiently skilled at interpreting pressure and waveform tracings (1,12,13).

Insertion Techniques

The pulmonary circulation can be monitored by percutaneous insertion of a balloon-tipped pulmonary artery catheter via the subclavian, internal jugular, external jugular, femoral, or antecubital vein. Catheterization can be done at the patient's bedside with only pressure waveform and amplitude and electrocardiographic monitoring. Fluoroscopy is not necessary, although the prescribed waveform must be displayed on the bedside oscilloscope. The pulmonary artery catheter used most frequently has four lumina plus a small thermistor near the tip for thermodilution cardiac output measurements. One lumen is used to inflate the balloon on the tip of the catheter. After the catheter is advanced into the thorax, the balloon is inflated. The flow-directed catheter then usually passes easily from the right atrium, across the tricuspid valve, through the right ventricle, and into the pulmonary artery (Fig. 25.1). If the catheter is advanced further with the balloon inflated, it will wedge in the pulmonary artery and occlude blood flow. The distal lumen, which opens at the tip of the catheter, will then record the downstream vascular pressure, the pulmonary arterial wedge pressure (see Fig. 25.1). When the balloon is deflated, the distal lumen records the phasic pulmonary arterial pressure. The proximal lumen, located 30 cm from the tip of the catheter, will then be positioned in the right atrium to measure central venous pressure when the tip of the catheter is in the pulmonary artery. This proximal lumen is also used to inject a bolus of indicator (10 mL of 5% dextrose) to determine cardiac output by thermodilution. The bolus is injected through the lumen in the right atrium so that the thermistor near the tip of the catheter in the pulmonary artery can

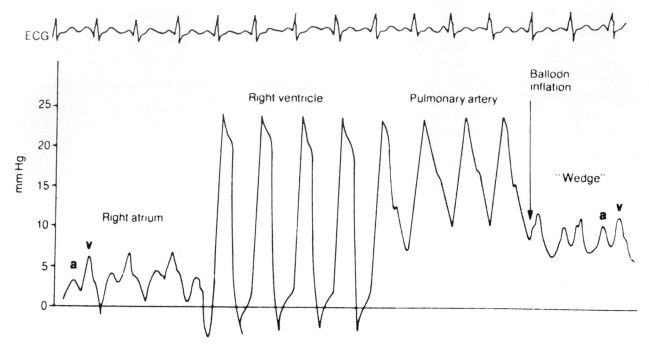

FIGURE 25.1. Representative recording of pressures as a Swan-Ganz catheter is inserted through an internal jugular vein through the right side of the heart into the pulmonary artery. The first recorded waveform is a right atrial tracing with characteristic *a* and *v* waves. In the right ventricle, note that end-diastolic pressure is zero. In the pulmonary artery, a normal pressure waveform is recorded. The catheter is then advanced to the wedge position with the balloon inflated. The wedge pressure tracing shows *a* and *v* waves transmitted from the left atrium. The wedge tracing is not always this clear, but it should not be overly damped. The pressures shown here are normal. (From Matthay MA. Invasive hemodynamic monitoring in critically ill patients. *Clin Chest Med* 1983;4(2):233–249, with permission.)

sense the change in temperature as the bolus flows into the pulmonary artery. A small bedside computer then integrates the time-temperature curve and prints out the cardiac output. The fourth lumen, located 31 cm from the tip of the catheter, is used for infusion of intravenous solutions. An introducer sheath that has an additional lumen is also available for the intravenous infusion of fluids.

Obtaining Reliable Pressure Measurements

Once the catheter is in place, the pressure is transmitted via the catheter through the fluid-filled tubing to the diaphragm of a transducer and then converted to an electronic signal. The signal is amplified, the pressure waveform is shown on an oscilloscope, and the pressure is shown on a digital display (see Fig. 25.1). Correct pressure measurements depend on accurately calibrated transducers, a fluid-filled catheter system without blood clots or air bubbles, and a monitor that displays the pressure tracing in an appropriate size to demonstrate the waveforms clearly. The pulmonary arterial and wedge pressure tracing in Figure 25.1 fulfills these requirements. Note that there is a single major pulmonary arterial pressure wave for each spike on the electrocardiogram. Correct amplitude settings are needed to dis-

play the waveform correctly. In general, amplitudes in the range of 0 to 30 or 0 to 60 mm Hg are appropriate for the pulmonary circulation. In addition, the contour of the tracing is important. Figure 25.2 illustrates the dampening effect of a small air bubble in the catheter system. The dampening of the tracing also can be caused by a clot on the end of the catheter.

Calibration of the transducer is important because transducers may not be linear over a wide range of pressures. Thus it is important that the transducer for the pulmonary artery catheter be calibrated for the lower pressures of the pulmonary circulation (0 to 40 mmHg) rather than for the higher pressure range of the systemic circulation (1,13). Another common pitfall is improper location of the zero reference point, particularly because patients are moving from side to side or the head of the bed is raised or lowered. In general, the proper zero reference is the midchest position.

Perhaps the most common source of error in making intrathoracic pressure measurements is failure to take into account the effects of respiration on these pressure measurements (1,12,14). Pleural pressure becomes negative during spontaneous inspiration and positive during the inspiratory cycle of mechanical ventilation (IPPV). Consequently, the pressure readout and the waveform on the oscilloscope will

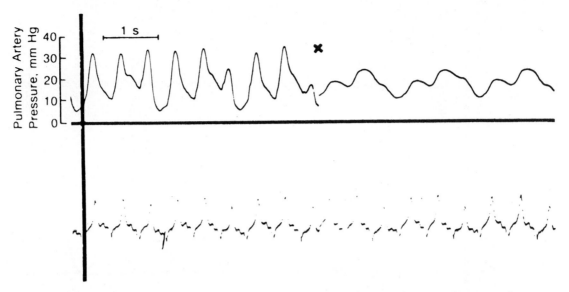

FIGURE 25.2. Pulmonary artery tracing after introduction of 0.5 cc of air into the connecting tubing at X, with the electrocardiogram recorded below. The phasic contour of the pulmonary artery tracing is damped out by the air bubble; the same pattern can be produced by clots in the catheter or on the catheter tip. (From Quinn K, Quebbeman EJ. Pulmonary artery pressure monitoring in the surgical intensive care unit. *Arch Surg* 1981;116:872–876, with permission.)

change, depending on the phase of respiration. In Figure 25.3, the recording of pulmonary arterial wedge pressure is interrupted by deep troughs in the tracing produced by the patient's spontaneous inspiratory efforts. During these troughs, the pressure reading is zero. Thus the problem is how to obtain a reliable transmural pressure measurement when the reference pressure (pleural pressure) is changing. To minimize the effects of changing pleural pressure, pulmonary arterial pressures should be measured at end-expiration when pleural pressures will be close to zero. In Figure 25.3, end-expiration can be clearly seen in both the pulmonary arterial pressure and the wedge pressure tracing. This approach enables the clinician to consider the measured pressure at end-expiration as a very close approximation of the true transmural pressure. This approach can be complicated if the patient is breathing so rapidly that the end-expiratory phase is very brief (Figure 25.4). In most circumstances, the best approach for obtaining a reliable pressure tracing is to obtain a printout of the actual pressure tracing, ideally on a strip-chart recorder, but alternatively on the oscilloscope's electrocardiographic monitor paper. First, the calibration lines for the pressure range are recorded on the paper, then the actual pressure tracing is recorded, and then the end-expiratory period can be noted on the paper. The pressure at end-expiration can then be measured from the tracing on the paper. When the patient's respiratory rate is rapid, the digital readout will not be accurate because the frequency response of the electronic system is usually too slow to detect the brief period of end-expiration.

Accurate measurements of pulmonary arterial pressures can be particularly difficult in patients with acute, severe airways obstruction. In order to overcome the high airway resistance, patients generate very positive intrathoracic pressures throughout expiration, and this leads to an elevated pulmonary arterial pressure or an elevated wedge pressure. During inspiration, the patient's pleural pressure may be markedly negative, and there will be a wide swing in the pulmonary arterial pressure tracing in the opposite direction. Similar problems occur when measuring pressures in patients on positive end–expiratory pressure (PEEP) and these are considered in the next section, after discussion of the relationship of wedge pressure to left atrial pressure.

Relation of Wedge Pressure to Left Arterial Pressure

The pulmonary arterial wedge pressure is used widely as an index of left atrial filling pressure. In general, most studies have demonstrated that the correlation between wedge pressure and left atrial pressure in patients is very good (1,14). The correlation of left atrial pressure to left ventricular end-diastolic pressure likewise is good, provided there is no mitral valve disease. The pulmonary arterial end-diastolic pressure provides an accurate indication of the pulmonary arterial wedge pressure except when there is an increase in pulmonary vascular resistance, in which case the end-diastolic pressure will be much higher than the wedge pressure. Pulmonary vascular resistance is elevated in several clinical conditions associated with acute or chronic pulmonary hypertension (see Chapters 10, Lung Transplantation

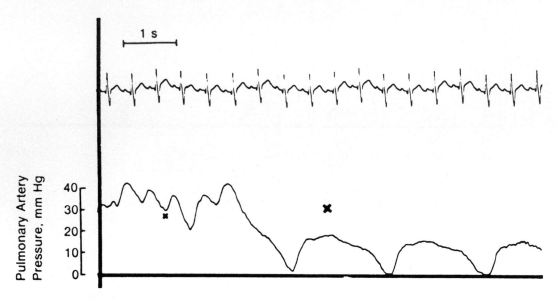

FIGURE 25.3. Continuous monitoring of the electrocardiogram and the phasic pulmonary artery pressure plus a segment of a pulmonary artery wedge tracing. Note that the troughs in the pulmonary artery and in the wedge tracings occur when the patient takes a spontaneous breath and pleural pressure becomes negative, thus causing a downward deflection in the tracing. The X marks indicate end-expiration in the respiratory cycle. AT end-expiration, pleural pressure is zero; therefore, the measured intraluminal pressure should be close to the real transmural pressure. Wedge pressure is about 15 mm Hg below the pulmonary artery end-diastolic pressure; the patient had pulmonary hypertension from acute pulmonary embolism which accounts for the gradient between the end-diastolic and the wedge pressures. (From Quinn K, Quebbeman EJ. Pulmonary artery pressure monitoring in the surgical intensive care unit. *Arch Surg* 1981;116: 872–876; with permission.)

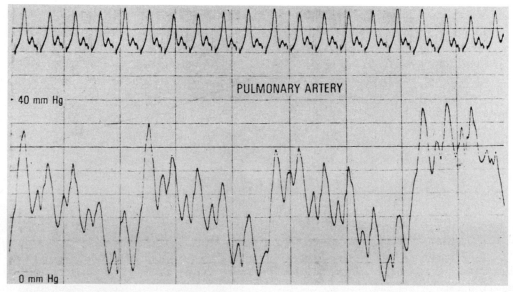

FIGURE 25.4. Example of how rapid, labored respirations can result in rapid oscillations of the pulmonary artery pressure tracing and highly variable pressure measurements. The patient's respiratory rate was 40 and the peak pulmonary artery pressure varied from 35 to 40 to 18 mm Hg. A brief period of end-expiration could be identified, but the electronic digital readout could not reflect that brief end-expiratory period alone. So the pulmonary artery tracing was recorded on calibrated paper and the pressures read off the paper at the point of end-expiration. Matthay MA. Invasive hemodynamic monitoring in critically ill patients. *Clin Chest Med* 1983;4(2):233–249, with permission.)

and Lung Volume Reduction Surgery, 11, Pulmonary Thromboembolism and Other Pulmonary Vascular Diseases, 13, Occupational and Environmental Lung Disease, 22, Acute Hypercapnic Respiratory Failure: Neuromuscular and Obstructive Disease).

Effect of PEEP on Wedge Pressure Measurements

Accurate transmural arterial and wedge pressure measurements may be more difficult to obtain in patients on PEEP in excess of 10 cm H_2O. PEEP may interfere with accurate measurements in two ways. First, it may result in an undetermined increase in pleural pressure. Second, the airway pressure generated by PEEP may be transmitted to the pulmonary microcirculation (14). Because PEEP prevents transpulmonary pressure from falling to zero at the end of expiration, this means the pleural pressure remains positive at the end of expiration; thus the reference pressure for the pulmonary arterial pressure measurement is not zero. Hence the recorded intraluminal pressure (central venous pressure, pulmonary arterial pressure, or wedge pressure) may be higher than the actual transmural pressure. One way to solve this problem is to measure esophageal pressure as an indicator of pleural pressure in order to obtain a more accurate reference pressure. However, reliable esophageal pressure measurements are difficult to obtain, especially in a supine patient in a critical care unit. One partial solution to the problem is to make an estimate of pleural pressure and subtract this value from the measured wedge pressure. In clinical studies in which pleural pressure was measured in patients with the acute respiratory distress syndrome (ARDS), pleural pressure did not usually become significantly positive with levels of PEEP below 10 cm H_2O (15,16). With levels of PEEP above 10 cm H_2O, pleural pressure was usually approximately 2 to 3 cm H_2O positive for every 5 cm H_2O increase in PEEP above 10 cm H_2O (15,16).

The other potential difficulty with levels of PEEP above 10 cm H_2O is that if alveolar pressure exceeds the pulmonary arterial pressure, the catheter tip may reflect airway pressure rather than vascular pressures. Theoretically, the wedge pressure will reflect left atrial pressure if the wedged catheter tip is located in a portion of the lung where pulmonary arterial and pulmonary venous pressures exceed the alveolar pressure (zone 3) (1,14). If the catheter tip is in an area where alveolar pressure exceeds venous pressure when pulmonary arterial flow is occluded with balloon inflation, the recorded pressure will be airway pressure rather than pulmonary artery pressure. If the catheter is located in zone 3, the wedged catheter can look through the pulmonary vasculature to sense left atrial pressure. Thus, to have an accurate indication of left atrial pressure, the pulmonary artery catheter must be in a zone 3 area.

Usually, the flow-directed pulmonary artery catheter migrates to zone 3 and the wedge pressure accurately reflects

TABLE 25.1. CHECKLIST FOR VERIFYING POSITION OF PULMONARY ARTERIAL CATHETER

Condition	Zone 3	Zone 1 or 2
Respiratory variation of PW	$\leq 1/2\ \Delta$ Palv	$> 1/2\ \Delta$ Palv
PW Contour	Cardiac ripple	Unnaturally smooth
Catheter tip location	LA level or below	Above LA level
Decrease PEEP trial	Δ PW ≤ 1.2 PEEP	Δ PW $> 1/2\ \Delta$ PEEP
PPAD vs. PW	PPAD $>$ PW	PPAD $\leq$ PW

PW, wedge pressure; Palv, static airway pressure; LA, left atrium; PEEP, positive end–expiratory pressure; PPAD, pulmonary artery diastolic pressure.
(Reproduced from Marini JJ. Obtaining meaningful data from the Swan-Ganz catheter. *Respir Care* 1985;30:572, with permission.)

left atrial pressure (1). If PEEP is increased, it is possible that the zone 3 area, where the catheter was initially placed, may become a zone 2 area, where alveolar pressure exceeds venous pressure. Although this does not happen very often, it has been shown experimentally that if the tip of the pulmonary artery catheter is at or below the left atrium, the mean wedge pressure at end-expiration still reflects left atrial pressure, even with levels of PEEP up to 30 cm H_2O (17). Therefore, it is reasonable to confirm the position of the catheter tip with an anteroposterior portable chest roentgenogram and, if necessary, a lateral chest radiograph (1). When a question arises concerning the location of the catheter tip, there are a few maneuvers that can be done to verify zone 3 conditions (Table 25.1) (18). For wedge pressure tracings outside zone 3, the wedge contour appears unusually smooth and the pulmonary artery end-diastolic pressure tends to be lower than the balloon-occlusion pressure. In zones 1 and 2, changes in the wedge pressure tend to follow alveolar rather than left atrial pressure.

Thus the swings in the wedge pressure during ventilation with positive pressure are unusually wide because only half or less of the change in static airway pressure (peak greater than plateau pressure) transmits to the pleural spaces, left atrium, and intrathoracic vessels. For the same reason, a trial of PEEP reduction causes a fall in the wedge pressure of unexpected magnitude (more than half the PEEP decrement) when the catheter tip is in zone 1 or 2 (see Table 25.1) (18).

One recent study reported that there is considerable interobserver variability in pressure measurement using pulmonary arterial catheter tracings (19). Nurse-physician differences were not substantially greater than physician-physician differences. Significant differences in measurement were more common in patients whose pulmonary arterial wedge pressure had a higher degree of respiratory variation, probably because of disagreement in identifying end-expiration on the tracings (19). The observed differences were likely to be clinically significant and potentially lead to inappropriate clinical decisions and clinical interventions.

PULMONARY ARTERY CATHETERIZATION: CLINICAL INDICATIONS

The most common clinical conditions for which pulmonary artery catheterization is used in intensive care units include acute pulmonary edema, shock, and management of patients after cardiac or major vascular surgery (1,9).

Acute Cardiogenic Pulmonary Edema

In general, acute cardiogenic pulmonary edema is accompanied by either systemic hypertension or hypotension. Indications for pulmonary artery catheterization depend mainly on the patient's systemic blood pressure. The diagnosis of cardiogenic pulmonary edema in the setting of systemic hypertension is nearly always accompanied by physical findings that point to left ventricular failure as the cause of the pulmonary edema (11). Treatment of the heart failure almost always results in prompt improvement, making it unnecessary to insert a pulmonary artery catheter for diagnosis or management. In fact, the pulmonary arterial wedge pressure may return to the normal range even before the pulmonary artery catheter can be inserted (20). Treatment of the acute pulmonary edema does not require pulmonary artery catheterization in these patients unless hemodynamic instability develops (11).

In contrast, patients with acute pulmonary edema in association with systemic hypotension secondary to an acute myocardial infarction present more difficult problems. A number of studies have documented that the hemodynamic profiles of patients within this group may vary considerably. Some patients will have markedly elevated left ventricular end-diastolic pressures in association with a very low cardiac output, while others may have a much more moderate elevation in the pulmonary arterial wedge pressure and better ventricular function (11,21). Occasionally, patients thought to have left ventricular failure will be found to have noncardiogenic pulmonary edema. Rational decisions regarding the use of vasopressors, vasodilators, and volume replacement can often be better made with knowledge of the left ventricular filling pressure and systemic vascular resistance (9,11), providing the measurements are accurate (19).

Acute Noncardiogenic Pulmonary Edema

There are several reasons why pulmonary arterial catheterization may be indicated in most patients with suspected noncardiogenic pulmonary edema. First, differentiation of cardiogenic from noncardiogenic pulmonary edema can be difficult both radiographically (22) and clinically. In one study, the clinical diagnosis of noncardiogenic pulmonary edema was substantiated on pulmonary artery catheterization in only 56% of patients (23). In addition, some patients who have primary lung injury also may have a mild elevation in the pulmonary arterial wedge pressure that contributes to the pulmonary edema (24). Therefore, in many patients with pulmonary edema that appears to be of a noncardiac origin, it is reasonable to obtain pulmonary hemodynamic measurements to be certain that the diagnosis is correct.

The management of certain patients with noncardiogenic pulmonary edema is facilitated by hemodynamic measurements (24). This is particularly true in patients with sepsis in whom systemic hypotension and acute respiratory failure occur together. In this setting, the goals of management are to produce optimal cardiac output and systemic perfusion with as little increase as possible in the pulmonary arterial wedge pressure. This balance can be achieved with the use of invasive hemodynamic monitoring, although there is no definite proof that measurement of these physiologic variables ultimately results in an improved patient outcome (9).

Most patients with ARDS should have their pulmonary artery catheter removed within three to four days in order to reduce the risk of secondary infection and to convert the central line onto a triple-lumen catheter that can be used for the administration of fluids, antibiotics, and hyperalimentation (see Chapter 26, Prevention of Nonpulmonary Complications of Intensive Care). There are some patients with ARDS who are very stable hemodynamically and in whom the oxygenation defect is not very severe. Some of these patients can be managed without pulmonary arterial catheterization (25,26).

Shock

One of the original justifications for pulmonary artery catheterization rests on the evidence that some patients with acute myocardial infarction may have a normal central venous pressure in the presence of an elevated pulmonary arterial wedge pressure (27). Also, some patients with an acute myocardial infarction and shock are found to have low left ventricular filling pressures that can be best treated with volume expansion to increase preload. Thus the argument has been that pulmonary arterial catheterization helps provide information that cannot be obtained by clinical examination alone. In fact, one study confirmed that clinical assessment of hemodynamic variables in patients with shock prior to insertion of a pulmonary artery catheter was poor (23). In patients with pulmonary arterial wedge pressures greater than 18 mm Hg, the wedge pressure was predicted correctly only 35% of the time. Similarly, in the same group of patients with a measured cardiac index of less than 2.2 L per minute per m^2, the cardiac index was predicted correctly only 55% of the time.

Management of Patients after Cardiac and Major Vascular Surgery

The indications for pulmonary artery catheterization in patients who have had cardiac surgery are controversial (9). In some institutions, for example, clinicians insert pulmonary artery catheters in all patients who undergo cardiac surgery, whereas in other institutions, even cardiac transplant patients do not have routine pulmonary artery pressure monitoring. However, available data regarding risks versus benefits of pulmonary artery catheterization after cardiac surgery support a more selective approach, reserving pulmonary artery catheterization for patients with a reduced left ventricular ejection fraction (9). Moreover, one study demonstrated that the pulmonary arterial wedge pressure was not a reliable indicator of left ventricular preload in the immediate period following coronary artery bypass surgery (28).

Patients who have undergone major vascular surgery often have coexistent cardiac and renal disease which places them at high risk for postoperative hemodynamic instability. In addition, it is common for these patients to have large collections of peritoneal fluid and a diffuse systemic capillary leak following cross-clamping of the aorta, so they have major fluid shifts postoperatively. Because these patients are at high risk of postoperative heart failure, volume overload respiratory failure, and renal failure, they may benefit from pulmonary artery catheterization, although the decision should be made on a case-by-case basis (9).

HOW TO DETERMINE THE PHYSIOLOGIC BASIS FOR SHOCK

Shock is present if evidence of multisystem organ hypoperfusion is apparent. Evidence of hypoperfusion obtained during the rapid initial clinical evaluation of a patient in shock may include tachycardia, a low mean blood pressure, an altered mental status, and a decreased urine output. There are several causes of shock that need to be differentiated as early as possible in the patient's clinical course.

A systematic approach to determining the etiology of shock is helpful in the initial diagnosis and management of the hypotensive patient. This approach acknowledges that shock is identified in most patients by systemic hypotension, and that mean arterial blood pressure is the product of cardiac output and the systemic vascular resistance (SVR) (29,30). Accordingly, hypotension may be due to reduced cardiac output or reduced system vascular resistance. Initial examination of the hypotensive patient seeks to determine if cardiac output is reduced or not. High-cardiac-output hypotension is most often signaled by a large pulse pressure, a low diastolic pressure, warm extremities, fever (or hypothermia), and leukocytosis (or leukopenia); these clinical findings strongly suggest a working diagnosis of septic shock, the initial treatment for which is antimicrobial therapy combined with adequate but not excessive expansion of the vascular volume (Table 25.2).

By contrast, a low cardiac output is indicated by a small pulse pressure and cool extremities with poor nail bed return. In this case, the clinical need is to determine if the heart is too full or not. A heart which is too full in a hypotensive patient is signaled by elevated jugular venous pressure

TABLE 25.2. CHARACTERISTICS OF SEPTIC, CARDIOGENIC, AND HYPOVOLEMIC SHOCK

Abnormalities in Shock	Septic	Cardiogenic	Hypovolemic
Blood pressure	↓	↓	↓
Heart rate	≥	≥	≤
Respiratory rate	>	≥	≤
Mentation	↓	↓	↓
Urine output	↓	↓	↓
Arterial pH	↓	↓	↓
Pulse pressure	↓	↓	↓
Diastolic pressure	↓↓↓	↓	↓
Extremities/digits	Warm	Cool	Cool
Temperature	≤ or ↓	↔	↔
White cell count	≤ or ↓	↔	↔
Site of infection	+ +	-	-
Is the Heart Too Full?	No	Yes	No
Symptoms/clinical context	Sepsis/liver failure	Ischemia/infarction	Hemorrhage/dehydration
Jugular venous pressure	↓	≥	↓
S$_3$, S$_4$, gallop rhythm	-	+ + +	-
Chest radiograph	Normal (early in course)	Large heart (sometimes) ≥ upper lobe flow Pulmonary edema	Normal
What Does Not Fit?			
Overlapping etiologies (septic + cardiogenic, septic + hypovolemic, cardiogenic + hypovolemic)			
Short list of other etiologies	High-output hypotension Thyroid storm Arteriovenous fistula Paget's disease	High-right-atrial-pressure hypotension Cardiac tamponade Right ventricular infarction Pulmonary hypertension	Nonresponsive hypovolemia Adrenal insufficiency Anaphylaxis Spinal shock
Obtain more information	Echocardiography, right-heart catheterization		

Hall JB, Schmidt GA, Wood LDH, eds. *Principles of critical care*, New York: McGraw-Hill, Inc., 1992;1393–1395, with permission.

(JVP), peripheral edema, crepitations on lung auscultation, a large heart with extra heart sounds (S_3,S_4), chest pain, ischemic changes on the electrocardiogram (ECG), and a chest radiograph showing a large heart with dilated upper-lobe vessels and pulmonary edema. These findings suggest cardiogenic shock, most often due to ischemic heart disease, and are generally absent when the low cardiac output is due to hypovolemia (see Table 25.2). Then, clinical examination reveals manifestations of blood loss (hematemesis, tarry stools, abdominal distention, reduced hematocrit), trauma, or manifestations of dehydration (reduced tissue turgor, vomiting or diarrhea, negative fluid balance). This distinction between cardiogenic and hypovolemic shock allows initial therapy to focus on vasoactive drugs or on volume infusions, respectively (see Table 25.2).

Whenever the clinical formulation is not obvious, it is helpful to determine what does not fit (30). Most often, the answer is that the hypotension is due to two or more etiologies of shock: (a) septic shock complicated by myocardial ischemia or hypovolemia; (b) cardiogenic shock complicated by hypovolemia or sepsis; and (c) hypovolemic shock masking as sepsis or ischemic heart disease. In these situations, more data is needed and it frequently can be obtained from echocardiography and pulmonary arterial catheterization. Proper interpretation of this data, along with response to initial therapy, frequently confirm that multiple etiologies for shock exist or it leads to a broader differential diagnosis of the etiologies of shock (see Table 25.2).

MULTIPLE ORGAN FAILURE

This section considers multiple organ failure (MOF) with a focus on definitions, epidemiology, pathogenesis, management, and prevention (31). One of the earliest descriptions of MOF was written by Baue in 1975:

> The sequence of events often begins with a period of shock or circulatory failure at some point during the initial injury, accompanied sooner or later by failure of ventilation and the need for ventilatory support. This may be followed by renal failure, hepatic failure (jaundice and decreasing albumin levels), gastrointestinal failure (stress ulcers and gastrointestinal bleeding), and metabolic failure (decrease in lean body mass and weakness due to progressive catabolism). Our ability to support a single system that has failed, transiently at least, is reasonably good. The support of two or more failed units, however, stresses our knowledge and capability. Survivors of multiple systems failure are infrequent (32).

Since this description, several medical and surgical studies have reported a high mortality rate associated with MOF in critically ill patients. Sepsis syndrome is clearly the most frequently encountered clinical problem associated with the development of MOF (32). Some patients who have MOF, however, do not seem to have a clear-cut infectious etiology.

For example, patients who have been treated with interleukin-2 for malignant disorders frquently develop renal failure, gastrointestinal failure, neurological disturbances, and sometimes even acute respiratory failure. These observations suggest that release of potent endogenous humoral factors during noninfectious disorders (e.g., severe hypovolemic shock) may produce the clinical features of the sepsis syndrome without necessarily being related to infection. Finally, it is also possible that primary lung injury itself can lead to the development of nonpulmonary organ failure (32). In any case, sepsis often complicates MOF, even if sepsis is not the initial clinical disorder (33,34).

In this section, the definition and epidemiology of MOF will be discussed, with an emphasis on specific guidelines for defining the failure or dysfunction of the respiratory, cardiovascular, renal, hepatic, central nervous, and hematologic systems. In the next section, the pathogenesis of MOF is considered. In the third section, guidelines are provided for the management of patients with MOF with an emphasis on guidelines for therapy with fluids, colloid, blood, and vasoactive agents, as well as antiinflammatory agents. In the final section, the prevention and early recognition of MOF and sepsis syndrome are reviewed.

Definition and Epidemiology

Multiple organ failure is often a major complication in patients with shock from sepsis, major trauma, severe pancreatitis, drug overdose, or thermal injury (31–36). The extent to which an individual organ is likely to be damaged in these clinical settings depends on numerous factors, including age, preexisting medical illnesses, severity of illness on admission to the intensive care unit, and the specific precipitating event (31,34,35). The clinical features of organ dysfunction in this patient group are also variable and have been defined by different criteria. Specifically, organ dysfunction in critically ill patients ranges in spectrum from minor biochemical abnormalities to irreversible organ failure. Nonetheless, the incidence of renal, gastrointestinal, hepatic, central nervous, and hematologic failure has been studied, especially in patients with acute respiratory failure. The definition and incidence of acute respiratory failure are discussed subsequently after considering criteria for failure of the nonpulmonary organ systems.

Cardiovascular Failure

The incidence of cardiovascular failure among critically ill patients varies from 10% to 23% (31). Although a uniform definition in critically ill patients has yet to be established, most clinicians agree that cardiovascular failure exists when one or more of the following are present: (a) mean arterial pressure less than or equal to 60 mm Hg, (b) cardiac index of 2 L minute per m^2 or less, or (c) reversible ventricular fibrillation or asystole. This definition could include a patient with an acute myocardial infarction and severe pump failure. It could also include a patient with septic shock who has a high cardiac output, a low systemic vascular resistance, and a low mean arterial blood pressure. Cardiovascular failure, therefore, includes those disturbances that cause a major decrease in myocardial function as well as those clinical disorders associated with abnormalities in the peripheral circulation.

Although human septic shock is usually characterized by elevated cardiac output and reduced systemic vascular resistance, it may also be associated with a decrease in the left ventricular ejection fraction. In addition, studies have shown that septic patients have increased left ventricular ejection fraction, increased end-systolic and end-diastolic volumes, normal or decreased stroke work, and decreased right ventricular ejection fraction. Among patients who survive, these cardiovascular parameters normalize (37).

The mechanism of myocardial dysfunction during sepsis is not entirely known (37,38). Nonetheless, serum obtained from patients with septic shock has been shown to depress myocardial cell contractility *in vitro*. Moreover, evidence suggests that tumor necrosis factor (TNF), an important humoral mediator of sepsis, is capable of depressing myocardial cell contractility. It is likely that one or more of these myocardial depressant substances are responsible for the reduction in ejection fracture and the ventricular volume changes that occur during sepsis.

Given the complexities associated with the diagnosis and management of cardiovascular dysfunction in acutely ill patients, the use of right-heart catheterization has become routine for many physicians caring for ICU patients. However, a recent prospective study suggested that the use of right-heart catheters was associated with an increase in both 30-day mortality (odds ratio = 1.24; 95% confidence interval = 1.03–1.49) and resource utilization (39). Although this study has been widely criticized on the basis of its design and conclusions, it has stimulated an intense dialogue on the role of these catheters in acutely ill patients. In addition, it has served as a catalyst for an upcoming prospective NIH-sponsored study on the role of right-heart catheterization in the management of critically ill patients.

Two other important features of sepsis syndrome are the abnormal vasodilatation of the systemic circulation and the abnormalities of peripheral oxygen uptake. These issues are discussed in the section on pathogenesis.

Renal Failure

Renal dysfunction is a frequent complication in critically ill patients (40% to 55% incidence) and is manifested by reductions in urine output and a rise in the serum urea and creatinine values (31,38). Specifically, renal failure may be defined in this patient group as a serum creatinine value in excess of 2 mg per dL and a urine output below 600 mL per 24 hours (34).

The three most important risk factors for the development of renal failure in critically ill patients are hypotension, sepsis, and nephrotoxic drugs (40,41). Acute nonoliguric renal failure, associated primarily with nephrotoxic drugs, has a better prognosis than acute oliguric renal failure that occurs with septic shock or after major cardiovascular surgery.

Gastrointestinal Failure

Alterations in gastrointestinal tract function are estimated to occur in 30% of critically ill patients (31,38). The pathologic basis for gastrointestinal dysfunction appears to be both an alteration in microvascular permeability and mucosal ischemia. For example, TNF causes necrosis of intestinal villi when infused into experimental animals. These morphologic observations suggest a pathologic basis for the functional abnormalities of the gastrointestinal tract that occur in critically ill patients (42).

The clinical features of gastrointestinal tract dysfunction are variable and include hemorrhage, ileus, malabsorption (e.g., inability to tolerate enteral feedings), and occasionally acalculous cholecystitis or pancreatitis. Among these complications, gastrointestinal bleeding is common but it is difficult to quantify. Gastrointestinal blood loss in excess of 1 g per dL of hemoglobin per 24 hours is generally accepted to be clinically significant, however (43).

An intact gastrointestinal tract mucosa provides an essential barrier to the entry of bacteria into the systemic circulation. Since mucosal integrity of the gastrointestinal tract is frequently impaired in critically ill patients, bacteria may translocate or migrate from the bowel lumen into the peritoneal cavity, or to regional gastrointestinal lymph nodes, and to the portosystemic circulation. To the extent that this occurs, the process of bacterial translocation may propagate septic shock and result in further organ dysfunction.

Clinical data in support of a central role for the gastrointestinal tract in the pathogenesis of MOF in acutely ill patients is increasing. In this regard, marked alterations in gastrointestinal permeability were demonstrated to occur in a prospectively studied group of ICU patients using monosaccharide and disaccharide probes (44). Perhaps even more significant, however, was the observation that the patients who developed MOF had significantly greater alterations in intestinal permeability upon ICU admission than those who did not ultimately develop MOF. Taken together, these observations suggest that altered gastrointestinal tract function plays an important if not central role in the pathogenesis of MOF in critically ill patients.

Hepatic Failure

Fulminant hepatic failure as a feature of organ failure in critically ill patients is uncommon and occurs in less than 10% of critically ill patients (31,38). By contrast, reversible elevations in serum transaminases and elevations in serum bilirubin or clotting parameters are common and may be found in as many as 95% of critically ill patients. Criteria for hepatic failure in critically ill patients are in a state of evolution. Nonetheless, elevations in serum bilirubin that exceed 4 to 5 mg per dL, a prothrombin time of more than 1.5 times control, and a serum albumin level below 2 g per dL are indicative of significant hepatic dysfunction (34,45).

As a complication of septic shock or other critical illnesses, hepatic dysfunction is of more than academic interest. The liver is an important reticuloendothelial organ whose function is also altered when the liver is damaged. For example, fibronectin, an opsonin that is important in the maintenance of host defense, is frequently decreased in critically ill patients. Mortality data indicate the importance of intact hepatic function to the outcome of critically ill patients. Mortality from septic shock approaches 100% in patients with severe hepatic damage. Also, when hepatic failure occurs in the setting of acute respiratory failure, the prognosis for recovery from the acute lung injury is poor (45). Thus evidence is accumulating to suggest that the various systemic organs are not merely targets of damage during critical illnesses. Rather, once these organs are damaged, their dysfunction has a substantial impact on host defense and the propagation of the underlying injury.

Central Nervous System Failure

Abnormalities of central nervous system (CNS) function have been frequently described in critically ill patients (35,38,46,47). For example, CNS dysfunction, including disorientation, confusion, agitation, obtundation, and seizures, occurs commonly in septic patients. One study reported a 9% incidence of CNS dysfunction, defined as an inability to follow simple commands, in 106 patients with intraabdominal sepsis. By contrast, another study, using an altered sensorium as the criteria for CNS dysfunction, reported a 33% incidence of CNS abnormalities in sepsis (31).

Use of the Glasgow Coma Scale helps to provide a more uniform, standard approach to defining CNS function (46). The Glasgow Coma Scale provides a measurement of visual, motor, and verbal (e.g., orientation) responsiveness (Table 25.3). The Glasgow Coma Scale can be used in intubated patients and is considered abnormal in critically ill patients with a score of less than 6 to 8 (maximal score = 15). Using these criteria, abnormalities of CNS function have been found to occur in 7% to 30% of critically ill patients. The factors that underlie CNS dysfunction in this patient population are unclear, but may include the production of false neurotransmitters, direct microvascular injury, and brain ischemia from global or regional reductions in cerebral blood flow (46,47).

Hematologic Failure

Hematologic abnormalities occur with a frequency that ranges from 0% to 26% among critically ill patients (31,38).

TABLE 25.3. GLASGOW COMA SCALE

Parameter	Score
Eye Opening	
Spontaneous	4
To speech	3
To pain	2
None	1
Motor Response	
Obeys verbal commands	6
Responds appropriately to painful stimuli (localizes pain)	5
Withdraws to pain	4
Decorticate posturing	3
Decerebrate posturing	2
No response	1
Verbal Responses	
Oriented and conversant	5
Disoriented but conversant	4
Inappropriate response	3
Incomprehensible sounds	2
No response	1

There is little clinical consensus regarding the definition of hematologic failure in this patient group. Several parameters, including the platelet count, the white blood cell count, fibrinogen levels, and coagulation parameters, have been used to assess the adequacy of the hematologic system in these patients. Despite some differences, most clinical studies employ criteria that include a platelet count less than or equal to 50,000 cells per μL, a white blood cell count less than or equal to 1,000 cells per μL, and a fibrinogen level below 100 mg per dL to define hematologic failure. Obviously, the presence of severe neutropenia decreases host resistance to infection, while thrombocytopenia increases the risk of bleeding and the need for transfusion of blood products. Disseminated intravascular coagulation is sometimes associated with acute lung injury (48).

Acute Respiratory Failure

The incidence of acute respiratory failure in critically ill patients varies considerably depending on the criteria used to define failure of the respiratory system. Although the term acute respiratory distress syndrome (ARDS) has been very useful for designating the clinical syndrome, a more quantitative definition is needed. A recent North American–European consensus conference proposed a simplified, uniform definition of acute lung injury and ARDS (49). Acute lung injury (ALI) is defined as a patient with a PaO_2/FiO_2 less than 300 with chest radiographic evidence of bilateral pulmonary infiltrates. Exclusion criteria include the presence of interstitial lung disease or left ventricular failure assessed by history, physical examination, or laboratory criteria. As previously noted, the role of right-heart catheterization in the management of patients with ARDS is controversial and will be the subject of an upcoming NIH-sponsored clinical trial. However, at the present time it appears prudent to recommend that a pulmonary arterial catheter be inserted only when it is clinically necessary to determine if the patient has a pulmonary arterial wedge pressure less than 18 mm Hg.

ARDS is defined with the same criteria as ALI except the PaO_2/FiO_2 ratio is less than 200. As such, the distinction between ALI and ARDS is based entirely on the severity of the gas exchange alterations. The clinical relevance of this distinction remains to be proven. Nonetheless, the notion that the distinction between ALI and ARDS may not be relevant was underscored by a recent study in which the overall mortality in medical patients with ALI was 58% and was identical to the mortality in the subset of these patients who had ARDS.

A quantitative scoring system for assessing ALI has also been used to evaluate the severity of lung injury (Table 25.4) (50). This system is based on the severity of hypoxemia and the extent of infiltrates on the chest radiograph. If the patient is mechanically ventilated, abnormalities in the compliance of the lungs and the level of positive end–expiratory pressure are also scored. Using these criteria, patients can be classified as having mild, moderate, or severe lung injury (50). Finally, newer definitions for diagnosis of ALI and ARDS may also be useful and are gaining acceptance (51) (see Chapter 23, Acute Hypoxemic Respiratory Failure: Pulmonary Edema and Acute Lung Injury).

Special Considerations

Although not unique to any particular organ system, a number of serious problems exist with respect to the MOF syndrome. Since there is a general lack of consensus regarding the criteria for individual organ system failure, the incidence of organ failure is variable among different study centers and contributes to the confusion in this area. Until uniform criteria are established, the true incidence and natural history of MOF will remain unclear. These problems are further compounded by the lack of uniform diagnostic criteria for the definition of septic shock and ALI. The net effect of this diagnostic imprecision is that patients with dissimilar critical illnesses are often inappropriately grouped together. However, a number of cooperative efforts have been undertaken to reach consensus on this issue and more precisely define the criteria for organ system failure in this patient group (52).

Despite the current uncertainties, several important issues regarding MOF among critically ill patients have been resolved. First, the number of involved organ systems impacts significantly on patient mortality (35). Mortality for a single organ failure ranges from 15% to 30%, and from 45% to 55% for failure of two organ systems. By contrast, mortality exceeds 80% when three or more organ systems

TABLE 25.4. COMPONENTS OF THE ACUTE LUNG INJURY SCORE

	Value
Chest Radiograph Score	
No alveolar consolidation	0
Alveolar consolidation in 1 quadrant	1
Alveolar consolidation in 2 quadrants	2
Alveolar consolidation in 3 quadrants	3
Alveolar consolidation in all 4 quadrants	4
Hypoxemia Score	
$PaO_2/FiO_2 \geq 300$	0
PaO_2/FiO_2 225–299	1
PaO_2/FiO_2 175–224	2
PaO_2/FiO_2 100–174	3
$PaO_2/FiO_2 < 100$	4
Respiratory System Compliance Score (When Ventilated)	
Compliance $\geq$ 80 mL/cm H_2O	0
Compliance 60–79 mL/cm H_2O	1
Compliance 40–59 mL/cm H_2O	2
Compliance 20–39 mL/cm H_2O	3
Compliance $\leq$ 19 mL/cm H_2O	4
Positive End–Expiratory Pressure (PEEP) Score (When Ventilated)	
PEEP $\leq$ 5 cm H_2O	0
PEEP 6–8 cm H_2O	1
PEEP 9–11 cm H_2O	2
PEEP 12–14 cm H_2O	3
PEEP $\geq$ 15 cm H_2O	4

The final value is obtained by dividing the aggregate sum by the number of components that were used.

	Score
No lung injury	0
Mild-to-moderate lung injury	0.1–2.5
Severe lung injury (ARDS)	>2.5

From Murray JF, Matthay MA, Luce J, et al. An expanded definition of the adult respiratory distress syndrome. *Am Rev Respir Dis* 1988; I38:720, with permission.)

have failed, and reaches 100% if the MOF persists beyond four hospital days (35). Second, certain organ systems (e.g., heart, kidney, lung, and liver) are involved more frequently than other organ systems. Third, although individual organs may be preferentially injured in specific situations (e.g., renal failure and respiratory failure in septic shock), MOF may occur after acute cardiorespiratory failure of any etiology. Finally, early detection and treatment of the underlying cause of the MOF may offer the best hope for treatment of this potentially fatal disorder (42,53,54).

Pathogenesis

The MOF syndrome occurs in a variety of clinical settings, including infection, severe hypotension, and multiple trauma. Prototypic among the risk factors for MOF is septic shock. Although a scientific consensus has yet to be established, there is evidence to suggest that MOF during sepsis,

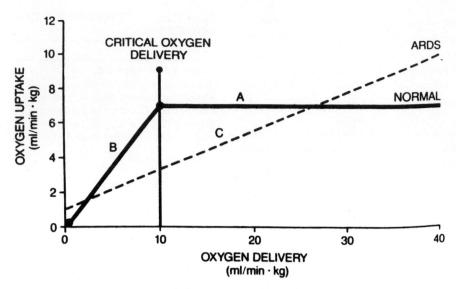

FIGURE 25.5. Oxygen uptake–oxygen delivery (VO_2-QO_2) relationships in normal subjects and in patients with ARDS. VO_2 is regulated by whole body metabolic demand and is normally constant over a wide range of QO_2. This is accomplished by local compensatory mechanisms, including increases in oxygen extraction and increases in the cross-sectional density of perfused capillaries. Once these compensatory mechanisms are exhausted, further reductions in QO_2 are accompanied by reductions in VO_2 (line B). The QO_2 below which VO_2 begins to decrease is termed the critical threshold for QO_2 (QO_{2c}). In contrast to the normal situation, VO_2 is dependent at nearly all levels of QO_2 in ARDS. This finding indicates that an oxygen supply-demand imbalance exists at all levels of QO_2 in ARDS patients. (Dorinsky PM, Gadek JE. Mechanisms of multiple nonpulmonary organ failure in ARDS. *Chest* 1989;96:885, with permission.)

and perhaps other critical illnesses, is due to widespread organ injury that is caused by activated inflammatory cells and a variety of humoral mediators (38,42,55,56). However, any theory regarding the pathogenesis of MOF during sepsis or other acute catastrophic illnesses must also take into account the abnormalities in systemic gas exchange that occur in these disorders and that are manifest as an abnormal relationship between oxygen uptake and oxygen delivery (QO_2).

As illustrated in Figure 25.5, whole-body oxygen uptake is normally maintained at a constant level over wide ranges of oxygen delivery (57). This is accomplished by means of local compensatory mechanisms, which include increases in oxygen extraction and increases in recruitable capillary reserves (e.g., the cross-sectional area of perfused capillaries within an individual organ). Once these mechanisms for the preservation of a constant oxygen uptake are exhausted, VO_2 falls in a manner that is directly related to the reductions in oxygen delivery. The level of oxygen delivery below which oxygen uptake begins to fall is termed QO_{2c} (i.e., critical threshold for oxygen delivery), and it signifies the level of QO_2 below which oxygen supply-demand imbalances exist (57,58).

In contrast to the situation described above for the normal VO_2/QO_2 relationship, the relationship between VO_2 and QO_2 in critically ill patients is often markedly altered

(59,60). For example, in many critically ill patients, VO_2 depends on QO_2 at nearly all levels of oxygen delivery, including levels that would normally be more than adequate to meet tissue metabolic demands. These abnormalities indicate that oxygen supply-demand imbalances exist at all levels of QO_2 in these patients.

In recent years, the concept that the VO_2-DO_2 relationship is altered in the critically ill patient has been challenged. In particular, whether VO_2 is calculated using the Fick equation [VO_2 = cardiac output $\times$ (A-VO_2 content difference)] or measured using a metabolic cart may affect whether or not an abnormal VO_2-DO_2 relationship is observed in these patients. The explanation for differences in measured versus calculated VO_2-DO_2 is not intuitively obvious. When both VO_2 and DO_2 are calculated, however, it is believed an artifactual mathematical coupling occurs because both VO_2 and DO_2 share the variables of cardiac output and arterial oxygen content. This problem may be avoided by measuring VO_2 directly, using a metabolic cart. However, an abnormal relationship between VO_2 and DO_2 can be observed whether or not VO_2 is measured using a metabolic cart or calculated using the Fick equation. As such, criticisms of the method by which VO_2 is determined do not negate the concept that VO_2-DO_2 relationships can be altered in the setting of sepsis or acute lung injury—a fact that has been well established experimentally. Rather, these observations underscore the notion that whole-body Vo_2-DO_2 relations in humans may be unreliable and that a better method for assessing oxygenation in individual tissues needs to be established.

There are several mechanisms that may explain both the nonpulmonary organ failure and the VO_2-QO_2 abnormalities that occur in this patient population. These may be divided into two broad categories: (a) altered blood flow distribution, and (b) endothelial or parenchymal injury (38).

Altered Blood Flow Distribution

Oxygenated blood that bypasses nutrient capillary beds could alter Vo_2-DO_2 relationships and cause organ damage. This sequence of events may result from: (a) a redistribution of cardiac output to organs with inherently low O_2 extraction fractions (e.g., skeletal muscle), (b) an increase in the fraction of cardiac output that bypasses nutrient capillaries through anatomic, precapillary arteriovenous channels (e.g., shunt flow), (c) local blood flow heterogeneities such that tissue oxygen supply and demand are imbalanced, or (d) a reduction in recruitable capillary reserves that would prevent effective compensation for reductions in oxygen supply (60).

Endothelial Or Parenchymal Injury

Endothelial injury may be accompanied by local edema formation, with subsequent increases in diffusion distances for oxygen or reductions in capillary surface area (e.g., reduced recruitable capillary reserves), or both. Alternatively, direct parenchymal cell injury may impair O_2 use at any level of oxygen delivery by impairing cellular oxidative metabolism.

Possible Mechanisms Of Injury

Little direct experimental evidence exists to support the idea that either MOF or the systemic VO_2-QO_2 alterations associated with ARDS, septic shock, and other critical illnesses are caused by primary alterations in the distribution of cardiac output (e.g., increased anatomic shunt flow or increased blood flow to organs with low oxygen extraction). However, there is evidence to indicate that nonpulmonary organs are damaged both structurally and functionally during critical illness, and this damage often includes alterations in individual organ VO_2-QO_2 matching (57–60).

The best studied experimental model for MOF has been septic shock that is produced either by live bacterial organisms or by endotoxin. In this context, structural studies of endothelial monolayers exposed to endotoxin show that these cells undergo contraction, become pyknotic, and finally die. Likewise, it is known that endotoxin or live bacteria can induce the release of various mediators, each of which can cause cell injury (56,61). Considerable experimental evidence indicates that both cyclooxygenase and lipoxygenase products of arachidonic acid metabolism participate in the hemodynamic, pathologic, and metabolic derangements that occur during sepsis. Also, complement is activated in sepsis, and there is some evidence to indicate that the elevated levels of a C5a derivative correlate with the severity of hypotension and metabolic acidosis during sepsis. There has also been considerable interest in the possible role of cytokines (e.g., TNF) in mediating systemic organ injury during sepsis (56,62). In this regard, antibodies to TNF are capable of preventing the development of endotoxin-mediated hypotension, fibrin deposition, and death in animals. Likewise, anti-TNF antibody prevented shock and death in baboons given live *Escherichia coli* organisms, but only if they were given two hours before the bacteremia (63). However, clinical studies using strategies to neutralize TNF-α in sepsis patients have not been effective (56).

Many studies (but not all) suggest a central role for neutrophils in mediating both the systemic and pulmonary injury from bacteria or endotoxin (42,51). Along this line, monoclonal antibodies to the adherence-promoting leukocyte glycoprotein complex (i.e., CD18) reduce systemic organ injury and improve survival from hemorrhagic shock in many species of animals. Although many schemes have been proposed to explain the mechanism by which neutrophils cause tissue injury, some work suggests that there may be important interactions between elastases and toxic oxygen radicals elaborated by neutrophils (56). Thus, in septic shock, endotoxin and bacteria may directly damage endothelial cells and promote the activation of polymorphonuclear leukocytes and mononuclear cells, as well as mediate the release of numerous proinflammatory agents (e.g., kinins, prostaglandins, complement, and monokines). Acting in concert, these events culminate in widespread organ injury.

Finally, evidence from several sources suggest there may also be a link between the organ injury that occurs during sepsis and other critical illnesses and the Vo_2-DO_2 alterations that occur in these settings. It has generally been presumed that the mechanism for the altered Vo_2-DO_2 relationships in these disorders is insufficient delivery of oxygen to metabolically active tissues. However, altered oxygen metabolism, especially during sepsis, cannot be totally accounted for by this proposed mechanism. This may explain the fact that several clinical trials have shown that augmentation of oxygen delivery in the setting of established sepsis or ALI failed to reduce mortality and, in some studies, actually increased mortality. This apparent clinical paradox may be reconciled by a hypothesis that proposes that both organ injury and Vo_2-DO_2 alterations during sepsis and other critical illnesses are the result of mitochondrial injury. Experimental data in support of this notion is increasing. However, future studies are needed to address more definitively the validity of this compelling hypothesis.

Management of the Patient with Multiple Organ Failure

Critically ill patients at risk for developing MOF generally present with one or more of the following clinical problems: shock (hypovolemic, cardiac, or septic), acute respiratory failure, or major alterations in mental status. These clinical problems initially require a prompt therapeutic response to stabilize the patient. In general, initial management is directed toward maintaining an adequate blood pressure and supporting gas exchange (24). For example, patients who present with hypovolemic shock, either from trauma or from gastrointestinal bleeding, require rapid intravascular volume expansion with blood. Likewise, patients who have severe alterations in mental status with failure to protect the airway and/or progressive respiratory failure require prompt endotracheal intubation and mechanical ventilation. It is important that the physician caring for critically ill patients recognize that the initial priority must be to stabilize the patient's circulatory and respiratory status. The decision, for example, to insert a pulmonary arterial catheter should not take precedence over initial management of the hypotension and respiratory failure (9,24). Once the patient is stabilized and appropriate support has been given to the circulatory and respiratory systems, a careful assessment of the likely cause of the patient's condition should be undertaken.

A logical starting point in the evaluation of critically ill patients is to search for the usual causes of shock, which include sepsis, cardiac failure (especially acute myocardial infarction), gastrointestinal bleeding, acute pancreatitis, drug overdose, and occult bleeding from recent trauma. One must always maintain a high index of suspicion for the presence of septicemia, however. There should be a low threshold for obtaining blood cultures and appropriate cultures of other possible sources of infection. In addition, patients with even presumptive evidence for infection should be promptly placed on broad-spectrum antibiotics. Given these general supportive measures, the remainder of this section is devoted to a discussion of specific issues related to support of the circulatory system.

Guidelines For Fluid And Blood Replacement

With the exception of patients with acute blood loss, for whom there is a need to transfuse blood to maintain the hematocrit between 25% and 30%, most patients also need crystalloid or colloid therapy (24). Most medical and surgical centers favor the use of crystalloid in preference to colloid for volume expansion. This preference is based, in part, on the fact that crystalloid, unlike colloid, can restore both the intravascular and the interstitial component of the extracellular fluid space. Some physicians do administer colloid in an attempt to maintain circulating plasma protein osmotic pressure, but large volumes of colloid are often needed to

achieve this objective, and the clearance of infused protein from the intravascular space is usually quite rapid (24). Despite the apparent advantages of crystalloid versus colloid, red blood cells remain the ideal volume expander because they have the advantage of both increasing oxygen transport to the tissues as well as maintaining intravascular volume. However, new evidence suggests that clinical criteria for transfusions in many critically ill patients have been higher than necessary. In one recent study, restrictive red cell transfusion criteria resulted in a better survival (64).

The appropriate guidelines for fluid therapy depend on the cause of the patient's shock. For the patient with an acute myocardial infarction, fluid replacement should be titrated to maintain the pulmonary arterial wedge pressure between 15 and 20 mm Hg. By contrast, for patients with hypovolemic shock, traumatic shock, or septic shock, an increase in the central venous pressure or pulmonary arterial wedge pressure to 15 to 20 mm Hg may not be optimal. For example, in one study that examined volume resuscitation in patients with septic shock, the investigators found that increases in pulmonary arterial wedge pressure beyond 11 to 12 mm Hg did not result in a higher cardiac output (24).

Ideally, optimal fluid resuscitation in any form of shock should include the restoration of euvolemia. Euvolemia is often difficult to define in critically ill patients. In addition, the adjustment of fluid therapy will depend on the use of vasoactive agents (24). Finally, although invasive hemodynamic monitoring with a pulmonary arterial catheter is frequently used to assist in the management of patients with septic shock, no evidence suggests that this kind of monitoring changes outcome (9,11). Given these uncertainties, the best indices for evaluating fluid replacement therapy are the patient's acid-base status, mental status, skin perfusion, and, perhaps most importantly, urine flow and renal function.

Vasoactive Agents

The most useful vasopressor for treating patients with septic shock may be dopamine (24). Dopamine improves cardiac output through a positive chronotropic effect, an increase in preload to the heart, and an increase in contractility. This agent is particularly efficacious in septic shock because it both increases cardiac output and improves blood flow to the kidneys when given at doses below 10 μg per kg per minute. Moreover, dopamine, in contrast to fluid replacement therapy, has the additional advantage of being able to increase cardiac output with only a small increase in pulmonary arterial wedge pressure (24). Finally, dopamine, unlike dobutamine, does not cause vasodilatation, thus making it preferable in treatment of shock caused by factors other than primary cardiac failure.

In some patients, septic shock will be unresponsive even to high doses of dopamine. In these patients, norepinephrine can be added to provide an increase in systemic arterial pressure. Epinephrine is another catecholamine that can be used for blood pressure support in severe septic shock. In doses of greater than 10 μg per minute, epinephrine causes primarily α-stimulation. High doses of any of these potent vasopressors will cause vasoconstriction that may maintain systemic blood pressure, but blood flow to the kidneys, the splanchnic bed, muscles, and skin may be markedly reduced.

It is often difficult to determine the level of mean arterial pressure or cardiac output that is optimal in septic shock. In general, it is best to try to adjust the mean arterial pressure and cardiac output to a level that stabilizes the metabolic acidosis associated with sepsis and improves tissue perfusion, particularly as indicated by urine flow. Some patients with severe septic shock will require high doses of dopamine, norepinephrine, and epinephrine to maintain even a barely adequate blood pressure. In most patients, vasodilator therapy is not appropriate in the setting of septic shock. In a minority of cases, patients with primary cardiac disease may present with hypotension and an elevation of systemic vascular resistance associated with septicemia. These patients may benefit from dobutamine and occasionally from low doses of afterload reduction with a vasodilator such as nitroprusside or nitroglycerin. With the exception of these patients, the use of vasodilators in the setting of multiple organ failure and septic shock remains experimental. There is no evidence that increasing cardiac output and oxygen delivery with fluids and vasoactive agents improves outcome in sepsis patients (65).

Antiinflammatory Agents

Large numbers of experimental animal model studies have demonstrated the potential value of various antiinflammatory agents for the treatment of septic shock. In many studies, however, the pharmacologic agents were effective only as prevention, not as treatment. In this regard, no antiinflammatory agents are clinically proven to decrease morbidity or improve mortality in patients with septicemia and MOF (56).

Corticosteroids were used for a number of years in the management of patients with septicemia and ARDS, based largely on the unproven clinical impression that they might be beneficial. In the past few years, however, a number of prospective well-controlled studies have demonstrated that corticosteroids are of no therapeutic value in patients with either ARDS or septic shock (51,56). Specifically, these clinical studies demonstrate that corticosteroids do not prevent the development of ARDS in patients with sepsis, nor do they prevent MOF, and they have no favorable effect on mortality (see Chapter 23, Acute Hypoxemic Respiratory Failure: Pulmonary Edema and Acute Lung Injury). Several agents are being evaluated in clinical trials currently, though none have yet been shown to be of clinical value (56).

Antibiotics

Selection of appropriate antibiotics for patients with septic shock and MOF is important. In general, a careful search for the likely source of sepsis should be undertaken and then appropriate broad-spectrum antibiotics administered. The antibiotic spectrum should include Gram-negative enteric bacteria as well as beta-lactamase producers. Effects of the agents on renal function should be considered and monitored.

Nutritional Support

Nutritional and metabolic support is an essential part of the management of patients with MOF. Hypermetabolism develops early in the syndrome, and severe malnutrition can become a prominent feature within days after the onset of illness. The characteristics of the hypermetabolic state include: (a) increases in resting energy expenditure and oxygen consumption, (b) increased use of carbohydrate, fat, and amino acids as energy substrates, and (c) increased loss of nitrogen in the urine. The hypermetabolic state results in profound protein catabolism, which is associated with a decrease in total-body protein synthesis. The mechanism for the alteration of metabolism observed in patients with multiple organ failure appears to be related to the inflammatory mediators and the hormonal response to injury. Unfortunately, these fundamental alterations in metabolism do not appear to be readily altered by therapy. However, if adequate nutritional support is not provided, then it is likely that organ dysfunction will be accelerated.

The goal of nutritional support in patients with or at risk for MOF is to prevent substrate-limited metabolism and to support, rather than attempt to alter, the hypermetabolism (see Chapter 20, Administrative, Nutritional, and Ethical Principles for the Management of Critically Ill Patients, for detailed discussion of nutritional support). In general, nutrition should be provided by the enteral route whenever possible. Enteral feedings eliminate cholestasis and reduce the risk of acalculous cholecystitis. Enteral alimentation may also offer some protection against gastrointestinal hemorrhage in mechanically ventilated patients.

Ethical Support

It is important for physicians to assess carefully the likelihood of meaningful recovery in each critically ill patient with MOF. This assessment will depend on the natural history of the patient's underlying disease, as well as on the extent and severity of his or her organ failure. There is a growing awareness among the medical community that reasonable limits should be exercised by physicians and patients' families in supporting patients with critical illnesses and MOF. Studies have demonstrated that some patient groups have a particularly poor prognosis for recovery. For example, patients with ARDS following bone marrow transplantation have a less than 10% chance for recovery, while patients with a combination of hepatic failure and acute lung injury have a nearly 100% mortality. In addition, one study in two intensive care units at the University of California Medical Center has shown that withdrawal of life support was the mechanism for death in about 50% of patients in the intensive care unit setting (66). As more information becomes available regarding prognostic indices for specific disease processes, it may help guide decisions to discontinue life support in patients who do not have a reasonable chance for meaningful recovery. See Chapter 20, Administrative, Nutritional, and Ethical Principles for the Management of Critically Ill Patients, for more discussion of ethical issues.

Early Recognition and Prevention of Multiple Organ Failure

Early Recognition

Several studies have been published that identify patients who are at the highest risk for developing MOF. Patients with multiple trauma and hypotension who require emergency surgery and multiple transfusions are one common group of patients at high risk. Other patients considered to be at high risk for the development of MOF include patients with septic shock, patients with advanced chronic diseases (e.g., chronic liver disease or chronic renal failure) who are hospitalized for cardiac failure or a primary infection, and patients with the acquired immunodeficiency syndrome. Finally, patients who are immunosuppressed due to an underlying malignancy or its treatment may be at particularly high risk for MOF, both from the toxic effects of the chemotherapy as well as the increased susceptibility to septicemia.

Some investigators have evaluated clinical factors as well as easily measurable plasma factors that might predict which patients with nonpulmonary sepsis syndrome would progress to develop ALI. In one study, the possible value of a product of endothelial cells for predicting ALI was studied (34). This study was based on the premise that endothelial cell injury is a ubiquitous early event in the pathogenesis of sepsis. In this regard, several *in vitro* and *in vivo* studies have shown that both pulmonary and systemic endothelial cell injury occurs during endotoxemia and septicemia. The investigators measured plasma levels of von Willebrand factor–antigen (VWF-Ag) because VWF-Ag has been shown to be released from endothelial cells *in vitro* when they are injured, and because two prior clinical studies demonstrated that plasma von Willebrand antigen levels are markedly elevated in patients with established acute respiratory failure. In this study, plasma von Willebrand antigen levels were increased twofold in patients with nonpulmonary sepsis who subsequently developed ALI compared with patients with nonpulmonary sepsis who did not progress to develop ALI. Moreover, of the 15 patients who developed

ALI from sepsis, 14 patients died (93% mortality). An elevated von Willebrand antigen level above 450 (percentage of control) was predictive of the development of acute lung injury (87% sensitivity, 77% specificity) and had a positive predictive value of 80% for identifying septic patients who were not likely to survive. Subsequent studies have explored the predictive value of several biologic markers, many of which have some pathogenetic and prognostic value (67,68).

More studies are needed to combine clinical factors and readily measurable plasma factors to identify those patients with sepsis syndrome who have the greatest risk of developing ALI and not surviving. These patients might be reasonable candidates for early treatment with immunotherapy, antiinflammatory agents, and other new treatments that may become available in the future. Unfortunately, a recent study testing administration of human growth hormone to critically ill patients had a deleterious effect on outcome, perhaps because of an adverse effect on host defense against infection (69).

Prevention

There has been a growing interest in various approaches to reducing the risk of MOF, particularly because the outcome is so poor once a patient develops MOF. Although specific treatment approaches have yet to be established, a number of general supportive measures are available. Perhaps the most important supportive measure is prevention of infection. Nosocomial infection can be reduced by good hand washing, removal of unnecessary intravascular and urinary catheters, and the prevention of skin ulcers. See Chapter 26, Prevention of Nonpulmonary Complications of Intensive Care, for a more complete discussion of these issues.

REFERENCES

1. Wiedemann HP, Matthay MA, Matthay RA. Cardiovascular-pulmonary monitoring in the intensive care unit. *Chest* 1984;85: 537–549[Part I],656–668[Part II].
2. Band JD, Maki DG. Infections caused by arterial catheters used for hemodynamic monitoring. *Am J Med* 1979;67:735–741.
3. Shinozaki T, Deane RS, Mazuzan JEJ Jr, et al. Bacterial contamination of arterial lines: a prospective study. *JAMA* 1983;249: 223–227.
4. Shapiro BA. Monitoring gas exchange in acute respiratory failure. *Respir Care* 1983;28:605–607.
5. Gardner RM, Schwartz R, Wong HC, et al. Percutaneous indwelling radial-artery catheters for monitoring cardiovascular function. *N Engl J Med* 1974;290:1227–1231.
6. Bedford RF. Long-term radial artery cannulation: effects on subsequent vessel function. *Crit Care Med* 1978;6:64–67.
7. Bedford RF. Radial arterial function following percutaneous cannulation with 18- and 20-gauge catheters. *Anesthesiology* 1977; 47:37–39.
8. Davis FM, Stewart JM. Radial artery cannulation. *Br J Anaesth* 1980;52:41–47.
9. Matthay MA, Chatterjee K. Bedside catheterization of the pul-

monary artery: risks compared with benefits. *Ann Intern Med* 1988;109:826–834.

10. Robin ED. The cult of the Swan-Ganz catheter: overuse and abuse of pulmonary flow catheters. *Ann Intern Med* 1985;103: 445–449.

11. Connors AF, Speroff T, Dawson NV, et al. The effectiveness of right heart catheterization in the initial care of critically ill patients. *JAMA* 1990;264:2928–2932.

12. Matthay MA. Invasive hemodynamic monitoring. *Clin Chest Med* 1983;4:233–249.

13. Quinn K, Quebbeman EJ. Pulmonary artery pressure, monitoring in the surgical intensive care unit. *Arch Surg* 1981;116: 872–876.

14. O'Quinn R, Marini JJ. Pulmonary artery occlusion pressure: clinical physiology measurement, and interpretation. *Am Rev Respir Dis* 1983;128:319–326.

15. Dhainault JF, Devaux J, Monsallier J. Mechanisms of decreased left ventricular preload during continuous positive pressure ventilation in ARDS. *Chest* 1986;90:74–80.

16. Jardin F, Farcot JC, Boisante L, et al. Influence of positive end–expiratory pressure on left ventricular performance. *N Engl J Med* 1981;304:387–392.

17. Tooker J, Huseby J, Butler J. The effect of Swan-Ganz catheter height on the wedge pressure relationship in edema during positive pressure ventilation. *Am Rev Respir Dis* 1978;117:721–725.

18. Marini JJ. Obtaining meaningful data from the Swan-Ganz catheter. *Respir Care* 1985;30:572–578.

19. Al-Kharrat T, Zarich S, Amoateng-Adjepong Y, et al. Analysis of observer variability in measurement of pulmonary artery occlusion pressures. *Am J Respir Crit Care Med* 1999;160:415–420.

20. Fein A, Goldberg S, Walhenstein M, et al. Is pulmonary artery catheterization necessary for the diagnosis of pulmonary edema? *Am Rev Respir Dis* 1984;129:1006–1009.

21. Chatterjee K, Swan HJ, Kaushik VS, et al. Effects of vasodilator therapy for severe pump failure in acute myocardial infarction on short-term and late prognosis. *Circulation* 1976;53:797–802.

22. Aberle DR. Hydrostatic versus increased permeability pulmonary edema: diagnosis based on radiographic criteria in critically ill patients. *Radiology* 1988;168:73–79.

23. Connors AF Jr, McCaffree DR, Gray BA. Evaluation of right-heart catheterization in the critically ill patient without acute myocardial infarction. *N Engl J Med* 1983;308:263–267.

24. Matthay MA, Broaddus VC. Fluid and hemodynamic management in acute lung injury. *Semin Respir Med* 1994;15:271–288.

25. Matthay MA, Eschenbacher WL, Goetzl EJ. Elevated concentrations of leukotriene D, in pulmonary edema fluid of patients with the adult respiratory distress syndrome. *J Clin Immunol* 1984;4:479–483.

26. Rinaldo JE. Indicators of risk, course, and prognosis in adult respiratory distress syndrome. *Annu Rev Respir Dis* 1986;133: 343–346.

27. Swan HJ, Ganz TW, Forrester J, et al. Catheterization of the heart in man with the use of a flow-directed balloon-tipped catheter. *N Engl J Med* 1970;283:447–451.

28. Hansen RM, Viquerat CE, Matthay MA, et al. Poor correlation between pulmonary arterial wedge pressure and left ventricular end-diastolic volume after coronary artery bypass surgery. *Anesthesiology* 1986;64:764–770.

29. Hall JB, Schmidt GA, Wood LDH, eds. *Principles of critical care*, New York: McGraw-Hill, Inc., 1992:1393–1395.

30. Tobin, MJ. *Principles and practice of intensive care monitoring*, New York: McGraw-Hill, Inc., 1998.

31. Dorinsky PM, Matthay MA. Management of the critically ill patient with multiple organ failure. In: Kelley WN, ed. *Textbook of internal medicine*, 2nd ed. Philadelphia: JR Lippincott Co., 1992:1850–1856.

32. Baue AE. Multiple, progressive, or sequential systems failure. *Arch Surg* 1975;110:779–781.

33. Bell RC, Coalson J, Smith JD, et al. Multiple organ failure and infection in adult respiratory distress syndrome. *Ann Intern Med* 1983;99:293–298.

34. Rubin DB, Wiener-Kronish JP, Murray JF, et al. Elevated von Willebrand factor antigen is an early plasma predictor of impending acute lung injury and death in non-pulmonary sepsis syndrome. *J Clin Invest* 1990;86:474–80.

35. Knaus WA, Wagner DP. Multiple systems organ failure: epidemiology and prognosis. *Crit Care Clin* 5(2):221–232, 1989.

36. Montgomery AB, Stager MA, Carrico CJ, et al. Causes of mortality in patients with the adult respiratory distress syndrome. *Am Rev Respir Dis* 1985;132:485–489.

37. Parillo JE, Parker MM, Natanson C, et al. Septic shock in humans. *Ann Int Med* 1990;113:227–242.

38. Dorinsky PM, Gadek JE. Mechanisms of multiple nonpulmonary organ failure in ARDS. *Chest* 1989;96:885–892.

39. Connors AF, Speroff T, Dawson NV, et al. The effectiveness of right heart catheterization in the initial care of critcally ill patients. *JAMA* 1996;276:889–897.

40. Kramar S, Khan F, Patel S, et al. Renal failure in the respiratory intensive care unit. *Crit Care Med* 1979;7:263–266.

41. Graber M, Chestnutt M. Acute renal failure and electrolyte disturbances in the intensive care unit. In: Matthay MA, Schwartz DE, eds. *Complications in the intensive care unit*. New York: Chapman and Hall, 1997:228–265.

42. St John RC, Dorinsky PM. Immunologic therapy for ARDS, septic shock and multiple organ failure. *Chest* 1993;103: 932–943.

43. Harris SK, Bone RC, Ruth WE. Gastrointestinal hemorrhage in a respiratory intensive care unit. *Chest* 1977;72:301–04.

44. Doig CJ, Sutherland LR, Sandham JD, et al. Increased intestinal permeability is associated with the development of multiple organ dysfunction syndrome in critically ill ICU patients. *Am J Respir Crit Care Med* 1998;158:444–451.

45. Schwartz DB, Bone RC, Balk RA, et al. Hepatic dysfunction in the adult respiratory distress syndrome. *Chest* 1989;95:871–875.

46. Prough DS, ed. Neurologic critical care. In: *Critical care clinics*, Vol. 5. Philadelphia: WB Saunders & Co, 1989.

47. Kelly BJ, Nicholau DK. Neurologic complications of intensive care medicine. In: Matthay MA, Schwartz DE, eds. *Complications in the intensive care unit*. New York: Chapman and Hall, 1997; 291–316.

48. Bone RC, Francis PB, Pierce AK. Intravascular coagulation associated with the adult respiratory distress syndrome. *Am J Med* 1976;61:585–589.

49. Artigas A, Bernard GR, Carlet J, et al. The American-European Consensus Conference on ARDS, Part 2. *Am J Respir Crit Care Med* 1998;157:1332–1347.

50. Murray JF, Matthay MA, Luce J, et al. An expanded definition of the adult respiratory distress syndrome. *Am Rev Respir Dis* 1988;138:720–723.

51. Ware LB, Matthay MA. Acute respiratory distress syndrome. *N Engl J Med* 2000;342:1334–1349.

52. Bone RC, Balk RA, Cerraf B, et al. Definitions for sepsis and organ failure and guidelines for the use of innovative therapies in sepsis. *Chest* 1992;101:1644–1655.

53. Macho JR, Luce JM. Rational approach to the management of multiple systems organ failure. *Crit Care Clin* 1989;5:379–392.

54. Pinsky MR, Matuschak GM, eds. Multiple systems organ failure. In: *Critical care clinics*, Vol. 5. Philadelphia: WB Saunders, 1989.

55. Goris RJA, Boekhorst TPA, Nuytinck JKS, et al. Multiple-organ failure: generalized autodestructive inflammation? *Arch Surg* 1985;120:1109–1115.

56. Wheeler AP, Bernard G. Treating patients with severe sepsis. *N Engl J Med* 1999;340:207–214.

57. Cain SM. Assessment of tissue oxygenation. *Crit Care Clin* 1986;2:537–550.

58. Cain SM. Oxygen delivery and uptake in dogs during anemic and hypoxic hypoxia. *J Appl Physiol* 1977;42:228–234.

59. Danek SJ, Lynch JP, Weg JG, et al. The dependence of oxygen uptake on oxygen delivery in the adult respiratory distress syndrome. *Am Rev Respir Dis* 1980;122:387–395.

60. Dorinsky PM, Costello JL, Gadek JE. Oxygen uptake–oxygen delivery relationship in non-ARDS respiratory failure. *Chest* 1988;93:103–111.

61. Baumgartner JD, Glauser MP, McCutchan JA, et al. Prevention of gram-negative shock and death in surgical patients by antibody to endotoxin core glycolipid. *Lancet* 1985;2:59–63.

62. Tracey KJ, Beutler B, Lowry SF, et al. Shock and tissue injury induced by recombinant human cachectin. *Science* 1986;234:470–474.

63. Tracey KJ, Fong Y, Hesse DG, et al. Anti-cachectin/TNF monoclonal antibodies prevent septic shock during lethal bacteraemia. *Nature* 1987;330:662–664.

64. Herbert P, Wells G, Blajchmann M, et al. A multicenter randomized controlled clinical trial of transfusion requirements in critical care. *N Engl J Med* 1999;340:409–417.

65. Gattinoni L, Brazzi L, Pelosi P, et al. A trial of goal-oriented hemodynamics in critically ill patients. *N Engl J Med* 1995;333:1025–1032.

66. Smedira N, Evans B, Grais L, et al. Withholding and withdrawing of life support from the critically ill. *N Engl J Med* 1990;1990;332:309–315.

67. Pittet JF, Mackersie RC, Martin TR, et al. Biological markers of acute lung injury: prognostic and pathogenetic significance. *Am J Respir Crit Care Med* 1997;155:1187–1205.

68. Parsons PE, Moss M. Early detection and markers of sepsis. *Clin Chest Med* 1996;17:199–212.

69. Takala J, Ruokonen E, Webster N, et al. Increased mortality associated with growth hormone treatment in critically ill adults. *N Engl J Med* 1999;341:705–792.

PREVENTION OF NONPULMONARY COMPLICATIONS OF INTENSIVE CARE

MARK D. EISNER
MICHAEL A. MATTHAY
SANJAY SAINT

INTRODUCTION

VENOUS THROMBOEMBOLISM
Prevalence and Risk Factors
Prevention
Recommendations

STRESS-RELATED UPPER GASTROINTESTINAL BLEEDING
Risk Factors
Prevention
Recommendations

VASCULAR CATHETER–RELATED INFECTION
Types of Infection
Risk Factors
Prevention
Recommendations

URINARY CATHETER–RELATED INFECTION
Risk Factors
Prevention
Recommendations

CONCLUSIONS

INTRODUCTION

As previously described in this critical care section, sophisticated supportive care is provided to critically ill medical and surgical patients in the intensive care unit (ICU) setting. A variety of invasive interventions occur, such as endotracheal intubation, mechanical ventilation, and central venous catheterization. As a result, patients may develop new medical problems resulting from intensive care. ICU-acquired infection, for instance, affects about 20% of critically ill patients and confers excess risk of mortality (1).

This chapter reviews four common, life-threatening, nonpulmonary complications of intensive care: venous thromboembolism, stress-related gastrointestinal bleeding, vascular catheter-related infection, and urinary catheter-related infection. For each complication, we review preventive strategies designed to reduce the risk posed to critically ill patients. We provide evidence-based recommendations for preventing these common ICU-related complications.

VENOUS THROMBOEMBOLISM

Hospitalized patients, especially those who are critically ill, are at risk for venous thromboembolism (2,3). Both deep venous thrombosis and pulmonary embolism are difficult to diagnose, presenting with nonspecific clinical manifestations (3,4). Pulmonary embolism, in particular, confers a substantial risk of mortality (10%) (4). Because of the silent and potentially lethal nature of this complication, prevention is paramount (5). Screening high risk patients is insensitive, impractical, and less cost-effective than preventive strategies (6–10).

Prevalence and Risk Factors

Critically ill patients often have risk factors for venous thromboembolism (Table 26.1). Although ICU patients have heterogeneous illnesses, they often have advanced age, malignancy, or prolonged immobility. Similarly, trauma and postoperative surgical patients are commonly encountered. As a result, the prevalence of venous thromboembolism is substantial in ICU patients (Table 26.2).

Although fewer studies have examined deep venous thrombosis in critically ill medical patients, numerous studies have documented a high prevalence in general surgical (25%) and trauma (51%) patients (11). In the few studies conducted in medical ICUs, about one-third of patients had documented deep venous thrombosis (12,13). Compared with medical ward patients, the risk of deep venous thrombosis was about threefold higher among ICU patients (12).

TABLE 26.1. RISK FACTORS FOR VENOUS THROMBOEMBOLISM

Age over 40 years
Previous venous thromboembolism
Malignancy
Obesity
Prolonged immobility or paralysis
Major surgery (abdomen, pelvis, lower extremity)
Congestive heart failure
Acute myocardial infarction
Stroke
Fracture (pelvic, hip, or leg)
Estrogen replacement therapy
Hypercoagulable states

Adapted from Saint SS, Matthay MA. Risk reduction in the intensive care unit. *Am J Med* 1998;105:515–523, with permission.

Prevention

Because pulmonary embolism is life-threatening, prevention of deep venous thrombosis is widely recommended for hospitalized patients (5). Some experts advocate prophylaxis for virtually all hospitalized patients (10). Although few studies have examined critically ill medical patients, the efficacy of venous thromboembolism prophylaxis has been well established in general surgical patients (5). A recent review of 70 randomized controlled clinical trials demonstrated a reduction of deep venous thrombosis from 25% in untreated controls to 7% to 8% in those receiving either unfractionated or low-molecular-weight heparin (11,14). Furthermore, these studies found a 50% reduction in fatal pulmonary embolism with heparin prophylaxis. Among general surgery patients, unfractionated and low-molecular-weight heparin appear equally effective (15,16). Intermittent pneumatic compression also reduces the risk of deep venous thrombosis by 50% (11). In higher-risk surgical pro-

TABLE 26.2. PREVALENCE OF VENOUS THROMBOEMBOLISM IN HOSPITALIZED PATIENTS

Patient Group	Deep Venous Thrombosis (%)	Pulmonary Embolism (%)
General surgery	25%	1.6%
Trauma	51%	0.5–2.0%
Ischemic stroke	63%	0.8%
Myocardial infarction	24%	N/A
Other medical conditions	9.1–26%	N/A
Medical ICU	29–33%	N/A

Data are summarized from the American College of Chest Physicians Consensus Conference. Clagett GP, Anderson FA, Geerts W, et al. Prevention of venous thromboembolism. *Chest* 1998; 114:531S–560S, with permission.
Prevalence for medical ICU patients is also derived from Hirsch DR, Ingenito EP, Goldhaber SZ. Prevalence of deep venous thrombosis among patients in medical intensive care. *JAMA* 1995;274:335–337, with permission.

cedures, especially orthopedic surgery involving total hip or knee replacement, low-molecular-weight heparin is more efficacious than low-dose unfractionated heparin (11). In postoperative patients, then, venous thromboembolism prophylaxis is clearly warranted.

Although less extensive, the available evidence supports preventive strategies targeted at venous thromboembolism in critically ill medical patients. The commonly employed prophylactic measures include low-dose unfractionated heparin, low-molecular-weight heparin, and intermittent pneumatic compression of the lower extremities.

Low-dose unfractionated heparin, usually administered in doses of 5,000 to 7,500 U every eight to twelve hours by subcutaneous injection, reduces the incidence of deep venous thrombosis in patients with myocardial infarction (17–19) and ischemic stroke (20,21). Fewer trials have assessed efficacy in other medical patients. In a randomized trial enrolling patients with congestive heart failure or respiratory infection, preventive treatment with low-dose unfractionated heparin (5,000 units SQ every eight hours) reduced the incidence of deep venous thrombosis from 26% to 4% (22). Only one randomized clinical trial examined venous thromboembolism in critically ill ICU patients, comparing low-dose unfractionated heparin (5,000 units SQ every 12 hours) with placebo (12). Investigators found a substantial reduction of deep venous thrombosis in patients receiving heparin (13%) compared to placebo (29%).

Nonrandomized studies have examined the impact of preventive therapy on pulmonary embolism and death. In a retrospective review of patients admitted to a respiratory intensive care unit, low-dose unfractionated heparin was associated with a reduced incidence of pulmonary embolism (23). Among 1,358 general medical ward patients nonrandomly assigned to low-dose unfractionated heparin or no prophylaxis, heparin treatment reduced mortality from 10.9% to 7.8% (24). Recently, an unblinded multicenter trial enrolling 11,693 subjects hospitalized with infectious diseases found that low-dose heparin reduced the incidence of nonfatal pulmonary embolism (25). There was, however, no significant difference in the risk of fatal pulmonary embolism or death (25). Taken together, the available evidence indicates that low-dose unfractionated heparin reduces the risk of deep venous thrombosis and pulmonary embolism in critically ill medical patients.

Although low-molecular-weight heparin is more efficacious than unfractionated heparin in orthopedic surgery, trauma, and high-risk general surgery patients (5,11,26–31), few trials have evaluated this agent in medical patients. In a randomized controlled trial of 270 hospitalized medical patients, low-molecular-weight heparin (enoxaparin 60 mg SQ daily) reduced the incidence of deep venous thrombosis threefold compared with placebo (9.1% versus 3.0%) (32). The risk of injection-site hematoma, however, was significantly increased in the low-molecular-weight heparin–treated group (32). Only two randomized controlled trials compared low-molecular-weight heparin with low-dose unfractionated heparin in hospitalized medical patients (33,34). A multicenter randomized trial of 442 elderly medical inpatients found no difference in the rate of venous thromboembolism between low-molecular-weight heparin (enoxaparin 20 mg SQ daily) and low-dose unfractionated heparin (5,000 units SQ twice daily) (4.8% versus 4.6%, respectively) (34). Similarly, another randomized trial of 166 hospitalized medical patients found no difference in the incidence of deep venous thrombosis between groups treated with low-molecular-weight heparin and low-dose unfractionated heparin (33).

Because randomized clinical trial data are scant, the relative efficacy of low-molecular-weight and unfractionated heparin remains uncertain among critically ill medical patients. In critically ill surgical or trauma patients, low-molecular-weight heparin is the superior strategy (11,35). Although it may be reasonable to generalize low-molecular-weight heparin data to medical ICU patients, further trials are necessary before conclusive recommendations can be provided.

Intermittent pneumatic compression has been extensively studied in surgical patients. In patients undergoing a variety of surgical procedures—general, neurological, orthopedic, cardiac, gynecological, and urologic surgery—pneumatic compression reduces the risk of venous thromboembolism (11,36–38). For example, five randomized clinical trials conducted in general surgical patients demonstrated a 60% reduction in the risk of deep venous thrombosis (11). Although we identified no randomized trials of intermittent pneumatic compression in medical patients, this strategy is likely to be efficacious. In critically ill medical patients with a contraindication to heparin, pneumatic compression may be the preferred preventive strategy.

Bleeding is a potentially important adverse effect of heparin. Evidence from surgical patients, however, indicates that both forms of heparin are relatively safe. No increase in major bleeding due to low-dose unfractionated heparin has been observed in individual trials, but two meta-analyses (39,40) found a statistically significant absolute increase (2%) in minor bleeding episodes (e.g., wound hematomas). Compared with low-dose unfractionated heparin, low-molecular-weight heparin probably causes less major and minor bleeding (27,41,42). In critically ill medical patients, the benefit of venous thromboembolism prophylaxis appears to outweigh the small excess of minor bleeding episodes.

Another potential risk is heparin-induced thrombocytopenia, an IgG-mediated effect associated with thrombotic complications (42). A recent randomized trial (43) in patients undergoing hip surgery found that low-molecular-weight heparin had a significantly lower incidence of heparin-induced thrombocytopenia than low-dose unfractionated heparin (0% versus 2.7%). Other trials have also demonstrated an approximately 3% incidence of heparin-induced thrombocytopenia in patients given low-dose unfractionated heparin (42).

Recommendations

1. Most critically ill patients are at moderate to high risk for venous thromboembolism and warrant prophylaxis.
2. Low-dose unfractionated heparin and low-molecular-weight heparin are probably both efficacious agents in critically ill medical patients. Although low-molecular-weight heparin is more effective in critically ill surgical and trauma patients, the preferred heparin strategy is uncertain among medical ICU patients.
3. Intermittent pneumatic compression has not been studied in critically ill medical patients, but may be the preferred strategy in patients at high risk of bleeding.

STRESS-RELATED UPPER GASTROINTESTINAL BLEEDING

Gastrointestinal bleeding is a well recognized complication in critically ill patients (44). Most of such bleeding results from stress ulceration of gastric or duodenal mucosa (45). Recent data indicates that gastrointestinal ulceration during critical illness is distinct in etiology from peptic ulcer disease presenting in ambulatory patients (44). In particular, critically ill patients with gastrointestinal ulceration have a lower prevalence of *Helicobacter pylori* infection and nonsteroidal antiinflammatory (NSAID) medication use than ambulatory patients with ulcer bleeding. Furthermore, hospitalized patients who develop gastrointestinal bleeding have worse outcomes than ambulatory patients, with higher transfusion requirements, rate of rebleeding, and duration of hospital stay (44). Mortality is also greater among hospitalized patients who develop gastrointestinal bleeding (25% to 50%) (46–48), compared with ambulatory patients (5% to 10%) (46,49). Because the morbidity and mortality from gastrointestinal hemorrhage in critically ill patients is substantial, many investigators have examined preventive strategies.

In critically ill patients, Cook and colleagues have proposed the following classification scheme (48). *Overt bleeding* is defined as hematemesis, gross blood or "coffee grounds" material in a nasogastric aspirate, hematochezia, or melena. *Clinically important* bleeding is overt bleeding complicated by any of the following within 24 hours: a spontaneous decrease in systolic blood pressure of more than 20 mm Hg; an increase in heart rate by at least 20 beats per minute or a decrease in systolic blood pressure of 10 mm Hg sitting upright; or a decrease in hemoglobin level by more than 2 g per dL.

Risk Factors

In modern intensive care units, a significant minority (less than 5%) of critically ill patients develop overt gastrointestinal bleeding (44,48,50). Patients who bleed, however, have a 12.5% excess mortality (50). As a result, investigators have attempted to define patient subgroups at higher risk of gastrointestinal bleeding. In a study of 179 critically ill medical patients, Schuster and colleagues (51) found that 14% had evidence of either occult or overt bleeding. Mechanical ventilation and the presence of a coagulopathy (defined as a platelet count less than 50,000 per mm^3 or a prolonged prothrombin or partial thromboplastin time) were independent risk factors for gastrointestinal bleeding (51). This result was confirmed in a larger prospective cohort study of 2,252 critically ill medical and surgical patients (48). Although 30% of patients received prophylaxis, investigators found a 4.2% incidence of overt bleeding and 1.5% clinically important bleeding. As before, respiratory failure requiring mechanical ventilation (for more than 48 hours) and coagulopathy were the only independent risk factors for gastrointestinal bleeding (48). Importantly, the presence of coagulopathy or mechanical ventilation identified nearly all patients who developed clinically important bleeding, with only 0.1% of the cases occurring among those with neither risk factor. Based on other studies, additional high-risk groups include surgical patients with extensive burns and those with head or multiple traumatic injuries (52).

Prevention

Because gastrointestinal bleeding is associated with increased mortality (53), investigators have developed preventive strategies for critically ill patients. These techniques include prophylaxis with histamine H_2-receptor antagonists, sucralfate, or antacids (48,54). Multiple randomized trials and four meta-analyses have addressed the prevention of stress ulceration (55–58). When assessing these studies, the impact of prophylaxis on three clinical outcomes must be considered. First, the rate of clinically important gastrointestinal bleeding, the target of prevention. Second, the incidence of nosocomial pneumonia. Many studies indicate that H_2-receptor antagonists and antacids may increase the probability of gastric bacterial colonization and late-onset nosocomial pneumonia (54,59–61). In particular, the risk of nosocomial pneumonia may be highest among patients who are mechanically ventilated longer than four days and are receiving H_2-receptor antagonist prophylaxis (60). Sucralfate, primarily a cytoprotective agent, may not have this disadvantage (54,59,62) and may have limited antibacterial activity (55,59,63). Third must be considered the impact of prophylaxis on mortality, which reflects the effects on both gastro-intestinal bleeding and nosocomial pneumonia.

Although many randomized controlled trials have been published, the clinical benefit of stress ulcer prophylaxis remains uncertain (44,55–58). A recent meta-analysis attempted to summarize prior clinical trials and meta-analyses, resolving discrepancies between these studies (56) (Table 26.3). Compared to placebo, H_2-receptor antagonists substantially reduce the incidence of clinically impor-

TABLE 26.3. COMPARISON OF RANDOMIZED TRIALS OF STRESS-RELATED UPPER GASTROINTESTINAL BLEEDING

Comparison	Number of trials	Pooled Odds Ratio (95% Confidence Interval)
H_2-receptor Antagonists versus Control/Placebo		
Clinically important bleeding	10	0.44 (0.22–0.88)
Pneumonia	8	1.25 (0.78–2.00)
Mortality	15	1.15 (0.86–1.53)
Sucralfate versus Control/Placebo		
Clinically important bleeding	1	1.26 (0.12–12.87)
Pneumonia	2	2.11 (0.82–5.44)
Mortality	4	1.06 (0.67–1.67)
Sucralfate vs H_2-receptor Antagonists		
Clinically important bleeding	4	1.28 (0.27–6.11)
Pneumonia	11	0.78 (0.60–1.01)
Mortality	11	0.83 (0.62–1.09)

Adapted from Cook DJ, Reeve BK, Guyatt GH, et al. Stress ulcer prophylaxis in critically ill patients. Resolving discordant meta-analyses. *JAMA* 1996;275(4):308–314, with permission.

tant gastrointestinal bleeding. However, H_2-receptor antagonists were associated with a trend toward higher rates of pneumonia and death. Fewer trials have compared sucralfate to placebo. Compared to placebo, sucralfate was not effective in reducing clinically important gastrointestinal bleeding. Also, sucralfate use may have increased the risk of nosocomial pneumonia. Finally, randomized trials have compared sucralfate to H_2-receptor antagonists. According to the most recent meta-analysis (56), there was no significant difference in gastrointestinal bleeding between sucralfate- and H_2-receptor antagonist–treated patients. However, a more recent randomized trial of 1,200 critically ill mechanically ventilated patients demonstrated that ranitidine reduced the risk of clinically important gastrointestinal bleeding compared to sucralfate (RR 0.44, 95% CI 0.21 to 0.92) (50). Ranitidine-treated patients had an 18% increased risk of ventilator-associated pneumonia, although the confidence interval did not exclude no effect (RR 1.18, 95% CI 0.92 to 1.51). There was no difference in mortality between the two treatment groups. Despite the relatively large sample size and excellent methodology, this trial may have been underpowered to detect a clinically important difference in nosocomial pneumonia, as suggested by the wide confidence interval. In fact, the data are compatible with a 51% increased risk of ventilator-associated pneumonia in those randomized to ranitidine (50).

Based on the available data, the decision to institute preventive therapy for gastrointestinal bleeding is complex. Unfortunately, the most effective agents for preventing gastrointestinal bleeding (H$_2$-receptor antagonists) are also associated with a greater risk of nosocomial pneumonia. Although sucralfate may carry a lower risk of pneumonia, clinical trials have not established its efficacy compared to placebo. Neither agent has an established mortality benefit.

Because the risk of clinically important gastrointestinal bleeding is low (0.1%) in patients without mechanical ventilation or coagulopathy, preventive therapy is usually not indicated. If prophylaxis is selected in higher risk patients, the choice between H$_2$-receptor antagonists and sucralfate should depend on the anticipated duration of mechanical ventilation. Nosocomial pneumonia related to H$_2$-receptor antagonists primarily occurs among patients ventilated for four or more days (60). In those who may require mechanical ventilation for less than four days, H$_2$-receptor antago-

nists may be used, because they have proven efficacy compared with placebo (whereas sucralfate has not). Because sucralfate may decrease the risk of nosocomial pneumonia compared to H$_2$-receptor antagonists, it may be the superior choice in when the clinician anticipates more prolonged mechanical ventilation. However, further clinical trials comparing sucralfate versus placebo are required to establish sucralfate's efficacy. One approach (64) to deciding whether prophylaxis is required and what agent to use is outlined in Figure 26.1.

Recommendations

1. In critically ill medical patients without mechanical ventilation or coagulopathy, prophylactic therapy is not in-

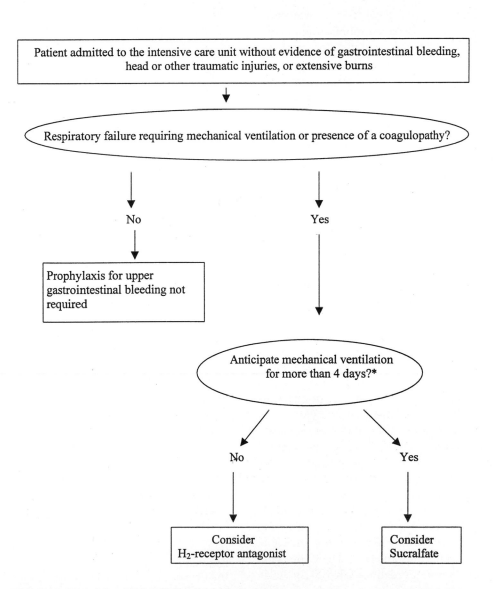

*This decision node is based on insufficient and conflicting data.

FIGURE 26.1. Stress-related upper gastrointestinal bleeding prophylaxis algorithm. Reprinted from Saint SS, Matthay MA. Risk reduction in the intensive care unit. *Am J Med* 1998;105:515–523, with permission.

dicated. In those with either risk factor, prophylaxis may be warranted.

2. Prophylaxis with H_2-receptor antagonists prevents clinically important upper gastrointestinal bleeding in critically ill patients, but a mortality benefit has not been shown.

3. If prophylaxis is selected, the choice between H_2-receptor antagonists and sucralfate may depend upon whether a prolonged (i.e., greater than four days) intubation is anticipated.

VASCULAR CATHETER–RELATED INFECTION

Central venous and pulmonary arterial (PA) catheters provide vascular access and hemodynamic monitoring in critically ill patients (65), but are associated with infectious complications. Each year, more than 200,000 cases of nosocomial bacteremia occur in the United States (66). Central venous catheters account for the majority of these episodes. The consequences of catheter-related bacteremia are substantial, resulting in longer hospital stays, increased medical costs, and an excess mortality of 10% to 35% (67–71). This section will focus on prevention of *short-term* central venous and PA catheter-related infection.

Types of Infection

The placement of central venous catheters can result in three major infectious syndromes (72). The first is local infection at the insertion site, manifested by regional warmth, erythema, swelling, or expression of purulent material. Untreated, this local skin infection can lead to other more advanced syndromes of catheter infection (72–74). The second is catheter colonization without evidence of systemic infection. Significant colonization is defined as a semiquantitative roll-plate catheter culture yielding more than 15 colony-forming units of bacterial growth (75) or quantitative catheter culture (sonication method) revealing more than 1,000 colony-forming units (76). Based on the landmark study by Maki and colleagues (75), this semiquantitative culture cutoff identified all cases that subsequently developed bloodstream infection. More recent reports indicate that the quantitative culture technique has even higher sensitivity for local and bacteremic catheter infection (76,77).

The third infectious syndrome is catheter-related bloodstream infection (CR-BSI) resulting in bacteremia and clinical manifestations of septic syndrome (72). The Centers for Disease Control and Prevention defines CR-BSI as: isolation of the same organism from cultures of both a catheter segment and peripheral blood cultures, clinical symptoms of BSI, and no other apparent source of infection (77). In the presence of bacteremia, defervescence after removal of a vascular catheter provides indirect evidence of CR-BSI in the absence of laboratory confirmation (77).

In recent studies, the incidence of central venous catheter colonization ranged from 13.7% to 71.4% (67). In two recent clinical trials, the rate of colonization was approximately 25 per 100 catheters (76,78). The incidence of CR-BSI is substantially lower, ranging from 2.1% to 11.7% (72). The best estimate is five BSIs per 100 catheters or seven BSIs per 1,000 catheter days (76–78).

Risk Factors

There have been numerous attempts to identify the clinical factors associated with a higher risk of central venous catheter-related infection (Table 26.4). The duration of central venous catheterization is an important risk factor for infection. Hampton and Sherertz (79) pooled data from 25 prospective trials to estimate the risk of local infection associated with different types of catheters. The risk for peripheral venous catheters was 1.3% per day and for central venous catheters it was 3.3% per day (79). The risk of infection over time, however, is nonlinear, with a markedly increased incidence after three days of catheterization (65,76,78,79). After seven days of central venous catheterization, the risk of bloodstream infection is increased nearly ninefold (80). Pooling data from four large prospective trials of PA catheter infection (nearly 1,000 catheters), Mermel and Maki found that the cumulative incidence of CR-BSI was very low (less than 1%) until day 4, when the risk of infection increased exponentially (72). Longer duration of central venous catheterization, then, appears to result in higher risk of infection.

The site of central venous catheterization affects the risk of infection. Studies of both central venous and PA catheters have documented an increased risk of infection for internal jugular vein compared to subclavian vein placement (76,80–83). Compared with subclavian vein catheterization, femoral vein catheter placement has also been associated with a higher risk of infection (76,80). There are several explanations for the increased infection risk with internal jugular vein catheterization, including anatomic proximity to the respiratory tract, presence of facial hair, and difficulty

TABLE 26.4. RISK FACTORS FOR VASCULAR CATHETER–RELATED INFECTION

Risk Factors
Longer duration of catheterization
Location of catheter
Use of transparent dressing
Lack of systemic antibiotic therapy
Less stringent barrier precautions during placement
Multilumen catheters (controversial)

maintaining tight-fitting dressings on the neck (82). Similarly, maintenance of groin catheter sites may be complicated by proximity to fecal flora. Although subclavian catheters have a lower infection risk, mechanical complications (e.g., pneumothorax) are more common than with internal jugular vein catheters (77).

Placement of PA catheters in the operating room, compared with the ICU, conferred increased risk of infection in a prospective, multivariate analysis (81). This increased risk was attributed to a less rigorous sterile technique employed by anesthesiologists in the operating room. A similar analysis demonstrated a higher risk of central venous catheter infection with placement outside the intensive care unit (76). Supporting the impact of setting and technique, a prospective randomized trial of maximal barrier precautions versus routine sterile procedure revealed a sixfold lower risk of central venous catheter infection with maximal precautions (72,84). A difficult catheter insertion has also been associated with higher risk of central venous catheter infection, supporting the impact of technique on the rate of catheter infection (74).

The type of dressing may also be important in determining the risk of central venous catheter–related infection. A meta-analysis of seven prospective randomized controlled trials comparing transparent polyurethane dressings with standard gauze dressings found a nearly twofold increased risk of central venous catheter tip infection with transparent dressings (85). There was a strong trend toward increased risk of catheter-related sepsis (RR 1.69, 95% CI 0.97 to 2.95) and bacteremia (RR 1.63, 95% CI 0.76 to 3.47), but the 95% confidence intervals did not exclude no association. Another more recent trial, however, found no significant difference between transparent or gauze dressing in local or bacteremic infection in 442 patients with PA catheters (86).

Many investigators have suggested that multilumen catheters increase the risk of CR-BSI, compared with single-lumen devices. Several nonrandomized trials (87–89) have found an association between multilumen catheter use and higher risk of infection. However, confounding by illness severity complicates interpretation of these studies—patients requiring multilumen catheters may have greater disease severity. Randomized trials have provided conflicting results, with some studies demonstrating an increased risk with multilumen catheters (90,91) and others finding no significant difference in risk of infection (92,93). As a practical consideration, many critically ill ICU patients require multilumen catheters to provide adequate medication and nutrition delivery.

Prevention

Strict adherence to proper hand-washing and aseptic technique during any catheter manipulation are crucial aspects of catheter infection prevention (94,95,95a). We review the other strongest evidence-based preventive strategies. A re-

cent Centers for Disease Control and Prevention guideline covers additional preventive techniques (77).

Site and Duration of Catheterization

Strict use of maximal barrier precautions during central venous catheter insertion is critical for infection prevention (77). Because the risk of central venous catheter infection increases with time, clinicians should minimize the duration of catheterization. Whenever possible, reducing duration of central venous catheterization to seven or fewer days is desirable. PA catheterization should not exceed four days, when the risk of infection increases exponentially. Although subclavian catheters have a lower risk of infection, they are associated with a higher rate of mechanical complications. Clinicians must weigh these relative risks when selecting a catheter insertion site.

Site Preparation And Maintenance

Most central venous catheter infections originate from cutaneous site colonization with microorganisms (72,96,97). Several investigators have examined whether site preparation with antiseptic compounds reduces the rate of central venous catheter colonization. Cleansing the insertion site with povidone-iodine solution modestly reduces the rate of catheter colonization (98,99). The best agent for suppressing cutaneous microorganisms, however, is 2% chlorhexidine gluconate. In a randomized trial of 668 central venous and arterial catheters, Maki and colleagues (98) found the incidence of local infection was significantly lower with chlorhexidine (2.3%) than with alcohol (7.1%) or povidone-iodine (9.3%). The investigators observed a trend toward less CR-BSI in the chlorhexidine group, but the confidence interval did not exclude no benefit (OR 0.23, 95% CI 0.03 to 1.8). A more recent randomized trial in critically ill surgical patients also found that an antiseptic solution containing chlorhexidine gluconate decreased the risk of local infection (RR = 0.4; 95% CI 0.1 to 0.9) and catheter-related sepsis (RR = 0.4; 95% CI 0.1 to 1.0) compared with povidone-iodine (100). Based on this evidence, chlorhexidine should be routinely used for central venous catheterization.

An important component of site maintenance is the dressing system. As discussed above, transparent dressings may be associated with a higher risk of local infection. However, transparent dressings have significant clinical advantages, such as permitting continuous visual inspection of the catheter site, less frequent dressing changes, and patient bathing without dressing disruption. Because the current evidence is conflicting, final recommendations regarding the use of transparent dressings must await further clinical trials.

Catheter Factors

Silver-impregnated cuffs may act as a mechanical and chemical barrier to organism migration from cutaneous insertion site to distal catheter tip, potentially reducing the incidence of infection (101). Though initial studies demonstrated a significant reduction in the incidence of local infection and CR-BSI (101,102), more recent studies—one randomized (103) and one observational (104)—found no reduction in catheter infection. Given the extra cost of these catheters (approximately $30 more per catheter) (103), efficacy should be clearly established before routine use can be recommended.

Recently, investigators have coated central venous catheters with antiseptic agents to prevent catheter-related infection. In a randomized controlled trial of 158 medical-surgical ICU patients, Maki and colleagues demonstrated that central venous catheters impregnated with chlorhexidine and silver sulfadiazine reduced the risk of central venous catheter colonization (RR 0.56, 95% CI 0.36 to 0.89) and bloodstream infection (RR 0.21, 95% CI 0.03 to 0.95) compared to control catheters (78). A recent meta-analysis of 11 randomized trials (2,603 catheters) comparing antiseptic impregnated central venous catheters with standard catheters found a decreased risk of colonization (OR 0.44, 95% CI 0.36 to 0.54) and CR-BSI (OR 0.56, 95% CI 0.37 to 0.84) (67). Therefore, central venous catheters impregnated with chlorhexidine and silver sulfadiazine are effective in reducing catheter colonization and bloodstream infection.

Using a similar strategy, other studies have examined the impact of antibiotic-coated central venous catheters on the incidence of infection. In a large randomized trial of surgical ICU patients, investigators demonstrated that a cefazolin-bonded catheter reduced the incidence of catheter colonization by sevenfold (105). More recently, Raad and colleagues conducted a multicenter randomized controlled trial comparing a minocycline and rifampin–coated central venous catheter with routine catheters (76). The antibiotic-coated catheter reduced the rate of colonization threefold and decreased the absolute risk of bloodstream infection by 5.2% (95% CI 0.2 to 12.4%).

Both antiseptic- and antibiotic-coated catheters reduce the risk of central venous catheter infection, but which strategy is superior? A recent multicenter randomized trial of 865 catheters compared minocycline/rifampin-impregnated catheters with chlorhexidine/silver sulfadiazine-coated catheters (80). The minocycline/rifampin catheters were one-third as likely to be colonized and one-twelfth as likely to result in bloodstream infection as the chlorhexidine/silver sulfadiazine catheters. Compared with the antiseptic-impregnated catheters, the antibiotic-coated catheters reduced the rate of CR-BSI from 4.1 per 1,000 catheter days to 0.3 per 1,000 catheter days. In both treatment groups, there were no local or systemic hypersensitivity reactions and no evidence of emerging antimicrobial resistance. Although formal cost-effectiveness analyses are required, preliminary analyses suggest that both antiseptic- and antibacterial-impregnated catheters are cost-beneficial strategies (76,78,106,106a).

Scheduled Catheter Replacement

Because the risk of infection increases with duration of catheterization, routine catheter replacement has been advocated by some investigators. Two randomized controlled trials have examined whether scheduled central venous and PA catheter replacement reduces infection, compared to catheter replacement for suspected infection or mechanical malfunction (107,108). In both studies, scheduled catheter replacement failed to reduce the incidence of catheter colonization or bloodstream infection. In fact, Cobb and colleagues (108) found that patients receiving replacement catheters at new insertion sites had no decrease in the risk of infection. These patients did, however, have an increased incidence of mechanical complications. Those undergoing routine replacement via guidewire exchange had a trend towards higher risk of bloodstream infection compared with patients who had catheter replacement only when clinically indicated. Therefore, routine replacement of central venous or PA catheters appears to increase, rather than decrease, the overall complication rate. Central venous catheters should be replaced only for well-defined clinical indications.

Prophylactic Antibiotics And Heparin

In two prospective multivariate analyses, use of systemic antibiotics was associated with a lower risk of central venous (76) and PA catheter colonization (97). The effectiveness of "prophylactic" systemic antibiotics has been mixed, but overall there seems to be no compelling evidence for reduction of central venous catheter infection rates (72,77,97,109). Given the problem of emerging antimicrobial resistance, prophylactic antibiotics cannot be recommended.

Catheter-related venous thrombosis may predispose to infection. Flushing central venous catheters with heparin may prevent thrombus formation and, as a result, infection. A recent meta-analysis of 12 randomized controlled trials (110) found that use of heparin flush reduced catheter-related deep venous thrombosis (RR 0.43, 95% CI 0.23 to 0.78), catheter colonization (RR 0.18, 95% CI 0.06 to 0.6), and bloodstream infection (RR 0.26, 95% CI 0.07 to 1.03). The complications of heparin-induced thrombocytopenia and bleeding may limit the benefit of this strategy. At present, further evaluation is necessary before heparin flushes can be routinely recommended (77).

Recommendations

1. Maximal barrier precautions should be used for central venous and PA catheter insertion. Strict adherence to proper hand-washing should be maintained during all phases of catheter care.
2. The duration of catheterization should be minimized. Whenever possible, PA catheter placement should be limited to four days.

3. The agent of choice for disinfecting the skin prior to and during catheterization is 2% chlorhexidine gluconate.
4. Transparent dressings may increase the risk of local infection compared with gauze dressing, but provide important benefits that may justify their use.
5. Central venous triple-lumen catheters impregnated with antiseptic or antibacterial agents should be used in all patients requiring prolonged central venous catheterization for more than two days.
6. Central venous and PA catheters should be changed only when clinically indicated. Routine, scheduled catheter replacement should not be employed.

URINARY CATHETER–RELATED INFECTION

Urinary catheters are widely utilized among hospitalized patients, with 25% receiving an indwelling urinary catheter (111). Unfortunately, indwelling urinary catheters are associated with a high incidence of nosocomial urinary tract infection (UTI) (5% per day) (111,112). A substantial proportion of patients with nosocomial UTI develop bloodstream infection (up to 4%) (113,114). Importantly, catheter related UTI is associated with longer hospital stay and a threefold greater mortality (115,116).

Among critically ill ICU patients, urinary catheter placement is even more common than in other hospitalized patients (117). After respiratory infection, UTI is the most common ICU-acquired infection, affecting 18% of patients (1). Controlling for other interventions, urinary catheterization increases the risk of ICU-acquired infection substantially (by 41%) (1). Because urinary catheter–related infection increases the risk of morbidity and mortality, preventive strategies should be employed in intensive care units.

Risk Factors

The definition of catheter-related UTI varies by investigator, with interchangeable use of the terms bacteriuria and UTI. Low-level growth from a catheterized specimen (i.e., 10^2 colony forming units (cfu) per mL) usually progresses to higher-grade bacteriuria (greater than 10^4 cfu per mL) within days (118). For patients with indwelling urinary catheters, most experts agree that culturing 10^2 or more cfu per mL of a predominant bacterial pathogen represents catheter-related UTI (119).

Several investigators have evaluated risk factors for urinary catheter–related UTI (Table 26.5). Over twenty-five years ago, Garibaldi and colleagues (112) prospectively followed 405 hospitalized patients who had indwelling catheters. Catheter-related UTI developed in a substantial proportion (23%) of patients. In univariate analyses, risk factors for catheter-related UTI were female gender (RR = 1.7), rapidly fatal underlying illness (RR = 2.5), age over 50 years (RR = 2), no receipt of systemic antibiotic therapy

TABLE 26.5. RISK FACTORS FOR DEVELOPING URINARY TRACT INFECTIONS IN PATIENTS WITH AN INDWELLING URINARY CATHETER

Risk Factors
Increasing duration of catheterization
Not receiving systemic antibiotic therapy
Female sex
Older age
Azotemia (serum creatinine concentration greater than 2.0 mg/ dL)
Diabetes mellitus
Rapidly fatal underlying illness
Nonsurgical disease
Faulty aseptic management of the indwelling catheter
Bacterial colonization of drainage bag

From Saint S, Lipsky BA. Preventing catheter-related bacteriuria: Should we? Can we? How? *Arch Intern Med* 1999;159:800–808, with permission.

(RR = 2), and nonsurgical disease (RR = 2.2). Another prospective study demonstrated that prolonged duration of urinary catheterization was a strong risk factor for UTI (RR 6.8 for seven or more days of catheterization) (120). In a further large-scale prospective cohort study of 1,458 adult inpatients (121), nearly 10% acquired UTIs during hospitalization. The investigators identified several independent risk factors for nosocomial UTI: longer duration of catheterization (OR = 2.3 to 22.4, depending on duration), no systemic antibiotic therapy (OR = 2.6), female gender (OR = 2.5), diabetes mellitus (OR = 2.3), and serum creatinine greater than 2 mg per dL at the time of catheterization (OR = 2.1) (121). Other prospective studies have confirmed the importance of longer duration of catheterization, female gender, and illness severity as risk factors for nosocomial catheter-related UTI (122,123).

Unfortunately, risk factors for UTI-related bloodstream infection have been less clearly defined (Table 26.6). Because fewer than 4% of patients with catheter-related UTI develop catheter-related bacteremia (113,114), most studies had low statistical power to examine risk factors. During a prospective 23-month hospital surveillance study, investigators identified 1,233 patients with nosocomial UTI (inci-

TABLE 26.6. RISK FACTORS FOR DEVELOPING BACTEREMIA IN PATIENTS WITH BACTERIURIA

Risk Factors
Male sex
Infection with *Serratia marcescens*
Older age
Noninfectious urinary tract disease (e.g., nephrolithiasis, prostatic hypertrophy)
Presence of an indwelling urinary catheter

From Saint S, Lipsky BA. Preventing catheter-related bacteriuria: Should we? Can we? How? *Arch Intern Med* 1999;159:800–808, with permission.

dence three cases per 100 admissions) (113). Nearly all patients with UTI had an indwelling urinary catheter (86%). Of the patients with UTI, 2.7% developed bloodstream infection. Risk factors for bloodstream infection were UTI due to *Serratia marcescens* (compared with other organisms, RR = 3.5) and male sex (RR = 2.0). No other factors (e.g., age, race, underlying disease, hospital service) were related to the risk of bacteremia.

A retrospective case-control study compared patients with community-acquired bacteremic UTI with nonbacteremic UTI (124). Risk factors for bacteremia were older age (mean age 74.7 versus 59.9 years), noninfectious urinary tract disease (e.g., nephrolithiasis, prostatic hypertrophy), and indwelling urinary catheter placement. Clearly, indwelling bladder catheters are the major risk factor for UTI-related bacteremia.

Prevention

Avoiding Indwelling Catheterization

Because the majority of nosocomial UTIs are related to indwelling urinary catheters (113,113a), the cornerstone of prevention is avoiding unnecessary catheterization. While urinary catheters may have important functions in critically ill patients, their use is often inappropriate. A recent prospective study found that medical ICU patients often underwent continued urinary catheterization for inappropriate indications (118). Of 597 patient-days of continued indwelling bladder catheterization, 41% were unjustified. Even when urinary catheter placement was initially indicated, catheters were often continued longer than necessary. When urinary catheters are no longer required, they should be removed immediately.

Intermittent Catheterization

If continued urinary collection is required, options other than indwelling catheterization should be considered. Intermittent catheterization, i.e., inserting and removing a sterile urinary catheter several times daily, may reduce the risk of UTI compared with an indwelling catheter. Because the incidence of bacteriuria is about 1% to 3% per insertion, however, most patients become bacteriuric within a few weeks (125).

External (Condom) Catheters

External urine collection systems may be associated with a lower risk of bacteriuria than indwelling catheters. Although devices have been developed for women, these systems are almost exclusively used with men. The proper role of condom catheters in hospitalized patients remains unclear. One prospective study conducted in a Department of Veterans Affairs (VA) Medical Center (126) demonstrated a low risk of UTI among men wearing condom catheters (approxi-

mately 12% per month). The rate was substantially higher, however, in those who frequently manipulated their catheters (126). In two parallel cohort studies in a VA nursing home, the incidence of symptomatic UTI was about 2.5 times greater in men with a chronic indwelling catheter compared to those wearing a condom catheter (127,128). On the other hand, a recent cross-sectional study in Denmark reported that the risk of UTI in hospitalized patients was higher in those wearing condom catheters than in those with indwelling catheters (129). Because these preventive efficacy data conflict, a randomized controlled trial comparing the safety and efficacy of these two devices is much needed (130). One of the authors (SS) is currently conducting such a clinical trial. In addition, condom catheters have recently been found to be less painful compared with indwelling catheters (130a).

Preventing UTI During Indwelling Catheterization

Asceptic Technique

Among critically ill patients, urinary catheterization may often be unavoidable. As a result, strategies to reduce infection in patients with indwelling catheters are paramount. The most important infection control advance is the closed catheter drainage system (131–134). Proper aseptic technique, including aseptic catheter insertion and maintenance, remains essential for preventing catheter-related UTI (119,135). When manipulating or emptying the urinary drainage bag, health care workers must wear gloves and wash their hands thoroughly between patient contacts.

Bladder Irrigation

Investigators have examined bladder irrigation with antiseptic (e.g., povidone-iodine, chlorhexidine) or antibacterial agents (e.g., neomycin, polymyxin) to prevent catheter-associated UTI. When modern closed drainage systems are used, this method has minimal efficacy (136–140). Because of the potential for local toxicity, bladder irrigation cannot be recommended.

Antimicrobial Agents in the Drainage Bag

In catheterized patients, UTIs may occur when bacterially colonized urine in a drainage bag refluxes into the patient's bladder. Several studies have evaluated addition of antibacterial agents (e.g., chlorhexidine, hydrogen peroxide, povidone-iodine) to the drainage bag. Although some studies suggested a reduction in catheter-related UTI (141–144), well-controlled randomized trials have demonstrated no significant benefit (145–147). Importantly, adding solutions to the drainage bag violates asceptic handling of the closed drainage system.

Rigorous Meatal Cleansing

Bacteria colonizing the urethral meatus may ascend along the urinary catheter's external surface and infect the urinary bladder. Reduction of urethral meatal colonization, then, might decrease the risk of UTI. Despite sound theoretical benefits (148), two large randomized trials have shown no impact of rigorous meatal cleansing on the risk of UTI (149,150). In one trial, investigators observed an increase prevalence of bacteriuria among patients undergoing meatal cleansing (149). As a result, rigorous meatal cleansing is not recommended.

Silver-Coated Catheters

Silver is a highly effective antibacterial substance that can be applied to various types of catheters. Unlike the above-mentioned interventions, silver-coated urinary catheters reduce the risk of catheter-related UTI. A recently published meta-analysis of eight randomized controlled trials found that silver-coated catheters significantly reduce the risk of UTI (OR 0.59, 95% CI 0.42 to 0.84) (151). While silver oxide–coated catheters were not effective, silver alloy-coated catheters significantly reduced the risk of UTI (OR 0.24, 95% CI 0.11 to 0.52). Although formal cost-effectiveness analyses have not been performed, we recommend using silver alloy-coated catheters in patients at high risk for UTI.

Systemic Antibiotic Therapy

Because systemic antibiotic therapy has been associated with a lower risk of catheter-related UTI (112,120,121,152), several investigators have studied this intervention. Evaluation of existing data is limited by retrospective study design, different definitions of UTI, and variation of antibiotic usage. Overall, clinical trials demonstrate that prophylactic systemic antibiotics modestly reduce the risk of catheter-related UTI. For instance, ciprofloxacin reduced the prevalence of UTI fourfold (153). In general, systemic antibiotic therapy appears to be most useful in patients requiring urinary catheterization for between three and 14 days (153–159). With shorter catheter duration, the risk of UTI is very low; longer duration is associated with near-universal bacteriuria regardless of therapy. However, most experts do not recommend routine prophylactic antibiotics in catheterized patients because of cost, potential adverse effects, and emerging antibacterial resistance (131,160). Supporting this contention, studies demonstrate a higher rate of resistant organisms among patients receiving antibiotic prophylaxis (153,155,159). Furthermore, most critically ill patients receive antibiotic therapy for other indications (122,123).

Recommendations

1. Avoid using a urinary catheter whenever possible. When catheters are placed, minimize the duration of use.
2. Always insert a catheter aseptically, use a closed drainage system, and properly maintain the catheter during use.
3. Consider using silver alloy–coated catheters in patients at high risk for UTI.

4. For incontinent men, a condom catheter may be preferable if they will not manipulate the device.
5. Bladder irrigation, antibacterial instillation in the drainage bag, and rigorous meatal cleaning should not be used.

CONCLUSIONS

The clinical outcomes of critically ill patients can be improved by reducing common complications of intensive care. In this chapter, we have reviewed the strategies that are most effective in reducing nonpulmonary complications. These complications are associated with longer duration of ICU stay, higher mortality, and increased cost. By rigorously employing these preventive strategies, the outcomes of critical illness will continue to improve.

ACKNOWLEDGMENTS

Dr. Eisner was supported by NIH grant F32 HL10054. This work was completed while Dr. Saint was a Robert Wood Johnson Clinical Scholar. Dr. Matthay was supported in part by NIH grant HL51856.

REFERENCES

1. Vincent JL, Bihari DJ, Suter PM, et al. The prevalence of nosocomial infection in intensive care units in Europe. *JAMA* 1995; 274:639–644.
2. Carter CJ. The natural history and epidemiology of venous thrombosis. *Prog Cardiovasc Dis* 1994;36(6):423–438.
3. Alpert JS, Dalen JE. Epidemiology and natural history of venous thromboembolism. *Prog Cardiovasc Dis* 1994;36(6):417–422.
4. Moser KM. Venous thromboembolism. *Am Rev Respir Dis* 1990;141(1):235–249.
5. Clagett GP, Anderson FA Jr, Heit J, et al. Prevention of venous thromboembolism. *Chest* 1995;108[4 Suppl]:312S–334S.
6. Oster G, Tuden RL, Colditz GA. Prevention of venous thromboembolism after general surgery. Cost-effectiveness analysis of alternative approaches to prophylaxis. *Am J Med* 1987;82(5): 889–899.
7. Oster G, Tuden RL, Colditz GA. A cost-effectiveness analysis of prophylaxis against deep-vein thrombosis in major orthopedic surgery. *JAMA* 1987;257(2):203–208.
8. Hull RD, Hirsh J, Sackett DL, et al. Cost-effectiveness of primary and secondary prevention of fatal pulmonary embolism in high-risk surgical patients. *Can Med Assoc J* 1982;127(10): 990–995.
9. Salzman EW, Davies GC. Prophylaxis of venous thromboembolism: analysis of cost effectiveness. *Ann Surg* 1980;191(2): 207–218.
10. Goldhaber SZ, Morpurgo M. Diagnosis, treatment, and prevention of pulmonary embolism. Report of the WHO/International Society and Federation of Cardiology Task Force. *JAMA* 1992;268(13):1727–1733.
11. Clagett GP, Anderson FA, Geerts W, et al. Prevention of venous thromboembolism. *Chest* 1998;114:531S–560S.

12. Cade JF. High risk of the critically ill for venous thromboembolism. *Crit Care Med* 1982;10(7):448–450.

13. Hirsch DR, Ingenito EP, Goldhaber SZ. Prevalence of deep venous thrombosis among patients in medical intensive care. *JAMA* 1995;274:335–337.

14. Collins R, Scrimgeour A, Yusuf S, et al. Reduction in fatal pulmonary embolism and venous thrombosis by perioperative administration of subcutaneous heparin. *N Engl J Med* 1988; 318:1162–1172.

15. Nuromohamed MT, Rosendaal FR, Buller HR, et al. Low molecular weight heparin versus standard heparin in general and orthopedic surgery: a meta-analysis. *Lancet* 1992;340:152–156.

16. Koch A, Boughes S, Ziegler S, et al. Low molecular weight heparin and unfractionated heparin in thrombosis prophylaxis after major surgical intervention: update of previous meta-analyses. *Br J Surg* 1997;84:750–759.

17. Warlow C, Terry G, Kenmure AC, et al. A double-blind trial of low doses of subcutaneous heparin in the prevention of deep-vein thrombosis after myocardial infarction. *Lancet* 1973; 2(835):934–936.

18. Gallus AS, Hirsh J, Tutle RJ, et al. Small subcutaneous doses of heparin in prevention of venous thrombosis. *N Engl J Med* 1973;288(11):545–551.

19. Handley AJ. Low-dose heparin after myocardial infarction. *Lancet* 1972;2(778):623–624.

20. McCarthy ST, Turner JJ, Robertson D, et al. Low-dose heparin as a prophylaxis against deep-vein thrombosis after acute stroke. *Lancet* 1977;2(8042):800–801.

21. Turpie AG, Gent M, Cote R, et al. A low-molecular-weight heparinoid compared with unfractionated heparin in the prevention of deep vein thrombosis in patients with acute ischemic stroke. A randomized, double-blind study. *Ann Intern Med* 1992;117(5):353–357.

22. Belch JJ, Lowe GD, Ward AG, et al. Prevention of deep vein thrombosis in medical patients by low-dose heparin. *Scott Med J* 1981;26(2):115–117.

23. Pingleton SK, Bone RC, Pingleton WW, et al. Prevention of pulmonary emboli in a respiratory intensive care unit: efficacy of low-dose heparin. *Chest* 1981;79(6):647–650.

24. Halkin H, Goldberg J, Modan M, et al. Reduction of mortality in general medical in-patients by low-dose heparin prophylaxis. *Ann Intern Med* 1982;96(5):561–565.

25. Gardlund B. Randomised, controlled trial of low-dose heparin for prevention of fatal pulmonary embolism in patients with infectious diseases. The Heparin Prophylaxis Study Group. *Lancet* 1996;347(9012):1357–1361.

26. Sevitt S, Gallagher N. Venous thrombosis and pulmonary embolism: a clinico-pathologic study in injured and burned patients. *Br J Surg* 1961;45:475–489.

27. Anderson DR, O'Brien BJ, Levine MN, Roberts R, et al. Efficacy and cost of low-molecular-weight heparin compared with standard heparin for the prevention of deep vein thrombosis after total hip arthroplasty. *Ann Intern Med* 1993;119(11): 1105–1112.

28. Turpie AG, Levine MN, Hirsh J, et al. A randomized controlled trial of a low-molecular-weight heparin (enoxaparin) to prevent deep-vein thrombosis in patients undergoing elective hip surgery. *N Engl J Med* 1986;315(15):925–929.

29. Levine MN, Hirsh J, Gent M, et al. Prevention of deep vein thrombosis after elective hip surgery. A randomized trial comparing low molecular weight heparin with standard unfractionated heparin. *Ann Intern Med* 1991;114(7):545–551.

30. Prins MH, Gelsema R, Sing AK, et al. Prophylaxis of deep venous thrombosis with a low-molecular-weight heparin (Kabi 2165/Fragmin) in stroke patients. *Haemostasis* 1989;19(5): 245–250.

31. Turpie AG, Levine MN, Hirsh J, et al. Double-blind randomised trial of Org 10172 low-molecular-weight heparinoid in prevention of deep-vein thrombosis in thrombotic stroke. *Lancet* 1987;1(8532):523–526.

32. Dahan R, Houlbert D, Caulin C, et al. Prevention of deep vein thrombosis in elderly medical in-patients by a low molecular weight heparin: a randomized double-blind trial. *Haemostasis* 1986;16(2):159–164.

33. Harenberg J, Kallenbach B, Martin U, et al. Randomized controlled study of heparin and low molecular weight heparin for prevention of deep-vein thrombosis in medical patients. *Thromb Res* 1990;59(3):639–650.

34. Bergman JF, Neuhart E. A multicenter randomized double-blind study of enoxaparin compared with unfractionated heparin in the prevention of venous thromboembolic disease in elderly inpatients bedridden for an acute medical illness. *Thromb Haemost* 1996;76:529–534.

35. Clagett GP, Anderson FA Jr, Geerts W. Prevention of venous thromboembolism. *Chest* 1998;102:391S–407S.

36. Coe NP, Collins REC, Klein LA, et al. Prevention of deep venous thrombosis in urological patients: a controlled, randomized trial of low-dose heparin and pneumatic compression boots. *Surgery* 1978;83:230–234.

37. Hull RD, Pineo GF. Intermittent pneumatic compression for the prevention of venous thromboembolism [Editorial; Comment]. *Chest* 1996;109(1):6–9.

38. Ramos R, Salem BI, De Pawlikowski MP, et al. The efficacy of pneumatic compression stockings in the prevention of pulmonary embolism after cardiac surgery. *Chest* 1996;109(1): 82–85.

39. Clagett GP, Reisch JS. Prevention of venous thromboembolism in general surgical patients. Results of meta-analysis. *Ann Surg* 1988;208(2):227–240.

40. Collins R, Scrimgeour A, Yusuf S, et al. Reduction in fatal pulmonary embolism and venous thrombosis by perioperative administration of subcutaneous heparin. Overview of results of randomized trials in general, orthopedic, and urologic surgery. *N Engl J Med* 1988;318(18):1162–1173.

41. Levine MN, Raskob G, Landefeld S, et al. Hemorrhagic complications of anticoagulant treatment. *Chest* 1995;108[4 Suppl]: 276S–290S.

42. Hirsh J, Raschke R, Warkentin TE, et al. Heparin: mechanism of action, pharmacokinetics, dosing considerations, monitoring, efficacy, and safety. *Chest* 1995;108[4 Suppl]:258S–275S.

43. Warkentin TE, Levine MN, Hirsh J, et al. Heparin-induced thrombocytopenia in patients treated with low-molecular-weight heparin or unfractionated heparin. *N Engl J Med* 1995; 332(20):1330–1335.

44. Terdiman JP. Gastrointestinal complications in the intensive care unit. In: Matthay MA, Schwartz DE, eds. *Complications in the intensive care unit.* New York: Chapman and Hall, 1997.

45. Schuster DP. Stress ulcer prophylaxis: in whom? With what? [Editorial; Comment]. *Crit Care Med* 1993;21(1):4–6.

46. Zimmerman J, Meroz Y, Siguencia J, et al. Upper gastrointestinal hemorrhage. Comparison of the causes and prognosis in primary and secondary bleeders. *Scand J Gastroenterol* 1994; 29(9):795–798.

47. Zimmerman J, Meroz Y, Arnon R, et al. Predictors of mortality in hospitalized patients with secondary upper gastrointestinal haemorrhage. *J Intern Med* 1995;237(3):331–337.

48. Cook DJ, Fuller HD, Guyatt GH, et al. Risk factors for gastrointestinal bleeding in critically ill patients. Canadian Critical Care Trials Group. *N Engl J Med* 1994;330(6):377–381.

49. Loperfido S, Monica F, Maifreni L, et al. Bleeding peptic ulcer occurring in hospitalized patients: analysis of predictive and risk

factors and comparison with out-of-hospital onset of hemorrhage. *Dig Dis Sci* 1994;39(4):698–705.

50. Cook D, Guyatt G, Marshall J, et al. A comparison of sucralfate and ranitidine for the prevention of upper gastrointestinal bleeding in patients requiring mechanical ventilation. Canadian Critical Care Trials Group. *N Engl J Med* 1998;338(12):791–797.

51. Schuster DP, Rowley H, Feinstein S, et al. Prospective evaluation of the risk of upper gastrointestinal bleeding after admission to a medical intensive care unit. *Am J Med* 1984;76(4):623–630.

52. Ben Menachem T, McCarthy BD, Fogel R, et al. Prophylaxis for stress-related gastrointestinal hemorrhage: a cost effectiveness analysis. *Crit Care Med* 1996;24(2):338–345.

53. Heyland DK, Gafini A, Griffith L, et al. The clinical and economic consequence of clinically important gastrointestinal bleeding in critically ill patients. *Clin Intensive Care* 1996;7:121–125.

54. Tryba M, Kulka PJ. Critical care pharmacotherapy. A review. *Drugs* 1993;45(3):338–352.

55. Cook DJ, Witt LG, Cook RJ, et al. Stress ulcer prophylaxis in the critically ill: a meta-analysis [published erratum appears in *Am J Med* 1991;91(6):670]. *Am J Med* 1991;91(5):519–527.

56. Cook DJ, Reeve BK, Guyatt GH, et al. Stress ulcer prophylaxis in critically ill patients. Resolving discordant meta-analyses. *JAMA* 1996;275(4):308–314.

57. Tryba M. Sucralfate versus antacids or H2-antagonists for stress ulcer prophylaxis: a meta-analysis on efficacy and pneumonia rate. *Crit Care Med* 1991;19(7):942–949.

58. Lacroix J, Infante Rivard C, Jenicek M, et al. Prophylaxis of upper gastrointestinal bleeding in intensive care units: a meta-analysis. *Crit Care Med* 1989;17(9):862–869.

59. Tryba M. Side effects of stress bleeding prophylaxis. *Am J Med* 1989;86(6A):85–93.

60. Prod'hom G, Leuenberger P, Koerfer J, et al. Nosocomial pneumonia in mechanically ventilated patients receiving antacid, ranitidine, or sucralfate as prophylaxis for stress ulcer. A randomized controlled trial. *Ann Intern Med* 1994;120(8):653–662.

61. Garvey BM, McCambley JA, Tuxen DV. Effects of gastric alkalization on bacterial colonization in critically ill patients. *Crit Care Med* 1989;17(3):211–216.

62. McCarthy DM. Sucralfate. *N Engl J Med* 1991;325(14):1017–1025.

63. Tryba M, Mantey Stiers F. Antibacterial activity of sucralfate in human gastric juice. *Am J Med* 1987;83(3B):125–127.

64. Saint S, Matthay MA. Risk reduction in the intensive care unit. *Am J Med* 1998;105:515–523.

65. Raad II, Bodey GP. Infectious complications of indwelling vascular catheters. *Clin Infect Dis* 1992;15(2):197–208.

66. Maki DG. Infections due to infusion therapy. In: Bennett JV, Brachman PS, eds. *Hospital infections.* Boston: Little, Brown, 1992;849–898.

67. Veenstra DL, Saint S, Saha S, et al. Efficacy of antiseptic-impregnated central venous catheters in preventing catheter-related bloodstream infection: a meta-analysis. *JAMA* 1999;281(3):261–267.

68. Corona ML, Peters SG, Narr BJ, et al. Infections related to central venous catheters. *Mayo Clin Proc* 1990;65(7):979–986.

69. Arnow PM, Quimosing EM, Beach M. Consequences of intravascular catheter sepsis. *Clin Infect Dis* 1993;16(6):778–784.

70. Pittet D, Tarara D, Wenzel RP. Nosocomial bloodstream infection in critically ill patients. Excess length of stay, extra costs, and attributable mortality. *JAMA* 1994;271(20):1598–1601.

71. Smith RL, Meixler SM, Simberkoff MS. Excess mortality in critically ill patients with nosocomial bloodstream infections. *Chest* 1991;100(1):164–167.

72. Mermel LA, Maki DG. Infectious complications of Swan-Ganz pulmonary artery catheters. *Am J Respir Crit Care Med* 1994;149:1020–1036.

73. Raad I, Gilbreath J, Suleimann N, et al. Maximal sterile barriers during the insertion of central venous catheters for the prevention of infections: a prospective randomized study. In: *Abstracts of the thirty-second interscience conference on antimicrobial agents and chemotherapy,* October, 1992. Washington, DC: American Society for Microbiology, 1992:264.

74. Maki DG, Will L. Risk factors for central venous catheter-related infection within the ICU [abstract]. A prospective study of 345 catheters. In: *Final program and abstracts of the third international conference on nosocomial infections,* July 31–August 3, 1990, Atlanta, GA: Centers for Disease Control, The National Foundation for Infectious Diseases, 1990;54.

75. Maki DG, Weise CE, Sarafin HW. A semiquantitative culture method for identifying intravenous-catheter-related infection. *N Engl J Med* 1977;296:1305–1309.

76. Raad I, Darouiche R, Dupuis J, et al. Central venous catheters coated with minocycline and rifampin for the prevention of catheter-related colonization and bloodstream infections. A randomized, double-blind trial. The Texas Medical Center Catheter Study Group. *Ann Intern Med* 1997;127(4):267–274.

77. Guideline for prevention of intravascular device-related infections. *Am J Infect Control* 1996;24(4):261–293.

78. Maki DG, Stolz SM, Wheeler S, et al. Prevention of central venous catheter-related bloodstream infection by use of an antiseptic-impregnated catheter. A randomized, controlled trial. *Ann Intern Med* 1997;127(4):257–266.

79. Hampton AA, Sherertz RJ. Vascular-access infections in hospitalized patients. *Surg Clin North Am* 1988;68(1):57–71.

80. Darouiche RO, Raad II, Heard SO, et al. A comparison of two antimicrobial-impregnated central venous catheters. *N Engl J Med* 1999;340(1):1–8.

81. Mermel LA, McCormick RD, Springman SR, et al. The pathogenesis and epidemiology of catheter-related infection with pulmonary artery Swan-Ganz catheters: a prospective study utilizing molecular subtyping. *Am J Med* 1991;91(3B):197S–205S.

82. Richet H, Hubert B, Nitemberg G, et al. Prospective multicenter study of vascular-catheter-related complications and risk factors for positive central-catheter cultures in intensive care unit patients. *J Clin Microbiol* 1990;28(11):2520–2525.

83. Gil RT, Kruse JA, Thill Baharozian MC, et al. Triple vs single-lumen central venous catheters. A prospective study in a critically ill population. *Arch Intern Med* 1989;149(5):1139–1143.

84. Raad II, Hohn DC, Gibreath BJ, et al. Prevention of central venous catheter-related infections by using maximal sterile barrier precautions during insertion. *Infect Control Hosp Epidemiol* 1994;15:231–238.

85. Hoffmann KK, Weber DJ, Samsa GP, et al. Transparent polyurethane film as an intravenous catheter dressing. A meta-analysis of the infection risks. *JAMA* 1992;267(15):2072–2076.

86. Maki DG, Stolz SS, Wheeler S, et al. A prospective, randomized trial of gauze and two polyurethane dressings for site care of pulmonary artery catheters: implications for catheter management. *Crit Care Med* 1994;22(11):1729–1737.

87. Pemberton LB, Lyman B, Lander V, et al. Sepsis from triple- vs single-lumen catheters during total parenteral nutrition in surgical or critically ill patients. *Arch Surg* 1986;121(5):591–594.

88. Yeung C, May J, Hughes R. Infection rate for single lumen vs triple lumen subclavian catheters. *Infect Control Hosp Epidemiol* 1988;9(4):154–158.

89. Hilton E, Haslett TM, Borenstein MT, et al. Central catheter infections: single- versus triple-lumen catheters. Influence of guide wires on infection rates when used for replacement of catheters. *Am J Med* 1988;84(4):667–672.

90. Clark Christoff N, Watters VA, Sparks W, et al. Use of triple-lumen subclavian catheters for administration of total parenteral nutrition. *JPEN J Parenter Enteral Nutr* 1992;16(5):403–407.

91. McCarthy MC, Shives JK, Robison RJ, et al. Prospective evaluation of single and triple lumen catheters in total parenteral nutrition. *JPEN J Parenter Enteral Nutr* 1987;11(3):259–262.

92. Farkas JC, Liu N, Bleriot JP, et al. Single- versus triple-lumen central catheter-related sepsis: a prospective randomized study in a critically ill population. *Am J Med* 1992;93(3):277–282.

93. Powell C, Fabri PJ, Kudsk KA. Risk of infection accompanying the use of single-lumen vs double-lumen subclavian catheters: a prospective randomized study. *JPEN J Parenter Enteral Nutr* 1988;12(2):127–129.

94. Nystrom B. Impact of handwashing on mortality in intensive care: examination of the evidence. *Infect Control Hosp Epidemiol* 1994;15(7):435–436.

95. Doebbeling BN, Stanley GL, Sheetz CT, et al. Comparative efficacy of alternative hand-washing agents in reducing nosocomial infections in intensive care units. *N Engl J Med* 1992; 327(2):88–93.

95a. Mermel LA. Prevention of catheter-related infections. *Ann Intern Med* 2000;132:391–402.

96. Henderson DK. Bacteremia due to percutaneous intravascular devices. In: Mandell GL, Bennett JE, Dolin R, eds. *Principles and practice of infectious diseases.* New York: Churchill Livingston Inc, 1995;2587–2599.

97. Rello J, Coll P, Net A, et al. Infection of pulmonary artery catheters: epidemiologic characteristics and multivariate analysis of risk factors. *Chest* 1993;103:132–136.

98. Maki DG, Ringer M, Alvarado CJ. Prospective randomized trial of povidone-iodine, alcohol, and chlorhexidine for prevention of infection associated with central venous and arterial catheters. *Lancet* 1991;338:339–343.

99. Levy JH, Nagle DM, Curling PE, et al. Contamination reduction during central venous catheterization. *Crit Care Med* 1988; 16:165–167.

100. Mimoz O, Pieroni L, Lawrence C, et al. Prospective, randomized trial of two antiseptic solutions for prevention of central venous or arterial catheter colonization and infection in intensive care unit patients. *Crit Care Med* 1996;24(11):1818–1823.

101. Maki DG, Cobb L, Garman JK, et al. An attachable silver-impregnated cuff for prevention of infection with central venous catheters: a prospective randomized multicenter trial. *Am J Med* 1988;85(3):307–314.

102. Flowers RH 3d, Schwenzer KJ, Kopel RF, et al. Efficacy of an attachable subcutaneous cuff for the prevention of intravascular catheter-related infection. A randomized, controlled trial. *JAMA* 1989;261(6):878–883.

103. Smith HO, DeVictoria CL, Garfinkel D, et al. A prospective randomized comparison of an attached silver-impregnated cuff to prevent central venous catheter-associated infection. *Gynecol Oncol* 1995;58(1):92–100.

104. Hasaniya NW, Angelis M, Brown MR, et al. Efficacy of subcutaneous silver-impregnated cuffs in preventing central venous catheter infections. *Chest* 1996;109(4):1030–1032.

105. Kamal GD, Pfaller MA, Rempe LE, et al. Reduced intravascular catheter infection by antibiotic bonding. A prospective, randomized, controlled trial. *JAMA* 1991;265(18):2364–2368.

106. Wenzel RP, Edmond MB. The evolving technology of venous access. N Engl J Med 1999;340:48–50.

106a. Veenstra DL, Saint S, Sullivan SD. Cost-effectiveness of antiseptic-impregnated central venous catheters for the prevention of catheter-related bloodstream infection. *JAMA* 1999;282: 544–560.

107. Eyer S, Brummitt C, Crossley K, et al. Catheter-related sepsis:

108. Cobb DK, High KP, Sawyer RG, et al. A controlled trial of scheduled replacement of central venous and pulmonary-artery catheters. *N Engl J Med* 1992;327(15):1062–1068.

109. Armstrong CW, Mayhall G, Miller K, et al. Prospective study of catheter replacement and other risk factors for infection of hyperalimentation catheters. *J Infect Dis* 1986;154:808–816.

110. Randolph AG, Cook DJ, Gonzales CA, et al. Benefit of heparin in central venous and pulmonary artery catheters. A meta-analysis of randomized controlled trials. *Chest* 1998;113:165–171.

111. Haley RW, Hooton TM, Culver DH, et al. Nosocomial infections in U.S. hospitals, 1975–1976: estimated frequency by selected characteristics of patients. *Am J Med* 1981;70:947–959.

112. Garibaldi RA, Burke JP, Dickman ML, et al. Factors predisposing to bacteriuria during indwelling urethral catheterization. *N Engl J Med* 1974;291:215–219.

112a. Saint S. Clinical and economic consequences of nosocomial catheter-related bacteriuria. *American Journal of Infection Control* 2000;28:68–75.

113. Krieger JN, Kaiser DL, Wenzel RP. Urinary tract etiology of bloodstream infections in hospitalized patients. *J Infect Dis* 1983;148:57–62.

113a. Saint S, Lipsky BA. Preventing catheter-related bacteriuria: Should we? Can we? How? *Arch Intern Med* 1999;159: 800–808.

114. Bryan CS, Reynolds KL. Hospital-acquired bacteremic urinary tract infection: epidemiology and outcome. *J Urol* 1984;132: 494–498.

115. Givens CD, Wenzel RP. Catheter-associated urinary tract infections in surgical patients: a controlled study on the excess morbidity and costs. *J Urol* 1980;124:646–648.

116. Green MS, Rubinstein E, Amit P. Estimating the effects of nosocomial infections on the length of hospitalization. *J Infect Dis* 1982;145:667–672.

117. Jain P, Parada JP, David A, et al. Overuse of the indwelling urinary tract catheter in hospitalized medical patients. *Arch Intern Med* 1995;155:1425–1429.

118. Stark RP, Maki DG. Bacteriuria in the catheterized patient. What quantitative level of bacteriuria is relevant? *N Engl J Med* 1984;311:560–564.

119. Stamm WE. Urinary tract infections. In: Bennett JV, Brachman PS, eds. *Hospital infections,* 4th ed. Philadelphia: Lippincott-Raven, 1998.

120. Shapiro M, Simchen E, Izraeli S, et al. A multivariate analysis of risk factors for acquiring bacteriuria in patients with indwelling urinary catheters for longer than 24 hours. *Infect Control* 1984; 5:525–532.

121. Platt R, Polk BF, Murdock B, et al. Risk factors for nosocomial urinary tract infection. *Am J Epidemiol* 1986;124:977–985.

122. Johnson JR, Roberts PL, Olsen RJ, et al. Prevention of catheter-associated urinary tract infection with a silver oxide–coated urinary catheter: clinical and microbiologic correlates. *J Infect Dis* 1990;162:1145–1150.

123. Riley DK, Classen DC, Stevens LE, et al. A large randomized clinical trial of a silver-impregnated urinary catheter: lack of efficacy and staphylococcal superinfection. *Am J Med* 1995;98: 349–356.

124. Jerkeman M, Braconier JH. Bacteremic and non-bacteremic febrile urinary tract infection—a review of 168 hospital-treated patients. *Infection* 1992;20:143–145.

125. Warren JW. Catheter-associated urinary tract infections. *Infect Dis Clin North Am* 1997;11:609–622.

126. Hirsh DD, Fainstein V, Musher DM. Do condom catheter collecting systems cause urinary tract infection? *JAMA* 1979; 242:340–341.

127. Ouslander JG, Greengold B, Chen S. Complications of chronic indwelling urinary catheters among male nursing home patients. a prospective study. *J Urol* 1987;138:1191–1195.

128. Ouslander JG, Greengold B, Chen S. External catheter use and urinary tract infections among incontinent male nursing home patients. *J Am Geriatr Soc* 1987;35:1063–1070.

129. Zimakoff J, Stickler DJ, Pontoppidan B, et al. Bladder management and urinary tract infections in Danish hospitals, nursing homes, and home care: a national prevalence study. *Infect Control Hosp Epidemiol* 1996;17:215–221.

130. Warren JW. Urethral catheters, condom catheters, and nosocomial urinary tract infections. *Infect Control Hosp Epidemiol* 1996;17:221–214.

130a. Saint S, Lipsky BA, Baker P, et al. Urinary catheters: What type do men and nurses prefer? *J Am G Soc* 1999;47:1453–1457.

131. Meares EM Jr. Current patterns in nosocomial urinary tract infections. *Urology* 1991;37:9–12.

132. Kunin CM, McCormack RC. Prevention of catheter-induced urinary-tract infections by sterile closed drainage. *N Engl J Med* 1966;274:1155–1161.

133. Thornton GF, Andriole VT. Bacteriuria during indwelling catheter drainage. II. Effect of a closed sterile drainage system. *JAMA* 1970;214:339–342.

134. Wolff G, Gradel E, Buchman B. Indwelling catheter and risk of urinary infection: a clinical investigation with a new closed-drainage system. *Urol Res* 1976;4:15–18.

135. Platt R, Polk BF, Murdock B, et al. Reduction of mortality associated with nosocomial urinary tract infection. *Lancet* 1983;1:893–897.

136. Dudley MN, Barriere SL. Antimicrobial irrigations in the prevention and treatment of catheter-related urinary tract infections. *Am J Hosp Pharm* 1981;38:59–65.

137. Bastable JR, Peel RN, Birch DM, et al. Continuous irrigation of the bladder after prostatectomy: its effect on post-prostatectomy infection. *Br J Urol* 1977;49:689–693.

138. Kirk D, Dunn M, Bullock DW, et al. Hibitane bladder irrigation in the prevention of catheter-associated urinary infection. *Br J Urol* 1979;51:528–531.

139. Warren JW, Platt R, Thomas RJ, et al. Antibiotic irrigation and catheter-associated urinary-tract infections. *N Engl J Med* 1978;299:570–573.

140. Gelman ML. Antibiotic irrigation and catheter-associated urinary tract infections [Editorial]. *Nephron* 1980;25:259.

141. Southampton Infection Control Team. Evaluation of aseptic techniques and chlorhexidine on the rate of catheter-associated urinary-tract infection. *Lancet* 1982;1:89–91.

142. Maizels M, Schaeffer AJ. Decreased incidence of bacteriuria associated with periodic instillations of hydrogen peroxide into the urethral catheter drainage bag. *J Urol* 1980;123:841–845.

143. Sujka SK, Petrelli NJ, Herrera L. Incidence of urinary tract infections in patients requiring long-term catheterization after abdominoperineal resection for rectal carcinoma: does Betadine in the Foley drainage bag make a difference? *Eur J Surg Oncol* 1987;13:341–343.

144. al Juburi AZ, Cicmanec J. New apparatus to reduce urinary drainage associated with urinary tract infections. *Urology* 1989;33:97–101.

145. Sweet DE, Goodpasture HC, Holl K, et al. Evaluation of H2O2 prophylaxis of bacteriuria in patients with long-term indwelling Foley catheters. a randomized controlled study. *Infect Control* 1985;6:263–266.

146. Thompson RL, Haley CE, Searcy MA, et al. Catheter-associated bacteriuria. Failure to reduce attack rates using periodic instillations of a disinfectant into urinary drainage systems. *JAMA* 1984;251:747–751.

147. Gillespie WA, Simpson RA, Jones JE, et al. Does the addition of disinfectant to urine drainage bags prevent infection in catheterised patients? *Lancet* 1983;1:1037–1039.

148. Garibaldi RA, Burke JP, Britt MR, et al. Meatal colonization and catheter-associated bacteriuria. *N Engl J Med* 1980;303:316–318.

149. Burke JP, Garibaldi RA, Britt MR, et al. Prevention of catheter-associated urinary tract infections. Efficacy of daily meatal care regimens. *Am J Med* 1981;70:655–658.

150. Burke JP, Jacobson JA, Garibaldi RA, et al. Evaluation of daily meatal care with poly-antibiotic ointment in prevention of urinary catheter–associated bacteriuria. *J Urol* 1983;129:331–334.

151. Saint S, Elmore JG, Sullivan SD, et al. The efficacy of silver alloy–coated urinary catheters in preventing urinary tract infection: a meta-analysis. *Am J Med* 1998;105(3):236–241.

152. Hustinx WN, Mintjes de Groot AJ, Verkooyen RP, et al. Impact of concurrent antimicrobial therapy on catheter-associated urinary tract infection. *J Hosp Infect* 1991;18:45–56.

153. van der Wall E, Verkooyen RP, Mintjes de Groot J, et al. Prophylactic ciprofloxacin for catheter-associated urinary-tract infection. *Lancet* 1992;339:946–951.

154. Vollaard EJ, Clasener HA, Zambon JV, et al. Prevention of catheter-associated gram-negative bacilluria with norfloxacin by selective decontamination of the bowel and high urinary concentration. *J Antimicrob Chemother* 1989;23:915–922.

155. Verbrugh HA, Mintjes de Groot AJ, Andriesse R, et al. Postoperative prophylaxis with norfloxacin in patients requiring bladder catheters. *Eur J Clin Microbiol Infect Dis* 1988;7:490–494.

156. Little PJ, Pearson S, Peddie BA, et al. Amoxicillin in the prevention of catheter-induced urinary infection. *J Infect Dis* 1974;129[suppl]:S241–242.

157. Catheter-acquired urinary tract infection [Editorial]. *Lancet* 1991;338:857–858.

158. Britt MR, Garibaldi RA, Miller WA, et al. Antimicrobial prophylaxis for catheter-associated bacteriuria. *Antimicrob Agents Chemother* 1977;11:240–243.

159. Mountokalakis T, Skounakis M, Tselentis J. Short-term versus prolonged systemic antibiotic prophylaxis in patients treated with indwelling catheters. *J Urol* 1985;134:506–508.

160. Platt R, Polk BF, Murdock B, et al. Prevention of catheter-associated urinary tract infection: a cost-benefit analysis. *Infect Control Hosp Epidemiol* 1989;10:60–64.

SUBJECT INDEX

Page numbers followed by f indicate figures; those followed by t indicate tables.

A

AA (arachidonic acid), metabolism of, 19–20, 19f
Abdominal muscles, 4, 5f
Abdominal surgery, pleural effusions after, 454
ABPA (allergic bronchopulmonary aspergillosis), 141–143
ABPF (allergic bronchopulmonary fungoses), 141
Abscess
 intraabdominal, pleural effusions with, 453–454
 lung, 379, 394f, 395, 395f
  pleural effusions with, 445–446
  sputum with, 62
  symptoms of, 60, 62, 63
Acanthosis nigricans, with lung cancer, 361
Accessory muscles, of inspiration, 4, 5f, 6
Accolate (zafirlukast), for asthma, 147t, 157
ACE (angiotensin-converting enzyme)
 in sarcoidosis, 292, 292t
 vasoactive properties of, 19, 20f
Acetaldehyde, inhalation injury due to, 323t
Acetazolamide (Diamox), for central sleep apnea, 494
Acetylcholine, in respiratory muscle function, 4
Acid aerosols, air pollution due to, 341, 341t
Acid-base abnormalities, in respiratory failure, 541–542
Acid-base analysis, 99
Acinus. See Terminal respiratory unit (TRU)
Acquired immunodeficiency syndrome (AIDS)
 aspergillosis in, 424
 bacterial infections in, 405–406, 405f, 436
 bronchoscopy in, 124
 coccidioidomycosis in, 438
 cryptococcosis in, 423, 437
 evaluation in, 434–435
 highly active antiretroviral therapy for, 434
 histoplasmosis in, 417, 418f, 437–438
 Mycobacterium avium complex in, 414, 415, 437

non-infectious pulmonary complications of, 434t
 open-lung biopsy in, 128
 pneumonia in, 389, 403–404, 404t, 436, 438
  Pneumocystis carinii, 405–406, 405f, 435–436, 438
 pneumothorax with bronchopleural fistula in, 436
 pulmonary effusion lymphoma in, 451
 respiratory infections in, 378
 tuberculosis in, 409, 410, 412, 436–437, 438
Acrylonitrile, carcinogenicity of, 337t, 339
Actinomycosis, pleural effusions due to, 447
Acute lung injury (ALI), 582–587, 582t, 583f–586f
 clinical course of, 584–585, 584f, 585f
 clinical disorders associated with, 582, 582t
 clinical manifestations of, 583–584, 583f–585f
 in critically ill patients, 630–631
 defined, 582
 diagnosis of, 587
 early recognition of, 636
 due to gastric aspiration, 583f, 585, 585f
 mechanism of, 585–586
 mortality in, 582–583
 pulmonary edema in, 582–587, 583f–586f
 scoring system for, 631, 631t
 due to sepsis, 583f, 585–586, 585f, 586f
 treatment for, 586–587
Acute lupus pneumonitis (ALP), 273
Acute rejection, after lung transplantation, 218–219, 219f, 219t
Acute respiratory distress syndrome (ARDS), 582–587
 clinical course of, 584–585, 584f, 585f
 clinical disorders associated with, 582, 582t
 clinical manifestations of, 583–584, 583f–585f
 in critically ill patients, 630–631, 631t
 defined, 582
 diagnosis of, 587
 due to gastric aspiration, 583f, 585, 585f
 mechanism of lung injury in, 585–586
 mortality in, 582–583

oxygen uptake in, 632, 632f
 due to pancreatitis, 584f
 pneumonia in, 378, 389, 389t, 401–402, 401f
 pulmonary artery catheterization for, 626
 pulmonary edema in, 582–587, 583f–586f
 right-to-left shunting in, 53
 due to sepsis, 583f, 585–586, 585f, 586f
 surfactant in, 31–32
 treatment for, 586–587
AC (assist-controlled) ventilation, 548, 549t
ADA (adenosine deaminase)
 in pleural fluid, 120–121
 in tuberculous pleuritis, 447
Adenocarcinoma, 352, 354, 354f
Adenoid cystic carcinoma, 356
Adenoma(s)
 alveolar, 356
 bronchial, 354–355
 pleomorphic, 356
Adenosine deaminase (ADA)
 in pleural fluid, 120–121
 in tuberculous pleuritis, 447
Adenosine triphosphatase (ATPase), in respiratory muscle function, 4–6
Adenosine triphosphate (ATP)
 for cystic fibrosis, 200
 in exercise, 101, 105
 in respiratory muscle function, 6
Adenovirus, pneumonia due to, 400t
ADH (antidiuretic hormone), syndrome of inappropriate secretion of, 359–360
Adhesion molecules, pulmonary endothelial cell, 14, 15f
Admission, to intensive care unit, 517–518
Adrenalin chloride. See Epinephrine (Medihaler-Epi, Adrenalin chloride)
Adult respiratory distress syndrome (ARDS). See Acute respiratory distress syndrome (ARDS)
Advair (salmeterol/fluticasone), for asthma, 147t
Advance directives, 508, 534
 for COPD, 195–196
Aeroallergens, 144
Aerobic capacity. See Work capacity (VO2max)
AeroBid (flunisolide)
 for asthma, 147t
 pharmacokinetics of, 154t, 155t

655

AFP (α-fetoprotein), with teratoma, 464
Aging. *See* Elderly
AHI (apnea-plus-hypopnea index), 482, 486, 488–489
AHR. *See* Airway hyperresponsiveness (AHR)
AIDS. *See* Acquired immunodeficiency syndrome (AIDS)
Air, distribution of, 7–11, 8f–11f
Air bronchograms, 82f
Air-conditioner lung, 296t
Air conduction system, 8f, 9, 9f
Air embolization, 246–247, 609–610
Airet (albuterol sulfate)
　for asthma, 135, 145, 146t, 150, 159, 572
　for COPD, 188t
Airflow
　effort dependent *vs.* effort independent, 34
　monitoring of, 482–483
　patterns of, 32–33, 32f
Airflow obstruction, reversible, in COPD, 180
Air pollution, 340, 341–342, 341t
　and lung cancer, 349
Airway(s)
　conducting, 8f, 9, 9f
　dynamic compression of, 35–36, 35f
　radiographic anatomy of, 69f–74f, 71–72, 72f
　total cross-sectional area of, 9, 9f
Airway conductance (Gaw), 33
　and lung volume, 33, 34f
　measurement of, 96–97
　specific, 33
Airway disorders, due to environmental exposure, 317–324, 318t, 320f, 323t, 324t
Airway hyperresponsiveness (AHR)
　in asthma, 138
　in COPD, 176–177
　measurement of, 93–94, 109
Airway infections, 384–387, 387f
Airway inflammation, in asthma, 136–137, 137f
Airway management, for respiratory failure, 546–548, 546t, 547f
Airway pressure release ventilation, 551
Airway resistance (Raw), 32–34, 32f
　defined, 32
　distribution of, 33
　factors influencing, 33–34, 34f
　lung volume and, 33, 34f
　measurement of, 96–97
　uses of, 110
Alanine metabolism, during stress, 520, 521f
Albendazole, for echinococcosis, 449
Albumin, serum, 523, 523t
Albuterol/ipratropium (Combivent), for asthma, 147t
Albuterol sulfate (Airet, Proventil)
　for asthma, 135, 145, 146t, 150, 159, 572
　for COPD, 188t

Alcoholism
　and lung transplantation, 211
　pneumonia with, 389, 389t
ALG (antilymphocyte globulin)
　for bronchiolitis obliterans, 220
　for lung transplantation, 215, 223
ALI. *See* Acute lung injury (ALI)
Allen's test, 620–621
Allergen avoidance, for asthma, 144
Allergic alveolitis, extrinsic, 296–299, 296t, 298t
Allergic angiitis, 281–282
Allergic bronchopulmonary aspergillosis (ABPA), 141–143
Allergic bronchopulmonary fungoses (ABPF), 141
Allergic granulomatosis, 281–282
Allergic reactions, to drugs, 287–290, 288t
Allergic rhinitis, 60, 63
ALP (acute lupus pneumonitis), 273
α_1-antitrypsin deficiency
　in COPD, 177–178, 189–190
　lung transplantation for, 209
α-fetoprotein (AFP), with teratoma, 464
Alpha waves, 478, 479f, 480f
Altitude, and arterial hypoxemia, 51
Aluminum pneumoconiosis, 335
Alupent (metaproterenol)
　for asthma, 145, 146t, 159, 572
　for COPD, 188t
Alveolar adenoma, 356
Alveolar air equation, 47, 51, 104
Alveolar-arterial oxygen gradient (P_{AO_2}-Pa_{O_2})
　in alveolar air equation, 45, 47
　in distribution of pulmonary blood flow, 16–17
　hypoxemia and, 51
　normal value for, 543, 543t
　in respiratory failure, 541
　and ventilation-perfusion mismatch, 52
　and work capacity, 104
Alveolar capillaries, 16, 16f, 577f, 578. *See also* Pulmonary capillaries
Alveolar-capillary barrier, 14, 15f
Alveolar-capillary membrane, 13, 14f
Alveolar carbon dioxide tension (P_{ACO_2})
　alveolar ventilation and, 45, 46f
　in COPD, 567
　normal, 45t
Alveolar dead space, 45
　with pulmonary embolism, 235
Alveolar ducts, functional anatomy of, 8f, 11
Alveolar-epithelial barrier, 14
Alveolar epithelial cells, 14, 14t
Alveolar hemorrhage, diffuse, 273
Alveolar hypoventilation, 45–46, 46f
　arterial hypoxemia due to, 51
　and hypercapnia, 541, 542f
Alveolar inflammatory diseases. *See* Diffuse interstitial lung diseases (DILDs)
Alveolar macrophages
　functional anatomy of, 22
　in idiopathic pulmonary fibrosis, 269
　in sarcoidosis, 293, 294f

Alveolar oxygen tension (P_{AO_2})
　in COPD, 567
　equation for, 47, 51, 104
　estimate of, 47
　mixed venous saturation and, 104, 104t
　normal, 45t
　and pulmonary vascular resistance, 18, 18f
Alveolar pressure, 27–28, 28f
　and pulmonary vascular resistance, 16, 16f
Alveolar proteinosis, pulmonary, 285–287, 285f
Alveolar recruitment, 549
Alveolar sacs, 11f
Alveolar ventilation ($\dot{V}A$), 45–47, 46f, 47f
　equation for, 45
　and minute ventilation, 51
　normal, 45
　work of breathing and, 41, 42f
Alveolitis
　cryptogenic fibrosing. *See* Idiopathic pulmonary fibrosis (IPF)
　CT of, 81f
　extrinsic allergic, 296–299, 296t, 298t
AMB. *See* Amphotericin B (AMB)
Ambient air pollution, 341, 341t
Amebiasis, pleural effusions in, 448
Amiloride, for cystic fibrosis, 200
Amines, biogenic, metabolism of, 19
Amino acids
　in parenteral nutrition, 531
　during stress, 519f, 521
Aminophylline
　for asthma, 147t, 150, 151t, 159–160
　for COPD, 569
Amiodarone
　pleural effusions due to, 455
　pulmonary reaction to, 289
Ammonia, inhalation injury due to, 323, 323t
Amniotic fluid embolism, 246
Amosite, 328, 350
Amoxicillin
　for acute bronchitis, 385
　for bronchiectasis, 386
Amoxicillin/clavulanate, for acute bronchitis, 385
Amphotericin B (AMB)
　for aspergillosis, 424, 433
　for blastomycosis, 420
　for coccidioidomycosis, 421, 438
　for cryptococcosis, 423, 437, 448
　for histoplasmosis, 418, 437
　after lung transplantation, 223
Amylase, in pleural fluid, 120, 453
Amyotrophic lateral sclerosis, respiratory failure with, 562t
ANA (antinuclear antibody), in systemic lupus erythematosus, 272
Anabolic state, 525
Anaerobic metabolism
　in exercise, 101, 105, 106f
　and work capacity, 105, 106f
Anaerobic threshold, 105, 106f
Analgesia, postoperative, 593

Anatomic dead space (V̇Danat), 45, 98

ANCA (antineutrophilic cytoplasmic antibody), in Wegener's granulomatosis, 277–278

Ancylostoma brasiliensis, eosinophilia due to, 299

Anesthesia
  with asthma, 593
  cardiopulmonary effects of, 592–593
  general *vs.* regional, 593
  for status asthmaticus, 162, 573

Aneurysm(s)
  of ascending aorta, 467f
  pulmonary artery, 257
  Rasmussen's, 411

Angiitis, allergic, 281–282

Angina pectoris, 61
  in pulmonary hypertension, 250
  surgical risk with, 600

Angiography, pulmonary, 85
  of chronic thromboembolic pulmonary hypertension, 244–245
  CT, 82–83, 82f
  of pulmonary embolism, 239t, 240

Angiotensin-converting enzyme (ACE)
  in sarcoidosis, 292, 292t
  vasoactive properties of, 19, 20f

Angiotensin II, vasoactive properties of, 17

Ankylosing spondylitis, 471
  respiratory failure with, 562t, 564

Anterior mandibular osteotomy, for obstructive sleep apnea, 490

Anthropometry, 522

Antibiotic-coated catheters, 646

Antibiotics
  for acute bronchitis, 384–385
  with asthma, 573
  for bronchiectasis, 386
  for COPD, 195
    with respiratory failure, 569–570
  for cor pulmonale, 254
  for cystic fibrosis, 201
  for epiglottitis, 383
  after lung transplantation, 215
  for multiple organ failure, 635
  for pharyngitis, 383
  for pneumonia, 408–409
    Chlamydia, 397
    Haemophilus influenzae, 396
    hospital-acquired, 402–403
    in immunocompromised host, 405
    Klebsiella pneumoniae, 399
    Legionella pneumophila, 393
    Mycoplasma pneumoniae, 397
    Pneumocystis carinii, 405–406
    Staphylococcus aureus, 399
    Streptococcus pneumoniae, 392
  for septic thromboembolism, 245
  for sinusitis, 382
  for urinary catheter-related infections, 648, 649
  for vascular catheter-related infection, 646

Antibody production, defective, drug-induced, 430t

Anticholinergic agents
  for asthma, 146t, 152, 160, 573
  for COPD, 186–187

Antidepressants, tricyclic, respiratory failure due to, 563

Antidiuretic hormone (ADH), syndrome of inappropriate secretion of, 359–360

Antiglomerular basement membrane (anti-GBM) antibody disease, 282–284, 283f

Antiinflammatory agents
  for asthma, 147t, 148t, 152–156, 153f, 154t, 155t
  for multiple organ failure, 635

Antileukotrienes, for asthma, 137, 147t, 156–158

Antilymphocyte globulin (ALG)
  for bronchiolitis obliterans, 220
  for lung transplantation, 215, 223

Antineutrophilic cytoplasmic antibody (ANCA), in Wegener's granulomatosis, 277–278

Antinuclear antibody (ANA), in systemic lupus erythematosus, 272

Antioxidants, in critical illness, 527

Antiretroviral therapy, highly active, for HIV infection, 434

Antiseptic-coated catheters, 646

Aortic aneurysm, 467f

Aortic dissection
  CT of, 82f
  MRI of, 84f
  pain of, 61

Aortic transection, 602

Aortography, 602

Apnea
  defined, 482
  sleep. *See* Sleep apnea

Apnea index, 482, 486

Apnea-plus-hypopnea index (AHI), 482, 486, 488–489

Apneic threshold, 488, 494

Apoptosis, in idiopathic pulmonary fibrosis, 269

Arachidonic acid (AA), metabolism of, 19–20, 19f

ARDS. *See* Acute respiratory distress syndrome (ARDS)

Arginine, in critical illness, 527

L-Arginine, vasoactive properties of, 19

Arousal(s), during sleep, 481
  in obstructive sleep apnea, 488
  respiratory-effort-related, 489, 489f

Arousal index, 481

Arrhythmias, in obstructive sleep apnea syndrome, 490

Arsenic, carcinogenicity of, 337t, 338, 350

Arterial-alveolar pressure difference. *See* Alveolar-arterial oxygen gradient (PAO$_2$-PaO$_2$)

Arterial blood gases
  in exercise testing, 108
  with pulmonary embolism, 237
  in respiratory failure, 540–541, 541f, 542f, 556

Arterial carbon dioxide tension (PaCO$_2$)
  alveolar ventilation and, 45
  in asthma, 140, 140f
  calculation of, 542–543
  normal, 44, 45t, 543t
  in respiratory failure, 541, 542f
  variables related to, 542–543

Arterial catheterization
  pulmonary, 621–627
    effect of PEEP on wedge pressure measurements in, 625
    indications for, 626–627
    infection related to, 644–647, 644t
    insertion techniques for, 621–622, 622f
    obtaining reliable pressure measurements with, 622–623, 623f, 624f
    relation of wedge pressure to left atrial pressure in, 623–625
    verifying catheter position in, 625, 625t
  systemic, 620–621

Arterial hemoglobin saturation. *See* Arterial oxygen saturation (SaO$_2$)

Arterial hypoxemia, 50–53, 50t
  with pulmonary embolism, 235

Arterial-mixed venous difference, in oxygen tension, 53

Arterial oxygen saturation (SaO$_2$), 44, 54, 483
  pH and, 54, 54f
  and work capacity, 104–105, 104f

Arterial oxygen tension (PaO$_2$)
  and arterial pH, 541, 542f
  calculation of, 543
  in cor pulmonale, 253
  normal, 44, 45t, 543t
  and oxygen delivery, 54–55
  and plasma bicarbonate, 541, 542f
  with pulmonary embolism, 237
  in respiratory failure, 541, 541f

Arterial venous oxygen difference, 50

Arterial-venous pressure gradient, 17

Arteriovenous malformations, 255t, 256f, 255, 257

Arteriovenous shunts, 256–257

Arthritis, rheumatoid, 274–275, 274t

Asbestos, 328
  in buildings, 340
  carcinogenicity of, 337t, 338, 340, 349–350
  and malignant mesothelioma, 340

Asbestosis, 328, 329–331, 330f, 331f

Asbestos pleural effusions, 324, 455

Asbestos-related pleural calcification, 458

Asbestos-related pleural disease, 328–329, 458

Asbestos-related pleural thickening, 329, 458

Asbestos-related pulmonary disease, nonmalignant, 328–331, 330f, 331f

Ascaris lumbricoides, Loeffler's syndrome due to, 299

Asmanex (mometasone furoate), for asthma, 147t, 154
Aspergillomas, 424
Aspergillosis, 423–425
  allergic bronchopulmonary, 141–143
  in immunocompromised patients, 431, 433
  after lung transplantation, 222–223, 223f
  pleural, 447–448
Aspiration, gastric
  acute lung injury and ARDS due to, 583f, 585, 585f
  perioperative, 596
Aspiration pneumonia, 393–395, 394f
Aspirin, asthma due to, 141
Assist-controlled (AC) ventilation, 548, 549t
Asthma, 133–163
  acute, 158–162
  airway hyperresponsiveness in, 138
    measurement of, 93–94, 109
  algorithm for management of, 143
  anesthesia with, 593
  classification of, 134
  clinical evaluation of, 137–143
  comorbid conditions with, 140–143
  cough in, 62, 138
  defined, 133–134
  diagnosis of, 138–139, 138f
  drug-induced, 141
  dynamic compliance in, 39
  dyspnea in, 61, 138
  environmental control for, 144
  epidemiology of, 134–136
  exercise-induced, 112, 139
  experimentally induced, 136
  experimental therapies for, 161, 162–163
  expiratory flow rate in, 37
  extrinsic, 134
  factitious, 139
  flow-volume loop in, 138–139, 138f
  gastroesophageal reflux disease and, 140–141
  glucocorticosteroids in, 145f
  goals of therapy for, 143
  grain, 322
  helium-oxygen gas for, 161
  hospitalization for, 139–140, 140t, 158–162
  hyperinflation of chest in, 64
  hypoxemia in, 140
  impairment with, 113–114
  incidence and prevalence of, 134
  inhalation anesthetics for, 162
  intravenous magnesium for, 161
  intrinsic, 134
  intubation for, 161
  mechanical ventilation for, 161–162
  mortality due to, 134–135
  natural history of, 135–136
  nocturnal, 496–497
  non-invasive ventilation for, 161
  occupational, 317–321, 318t, 320f
  PaCO2 in, 140, 140f

  pathology and pathogenesis of, 136–137, 136f, 137f
  patient education for, 143–144
  peak expiratory flow in, 139
    monitoring of, 144
  pharmacotherapy for, 144–158, 145f, 146t–148t
    with anticholinergic agents, 146t, 152, 160
    with antileukotrienes, 137, 147t, 156–158
    with β-adrenergic agonists, 135, 145–150, 146t–147t, 158–159
    with bronchodilators, 145–152, 146t–148t, 151t
    with combination products, 147t
    with corticosteroids
      inhaled, 147t, 152–156, 153f, 154t, 155t
      systemic, 148t, 160
    with cromoglycates, 147t, 156
    with cyclosporine A, 163
    with dry powder inhalers, 149
    with gold preparations, 162–163
    intravenous administration of, 159
    with metered dose inhalers, 144, 149, 150, 154, 158–159
    with methotrexate, 162
    with methylxanthines, 147t–148t, 150–152, 151t
    with nebulizer, 149, 158–159
    with troleandomycin, 163
    via subcutaneous injection, 159
  pulmonary eosinophilia with, 300
  pulmonary function testing in, 110–111
  respiratory failure in, 570–573, 570t, 572t
  severe, management of, 145, 155t
  severity of
    assessment of, 139–140, 140f, 140t, 570, 570t
    classification of, 148t
  sleep and, 496–497
  steroid-dependent, 162–163
  surgical considerations in, 598
  vs. upper airway obstruction, 138–139, 138f
  upper respiratory tract symptoms in, 60
  wheezing in, 138
Asthmatic bronchitis, 175
Asthmatic constitution, 176
Atelectasis
  with anesthesia, 592–593
  basilar, in systemic lupus erythematosus, 272
  patterns of, 72, 73f, 74f
  postoperative, 594–595
  rounded, asbestos-related, 329
Atmospheric pollution, 340, 341–342, 341t
  and lung cancer, 349
Atopy, and occupational asthma, 317–319
ATP (adenosine triphosphate)
  for cystic fibrosis, 200
  in exercise, 101, 105
  in respiratory muscle function, 6

ATPase (adenosine triphosphatase), in respiratory muscle function, 4–6
Atropine sulfate
  for asthma, 146t, 152, 160
  for COPD, 186–187
Atrovent. *See* Ipratropium bromide (Atrovent)
Attapulgite pneumoconiosis, 335
Auranofin, for asthma, 163
Auscultation, 65–66, 65t
Autonomic nervous system, regulation of pulmonary circulation by, 17
Autonomic nervous system abnormalities, due to lung cancer, 360
Auto-PEEP, 550, 568, 572
Azathioprine
  for Churg-Strauss syndrome, 282
  for idiopathic pulmonary fibrosis, 270
  for lung transplantation, 215, 219, 223, 224, 224t, 225
  for Wegener's granulomatosis, 279
Azmacort (triamcinolone acetonide)
  for asthma, 147t
  pharmacokinetics of, 154t, 155t
Azygos node, 23

B

Baclofen, for hiccups, 474
Bacterial adherence, in pneumonia, 387–388, 387f
Bacterial infections, 381–399
  in AIDS, 405–406, 405f, 436
  in bronchiectasis, 386–387, 387f
  bronchiolitis due to, 385
  bronchitis due to, 384–385
  in COPD, 177, 177f, 195, 196f
  in immunocompromised host, 403–405, 404t, 432–433
  lung abscess due to, 394f, 395, 395f
  pneumonia due to, 387–399, 401–409
    in AIDS, 405–406, 405f
    approach to patient with, 406–408
    aspiration, 393–395, 394f
    atypical, 398t
    clinical features of, 389–391, 390f
    community-acquired, 389–399
    hospital-acquired, 401–403, 401f, 403f
    in immunocompromised host, 403–405, 404t
    after lung transplantation, 221
    pathogenesis of, 387–389, 387f, 388t, 389t
    specific pathogens in, 391–399, 392f, 394f–396f, 398t, 399f
    therapy for, 408–409
  of upper respiratory tract, 381–384
Bacterial interference, 387
Bacterial translocation, 526
Bacteriology, of respiratory tract, 379–381, 380t
Bagassosis, 60, 296t
BAL. *See* Bronchoalveolar lavage (BAL)
BALT (bronchus-associated lymphoid tissue), 23
Baltomas, 357, 358
Barbiturates, cardiovascular effects of, 593

Barium swallow, 85
Barometric pressure, and arterial
  hypoxemia, 51
Barrel chest, in COPD, 179
Basal cells, functional anatomy of, 10
Basilar atelectasis, in systemic lupus
  erythematosus, 272
B-cell defects
  causes of, 430t
  pneumonia with, 403, 404t
BCME (bischloromethyl ether),
  carcinogenicity of, 337t, 339
Beclomethasone dipropionate (Beclovent,
  HFA-BDP, Qvar, Vanceril)
  for asthma, 147t, 154
  pharmacokinetics of, 154t, 155t
Beclomethasone monopropionate (BMP),
  pharmacokinetics of, 154t
Bell's palsy, 64
Beneficence, in medical decision-making,
  533
Benign neoplasms
  alveolar adenoma, 356
  chondroma and osteochondroma, 357
  hamartoma, 357
  leiomyoma, 357
  lipoma, 357
  sclerosing hemangioma, 356
  solitary peripheral parenchymal mass as,
    368, 368t
Beryllium
  carcinogenicity of, 337t, 338–339
  inhalation injury due to, 323, 323t
  interstitial lung disease due to, 332–334,
    333f
β-adrenergic agonists
  for asthma, 135, 145–150, 146t–147t,
    158–159, 572, 573
  for COPD, 187–188, 188t, 194
  for cor pulmonale, 254
  side effects of, 187–188
Beta-carotene, and lung cancer, 350, 351f
BIA (bioelectrical impedance), 523
Bicarbonate (HCO$_3$⁻), plasma, PaCO$_2$ and,
    541, 542f
Bilateral lung transplantation (BLT). *See
    also* Lung transplantation (LT)
  indications for, 209, 210t
Bioelectrical impedance (BIA), 523
Biogenic amines, metabolism of, 19
Biomass fuels, exposure to, 342
Biopsy
  lung
    in asbestosis, 330, 331f
    for idiopathic pulmonary fibrosis, 265,
      267
    in immunocompromised patient, 432
    for occupational interstitial lung
      disease, 326
    open-, 127–128
    for pneumonia, 407
    transbronchial, 121
    for Wegener's granulomatosis, 279
  lymph node, in lung cancer, 365
  needle aspiration
    endoscopic ultrasound-guided, 127
    in immunocompromised patient, 432

in lung cancer, 362–363, 365
  of mediastinal mass, 461
  transbronchial, 122
  transthoracic, 125
  pleural, 121
    in immunocompromised patient, 432
    in lung cancer, 363
    in tuberculous pleuritis, 447
Biphasic positive airway pressure, 544, 544f
Bird breeder's lung, 296t, 297
Bischloromethyl ether (BCME),
  carcinogenicity of, 337t, 339
Bitolterol mesylate (Tornalate)
  for asthma, 146t
  for COPD, 188t
Bladder irrigation, 648
Blastomycosis, 419–420, 419f, 420f
  pleural effusions in, 448
Bleeding. *See* Hemorrhage
Bleomycin, pulmonary reaction to,
    288–289
Blood cultures, in immunocompromised
    patients, 432
Blood doping, 103
Blood flow distribution, 12–14, 13f, 14f,
    14t
  in critically ill patients, 633
  in oxygen delivery, 53
  pulmonary, 16–17, 16f
Blood gas analysis, 99
Blood gas tensions, normal, 44–45, 45t
Blood transfusion, for multiple organ
    failure, 633
BLT (bilateral lung transplantation). *See
    also* Lung transplantation (LT)
  indications for, 209, 210t
Blum-Singer valve, 547
BMP (beclomethasone monopropionate),
    pharmacokinetics of, 154t
BMT (bone marrow transplant),
    pulmonary complications of,
    430–434, 430t–432t
Body weight, assessment of, 522
Boerhaave's syndrome, 453
Bohr effect, 54f
Bohr equation, 46–47, 46f, 47f
Bolus feedings, 529
Bone marrow emboli, 246
Bone marrow transplant (BMT),
    pulmonary complications of,
    430–434, 430t–432t
Bone scan, for lung cancer, 367
BOOP. *See* Bronchiolitis obliterans with
    organizing pneumonia (BOOP)
BOS (bronchiolitis obliterans syndrome),
    after lung transplantation,
    219–220, 220f, 220t
Boyden system, 72f, 72t
Brachytherapy, for lung cancer, 370
Bradykinin, vasoactive properties of, 19
Breathing
  active, 4, 5f
  Cheyne-Stokes, 493t, 494, 494t,
    495–496, 496f
  deep, postoperative, 595
  diaphragmatic, for COPD, 192

dynamics of, 32–42, 32f, 34f, 35f, 37f,
    38f, 40f–42f
  mouth, during exercise, 7
  oxygen cost of, 41–42
  pursed-lip, for COPD, 192
  quiet, 4, 5f
  rapid shallow, 506f, 552
  re-, 100
  resting tidal, 6
  spontaneous, trial of, 551
  work of, 40–42, 41f, 42f, 555
Breathing retraining, for COPD, 192
Breathlessness, 61
Breath sounds, 65–66, 65t
Brethaire. *See* Terbutaline sulfate
    (Brethaire, Bricanyl)
Bricanyl. *See* Terbutaline sulfate (Brethaire,
    Bricanyl)
British hypothesis, of COPD, 177, 177f
Bromocriptine, pleural effusions due to,
    455
Bronchial adenoma, 354–355
Bronchial asthma. *See* Asthma
Bronchial stenosis, after lung
    transplantation, 217–218
Bronchial strictures, after lung
    transplantation, 217–218
Bronchial tumors, of salivary gland type,
    356
Bronchial washing, 122
Bronchiectasis, 197–198
  causes of, 386
  classification of, 197
  clinical presentation of, 197, 386
  conditions associated with development
    of, 197t
  cystic fibrosis with, 386–387
  defined, 197
  dry *vs.* wet, 197
  evaluation of, 197–198, 387, 387f
  hemoptysis in, 63, 63t
  immotile cilia syndrome and, 198
  immunodeficiency with, 198
  infection in, 380t, 386–387, 387f
  lung transplantation for, 209
  pleural effusions with, 445–446
  treatment of, 198
Bronchioalveolar tumor, intravascular, 356
Bronchioles
  functional anatomy of, 11, 11f
  metabolic and secretory functions of,
    11–12
  nonrespiratory, 8f, 11
  respiratory, 8f, 11, 11f
  terminal, 11, 11f
Bronchiolitis, 378, 380t, 385
  respiratory, 271–272
Bronchiolitis obliterans syndrome (BOS),
    after lung transplantation,
    219–220, 220f, 220t
Bronchiolitis obliterans with organizing
    pneumonia (BOOP), 271, 385
  clinical presentation of, 271
  diagnosis of, 268, 271
  after lung transplantation, 219
  with rheumatoid arthritis, 275
  treatment of, 271

Bronchitis
acute, 378, 380t, 384–385
asthmatic, 175
chronic. *See also* Chronic obstructive
pulmonary disease (COPD)
acute exacerbations of, 384–385
defined, 174–175
vs. emphysema, 179, 179t
expiratory flow rate in, 37, 38
hemoptysis in, 63, 63t, 179
obstructive, 175
pneumonia with, 389, 389t
pulmonary function testing in,
110–111
radiographic criteria for, 181, 182f
simple, 175
occupational or industrial, 335–337,
336t
from coal dust, 331
silica associated, 328
Bronchoalveolar lavage (BAL)
in hypersensitivity pneumonitis, 298,
298t
in idiopathic pulmonary fibrosis, 267,
268, 268t
in immunocompromised patients, 432
indications for, 124
in occupational interstitial lung disease,
326
in *Pneumocystis carinii* pneumonia, 435
for pulmonary alveolar proteinosis, 287
in sarcoidosis, 292–293, 293t
technique of, 122
Bronchoconstriction, with pulmonary
embolism, 235
Bronchodilators
for asthma, 145–152, 146t–148t, 151t,
572
for COPD, 186–189, 188t
for cor pulmonale, 254
Bronchodilator testing, 110
Bronchogenic carcinoma, 351–354
classification of, 351
clinical manifestations of, 358–361, 359t
diagnosis of, 361–363
epidemiology of, 346–347, 347f
etiology of, 347–351, 348f, 349f, 349t,
351f
hemoptysis in, 63, 63t
histology of, 352–354, 352f–355f, 354t
pathogenesis of, 351–352
pleural effusions due to, 449
staging of, 363–367, 363t, 364t, 366f,
367f
treatment for, 368–371, 371f
Bronchogenic cysts, 462f, 466
Bronchography, 85
air, 82f
of bronchiectasis, 197–198
Bronchophony, 65
Bronchopleural fistula, with HIV infection,
436
Bronchoprovocation tests, 93–94, 109, 111
Bronchopulmonary lymph nodes, 23
Bronchopulmonary segments
anatomy of, 9, 10f
classification of, 9

radiographic anatomy of, 69f, 70f, 72,
72f–74f, 72t
Bronchoscopic ultrasonography, 122
Bronchoscopy, 121–125
of bronchiectasis, 198
of chest trauma, 602
complications of, 122–123
with HIV infection, 435
of idiopathic pulmonary fibrosis, 267
in immunocompromised patients, 432
indications for, 123–125
of lung cancer, 123–124, 362, 365
after lung transplantation, 216–217
of occupational interstitial lung disease,
326
of pneumonia, 407–408, 409
Pneumocystis carinii, 435
techniques of, 121–122
of tracheobronchial disruption, 612
transbronchial, 121
Bronchospasm, postinfectious, 384
Bronchus(i)
functional anatomy of, 8f, 9–10, 10f,
11f
intermediate, 9
lobar, 9
main
left and right, 9
radiographic anatomy of, 69f, 70f,
71–72, 72f
metabolic and secretory functions of,
11–12
papillomas of, 356
segmental, 9
Bronchus-associated lymphoid tissue
(BALT), 23
Bronkometer (isoetharine HCl)
for asthma, 145, 146t, 159
for COPD, 188t
Brugia malayi, tropical pulmonary
eosinophilia due to, 300
Brush cells, functional anatomy of, 10
Budesonide (Pulmicort)
for asthma, 147t, 153–154
for COPD, 189
pharmacokinetics of, 154t, 155t
Budoxis (formoterol/budesonide), for
asthma, 147t
Bupropion hydrochloride (Zyban), for
smoking cessation, 185
Busulfan, pulmonary reaction to, 289
Byssinosis, 321–322

C

CABP (coronary artery bypass graft)
with COPD, 597–598
pleural effusions after, 454, 456
Cadherins, 14
Cadmium
carcinogenicity of, 337t, 339
inhalation injury due to, 323, 323t
Calcium, in respiratory muscle function, 4
Calcium channel blockers, for primary
pulmonary hypertension, 251
Caloric stores, normal, 519, 519t
Calorimetry, indirect, 524

Canals of Lambert, 11, 40
Cancer. *See* Lung cancer
Candidiasis
after lung transplantation, 222, 223
oropharyngeal, 63
CaO$_2$, normal value for, 543t
CAP. *See* Community-acquired pneumonia
(CAP)
Capillaries. *See* Pulmonary capillaries
Capillaritis, 273
Capillary-endothelial barrier, 14, 15f
Capillary recruitment, 16, 17
Caplan's syndrome, 274–275
with coal workers' pneumoconiosis, 332
with silicosis, 328
Carbidopa, for periodic limb movements,
486
Carbohydrate metabolism, during stress,
519f–521f, 520–521
Carbon dioxide (CO$_2$)
environmental, 342
inspired and expired, 46, 46f
Carbon dioxide (CO$_2$) dissociation curve,
46, 47f
Carbon dioxide (CO$_2$) production (V̇CO$_2$),
45–46, 556
Carbon dioxide (CO$_2$) tension (PCO$_2$)
alveolar. *See* Alveolar carbon dioxide
tension (PACO$_2$)
arterial. *See* Arterial carbon dioxide
tension (PaCO$_2$)
in central sleep apnea, 493–494, 493t
with Cheyne-Stokes breathing, 495
in COPD, 497–498
in obesity hypoventilation syndrome,
489
in overlap syndrome, 489
during sleep, 481
transcutaneous, 556
venous, 543t
Carbon monoxide (CO)
air pollution due to, 341, 341t
and oxygen delivery, 54
Carbon monoxide (CO) diffusing capacity
(DLCO), 47, 99–100, 99f
in emphysema, 110
in Goodpasture's syndrome, 283
in sarcoidosis, 291
Carboxyhemoglobin, and oxygen delivery,
54
Carcinogens, occupational, 337–340, 337t,
349–350, 349f, 349t
Carcinoid syndrome, 360
Carcinoid tumor, 354–355
Carcinoma
adeno-, 352, 354, 354f
adenoid cystic, 356
bronchogenic, 351–354
classification of, 351
clinical manifestations of, 358–361,
359t
diagnosis of, 361–363
epidemiology of, 346–347, 347f
etiology of, 347–351, 348f, 349f,
349t, 351f
hemoptysis in, 63, 63t
histology of, 352–354, 352f–355f,
354t

pathogenesis of, 351–352
pleural effusions due to, 449
staging of, 363–367, 363t, 364t, 366f, 367f
treatment for, 368–371, 371f
giant cell, 354
large cell (undifferentiated), 354, 355f
neuroendocrine, 355
mucoepidermoid, 356
oat cell (lymphocyte-like), 352–353
small cell, 352–353, 353f, 354t
squamous cell, 351–352, 352f, 353f
Carcinomatosis, lymphangitic, 81f
Cardiac disease, pneumonia with, 389, 389t
Cardiac output (Q̇), 45, 49
with exercise, 106
and oxygen delivery, 53
and work capacity, 103
Cardiac surgery
mediastinitis after, 468
pulmonary artery catheterization after, 626–637
Cardiogenic pulmonary edema, high-pressure, 579–581, 579f, 580f
pulmonary artery catheterization for, 626
Cardiogenic shock, 627t
Cardiopulmonary risk index (CPRI), for lung resection, 510, 599–600, 599t
Cardiovascular consequences, of obstructive sleep apnea syndrome, 489–490
Cardiovascular dysfunction, exercise testing with, 112
Cardiovascular exercise testing. *See* Exercise testing
Cardiovascular failure, in multiple organ failure, 628–629
Cardiovascular monitoring, 620–627
via pulmonary arterial catheterization, 621–627
effect of PEEP on wedge pressure measurements in, 625
indications for, 626–627
insertion techniques for, 621–622, 622f
obtaining reliable pressure measurements with, 622–623, 623f, 624f
relation of wedge pressure to left atrial pressure in, 623–625
verifying catheter position in, 625, 625t
via systemic arterial catheterization, 620–621
Carina, position of, 9
Castleman's disease, 465
Catabolic state, 525
Cataplexy, 484, 485
Catecholamines
for asthma, 145
regulation of pulmonary circulation by, 17
Catheter colonization, 644
Catheterization
central venous, infection related to, 644–647, 644t
pulmonary artery, 621–627

effect of PEEP on wedge pressure measurements in, 625
indications for, 626–627
infection related to, 644–647, 644t
insertion techniques for, 621–622, 622f
obtaining reliable pressure measurements with, 622–623, 623f, 624f
relation of wedge pressure to left atrial pressure in, 623–625
verifying catheter position in, 625, 625t
systemic arterial, 620–621
urinary, infection related to, 647–649, 647t
Catheter-related bloodstream infection (CR-BSI), 644
Catheter-related venous thrombosis, 646
Causal relationship, for environmental lung disease, 315
Caveolae intracellulare, 20, 20f
CBD (chronic beryllium disease), 332–334, 333f
CC (closing capacity), 98
CD4 cell count, with HIV infection, 434
and *Pneumocystis carinii* pneumonia, 435, 438
Central nervous system (CNS) failure, in multiple organ failure, 630, 630t
Central sleep apnea (CSA), 493–496
with Cheyne-Stokes breathing, 493t, 494, 494t, 495–496, 496f
in congestive heart failure, 493t, 494, 494f, 495–496, 496f
defined, 482, 482f, 486, 493
hypercapnic, 493–494, 493t
idiopathic, 494–495, 494f
nonhypercapnic, 493t, 494, 494f
Central sleep apnea syndrome (CSAS). *See* Central sleep apnea (CSA)
Central venous catheter, infection related to, 644–647, 644t
Cerebellar degeneration, due to lung cancer, 360
Cervical lymph node tuberculosis, 411
CF. *See* Cystic fibrosis (CF)
CFCs (chlorofluorocarbons), in metered dose inhalers, 149
Cheese worker's lung, 296t
Chemical workers lung, 296t
Chemotherapy
for lung cancer, 369–370
pulmonary complications of, 430–434, 430t–432t
Chest
flail, 472, 605–606
fluoroscopy of, 77–78
funnel, 471
hyperinflation of, 64
percussion of, 65
Chest barrel, 179
Chest pain, 60–61
in lung cancer, 358
in malignant mesothelioma, 451
pleuritic, 7, 61, 442

with pleural effusions, 442
with pulmonary embolism, 237, 237t
due to tuberculosis, 411
Chest physiotherapy (CPT)
for cystic fibrosis, 201
for pneumonia, 409
postoperative, 595
Chest radiography, 68–78
of ARDS, 583, 583f, 585f
of asbestosis, 329, 330, 330f
of asthma, 140, 571
of BOOP, 271
of bronchiectasis, 197–198
of Churg-Strauss syndrome, 281
of COPD, 180–181, 180t, 181f, 182f, 566–567, 566f
of cor pulmonale, 252–253, 253f
of cystic fibrosis, 199
of diaphragmatic rupture, 610, 611f
of drug-induced pulmonary disease, 287–288
of eosinophilic granuloma, 301, 302f
of esophageal injury, 611
of Goodpasture's syndrome, 282–283, 283f
hila on, 72–75, 75f, 76f
of HIV infection, 435
identification of structures in, 69f, 70f, 71–75
of idiopathic pulmonary fibrosis, 265, 266, 266f
of idiopathic pulmonary hemosiderosis, 284–285
in immunocompromised patients, 431–432, 432t
lobar bronchial segments on, 69f, 70f, 72, 72f–74f, 72t
of lung cancer, 361–362, 364
of lymphomatoid granulomatosis, 280, 280f
main bronchi on, 69f, 70f, 71–72, 72f
observer error in, 71
of occupational interstitial lung disease, 325
of pleural effusions, 443
of pneumonia, 406–407
Pneumocystis carinii, 435
portable, 71
of progressive systemic sclerosis, 275
of pulmonary alveolar proteinosis, 285f, 286
of pulmonary contusion, 608, 608f
of pulmonary embolism, 238
of pulmonary hypertension, 250
pulmonary vascular system on, 69f, 70f, 72–75, 75f, 76f
of rheumatoid arthritis, 274
routine projections on, 69f, 70, 70f
of sarcoidosis, 290–291, 291f
special view on, 75–77, 77f
of systemic lupus erythematosus, 272, 272f, 273f
technique of, 68
trachea on, 69f, 70f, 71–72
of trauma, 601, 604f, 607f, 608f
of tuberculosis, 412
of Wegener's granulomatosis, 278, 278f

Chest tightness, in byssinosis, 321
Chest trauma, 600–613
  air embolization due to, 609–610
  to chest wall, 603–607, 603f, 607f
    respiratory failure due to, 564
  contusion due to, 607–609, 608f
  diagnostic and therapeutic modalities for, 601–603, 602t, 603t
  to diaphragm, 610, 611f
  esophageal injury due to, 610–612, 611f
  flail chest due to, 605–606
  hematoma due to, 609
  hemothorax due to, 607, 607f
  incidence of, 600
  initial evaluation of, 600–601, 601t
  laceration due to, 609–610
  to mediastinum, 610–613, 611f, 613t
  pneumothorax due to, 458, 606–607
  to pulmonary parenchyma, 607–610, 608f
  rib fractures due to, 601, 603–605, 604f
  sternal fractures due to, 601, 603, 604f
  tracheal and bronchial disruption due to, 612–613, 613t
Chest tube
  for hemothorax, 607
  for pneumothorax, 606
Chest wall
  abnormalities of, respiratory failure due to, 562t, 564
  diseases of, 470–472
  distending pressure of, 27, 27f
  examination of, 64
  factors holding lung against, 29–30
  functional anatomy of, 4, 4f, 5f
  injuries to, 603–607, 603f, 607f
    respiratory failure due to, 564
  pressure-volume curve for, 27, 28f
  resting volume of, 27
Chest wall pain, 61
Cheyne-Stokes breathing (CSB), 493t, 494, 494t, 495–496, 496f
Chief complaint, 59
China clay pneumoconiosis, 334
Chlamydia pneumoniae, 397, 398t
Chlamydia psittaci, 397, 398t
Chloride channels, 12, 12f
  cystic fibrosis transmembrane conductance regulator (CFTR), 12, 12f
Chlorine, inhalation injury due to, 323, 323t
Chlorofluorocarbons (CFCs), in metered dose inhalers, 149
Chloromethyl ether, carcinogenicity of, 337t, 339
Chlorpromazine, for hiccups, 474
Cholestasis, due to parenteral nutrition, 532
Chondroma, 357
Chromium
  carcinogenicity of, 337t, 339, 350
  inhalation injury due to, 323t
Chronic beryllium disease (CBD), 332–334, 333f

Chronic obstructive pulmonary disease (COPD), 174–196. *See also* Bronchitis, chronic; Emphysema
  acute exacerbations of, 194–195, 194t, 196f
  advance directives for, 195–196
  airway hyperresponsiveness in, 176–177
  α_1-antitrypsin deficiency in, 177–178, 189–190
  breathing retraining for, 192
  British hypothesis of, 177, 177f
  bronchodilators for, 186–189, 188t
  cigarette smoking and, 176
  clinical course of, 182–183, 183f, 195–196, 196t
  clinical presentation of, 179, 179t
  defined, 174
  Dutch hypothesis of, 176
  dyspnea in, 61, 179, 183
  elastase-antielastase theory of, 177–178
  epidemiology of, 175–176
  exercise for, 106–107, 191–192
  exercise testing in, 111–112
  hospitalization for, 194, 194t
  hyperinflation of chest in, 64
  hypoxic vasoconstriction in, 18
  infections in, 177, 177f, 183, 195, 196f
  laboratory assessment of, 179
  late stages of, 183
  lung transplantation for, 209, 211–212, 212t
  mucus hypersecretion in, 62, 177
  nutritional assessment for, 191
  obstructive sleep apnea with, 489, 497, 498
  oxidants in, 177–178
  oxygen therapy for, 193–194, 195
  pathogenesis of, 176–178, 177f
  patient education for, 191
  pneumothorax due to, 459
  and postoperative pulmonary complications, 509, 509t, 510
  prediction of, 111
  prevention of, 183–186, 184f, 184t
  prognosis for, 195, 196t
  protease-antiprotease hypothesis of, 177–178
  psychosocial support for, 192
  pulmonary function testing in, 111, 180
  pulmonary rehabilitation for, 190–193, 190t, 191t
  radiographic signs of, 180–182, 180t, 181f, 182f, 566–567, 566f
  respiratory failure due to, 565–570, 566f, 567f
  risk factors for, 176
  severe, prognosis for, 195–196, 196t
  sleep and, 497–498
  smoking and, 176
  smoking cessation for, 182–183, 183f, 184–185, 184f, 184t
  sputum in, 62, 177, 566
  stable, management of, 186–190, 186f, 187f
  surgical considerations in, 597–598, 598t

  types of, 174–175
  vicious circle hypothesis of, 177, 177f
  weight loss in, 179, 183
Chronic thromboembolic pulmonary hypertension, 244–245
Chrysotile, 328, 349–350
Churg-Strauss syndrome, 281–282
  with antileukotrienes, 157
  pleural effusions with, 452
Chyliform pleural effusion, 457
Chylothorax, 456–457
  in pulmonary lymphangiomyomatosis, 455
Chylous pleural effusion, 457
Cigarette smoking. *See* Smoking
Cilia
  defects in, 22
  immotile, 22
  in sinus cavities, 7
Ciliated cells
  functional anatomy of, 10, 11f
  in mucociliary escalator, 21, 21f, 22
Circulatory system, 12–14, 13f, 14f, 14t
  in critically ill patients, 633
  in oxygen delivery, 53
  pulmonary, 16–17, 16f
Cirrhosis, pleural effusions with, 444
Clara cell(s), functional anatomy of, 10, 11
Clara cell protein, 11–12
Clindamycin, for aspiration, 394
Clonazepam, for periodic limb movements, 486
Closed-circuit helium method, 94–95, 95f
Closing capacity (CC), 98
Closing volume (CV), 98, 594
Clubbing, 66, 66f
  in idiopathic pulmonary fibrosis, 266
  in lung cancer, 361
  in respiratory failure, 540
CMV. *See* Cytomegalovirus (CMV)
CMV (controlled mechanical ventilation), 548
CNS (central nervous system) failure, in multiple organ failure, 630, 630t
CO. *See* Carbon monoxide (CO)
CO_2. *See* Carbon dioxide (CO_2)
Coagulation system, in acute lung injury, 585–586
Coal workers' pneumoconiosis (CWP), 331–332, 332f
Cobalt-related lung disease, 332, 334
Cobb measure, of scoliosis curves, 470–471, 470f
Coccidioidal meningitis, 422
Coccidioidomycosis, 420–422, 421f, 438
  pleural effusions in, 448
Coin lesions
  appropriate investigation of, 368, 368t
  due to histoplasmosis, 415
Cold, common, 377, 380t, 381
Collagen vascular disease, 272–276, 272f, 272t, 273f, 274t
  pleural effusions with, 452
Collapsible segment, 36, 37f
Collateral ventilation, 11, 40

Columnar cells, functional anatomy of, 10, 11f
Coma scale, 630, 630t
Combivent (albuterol/ipratropium), for asthma, 147t
Common cold, 377, 380t, 381
Community-acquired pneumonia (CAP), 389–401
　antibiotics for, 408–409
　bacterial, 391–399, 392f, 394f–396f, 397t, 398f
　clinical features of, 389–391, 390f
　hospitalization for, 408
　viral, 399–401, 400f, 400t
Complement disorders, pneumonia with, 404t
Compliance, 27
　dynamic, 39–40, 40f
　frequency dependence of, 39–40, 40f
　measurement of, 97, 97f
　specific, 97
　static, 97, 97f
　total, 97
Computed tomography (CT), 78–83
　of bronchiectasis, 198
　of chest trauma, 601–602
　of esophageal injury, 611f
　helical, 80–83, 82f
　high-resolution
　　of emphysema, 181–182, 182f
　　of idiopathic pulmonary fibrosis, 265, 266, 266f
　　of progressive systemic sclerosis, 275
　in immunocompromised patients, 432
　indications for, 79–80, 80f–82f
　of lung cancer, 361, 364–365, 367
　of mediastinal masses, 79, 80f, 461, 462f
　of occupational interstitial lung disease, 325–326
　of pulmonary contusion, 608, 608f
　of pulmonary embolism, 240
　spiral, of pulmonary embolism, 240
　technique of, 78–79, 79f
Computed tomography (CT) pulmonary angiography, 82–83, 82f
Condom catheters, 648
Conducting airways, 8f, 9, 9f
　total cross-sectional area of, 9, 9f
Congenital pulmonary vascular disorders, 255–257, 255t, 256f
Congestive heart failure
　pleural effusions in, 444
　sleep apnea in, 493t, 494, 494t, 495–496, 496f
Conjunctivitis, 60
Connective tissue diseases, 272–276, 272f, 272t, 273f, 274t
Consent, informed, 533–534
Conservators, for medical decision-making, 533
Constipation, from tube feeding, 530
Continuous ambulatory peritoneal dialysis, pleural effusions with, 444
Continuous feedings, 529
Continuous positive airway pressure (CPAP), 544, 544f

for Cheyne-Stokes breathing, 495
for sleep apnea
　central, 495
　obstructive, 490, 491–493
for status asthmaticus, 161
for weaning, 553
　with COPD, 569
Contrast examinations, 84–85
Controlled mechanical ventilation (CMV), 548
Contusion, pulmonary, 607–609, 608f
Copper fumes, exposure to, 323–324
Cori cycle, 520, 520f
Coronary artery bypass graft (CABG)
　with COPD, 597–598
　pleural effusions after, 454, 456
Coronavirus, pneumonia due to, 400t
Cor pulmonale, 252–255
　chest radiography of, 252–253, 253f
　in COPD, 179
　defined, 252
　electrocardiographic abnormalities in, 252
　evaluation of, 252–253, 253f
　incidence of, 252
　long-term management of, 255
　symptoms and signs of, 252
　therapy for, 253–254
Corticosteroids
　for acute pulmonary rejection, 219
　for asthma
　　inhaled, 147t, 152–156, 153f, 154t, 155t
　　nocturnal, 497
　　systemic, 148t, 160, 573
　　in asthma, 145f
　for bronchiolitis obliterans, 220
　　with organizing pneumonia, 271
　for COPD, 188–189, 194–195
　　with respiratory failure, 569
　for cor pulmonale, 254
　for cystic fibrosis, 201
　for idiopathic pulmonary fibrosis, 269–270
　and lung transplantation, 211, 215, 225
　for multiple organ failure, 635
　for *Pneumocystis carinii* pneumonia, 436
　pneumonia with, 404t
　for sarcoidosis, 295
　for tuberculous pleuritis, 447
　for Wegener's granulomatosis, 279
Cortisone, for asthma, 160
Costochondritis, 61
Costophrenic angles, with pleural effusions, 443
Cotton dust-related disease, 321–322
Cough, 61–62
　in asbestosis, 329
　in asthma, 62, 138
　　occupational, 319
　in BOOP, 271
　bronchoscopy of, 125
　in chronic bronchitis, 174, 179, 180
　in cystic fibrosis, 199
　in idiopathic pulmonary fibrosis, 265
　in lung cancer, 358

mechanism of, 8
in pulmonary alveolar proteinosis, 286
smoker's, 62
in tuberculosis, 410
Coumarin, for deep venous thrombosis, 243
CPAP. *See* Continuous positive airway pressure (CPAP)
CPRI (cardiopulmonary risk index), for lung resection, 510, 599–600, 599t
CPT. *See* Chest physiotherapy (CPT)
Crackles, 65, 65t
　in BOOP, 271
　in idiopathic pulmonary fibrosis, 266
CR-BSI (catheter-related bloodstream infection), 644
Critical closing pressure of collapsible segment (Ptm'), 36, 37f
Critically ill patients
　admission and discharge of, 517–518
　bronchoscopy in, 125
　death of, 535–536
　ethical principles for, 533–536
　informed consent for, 533–534
　life support for, 534–535
　medical decision-making for, 533
　nutrition for, 518–533
　　assessment of, 522–523, 523t
　　enteral, 518–519, 527–530, 528t
　　fuel utilization and, 519–521, 519f–522f, 519t
　　goals of, 525–526
　　modalities for, 527–532
　　parenteral, 530–532, 531t
　　requirements for, 523–525, 523t, 524t
　　role of gut in, 526–527, 526t
　pneumonia in, 378
　quality assurance for, 518
　stress-related upper gastrointestinal bleeding in, 641–644, 642t, 643f
　urinary catheter-related infection in, 647–649, 647t
　vascular catheter-related infection in, 644–647, 644t
　venous thromboembolism in, 639–641, 640t
Crocidolite, 328, 350
Cromoglycates, for asthma, 147t, 156
Cromolyn sodium (Intal), for asthma, 147t, 156
Croup, 380t, 383–384
　respiratory failure with, 564
Cryptococcal meningitis, 423, 437
Cryptococcosis, 422–423, 437
　pleural effusions in, 448
Cryptogenic fibrosing alveolitis. *See* Idiopathic pulmonary fibrosis (IPF)
CSA. *See* Central sleep apnea (CSA)
CsA (cyclosporine A)
　for asthma, 163
　for lung transplantation, 215, 223, 224, 224t, 225
CSAS (central sleep apnea syndrome). *See* Central sleep apnea (CSA)

CSB (Cheyne-Stokes breathing), 493t, 494, 494t, 495–496, 496f
CT. *See* Computed tomography (CT)
Cushing's syndrome, paraneoplastic, 359
CV (closing volume), 98, 594
CWP (coal workers' pneumoconiosis), 331–332, 332f
Cyanosis, 66
Cyclophosphamide
    for Churg-Strauss syndrome, 282
    for idiopathic pulmonary fibrosis, 270
    pulmonary reaction to, 289
    for Wegener's granulomatosis, 279
Cyclosporine A (CsA)
    for asthma, 163
    for lung transplantation, 215, 223, 224, 224t, 225
Cyst(s)
    bronchogenic, 462f, 466
    dermoid, of mediastinum, 463
    gastroenteric, 467–468
    mesothelial (pericardial, pleuropericardial, spring water), 466
Cystic fibrosis (CF), 198–202
    atypical or difficult cases of, 200, 200t
    with bronchiectasis, 386–387
    clinical manifestations of, 199, 199t
    complications of, 202
    diagnosis of, 199–200
    infections of, 201
    lung transplantation for, 209, 212–213, 212t
    pneumonia with, 389, 389t
    treatment of, 200–202
Cystic fibrosis (CF) gene, 199
Cystic fibrosis transmembrane conductance regulator (CFTR), 199
Cystic fibrosis transmembrane conductance regulator (CFTR) chloride channels, 12, 12f
Cytokines
    in acute lung injury, 586
    release of, by alveolar macrophages, 22
Cytology, pleural fluid, 120
Cytomegalovirus (CMV)
    in immunocompromised patients, 431, 433
    after lung transplantation, 221–222, 222f
    pneumonia due to, 400t
Cytotoxic drugs, pulmonary reactions to, 288–289, 288t

D

Dantrolene, pleural effusions due to, 455
Dead space
    alveolar, 45
    anatomic, 45, 98
    physiologic, 45
Dead space fraction, 556
Dead space ventilation (V̇D), 46, 46f, 543, 543t
Death, management of, 535–536
Decortication, for parapneumonic effusions, 446

Deep-breathing exercises, postoperative, 595
Deep venous thrombosis (DVT)
    clinical manifestations of, 236–237
    conditions predisposing to, 234t
    in critically ill patients, 639–641, 640t
    incidence of, 234, 234t, 241
    prophylaxis of, 241, 242t, 640–641
    risk factors for, 640t
    treatment of, 241–243, 242t
Defense mechanisms, of lungs, 21–23, 21f
Delta waves, 480
Dental devices, for obstructive sleep apnea, 492, 492f
Deoxyribonuclease (DNAse), for cystic fibrosis, 200–201
Derivation, in EEG, 478
Dermatologic manifestations, of lung cancer, 361
Dermatomyositis (DM), 276
Dermoid cysts, of mediastinum, 463
Desaturations, 482, 487
Desert rheumatism, 420
Desmosomes, functional anatomy of, 10
Desquamative interstitial pneumonitis (DIP), 265
Dexamethasone, pharmacokinetics of, 154t
Dextrose, in parenteral nutrition, 530–531
Dialysis, peritoneal, pleural effusions with, 444
Diamox (acetazolamide), for central sleep apnea, 494
Diaphragm
    in chronic bronchitis, 182f
    costal, 6
    crural, 6
    diseases of, 472–474
    in emphysema, 180t, 181f
    eventration of, 473–474
    fatigue of, 6
    during hyperinflation, 6
    impairment of, respiratory failure due to, 563
    injuries to, 610, 611f
    innervation of, 6
    during inspiration, 4, 5f, 6
    paralysis of, 472–473
    percussion of, 65
Diaphragmatic breathing, for COPD, 192
Diaphragmatic function, surgical incision site and, 594
Diaphragmatic pacing, 473
Diaphragmatic rupture, 610, 611f
Diarrhea, from tube feeding, 530
Diet(s). *See also* Nutrition
    and lung cancer, 337, 350, 351f
    peptide-based, 527
Dietary fiber, 526–527, 526t
Diffuse alveolar hemorrhage, 273
Diffuse interstitial lung diseases (DILDs), 262–302
    allergic angiitis and granulomatosis (Churg-Strauss syndrome), 281–282
    bronchiolitis obliterans organizing pneumonia, 271
    classification of, 265, 265t

drug-induced pulmonary disease, 287–290, 288t
    eosinophilic granuloma (Langerhans cell granulomatosis), 301–302, 302f
    eosinophilic syndromes, 299–301
    Goodpasture's syndrome (antiglomerular basement membrane disease), 282–284, 283f
    hypersensitivity pneumonitis (extrinsic allergic alveolitis), 296–299, 296t, 298t
    idiopathic pulmonary fibrosis (cryptogenic fibrosing alveolitis), 265–271, 266f, 268t
    idiopathic pulmonary hemosiderosis, 284–285
    lymphangioleiomyomatosis, 302
    lymphoid granulomatosis, 279–281, 280f
    lymphoid interstitial pneumonitis, 299
    pathophysiology of, 264–265, 264f
    polymyositis-dermatomyositis, 276
    progressive systemic sclerosis (scleroderma), 275–276
    pulmonary alveolar proteinosis, 285–287, 285f
    respiratory bronchiolitis, 271–272
    rheumatoid arthritis, 274–275, 274t
    sarcoidosis, 290–296, 290t, 291f, 292t, 293t, 294f
    systemic lupus erythematosus, 272–274, 272f, 272t, 273f
    Wegener's granulomatosis, 276–279, 277t, 278f
Diffusing capacity (DL), 99–100, 99f
    in occupational interstitial lung disease, 326
    and work capacity, 104
Diffusion, 47–48
Diffusion defect, arterial hypoxemia due to, 52
Digital clubbing. *See* Clubbing
Digitalis
    for cor pulmonale, 254
    for pulmonary edema, 581
DILDs. *See* Diffuse interstitial lung diseases (DILDs)
Diltiazem, for primary pulmonary hypertension, 251
DIP (desquamative interstitial pneumonitis), 265
2,3-Diphosphoglycerate (2,3-DPG), and oxygen delivery, 54
Directed search, 71
"Dirty lungs," in chronic bronchitis, 181, 182f
Disability, evaluation of, 113–114, 114f
Discharge, from intensive care unit, 518
Distending pressures, 26–27, 27f
Diuretics
    for cor pulmonale, 254
    for pulmonary edema, 581
Diverticula, esophageal (Zenker's), 468
DL (diffusing capacity), 99–100, 99f
    in occupational interstitial lung disease, 326
    and work capacity, 104

DLCO. *See* Carbon monoxide (CO) diffusing capacity (DLCO)
DM (dermatomyositis), 276
DNAse (deoxyribonuclease), for cystic fibrosis, 200–201
DO₂ (oxygen diffusing capacity), 47
Dobutamine, for pulmonary edema, 581
Do-not-resuscitate (DNR) orders, 507, 508
Dopamine
    for multiple organ failure, 633
    for pulmonary edema, 581
Double lung transplantation (DLT). *See also* Lung transplantation (LT)
    indications for, 209, 210t
Doxycycline
    for malignant pleural effusions, 450
    for pneumothorax, 459
2,3-DPG (2,3-diphosphoglycerate), and oxygen delivery, 54
Dressler's syndrome, 456
Drug abuse, and lung transplantation, 211
Drug-induced asthma, 141
Drug-induced pulmonary disease, 287–290, 288t
Drug-induced pulmonary eosinophilic syndromes, 299–300
Drug overdoses, respiratory failure due to, 563–564
Drug reactions, pleural effusions due to, 454–455
Dry powder inhalers (DPIs), for asthma, 149
Dust(s), hypersensitivity to, 296–299, 296t, 298t
Dust-induced diseases. *See* Pneumoconiosis(es)
Dutch hypothesis, of COPD, 176
DVT. *See* Deep venous thrombosis (DVT)
Dynamic compression, of airways, 35–36, 35f
Dysphagia, in lung cancer, 358
Dyspnea, 61
    in byssinosis, 321
    in chronic beryllium disease, 333
    in COPD, 179, 183
    due to fatigue of inspiratory muscles, 6
    in idiopathic pulmonary fibrosis, 265
    in occupational asthma, 319
    in occupational interstitial lung disease, 326
    in pulmonary alveolar proteinosis, 285, 286
    in pulmonary embolism, 237, 237t
    in pulmonary hypertension, 250
    in respiratory failure, 539
    in sarcoidosis, 291
    in silicosis, 327
    in tuberculosis, 411

E

Ear(s), examination of, 63
Early asthmatic response (EAR), 136, 136f
ECG (electrocardiogram)
    in COPD, 179
    in cor pulmonale, 252
    in pulmonary embolism, 238

Echinococcosis, pleural effusions in, 449
Echocardiography, 602
Edema, pulmonary. *See* Pulmonary edema
EDS (excessive daytime sleepiness). *See* Sleep disorders
EEG (electroencephalography), during sleep, 478–480, 479f–481f
EFA (essential fatty acids), in parenteral nutrition, 531
Effusions, pleural. *See* Pleural effusions
EG (eosinophilic granuloma), 301–302, 302f
Egophony, 65
Eicosanoids, metabolism of, 19–20, 19f
Eisenmenger's syndrome, lung transplantation for, 209
Elastase-antielastase theory, of COPD, 177–178
Elastic recoil, of lungs, 30–32, 30f, 31f
    in emphysema, 180
Elastic recoil pressure (Pst(L)), 30
Elderly, 503–511
    exercise performance in, 107–108
    intensity of care for, 503, 504f
    mechanical ventilation in, 503–507, 504f–506f, 505t
        ethical decisions regarding, 507–508
        weaning from, 506–507, 506f, 507t
    pneumonia in, 378, 389, 389t, 390t
    postoperative pulmonary complications in, 508–511, 509t, 511t
    preoperative pulmonary evaluation in, 508–511, 509t, 511t
    surgical considerations in, 597
Electrocardiogram (ECG)
    in COPD, 179
    in cor pulmonale, 252
    in pulmonary embolism, 238
Electroencephalography (EEG), during sleep, 478–480, 479f–481f
Electrolytes, in parenteral nutrition, 531
Electrolyte transport, through respiratory epithelium, 12, 12f
Electromyography (EMG), during sleep, 478, 479f–481f, 480
Electrooculography (EOG), during sleep, 478–480, 479f–481f
Elixophyllin. *See* Theophylline (Slo-Phylline, Theolair, Quibron, Elixophyllin, Theo-24, Uniphyl)
EMB (ethambutol), for tuberculosis, 436
Embolectomy, surgical, 244
Embolism
    fat, 246, 613–614, 613t
    pulmonary. *See* Pulmonary embolism (PE)
    from systemic arterial catheterization, 621
Embolization
    air, 246–247, 609–610
    of arteriovenous malformation, 257
    paradoxical, 609–610
Embolus(i)
    CT of, 82–83, 82f
    foreign body, 246
    tumor, 257

Emergencies, in ventilated patient, 553–555, 554f
EMG (electromyography), during sleep, 478, 479f–481f, 480
Emphysema. *See also* Chronic obstructive pulmonary disease (COPD)
    α₁-antitrypsin deficiency in, 177–178, 189–190
    centrilobular (proximal), 175
    vs. chronic bronchitis, 179, 179t
    in coal miners, 336
    computed tomography of, 181–182, 182f
    CT of, 81f
    defined, 175
    elastic recoil in, 30, 30f
    expiratory flow rate in, 37, 38
    flow-volume loop in, 138–139, 138f
    high-resolution computed tomography of, 181–182, 182f
    lung transplantation for, 209
    lung volume reduction surgery for, 225–227, 226t
    mediastinal, 469–470
    panacinar, 175
    paraseptal (distal), 175
    pulmonary function testing in, 110–111, 180
    radiographic signs of, 180–181, 180t, 181f, 182f
Empyema, 379, 394f, 395
    symptoms of, 60, 63
    tuberculous, 411
Empyema necessitatis, 445
Endobronchial lesions, bronchoscopy of, 123
Endobronchial prostheses, for lung cancer, 370
Endobronchial ultrasound, 122
Endocarditis, with lung cancer, 361
End-of-life care, quality, 507–508, 535
Endoscopic ultrasound-guided fine needle aspiration (EUS-FNA), 127
Endoscopic variceal sclerotherapy, pleural effusions after, 454
Endothelial-derived relaxing factor, 17–18
Endothelial-derived vasoactive factors, 17–18, 20
Endothelial injury, in critically ill patients, 633
Endothelins (ETs)
    metabolism of, 20
    vasoactive properties of, 17
Endotracheal intubation
    for asthma, 571
    for flail chest, 605
    for pneumonia, 409
    for pulmonary edema, 581
    for respiratory failure, 546–548, 546t, 547f
        in COPD, 567–568
    respiratory resistance after, 593
    for status asthmaticus, 161
    with tracheobronchial disruption, 612
Energy expenditure, 524

Energy requirements, 101, 101t, 523–524, 524t
Enflurane, cardiovascular effects of, 593
Entamoeba histolytica, pleural effusions with, 448
Enteral formulas, 528–529, 528t
Enteral nutrition, 518–519, 527–530, 528t
Environmental control, for asthma, 144
Environmental exposure, assessment of, 316
Environmental lung disease
   acute pleural, 324
   due to air pollution, 341–342, 341t
   airway disorders, 317–324, 318t, 320f, 323t, 324t
   aluminum pneumoconiosis, 335
   asthma, 317–321, 318t, 320f
   beryllium and hard metal-related, 332–334, 333f
   byssinosis, 321–322
   chronic bronchitis, 335–337, 336t
   classification of, 316, 317t
   clinical approach to, 315
   coal workers' pneumoconiosis, 331–332, 332f
   diagnostic criteria for, 315–316
   exposure assessment for, 316
   flock worker's lung, 335
   Fuller's earth-associated, 335
   due to grain dust, 322
   graphite pneumoconiosis, 335
   inhalation injury, 322–324, 324t
   interstitial fibrosing, 324–335, 325t
   kaolin pneumoconiosis, 334
   malignancies due to, 337–340, 337t
   due to manmade vitreous fibers, 335
   mica-associated, 335
   mixed-dust pneumoconiosis, 335
   nonmalignant asbestos-related, 328–331, 330f, 331t
   principles of, 314–316
   silicosis, 326–328, 327f, 328f
   talcosis, 334
   upper respiratory tract irritation, 316
Environmental tobacco smoke (ETS), 340, 343, 348
EOG (electrooculography), during sleep, 478–480, 479f–481f
Eosinophilia, pulmonary
   with asthma, 300
   simple, 299
   tropical, 300
Eosinophilia-myalgia syndrome, L-tryptophan, 300
Eosinophilic granuloma (EG), 301–302, 302f
Eosinophilic pneumonia, 299, 300
Eosinophilic syndromes, 299–301
EPAP (expiratory positive airway pressure), for obstructive sleep apnea, 491
Epiglottis, 7
Epiglottitis, 380t, 382–383
   respiratory failure with, 564
Epinephrine (Medihaler-Epi, Adrenalin chloride)

for asthma, 146t, 159
   for multiple organ failure, 634
   vasoactive properties of, 17
Epistaxis, 60
Epithelial cells
   alveolar, 14, 14t
   functional anatomy of, 9–10, 11f
   metabolic and secretory functions of, 11–12
Epochs, 478
Epoprostenol, for primary pulmonary hypertension, 251
Equal-pressure point (EPP), 35–38, 35f, 37f
Ergometry, 108
ERV (expiratory reserve volume), 26, 27f, 94, 94f
Erythromycin
   for *Legionella* pneumonia, 393
   for *Mycoplasma pneumoniae,* 397
Erythropoietic system, in oxygen delivery, 53–54, 54f
Esophageal dilation, 468
Esophageal diverticula, 468
Esophageal injury, 610–612, 611f
Esophageal pain, 61
Esophageal perforations, pleural effusions with, 453
Esophageal pressure(s), 29
   changes in, 483
Essential fatty acids (EFA), in parenteral nutrition, 531
Ethambutol (EMB), for tuberculosis, 436
Ethics, 533–536
   of death and dying, 535–536
   of foregoing life-sustaining therapy, 534–535
   of informed consent, 533–534
   of mechanical ventilation
      in COPD, 569
      in elderly, 507–508
   of medical decision-making, 533
   of multiple organ failure, 635–636
ETs (endothelins)
   metabolism of, 20
   vasoactive properties of, 17
ETS (environmental tobacco smoke), 340, 343, 348
EUS-FNA (endoscopic ultrasound-guided fine needle aspiration), 127
Eventration, of diaphragm, 473–474
Excessive daytime sleepiness (EDS). *See* Sleep disorders
Exercise, 100–108
   aging and, 107–108
   for COPD, 191–192
   intensity, duration, and frequency of, 106, 107t
   maximum, 101–105
      determinants of, 102–105, 104t, 106f
      measures of, 101–102, 102f, 102t
      physiology and pathophysiology of, 101, 101t, 106–107, 107f, 107t
Exercise-induced asthma, 112, 139
Exercise intolerance
   in COPD, 179

evaluation of, 111–113
   in idiopathic pulmonary fibrosis, 265
Exercise testing
   with cardiovascular dysfunction, 112
   for evaluation of disability, 113, 114f
   with idiopathic pulmonary fibrosis, 267
   with lack of fitness, 112
   with malingering, 112–113
   with obstructive ventilatory dysfunction, 111–112
   with occupational interstitial lung disease, 326
   performance of, 108
   preoperative, 599–600, 599t
   with pulmonary hypertension, 112
   rationale for, 100–101
   with restrictive ventilatory dysfunction, 112
   use of, 109–114, 114f
Exercise tolerance, after lung volume reduction surgery, 226
Expiration
   limitation of flow on, 34–35, 35f
   movement of chest wall and lungs during, 4, 5f
   muscles of, 4, 5f
Expiration film, 77
Expiratory film, 77
Expiratory flow rates, 36–38, 37f
   measurement of, 91–93, 92f, 93f
Expiratory positive airway pressure (EPAP), for obstructive sleep apnea, 491
Expiratory pressure, maximal, 27–28, 28f
Expiratory reserve volume (ERV), 26, 27f, 94, 94f
Expired carbon dioxide (PE_{CO_2}), 46, 46f, 556
Exposure history, 60
Extensive disease, 364
External oblique muscles, 5f
External urine collection systems, 648
Extramedullary hematopoiesis, mediastinal masses due to, 468
Extrapulmonary signs, 66, 66f
Extrinsic allergic alveolitis, 296–299, 296t, 298t
Exudates, in pleural fluid, 119

F

Face masks, 543, 544–545
Face tents, 543
Familial Mediterranean fever, pleural effusions with, 452
Family history, 60
Farmer's lung, 60, 296t, 297–298
Fat(s), in parenteral nutrition, 531
Fat embolism syndrome (FES), 246, 613–614, 613t
Fatigue, muscle, functional anatomy of, 4, 6
Fat metabolism
   in nonstressed starvation, 520
   during stress, 519f, 521
Fatty acids, essential, in parenteral nutrition, 531
Fatty liver, due to parenteral nutrition, 532

5-FC (5-fluorocytosine), for cryptococcosis, 423
Febrile tracheobronchitis, 385
Feeding tubes, 518–519, 527–550, 528t
FEFs (forced expiratory flows), 92, 92f
Fenoterol, for asthma, 135, 145
FES (fat embolism syndrome), 246, 613–614, 613t
FET (forced expiratory time), and postoperative pulmonary complications, 510
FEV. *See* Forced expiratory volume (FEV)
Fever, grain, 322
Fiber, dietary, 526–527, 526t
Fibrinogen, in acute lung injury, 585–586
Fibroblasts, in idiopathic pulmonary fibrosis, 269
Fibrosis, mediastinal, 469
Fibrothorax, 458
    respiratory failure with, 562t, 564
Fibrous histiocytoma, malignant, 357
Fick equation, 49, 524, 524t
Filarial infection, tropical pulmonary eosinophilia due to, 300
Fine needle aspiration, endoscopic ultrasound-guided, 127
FIO_2. *See* Inspired oxygen content (FIO_2)
Fistula
    bronchopleural, with HIV infection, 436
    tracheoesophageal, 555, 613
Flail chest, 472, 605–606
Flock worker's lung, 335
Flovent (fluticasone propionate)
    for asthma, 147t, 154
    pharmacokinetics of, 154t, 155t
Flow cytometry, of pleural fluid, 120
Flow limitation, 36–38, 37f
Flow-volume loop, 35, 92–93, 93f
    in asthma, 138–139, 138f
    in emphysema, 138–139, 138f
    $He-O_2$, 38–39, 38f
    in upper airway obstruction, 138–139, 138f
Fluconazole
    for candidiasis, 223
    for coccidioidomycosis, 421–422, 438
    for cryptococcosis, 437
5-Flucytosine, for cryptococcosis, 437, 448
Fluid balance, in lung, 12
Fluid exchange, in lung, 576–579, 577f, 577t, 578f
Fluid resuscitation
    for multiple organ failure, 633
    for pulmonary contusion, 608–609
Flunisolide (AeroBid)
    for asthma, 147t
    pharmacokinetics of, 154t, 155t
5-Fluorocytosine (5-FC), for cryptococcosis, 423
Fluoroscopy, 77–78
Fluoxetine
    for cataplexy, 485
    for obstructive sleep apnea, 491
Fluticasone propionate (Flovent)
    for asthma, 147t, 154
    pharmacokinetics of, 154t, 155t

Foradil (formoterol), for asthma, 146t
Foramen of Bochdalek, hernia through, 468
Foramen of Morgagni, hernia through, 465
Forced expiratory flows (FEFs), 92, 92f
Forced expiratory spirogram, 35
Forced expiratory time (FET), and postoperative pulmonary complications, 510
Forced expiratory volume in 0.5 second ($FEV_{0.5}$), 91, 92f
Forced expiratory volume in 1 second (FEV_1), 91, 92f
    in asthma, 139, 571
        occupational, 319
    in emphysema, 180
    after lung volume reduction surgery, 226–227
    with obstructive ventilatory dysfunction, 109, 109t
    postoperative, 598–599
    and response to therapy, 111
    with restrictive ventilatory dysfunction, 110
    smoking and, 182–183, 183f, 184, 184f
Forced expiratory volume in 1 second/forced vital capacity (FEV_1/FVC), 91
    with mixed ventilatory dysfunction, 110
    with obstructive ventilatory dysfunction, 109, 109t
    with respiratory failure, 542
    with restrictive ventilatory dysfunction, 110
Forced expiratory volume in 3 seconds (FEV_3), 91, 92f
Forced vital capacity (FVC), 91, 92, 92f
    and response to therapy, 111
    with restrictive ventilatory dysfunction, 110
Foreign body emboli, 246
Formaldehyde, carcinogenicity of, 337t, 339
Formoterol (Foradil), for asthma, 146t
Formoterol/budesonide (Budoxis), for asthma, 147t
Formula
    for enteral nutrition, 528–529, 528t
    for parenteral nutrition, 530–532, 531t
Fossil fuels, exposure to, 342
Fractures
    rib, 471–472, 601, 603–605, 604f
        pain of, 61, 472
    scapular, 601
    sternal, 601, 603, 604f
    vertebral, 601
Free search, 71
Freons, in metered dose inhalers, 149
Friction rubs, 66
Friedlander's pneumonia, 397–399
Fuel utilization, during critical illness, 519–521, 519f–522f, 519t
Fuller's earth pneumoconiosis, 335
Functional residual capacity (FRC), 26, 27f
    closed circuit helium dilution method for, 94–95, 95f, 96f

in emphysema, 180
    nitrogen washout technique for, 95, 96f
    in spirometric volume determinations, 94f
Fungal infections, 415–423, 416f, 418f–421f
    with HIV infection, 437–438
    in immunocompromised host, 423–425, 433
    after lung transplantation, 222
    opportunistic, 423–425
    of pleura, 447–448
Fungoses, allergic bronchopulmonary, 141
Fungus balls, 424
Funnel chest, 471
Furosemide, for pulmonary edema, 581
Futility, and withdrawal of care, 508
FVC (forced vital capacity), 91, 92, 92f
    and response to therapy, 111
    with restrictive ventilatory dysfunction, 110
f/VT (respiratory rate to tidal volume ratio), 6

G

GALT (gut-associated lymphoid tissue), 526
Gamma camera, 86
Gamma-interferon
    in pleural fluid, 121
    in sarcoidosis, 294
    in tuberculous pleuritis, 447
Ganciclovir, for cytomegalovirus, 222
Gap junctions, functional anatomy of, 10
Gas(es), irritant, 322, 323, 323t
Gas density, 38–39, 38f
Gas dilution, measurement of, 94–95, 95f
Gas distribution, tests of, 97–99, 98f
Gas exchange, 44, 99–100, 99f
Gas exchange area, 20, 21f
Gas exchange surface, 8f, 9, 9f
Gas transfer, 47–48, 99–100, 99f
Gastric aspiration
    acute lung injury and ARDS due to, 583f, 585, 585f
    perioperative, 596
Gastroenteric cysts, 467–468
Gastroesophageal reflux disease (GERD), and asthma, 140–141
Gastrointestinal bleeding, 629, 641–644, 642t, 643f
Gastrointestinal failure, in multiple organ failure, 629
Gas viscosity, 38
Gaw. *See* Airway conductance (Gaw)
GCS (glucocorticosteroids). *See* Corticosteroids
G-CSF (granulocyte colony-stimulating factor), in immunocompromised patients, 434
Gender differences, in lung cancer, 346, 347f, 348–349
Gene therapy, for cystic fibrosis, 200
Genetic factors, in lung cancer, 350–351
Genital tuberculosis, 411

GERD (gastroesophageal reflux disease), and asthma, 140–141

Germ cell tumors, of mediastinum, 463–464

Ghon complex, 410

Giant cell carcinoma, 354

Giant lymph node hyperplasia, 465

Glasgow Coma Scale, 630, 630t

Glucocorticoids. *See* Corticosteroids

Glucocorticosteroids (GCS). *See* Corticosteroids

Glucose, in pleural fluid, 119

Glucose-alanine cycle, during stress, 520, 521f

Glucose metabolism
in nonstressed starvation, 519–520
during stress, 519f–521f, 520–521

Glutamine, in critical illness, 526

Glycerol metabolism, during stress, 520

Glycogen, in nonstressed starvation, 520

GM-CSF (granulocyte-macrophage colony-stimulating factor), in immunocompromised patients, 434

Goblet cells
functional anatomy of, 10
in mucociliary escalator, 21

Goiter, intrathoracic, 464, 464f

Goldman Index, 600, 600t

Gold preparations, for asthma, 162–163

Gonadotropin, ectopic, due to lung cancer, 360

Goodpasture's syndrome, 282–284, 283f

Graft failure, after lung transplantation, 215, 216

Graft rejection, after lung transplantation, 215, 216, 218–219, 219f, 219t

Graft-*versus*-host disease (GVHD), 433

Grain asthma, 322

Grain dust exposure, 322

Grain fever, 322

Grain handler's lung, 296t

Gram-negative organisms
hospital-acquired pneumonia due to, 401
in oropharynx, 380, 387–388, 388t
in tracheobronchial tree, 380–381, 388, 388t

Gram stain, in pneumonia, 407

Granulocyte colony-stimulating factor (G-CSF), in immunocompromised patients, 434

Granulocyte-macrophage colony-stimulating factor (GM-CSF), in immunocompromised patients, 434

Granulocytopenia, 430t

Granuloma(s)
in chronic beryllium disease, 333, 333f
eosinophilic, 301–302, 302f
mediastinal, 469

Granulomatosis
allergic, 281–282
Langerhans cell, 301–302, 302f
lymphomatoid, 279–281, 280f, 357–358
Wegener's. *See* Wegener's granulomatosis (WG)

Granulomatous mediastinitis, lymph node involvement in, 465, 465f

Graphite pneumoconiosis, 335

Ground-glass opacity, 81f

Guillain-Barré syndrome, respiratory failure in, 561–562

Gut, in nutrition, 526–527, 526t

Gut-associated lymphoid tissue (GALT), 526

Gut fuels, 526–527, 526t

GVHD (graft-*versus*-host disease), 433

H

H_2-receptor antagonists, for stress-related gastrointestinal ulceration, 642–643, 642t, 643f

HAART (highly active antiretroviral therapy), for HIV infection, 434

Haemophilus influenzae
in cystic fibrosis, 201
epiglottitis due to, 382, 383
pneumonia due to, 395–396, 396f

Haldane effect, 47f

Hallucinations, hypnagogic and hypnopompic, 484

Halothane
for asthma, 573
with asthma, 593
cardiovascular effects of, 593

Hamartoma, 357

Hamman's sign, 469, 540

Hand-Schüller-Christian disease, 301

Hard metal disease, 332, 334

Harris-Benedict equation, 523–524, 524t

HCG (human chorionic gonadotropin), with teratoma, 464

HCO_3^- (bicarbonate), plasma, $Paco_2$ and, 541, 542f

Heart, "shaggy," in asbestosis, 330, 330f

Heart disease, pulmonary. *See* Cor pulmonale

Heart failure
congestive
pleural effusions in, 444
sleep apnea in, 493t, 494, 494t, 495–496, 496f
left ventricular, pulmonary edema due to, 579–581, 579f, 580f
right, in COPD, 179

Heart-lung transplantation (HLT). *See also* Lung transplantation (LT)
indications for, 209–210, 210t

Heart sounds
in cor pulmonale, 252
in idiopathic pulmonary fibrosis, 266
in pulmonary embolism, 237, 237t

Helium-oxygen (He-O_2) flow-volume loops, 38–39, 38f

Helium-oxygen (He-O_2) gas (heliox), for status asthmaticus, 161

Hemangioma, sclerosing, 356

Hematemesis, 63

Hematite, carcinogenicity of, 350

Hematocrit, in respiratory failure, 540

Hematologic failure, in multiple organ failure, 630

Hematoma, pulmonary, 609

Hematopoiesis, extramedullary, mediastinal masses due to, 468

Hemoglobin (Hg)
affinity for oxygen of, 54, 54f
arterial saturation of, 44, 54
pH and, 54, 54f

Hemoglobin (Hg) concentration
normal, 45, 53–54
in respiratory failure, 540
and work capacity, 103

Hemoptysis, 63, 63t
in bronchiectasis, 197
bronchoscopy of, 124
in carcinoid tumor, 355
in COPD, 63, 63t, 179
in cystic fibrosis, 202
in Goodpasture's syndrome, 282
in idiopathic pulmonary hemosiderosis, 284
in lung cancer, 358
in pulmonary embolism, 237, 237t
in tuberculosis, 410–411

Hemorrhage
diffuse alveolar, 273
gastrointestinal, 629, 641–644, 642t, 643f
due to heparin, 641

Hemorrhagic telangiectasia, hereditary, 255–256

Hemosiderosis, idiopathic pulmonary, 284–285

Hemothorax, 457–458
due to chest trauma, 607, 607f
clotted, 607

Henderson-Hasselbalch equation, 541

Heparin
for deep venous thrombosis, 241–243, 242t, 640–641
for septic thromboembolism, 245
for vascular catheter-related infection, 646

Hepatic failure, in multiple organ failure, 629–630

Hepatobiliary abnormalities, due to parenteral nutrition, 532

Hereditary hemorrhagic telangiectasia (HHT), 255–256

Hernia
hiatal, 468
through foramen of Bochdalek, 468
through foramen of Morgagni, 465

Heroin, respiratory failure due to, 563

Herpes simplex virus (HSV), pneumonia due to, 400t

HFA-BDP (beclomethasone dipropionate)
for asthma, 147t, 154
pharmacokinetics of, 154t, 155t

HFAs (hydrofluoroalkanes), in metered dose inhalers, 154

Hg. *See* Hemoglobin (Hg)

HHT (hereditary hemorrhagic telangiectasia), 255–256

Hiatal hernia, 468

Hiccups, 474

High-frequency oscillatory ventilation, 551

Highly active antiretroviral therapy (HAART), for HIV infection, 434

High-pressure cardiogenic pulmonary edema, 579–581, 579f, 580f
    pulmonary artery catheterization for, 626
High-resolution computed tomography (HRCT)
    of emphysema, 181–182, 182f
    of idiopathic pulmonary fibrosis, 265, 266, 266f
    of progressive systemic sclerosis, 275
Hila, radiographic anatomy of, 72–75, 75f, 76f
Hilar adenopathy, in sarcoidosis, 290–291, 291f
Hilar lymph nodes, 23
    eggshell calcification of, 327, 328f
Histamine, vasoactive properties of, 17, 19
Histiocytoma, malignant fibrous, 357
Histiocytoses, 301–302, 302f
Histoplasmosis, 415–419, 416f, 418f, 437–438
    pleural effusions in, 448
History
    nutritional, 522
    respiratory, 59–60
HIV (human immunodeficiency virus). *See* Acquired immunodeficiency syndrome (AIDS)
HLT (heart-lung transplantation). *See also* Lung transplantation (LT)
    indications for, 209–210, 210t
Hoarseness, 60
    in lung cancer, 358
Hodgkin's lymphoma, mediastinal, 462–463
Honeycombing, 81f
Hoover's sign, 6, 64, 179, 473
Horner's syndrome, 66
Hospital-acquired pneumonia, 377, 378, 401–403, 401f, 403f
    in immunocompromised patients, 431
Hospitalization
    for asthma, 139–140, 140t, 158–162
    for community-acquired pneumonia, 408
    for COPD, 194, 194t
HP (hypersensitivity pneumonitis), 296–299, 296t, 298t
HRCT. *See* High-resolution computed tomography (HRCT)
HSV (herpes simplex virus), pneumonia due to, 400t
Human chorionic gonadotropin (HCG), with teratoma, 464
Human immunodeficiency virus (HIV). *See* Acquired immunodeficiency syndrome (AIDS)
Humidifier lung, 296t
Humoral hypercalcemia of malignancy, 360
Hydrocortisone sodium succinate (Solu-Cortef), for asthma, 148t, 160
Hydrofluoroalkanes (HFAs), in metered dose inhalers, 154
Hydrogen fluoride, inhalation injury due to, 323t
Hydrogen sulfide, inhalation injury due to, 323t

Hydropneumothorax(ces)
    with coccidioidomycosis, 448
    with esophageal perforations, 453
Hydrostatic pressure
    and lung blood flow, 16–17, 16f, 577, 577t
    in pleural fluid, 442, 442f
5-Hydroxytryptamine, vasoactive properties of, 17, 19
Hyperacute rejection, after lung transplantation, 218
Hypercalcemia, of malignancy, 360
Hypercapnia
    with central sleep apnea, 493–494, 493t
    daytime, obstructive sleep apnea syndrome and, 489
    permissive, 550
    in respiratory failure, 541, 542f, 561–573
Hypercarbia, in respiratory failure, 540
Hypereosinophilic syndrome, idiopathic, 300–301
Hyperglycemia
    due to parenteral nutrition, 532
    during stress, 520–521, 520f, 521f
Hyperinfection syndrome, 299
Hyperinflation, 6
    in COPD, 179, 181, 182f
Hypermetabolic hypercatabolic stress response, 519, 519f, 519t
Hypermetabolism, in multiple organ failure, 635
Hyperresponsiveness, airway
    in asthma, 138
    in COPD, 176–177
    measurement of, 93–94, 109
Hypersensitivity
    to drugs, 287–290, 288t
    summer type, 296t
Hypersensitivity pneumonitis (HP), 296–299, 296t, 298t
Hypersomnia, idiopathic, 485
Hypertension
    pulmonary, 247–251
        arterial, 249
        chronic thromboembolic, 244–245
        classification of, 248t
        clinical manifestations of, 250–251
        defined, 247
        diagnosis of, 250–251
        differential diagnosis of, 251
        exercise testing with, 112
        hemodynamic studies in, 251
        due to high altitude, 249
        due to increased flow, 248
        due to mitral stenosis, 249–251
        in obstructive sleep apnea syndrome, 490
        pathogenesis of, 247–248, 248t
        pathologic characteristics of, 247
        porto-, 251
        postcapillary, 248t, 249–250
        precapillary, 248–249, 248t
        primary
           clinical manifestations of, 250
           lung transplantation for, 209, 212t, 213

        pathogenesis of, 248–249, 248t
        treatment of, 251
        due to primary pleuropulmonary disease, 249
        in rheumatoid arthritis, 275
        in systemic lupus erythematosus, 273
        due to thromboses, 249
        treatment of, 251
        venous, 250
    systemic, in obstructive sleep apnea syndrome, 490
Hypertrophic pulmonary osteoarthropathy
    with benign fibrous mesothelioma, 451
    with lung cancer, 361
Hyperventilation syndrome, 61
Hypnagogic hallucinations, 484
Hypnopompic hallucinations, 484
Hypochloremia, in respiratory failure, 540
Hypoglycemia, in lung cancer, 360
Hypokalemia, in respiratory failure, 540
Hypophosphatemia, in respiratory failure, 540
Hypopneas, 482, 482f
Hypoventilation, 45–46, 46f
    arterial hypoxemia due to, 51
    central alveolar, 493–494, 493t
    daytime, 489
Hypovolemic shock, 627t
Hypoxemia
    arterial, 50–53, 50t
        with pulmonary embolism, 235
    in COPD, 179
    postoperative, 594–595, 594t
    in respiratory failure, 541, 541f, 576–587
Hypoxia, resting, in emphysema, 180
Hypoxic vasoconstriction, regulation of pulmonary circulation by, 18, 18f
Hysteresis, 30

I

IC (inspiratory capacity), 26, 27f, 94, 94f
ICH. *See* Immunocompromised host (ICH)
ICSD (International Classification of Sleep Disorders), 484
ICU (intensive care unit). *See also* Critically ill patients
    administration of, 517–518
Idiopathic hypereosinophilic syndrome (IHS), 300–301
Idiopathic pulmonary fibrosis (IPF), 264–271
    vs. BOOP, 271
    clinical presentation and evaluation of, 265–267, 266f
    CT of, 81f
    epidemiology of, 266
    immunopathogenic concepts of, 268–269
    lung histology and staging of, 267–268, 268t
    lung transplantation for, 209, 212, 212t
    vs. respiratory bronchiolitis, 271–272
    treatment and prognosis for, 269–271
Idiopathic pulmonary hemosiderosis (IPH), 284–285

IgA (immunoglobulin A), secretory, in intestine, 526

IHS (idiopathic hypereosinophilic syndrome), 300–301

ILs (interleukins), in sarcoidosis, 293, 294

Imipramine (Tofranil), for cataplexy, 485

Immotile cilia syndrome, 22
  and bronchiectasis, 198

Immunoblastic lymphadenopathy, pleural effusions with, 452

Immunocompromised host (ICH). *See also* Acquired immunodeficiency syndrome (AIDS)
  bronchoscopy in, 124
  graft-*versus*-host disease in, 433
  due to immune defects, 430t
  interstitial pneumonitis in, 433–434
  due to medications, 430t
  noninfectious conditions in, 431t
  respiratory infections in
    bacterial, 432–433
    epidemiology of, 378, 430
    evaluation of, 431–432, 432t
    fungal, 433
    pneumonia, 403–406, 404t, 405f
    prevention of, 434
    viral, 433

Immunodeficiency, with bronchiectasis, 198

Immunoglobulin(s)
  in hypersensitivity pneumonitis, 298, 298t
  in sarcoidosis, 292, 292t

Immunoglobulin A (IgA), secretory, in intestine, 526

Immunoglobulin deficiency, with bronchiectasis, 198

Immunohistochemical testing, of pleural fluid, 120

Immunosuppression, for lung transplantation, 215, 219, 223–225, 224t

Impairment, evaluation of, 113–114, 114f

Implosion effect, in pulmonary contusion, 608

IMV (intermittent mandatory ventilation), 548–549, 549f
  synchronized, 548–549, 549f
  for weaning, 553

Incentive spirometry, postoperative, 595

Increased-permeability pulmonary edema, 582–587, 582t, 583f–586f
  pulmonary artery catheterization for, 626

Indirect calorimetry, 524

Indoor air pollution, 340, 341–342

Industrial bronchitis, 335–337, 336t

Indwelling urinary catheters, 648

Inertial effect, in pulmonary contusion, 608

Infant, respiratory distress syndrome in, 31–32

Infarction
  myocardial. *See* Myocardial infarction (MI)
  pulmonary, 236, 241

Infection(s), 377–425
  with AIDS, 378, 405–406, 405f, 414–415

airway, 384–387, 387f
bacterial, 381–399
  in AIDS, 405–406, 405f, 436
  in bronchiectasis, 386–387, 387f
  bronchiolitis due to, 385
  bronchitis due to, 384–385
  in COPD, 177, 177f, 195, 196f
  in immunocompromised host, 403–405, 404t, 432–433
  lung abscess due to, 394f, 395, 395f
  pneumonia due to, 387–399, 401–409. *See also* Pneumonia
  of upper respiratory tract, 381–384
bronchiectasis due to, 380t, 386–387, 387f
bronchiolitis due to, 378, 380t, 385
bronchitis due to, 378, 380t, 384–385
bronchoscopy of, 124
common cold due to, 377, 380t, 381
in COPD, 177, 177f, 183, 195, 196f
in cor pulmonale, 254
croup due to, 380t, 383–384
in cystic fibrosis, 201
definitions for, 378–379
epidemiology of, 377–378
epiglottitis due to, 380t, 382–383
fungal, 415–423, 416f, 418f–421f
  with HIV infection, 437–438
  in immunocompromised host, 423–425, 433
  after lung transplantation, 222
  opportunistic, 423–425
  of pleura, 447–448
and idiopathic pulmonary fibrosis, 265–266, 268–269
in immunocompromised host, 378, 403–406, 404t, 405f, 414–415
influenza due to, 385–386
lower respiratory tract, 379, 380–381, 380t, 384–415
lung abscess due to, 379, 394f, 395, 395f
after lung transplantation, 221–223, 222f, 223f
mycobacterial, 378, 414–415, 414f
  with silicosis, 327–328
parasitic
  eosinophilic syndromes due to, 299
  of pleura, 448–449
parenchymal, 379, 387–415. *See also* Pneumonia
pharyngitis due to, 380t, 383
pneumonia due to. *See* Pneumonia
in pulmonary alveolar proteinosis, 286
sinusitis due to, 380t, 381–382
from systemic arterial catheterization, 621
tuberculosis due to, 378, 409–414, 411f
upper respiratory tract, 379–380, 380t, 381–384
urinary catheter-related, 647–649, 647t
vascular catheter-related, 644–647, 644t
viral
  in bronchiolitis, 385
  bronchitis due to, 384
  common cold due to, 377, 380t, 381

and idiopathic pulmonary fibrosis, 265–266, 268–269
  in immunocompromised host, 433
  influenza due to, 385–386
  pneumonia due to, 399–401, 400f, 400t

Infection control, in intensive care unit, 518

Inferior vena cava interruption, 244

Inflammatory cascade, in asthma, 136–137, 137f

Inflammatory diseases, alveolar. *See* Diffuse interstitial lung diseases (DILDs)

Influenza, 385–386
  in immunocompromised host, 433

Influenza vaccines, for COPD prevention, 185–186

Influenza virus, pneumonia due to, 400t

Informed consent, 533–534

INH (isoniazid), for tuberculosis, 413, 436–437, 438

Inhalation challenge tests, 93–94, 109, 111
  for occupational asthma, 319

Inhalation injury, 322–324, 324t

Injury. *See* Acute lung injury (ALI); Chest trauma

Insomnia. *See* Sleep disorders

Inspection, 63–65, 64f

Inspiration
  movement of chest wall and lungs during, 4, 5f
  muscles of, 4, 5f, 6
    fatigue of, 6

Inspiratory capacity (IC), 26, 27f, 94, 94f

Inspiratory positive airway pressure (IPAP), for obstructive sleep apnea, 491

Inspiratory pressure, maximal, 27–28, 28f, 552

Inspiratory reserve volume (IRV), 26, 27f, 94, 94f

Inspired carbon dioxide ($PICO_2$), 46, 46f

Inspired oxygen content (FIO_2)
  low, arterial hypoxemia due to, 51
  with supplemental oxygen, 543
    for COPD, 567, 567f

Insufficient sleep syndrome, 485

Insulin, in nonstressed starvation, 520

Intal (cromolyn sodium), for asthma, 147t, 156

Intensive care unit (ICU). *See also* Critically ill patients
  administration of, 517–518

Interbronchiolar communications of Martin, 40

Intercartilaginous muscles, parasternal, 5f

Intercostal muscles
  external, 5f
  inspiratory, 4, 5f
  internal, 4, 5f

Intercostal nerves, innervation of diaphragm by, 6

Interdependence, tissue, 40

Interleukins (ILs), in sarcoidosis, 293, 294

Interlobular septum, 20

Intermittent catheterization, 648

Intermittent feedings, 529

Intermittent mandatory ventilation (IMV), 548–549, 549f
  synchronized, 548–549, 549f
  for weaning, 553
Intermittent pneumatic compression, for deep venous thrombosis, 641
Intermittent positive pressure ventilation (IPPV)
  for asthma, 571
  for COPD, 568
Internal oblique muscles, 5f
International Classification of Sleep Disorders (ICSD), 484
Interruptor technique, 555
Interstitial fibrosing diseases, occupational and environmental, 324–335, 325t
  aluminum pneumoconiosis, 335
  asbestos-related, 328–331, 330f, 331f
  beryllium and hard metal-related, 332–334, 333f
  bronchoscopy of, 326
  cardiovascular exercise testing for, 326
  causes of, 325, 325t
  chest radiography of, 325
  coal workers' pneumoconiosis, 331–332, 332f
  computed tomography of, 325–326
  epidemiology of, 325
  flock worker's lung, 335
  Fuller's earth-related, 335
  graphite pneumoconiosis, 335
  kaolin pneumoconiosis, 334
  lung biopsy for, 326
  due to manmade vitreous fibers, 335
  mica-related, 335
  due to miscellaneous dusts, 335
  mixed-dust pneumoconiosis, 335
  overview of, 324–326, 325t
  pulmonary function testing for, 326
  silicosis, 326–328, 327f, 328f
  talcosis, 334
Interstitial fibrosis, elastic recoil in, 30, 30f
Interstitial lung diseases
  bronchoscopy of, 125
  diffuse. *See* Diffuse interstitial lung diseases (DILDs)
  thoracoscopy of, 126
Interstitial pneumonitis
  after bone marrow transplant, 433–434
  desquamative, 265
  nonspecific, 265
  usual, 265
Interstitium, of lungs, 263
Interview, 59
Intestine, in nutrition, 526–527, 526t
Intraabdominal abscess, pleural effusions with, 453–454
Intraoperative risk reduction strategies, 511t
Intravascular bronchioalveolar tumor, 356
Intrinsic PEEP, 550, 568, 572
Intubation. *See* Endotracheal intubation
Inverse ratio (IR) ventilation, 549
Ion transport, through respiratory epithelium, 12, 12f

IPAP (inspiratory positive airway pressure), for obstructive sleep apnea, 491
IPF. *See* Idiopathic pulmonary fibrosis (IPF)
IPH (idiopathic pulmonary hemosiderosis), 284–285
IPPV (intermittent positive pressure ventilation)
  for asthma, 571
  for COPD, 568
Ipratropium bromide (Atrovent)
  for asthma, 146t, 152, 160
    nocturnal, 497
  for COPD, 187, 194
    with central sleep apnea, 498
Ireton-Jones predictive equation, 524, 524t
Iron, carcinogenicity of, 350
Irritant gases, 322, 323, 323t
Irritant metals, 322, 323–324, 323t
IRV (inspiratory reserve volume), 26, 27f, 94, 94f
IR (inverse ratio) ventilation, 549
Ischemia, from systemic arterial catheterization, 621
Isoetharine HCl (Bronkometer)
  for asthma, 145, 146t, 159
  for COPD, 188t
Isoflow volume, 38, 38f
Isoflurane
  for asthma, 573
  with asthma, 593
  cardiovascular effects of, 593
Isoniazid (INH), for tuberculosis, 413, 436–437, 438
Isoproterenol HCl (Medihaler-150, Isuprel Mistometer)
  for asthma, 145, 146t
  for COPD, 188t
Isovolume pressure-flow curves, 34, 35f
Itraconazole
  for aspergillosis, 424–425
  for blastomycosis, 420
  for coccidioidomycosis, 421
  for histoplasmosis, 418, 437–438
  for paracoccidioidomycosis, 422

J
Jackson-Huber system, 72t
Jet ventilation, 551
Job-related lung disease. *See* Occupational lung disease

K
Kaolin pneumoconiosis, 334
K complexes, 480, 480f
Kerley B lines, 20
  in pulmonary edema, 579, 579f
  in pulmonary hypertension, 250–251
Ketoconazole
  for blastomycosis, 420
  for histoplasmosis, 418
  for paracoccidioidomycosis, 422
Ketone bodies
  in nonstressed starvation, 519f, 520
  during stress, 519f, 521

Klebsiella pneumoniae, 397–399
Koch's bacillus, 409
Kveim test, for sarcoidosis, 291–292
Kyphoscoliosis, 64, 470–471, 470f

L
Laceration, pulmonary, 609–610
Lactate, blood, 6
Lactic acid, production of, 105
Lactic acid dehydrogenase (LDH)
  in pleural fluid, 119
  in pulmonary alveolar proteinosis, 286
LAM (lymphangioleiomyomatosis), 302
Lambertosis, 11
Laminagram, 78
Laminar flow, 32–33, 32f
Langerhans cell granulomatosis, 301–302, 302f
Lansoprazole, for gastroesophageal reflux disease, 141
LAO (left anterior oblique) view, 76
LAP (laser-assisted palatoplasty), for obstructive sleep apnea, 490
Laparoscopic surgery, 594
Laplace's equation, 31
LAR (late asthmatic response), 136, 136f
Large airway obstruction, pulmonary function testing in, 110–111
Large cell carcinoma, 354, 355f
Large cell neuroendocrine carcinoma (LCNEC), 355
Laryngeal nerve, left recurrent, 8
Laryngotracheobronchitis, 383–384
Larynx
  carcinoma of, 8–9
  functional anatomy of, 8–9
Laser-assisted palatoplasty (LAP), for obstructive sleep apnea, 490
Laser therapy, for lung cancer, 370
Late asthmatic response (LAR), 136, 136f
Lateral chest radiography, 70, 70f
Lateral decubitus views, 76
LCNEC (large cell neuroendocrine carcinoma), 355
LDH (lactic acid dehydrogenase)
  in pleural fluid, 119
  in pulmonary alveolar proteinosis, 286
Lead, air pollution due to, 341t
Left anterior oblique (LAO) view, 76
Left atrial pressure
  and pulmonary edema, 579–581, 579f, 580f
  relation of wedge pressure to, 623–625
Left outer canthus (LOC) electrode, 478, 479f
Left ventricular heart failure, pulmonary edema due to, 579–581, 579f, 580f
Legionnaires' disease, 392–393, 398t
  in immunocompromised patients, 431
Leg movements, periodic, 483, 485–486
Leiomyoma, 357
Leiomyosarcoma, 357
Letterer-Siwe disease, 301
Leukopenia, in sarcoidosis, 292, 292t
Leukoprotease, for cystic fibrosis, 201

Leukotrienes
  in asthma, 137, 156–157
  vasoactive properties of, 17, 20
Leuprolide, pulmonary reaction to, 290
Levalbuterol (Xopenex), for asthma, 146t, 150
Levodopa, for periodic limb movements, 486
Life support
  foregoing of, 534–535
  withdrawal of, 507–508, 534–535
Limb movements, periodic, 483, 485–486
Limited disease, 364
Lingula, 9, 10f
LIP (lymphoid interstitial pneumonitis), 299
Lipoma, 357
Liver, fatty, due to parenteral nutrition, 532
Liver scan, for lung cancer, 367
Liver transplantation
  for α_1-antitrypsin deficiency, 189
  pleural effusions after, 454
Lobar bronchial segments, radiographic anatomy of, 69f, 70f, 72, 72f–74f, 72t
Lobule
  primary, 8f, 9, 20, 21f
  pulmonary, 20
LOC (left outer canthus) electrode, 478, 479f
Loeffler's syndrome, 299
Lordotic view, 76–77, 77f
Lower respiratory tract, functional anatomy of, 8f–11f, 9–11
Lower respiratory tract infections, 380–381, 381t, 384–415
  bronchiectasis, 380t, 386–387, 387f
  bronchiolitis, 378, 380t, 385
  bronchitis, 378, 380t, 384–385
  epidemiology of, 379
  fungal, 415–423, 416f, 418f–421f
    opportunistic, 423–425
  influenza, 385–386
  lung abscess, 394f, 395, 395f
  with mycobacteria other than tuberculosis, 378, 414–415, 414f
  pneumonia. *See* Pneumonia
  tuberculosis, 378, 409–414, 411f
LT. *See* Lung transplantation (LT)
L-tryptophan eosinophilia-myalgia syndrome, 300
Lung(s)
  air-conditioner, 296t
  air conduction system of, 8f, 9, 9f
  bird breeder's, 296t, 297
  in blood flow distribution, 12, 16–17, 16f
  cheese worker's, 296t
  chemical workers, 296t
  clearance and defenses of, 21–23, 21f
  diffusing capacity of, 99–100, 99f
    and work capacity, 104
  "dirty," in chronic bronchitis, 181, 182f
  distending pressure of, 26, 27f
  elastic recoil of, 30–32, 30f, 31f
  farmer's, 60, 296t, 297–298
  flock worker's, 335

  fluid balance of, 12
  fluid exchange in, 576–579, 577f, 577t, 578f
  grain handler's, 296t
  held against chest wall, 29–30
  humidifier, 296t
  interstitium of, 263
  lobes of, normal location of, 63, 64f
  malt workers,' 296t
  maple bark stripper's, 296t
  metabolic, nonrespiratory functions of, 18–20, 19f, 19t
  pressure-volume curve of, 27, 28f
    factors influencing, 30–32, 30f, 31f
    normal, 29f
  resting volume of, 27
  terminal respiratory unit of, 8f, 9, 20, 21f
  transport systems of, 21–23, 21f
  trapped, 456
  vanishing, in systemic lupus erythematosus, 272
Lung abscess, 379, 394f, 395, 395f
  pleural effusions with, 445–446
  sputum in, 62
  symptoms of, 60, 62, 63
Lung biopsy
  in asbestosis, 330, 331f
  for idiopathic pulmonary fibrosis, 265, 267
  in immunocompromised patient, 432
  for occupational interstitial lung disease, 326
  open-, 127–128
  for pneumonia, 407
  transbronchial, 121
  for Wegener's granulomatosis, 279
Lung cancer, 346–371
  adenocarcinoma, 354, 354f
  atmospheric pollution and, 349
  bronchial adenoma, 354–355
  bronchial papillomas, 356
  bronchial tumors of salivary gland type, 356
  bronchogenic carcinoma, 351–354, 352f–355f, 354t
  bronchoscopy of, 123–124
  carcinoid tumor, 354–355
  classification of, 351
  clinical manifestations of, 358–361, 359t
  dermatologic manifestations of, 361
  diagnosis of, 361–363
  diet and, 337, 350, 351f
  epidemiology of, 346–347, 347f
  etiology of, 347–351, 348f, 349f, 349t, 351f
  gender differences in, 346, 347f, 348–349
  genetic factors in, 350–351
  histology of, 351–354, 352f–355f, 354t
  intravascular bronchioalveolar tumor, 356
  investigation of solitary peripheral parenchymal mass for, 368, 368t
  large cell carcinoma, 354, 355f
  lymphoma, 357–358
  metabolic manifestations of, 359–360

  metastases of
    evaluation for, 367
    signs and symptoms of, 358–359
    in staging, 363–364, 363t, 364t
  neuromuscular manifestations of, 360
  occupational and environmental factors in, 337–340, 337t, 349–350, 349f, 349t
  paraneoplastic syndromes with, 359–361, 359t
  pathogenesis of, 351–352
  pathology of, 351–358, 352f–355f, 354t
  radioactive materials and, 349, 349f
  sarcoma, 357
  screening for, 361
  skeletal manifestations of, 361
  small cell carcinoma, 352–353, 353f, 354t
  smoking and, 346, 347–348, 348f
  squamous cell carcinoma, 352, 352f, 353f
  staging of, 363–367
    bronchoscopy for, 123–124, 365
    classification system for, 363–364, 363t, 364t
    lymph node biopsy for, 365
    mediastinoscopy and mediastinotomy for, 365–367, 366f, 367f
    needle aspiration biopsy for, 365
    thoracic imaging for, 364–365
    thoracotomy for, 367
  symptoms and signs of, 358–359, 359t
  treatment of, 368–371, 371f
  vascular manifestations of, 361
Lung capacity, total, 26, 27f, 28, 94f
  with restrictive ventilatory dysfunction, 109–110, 110t
Lung compliance. *See* Compliance
Lung function tests. *See* Pulmonary function tests (PFTs)
Lung injury
  acute. *See* Acute lung injury (ALI)
  toxic, 322
Lung resection
  cardiac considerations for, 600, 600t
  cardiopulmonary risk index for, 510, 599–600, 599t
  contraindications to, 598, 598t
  evaluation of suitability for, 598–600, 598t–600t
  for lung cancer, 368–369
  postoperative pulmonary function and complications after, 598–600, 599t
Lung scanning, 85–88, 86f, 87f
  for chronic thromboembolic pulmonary hypertension, 244
  for idiopathic pulmonary fibrosis, 267
  preoperative, 598–599
  for pulmonary embolism, 238–240, 239t, 240f
Lung transplantation (LT), 208–225
  for α_1-antitrypsin deficiency, 190
  bilateral, indications for, 209, 210t
  complications of, 217–223
    airway, 217–218
    graft rejection, 218–219, 219f, 219t
    infectious, 221–223, 222f, 223f

lymphoproliferative disorders, 223
  obliterative bronchiolitis, 219–220,
    220f, 220t
  pleural effusions, 454
contraindications to, 210–211, 210t
for COPD, 209, 211–212, 212t
for cystic fibrosis, 201–202, 209,
    212–213, 212t
donor selection for, 213–214, 213t
evaluation for, 213
heart-, indications for, 209–210, 210t
historical background of, 208–209
for idiopathic pulmonary fibrosis, 209,
    212, 212t
immunosuppression for, 215, 219,
    223–225, 224t
indications for, 209–210, 210t
outcome of, 217
postoperative management of, 215–217,
    216f
for primary pulmonary hypertension,
    209, 212t, 213, 251
recipient selection for, 210–211, 210t
single
    for idiopathic pulmonary fibrosis,
      270–271
    indications for, 209, 210t
    surgical technique for, 214
  surgical technique for, 214
  timing of, 211–213, 212t
Lung volume(s), 26, 27f
  and airway conductance, 33, 34f
  and airway resistance, 33, 34f
  measurement of, 94–96, 94f–97f
  and pulmonary vascular resistance, 16,
    16f
Lung volume reduction surgery (LVRS),
    225–227, 226t
Lupus erythematosus, systemic, 272–274,
    272f, 272t, 273f
  pleural effusions with, 452
Lupus pleuritis, 452
Lupus pneumonitis, acute, 273
LYG (lymphomatoid granulomatosis),
    279–281, 280f, 357–358
Lymphadenopathy
  immunoblastic, pleural effusions with,
    452
  in sarcoidosis, 290–291, 291f
Lymphangioleiomyomatosis (LAM), 302
Lymphangiomyomatosis, pulmonary,
    455–456
Lymphangitic carcinoma, metastatic, 257
Lymphangitic carcinomatosis, 81f
Lymphatics, pulmonary, 22–23
Lymph flow, in pulmonary edema, 579,
    579f, 580
Lymph node(s)
  functional anatomy of, 23
  mediastinoscopy and mediastinotomy of,
    365–366, 366f, 367f
  in staging of lung cancer, 363–364,
    363t, 364t
Lymph node biopsy, in lung cancer, 365
Lymph node enlargement, metastatic,
    465–466, 466f
Lymph node hyperplasia, giant, 465

Lymph node involvement, in
    granulomatous mediastinitis, 465,
    465f
Lymphocyte(s), 23
  in hypersensitivity pneumonitis, 298,
    298t
  in sarcoidosis, 292–295, 293t, 294f
Lymphocyte dysfunction, drug-induced,
    430t
Lymphocyte-like carcinoma, 352–353
Lymphohematogenous drainage, 22–23
Lymphoid interstitial pneumonitis (LIP),
    299
Lymphoid tissue
  bronchus-associated, 23
  gut-associated, 526
Lymphoma(s), 357–358
  mediastinal, 462–463, 463f
  pneumonia with, 403, 404t
  primary effusion, 451
  pyothorax-associated, 451–452
Lymphomatoid granulomatosis (LYG),
    279–281, 280f, 357–358
Lymphoproliferative disorders, after lung
    transplantation, 223
Lysozyme, in sarcoidosis, 292, 292t

M

MAC (*Mycobacterium avium* complex),
    414, 414f, 415, 437
Macrophage(s), alveolar
  functional anatomy of, 22
  in idiopathic pulmonary fibrosis, 269
  in sarcoidosis, 293, 294f
Macrophage dysfunction, drug-induced,
    430t
Magnesium, intravenous, for status
    asthmaticus, 161
Magnetic resonance imaging (MRI),
    83–84, 84f
  of chest trauma, 602
  of lung cancer, 365
Magnification radiographs, 77
Mainstream smoke (MS), 340
Maintenance of wakefulness test (MWT),
    483
Malignancy(ies). *See also* Lung cancer
  hypercalcemia of, 360
  due to occupational and environmental
    exposure, 337–340, 337t
  pleural fluid tests for, 120
Malignancy-associated phlebitis, 235
Malignant fibrous histiocytoma, 357
Malingering, exercise testing with,
    112–113
Malnutrition. *See also* Nutrition
  in critical illness and injury, 518,
    522–523
Malt workers' lung, 296t
Mandibular osteotomy, for obstructive
    sleep apnea, 490
Manganese, inhalation injury due to, 323,
    323t
Manmade vitreous fibers (MMVFs)
  carcinogenicity of, 337t, 339
  pneumoconiosis due to, 335
Mantoux test, 412

Maple bark stripper's lung, 296t
Masson bodies, 271
Material Safety Data Sheets (MSDSs), 316
Maxair (pirbuterol acetate)
  for asthma, 146t
  for COPD, 188t
Maxillary mandibular osteotomy (MMO),
    for obstructive sleep apnea, 490
Maximal air flow, density dependence of,
    38–39, 38f
Maximal expiratory pressure ($Pmax_{exp}$),
    27–28, 28f
Maximal inspiratory pressure ($Pmax_{insp}$,
    MIP), 27–28, 28f, 552
Maximal midexpiratory flow rate (MMF),
    92
Maximal volume ($\dot{V}max$), 36, 37
Maximal voluntary ventilation (MVV), 93
  and work capacity, 105
Maximum oxygen consumption. *See* Work
    capacity ($\dot{V}O_2max$)
MDIs (metered dose inhalers), 144, 149,
    150, 154, 158–159
MDR-TB (multidrug-resistant
    tuberculosis), 409, 413–414
  with HIV infection, 437
Mechanical ventilation (MV)
  airway pressure release, 551
  for ARDS, 587
  for asthma, 571–572, 572t
  controlled, 548
  conventional, 550, 550t
  in elderly, 503–507, 504f–506f, 505t
    ethical decisions regarding, 507–508
    weaning from, 506–507, 506f, 507t
  emergencies with, 553–555, 554f
  for flail chest, 605
  high-frequency oscillatory, 551
  indications for, 546t, 548
  and lung transplantation, 211
  modes of, 548–549, 549f, 551
  nutritional support with, 525–526
  PEEP with, 549–550
  for pneumonia, 409
  pneumonia with, 378, 389, 389t
  pressure-cycled, 549
  pressure-regulated-volume-controlled,
    551
  pressure support, 549
  for pulmonary contusion, 608
  for pulmonary edema
    high-pressure cardiogenic, 581
    increased-permeability
      (noncardiogenic), 587
  for respiratory failure, 548–555
    in COPD, 567–568
  respiratory monitoring with, 555–557,
    556f
  for status asthmaticus, 161–162
  strategies for, 550, 550t
  variable pressure-support and volume-
    support, 551
  ventilator features for, 548
  volume-cycled, 548–549, 549f
  weaning from, 551–553, 552t
    in COPD, 568–569
    in elderly, 506–507, 506f, 507t

Mediastinal crunch, 66
Mediastinal disease, 459–470, 460t
  thoracoscopy of, 126
Mediastinal emphysema, 469–470
Mediastinal fibrosis, 469
  due to histoplasmosis, 415, 416f
Mediastinal granuloma, 469
Mediastinal masses, 460–468
  in anterior compartment, 460t,
    461–466, 462f–464f
  CT of, 79, 80f, 461, 462f
  differential diagnosis of, 460–461, 460t,
    461t
  evaluation of, 460–461
  in middle compartment, 460t, 465–466,
    465f–467f
  in posterior compartment, 466–468
  of vascular origin, 466, 467f
Mediastinitis, 468–469
  acute, 468
  after cardiac surgery, 468
  fibrosing, 469
  granulomatous, 468–469
    lymph node involvement in, 465,
      465f
Mediastinoscopy, 127
  in lung cancer, 365–366, 366f
Mediastinotomy, in lung cancer, 365,
    366–367, 367f
Mediastinum, 459–460, 460f, 460t
  computed tomography of, 461, 462f
  injuries to, 610–613, 611f, 613t
Medical decision-making, 533
Medihaler-150 (isoproterenol HCl)
  for asthma, 145, 146t
  for COPD, 188t
Medihaler-Epi. *See* Epinephrine
    (Medihaler-Epi, Adrenalin
    chloride)
Mediterranean fever, familial, pleural
    effusions with, 452
Medrol. *See* Methylprednisolone sodium
    succinate (Medrol, Solu-Medrol)
Medroxyprogesterone (Provera)
  for obstructive sleep apnea, 491
  for pulmonary lymphangiomyomatosis,
    456
Meigs' syndrome, 455
Meningeal coccidioidomycosis, 422
Meningitis
  coccidioidal, 422
  cryptococcal, 423, 437
  tuberculous, 411
Meningocele, mediastinal, 467
Meningomyelocele, mediastinal, 467
Mental abnormalities, due to lung cancer,
    360
Mercury, inhalation injury due to, 323,
    323t
Mesenchymal tumors, mediastinal, 465
Mesodermal tumors, 356–357
Mesothelial cysts, 466
Mesothelioma
  localized benign pleural, 451
  malignant, 451
    asbestos and, 340

Metabolic acidosis, in respiratory failure,
    542
Metabolic alkalosis, in respiratory failure,
    542
Metabolic complications, of tube feeding,
    530
Metabolic equivalents (METs), 102
Metabolic manifestations, of lung cancer,
    359–360
Metal(s), irritant, 322, 323–324, 323t
Metal fume fever, 323–324
Metaproterenol (Alupent, Metaprel)
  for asthma, 145, 146t, 159, 572
  for COPD, 188t
Metastases
  evaluation for, 367
  pulmonary, CT of, 79f
  signs and symptoms of, 358–359
  in staging of lung cancer, 363–364,
    363t, 364t
Metastatic lymph node enlargement,
    465–466, 466f
Metered dose inhalers (MDIs), 144, 149,
    150, 154, 158–159
Methotrexate
  for asthma, 162
  pulmonary reaction to, 289
  for Wegener's granulomatosis, 279
Methylisocyanate, inhalation injury due to,
    323t
Methylphenidate (Ritalin), for narcolepsy,
    485
Methylprednisolone sodium succinate
    (Medrol, Solu-Medrol)
  for acute pulmonary rejection, 219
  for asthma, 148t, 160, 573
  for bronchiolitis obliterans, 220
  for COPD, 194–195
  for lung transplantation, 215
Methylxanthines
  for asthma, 147t–148t, 150–152, 151t
  for COPD, 188, 188t
Methysergide, pleural effusions due to, 455
Metronidazole, for amebiasis, 448
MI. *See* Myocardial infarction (MI)
Mica-associated lung disease, 335
Midexpiratory flow rate, maximal, 92
Miliary tuberculosis, 412
Minerals, in parenteral nutrition, 531–532,
    531t
Minute ventilation (V̇E)
  and alveolar ventilation, 51
  with exercise, 6
  normal, 6, 543t
  total, 46, 46f, 543
  and work capacity, 105, 106f
MIP (maximal inspiratory pressure),
    27–28, 28f, 552
Mitomycin C, pulmonary reaction to, 289
Mitral stenosis, pulmonary hypertension
    due to, 249–251
Mixed-dust pneumoconiosis, 335
Mixed venous saturation (S V̄O₂), 53
  exercise and, 106
  and work capacity, 103–104, 104t
Mixed ventilatory dysfunction, pulmonary
    function testing with, 110

MMF (maximal midexpiratory flow rate),
    92
MMF (mycophenolate mofetil)
  for bronchiolitis obliterans, 220
  for lung transplantation, 215, 219, 223,
    224, 224t, 225
MMO (maxillary mandibular osteotomy),
    for obstructive sleep apnea, 490
MMVFs (manmade vitreous fibers)
  carcinogenicity of, 337t, 339
  pneumoconiosis due to, 335
Modafinil, for narcolepsy, 485
MOF. *See* Multiple organ failure (MOF)
Mometasone furoate (Asmanex), for
    asthma, 147t, 154
Monge's disease, 249
Monitoring
  airflow, 482–483
  cardiovascular, 620–627
  of peak expiratory flow, 144
  respiratory, 555–557, 556f
  of sleep, 478–481, 479f–481f,
    482–483, 483t
Monoclonal anti-T lymphocyte antibodies,
    for lung transplantation,
    223–224
Monokines, in sarcoidosis, 294
Montelukast (Singulair), for asthma, 147t,
    157–158
Moraxella spp, bronchitis due to, 384
Morphine sulfate
  cardiovascular effects of, 593
  for pulmonary edema, 581
Motor neuropathy, due to lung cancer, 360
MOTT (mycobacteria other than
    tuberculosis), 414–415, 414f,
    437
Mountain sickness, chronic, 249
Mouth breathing, during exercise, 7
MRI (magnetic resonance imaging),
    83–84, 84f
  of chest trauma, 602
  of lung cancer, 365
MS (mainstream smoke), 340
MSDSs (Material Safety Data Sheets), 316
MSLT (multiple sleep latency test), 483,
    483t
  in obstructive sleep apnea syndrome, 488
Mucin-associated antigens, 12
Mucociliary escalator, 21–22, 21f
Mucoepidermoid carcinoma, 356
Mucolytic therapy
  for COPD, 189
  for pneumonia, 409
Mucormycosis, 425
Mucosa, respiratory, metabolic and
    secretory functions of, 11–12,
    12f
Mucous cells, functional anatomy of, 10
Mucous glands
  functional anatomy of, 10
  hypertrophy of, 10
  in mucociliary escalator, 21, 21f
Mucus
  formation of, 12, 21
  gel layer of, 21–22, 21f
  sol layer of, 21f, 22

Mucus secretion
  in chronic bronchitis, 174, 179
  in COPD, 177
  in idiopathic pulmonary fibrosis, 265
Multibreath nitrogen washout, 95, 96f, 98
Multidrug-resistant tuberculosis (MDR-TB), 409, 413–414
  with HIV infection, 437
Multiple organ failure (MOF), 628–636
  cardiovascular failure in, 628–629
  CNS failure in, 630, 630t
  defined, 628
  early recognition of, 636
  epidemiology of, 628–631
  gastrointestinal failure in, 629
  hematologic failure in, 630
  hepatic failure in, 629–630
  management of, 634–636
  mortality with, 631
  pathogenesis of, 631–633, 632f
  prevention of, 636
  renal failure in, 629
  respiratory failure in, 630–631, 631t
Multiple sclerosis, respiratory failure with, 562t
Multiple sleep latency test (MSLT), 483, 483t
  in obstructive sleep apnea syndrome, 488
Muromonab-CO3 (Orthoclone OKT3)
  for bronchiolitis obliterans, 220
  for lung transplantation, 215, 223
Muscle(s), respiratory. *See* Respiratory muscle(s)
Muscle fatigue, functional anatomy of, 4, 6
Muscular dystrophies, respiratory failure with, 562t
Muscular efforts, volume-pressure relations during, 27–32, 28f, 31f
Mustard gas, carcinogenicity of, 337t, 339
MV. *See* Mechanical ventilation (MV)
MVV (maximal voluntary ventilation), 93
  and work capacity, 105
MWT (maintenance of wakefulness test), 483
Myasthenia gravis
  respiratory failure in, 562–563, 562t
  with thymoma, 461
Mycobacterial infections, 378, 414–415, 414f
  with silicosis, 327–328
Mycobacteria other than tuberculosis (MOTT), 414–415, 414f, 437
Mycobacterium avium complex (MAC), 414, 414f, 415, 437
Mycobacterium tuberculosis, 409. *See also* Tuberculosis (TB)
Mycophenolate mofetil (MMF)
  for bronchiolitis obliterans, 220
  for lung transplantation, 215, 219, 223, 224, 224t, 225
Mycoplasma pneumoniae, 396–397, 398t
Myeloma, pneumonia with, 403, 404t
Myocardial infarction (MI)
  pleural effusions after, 456
  pulmonary artery catheterization for, 626
  surgery after, 600

Myopathy, due to lung cancer, 360
Myxedema, pleural effusions with, 444

N

Narcolepsy, 484–485
Narcotics, respiratory failure due to, 563
Nasal CPAP
  for central sleep apnea, 495
  for Cheyne-Stokes breathing, 495
  for obstructive sleep apnea, 490, 491–493
Nasal masks, 544, 545
Nasal mucosa, 7
Nasal polyps, 63
Nasal prongs, 543
Nasoenteric feeding tubes, 518–519, 527–530, 528t
Nasopharynx, 7
Nasotracheal intubation, for respiratory failure, 546–548, 546t, 547f
Nebulizer therapy, for asthma, 149, 158–159
Neck veins, examination of, 64
Nedocromil sodium (Tilade), for asthma, 147t, 156
Needle aspiration biopsy
  endoscopic ultrasound-guided, 127
  in immunocompromised patient, 432
  in lung cancer, 362–363, 365
  of mediastinal mass, 461
  transbronchial, 122
  transthoracic, 125
Neoplasms
  benign
    alveolar adenoma, 356
    chondroma and osteochondroma, 357
    hamartoma, 357
    leiomyoma, 357
    lipoma, 357
    sclerosing hemangioma, 356
    solitary peripheral parenchymal mass as, 368, 368t
  bronchial, of salivary gland type, 356
  intravascular bronchioalveolar, 356
  malignant. *See* Lung cancer
  pleural effusions secondary to, 449–451
  of pulmonary vascular bed, 257
Nephrotic syndrome, pleural effusions in, 444
Net transvascular fluid flow, 577, 577t
Neuroendocrine carcinoma, large cell, 355
Neurofibromas, mediastinal, 466–467
Neurogenic tumors, of mediastinum, 466–467
Neuromuscular disorders, respiratory failure due to, 561–563, 562t
Neuromuscular manifestations, of lung cancer, 360
Neutropenia
  pneumonia with, 389, 389t, 403, 404t
  pulmonary complications of, 430–434, 430t–432t
Neutrophil(s)
  in acute lung injury, 585
  in septic shock, 633

Neutrophil dysfunction, drug-induced, 430t
Nickel
  carcinogenicity of, 337t, 339, 350
  inhalation injury due to, 323t
Nicotine replacement therapy, 185
Nifedipine, for primary pulmonary hypertension, 251
Nilutamide, pulmonary reaction to, 290
NIPPV (noninvasive positive pressure ventilation), 544–546, 544f, 545t
  for COPD, 568
  for status asthmaticus, 161
Nitric oxide (NO), vasoactive properties of, 17–18
Nitrofurantoin
  pleural effusions due to, 454–455
  pulmonary reaction to, 289
Nitrogen balance, 525
Nitrogen dioxide, air pollution due to, 341t
Nitrogen elimination test, single-breath, 98, 98f
Nitrogen excretion
  in nonstressed starvation, 520
  during stress, 521, 522f
Nitrogen oxides, inhalation injury due to, 323, 323t
Nitrogen washout technique, 95, 96f, 98
Nitroglycerin, for pulmonary edema, 581
Nitroprusside, for pulmonary edema, 581
Nitrous oxide, cardiovascular effects of, 593
NO (nitric oxide), vasoactive properties of, 17–18
Nocardiosis
  in immunocompromised patients, 431
  pleural effusions due to, 447
Nodules. *See* Pulmonary nodules
Nonadherence, in asthma, 143
Noncompliance, in asthma, 143
Non-Hodgkin's lymphoma, mediastinal, 462–463
Noninvasive positive pressure ventilation (NIPPV), 544–546, 544f, 545t
  for COPD, 568
  for status asthmaticus, 161
Non-rapid eye movement (NREM) sleep, 478, 480, 481, 482
Nonspecific interstitial pneumonitis (NSIP), 265
Nonsteroidal anti-inflammatory drugs (NSAIDs), asthma due to, 141
Nonstressed starvation, 519–520, 519f, 519t
Norepinephrine
  for multiple organ failure, 633–634
  vasoactive properties of, 17, 19
Nose
  examination of, 63
  functional anatomy of, 7
Nosebleeds, 60
Nosocomial pneumonia, 377, 378, 401–403, 401f, 403f
  in immunocompromised patients, 431
NREM (non-rapid eye movement) sleep, 478, 480, 481, 482

NSAIDs (nonsteroidal anti-inflammatory drugs), asthma due to, 141

NSIP (nonspecific interstitial pneumonitis), 265

Nucleotides, vasoactive, 20, 20f

Nutrition. *See also* Diet(s)
in critical illness and injury, 518–533
assessment of, 522–523, 523t
enteral, 518–519, 527–530, 528t
fuel utilization and, 519–521, 519f–522f, 519t
goals of, 525–526
modalities for, 527–532
parenteral, 530–532, 531t
requirements for, 523–525, 523t, 524t
role of gut in, 526–527, 526t
for cystic fibrosis, 201

Nutritional assessment
for COPD, 191
for critically ill patients, 522–523, 523t
serum proteins in, 523, 523t

Nutritional history, 522

Nutritional requirements, 523–525, 523t, 524t

Nutritional status
evaluation of. *See* Nutritional assessment
and lung transplantation, 211

Nutritional support
goals of, 525–526
modalities for, 527–532
for multiple organ failure, 635
of ventilator-dependent patients, 525–526

Nylon flock, interstitial lung disease due to, 335

O

OA (oral appliances), for obstructive sleep apnea, 492, 492f

Oat cell carcinoma, 352–353

Obesity hypoventilation syndrome (OHS), 489
respiratory failure with, 562t, 564

Oblique views, 75–76

Obliterative bronchiolitis (OB), after lung transplantation, 219–220, 220f, 220t

Obstructive sleep apnea (OSA), 486–493
apnea termination and arousal in, 488
automobile accidents with, 493
cardiovascular consequences of, 489–490
clinical manifestations of, 486
and daytime hypercapnia, 489
defined, 482, 482f
impaired sleep and daytime sleepiness in, 488–489
incidence of, 486
obesity hyperventilation syndrome in, 489
overlap syndrome in, 489, 497, 498
pathophysiology of, 487–488
polysomnography in, 486–487, 487f
predisposing conditions for, 486
prognosis and mortality with, 493
treatment of, 490–493, 492f, 492t

upper airway resistance syndrome in, 489, 489f

Obstructive sleep apnea syndrome (OSAS). *See* Obstructive sleep apnea (OSA)

Obstructive ventilatory dysfunction
exercise testing with, 111–112
pulmonary function testing with, 109, 109t

Occludin, 14

Occupational asthma, 317–321, 318t, 320f

Occupational bronchitis, 335–337, 336t

Occupational exposure
assessment of, 316
in hypersensitivity pneumonitis, 296–299, 296t, 298t
in interstitial lung disease, 264
in lung cancer, 349–350, 349f, 349t
in pulmonary alveolar proteinosis, 285

Occupational history, 60

Occupational lung disease, 314–342
acute pleural, 324
airway disorders, 317–324, 318t, 320f, 323t, 324t
aluminum pneumoconiosis, 335
asthma, 317–321, 318t, 320f
beryllium and hard metal-related, 332–334, 333f
byssinosis, 321–322
chronic bronchitis, 335–337, 336t
classification of, 316, 317t
clinical approach to, 315
coal workers' pneumoconiosis, 331–332, 332f
diagnostic criteria for, 315–316
exposure assessment for, 316
flock worker's lung, 335
Fuller's earth-associated, 335
due to grain dust, 322
graphite pneumoconiosis, 335
inhalation injury, 322–324, 324t
interstitial fibrosing, 324–335, 325t
kaolin pneumoconiosis, 334
malignancies due to, 337–340, 337t
due to manmade vitreous fibers, 335
mica-associated, 335
mixed-dust pneumoconiosis, 335
nonmalignant asbestos-related, 328–331, 330f, 331t
principles of, 314–316
silicosis, 326–328, 327f, 328f
talcosis, 334
upper respiratory tract irritation, 316

OHS (obesity hypoventilation syndrome), 489
respiratory failure with, 562t, 564

OKT3 (muromonab-CO3)
for bronchiolitis obliterans, 220
for lung transplantation, 215, 223

Omega-3 fatty acids, in critical illness, 527

Omeprazole, for gastroesophageal reflux disease, 141

Oncotic pressure, in pleural fluid, 442, 442f

Open lung approach, to mechanical ventilation, 550

Open-lung biopsy, 127–128

Opportunistic infections
fungal, 423–425, 433
after lung transplantation, 221–223, 222f, 223f

Oral appliances (OA), for obstructive sleep apnea, 492, 492f

Organic dusts, hypersensitivity to, 296–299, 296t, 298t

Organ transplants, pneumonia with, 404

Oriental lung fluke, 448–449

Oropharynx, 7, 8
bacteriology of, 379–380, 380t

Orthoclone OKT3 (muromonab-CO3)
for bronchiolitis obliterans, 220
for lung transplantation, 215, 223

Orthopnea, 61

OSA. *See* Obstructive sleep apnea (OSA)

OSAS (obstructive sleep apnea syndrome). *See* Obstructive sleep apnea (OSA)

Oscillating bed, for pneumonia, 409

Osler-Weber-Rendu disease, 255–256

Osmium, inhalation injury due o, 323t

Osteoarthropathy, hypertrophic pulmonary
with benign fibrous mesothelioma, 451
with lung cancer, 361

Osteochondroma, 357

Osteoporosis, and lung transplantation, 211

Osteotomy, mandibular, for obstructive sleep apnea, 490

Overlap syndrome
of COPD and obstructive sleep apnea, 489, 497, 498
of systemic vasculitides, 281–282

Overpenetrated grid radiograph, 77

"Owl's eye" inclusions, in cytomegalovirus, 222, 222f

Oxidants, in acute lung injury, 586

Oximetry, 67
pulse, 556–557

Oxygenation, variables related to, 543

Oxygen consumption ($\dot{V}O_2$), 41–42
equation for, 102, 543
exercise and, 101, 101t
maximum. *See* Work capacity ($\dot{V}O_2$max)
normal, 45, 543t
and other measures of work, 102, 102t

Oxygen content, 49–50
inspired. *See* Inspired oxygen content (FIO_2)

Oxygen cost, of breathing, 41–42

Oxygen delivery, systemic, 53–55, 54f

Oxygen diffusing capacity (DO_2), 47

Oxygen extraction, 53
peripheral, and work capacity, 103–104

Oxygen requirements, 101, 101t

Oxygen saturation
arterial, 44, 54, 483
pH and, 54, 54f
and work capacity, 104–105, 104f
normal value for, 543t

Oxygen tension (PO_2)
alveolar. *See* Alveolar oxygen tension (PAO_2)
arterial. *See* Arterial oxygen tension (PaO_2)
mixed venous difference in, 53

transcutaneous, 556
venous
  arterial hypoxemia due to low mixed, 53
  normal value for, 543t
Oxygen therapy
  for asthma, 571
  for central sleep apnea, 494, 495
  for Cheyne-Stokes breathing, 495
  for COPD, 193–194, 195, 497–498, 567, 567f
  for cor pulmonale, 254, 255
  for idiopathic pulmonary fibrosis, 270
  for obstructive sleep apnea, 491
  for pneumonia, 409
  for pulmonary contusion, 608
  for respiratory failure, 543–544
Oxygen transport, 49–50, 49f
Oxygen uptake, in ARDS, 632, 632f
Oxyhemoglobin dissociation curve, 49–50, 49f, 54f
Ozone
  air pollution due to, 341, 341t
  inhalation injury due to, 323, 323t

P
P_{50}, 54
PA catheterization. *See* Pulmonary artery (PA) catheterization
PA (posteroanterior) chest radiograph, 69f, 70
P_{ACO_2}. *See* Alveolar carbon dioxide tension (P_{ACO_2})
Pa_{CO_2}. *See* Arterial carbon dioxide tension (Pa_{CO_2})
PAHs (polyaromatic hydrocarbons), carcinogenicity of, 337t, 339
Pain
  of aortic dissection, 61
  chest, 60–61
    in lung cancer, 358
    in malignant mesothelioma, 451
    due to tuberculosis, 411
  esophageal, 61
  pericardial, 61
  pleuritic, 7, 61, 442
    with pleural effusions, 442
    with pulmonary embolism, 237, 237t
  of rib fractures, 61, 472
Palatoplasty, laser-assisted, for obstructive sleep apnea, 490
Palpation, 63–65, 64f
Pancoast tumor, MRI of, 84f
Pancreatic pseudocyst, pleural effusions with, 453
Pancreatitis, pleural effusions with, 453
Panhypogammaglobulinemia, with bronchiectasis, 198
P_{AO_2}. *See* Alveolar oxygen tension (P_{AO_2})
Pa_{O_2}. *See* Arterial oxygen tension (Pa_{O_2})
P_{AO_2}-Pa_{O_2}. *See* Alveolar-arterial oxygen gradient (P_{AO_2}-Pa_{O_2})
PAP. *See* Positive airway pressure (PAP)
Papillomas, of bronchus, 356
Paracoccidioidomycosis, 422
Paradoxical embolization, 609–610

Paradoxical respiration, 6
Paragonimiasis, pleural effusions in, 448–449
Parainfluenza virus, pneumonia due to, 400t
Paralysis
  of diaphragm, 472–473
  sleep, 484
Paranasal sinuses, functional anatomy of, 7
Paraneoplastic syndromes, 66, 359–361, 359t
  with thymoma, 461
Parapneumonic effusion, 445–446
Parasitic infections
  eosinophilic syndromes due to, 299
  of pleura, 448–449
Parathyroid tumors, mediastinal, 464–465
Paratracheal nodes, 23
Parenchymal infection, 379, 387–415. *See also* Pneumonia
Parenchymal injuries, 607–610, 608f
  in critically ill patients, 633
Parenteral nutrition (PN), 530–532, 531t
Parietal pleura, 7, 441
Paroxetine, for obstructive sleep apnea, 491
Particle deposition, in respiratory tract, 21
Particle removal, from respiratory tract, 21–23, 21f
Particulate matter, air pollution due to, 341, 341t
Passey-Muir valve, 547
Passive smoking, 340, 342, 348
Patient education
  for asthma, 143–144
  for COPD, 191
Patient Self-Determination Act, 535
P_{CO_2}. *See* Carbon dioxide (CO_2) tension (P_{CO_2})
PCP (*Pneumocystis carinii* pneumonia)
  with HIV infection, 405–406, 405f, 435–436, 438
  after lung transplantation, 221
PCR (polymerase chain reaction) tests, of pleural fluid, 121
PC (pressure controlled) ventilation, 549
PDH (progressive disseminated histoplasmosis), 417, 418f
PE. *See* Pulmonary embolism (PE)
Peak expiratory flow rate (PEFR), 93
  in asthma, 139
    monitoring of, 144
    occupational, 319, 320f
  in respiratory failure, 542
Peak flow meters, 67
PE_{CO_2} (expired carbon dioxide), 46, 46f, 556
Pectoralis major muscle, 4, 5f
Pectus carinatum, 471
Pectus excavatum, 471
PEEP. *See* Positive-end-expiratory pressure (PEEP)
PEFR. *See* Peak expiratory flow rate (PEFR)
Pendelluft, 39
Penicillin G, for aspiration, 394

Penicillin-resistant *Streptococcus pneumoniae* (PRSP), 390, 392
Penicillin VK, for streptococcal pharyngitis, 383
Pentamidine, for *Pneumocystis carinii* pneumonia, 406
Peptide(s), vasoactive, 19
Peptide-based diets, 527
Percussion, of chest, 65
Percutaneous dilational tracheostomy, 547
Percutaneous needle biopsy, of mediastinal mass, 461
Perfusion lung scans, 85–88, 86f, 87f
  of chronic thromboembolic pulmonary hypertension, 244
  of pulmonary embolism, 238–240, 239t, 240f
Peribronchiolar metaplasia, 11
Pericardial cysts, 466
Pericardial disease, pleural effusions in, 444
Pericardial friction rubs, 66
Pericardial pain, 61
Periodic limb movements (PLMs), 483, 485–486
Peripheral oxygen extraction, and work capacity, 103–104
Peripheral parenteral nutrition (PPN), 530
Peripheral vessels, in emphysema, 180t
Peritoneal dialysis, pleural effusions with, 444
Peritonitis, tuberculous, 411
Permissive hypercapnia, 550
PET (positron emission tomography), 88
  of lung cancer, 365, 367
PFTs. *See* Pulmonary function tests (PFTs)
PGF (primary graft failure), after lung transplantation, 215, 216
PGI_2 (prostacyclin)
  for primary pulmonary hypertension, 251
  vasoactive properties of, 17, 20
pH
  arterial
    normal, 543t
    Pa_{CO_2} and, 541, 542f
  in asthma, 571
  in COPD, 566
  pleural fluid, 120
Phagocytosis, 388
  by alveolar macrophages, 22
Pharyngitis, 380t, 383
Pharynx, functional anatomy of, 7–8
Phase III slope, 98
Phasic activity, 487
Phasic REM sleep, 481–482
Phlebitis, malignancy-associated, 235
Phlebotomy, for cor pulmonale, 254
Phlegm, in chronic bronchitis, 174, 179
Phosgene, inhalation injury due to, 323, 323t
Phrenic nerve, innervation of diaphragm by, 6
Physical examination, 63–66, 64f, 65t, 66f
Physical training, 106–107, 107f
Physiologic dead space, 45
PI_{CO_2} (inspired carbon dioxide), 46, 46f

Pigeon breast, 471
Pigeon breeder's lung, 296t, 297
Pipe smoking, and lung cancer, 348
Pirbuterol acetate (Maxair)
    for asthma, 146t
    for COPD, 188t
Pixels, 78
PL (transpulmonary pressure), 26, 27f, 97, 97f
Plaques, pleural, asbestos-related, 329
Plasmapheresis
    for Goodpasture's syndrome, 283–284
    for Guillain-Barré syndrome, 562
Plasmin byproducts, with pulmonary embolism, 238
Pleomorphic adenomas, 356
Plethysmography, 96–97, 98f
    respiratory inductance, 483, 555
Pleura
    fungal diseases of, 447–448
    parasitic diseases of, 448–449
    parietal, 7, 441
    physiology of, 7, 441–442, 442f
    viral diseases of, 448
    visceral, 7, 441
Pleural biopsy, 121
    in immunocompromised patient, 432
    in lung cancer, 363
    in tuberculous pleuritis, 447
Pleural calcification, asbestos-related, 458
Pleural disease, 441–459
    asbestos-related, 324, 328–329, 455, 458
    chylothorax and pseudochylothorax, 456–457
    fibrothorax, 458
    hemothorax, 457–458
    pleural effusions. *See* Pleural effusions
    pneumothorax, 458–459
Pleural effusions, 442–456
    after abdominal surgery, 454
    with actinomycosis, 447
    with amebiasis, 448
    approach to patient with, 443–444, 443t
    asbestos-induced, 324, 455
    with aspergillosis, 447–448
    with blastomycosis, 448
    bronchoscopy of, 125
    chyliform, 457
    due to chylothorax and pseudochylothorax, 456–457
    chylous, 457
    in cirrhosis, 444
    clinical manifestations of, 442–443
    with coccidioidomycosis, 448
    in collagen vascular disease, 452
    in congestive heart failure, 444
    after coronary artery bypass surgery, 454, 456
    in cor pulmonale, 253
    with cryptococcosis, 448
    CT of, 82f
    differential diagnosis of, 443–444, 443t
    due to drug reactions, 454–455
    with echinococcosis, 449
    after endoscopic variceal sclerotherapy, 454

with esophageal perforations, 453
exudative, 119, 442, 443–444, 443t, 445–456
    due to fungal diseases, 447–448
    with gastrointestinal conditions, 453–454
    due to hemothorax, 457–458
    with histoplasmosis, 448
    with intraabdominal abscess, 453–454
lateral decubitus radiograph of, 117, 118f
after liver transplantation, 454
loculated, 443, 445–446
in lung cancer, 358
after lung transplantation, 454
with lymphomas, 451–452
malignant, 449–451
in Meigs' syndrome, 455
with mesothelioma, 451
with myxedema, 444
in nephrotic syndrome, 444
with nocardiosis, 447
with pancreatic pseudocyst, 453
with pancreatitis, 453
with paragonimiasis, 448–449
parapneumonic, 445–446
due to parasitic diseases, 448–449
pathophysiology of, 442
due to pericardial disease, 444
with peritoneal dialysis, 444
in post-cardiac injury (Dressler's) syndrome, 456
postsurgical, 454
in pulmonary edema, 580
with pulmonary embolism, 237, 237t, 452–453
in pulmonary lymphangiomyomatosis, 455–456
radiographic appearance of, 443
in rheumatoid pleuritis, 452
in sarcoidosis, 456
in systemic lupus erythematosus, 272, 272f, 452
thoracoscopy of, 126
transudative, 119, 442, 443, 443t, 444
in trapped lung, 456
tuberculous, 411, 446–447
ultrasound of, 84
in uremia, 456
with urinary tract obstruction, 456
due to viral diseases, 448
in yellow nail syndrome, 456
Pleural fluid
    absorption of, 7, 441–442, 442f
    adenosine deaminase levels in, 120–121
    amylase in, 120, 453
    appearance of, 118–119
    bacteriology of, 120
    cell count and differentials for, 119
    chemistries for, 119–120
    "chocolate sauce," 448
    with chylothorax, 457
    cytology of, 120
    diagnostic tests on, 118, 118t
    flow cytometry of, 120
    formation of, 7, 441–442, 442f

gamma interferon levels in, 121
glucose in, 119
hematocrit of, 118–119
immunohistochemical testing of, 120
lactic acid dehydrogenase in, 119
pH of, 120
polymerase chain reaction tests of, 121
protein in, 119
separation of transudates from exudates in, 119
tests for malignancy in, 120
triglycerides in, 457
tuberculosis markers in, 120–121
in tuberculous pleuritis, 447
tumor markers in, 120
Pleural friction rub, 66
    with pulmonary embolism, 237, 237t
Pleural peel, 445, 446, 456
Pleural plaques, asbestos-related, 329
Pleural pressure (Ppl), 26, 27, 27f
    gradients in, 29, 29f
    measurement of, 28–29
    negative, 7
Pleural space
    anatomy of, 7, 441
    defined, 441
    gases in, 29–30
    liquid in, 30
    maintenance of, 29–30
    physiology of, 7, 441–442, 442f
Pleural thickening, asbestos-related, 329, 458
Pleuritic pain, 7, 61, 442
    with pleural effusions, 442
    with pulmonary embolism, 237, 237t
Pleuritis
    lupus, 452
    rheumatoid, 452
    tuberculous, 411, 446–447
    uremic, 456
Pleurodesis
    for malignant mesothelioma, 451
    for malignant pleural effusions, 450
    for pneumothorax, 459
Pleuropericardial cysts, 466
Pleuroperitoneal shunt, for malignant pleural effusions, 451
PLMs (periodic limb movements), 483, 485–486
Pmax_exp (maximal expiratory pressure), 27–28, 28f
Pmax_insp (maximal inspiratory pressure), 27–28, 28f, 552
PM-DM (polymyositis-dermatomyositis), 276
PMF (progressive massive fibrosis)
    in coal workers' pneumoconiosis, 332, 332f
    in silicosis, 327
PMNs (polymorphonuclear cells)
    in idiopathic pulmonary fibrosis, 269
    in sarcoidosis, 295
PN (parenteral nutrition), 530–532, 531t
Pneumatic compression, intermittent, for deep venous thrombosis, 641
Pneumococcal pneumonia, 390–392, 392f

Pneumococcal vaccine, 392
  for COPD prevention, 185
  with HIV infection, 438
Pneumoconiosis(es), 324–335
  aluminum, 335
  asbestos-related, 328–331, 330f, 331f
  attapulgite, 335
  beryllium and hard metal-related,
      332–334, 333f
  bronchoscopy of, 326
  cardiovascular exercise testing for, 326
  causes of, 325, 325t
  chest radiography of, 325
  coal workers', 331–332, 332f
  CT of, 325–326
  defined, 324
  epidemiology of, 325
  flock worker's lung, 335
  Fuller's earth-related, 335
  graphite, 335
  kaolin (China clay), 334
  lung biopsy for, 326
  due to manmade vitreous fibers, 335
  mica-related, 335
  due to miscellaneous dusts, 335
  mixed-dust, 335
  overview of, 324–326, 325t
  pulmonary function testing for, 326
  rheumatoid, 274–275
  silicosis, 326–328, 327f, 328f
  talcosis, 334
Pneumocystis carinii pneumonia (PCP)
  with HIV infection, 405–406, 405f,
      435–436, 438
  after lung transplantation, 221
Pneumomediastinum, 469–470, 540
Pneumonia, 387–409
  with AIDS, 389, 403–404, 404t,
      405–406, 405f, 436
  with alcoholism, 389, 389t
  approach to patient with, 406–408
  with ARDS, 389, 389t
  aspiration, 393–395, 394f
  atypical, 389, 398t
  after bone marrow transplant, 433
  bronchiolitis obliterans with organizing.
      See Bronchiolitis obliterans with
      organizing pneumonia (BOOP)
  with cardiac disease, 389, 389t
  cavitary, 394f, 395, 395f
  chest radiograph of, 406–407
  chlamydial, 397, 398t
  with chronic bronchitis, 389, 389t
  clinical features of, 389–391, 390f
  common pathogens in, 380t
  community-acquired, 389–401
    antibiotics for, 408–409
    bacterial, 391–399, 392f, 394f–396f,
        397t, 398f
    clinical features of, 389–391, 390f
    hospitalization for, 408
    viral, 399–401, 400f, 400t
  in critically ill patients, 378
  with cystic fibrosis, 389, 389t
  diagnosis of, 406–408
  in elderly, 378, 389, 389t, 390t

eosinophilic, 299, 300
epidemiology of, 377–378
Friedlander's, 397–399
Haemophilus influenzae, 395–396, 396f
history and physical examination of, 406
hospital-acquired (nosocomial), 377,
      378, 401–403, 401f, 403f
in immunocompromised host, 403–406,
      404t, 405f
Klebsiella pneumoniae, 397–399
Legionella pneumophila, 392–393, 398t
  after lung transplantation, 221
  with lymphoma, 403, 404t
  with mechanical ventilation, 389, 389t
Mycoplasma pneumoniae, 396–397, 398t
  with myeloma, 403, 404t
  with neutropenia, 389, 389t, 403, 404t
  with organ transplants, 404
  pathogenesis of, 387–389, 387f,
      388t–390t
  pleural effusions with, 445–446
  pneumococcal, 390–392, 392f
Pneumocystis carinii, 405–406, 405f,
      435–436, 438
  pneumothorax due to, 459
  postinfluenza, 389, 389t
  postoperative, 596–597, 597t
Pseudomonas aeruginosa, 403, 403f
  risk factors for, 378, 388–389, 388t,
      389t
  severe, 391, 406
  with splenectomy, 389, 389t, 403, 404t
  sputum in, 62
Staphylococcus aureus, 399, 399f
Streptococcus pneumoniae, 391–392, 392f
    penicillin-resistant, 390, 392
  symptoms of, 63
  therapy of, 408–409
  typical, 389, 391
  viral, 399–401, 400f, 400t
Pneumonitis
  acute lupus, 273
  hypersensitivity, 296–299, 296t, 298t
  interstitial
    after bone marrow transplant,
        433–434
    desquamative, 265
    lymphoid, 299
    nonspecific, 265
    usual, 265
  radiation, 370, 371f
  toxic, 322
Pneumotachograph, 67
Pneumothorax, 458–459
  in cystic fibrosis, 202
  defined, 458
  with HIV infection, 436
  with mechanical ventilation, 554, 554f
  open, 606
  pathogenesis of, 458
  physical examination of, 64–65
  in pulmonary lymphangiomyomatosis,
      455–456
  respiratory failure due to, 540
  simple, 606

spontaneous, 458–459
  primary, 458–459
  secondary, 458, 459
  tension, 458, 459
    due to chest trauma, 606–607
    hyperinflation of chest in, 64
    with mechanical ventilation, 554, 554f
  due to transthoracic needle aspiration,
      363
  traumatic, 458, 606–607
PO_2. *See* Oxygen tension (PO_2)
Poiseuille's equation, 32
Poliomyelitis, respiratory failure with, 562t
Pollution, air, 340, 341–342, 341t
  and lung cancer, 349
Polyaromatic hydrocarbons (PAHs),
      carcinogenicity of, 337t, 339
Polymerase chain reaction (PCR) tests, of
      pleural fluid, 121
Polymer fume fever, 324
Polymorphonuclear cells (PMNs)
  in idiopathic pulmonary fibrosis, 269
  in sarcoidosis, 295
Polymyositis, due to lung cancer, 360
Polymyositis-dermatomyositis (PM-DM),
      276
Polyneuritis, due to lung cancer, 360
Polyps, nasal, 63
Polysomnography, 482–483
  in obstructive sleep apnea syndrome,
      486–487, 487f
POPC. *See* Postoperative pulmonary
      complications (POPC)
Pores of Kohn, 11, 40
Porto-pulmonary hypertension, 251
Positional apnea, 487
Positive airway pressure (PAP)
  biphasic, 544, 544f
  continuous. *See* Continuous positive
      airway pressure (CPAP)
  expiratory, for obstructive sleep apnea,
      491
  inspiratory, for obstructive sleep apnea,
      491
Positive-end-expiratory pressure (PEEP),
      549–550
  for ARDS, 587
  intrinsic (auto-), 550, 568, 572
  and wedge pressure, 625, 625t
Positive pressure ventilation, noninvasive,
      544–546, 544f, 545t
  for COPD, 568
  for status asthmaticus, 161
Positron emission tomography (PET), 88
  of lung cancer, 365, 367
Post-cardiac injury syndrome, 456
Posteroanterior (PA) chest radiograph, 69f,
      70
Postinfluenza pneumonia, 389, 389t
Postnasal drip, 7, 60
Postoperative period
  analgesia in, 593
  chest physiotherapy in, 595
  diaphragmatic function in, 594
  hypoxemia in, 594–595, 594t

Postoperative pulmonary complications (POPC), 594–595, 594t, 596–597, 597t
  atelectasis, 594–595
  with COPD, 597–598, 598t
  in elderly, 508–511, 509t, 511t, 597
  hypoxemia, 594–595, 594t
  after lung resection, 598–600, 598t–600t
  pneumonia, 596–597, 597t
Postoperative risk reduction strategies, 511t
Postpoliomyelitis, respiratory failure with, 562t
Posttransplant lymphoproliferative disorders (PTLDs), 223
PPD (purified protein derivative) test, 412, 446
PPH. *See* Primary pulmonary hypertension (PPH)
Ppl. *See* Pleural pressure (Ppl)
PPN (peripheral parenteral nutrition), 530
Praziquantel, for paragonimiasis, 449
Prealbumin, serum, 523, 523t
Prednisolone, for COPD, 189
Prednisone
  for acute pulmonary rejection, 219
  for allergic bronchopulmonary aspergillosis, 142–143
  for asthma, 148t, 160
  for BOOP, 271
  for Churg-Strauss syndrome, 282
  for cystic fibrosis, 201
  for idiopathic pulmonary fibrosis, 269–270
  for lung transplantation, 223, 224, 224t
  for *Pneumocystis carinii* pneumonia, 406, 436
  for sarcoidosis, 295
  for tuberculous pleuritis, 447
Pregnancy, pulmonary embolism in, 240
Premature ventricular contractions (PVCs), in obstructive sleep apnea syndrome, 490
Preoperative period
  pulmonary function testing in, 595
  smoking in, 595–596
Preoperative pulmonary evaluation, in elderly, 508–511, 509t, 511t
Preoperative risk reduction strategies, 511t
Pressure controlled (PC) ventilation, 549
Pressure-cycled ventilation, 549, 550t
Pressure-flow relationships, 34–38, 35f, 37f
Pressure-regulated-volume-controlled (PRVC) ventilation, 551
Pressure support (PS) ventilation, 544, 544f, 545, 549
  variable, 551
  for weaning, 551
Pressure-volume curve(s)
  factors influencing, 30–32, 30f, 31f
  normal, 29f
  static, 27, 28f
Primary effusion lymphoma, 451
Primary graft failure (PGF), after lung transplantation, 215, 216
Primary lobule, 8f, 9, 20, 21f

Primary pulmonary hypertension (PPH)
  clinical manifestations of, 250
  lung transplantation for, 209, 212t, 213, 251
  pathogenesis of, 248–249, 248t
  treatment of, 251
Procarbazine, pleural effusions due to, 455
Progressive disseminated histoplasmosis (PDH), 417, 418f
Progressive massive fibrosis (PMF)
  in coal workers' pneumoconiosis, 332, 332f
  in silicosis, 327
Progressive systemic sclerosis, 275–276
Prophylaxis
  for deep vein thrombosis, 241, 242t, 640–641
  with HIV infection, 438
  in immunocompromised patients, 434
  for influenza, 386
  for tuberculosis, 413
Propofol, and parenteral nutrition, 531
Prostacyclin (PGI₂)
  for primary pulmonary hypertension, 251
  vasoactive properties of, 17, 20
Prostaglandins
  in asthma, 137
  vasoactive properties of, 17, 20
Protease-antiprotease hypothesis, of COPD, 177–178
Protected specimen brushing (PSB), 124
Protective ventilation, 550
Protein(s)
  in pleural fluid, 119
  serum, for nutritional assessment, 523, 523t
  vasoactive, 19
Protein metabolism
  in nonstressed starvation, 520
  during stress, 519f, 521, 522f
Proteinosis, pulmonary alveolar, 285–287, 285f
Protein osmotic pressure, 577–578
  in pulmonary edema, 580
Protein requirements, 524–525, 524t
Protriptyline (Vivactil)
  for cataplexy, 485
  for obstructive sleep apnea, 491
Proventil (albuterol sulfate)
  for asthma, 135, 145, 146t, 150, 159, 572
  for COPD, 188t
Provera (medroxyprogesterone)
  for obstructive sleep apnea, 491
  for pulmonary lymphangiomyomatosis, 456
PRP (pulmonary reimplantation response), after lung transplantation, 215–216, 216f
PRSP (penicillin-resistant *Streptococcus pneumoniae*), 390, 392
PRVC (pressure-regulated-volume-controlled) ventilation, 551
PSB (protected specimen brushing), 124
P-selection, 15f

P-selection glycoprotein ligand (PSGL-1), 15f
Pseudallescheriasis, 425
Pseudochylothorax, 456–457
Pseudocyst, pancreatic, pleural effusions with, 453
Pseudomonas aeruginosa
  in cystic fibrosis, 199, 201
  in immunocompromised patients, 431
  after lung transplantation, 221
  nosocomial pneumonia due to, 403, 403f
Pseudomonas cepacia, in cystic fibrosis, 201
Pseudostratified columnar epithelial cells, functional anatomy of, 10, 11f
PSGL-1 (p-selection glycoprotein ligand), 15f
Psittacosis, 397, 398t
Pst(L) (elastic recoil pressure), 30
PS (pressure support) ventilation, 544, 544f, 545, 549
  variable, 551
  for weaning, 551
Psychosocial support, for COPD, 192
PTLDs (posttransplant lymphoproliferative disorders), 223
Ptm' (critical closing pressure of collapsible segment), 36, 37f
Ptm (transmural pressure of collapsible segment), 36, 37f
Pulmicort. *See* Budesonide (Pulmicort)
Pulmonary alveolar proteinosis, 285–287, 285f
Pulmonary angiography. *See* Angiography
Pulmonary arteries
  aneurysms of, 257
  in cor pulmonale, 252–253, 253f
  enlarged, 467f
  functional anatomy of, 13
  radiographic anatomy of, 69f, 70f, 74, 75f, 76f
Pulmonary arteriogram, 75f
Pulmonary artery (PA) catheterization, 621–627
  effect of PEEP on wedge pressure measurements in, 625
  indications for, 626–627
  infection related to, 644–647, 644t
  insertion techniques for, 621–622, 622f
  obtaining reliable pressure measurements with, 622–623, 623f, 624f
  relation of wedge pressure to left atrial pressure in, 623–625
  verifying catheter position in, 625, 625t
Pulmonary artery pressure
  in obstructive sleep apnea syndrome, 490
  with pulmonary embolism, 236
  and pulmonary vascular resistance, 15–16, 16f
Pulmonary artery wedge pressure, 577, 622f
  and left atrial pressure, 623–625
  obtaining reliable measurements of, 622–623, 623f, 624f
  PEEP effect on, 625, 625t
  in pulmonary edema, 587

Pulmonary aspiration, 393–395, 394f
Pulmonary capillaries
  alveolar, 16, 16f, 577f, 578
  distention of, 16, 17
  extra-alveolar, 16, 16f
  functional anatomy of, 12f, 12t, 13–14, 13f
  hydrostatic pressure gradient in, 16–17, 16f
  and pulmonary vascular resistance, 16, 16f
Pulmonary circulation
  distribution of blood in, 12–14, 13f, 14f, 14t, 16–17, 16f
  physiology of, 14–18, 15f, 16f, 18f
  radiographic anatomy of, 69f, 70f, 72–75, 75f, 76f
  regulation of, 17–18, 18f
Pulmonary complications, postoperative, 594–595, 594t, 596–597, 597t
  atelectasis in, 594–595
  with COPD, 597–598, 598t
  in elderly, 508–511, 509t, 511t, 597
  hypoxemia in, 594–595, 594t
  after lung resection, 598–600, 598t–600t
  pneumonia in, 596–597, 597t
Pulmonary edema, 576–587
  high-pressure cardiogenic, 579–581, 579f, 580f
  increased-permeability (noncardiogenic), 582–587, 582t, 583f–586f
  physiologic and structural basis for, 576–579, 577f, 577t, 578f
  pulmonary artery catheterization for, 626
Pulmonary embolism (PE), 233–247
  angiography of, 85, 239, 239t, 240
  arterial blood gases with, 237
  chest radiograph of, 238
  chronic thromboembolic pulmonary hypertension due to, 244–245
  clinical manifestations of, 236–238, 237t
  conditions predisposing to, 234t
  CT of, 82–83, 82f, 240
  differential diagnosis of, 241
  electrocardiogram in, 238
  hemodynamic consequences of, 235–236
  incidence of, 234, 234t
  lung scan of, 85, 86, 87f, 238–240, 239t, 240f
  pathogenesis of, 234–236
  pleural effusions with, 237, 237t, 452–453
  in pregnant patient, 240
  prevention of, 241–243, 242t, 640–641
  resolution of, 236
  respiratory consequences of, 235
  septic, 245
  in systemic lupus erythematosus, 274
  thoracentesis of, 238
  thrombin and plasmin byproducts in, 238
  treatment of, 243–244
  tumor, 257
  types of, 245–247, 245t

Pulmonary fibrosis, idiopathic. *See* Idiopathic pulmonary fibrosis (IPF)
Pulmonary function tests (PFTs), 91–100
  of airway hyperresponsiveness, 93–94
  of airway resistance, 96–97
  in asbestosis, 330
  in chronic thromboembolic pulmonary hypertension, 244
  in coal workers' pneumoconiosis, 332
  in COPD, 180
  in cystic fibrosis, 199
  of distribution of ventilation, 97–99, 98f
  for evaluation of disability, 113
  of expiratory flow rates, 91–93, 92f, 93f
  of gas transfer and exchange, 99–100, 99f
  in Goodpasture's syndrome, 283
  in hypersensitivity pneumonitis, 297
  in idiopathic pulmonary fibrosis, 267
  of lung compliance, 97, 97f
  after lung transplantation, 216, 218
  after lung volume reduction surgery, 226–227
  of lung volumes, 94–96, 94f–97f
  in occupational interstitial lung disease, 326
  preoperative, 510, 595
  in progressive systemic sclerosis, 275
  in pulmonary alveolar proteinosis, 286
  in respiratory failure, 542
  in sarcoidosis, 291
  use of, 109–114, 109t, 110t
Pulmonary heart disease. *See* Cor pulmonale
Pulmonary hypertension. *See* Hypertension, pulmonary
Pulmonary infarction, 236, 241
Pulmonary infiltrates, in systemic lupus erythematosus, 273
Pulmonary lobule, 20
Pulmonary lymphangiomyomatosis, 455–456
Pulmonary lymphatics, 22–23
Pulmonary nodules
  in lymphoid granulomatosis, 280, 280f
  in pulmonary alveolar proteinosis, 285
  solitary
    appropriate investigation of, 368, 368t
    benign causes of, 368, 368t
    bronchoscopy of, 123
    CT of, 83
    thoracoscopy of, 126
    in Wegener's granulomatosis, 278, 278f
Pulmonary rehabilitation, for COPD, 190–193, 190t, 191t
Pulmonary reimplantation response (PRP), after lung transplantation, 215–216, 216f
Pulmonary vascular bed, neoplasia of, 257
Pulmonary vascular disease
  acquired, 257
  congenital, 255–257, 255t, 256f
  lung transplantation for, 209
Pulmonary vascular pressures, 14–15, 15f
Pulmonary vascular resistance (PVR), 15–16, 15f, 16f

alveolar oxygen tension and, 18, 18f
alveolar pressure and, 16, 16f
lung volume and, 16, 16f
normal values for, 543t
preoperative, 599
pulmonary artery or venous pressure and, 15–16, 16f
with pulmonary embolism, 236
Pulmonary vascular system. *See* Pulmonary circulation
Pulmonary veins
  functional anatomy of, 13
  radiographic anatomy of, 69f, 70f, 74, 75f, 76f
Pulmonary veno-occlusive disease, 250
Pulmonary venous pressure, and pulmonary vascular resistance, 15–16, 16f
Pulse oximetry, 556–557
Pulsus paradoxus, in asthma, 139
Purified protein derivative (PPD) test, 412, 446
Pursed-lip breathing, for COPD, 192
$PVCO_2$ (venous carbon dioxide tension), 543t
PVCs (premature ventricular contractions), in obstructive sleep apnea syndrome, 490
PVO_2 (venous oxygen tension)
  arterial hypoxemia due to low mixed, 53
  normal value for, 543t
PVR. *See* Pulmonary vascular resistance (PVR)
Pyothorax-associated lymphoma, 451–452
Pyrazinamide (PZA), for tuberculosis, 413, 436

Q
$\dot{Q}$. *See* Cardiac output ($\dot{Q}$)
Q fever, 398t
$\dot{Q}s/\dot{Q}t$ (shunt fraction), 50, 543t
$\dot{Q}t$, 543t
Quality assurance, in intensive care unit, 518
Quality end-of-life care, 507–508, 535
Quibron. *See* Theophylline (Slo-Phylline, Theolair, Quibron, Elixophyllin, Theo-24, Uniphyl)
Qvar (beclomethasone dipropionate)
  for asthma, 147t, 154
  pharmacokinetics of, 154t, 155t

R
Radiation pneumonitis, 370, 371f
Radiation therapy, for lung cancer, 369, 370f
Radioactive materials, and lung cancer, 349, 349f
Radioactive xenon distribution, 98–99
Radiography, chest. *See* Chest radiography
Radionuclide ventriculography, of cor pulmonale, 253
Radon, carcinogenicity of, 337t, 339–340
RADS (reactive airways dysfunction syndrome), 320–321
Rales, 65
  in idiopathic pulmonary fibrosis, 266

RAO (right anterior oblique) view, 76
Rapid eye movement (REM) latency, 480
Rapid eye movement (REM) sleep, 478,
    479f, 480, 481–482, 481f
  phasic *vs.* tonic, 481–482
  sleep-onset, 480, 484
Rapid Shallow Breathing Index (RSBI),
    506f, 552
Rasmussen's aneurysm, 411
Raw. *See* Airway resistance (Raw)
RB (respiratory bronchiolitis), 271–272
RDI (respiratory disturbance index), 482
RE (Reynolds number), 33
Reactive airways dysfunction syndrome
    (RADS), 320–321
Rebreathing method, for diffusing capacity,
    100
Recoil pressure, 30
Rectus abdominis muscle, 5f
Reid index, 10, 174
Reimplantation injury, with lung
    transplantation, 215
Rejection, after lung transplantation,
    218–219, 219f, 219t
Relaxation, volume-pressure relations
    during, 26–27, 27f, 28f
REM (rapid eye movement) latency, 480
REM (rapid eye movement) sleep, 478,
    479f, 480, 481–482, 481f
  phasic *vs.* tonic, 481–482
  sleep-onset, 480, 484
Renal failure, in multiple organ failure, 629
Renal tuberculosis, 411
RERAs (respiratory-effort-related arousals),
    489, 489f
Residual volume (RV), 26, 27f, 28, 92, 94f
  in emphysema, 180
Resorcinols, for asthma, 145
Respiration
  mechanics of, 26–42
  paradoxical, 6
Respiratory alkalosis, in respiratory failure,
    542
Respiratory alternans, 6
Respiratory arousal index, 489
Respiratory bronchiolitis (RB), 271–272
Respiratory disease(s)
  office and home testing for, 66–67
  symptoms of, 60–63, 63t
Respiratory distress syndrome
  acute (adult). *See* Acute respiratory
      distress syndrome (ARDS)
  infant, surfactant in, 31–32
Respiratory disturbance index (RDI), 482
Respiratory effort, monitoring of, 483
Respiratory-effort-related arousals (RERAs),
    489, 489f
Respiratory exchange ratio ($\dot{V}CO_2/\dot{V}O_2$),
    45, 543t
Respiratory failure
  acid-base abnormalities in, 541–542
  airway management for, 546–548, 546t,
      547f
  arterial blood gases in, 540–541, 541f,
      542f
  assessment of, 539–543

in asthma, 570–573, 570t, 572t
calculation of respiratory variables in,
    542–543, 543t
due to chest wall abnormalities, 562t,
    564
clinical manifestations of, 539–540
due to COPD, 565–570, 566f, 567f
in critically ill patients, 630–631, 631t
due to drug overdoses, 563–564
hypercapnic, 541, 542f, 561–573
hypoxemic, 541, 541f, 576–587
laboratory evaluation of, 540
lung function measurement in, 542
mechanical ventilation for, 548–555
  airway pressure release, 551
  emergencies with, 553–555, 554f
  features of ventilators for, 548
  high-frequency oscillatory, 551
  indications for, 546t, 548
  modes of, 548–549, 549f, 551
  PEEP with, 549–550
  pressure-cycled, 549
  pressure-regulated-volume-controlled,
      551
  pressure support, 549
  strategies for, 550, 550t
  variable pressure-support and volume-
      support, 551
  volume-cycled, 548–549, 549f
  weaning from, 551–553, 552t
monitoring of, 555–557, 556f
in multiple organ failure, 630–631, 631t
neuromuscular etiologies of, 561–563,
    562t
noninvasive ventilation for, 544–546,
    544f, 545t
supplemental oxygen for, 543–544
treatment of, 543–557
due to upper airway obstruction,
    564–565
Respiratory history, 59–60
Respiratory inductance plethysmography
    (RIP), 483, 555
Respiratory infections. *See* Infection(s)
Respiratory monitoring, 555–557, 556f
Respiratory mucosa, metabolic and
    secretory functions of, 11–12,
    12f
Respiratory muscle(s)
  fatigue of, 4, 6
  functional anatomy of, 4–6, 5f
  weakness of, 4
Respiratory muscle function, 6, 555, 556f
Respiratory quotient (RQ), 524
Respiratory rate
  in critically ill patient, 555
  with mechanical ventilation, 555
  normal value for, 543t
Respiratory rate to tidal volume ratio (f/
    VT), 6
Respiratory syncytial virus (RSV)
  in immunocompromised host, 433
  pneumonia due to, 400t
Respiratory system
  dimensions of, 26, 27f
  dynamics of, 32–42, 32f, 34f, 35f, 37f,
      38f, 40f–42f

functional anatomy of, 3–23, 4t
  as alveolar-capillary barrier, 14, 15f
  for distribution of air, 7–11, 8f–11f
  for distribution of blood, 12–14, 13f,
      14f, 14t
  as gas exchange area, 20, 21f
  for lung clearance and defenses,
      21–23, 21f
  metabolic, nonrespiratory functions of
      lung in, 18–20, 19f, 19t, 20f
  metabolic and secretory functions of
      respiratory mucosa in, 11–12,
      12f
  physiology of pulmonary circulation
      in, 14–18, 15f, 16f, 18f
  as ventilatory pump, 3–7, 4f, 5f
in oxygen delivery, 54–55
pressure-volume curve for, 27, 28f
resting volume of, 27
volume-pressure relations of
  during muscular efforts, 27–32, 28f,
      31f
  during relaxation, 26–27, 27f, 28f
Respiratory tract
  bacteriology of, 379–381, 380t
  lower, functional anatomy of, 8f–11f,
      9–11
  particle deposition in, 21
  upper, functional anatomy of, 7–9, 8f
Respiratory tract infections. *See* Infection(s)
Respiratory unit
  terminal, 8f, 9, 20, 21f
  time constant of, 39–40, 40f
Respiratory variables, calculation of,
    542–543, 543t
Resting hypoxia, in emphysema, 180
Resting vascular tone, 17
Resting volumes, 27
Restless leg syndrome (RLS), 485, 486
Restrictive ventilatory dysfunction
  exercise testing with, 112
  pulmonary function testing with,
      109–110, 110t
Retinol-binding protein, serum, 523, 523t
Retrosternal space, in emphysema, 180t
Reynolds number *(Re)*, 33
Rheumatoid arthritis, 274–275, 274t
Rheumatoid pleuritis, 452
Rheumatoid pneumoconiosis, 274–275
Rhinitis, allergic, 60, 63
Rhinorrhea, 60
Rhinovirus, common cold due to, 381
Rhonchi, 65–66
Rib belts, 604–605
Rib fractures, 471–472, 601, 603–605,
    604f
  pain of, 61, 472
Rifampin (RIF)
  for *Legionella* pneumonia, 393
  for tuberculosis, 413, 436–437
Right anterior oblique (RAO) view, 76
Right heart failure, in COPD, 179
Right outer canthus (ROC) electrode, 478,
    479f
Right-to-left shunt
  arterial hypoxemia due to, 52–53

in respiratory failure, 541, 541f
venous admixture due to, 49
Right ventricle, functional anatomy of, 12–13, 13f
Right ventricular work, with pulmonary embolism, 236
RIP (respiratory inductance plethysmography), 483, 555
Ritalin (methylphenidate), for narcolepsy, 485
RLS (restless leg syndrome), 485, 486
ROC (right outer canthus) electrode, 478, 479f
Rounded atelectasis, asbestos-related, 329
RQ (respiratory quotient), 524
RSBI (Rapid Shallow Breathing Index), 506f, 552
RSV (respiratory syncytial virus)
in immunocompromised host, 433
pneumonia due to, 400t
RV (residual volume), 26, 27f, 28, 92, 94f
in emphysema, 180

S

Saber sheath trachea, in emphysema, 180
Saligenins, for asthma, 145
Salivary-gland-type tumors, 356
Salmeterol/fluticasone (Advair), for asthma, 147t
Salmeterol xinafoate (Serevent)
for asthma, 145, 147t, 149
nocturnal, 497
for COPD, 188t
with central sleep apnea, 498
SaO2. *See* Arterial oxygen saturation (SaO2)
Sarcoidosis, 290–296
clinical presentation of, 290, 290t
course of, 295–296
immunologic concepts in, 293–295
laboratory findings in, 291–293, 292t, 293t, 294f
mediastinal, 465f
pleural effusions in, 456
radiographic findings in, 290–291, 291f
symptoms of, 63–64
therapy for, 295–296
Sarcoma, 357
of pulmonary arteries, 257
Sawtooth waves, 480, 481f
SBS (sick building syndrome), 296, 342
Scalenus muscle, during inspiration, 4, 5f
Scapular fractures, 601
Scleroderma, 275–276
with silicosis, 328
Sclerosing hemangioma, 356
Sclerotherapy, endoscopic variceal, pleural effusions after, 454
Scoliosis, 470–471, 470f
respiratory failure with, 562t, 564
Screening, for lung cancer, 361
Scrofula, 411
Secretory immunoglobulin A, in intestine, 526
Sedative hypnotics, overdoses of, respiratory failure due to, 563

Selective serotonin reuptake inhibitors (SSRIs), for obstructive sleep apnea, 491
Sensitizing agents, in occupational asthma, 317–319, 318t, 320, 321
Sensory neuropathy, due to lung cancer, 360
Sepsis, acute lung injury and ARDS due to, 583f, 585–586, 585f, 586f
Sepsis syndrome, in multiple organ failure, 628
Septic shock, 627t
cardiovascular failure in, 629
hepatic failure in, 630
management of, 634–635
multiple organ failure in, 631–632, 633, 634
Septic thromboembolism, 245
Sequoiosis, 296t
Serevent. *See* Salmeterol xinafoate (Serevent)
Serotonin, vasoactive properties of, 17, 19
Serous cells, functional anatomy of, 10
Serratus anterior muscle, 4, 5f
Serum proteins, for nutritional assessment, 523, 523t
Sevoflurane, with asthma, 593
SGA (subjective global assessment), 522
SGaw (specific airway conductance), 33
"Shaggy heart," in asbestosis, 330, 330f
Shaver's disease, 335
Shock
cardiogenic, 627t
defined, 627
hypovolemic, 627t
physiologic basis for, 627–628, 627t
pulmonary artery catheterization for, 626
septic, 627t
cardiovascular failure in, 629
hepatic failure in, 630
management of, 634–635
multiple organ failure in, 631–632, 633, 634
Shunt(s)
arteriovenous, 256–257
pleuroperitoneal, for malignant pleural effusions, 451
right-to-left
arterial hypoxemia due to, 52–53
in respiratory failure, 541, 541f
venous admixture due to, 49
Shunt equation, 50
Shunt fraction (Qs/Qt), 50, 543t
Shuttle walk, 108
SIADH (syndrome of inappropriate antidiuretic hormone secretion), due to lung cancer, 359–360
Sick building syndrome (SBS), 296, 342
Sidestream smoke (SS), 340, 343, 348
Signet-ring appearance, 81f
Silica, 326
carcinogenicity of, 337t, 339, 350
Silicates, 326
Silicon dioxide, 326
Silicosis, 326–328, 327f, 328f
Silicotuberculosis, 328

Silo filler's disease, 60
Silver-coated catheters
urinary, 649
vascular, 645–646
Single-breath carbon monoxide test, 99–100, 99f
Single-breath nitrogen elimination test, 98, 98f
Single lung transplantation (SLT). *See also* Lung transplantation (LT)
for idiopathic pulmonary fibrosis, 270–271
indications for, 209
surgical technique for, 214
Singulair (montelukast), for asthma, 147t, 157–158
Sinus(es), paranasal, functional anatomy of, 7
Sinus arrhythmia, in obstructive sleep apnea syndrome, 490
Sinusitis, 63, 380t, 381–382
Sinus radiographs, 382
Skeletal manifestations, of lung cancer, 361
Skinfold measurements, 522–523
Skin test, for tuberculosis, 412–413
Skin test anergy, in sarcoidosis, 292, 292t
SLE (systemic lupus erythematosus), 272–274, 272f, 272t, 273f
pleural effusions with, 452
Sleep
architecture of, 478–481, 479f–481f
and asthma, 496–497
and chronic obstructive pulmonary disease, 497–498
deep (slow-wave), 478
insufficient, 485
light, 478
monitoring of, 478–481, 479f–481f, 482–483, 483t
non-rapid eye movement, 478, 480, 481, 482
rapid eye movement, 478, 479f, 480, 481–482, 481f
phasic *vs.* tonic, 481–482
sleep-onset, 484
ventilation and, 481–482
Sleep apnea, 486–496
central, 493–496
with Cheyne-Stokes breathing, 493t, 494, 494t, 495–496, 496f
in congestive heart failure, 493t, 494, 494t, 495–496, 496f
defined, 482, 482f, 486, 493
hypercapnic, 493–494, 493t
idiopathic, 494–495, 494f
nonhypercapnic, 493t, 494, 494f
mixed, 482, 482f, 496, 496f
obstructive, 486–493
apnea termination and arousal in, 488
automobile accidents with, 493
cardiovascular consequences of, 489–490
clinical manifestations of, 486
and daytime hypercapnia, 489
defined, 482, 482f

Sleep apnea (*contd.*)
impaired sleep and daytime sleepiness
in, 488–489
incidence of, 486
obesity hyperventilation syndrome in,
489
overlap syndrome in, 489, 497, 498
pathophysiology of, 487–488
polysomnography in, 486–487, 487f
predisposing conditions for, 486
prognosis and mortality with, 493
treatment of, 490–493, 492f, 492t
upper airway resistance syndrome in,
489, 489f
positional, 487
Sleep attacks, 484
Sleep cycles, 480
Sleep disorders, 484–498, 484t
Cheyne-Stokes breathing, 494, 494f, 495
with congestive heart failure, 495–496,
496f
definitions used in, 482
idiopathic hypersomnia, 485
insufficient sleep syndrome, 485
International Classification of, 484
narcolepsy, 484–485
periodic limb movement disorder, 483,
485–486
sleep apnea syndromes. *See* Sleep apnea
Sleep efficiency, 480
Sleep fragmentation, 488–489
Sleep latency, 480
Sleep latency test, multiple, 483, 483t
in obstructive sleep apnea syndrome, 488
Sleep-onset REM (SOREM), 480, 484
Sleep paralysis, 484
Sleep period time (SPT), 480
Sleep spindles, 480, 480f
Sleep time, total, 480
Slo-Phylline. *See* Theophylline (Slo-
Phylline, Theolair, Quibron,
Elixophyllin, Theo-24, Uniphyl)
Slow eye movements, 478–480, 479f, 480f
Slow-wave sleep, 478
SLT. *See* Single lung transplantation (SLT)
Small cell carcinoma, 352–353, 353f, 354t
Smoke, environmental tobacco
(sidestream), 340, 342, 348
Smoke inhalation, 324, 324t
Smokers
He-O$_2$ flow-volume loops for, 38f, 39
sputum in, 62
Smoker's cough, 62
Smoking
and asbestosis, 330–331
and asbestos-related lung cancer, 338,
350
and COPD, 176
and eosinophilic granuloma, 302
and FEV$_1$, 182–183, 183f, 184, 184f
history of, 60
and lung cancer, 346, 347–348, 348f
and occupational bronchitis, 336
passive, 340, 342, 348
and pneumothorax, 458
in preoperative period, 595–596

and radon-related lung cancer, 339
and respiratory bronchiolitis, 271–272
and work capacity, 103
Smoking cessation
for COPD, 182–183, 183f, 184–185,
184f, 184t
for eosinophilic granuloma, 302, 302f
and lung cancer, 348
prior to surgery, 596
Sneezing, 60
Sniff test, 77, 472–473
Sodium nitroprusside, for pulmonary
edema, 581
Sodium transport
in pulmonary edema, 581
through respiratory epithelium, 12, 12f
Solitary pulmonary nodule (SPN)
appropriate investigation of, 368, 368t
benign causes of, 368, 368t
bronchoscopy of, 123
CT of, 83
thoracoscopy of, 126
Solu-Cortef (hydrocortisone sodium
succinate), for asthma, 148t, 160
Solu-Medrol. *See* Methylprednisolone
sodium succinate (Medrol, Solu-
Medrol)
Somnoplasty, for obstructive sleep apnea,
490
SOREM (sleep-onset REM), 480, 484
Spalling effect, in pulmonary contusion,
608
Specific airway conductance (SGaw), 33
Spinal cord injury, respiratory failure with,
561, 562t
Spirometry, 91–92, 92f
forced expiratory, 35, 91–92, 92f
after lung transplantation, 216
postoperative incentive, 595
preoperative, 595
simple, 91–92, 92f
uses of, 109
volume determination by, 94, 94f
Splenectomy, pneumonia with, 389, 389t,
403, 404t
SPN. *See* Solitary pulmonary nodule (SPN)
Spondylitis, ankylosing, 471
respiratory failure with, 562t, 564
Spontaneous breathing trial, 551
Sporotrichosis, 422
Spring-water cysts, 466
SPT (sleep period time), 480
Sputum
in bronchiectasis, 197
"chocolate sauce," 448
in chronic bronchitis, 174, 179
in COPD, 62, 177, 566
in cystic fibrosis, 199
expectoration of, 62–63
in HIV infection, 435
in idiopathic pulmonary fibrosis, 265
in immunocompromised patients, 432
induction of, 62–63
in lung cancer, 361, 362
in pneumonia, 407
Pneumocystis carinii, 435
in tuberculosis, 412

Squamous cell carcinoma, 351–352, 352f,
353f
MRI of, 84f
SS (sidestream smoke), 340, 343, 348
SSRIs (selective serotonin reuptake
inhibitors), for obstructive sleep
apnea, 491
Staging, of lung cancer, 363–367
bronchoscopy for, 123–124, 365
classification system for, 363–364, 363t,
364t
lymph node biopsy for, 365
mediastinoscopy and mediastinotomy
for, 365–367, 366f, 367f
needle aspiration biopsy for, 365
thoracic imaging for, 364–365
thoracotomy for, 367
Staphylococcus aureus, 399, 399f
in cystic fibrosis, 201
Staphylococcus spp, after lung
transplantation, 221
Starling equation, 576–577, 577t
Starvation, nonstressed, 519–520, 519f,
519t
Status asthmaticus, 158–162
respiratory failure in, 570–573, 570t,
572t
Steady-state method, for diffusing capacity,
100
Steatosis, due to parenteral nutrition, 532
Sternal fractures, 601, 603, 604f
Sternocleidomastoid muscle, during
inspiration, 4, 5f
Steroid(s). *See* Corticosteroids
Steroid-dependent asthma, 162–163
Stramonium, for asthma, 152
Streptococcal pharyngitis, 383
Streptococcus pneumoniae, 391–392, 392f
penicillin-resistant, 390, 392
Streptokinase
for deep venous thrombosis, 243
for loculated pleural fluid, 445–446
for pulmonary embolism, 244
Stress
fat metabolism during, 519f, 521
glucose metabolism during, 519f–521f,
520–521
hypermetabolic hypercatabolic response
to, 519, 519f, 519t
protein metabolism during, 519f, 521,
522f
Stress-related gastrointestinal bleeding,
641–644, 642t, 643f
Strictures, bronchial, after lung
transplantation, 217–218
Strongyloides stercoralis
eosinophilia due to, 299
in immunocompromised host, 431, 433
Study to Understand Prognoses and
Preference for Outcomes and
Risks of Treatment (SUPPORT),
503, 508, 535
Subcarinal nodes, 23
Suberosis, 296t
Subjective global assessment (SGA), 522
Substance abuse, and lung transplantation,
211

Sucralfate, for stress-related gastrointestinal ulceration, 642–643, 642t, 643f

Sulfur dioxide, inhalation injury due to, 323, 323t

Sulfur oxides, air pollution due to, 341, 341t

Summer type hypersensitivity, 296t

Superior vena caval syndrome, in lung cancer, 358

Supplemental oxygen. *See* Oxygen therapy

SUPPORT (Study to Understand Prognoses and Preference for Outcomes and Risks of Treatment), 503, 508, 535

Surface tension *(T),* 31

Surfactant
composition of, 31
functions of, 31–32
in mucociliary escalator, 21
production of, 11
properties of, 11, 31
and pulmonary edema, 578–579
with pulmonary embolism, 235
and surface tension, 31–32, 31f

Surfactant proteins, 11

Surgery
analgesia after, 593
anesthesia for, 592–593
with angina pectoris, 600
aspiration of gastric contents during, 596
with asthma, 598
with COPD, 597–598, 598t
in elderly, 597
after myocardial infarction, 600
pneumonia after, 596–597, 597t
pulmonary artery catheterization after, 626–637
pulmonary complications after, 594–595, 594t
pulmonary function testing prior to, 595
smoking prior to, 595–596

Surgical incision site, and diaphragmatic function, 594

Surrogate, for medical decision-making, 533

$S\bar{V}O_2$ (mixed venous saturation), 53
exercise and, 106
and work capacity, 103–104, 104t

SVR, 543t

Sweat chloride test, 199–200

Symptoms, of respiratory diseases, 60–63, 63t

Synchronized intermittent mandatory ventilation, 548–549, 549f

Syncope, in pulmonary hypertension, 250

Syndrome of inappropriate antidiuretic hormone secretion (SIADH), due to lung cancer, 359–360

Systemic arterial catheterization, 620–621

Systemic lupus erythematosus (SLE), 272–274, 272f, 272t, 273f
pleural effusions with, 452

T

T (surface tension), 31

Tachycardia, with pulmonary embolism, 237, 237t

Tachypnea
in idiopathic pulmonary fibrosis, 266
with pulmonary embolism, 237, 237t

Tacrolimus
for bronchiolitis obliterans, 220
for lung transplantation, 215, 223, 224, 224t, 225

Talcosis, 334

TB. *See* Tuberculosis (TB)

TBB (transbronchial biopsy), 121
after lung transplantation, 218, 219f, 220, 220f
for Wegener's granulomatosis, 279

TBNA (transbronchial needle aspiration), 122
for lung cancer, 362–363

T cells. *See* T lymphocytes

TEE (transesophageal echocardiography), 602

Telangiectasia, hereditary hemorrhagic, 255–256

Tension pneumothorax, 458, 459
due to chest trauma, 606–607
hyperinflation of chest in, 64
with mechanical ventilation, 554, 554f

Teratomas, of mediastinum, 463–464

Terbutaline sulfate (Brethaire, Bricanyl)
for asthma, 145, 147t, 153–154, 159, 572
for COPD, 188t, 189
for cor pulmonale, 254

Terminal respiratory unit (TRU), 8f, 9, 20, 21f

Testing, for respiratory disease, 66–67

Tetracycline
for chlamydial pneumonia, 397
for pneumothorax, 459

Textile dust-related disease, 321–322

Theophylline (Slo-Phylline, Theolair, Quibron, Elixophyllin, Theo-24, Uniphyl)
for asthma, 148t, 150–152, 151t, 159, 573
nocturnal, 497
for COPD, 188, 188t, 194, 569
with central sleep apnea, 498
for cor pulmonale, 254
factors that alter metabolism of, 188t

Thoracentesis, 117–118, 118t
for parapneumonic effusions, 445
for pleural effusions, 444
of pulmonary embolism, 238

Thoracic gas volume (V_{TG}), 95–96, 97f

Thoracic spine disease, mediastinal masses due to, 468

Thoracic trauma. *See* Chest trauma

Thoracoplasty, respiratory failure with, 562t, 564

Thoracoscopic surgery, video assisted, 125–127, 594

Thoracoscopy, 125–127
for chest trauma, 602–603
for loculated pleural effusions, 446
for malignant mesothelioma, 451
for pneumothorax, 459

Thoracostomy
for chest trauma, 602, 602t

for hemothorax, 607
for malignant mesothelioma, 451

Thoracotomy
for chest trauma, 603, 603t
for lung cancer, 367
for parapneumonic effusions, 446
for pneumothorax, 459

Thorax, functional anatomy of, 4, 4f

Throat, examination of, 63

Thrombin byproducts, with pulmonary embolism, 238

Thrombocytopenia, heparin-induced, 641

Thromboembolic pulmonary hypertension, chronic, 244–245

Thromboembolism
pulmonary. *See* Pulmonary embolism (PE)
septic, 245
venous, in critically ill patients, 639–641, 640t

Thrombolytic therapy
for deep venous thrombosis, 243
for loculated pleural fluid, 445–446
for pulmonary embolism, 244

Thrombophlebitis, with lung cancer, 361

Thrombosis(es)
deep venous. *See* Deep venous thrombosis (DVT)
pulmonary hypertension due to, 249
from systemic arterial catheterization, 621

Thrombus, CT of, 82–83, 82f

Thrush, 63

Thymoma, of mediastinum, 461–462, 463f

Thyroid masses, intrathoracic, 464, 464f

Thyroxine-binding prealbumin, serum, 523, 523t

TIB (time in bed), 480

Tidal flow, 4

Tidal volume (V_T), 26, 27f, 94, 94f, 543t
respiratory rate to, 6

Tietze's syndrome, 61

Tight junctions, functional anatomy of, 10

Tilade (nedocromil sodium), for asthma, 147t, 156

Time constant, of respiratory unit, 39–40, 40f

Time in bed (TIB), 480

Tissue interdependence, 40

Tissue plasminogen activator
for deep venous thrombosis, 243
for pulmonary embolism, 244

Tissue tropism, 380

TLC (total lung capacity), 26, 27f, 28, 94f
with restrictive ventilatory dysfunction, 109–110, 110t

T lymphocytes
in asthma, 136–137
defective
causes of, 430t
pneumonia with, 403, 404t
in hypersensitivity pneumonitis, 298, 298t
in sarcoidosis, 292–295, 293t, 294f

TMP/SMX (trimethoprim/
  sulfamethoxazole)
  for *Pneumocystis carinii* pneumonia, 406,
    435–436, 438
  for Wegener's granulomatosis, 279
TNF (tumor necrosis factor), in septic
  shock, 633
TNM (tumor-node-metastasis)
  classification, 363–364, 363t,
  364t
Tobacco smoke, environmental, 340, 342
Tobacco smoking. *See* Smoking
Tofranil (imipramine), for cataplexy, 485
Tomogram, 78
Tomography, 78–83
  computed. *See* Computed tomography
    (CT)
  conventional, 78, 79f
  indications for, 78
  of lung cancer, 364
  positron emission, 88
    of lung cancer, 365, 367
T1-weighted images, 83
Tongue retaining devices (TRDs), for
  obstructive sleep apnea, 492,
  492f
Tonic activity, 487
Tonic REM sleep, 481–482
Tornalate (bitolterol mesylate)
  for asthma, 146t
  for COPD, 188t
Total lung capacity (TLC), 26, 27f, 28, 94f
  with restrictive ventilatory dysfunction,
    109–110, 110t
Total parenteral nutrition (TPN),
    530–532, 531t
Total sleep time (TST), 480
Toxic lung injury, 322
Toxic pneumonitis, 322
Toxocara canis, eosinophilia due to, 299
TPE (tropical pulmonary eosinophilia), 300
T-piece weaning, 551–552
  in COPD, 568–569
TPN (total parenteral nutrition), 530–532,
    531t
Trace elements, in parenteral nutrition,
    531–532, 531t
Trachea
  examination of, 64
  functional anatomy of, 8f, 9
  radiographic anatomy of, 69f, 70f,
    71–72
  saber sheath, 180
Tracheal intubation. *See* Endotracheal
    intubation
Tracheal traction, 488
Tracheobronchial toilet, for pneumonia,
    409
Tracheobronchial tree
  bacteriology of, 380–381, 380t
  traumatic disruption of, 612–613, 613t
Tracheobronchitis, febrile, 385
Tracheoesophageal fistula, 555, 613
Tracheostomy
  with endotracheal intubation, 547
  for obstructive sleep apnea, 490
  percutaneous dilational, 547
Training, 106–107, 107f

Tramlines, in chronic bronchitis, 181, 182f
Transbronchial biopsy (TBB), 121
  after lung transplantation, 218, 219f,
    220, 220f
  for Wegener's granulomatosis, 279
Transbronchial needle aspiration (TBNA),
    122
  for lung cancer, 362–363
Transdiaphragmatic pressure, 473
Transesophageal echocardiography (TEE),
    602
Transferrin, serum, 523, 523t
Transforming growth factor-β, in
    idiopathic pulmonary fibrosis,
    269
Transillumination, of sinuses, 382
Transitional flow, 32f, 33
Transmural pressure of collapsible segment
    (Ptm), 36, 37f
Transplantation. *See* Lung transplantation
    (LT)
"Transplant window," 211
Transpulmonary pressure (PL), 26, 27f, 97,
    97f
Transpyloric feedings, 528
Transthoracic needle aspiration (TTNA),
    125
  in immunocompromised patient, 432
  in lung cancer, 362–363
Transthyretin, serum, 523, 523t
Transudates, in pleural fluid, 119
Transvascular fluid flow, 577, 577t
Transversus abdominis muscle, 5f
Trapped lung, 456
Trauma, chest. *See* Chest trauma
TRDs (tongue retaining devices), for
    obstructive sleep apnea, 492,
    492f
Trial of spontaneous ventilation, 551
Triamcinolone acetonide (Azmacort)
  for asthma, 147t
  pharmacokinetics of, 154t, 155t
Triazolam, for COPD, 498
Tricyclic antidepressants, respiratory failure
    due to, 563
Triglycerides, in pleural fluid, 457
Trimethoprim/sulfamethoxazole (TMP/
    SMX)
  for *Pneumocystis carinii* pneumonia, 406,
    435–436, 438
  for Wegener's granulomatosis, 279
Triphosphate nucleotides, for cystic
    fibrosis, 200
Tripod sign, in COPD, 179
Troleandomycin, for asthma, 163
Tropical pulmonary eosinophilia (TPE),
    300
Trousseau's syndrome, 235
TRU (terminal respiratory unit), 8f, 9, 20,
    21f
TST (total sleep time), 480
TTNA (transthoracic needle aspiration),
    125
  in immunocompromised patient, 432
  in lung cancer, 362–363
T2-weighted images, 83
Tube feedings, 518–519, 527–530, 528t
Tuberculin test, 412–413

Tuberculoma, 412
Tuberculosis (TB), 409–414, 411f
  with AIDS, 409, 410, 412, 436–437,
    438
  cervical lymph node, 411
  clinical features of, 410–412
  diagnosis of, 412–413
  epidemiology of, 378, 409
  extrapulmonary disease in, 411–412
  genital, 411
  hemoptysis in, 63, 63t, 410–411
  miliary, 412
  multidrug-resistant, 409, 413–414
    with HIV infection, 437
  mycobacteria other than, 414–415, 414f
  pathogenesis of, 409–410, 411f
  pleural effusions in, 411, 446–447
  pleural fluid tests for, 120–121
  pneumothorax due to, 459
  primary, 410
  progressive, 410, 411f
  reactivation, 410, 411f
  renal, 411
  risk factors for, 409
  with silicosis, 327–328
  sputum in, 62
  treatment of, 413–414
Tuberculous meningitis, 411
Tuberculous peritonitis, 411
Tube thoracostomy
  for chest trauma, 602, 602t
  for hemothorax, 607
Tularemia, 398t
Tumor(s). *See* Lung cancer; Neoplasms
Tumor emboli, 257
Tumor markers, in pleural fluid, 120
Tumor necrosis factor (TNF), in septic
    shock, 633
Tumor-node-metastasis (TNM)
    classification, 363–364, 363t,
    364t
Turbinates, 7
Turbulent flow, 32f, 33
TWAR agent, 397, 398t

U
UAO. *See* Upper airway obstruction
    (UAO)
UARS (upper airway resistance syndrome),
    489, 489f
UIP (usual interstitial pneumonitis), 265
Ulceration, stress-related gastrointestinal,
    641–644, 642t, 643f
Ultrasonography, 84
  bronchoscopic (endobronchial), 122
  of chest trauma, 602
Undifferentiated carcinoma, 354, 355f
Uniphyl. *See* Theophylline (Slo-Phylline,
    Theolair, Quibron, Elixophyllin,
    Theo-24, Uniphyl)
Upper airway obstruction (UAO)
  vs. asthma, 138–139, 138f
  pathophysiology of, 487–488
  pulmonary function testing in, 110–111
  respiratory failure due to, 564–565
Upper airway resistance syndrome (UARS),
    489, 489f

Upper respiratory tract, functional anatomy of, 7–9, 8f

Upper respiratory tract infections, 379–380, 380t, 381–384

Upper respiratory tract irritation, due to environmental exposure, 316

Upper respiratory tract symptoms, 60

UPPP (uvulopalatopharyngoplasty), for obstructive sleep apnea, 490

Uranium exposure, and lung cancer, 349, 349f

Uremic pleuritis, 456

Uridine triphosphate, for cystic fibrosis, 200

Urinary catheter-related infection, 647–649, 647t

Urinary tract infection (UTI), catheter-related, 647–649, 647t

Urinary tract obstruction, pleural effusions due to, 456

Urokinase
for deep venous thrombosis, 243
for loculated pleural fluid, 445–446
for pulmonary embolism, 244

Usual interstitial pneumonitis (UIP), 265

UTI (urinary tract infection), catheter-related, 647–649, 647t

Uvulopalatopharyngoplasty (UPPP), for obstructive sleep apnea, 490

V

$\dot{V}A$. *See* Alveolar ventilation $(\dot{V}A)$

Vaccine
influenza, for COPD prevention, 185–186
pneumococcal, 392
for COPD prevention, 185–186
with HIV infection, 438

Valley fever, 420

Vanadium, inhalation injury due to, 323t

Vanceril (beclomethasone dipropionate)
for asthma, 147t, 154
pharmacokinetics of, 154t, 155t

Vanishing lung syndrome, in systemic lupus erythematosus, 272

Variable pressure-support and volume-support ventilation, 551

Variceal sclerotherapy, endoscopic, pleural effusions after, 454

Varicella zoster virus (VZV), pneumonia due to, 400f, 400t

Vascular. *See also* entries under Pulmonary vascular

Vascular catheter-related infection, 644–647, 644t

Vascular manifestations, of lung cancer, 361

Vascular resistance, pulmonary. *See* Pulmonary vascular resistance (PVR)

Vascular surgery, pulmonary artery catheterization after, 627

Vascular tone, resting, 17

Vasoactive agents, for multiple organ failure, 633–634

Vasoactive substances, 17, 19–20, 19f
modification of, 18–19, 19t

Vasoconstriction, hypoxic, regulation of pulmonary circulation by, 18, 18f

Vasodilators, for primary pulmonary hypertension, 251

Vasopressors
for multiple organ failure, 633–634
for pulmonary edema, 581

VATS (video-assisted thoracoscopic surgery), 125–127, 594

VC (vital capacity), 26, 27f, 94, 94f
in emphysema, 180
in respiratory failure, 542
with restrictive ventilatory dysfunction, 110t

$\dot{V}CO_2$ (carbon dioxide production), 45–46, 556

$\dot{V}CO_2/\dot{V}O_2$ (respiratory exchange ratio), 45, 543t

$\dot{V}D$ (dead space ventilation), 46, 46f, 543, 543t

$\dot{V}Danat$ (anatomic dead space), 45, 98

$\dot{V}D/\dot{V}T$ (wasted ventilation fraction)
in exercise testing, 108
and work capacity, 105

$\dot{V}E$. *See* Minute ventilation $(\dot{V}E)$

Venodilators, for pulmonary edema, 581

Veno-occlusive disease, pulmonary, 250

Venous admixture, 46
estimation of, 50
due to right-to-left shunts, 49

Venous carbon dioxide tension (PVCO₂), 543t

Venous oxygen tension (PVO₂)
arterial hypoxemia due to low mixed, 53
normal value for, 543t

Venous pressure, pulmonary, and pulmonary vascular resistance, 15–16, 16f

Venous thromboembolism, in critically ill patients, 639–641, 640t

Venous thrombosis
catheter-related, 646
deep. *See* Deep venous thrombosis (DVT)

Ventilation
airway pressure release, 551
alveolar, 45–47, 46f, 47f
equation for, 45
and minute ventilation, 51
normal, 45
work of breathing and, 41, 42f
assist-controlled, 548, 549t
collateral, 11, 40
dead space ("wasted"), 46, 46f
distribution of, 39–40, 40f, 97–99, 98f
high-frequency oscillatory, 551
hypo-, 45–46, 46f
arterial hypoxemia due to, 51
central alveolar, 493–494, 493t
daytime, 489
intermittent mandatory, 548–549, 549f
synchronized, 548–549, 549f
for weaning, 553
inverse ratio, 549

jet, 551
maximal voluntary, 93
mechanical. *See* Mechanical ventilation (MV)
minute
and alveolar ventilation, 51
with exercise, 6
normal, 6, 543t
total, 46, 46f, 543
and work capacity, 105, 106f
noninvasive positive pressure, 544–546, 544f, 545f
for COPD, 568
for status asthmaticus, 161
pressure controlled, 549
pressure-cycled, 549, 550t
pressure-regulated-volume-controlled, 551
pressure support, 544, 544f, 545, 549
protective, 550
and sleep, 481–482
trial of spontaneous, 551
variable pressure-support and volume-support, 551
volume-cycled, 545, 548–549, 549f, 550t

Ventilation-perfusion $(\dot{V}/\dot{Q})$ lung scanning, 85–88, 86f, 87f
of chronic thromboembolic pulmonary hypertension, 244
for idiopathic pulmonary fibrosis, 267
preoperative, 598–599
for pulmonary embolism, 238–240, 239t, 240f

Ventilation-perfusion $(\dot{V}/\dot{Q})$ mismatch, 48, 49
arterial hypoxemia due to, 52
in chronic thromboembolic pulmonary hypertension, 244
in pulmonary alveolar proteinosis, 286
in pulmonary embolism, 239
in respiratory failure, 541

Ventilation-perfusion $(\dot{V}/\dot{Q})$ ratio, 48, 48f
normal, 45
and work capacity, 104–105

Ventilation-perfusion $(\dot{V}/\dot{Q})$ relationships, 48–49, 48f

Ventilator-dependent patients. *See* Mechanical ventilation (MV)

Ventilatory dysfunction, type of, 109–110, 109t, 110t

Ventilatory function, measurements of, 91–100, 92f–99f

Ventilatory limitation, and work capacity, 105

Ventilatory pump, 3–7, 4f, 5f

Ventolin (Volmax), for asthma, 146t

Ventricle, right, functional anatomy of, 12–13, 13f

Ventriculography, radionuclide, of cor pulmonale, 253

Vertebral fractures, 601

Vicious circle hypothesis, of COPD, 177, 177f

Video-assisted thoracoscopic surgery (VATS), 125–127, 594

Vinyl chloride monomer, carcinogenicity
   of, 337t, 339
Viral infections
   bronchiolitis due to, 385
   bronchitis due to, 384
   common cold due to, 377, 380t, 381
   and idiopathic pulmonary fibrosis,
      265–266, 268–269
   in immunocompromised host, 433
   influenza due to, 385–386
   of pleura, 448
Viral pneumonia, 399–401, 400f, 400t
Visceral chest pain, 61
Visceral larva migrans, eosinophilia due to,
   299
Visceral pleura, 7, 441
Vital capacity (VC), 26, 27f, 94, 94f
   in emphysema, 180
   in respiratory failure, 542
   with restrictive ventilatory dysfunction,
      110t
Vitamins, in parenteral nutrition, 531,
   531t
Vivactil (protriptyline)
   for cataplexy, 485
   for obstructive sleep apnea, 491
$\dot{V}$max (maximal volume), 36, 37
$\dot{V}O_2$. *See* Oxygen consumption ($\dot{V}O_2$)
$\dot{V}O_2$-DO_2, in critically ill patients,
   632–633
$\dot{V}O_2$max. *See* Work capacity ($\dot{V}O_2$max)
Vocal cords
   functional anatomy of, 8
   paralysis of, 8
Volmax (ventolin), for asthma, 146t
Volume-cycled ventilation, 545, 548–549,
   549f, 550t
Volume-pressure relations
   during muscular efforts, 27–32, 28f, 31f
   during relaxation, 26–27, 27f, 28f

von Recklinghausen's disease, mediastinal
   neurofibromas in, 467
von Willebrand factor-antigen (VWF-Ag),
   in acute lung injury, 636
$\dot{V}/\dot{Q}$. *See* Ventilation-perfusion
V_T (tidal volume), 26, 27f, 94, 94f, 543t
   respiratory rate to, 6
V_{TG} (thoracic gas volume), 95–96, 97f
VZV (varicella zoster virus), pneumonia
   due to, 400f, 400t

W

Wakefulness stimulus, 481, 487
Walking tests, self-paced, 108
Warfarin, for deep venous thrombosis, 243
Wasted ventilation fraction ($\dot{V}D/\dot{V}T$)
   in exercise testing, 108
   and work capacity, 105
WBC (white blood cell count), in pleural
   effusions, 119
Weaning, from mechanical ventilation,
   551–553, 552t
   in COPD, 568–569
   in elderly, 506–507, 506f, 507t
Wedge pressure, 577, 622f
   and left atrial pressure, 623–625
   obtaining reliable measurements of,
      622–623, 623f, 624f
   PEEP effect on, 625, 625t
   in pulmonary edema, 587
Wegener's granulomatosis (WG), 276–279
   chest radiograph of, 278, 278f
   clinicopathologic features of, 60,
      277–278, 277t
   diagnosis and pathologic findings in,
      278–279
   vs. lymphomatoid granulomatosis, 280
   pleural effusions with, 452
   treatment and prognosis for, 279
Weight, assessment of, 522
Weight loss, in COPD, 179, 183

Wheat weevil disease, 296t
Wheezing, 65
   in airway obstruction, 540
   in asthma, 138
      occupational, 319
   in COPD, 179
   in cystic fibrosis, 199
Whispered pectoriloquy, 65
White blood cell count (WBC), in pleural
   effusions, 119
Work capacity ($\dot{V}O_2$max), 101–105
   with aging, 107–108
   with cardiovascular dysfunction, 112
   determinants of, 102–105, 104t, 106f
   and impairment, 113, 114f
   measures of, 101–102, 102f, 102t
   predicted values for, 108
   preoperative, 599
Work of breathing, 40–42, 41f, 42f, 555
Work-related lung disease. *See*
   Occupational lung disease

X

Xenon distribution, radioactive, 98–99
Xopenex (levalbuterol), for asthma, 146t,
   150
X-rays. *See* Chest radiography

Y

Yellow nail syndrome, 456

Z

Zafirlukast (Accolate), for asthma, 147t,
   157
Zenker's diverticulum, 468
Zileuton (Zyflo), for asthma, 147t, 157
Zinc, inhalation injury due to, 323–324,
   323t
Zolpidem, for COPD, 498
Zyban (bupropion hydrochloride), for
   smoking cessation, 185